Postoperative Orthopaedic Rehabilitation

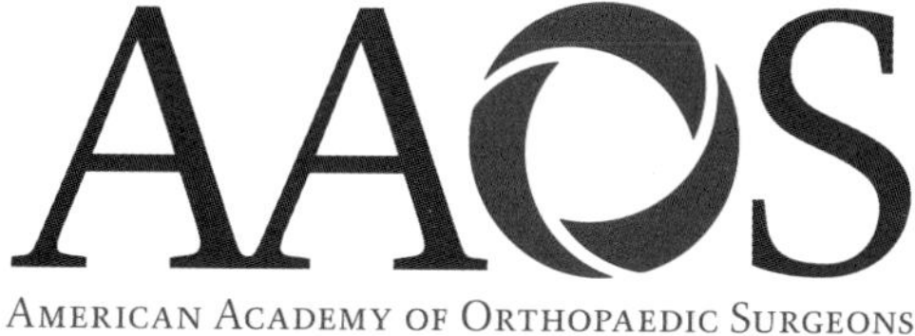

Postoperative Orthopaedic Rehabilitation

Editors

Andrew Green, MD
Associate Professor, Orthopaedic Surgery
Chief of Shoulder and Elbow Surgery
Department of Orthopaedic Surgery
Warren Alpert School of Medicine, Brown University
Providence, Rhode Island

Roman Hayda, MD, COL (ret)
Associate Professor, Orthopaedic Surgery
Warren Alpert School of Medicine, Brown University
Director, Orthopaedic Trauma
Rhode Island Hospital
Providence, Rhode Island

Andrew C. Hecht, MD
Chief, Spine Surgery
Mount Sinai Hospital and Mount Sinai Health System
Director, Mount Sinai Spine Center
Associate Professor, Orthopaedic and Neurosurgery
Mt. Sinai Medical Center and Icahn School of Medicine
New York, New York

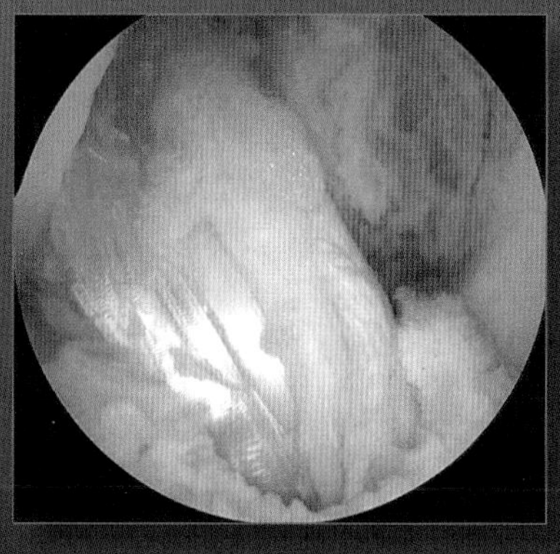

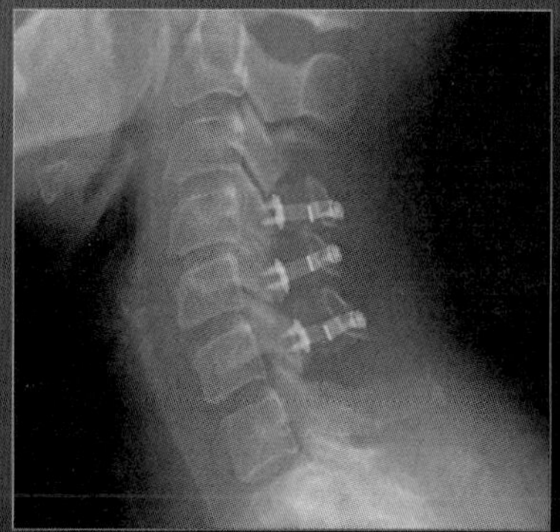

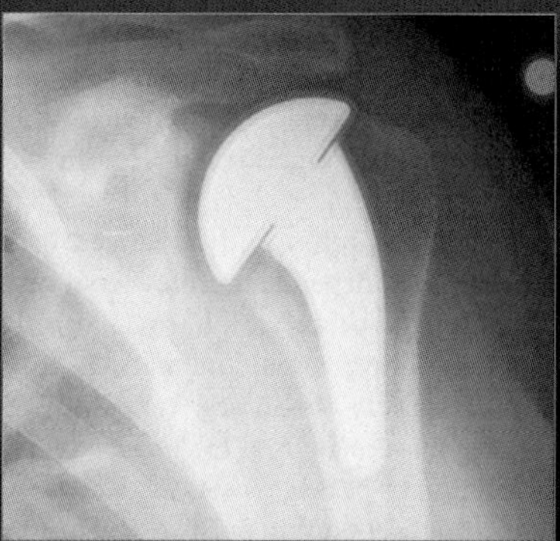

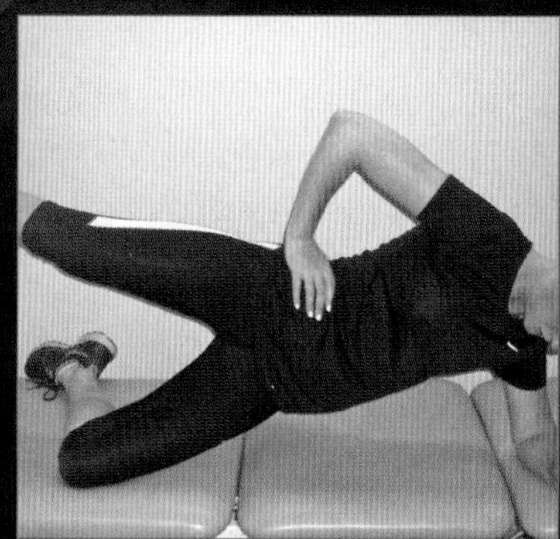

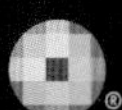
Wolters Kluwer

Philadelphia • Baltimore • New York • London
Buenos Aires • Hong Kong • Sydney • Tokyo

AAOS
American Academy of Orthopaedic Surgeons

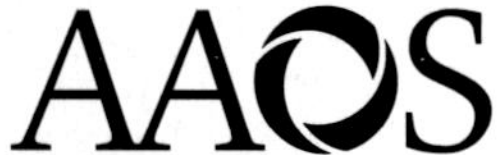

American Academy of
Orthopaedic Surgeons

American Academy of Orthopaedic Surgeons Board of Directors, 2017–2018

William J. Maloney, MD
President

David A. Halsey, MD
First Vice President

Kristy L. Weber, MD
Second Vice President

M. Bradford Henley, MD, MBA, FACS
Treasurer

Gerald R. Williams, Jr, MD
Past President

Dirk H. Alander, MD

James J. Balaschak

Basil R. Besh, MD

Robert H. Brophy, MD

Jacob M. Buchowski, MD, MS

Lisa K. Cannada, MD

Brian J. Galinat, MD, MBA

Daniel K. Guy, MD

Amy L. Ladd, MD

Ronald A. Navarro, MD

Robert M. Orfaly, MD

Thomas E. Arend, Jr, Esq., CAE *(ex officio)*

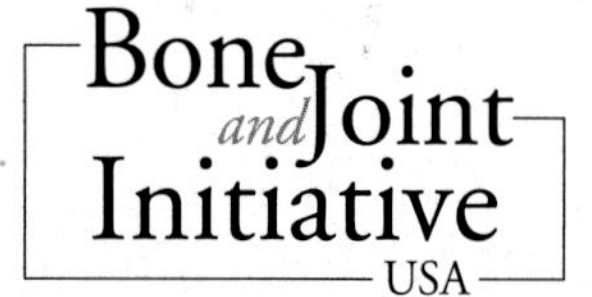

Acquisitions Editor: Brian Brown
Product Development Editor: Kate Heaney
Production Project Manager: David Orzechowski
Design Coordinator: Elaine Kasmer
Manufacturing Coordinator: Beth Welsh
Marketing Manager: Dan Dressler
Prepress Vendor: Aptara, Inc.

Copyright © 2018 American Academy of Orthopaedic Surgeons

All rights reserved. This book is protected by copyright. No part of this book may be reproduced or transmitted in any form or by any means, including as photocopies or scanned-in or other electronic copies, or utilized by any information storage and retrieval system without written permission from the copyright owner, except for brief quotations embodied in critical articles and reviews. Materials appearing in this book prepared by individuals as part of their official duties as U.S. government employees are not covered by the above-mentioned copyright. To request permission, please contact Wolters Kluwer at Two Commerce Square, 2001 Market Street, Philadelphia, PA 19103, via email at permissions@lww.com, or via our website at lww.com (products and services).

9 8 7 6 5 4 3 2 1

Printed in China

Library of Congress Cataloging-in-Publication Data

Names: Green, Andrew, MD, editor. | Hayda, Roman A., editor. | Hecht, Andrew C. MD, editor
Title: Postoperative orthopaedic rehabilitation / [edited by] Andrew Green, Roman Hayda, and Andrew Hecht.
Description: Philadelphia : Wolters Kluwer, [2017] | Includes bibliographical references.
Identifiers: LCCN 2017011918 | ISBN 9781496360281
Subjects: | MESH: Orthopedic Procedures–rehabilitation | Rehabilitation–methods | Recovery of Function
Classification: LCC RD755 | NLM WE 168 | DDC 617.9–dc23
LC record available at https://lccn.loc.gov/2017011918

This work is provided "as is," and the publisher disclaims any and all warranties, express or implied, including any warranties as to accuracy, comprehensiveness, or currency of the content of this work.

This work is no substitute for individual patient assessment based upon healthcare professionals' examination of each patient and consideration of, among other things, age, weight, gender, current or prior medical conditions, medication history, laboratory data and other factors unique to the patient. The publisher does not provide medical advice or guidance and this work is merely a reference tool. Healthcare professionals, and not the publisher, are solely responsible for the use of this work including all medical judgments and for any resulting diagnosis and treatments.

Given continuous, rapid advances in medical science and health information, independent professional verification of medical diagnoses, indications, appropriate pharmaceutical selections and dosages, and treatment options should be made and healthcare professionals should consult a variety of sources. When prescribing medication, healthcare professionals are advised to consult the product information sheet (the manufacturer's package insert) accompanying each drug to verify, among other things, conditions of use, warnings and side effects and identify any changes in dosage schedule or contraindications, particularly if the medication to be administered is new, infrequently used or has a narrow therapeutic range. To the maximum extent permitted under applicable law, no responsibility is assumed by the publisher for any injury and/or damage to persons or property, as a matter of products liability, negligence law or otherwise, or from any reference to or use by any person of this work.

LWW.com

RRS1705

Contributors

Joseph A. Abboud, MD
Associate Professor of Orthopedics, Division of Shoulder and Elbow Surgery
Rothman Institute for Orthopedics
Thomas Jefferson University Hospital
Philadelphia, Pennsylvania

Christopher S. Ahmad, MD
Professor of Clinical Orthopaedic Surgery
Orthopaedic Surgery Department
Columbia University Medical Center
New York, New York

Jeffrey Algra, MD, MS
Resident
Physical Medicine & Rehabilitation Department
Montefiore Medical Center
New York, New York

Abigail K. Allen, MD
Chief of Pediatric Orthopaedic Surgery
Icahn School of Medicine at Mount Sinai
New York, New York

April Armstrong, BSc(PT), MSc, MD, FRCSC
Professor, Chief Shoulder and Elbow Surgery
Bone and Joint Institute
Penn State Milton S. Hershey Medical Center
Hershey, Pennsylvania

Annie Ashok, MD
Resident
Orthopaedic Surgery
Drexel University
Philadelphia, Pennsylvania

Mathieu Assal, MD, PD Dr.
Center for Surgery of the Foot & Ankle
Clinique La Colline
Geneva, Switzerland

George S. Athwal, MD, FRCSC
Associate Professor
Roth McFarlane Hand and Upper Limb Center
Western University
London, Ontario, Canada

Rahul Banerjee, MD
Assistant Professor
Orthopaedic Surgery Department
University of Texas Southwestern Medical Center
Dallas, Texas

Jenna Baynes, MD
Physical Therapist
Orthopaedics Department
Columbia University Medical Center, Department of Orthopaedic Surgery
New York, New York

Katherine Barnum Baynes, MS, OTR, CHT
Occupational Therapist, Certified Hand Therapist
Occupational Therapy Department
University of Colorado Hospital
Aurora, Colorado

Kathleen Beaulieu, OTR/L, CHT
Occupational Therapist, Certified Hand Therapist
Penn State Hershey Medical Center
Hershey, Pennsylvania

John-Erik Bell, MD, MS
Associate Professor
Department of Orthopaedic Surgery, Shoulder, Elbow and Sports Medicine
Dartmouth-Hitchcock Medical Center
Lebanon, New Hampshire

Jessica Bloch, MS, OTR/L
Occupational Therapist
Rehabilitation Department
Hospital for Special Surgery
New York, New York

Eric M. Bluman, MD, PhD
Assistant Professor
Orthopedic Surgery
Harvard University
Boston, Massachusetts

Friedrich Boettner, MD
Attending Orthopaedic Surgeon
Orthopaedic Surgery Department
Hospital for Special Surgery
New York, New York

Eugene W. Brabston III, MD
Fellow
Center for Shoulder, Elbow, and Sports Medicine
Columbia Presbyterian Medical Center
New York, New York

Brett A. Braly, MD
Orthopaedic Spine Surgery
Oklahoma Sports, Science and Orthopaedics
Oklahoma City, Oklahoma

David M. Brogan, MD, MSc
Resident
Department of Orthopedic Surgery
Mayo Clinic
Rochester, Minnesota

Ryan P. Calfee, MD, MSc
Associate Professor
Department of Orthopaedic Surgery
Washington University School of Medicine
St. Louis, Missouri

Caleb Campbell, MD
Orthopedic Surgeon
Brown University
Providence, Rhode Island

Shannon R. Carpenter, MD
Shoulder and Elbow Fellowship Trained Orthopedic Surgeon
Overland Park Regional Medical Center
Overland Park, Kansas

John Cavanaugh, PT, ATC, SCS
Clinical Supervisor
Sports Rehabilitation and Performance Center
Hospital for Special Surgery
New York, New York

Kevin Chan, MD, MSc, FRCSC
Chief Orthopaedic Surgery Resident
Division of Orthopaedic Surgery
McMaster University
Hamilton, Ontario, Canada

Lan Chen, MD
Department of Orthopedic Surgery
Northshore Medical Group
Evanston, Illinois

David S. Cheng, MD
Assistant Professor
Physical Medicine
Rush University Medical Center
Chicago, Illinois

Shrikant J. Chinchalkar, MThO, BScOT, OTR, CHT
Hand Therapist
Hand Therapy Division
Roth-McFarlane Hand and Upper Limb Center
St. Joseph's Health Care
London, Ontario, Canada

Samuel K. Cho, MD
Assistant Professor
Department of Orthopedic Surgery
Mount Sinai Hospital
New York, New York

Joseph L. Ciccone, PT, DPT, SCS, CIMT, CSCS
Associate Director
Columbia Sports Therapy
Columbia University
New York, New York

Brian J. Cole, MD, MBA
Professor of Orthopedics
Midwest Orthopedics at Rush
Rush University Medical Center
Chicago, Illinois

Mark P. Cote, PT, DPT, MSCTR
Sports Medicine Clinical Outcomes Research Facilitator
Orthopaedic Surgery
University of Connecticut Health Center
Farmington, Connecticut

Charles L. Cox, MD, MPH
Assistant Professor
Orthopaedics and Rehabilitation
Vanderbilt University Medical Center
Nashville, Tennessee

Xavier Crevoisier, MD
Assistant Professor
Orthopedics & Traumatology Department
CHUV
Lausanne, Switzerland

Anthony D'Angelo, MS, PT, ACT, CSCS
Practice Owner
Physical Therapy Department
Professional Orthopedics and Sports Physical Therapy
New York, New York

Alan H. Daniels, MD
Assistant Professor, Director of Adult Spinal Deformity
Division of Spine Surgery, Department of Orthopaedic Surgery
Warren Alpert Medical School of Brown University
Providence, Rhode Island

Agnes Z. Dardas, MD, MSc
Department of Orthopaedic Surgery
Washington University School of Medicine in St. Louis
Saint Louis, MO

Michael Darowish, MD
Assistant Professor
Department of Orthopaedics and Rehabilitation
Penn State Milton S. Hershey Medical Center
Hershey, Pennsylvania

Daniel DeBottis, MD
Division of Shoulder and Elbow
Orthopaedic Specialty Institute
Orange County, California

 © 2018 American Academy of Orthopaedic Surgeons

Alejandro Della Valle, MD
Orthopaedic Surgeon
Orthopaedic Surgery Department
Hospital for Special Surgery
New York, New York

Stephanie Dickason, PT
Physical Therapist III
Department of Physical Medicine & Rehabilitation
Parkland Hospital
Dallas, Texas

Thomas C. Dowd, MD
Associate Program Director
SAUSHEC Orthopedic Surgery Residency
San Antonio Military Medical Center
Fort Sam Houston, Texas

Charles Eaton, MD
Executive Director
Dupuytren Research Group
West Palm Beach, Florida

David Ebaugh, PT, PhD
Clinical Professor
Physical Therapy and Rehabilitation Sciences Department
Health Sciences Department
College of Nursing and Health Professions
Drexel University
Philadelphia, Pennsylvania

Todd S. Ellenbecker, DPT, MS, SCS, OCS, CSCS
Clinic Director
Physiotherapy Associates Scottsdale Sports Clinic
Scottsdale, Arizona

Adam E.M. Eltorai, MD
Medical Student
Warren Alpert Medical School of Brown University
Providence, Rhode Island

Daniel C. Farber, MD
Assistant Professor of Clinical Orthopaedic Surgery
Department of Orthopaedic Surgery
University of Pennsylvania
Philadelphia, Pennsylvania

Austin T. Fragomen, MD
Associate Professor Orthopedics
Limb Lengthening Complex Reconstruction
Hospital for Special Surgery
New York, New York

Samantha Francucci, PT, DPT
Physical Therapist
Physical Therapy Department
Lahey Hospital and Medical Center
Danvers, Massachusetts

Erik Freeland, PT, DO
Fellow
University of Pennsylvania
Department of Orthopedic Surgery
Philadelphia, Pennsylvania

H. Michael Frisch, MD
Orthopaedic Trauma Services
Mission Hospitals
Asheville, North Carolina

Charles L. Getz, MD
Associate Professor
Rothman Institute
Department of Orthopaedics
Thomas Jefferson University
Philadelphia, Pennsylvania

Christopher Got, MD
Assistant Professor of Orthopedics
Brown University/University Orthopedics
Providence, Rhode Island

Andrew Green, MD
Associate Professor, Orthopaedic Surgery
Chief of Shoulder and Elbow Surgery
Department of Orthopaedic Surgery
Warren Alpert School of Medicine, Brown University
Providence, Rhode Island

Justin K. Greisberg, MD
Associate Professor of Orthopaedic Surgery
Columbia University
New York, New York

Steven B. Haas, MD
Chief Knee Service
Orthopedics Department
Hospital for Special Surgery
New York, New York

Marc S. Haro, MD, MSPT
Assistant Professor
Department of Orthopaedics
Medical University of South Carolina
Charleston, South Carolina

Roman Hayda, MD, COL (ret)
Associate Professor, Orthopaedic Surgery
Warren Alpert School of Medicine, Brown University
Director, Orthopaedic Trauma
Rhode Island Hospital
Providence, Rhode Island

© 2018 American Academy of Orthopaedic Surgeons

Andrew C. Hecht, MD
Chief, Spine Surgery
Mount Sinai Hospital and Mount Sinai Health System
Director, Mount Sinai Spine Center
Associate Professor, Orthopaedic and Neurosurgery
Mt. Sinai Medical Center and Icahn School of Medicine
New York, New York

Heather E. Hensl, PA-C, MPH
Physician Assistant
NY Downtown Orthopaedic Associates
NY Presbyterian—Lower Manhattan Hospital
New York, New York

Todd R. Hooks, PT, ATC
Physical Therapist
Champion Sports Medicine
Birmingham, Alabama

Jerry I. Huang, MD
Assistant Professor
Department of Orthopaedics and Sports Medicine
University of Washington Medical Center
Seattle, Washington

Seth Jerabek, MD
Assistant Professor
Orthopaedic Surgery Department
Hospital for Special Surgery
New York, New York

Christopher H. Judson, MD
Physician
Orthopaedics Department
University of Connecticut Health Center
Farmington, Connecticut

Sanjeev Kakar, MD, MRCS
Associate Professor of Orthopedics
Orthopedic Surgery
Mayo Clinic
Rochester, Minnesota

Stephanie Kannas, OTR/L, CHT, CLT-LANA
Lead Clinical Hand Therapist
Department of Physical Medicine
Mayo Clinic
Rochester, Minnesota

Jay D. Keener, MD
Assistant Professor
Department of Orthopaedic Surgery
Washington University
St. Louis, Missouri

Bryan T. Kelly, MD
Chief of Hip Preservation Service
Center for Hip Preservation
Hospital for Special Surgery
New York, New York

Michelle Kenny, MS, PT
Physical Therapist
Department of Physical Medicine and Rehabilitation
MetroHealth Medical Center
Cleveland, Ohio

W. Ben Kibler, MD
Medical Director
Shoulder Center of Kentucky
Lexington Clinic
Lexington, Kentucky

H. Mike Kim, MD
Assistant Professor
Department of Orthopaedics and Rehabilitation
Penn State College of Medicine
Hershey, Pennsylvania

Soo Yeon Kim, MD
Assistant Professor
Physical Medicine and Rehabilitation
Montefiore Medical Center
Bronx, New York

Graham J.W. King, MD, MSc, FRCSC
Medical Director
Roth | McFarlane Hand and Upper Limb Centre
St. Joseph's Health Centre, Western University
London, Ontario, Canada

Kevin L. Kirk, DO
Clinical Associate Professor
Department of Orthopedic Surgery
Rutgers/Robert Wood Johnson Medical School
New Brunswick, New Jersey

Elisa J. Knutsen, MD
Assistant Professor of Orthopaedic Surgery
Department of Orthopaedic Surgery
The GW Medical Faculty Associates
Washington, District of Columbia

Rebekah L. Lawrence, PT, DPT, OCS
PhD Student
Department of Physical Medicine and Rehabilitation
University of Minnesota
Minneapolis, Minnesota

Margaret J. Lobo, MD
Orthopaedic Surgeon, Director, Foot and Ankle
Lahey Health Medical Center
Burlington, Massachusetts

 © 2018 American Academy of Orthopaedic Surgeons

Paula M. Ludewig, PT, PhD
Associate Professor
Department of Physical Medicine and Rehabilitation
University of Minnesota
Minneapolis, Minnesota

May Fong Mak, FRCSEd (Ortho)
Department of Orthopaedic Surgery
Khoo Teck Puat Hospital
Singapore

Maya C. Manning, PT, DPT
Clinical Supervisor of Acute Care Rehabilitation
Hospital for Special Surgery—Rehabilitation
New York, New York

Alejandro Marquez-Lara, MD
Research Coordinator
Department of Orthopaedic Surgery
Rush University Medical Center
Chicago, Illinois

Jun Matsui, MD
Fellow, Hand and Upper Extremity Surgery
Department of Orthopaedic Surgery
Washington University School of Medicine
St. Louis, Missouri

David J. Mayman, MD
Assistant Attending Orthopaedic Surgeon
Department of Adult Reconstruction and Joint Replacement
Hospital for Special Surgery
New York, New York

Augustus D. Mazzocca, MS, MD
Director, New England Musculoskeletal Institute
Professor and Chairman
Department of Orthopaedic Surgery
University of Connecticut Health Center
Farmington, Connecticut

Rowena McBeath, MD, PhD
Attending Hand Surgeon, The Philadelphia Hand Center
Assistant Professor, Thomas Jefferson University
Philadelphia, Pennsylvania

Phillip W. McClure, PT, PhD
Professor
Department of Physical Therapy
Arcadia University
Glenside, Pennsylvania

Corey McGee, PhD, MS, OTR/L, CHT
Assistant Professor
Program in Occupational Therapy
University of Minnesota
Minneapolis, Minnesota

Sarah E. McLean, PT, MSPT
Physical Therapist
Sports Rehabilitation and Performance Center
Hospital for Special Surgery
New York, New York

Gleb Medvedev, MD
Resident
Department of Orthopaedics
George Washington University
Washington, District of Columbia

CarolLynn Meyers, PT
Physical Therapist
Illinois Bone and Joint Physical Therapy
Glenview, Illinois

Lori A. Michener, PhD, PT, ATC
Professor
Department of Physical Therapy
Virginia Commonwealth University
Richmond, Virginia

Bradley Moatz, MD
Resident Physician
Orthopaedics
Medstar Union Memorial Hospital
Baltimore, Maryland

Jacqueline Munch, MD
Fellow
Department of Sports Medicine and Shoulder Surgery
Hospital for Special Surgery
New York, New York

Anand M. Murthi, MD
Attending, Chief, Shoulder and Elbow Surgery
Department of Orthopaedics
MedStar Union Memorial Hospital
Baltimore, Maryland

Surena Namdari, MD, MSc
Assistant Professor of Orthopaedic Surgery
Rothman Institute—Jefferson Medical College
Philadelphia, Pennsylvania

Sreeharsha V. Nandyala, BA
Medical Student
University of Missouri Kansas City School of Medicine
Kansas City, Missouri

Kerellos Nasr, MD
Fellow
Orthopaedic Surgery
University of Texas Southwestern Medical Center
Dallas, Texas

Gregory N. Nelson, Jr, MD
Clinical Fellow, Shoulder and Elbow Department
Rothman Institute for Orthopedics
Thomas Jefferson University Hospital
Philadelphia, Pennsylvania

© 2018 American Academy of Orthopaedic Surgeons

Lucy Oliver-Welsh, MBChB
Foundation Doctor
Tunbridge Wells Hospital
Kent, United Kingdom

Eilish O'Sullivan, PT, DPT, OCS, SCS
Physical Therapist
Centers of Hip Preservation
Hospital for Special Surgery
New York, New York

Samuel C. Overley, MD
Resident
Department of Orthopaedic Surgery
The Mount Sinai Icahn School of Medicine
New York, New York

Brett D. Owens, MD
Professor of Orthopaedic Surgery
Department of Orthopaedic Surgery
Warren Alpert Medical School Brown University
Providence, Rhode Island

Johnny Owens, MPT
Chief, Human Performance Optimization Program
Department of Orthopedics and Rehabilitation
Center for the Intrepid, Joint Base San Antonio
San Antonio, Texas

Michael Lloyd Parks, MD
Hospital for Special Surgery
New York, New York

E. Scott Paxton, MD
Division of Shoulder and Elbow Surgery
Department of Orthopaedic Surgery
Warren Alpert Medical School Brown University
Providence, Rhode Island

James J. Perry, OT/L, OTR, CHT, RNCST
Occupational Therapist, Hand Therapist
Department of Rehabilitation Medicine
Dartmouth Hitchcock Medical Center
Lebanon, New Hampshire

David Pezzullo, MS, PT, SCS, ATC
Director of Physical Therapy
University Orthopedics, Inc.
Providence, Rhode Island

Joey G. Pipicelli, PhD Student, MScOT, CH
Occupational Therapist, Certified Hand Therapist
Division of Hand Therapy, Roth McFarlane Hand and Upper Limb Centre
London, Ontario, Canada

Karen Pitbladdo, MS, OTR/L, CHT
Senior Occupational Therapist
San Francisco General Hospital
San Francisco, California

Benjamin K. Potter, MD
Chief Orthopaedic Surgeon, Amputee Patient Care Program
Department of Orthopaedics
Walter Reed National Military Medical Center
Bethesda, Maryland

Rhonda K. Powell, OTD, OTR/L, CHT
Senior Therapist
Milliken Hand Rehabilitation Center
The Rehabilitation Institute of St. Louis
St. Louis, Missouri

Sheeraz Qureshi, MD
Associate Professor
Orthopaedic Spine Surgery
The Mount Sinai Icahn School of Medicine
New York, New York

Craig S. Radnay, MD, MPH
Orthopedic Surgeon
Insall Scott Kelly Institute for Orthopaedics and Sports Medicine
St Francis Hospital
NYU/Hospital for Joint Diseases
New York, New York

Anil S. Ranawat, MD
Sports Medicine Surgeon
Sports Medicine
Hospital for Special Surgery
New York, New York

Carol Recor, OTR/L, CHT
OT Specialist
Exercise Training Center
University of Washington Medical Center
Seattle, Washington

Saqib Rehman, MD
Associate Professor, Director of Orthopaedic Trauma
Department of Orthopaedic Surgery
Temple University
Philadelphia, Pennsylvania

Davis V. Reyes, PT, DPT, OCS
Physical Therapist III
Outpatient Therapy Services
Goleta Valley Cottage Hospital
Goleta, California

John M. Rhee, MD
Orthopaedic Spine Surgery
Emory Orthopaedics and Spine
Atlanta, Georgia

Benjamin F. Ricciardi, MD
Assistant Professor, Division of Adult Reconstruction
Department of Orthopedic Surgery
University of Rochester School of Medicine
Rochester, New York

© 2018 American Academy of Orthopaedic Surgeons

Brian E. Richardson, PT, MS, SCS, CSCS
Physical Therapist
Orthopaedics and Rehabilitation
Vanderbilt University Medical Center
Nashville, Tennessee

Bradley M. Ritland, MD
Chief, Amputee Physical Therapy
Rehabilitation/Physical Therapy
Walter Reed National Military Medical Center
Bethesda, Maryland

Scott Alan Rodeo, MD
Co-Chief, Sports Medicine and Shoulder Service
Professor, Orthopaedic Surgery
Hospital for Special Surgery
New York, New York

Craig M. Rodner, MD
Physician
Department of Orthopaedics
University of Connecticut Health Center
Farmington, Connecticut

Madeline C. Rodriguez, PT, MS, DPT
Physical Therapist
Private Practice
Medfield, Massachusetts

S. Robert Rozbruch, MD
Service Chief
Limb Lengthening and Complex Reconstruction Service
Hospital for Special Surgery
New York, New York

Joaquin Sanchez-Sotelo, MD, PhD
Consultant and Professor
Department of Orthopedic Surgery
Mayo Clinic
Rochester, Minnesota

Andrew K. Sands, MD
Chief, Foot & Ankle Surgery
NY Downtown Orthopedic Associates
Clinical Associate Professor of Orthopedic Surgery
Weill Cornell Medical College
New York, New York

Vikram M. Sathyendra, MD
Fellow
Department of Orthopaedics
MedStar Union Memorial Hospital
Baltimore, Maryland

Oliver Schipper, MD
Resident Physician
Orthopaedic Surgery and Rehabilitation
University of Chicago Medical Center
Chicago, Illinois

Tom Schmidt-Braekling, MD
Research Fellow
Department of Orthopedic Surgery
Hospital for Special Surgery
New York, New York

Nicole S. Schroeder, MD
Assistant Clinical Professor
Department of Orthopaedic Surgery
University of California, San Francisco
San Francisco, California

Alok D. Sharan, MD, MHCDS
Chief, Orthopedic Spine Service
Department of Orthopedic Surgery
Montefiore Medical Center
Bronx, New York

Kern Singh, MD
Associate Professor
Department of Orthopaedic Surgery
Rush University Medical Center
Chicago, Illinois

Ernest L. Sink, MD
Associate Professor
Orthopaedic Surgery
Hospital for Special Surgery
New York, New York

Scott K. Siverling, PT, OCS
Physical Therapist
Integrative Care Center
Hospital for Special Surgery
New York, New York

Terri Skirven, OTR/L, CHT
Director of Therapy
The Philadelphia Hand Center
Philadelphia, Pennsylvania

Kathleen E. Snelgrove, OTR/L, CHT
Director of Hand Therapy
University Orthopedics Inc.
Providence, Rhode Island

Mark K. Solarz, MD
Resident
Department of Orthopaedic Surgery
Temple University
Philadelphia, Pennsylvania

Bryan A. Spinelli, PT, PhD, OCS, CLT-LANA
Clinical Rehabilitation Specialist
Rhode Island Hospital
Providence, Rhode Island

© 2018 American Academy of Orthopaedic Surgeons

Daniel J. Stinner, MD
Orthopaedic Trauma Surgeon
Department of Orthopaedics and Rehabilitation
San Antonio Military Medical Center
San Antonio, Texas

David Alex Stroh, MD
Resident
Department of Orthopaedic Surgery
Union Memorial Hospital
Baltimore, Maryland

Edwin P. Su, MD
Orthopaedic Surgeon
Department of Adult Reconstruction and Joint Replacement
Hospital for Special Surgery
New York, New York

Maureen Suhr, PT, DPT, PCS
Manager
Department of Rehabilitation
Hospital for Special Surgery
New York, New York

Michael Szekeres, OT Reg (Ont.), CHT
Occupational Therapist
Hand & Upper Limb Centre
St. Joseph's Health Care
London, Ontario, Canada

Robert Z. Tashjian, MD
Associate Professor
Department of Orthopaedics
University of Utah School of Medicine
Salt Lake City, Utah

Samuel Arthur Taylor, MD
Sports Medicine Fellow
Department of Sports Medicine
Hospital for Special Surgery
New York, New York

Matthew P. Titmuss, PT, DPT
Director, Acute Care Orthopedic Rehabilitation
HSS Rehabilitation
Hospital for Special Surgery
New York, New York

P. Justin Tortolani, MD
Director of Spine Education and Research
MedStar Union Memorial Hospital
Baltimore, Maryland

Andrea Tychanski, PT, DPT, SCS, ATC, CSCS
Physical Therapist
Sports Rehabilitation and Performance Center
Hospital for Special Surgery
New York, New York

Sarah Tyndall, MPT, OCS
Physical Therapist
NovaCare Rehabilitation
Philadelphia, Pennsylvania

Heather A. Vallier, MD
Professor of Orthopaedic Surgery
Department of Orthopaedic Surgery
MetroHealth Medical Center
Cleveland, Ohio

Vivek Venugopal, MD
Resident Physician
Department of Surgery
Beth Israel Deaconess Medical Center
Boston, Massachusetts

Mandeep Singh Virk, MD, MBBS
Resident
Department of Orthopaedic Surgery
University of Connecticut School of Medicine
Farmington, Connecticut

J. Turner Vosseller, MD
Assistant Professor
Department of Orthopaedic Surgery
Columbia University Medical Center
New York, New York

John J. Walker, PT, DPT, MBA
Senior Physical Therapist
Orthopaedics and Sports Medicine
Temple University
Philadelphia, Pennsylvania

Lindley B. Wall, MD
Assistant Professor
Department of Orthopaedic Surgery
Washington University
St. Louis, Missouri

Kempland C. Walley, BSc
Biomedical Engineer and Research Fellow
Department of Orthopedic Surgery
Beth Israel Deaconess Medical Center, Harvard Medical School
Boston, Massachusetts

Laura Walsh, MS, OTR/L, CHT
Hand Therapy Team Leader
University of Pennsylvania Therapy and Fitness Upper Extremity Center
Penne Presbyterian Medical Center
Philadelphia, Pennsylvania

Mark E. Warren, OTR/L, CHT
Department of Orthopaedics
University of Connecticut Health Center
Farmington, Connecticut

 © 2018 American Academy of Orthopaedic Surgeons

Cynthia Watkins, PT, DPT, CHT
Manager of Hand Therapy
Hand Therapy
Rothman Institute
Philadelphia, Pennsylvania

Alicia Faye White, PT, ATC, DPT
Physical Therapist
Department of Orthopaedics and Rehabilitation
San Antonio, Texas

Kevin E. Wilk, DPT, FAPTA
Clinical Director
Physical Therapy
Champion Sports Medicine
Birmingham, Alabama

Trevor W. Wilkes, MD
Orthopedic Surgeon
Orthopedics-Sports Medicine
Lexington Clinic
Lexington, Kentucky

Gerald R. Williams, Jr, MD
Professor, Chief—Shoulder and Elbow Surgery
The Rothman Institute
Jefferson Medical College
Philadelphia, Pennsylvania

Richard D. Wilson, MD, MS
Assistant Professor of Physical Medicine and Rehabilitation
MetroHealth Rehabilitation Institute
Case Western Reserve University
Cleveland, Ohio

John J. Wixted, MD
Orthopaedic Trauma Surgeon
Department of Orthopaedic Surgery
Beth Israel Deaconess Medical Center
Boston, Massachusetts

Jennifer Moriatis Wolf, MD
Associate Professor
Department of Orthopaedic Surgery
University of Connecticut Health Center
Farmington, Connecticut

Adrian James Yenchak, DPT, PT
Director
Columbia Sports Therapy
Columbia Doctors Orthopedics
Columbia University
New York, New York

Elizabeth Zhu, MD
Medical Student
Orthopaedic Surgery
Icahn School of Medicine at Mount Sinai
New York, New York

© 2018 American Academy of Orthopaedic Surgeons

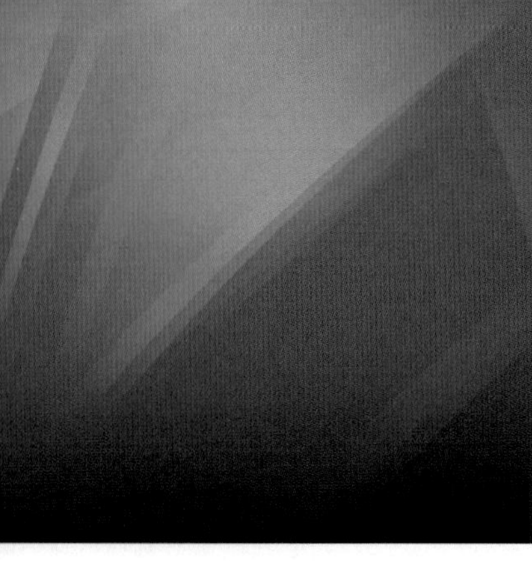

Foreword

It gives me great pleasure and much pride to write a foreword to this very impressive book. I served as Chair of the Publications Committee for the AAOS when Dr. Green first proposed the concept and recruited Drs. Hayda and Hecht as co-editors. Now as Chair of the Council on Education, I have been privileged to follow the outstanding efforts of this team as they expertly guided the authors, acclaimed orthopaedic educators and skilled surgeons, through the arduous process of completing this vital work.

My mentor, Charles Neer, routinely told his patients that he would do his part of the treatment by replacing their shoulder or repairing their rotator cuff, but they would do the major work of rehabilitating their shoulder afterward. Indeed, I learned as much or more in his office watching him guide his patients and interact with their physical and occupational therapists as I did assisting at surgery. While we all acknowledge how crucial postoperative rehabilitation is to the final result, too often lectures and book chapters focus lovingly on every step of the surgery with only a brief and sometimes perfunctory summary of postoperative care at the end. Not in this book, which carefully describes the theory and practice of postoperative rehabilitation after most of the common orthopaedic procedures.

The authors and editors, each a renowned authority in his or her field, have thoughtfully explained the principles, for each procedure, of postoperative care: what structures must be protected during healing, what exercises will help prevent stiffness and adhesions, and how best to reeducate the muscles and control mechanisms to return patients to sports and everyday life. Most importantly, they sketch out the subtle variations in anatomy and procedures that require modification of the regimen. These priceless lessons will undoubtedly be pored over again and again by the many therapists and surgeons who work so hard together to advance the care of their patients.

Evan L. Flatow, MD
President, Mount Sinai West
Lasker Professor of Orthopaedic Surgery
New York, New York

© 2018 American Academy of Orthopaedic Surgeons

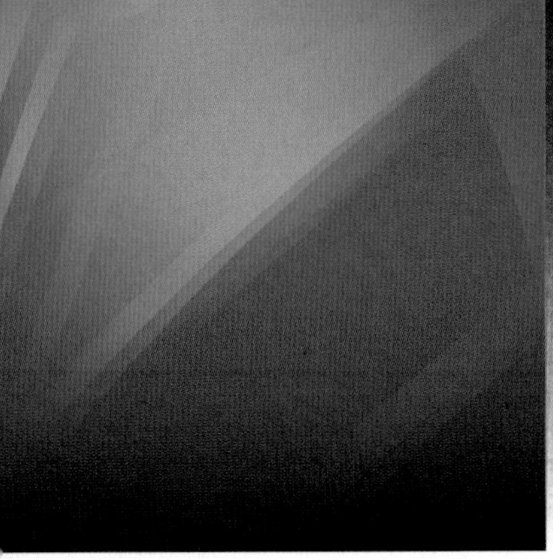

Preface

ADULT ORTHOPAEDIC POSTOPERATIVE REHABILITATION

Postoperative rehabilitation is a critical component of the successful surgical management of all orthopaedic conditions. The relationship between the surgeon, rehabilitation specialist, and patient must include a detailed understanding of the anatomy, pathology, pathophysiology, surgical procedure, healing responses, and rehabilitation techniques and modalities. Traditional orthopaedic education and training rarely devoted sufficient exposure to rehabilitation beyond the immediate postoperative period. In clinical practice, the interactions between surgeons and rehabilitation specialists are variable. Greater understanding and exposure of surgeons to rehabilitation principles and techniques can improve outcomes. Similarly, an enhanced understanding of the surgical procedure and its nuances will assist the therapist to provide expert care tailored to each individual patient. The coordination of surgery and rehabilitation can have a tremendous positive effect on achieving successful outcomes. In addition, the role and experience of the patient, who often has more questions about after care and rehabilitation than the procedure itself, must be considered.

The personal experiences of the editors of this text in their clinical practices provided the impetus to undertake this project. In the ideal setting, the surgeon and rehabilitation specialist work together to manage the postoperative recovery after orthopaedic surgery. However, in reality, it is not uncommon that the only interaction and communication between surgeon and rehabilitation specialist is a referral, often only noting the procedure with instructions to evaluate and treat. The primary objective of this text is to demonstrate that the surgery and rehabilitation must be linked for there to be a successful result.

The goal of this text is to provide a comprehensive resource for all individuals involved in the postoperative rehabilitation after orthopaedic surgery including surgeons, nonoperative musculoskeletal providers, midlevel providers (physician assistants and nurse practitioners), physiatrists, physicians in training, and physical and occupational therapists. The text is divided into sections that address the most common surgical procedures of the upper extremity, lower extremity, pelvis, spine, and trauma. Each chapter is co-authored by expert surgeons and physical and occupational therapists and provides information about the relevant anatomy, surgical indications and technique, rehabilitation protocols, and specific tips and pearls explaining the rationale behind the rehabilitation protocol. The intention is to provide the professionals tasked to rehabilitate orthopaedic surgical patients with a clear understanding and basis for guiding the rehabilitation of the patient to their final outcome.

We would be remiss if we did not acknowledge the many individuals who were involved in the conception, development, and production of this work. A special note of gratitude goes to Evan Flatow, MD and the physician members of the American Academy of Orthopaedic Surgeons Publications Committee who approved the initial proposal for this project several years ago. We are also forever grateful to the Academy staff (Laurie Braun, Marilyn Fox, PhD, Joan Golembiewski, Hans Koelsch, PhD, Howard Mevis, Lisa Moore, Sylvia Orellana, and Rachel Winokur) who assisted along the way, as well as the staff from Wolters Kluwer Publishing (Kate Heaney, Brendan Huffman, and David Orzechowski) and Indu Jawwad, our production manager, who guided us through the final phases of production. We also thank the section editors for their efforts to organize the chapter authors and their assistance in the editorial process.

We hope that you enjoy the text and find it to be a helpful resource in the care of your patients.

Andrew Green, MD
Roman Hayda, MD
Andrew C. Hecht, MD

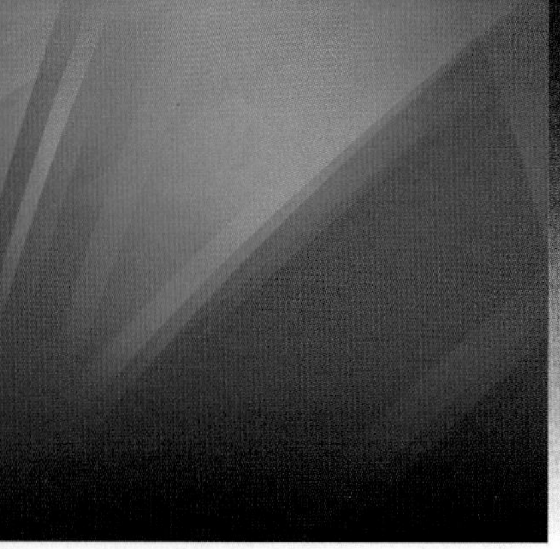

Introduction

Todd S. Ellenbecker, DPT, MS, SCS, OCS, CSCS

The importance of postoperative rehabilitation is agreed upon by both the orthopaedic surgeons who order it and the physical therapists who provide it. The primary goal of restoring anatomy during a surgical procedure is further enhanced by progressive rehabilitation procedures meant to restore the physiology that creates function and ultimately ensures an enhanced outcome for the patient. This comprehensive text couples the two specialties (surgery and therapy) in an effort to increase the awareness of the extent of surgical exposure and technical procedures inherent in specific surgical procedures with the depth and progression of rehabilitation exercise and therapeutic techniques used to restore function and improve outcomes during postoperative rehabilitation. This introduction will address communication between the surgeon and therapist, the roles of each in the rehabilitation process, highlight specific examples of the interaction, and discuss the role and application of rehabilitation protocols.

COMMUNICATION ISSUES

This introductory chapter will provide points that will highlight the importance of high-level understanding of both the surgical procedure and extent of tissue involvement and the stresses, activation levels, and ultimate demands of the evidence-based rehabilitation procedures present in current state-of-the-art rehabilitation programs. The most basic point is the critical importance of collegial communication between the referring surgeon and the physical or occupational therapist. Challenges in all aspects of medical practice can decrease effective communication channels between the surgeon and therapist that ultimately can jeopardize patient care. A perfect example can be demonstrated by a typical postoperative prescription for physical therapy following an arthroscopic shoulder surgery (Figure 1). Despite the basic information provided regarding duration and general goals to increase strength and range of motion (ROM), information regarding the type of surgical repair is missing, leaving the treating therapist with limited information, which will impact many aspects of the early postoperative rehabilitation. Factors relating to surgical technique, tissue quality, and anticipated patient demands may have substantial ramifications on the types of physical therapy procedures used and the progression rate of the methods applied.

In general, a surgeon's role in postoperative rehabilitation is to surgically optimize the anatomy; communicate the anatomic status; know the general principles, stages, and progression of the rehabilitation process; and assist in the determination of the return to activity of the patient. The surgeon should provide "red light" criteria that disallow certain motions or loading and "green light" criteria that allow progression. The surgeon provides information that the therapist utilizes to determine and implement the specific exercises and progressions. The therapist's role is to understand the relevant anatomy, pathophysiology of the condition, and the surgical procedure while providing knowledge of the exercises and directing the execution of the exercise protocol throughout

Physical Therapy Prescription

℞

STATUS POST LABRAL REPAIR LEFT SHOULDER

EVALUATE AND TREAT – MODALITIES, RANGE OF MOTION, STRENGTENING

THREE TIMES A WEEK FOR 6 WEEKS

SUBSTITUTION PERMISSABLE　　DISPENSE AS WRITTEN

Figure 1 Example of prescription for physical therapy with nonessential information between therapist and surgeon.

© 2018 American Academy of Orthopaedic Surgeons

the course of postoperative management. The therapist is also responsible for determining and recommending readiness for progression through the protocol and developing activity-specific or sport-specific functional exercises for the return to activity or sport following surgery. A coordinated collaboration between the surgeon to optimize the anatomy and the therapist to optimize the physiology and function leads to an optimized outcome.

A specific example of a type of therapy (a patient status postarthroscopic glenoid labral repair) can be used to illustrate several concepts to highlight the importance of professional interaction between the therapist and surgeon.

One of the major factors guiding progression of ROM following labral repair is the anatomic location of the labral repair. Based on the location of the labral repair (anterior, superior, posterior) and the underlying pathophysiology (traumatic instability, repetitive overload, or degenerative), therapeutic progressions and treatments may be altered. The identification of a low tension zone in the anterior capsule by Black et al and the findings by Penna et al of the effects of combined abduction and external rotation versus the effects of external rotation in adduction provide important guidance regarding the extent and combined effects of glenohumeral joint ROM following anterior inferior labral repair. Without the knowledge of the anatomic location of the repair, the application of evidence-based exercises and joint ROM by the therapist would not optimally protect the labral repair by minimizing or appropriately loading the glenohumeral capsular tissue during ROM. Additionally, without detailed information on labral repair location, the therapist would likely approach the patient with a much less aggressive ROM program to be protective of the capsulolabral tissue globally. The therapist, in that case, might not provide the optimal early ROM, which can lead to stiffness and loss of motion and a more complicated rehabilitation. Awareness of each other's roles and expertise coupled with effective communication strategies can lead to optimal functional results for the patient.

APPLICATION OF BASIC SCIENCE RESEARCH IN REHABILITATION

In addition to the critically important communication about the surgical procedure between the surgeon and therapist, optimal high-level postoperative rehabilitation should be based as much as possible on evidence-based methods. This can facilitate agreement and coordination of the patient's care. This can be illustrated for the purposes of this chapter in the rehabilitation of patients following rotator cuff repair.

Early ROM (optimal physiology) is a key initial goal to minimize disuse atrophy, minimize capsular contracture, and improve both short-term and long-term outcomes following rotator cuff repair. This has been a topic of much research, with some studies showing no difference in shoulder ROM at long-term follow-up with delayed motion protocol following rotator cuff repair. Conversely, several studies show no increase in rotator cuff re-tear rates when early passive motion is applied, implying that early ROM does not harm the rotator cuff repair. However, motion has to be performed within safe ranges that do not place undue loads on the repaired tendon and jeopardize the anatomic repair. For example, there are clearly differences between small, stable rotator cuff repairs and repairs of larger and massive tears with poorer quality tissue. Research provides direct guidance on safe, low-tension ROMs for the repaired rotator cuff while allowing glenohumeral joint motion and capsular elongation. Basic science biomechanical studies demonstrate that in 30° of elevation in the scapular plane, up to 60° of external rotation does not place significant increases in tension on the supraspinatus as compared to the position of adduction and neutral rotation. However, movement to the position of 60° of internal rotation does increase stress on the supraspinatus tendon over the neutral position. These results indicate that shoulder motion during the early phases of rehabilitation using 30° of elevation in the scapular plane into internal and external rotation can optimize physiology without jeopardizing anatomy.

Park et al published an experimental cadaver study applying loads to transosseous equivalent (TOE) rotator cuff repairs. Their study shows that loads expected during early rehabilitative activities, such as side-lying external rotation exercise and passive external rotation ROM (which range between 15–90 Newtons), would be far less than loads producing excessive stress on the supraspinatus tendon repair using the TOE repair construct.

A number of studies that estimated the load generated by passive and active assisted external rotation motion demonstrate that the loads encountered during such rehabilitation are unlikely to jeopardize the anatomic integrity of a supraspinatus repair. Knowledge and application of these types of studies can assist the surgeon and therapist to collaboratively develop a protocol for early safe ROM and exercise while not jeopardizing repair integrity or provide loading that would negatively affect healing.

PROTOCOL-BASED REHABILITATION

The use of established and written postoperative protocols is common in orthopaedic and sports physical therapy; many such protocols will be discussed throughout this text. Many protocols contain detailed procedures that are based on time points since surgery and on the patient achieving certain preselected goals or activities prior to progressing to the next phase of rehabilitation. The main point of emphasis is that each protocol must be applied individually to the patient and must be based on evaluation and reevaluation of patient signs and symptoms and responses to ongoing treatment. For example, research clearly shows the need for differing rates of progression with rehabilitation and return to functional activities in patients with various sizes of rotator cuff tears (i.e., small vs. large vs. massive), quality of tendon tissue at time of repair (retracted tendon, fatty infiltration), and other factors (smoker vs. nonsmoker). It is critical when applying

© 2018 American Academy of Orthopaedic Surgeons

the information in this text that readers understand that the protocols and recommendations provided here are the authors' preferred techniques and rehabilitation recommendations, that these should be used as guidelines to be applied to individual patients, and that each patient requires specific evaluation and consideration regarding the application of rehabilitation progressions and techniques. That being said, the chapters in this book provide extensive details and evidence regarding the rehabilitation protocols and guidelines recommended for each joint or body segment.

SUMMARY

Expert surgeons and rehabilitation specialists have worked together on the chapters in this text to describe common surgical procedures and postoperative rehabilitation of the upper and lower extremities and axial skeleton and spine. The information contained here can be used to advance physician and therapist interaction, improve the development and modification of evidence-based postoperative rehabilitation protocols, and ultimately produce improved surgical outcomes. The ultimate goal is for surgeon and therapist to combine efforts to optimize and restore the anatomy and address the physiologic and functional deficiencies through evidence-based rehabilitation. The future focus lies in improving outcomes and ensuring that objective methods to evaluate outcomes are ultimately part of the entire process of surgical management and postoperative rehabilitation in orthopaedics.

BIBLIOGRAPHY

Black KP, Lim TH, McGrady LM, Raasch W: In vitro evaluation of shoulder external rotation after a Bankart reconstruction. *Am J Sports Med* 1997;25:449–453.

Chen M, Xu W, Dong Q, Huang Q, Xie Z, Mao Y: Outcomes of single-row versus double-row arthroscopic rotator cuff repair: A systematic review and meta-analysis of current evidence. *Arthroscopy* 2013;29(8):1437–1449.

Ellenbecker TS, Bailie DS, Kibler WB: Rehabilitation following rotator cuff repair, in Manske R, ed: *Postsurgical Orthopedic Sports Rehabilitation: Knee & Shoulder*. Philadelphia, PA, Elsevier Science, 2006.

Ghodadra NS, Provencher MT, Verma NN, Wilk KE, Romeo AA: Open, mini-open and all arthroscopic rotator cuff repair surgery: indications and implications for surgery. *J Orthop Sports Phys Ther* 2009;39(2):81–89.

Hatakeyama Y, Itoi E, Urayama M, Pradham RL, Sato K: Effect of superior capsule and coracohumeral ligament release on strain in the repaired rotator cuff tendon. *Am J Sports Medicine* 2001;29(5):633–640.

Mazzocca AD, Bollier M, Fehsenfeld D, Romeo AA, Stephens K, Solovyoya O, Obopilwe E, Cimineiello A, Nowak MD, Arciero R: Biomechanical evaluation of margin convergence. *Arthroscopy* 2011;27(2):330–338.

Park MC, Idjadi JA, ElAttrache NS, Tibone JE, McGarry MH, Lee TQ: The effect of dynamic external rotation comparing 2 footprint-restoring rotator cuff repair techniques. *Am J Sports Med* 2008;36:893–900.

Penna J, Deramo D, Nelson CO, Sileo MJ, Levin SM, Tompkins B, Ianuzzi A: Determination of anterior labral repair stress during passive arm motion in a cadaveric model. *Arthroscopy* 2008;24(8):930–935.

Riboh JC, Garrigues GE: Early passive range of motion versus immobilization after arthroscopic rotator cuff repair. *Arthroscopy* 2014;30(8):997–1005.

Van Der Meijden OA, Westgard P, Chandler Z, Gaskill TR, Kokmeyer D, Millett PJ: Rehabilitation after arthroscopic rotator cuff repair: Current concepts review and evidence-based guidelines. *Int J Sports Physical Therapy* 2012;7(2): 197–218.

© 2018 American Academy of Orthopaedic Surgeons

Contents

© 2018 American Academy of Orthopaedic Surgeons

 © 2018 American Academy of Orthopaedic Surgeons

© 2018 American Academy of Orthopaedic Surgeons

 © 2018 American Academy of Orthopaedic Surgeons

© 2018 American Academy of Orthopaedic Surgeons

 © 2018 American Academy of Orthopaedic Surgeons

© 2018 American Academy of Orthopaedic Surgeons

SECTION 1

Shoulder

1 Anatomic and Physiologic Basis for Postoperative Rehabilitation for the Shoulder

Trevor W. Wilkes, MD, David Ebaugh, PT, PhD, Bryan A. Spinelli, PT, PhD, OCS, CLT-LANA, Rebekah L. Lawrence, PT, DPT, OCS, Paula M. Ludewig, PT, PhD, and W. Ben Kibler, MD

INTRODUCTION

The foundation of all shoulder rehabilitation interventions is a thorough understanding of the anatomy, complex three-dimensional movement patterns, and multiple functional task demands at the shoulder girdle. The skeletal, articular, and muscular structure and resultant kinesiology support the two key requirements of mobility and dynamic stability that ultimately facilitate the functional achievement of task demands.

Optimal mobility, which is necessary to allow coordinated and sequential movements of the bones and joints to respond to varied task demands, is directly related to joint congruity, the pliability of the joint capsules and ligaments, and the flexibility of the surrounding muscles. Dynamic stability is necessary to convert the relatively unstable joint articulations, especially the glenohumeral joint, into a closed chain that allows for the transfer of forces between the trunk and the arm, minimizes intra-articular forces and loads, and creates ball-and-socket kinematics at the glenohumeral joint.

Rehabilitation interventions can affect many of these mobility and stability factors to create optimal shoulder function. This chapter will review the anatomic, physiologic, and mechanical concepts and principles to provide the foundation for postoperative rehabilitation of the shoulder.

JOINT ARTICULATIONS

Shoulder girdle motion is based on the complex interaction of the sternoclavicular (SC), acromioclavicular (AC), and glenohumeral (GH) joints, as well as the scapulothoracic (ST) articulation. The SC joint is a saddle-shaped synovial joint formed by the medial end of the clavicle and the superolateral aspect of the manubrium; it is the only skeletal articulation that links the upper extremity with the axial skeleton. It is supported by strong ligamentous structures, including the intra-articular disk ligament, the costoclavicular (rhomboid) ligament, the interclavicular ligament, and the capsular ligaments. Sternoclavicular joint motion is described as elevation/depression, protraction/retraction, and posterior/anterior rotation (Figure 1.1). Elevation/depression occurs around a anterior-posterior directed axis and results in raising and lowering of the lateral end of the clavicle. Protraction (forward motion of the lateral end of the clavicle) and retraction (backward motion of the clavicle) occurs around an vertically directed axis. Posterior/anterior rotation occurs along the long axis of the clavicle and results in the anterolateral aspect of the clavicle rotating up and back, and down and forward, respectively.

The AC joint is a diathrodial synovial joint formed by the distal clavicle, acromion, the surrounding capsule, and an intra-articular fibrocartilaginous meniscal disc. It is a stable pivot for coordinated movements of the clavicle and scapula. The AC capsular ligaments attach 3 to 5 mm medial to the distal end of the clavicle and provide the primary restraint of anterior-posterior translation. The coracoclavicular (CC) ligaments, the conoid and trapezoid, are the primary restraint to superior translation of the distal clavicle, and also provide some rotational control. The CC ligaments extend from the undersurface of the clavicle to the base of the coracoid process.

Dr. Ludewig or an immediate family member has received nonincome support (such as equipment or services), commercially derived honoraria, or other non-research–related funding (such as paid travel) from Innovative Sports Training. Dr. Wilkes or an immediate family member is a member of a speakers' bureau or has made paid presentations on behalf of Arthrex. Neither of the following authors nor any immediate family member has received anything of value from or has stock or stock options held in a commercial company or institution related directly or indirectly to the subject of this article: Dr. Ebaugh, Dr. Lawrence, and Dr. Spinelli.

© 2018 American Academy of Orthopaedic Surgeons

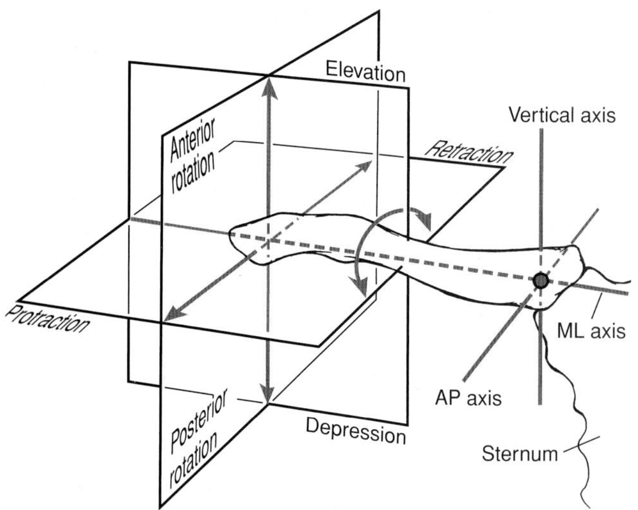

Figure 1.1 Sternoclavicular motions; elevation/depression around an A-P axis; protraction/retraction around a vertical axis; posterior rotation around medial/lateral axis. (From Oatis, Carol A. *Kinesiology: The Mechanics & Pathomechanics of Human Movement*, 3e. Philadelphia: Wolters Kluwer, 2016.)

The conoid ligament is more medial, attaching slightly posterior and, on average, 45 mm from the AC joint; it is mainly responsible for inferior/superior joint stability. The trapezoid ligament inserts roughly 15 mm laterally and more centrally on the clavicle, and provides restraint to inferior/superior as well as lateral translation.

The AC joint is inherently very stable and has medial-lateral limited motion. Three rotary motions available at this joint include upward/downward rotation, anterior/posterior tilt, and internal/external rotation (Figure 1.2). These motions are best understood if one considers the direction in which the glenoid fossa and posterior acromion move with each motion. Upward/downward rotation occurs around an axis that is roughly perpendicular to the body of the scapula. During upward rotation, the glenoid fossa rotates in a superior direction. As the scapula downwardly rotates, the glenoid fossa moves in an inferior direction. Anterior/posterior tilting occurs around a medial-lateral axis that runs through the scapular spine. During anterior tilt the posterior acromion moves in an anterior-superior direction, and duinrg posterior tilt it moves in a posterior-inferior direction. Internal/external rotation occurs around a vertical axis. As the scapula moves into internal rotation (IR), the glenoid fossa rotates in an anteromedial direction; during external rotation (ER), the glenoid fossa rotates in a posterolateral direction.

The GH joint is formed by the shallow glenoid and articular segment of the humeral head. The glenoid, covered in hyaline articular cartilage, is surrounded by the fibrocartilaginous labrum. The labrum extends and deepens the glenoid fossa both spreading joint loads and providing restraint to humeral head translation. The capsule has a synovial lining and arises from the margin of the labrum, attaching along the humeral anatomic neck. The labrum is the site of origin of the superior, middle, and inferior GH ligaments. The superior labrum is also the origin of the long head biceps tendon.

The glenohumeral ligaments are discrete thickenings within the capsule that control rotation and translation of the humeral head, especially at the extremes of glenohumeral motion. The superior and middle GH ligaments arise from the anterior glenoid and insert laterally on the humerus. The inferior glenohumeral ligament complex is comprised of anterior and posterior bands that support the inferior capsule and provides stability in varying positions of arm elevation and rotation. The rotator cuff interval is comprised of the coracohumeral ligament, the superior glenohumeral ligament, and rotator cuff interval capsule. The coracohumeral ligament arises from the lateral coracoid, is contained in the rotator cuff interval, and inserts on the lesser and greater tuberosities. The entire capsulolabral complex is essential to glenohumeral stability.

The GH joint has six degrees of freedom with three rotary and three translatory motions. Together with ST, SC, and AC joint motion, the GH joint enables a large range of shoulder, which is important for performing a wide range of functional activities. Flexion/extension occurs about a medial-lateral axis, IR/ER about a vertical axis along the shaft of the humerus, and abduction/adduction about an anterior-posterior axis. Functional elevation typically occurs in the scapular plane. Translatory motions are generally small (1–2 mm superior/inferior, 3–5 mm anterior/posterior), and are important for normal glenohumeral motion.

The relatively shallow glenoid "socket" allows substantial mobility of the GH joint, yet provides limited stability. The bony stability can be further altered by pathology, including glenoid deficiency (bony Bankart lesions) and humeral head defects (Hill-Sachs and reverse Hill-Sachs). When the arm is positioned at the side, the superior GH ligament and coracohumeral ligament provide some resistance to inferior subluxation. The coracohumeral ligament also resists humeral ER and the superior GH ligament contributes to anterior stability. As the arm is progressively elevated, the capsular contributions to anterior stability progressively shift to the middle GH ligament, and eventually the inferior GH ligament complex. At higher angles of arm elevation, the inferior GH ligament complex functions as a "sling" or hammock, contributing to inferior stability, as well as anterior stability when the arm is externally rotated, and posterior stability when the arm is internally rotated. Capsular or labral injuries inherently reduce stability, and increase reliance on the secondary constraints of the dynamic activation of the rotator cuff.

The rotator cuff plays a critical role in maximizing glenohumeral joint stability by centering the humeral head in the glenoid and providing medial compressive force throughout motion. In the presence of capsular or labral injuries, it is even more critical to ensure optimal activation, control, and endurance from the rotator cuff muscle group. While the supraspinatus—which provides a medial compressive line of action and functions as an accessory abductor—often receives the greatest attention, the remainder of the cuff musculature (subscapularis, infraspinatus, teres minor) is more important

© 2018 American Academy of Orthopaedic Surgeons

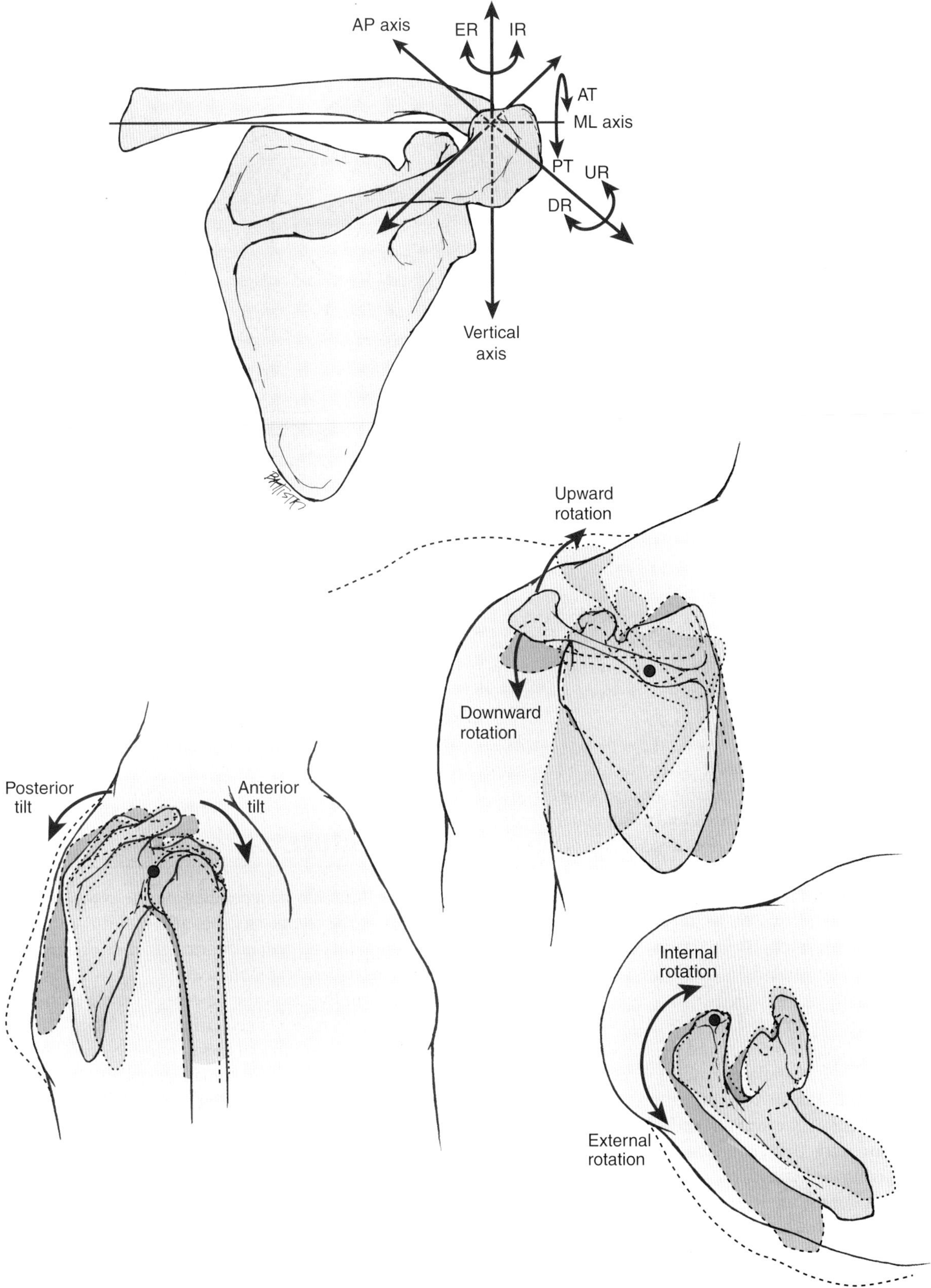

Figure 1.2 Acromioclavicular joint motions; upward/downward rotation about an A-P axis; anterior/posterior tilt about a medial/lateral axis; internal/external rotation about a vertical axis. (From Oatis, Carol A. *Kinesiology: The Mechanics & Pathomechanics of Human Movement,* 3e. Philadelphia: Wolters Kluwer, 2016.)

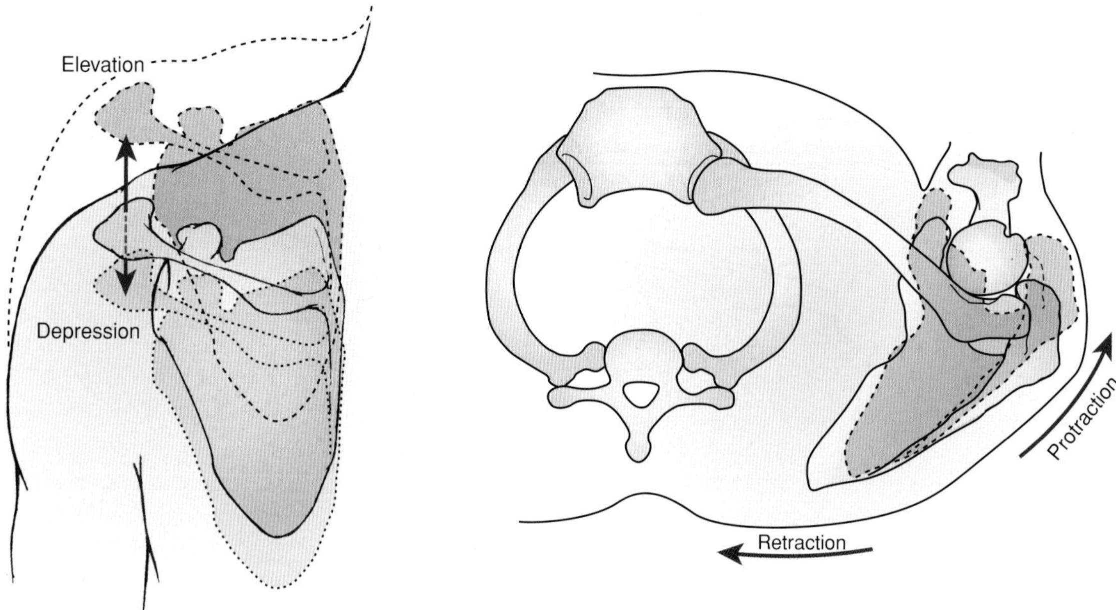

Figure 1.3 Scapulothoracic motions; elevation/depression and protraction/retraction around the thoracic wall. (From Oatis, Carol A. *Kinesiology: The Mechanics & Pathomechanics of Human Movement,* 3e. Philadelphia: Wolters Kluwer, 2016.)

in offsetting the superior translatory component of the deltoid during arm elevation. The subscapularis, infraspinatus, and teres minor also play key roles in preventing excessive translation by controlling anterior and posterior humeral head motion.

The ST articulation occurs at two fascial plane interfaces between the scapula and thorax. These fascial planes are located between the subscapularis and serratus anterior muscles, and the serratus anterior muscle and posterolateral aspect of the thorax. Although ST motion describes movement of the scapula on the thorax, this motion is a composite motion controlled and constrained by the SC and AC joint motions. ST motion consists of two translatory motions (elevation/depression and protraction/retraction) and three rotary motions (upward/downward, internal/external, and anterior/posterior tilt).

Elevation and depression of the scapula are directly linked with clavicular elevation and depression respectively (Figure 1.3). As the scapula elevates and depresses on the thorax, small amounts of AC joint motion occur to ensure optimal alignment of the scapula with the thorax. Scapular protraction and retraction are linked with clavicular protraction and retraction, respectively (Figure 1.3). Additionally, during these motions, small amounts of scapular IR and ER occur at the AC joint, which facilitates optimal positioning of the scapula on the thoracic wall. ST rotations include upward/downward rotation, anterior/posterior tilt, and IR/ER. It is important to recognize that during most functional activities involving the shoulder girdle, these ST rotations do not occur as isolated motions. For example, as the arm is raised over the head, the typical pattern of ST motion includes elevation, retraction, upward rotation, posterior tilt, and ER or IR depending on the primary plane of arm elevation (ER if the arm is raised closer to the frontal plane, i.e., abduction). These ST motions are important for maintaining optimal alignment between the humeral head and glenoid fossa, optimal size of the subacromial space, ideal length tension relationship of the rotator cuff muscles, and contributing to the range of arm elevation.

MUSCULATURE

Shoulder function is dependent on the complex recruitment patterns of the 18 muscles that attach to the scapula and arm. These muscles can generally be categorized as thoracohumeral, axioscapular, and scapulohumeral.

The main thoracohumeral muscles are the latissimus dorsi and pectoralis major. Their primary functions are to produce large range of motion and power movements of the arm. They also indirectly produce scapular movements by their effect on the arm through the GH joint. The latissimus dorsi is innervated by the thoracodorsal nerve and is a powerful adductor and internal rotator of the arm, especially in positions of arm abduction greater than 90° due to the wide origin on the spine and dorsolumbar fascia, long length, and the insertion posterior to the biceps groove. The pectoralis major is innervated by the lateral and medial pectoral nerves and is also an adductor and internal rotator, with additional functions as a flexor of the arm. It is most effective at lower arm elevations. Both of these thoracohumeral muscles can become tight and can restrict both GH joint and scapular motion.

The axioscapular muscles anchor the scapula to the axial skeleton and support its role as the platform of the shoulder

 © 2018 American Academy of Orthopaedic Surgeons

while guiding the scapula through the requisite degrees of freedom. These muscles include the serratus anterior, levator scapula, pectoralis minor, rhomboids, and trapezius.

The trapezius muscle is the largest and most superficial axioscapular muscle, and is innervated by the spinal accessory nerve (11th cranial nerve). The expansive muscle originates from the occiput, nuchal ligament, and spinous processes of C7 through T12. The upper trapezius inserts on the distal third of the clavicle and the acromion, the middle trapezius inserts along the scapular spine, and the lower trapezius inserts at the base of the scapular spine. This broad muscle is precisely oriented to allow the complex functions of scapular retraction, elevation, and posterior tilting based on the selective recruitment pattern. The upper and lower trapezius appear to be activated as separate but complementary muscles.

The rhomboid minor muscle is innervated by the dorsal scapular nerve (C5), originates from the spinous processes of C7 through T1, and inserts at the medial scapular border at the base of the scapular spine. The rhomboid major is also innervated by the dorsal scapular nerve, and the muscle originates from T2 through T5 and inserts along the posterior aspect of the medial border from the base of the scapular spine, to the inferior angle. This orientation facilitates the contribution of the rhomboid major to scapular retraction.

The serratus anterior muscle is innervated by the long thoracic nerve and is comprised of three divisions, originating from the anterolateral aspect of the first through ninth ribs. The serratus anterior protracts and upwardly rotates the scapula in association with arm elevation while providing a critical stabilization function against excessive ST IR throughout nearly all positions of arm forward flexion and elevation. The levator scapula muscle is innervated by deep branches of C3 and C4, originates from the transverse processes of C1 through C3 (and at times C4), inserts at the superior medial angle of the scapula, and functions in concert with the serratus anterior, serving to elevate and upwardly rotate the scapula. The pectoralis minor, which is often overlooked in its role in scapular positioning, originates from the anterior aspect of the second through fifth ribs, coursing superolaterally to insert on the medial aspect of the coracoid process, and is innervated by both the medial and lateral pectoral nerves. Chronic tightness can contribute to a protracted, anteriorly tilted scapular position.

The scapulohumeral muscles include the deltoid, supraspinatus, infraspinatus, subscapularis, teres minor, and teres major muscles, and primarily produce glenohumeral motion. The deltoid originates broadly from the lateral clavicle, the entire acromion, and the scapular spine while inserting on the deltoid tubercle of the humerus. This structural arrangement allows it to contribute to arm elevation in multiple planes. The suprapinatus and infraspinatus muscles originate from the medial two-thirds of their respective scapular fossae while inserting in a complex, but reasonably consistent, arrangement on the greater tuberosity. The subscapularis muscle originates from the anterior aspect of the scapula and inserts on the lesser tuberosity. The teres minor muscle originates from the middle section of the lateral scapula and is innervated by the posterior branch of the axillary nerve. The footprint of the posterior-superior rotator cuff on the greater tuberosity is the insertion site of interdigitating tendon fibers, with the infraspinatus wrapping around the supraspinatus from posterior to anterior. The teres major muscle originates on the inferior lateral scapula and inserts with the latissimus on the medial biceps groove, is innervated by the subscapular nerve, and functions in humeral IR, adduction, and extension.

MOVEMENT PATTERNS

Normal shoulder girdle kinematics are dependent on optimal motions and stability of the SC, AC, and GH joints as well as the ST articulation, and coordinated, sequential activation of the muscles in force couples. Motion is required at each joint of the shoulder complex to produce composite functional movement. The required motions are task specific. The largest amount of normal shoulder girdle motion occurs at the ST articulation and the GH joints. Although SC and AC joint motions are component motions of the resulting ST motion, they are still critical to normal motion (Table 1.1).

ST motion is needed to maximize available motion, clear the subacromial soft tissues, and maintain dynamic GH joint stability. Stabilized GH motion is needed to allow required arm mobility to place the arm and hand in effective positions. ST joint motion is constrained by contact with the thorax and the

Table 1.1 SUMMARY OF MOTION DURING FUNCTIONAL SHOULDER ELEVATION

Joint Rotation	Motion (Degrees)
Sternoclavicular Joint	
Posterior rotation	24
Retraction	13
Elevation	6
Acromioclavicular Joint	
Posterior tilt	15
Upward rotation	11
Internal rotation	6
Scapulothoracic Articulation	
Upward rotation	54
Posterior tilt	16
Internal/external rotation	0.2
Glenohumeral Joint	
Elevation	74
External rotation	27

Note: Functional motion is defined as rest to 120° of elevation in the scapular plane.
(Data from Ludewig PM, Phadke V, Braman JP, Hassett DR, Cieminski CJ, LaPrade RF. Motion of the shoulder complex during multiplanar humeral elevation. *J Bone Joint Surg Am* 2009;91(2):378–389.)

© 2018 American Academy of Orthopaedic Surgeons

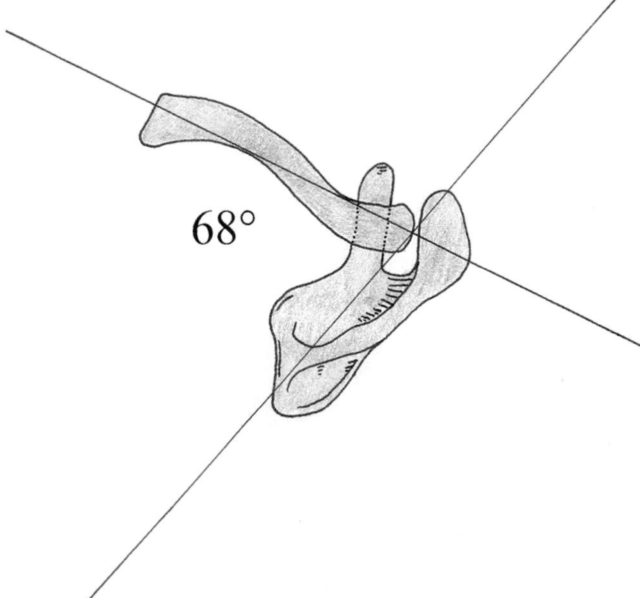

Figure 1.4 The angle between the clavicle and the scapula, representing acromioclavicular internal rotation, helps define the patterns of coupling between the sternoclavicular, acromioclavicular, and scapulothoracic joints. (From Teece RM, Lunden JB, Lloyd AS, Kaiser AP, Cieminski CJ, Ludewig PM: Three-dimensional acromioclavicular joint motions during elevation of the arm. *J Orthop Sports Phys Ther* 2008;38(4):181–190.)

SC and AC joints. ST motion requires substantial motion at the SC and AC joints (see Table 1.1). The degree to which SC and AC motion contributes to ST motion is influenced by the magnitude of the angle between the clavicle and the scapula in the transverse plane, representing AC IR (Figure 1.4). When observed three-dimensionally, upward rotation of the AC joint and posterior rotation of the SC joint in combination results in upward rotation of the scapula on the thorax. SC elevation also produces a small amount of ST upward rotation. In addition to upward rotation, SC elevation produces ST anterior tilt that slightly offsets the AC posterior tilt, which occurs concomitantly. The result is a net posterior tilt of the scapula on the thorax.

Recognizing the fact that ST motion is a composite motion produced through the SC and AC joint motions, it is important to understand that, unlike other muscles of the body, the muscles responsible for these motions do not directly cross the SC and AC joints, and their origin and/or insertion are onto bones other than the manubrium, clavicle, or acromion process. For example, the pectoralis minor muscle, which has the capability of protracting and depressing the clavicle and scapula through the SC joint, attaches to ribs 3 to 5 and the coracoid process. Such an arrangement illustrates the importance of normally functioning AC and SC joints for ST motion.

The scapula plays a complex role in stabilizing the GH joint while also preserving rotator cuff clearance relative to the glenoid and beneath the coracoacromial arch. As such, it must be both mobile and stable over the curved rib cage. Scapular upward rotation is typically accompanied by posterior tilt and AC ER, motions that help to keep the inferior angle and medial border of the scapula against the thoracic wall. Therefore, the scapula should remain flat against the thoracic wall and neither the medial border nor inferior angle of the scapula should be prominent. The serratus anterior, with large moment arms and attachment across the medial border of the scapula, is both the prime mover into upward rotation as well as a major contributor to preventing excess scapular IR (winging or medial border prominence). The upper trapezius plays a prominent role in positioning the scapula through SC retraction and elevation. The middle and lower trapezius are also critical scapular stabilizers to minimize excess IR at the AC joint, and the lower trapezius further assists in providing scapular upward rotation. Based on the line of action of these muscles, normal serratus anterior function is more critical to optimal scapular control during shoulder flexion, and the trapezius more aligned to contribute to coronal plane abduction. Any deviation from this typical movement pattern is called scapular dyskinesis, and is indicative of underlying neuromusculoskeletal impairment.

The muscles that are primarily responsible for producing and controlling ST motion can be separated into anterior and posterior groups. The trapezius, levator scapulae, rhomboids, and latissimus dorsi muscles comprise the posterior muscle group. The pectoralis major, pectoralis minor, and serratus anterior muscles make up the anterior group. Collectively, these muscles are primarily responsible for producing and controlling ST motion.

The upper portion of the trapezius, levator scapula, and rhomboid muscles produce elevation of the scapula, otherwise known as a shoulder shrug (Figure 1.5, A). Since the levator scapula and rhomboid muscles' attachment sites to the scapula are medial to the axis of upward/downward rotation, they also downwardly rotate the scapula. By elevating the lateral end of the clavicle, the upper trapezius also has the potential to play a minor role in upwardly rotating the scapula.

Forceful depression of the scapula is produced by the latissimus dorsi, lower trapezius, pectoralis minor, and lower portion of the pectoralis major muscle (Figure 1.5, B). Additionally, the latissimus dorsi, pectoralis major, and pectoralis minor muscles have the potential to downwardly rotate the scapula as the line of action of these muscles is lateral to the axis of upward/downward rotation. Whether the scapula protracts, retracts, or remains in a neutral position with depression depends on the relative balance in the activity levels between the anteriorly located pectoral muscles and the posteriorly located latissimus dorsi and trapezius muscles.

The pectoralis major, pectoralis minor, and serratus anterior muscles produce scapular protraction. In addition to scapular protraction and downward rotation, the pectoral muscles can also produce scapular anterior tilting and IR. The serratus anterior muscle can upwardly rotate, externally rotate, and posteriorly tilt the scapula. Therefore, scapular protraction may be accompanied by upward rotation, posterior tilt, and ER if dominated by serratus anterior activity. Likewise, the scapula

 © 2018 American Academy of Orthopaedic Surgeons

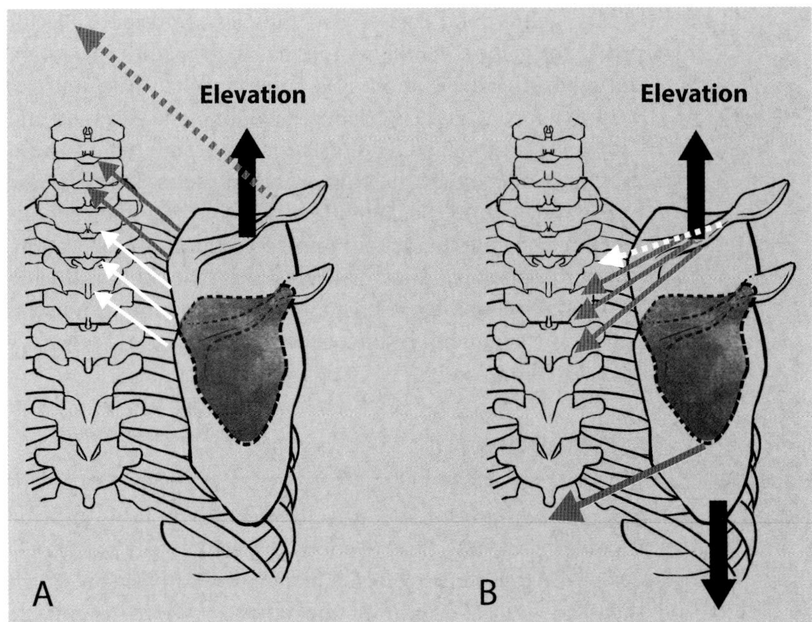

Figure 1.5 **A**, Muscles responsible for producing scapular elevation. Dashed red line = upper trapezius; solid purple lines = levator scapulae; solid white lines = rhomboids. **B**, Muscles responsible for producing scapular depression. Dashed white line = pectoralis major and minor; solid red lines = lower trapezius; solid purple line = latissimus dorsi.

will move into IR and anterior tilt as it protracts if the motion is dominated by pectoral muscle activity.

Scapular retraction is produced by the trapezius, rhomboids, and latissimus dorsi muscles. As the rhomboids and latissimus dorsi muscles retract the scapula, there is also scapular downward rotation. This motion could be offset by the tendency of the trapezius muscle to upwardly rotate the scapula, thereby allowing the scapula to retract and remain in a neutral upward/downwardly rotated position.

Raising the arm to an overhead position requires coordinated activity of the ST and GH musculature. Many overhead motions take place in the plane of the scapula (scaption), which is approximately 30° to 45° anterior to the coronal body plane. As the arm is raised over the head, the primary ST motion is upward rotation. The upper and lower trapezius, along with the serratus anterior muscles, have been described as forming a force couple to produce this motion. However, the role of the upper trapezius muscle in upward rotation of the scapula is somewhat controversial. The serratus anterior and middle trapezius muscles then continue to work in a force couple to upwardly rotate the scapula as the arm is raised over the head (Figure 1.6). The role of the lower trapezius is felt to be one of a scapular stabilizer, offsetting scapular protraction and elevation produced by the serratus anterior and upper trapezius muscles, respectively.

During scapular plane elevation the scapula tilts posteriorly and externally rotators at the end range. The serratus anterior, rhomboids, and trapezius muscles work together in force couples to produce these motions. Due to the large attachment to the inferior angle of the scapula the lower portion of the serratus anterior muscle is ideally positioned to produce posterior tilt of the scapula. The lower trapezius muscle attaches to the lower thoracic spinous processes and the deltoid tubercle on the scapular spine, and works with the lower portion of the serratus anterior is thought to produce scapular posterior tilt (Figure 1.7). The serratus anterior and rhomboid muscles attach to the vertebral border of the scapula, forming a force couple that is capable of producing scapular ER (Figure 1.8).

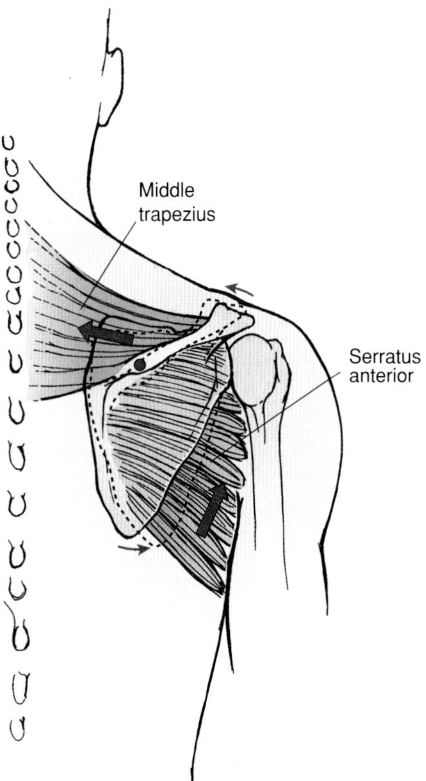

Figure 1.6 Muscles responsible for producing scapula upward rotation (middle trapezius; lower portion of serratus anterior). (From Oatis, Carol A. *Kinesiology: The Mechanics & Pathomechanics of Human Movement,* 3e. Philadelphia: Wolters Kluwer, 2016.)

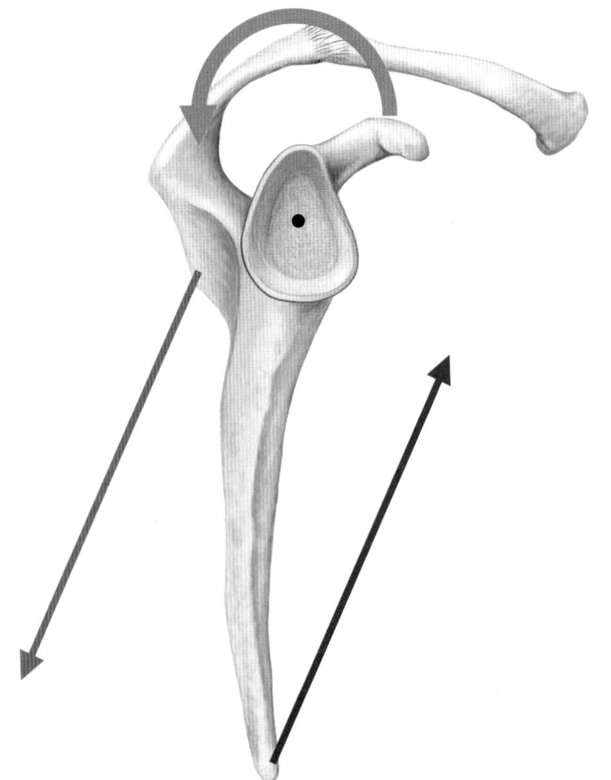

Figure 1.7 Muscles responsible for producing scapula posterior tilt. Black dot = axis of rotation; green arrow = posterior tilt motion; purple arrow = serratus anterior; red arrow = lower trapezius. (From Oatis, Carol A. *Kinesiology: The Mechanics & Pathomechanics of Human Movement,* 3e. Philadelphia: Wolters Kluwer, 2016.)

The deltoid and rotator cuff muscles are responsible for producing glenohumeral motion that accompanies ST motion during overhead elevation. It is important that these muscles work as a force couple to produce glenohumeral elevation and ER while minimizing GH translations to ensure full overhead motion. Collectively, the rotator cuff muscles compress the humeral head into the glenoid fossa, stabilizing the glenohumeral joint while the deltoid muscle produces arm elevation. The supraspinatus muscle will assist the deltoid in producing arm elevation, and the infraspinatus and teres minor muscles will produce humeral ER that occurs toward the end ranges of arm elevation.

SUMMARY

Understanding how SC, AC, GH, and ST motions and the shoulder girdle muscle activations contribute to overall shoulder girdle motion provides clinicians with a basis on which they can evaluate aberrant movement patterns or muscle weakness that may be associated with pathologic shoulder conditions and injuries as well as postsurgical conditions that need to be addressed in rehabilitation. Many of these alterations can be observed in the variety of shoulder injuries and conditions that are managed and rehabilitated after surgery. The purpose of this overview is to highlight the interaction of motion and strength over several body segments to produce stability and mobility and to stress the importance of restoration of all of these areas in postoperative rehabilitation to serve as the basis for successful return to functional activity.

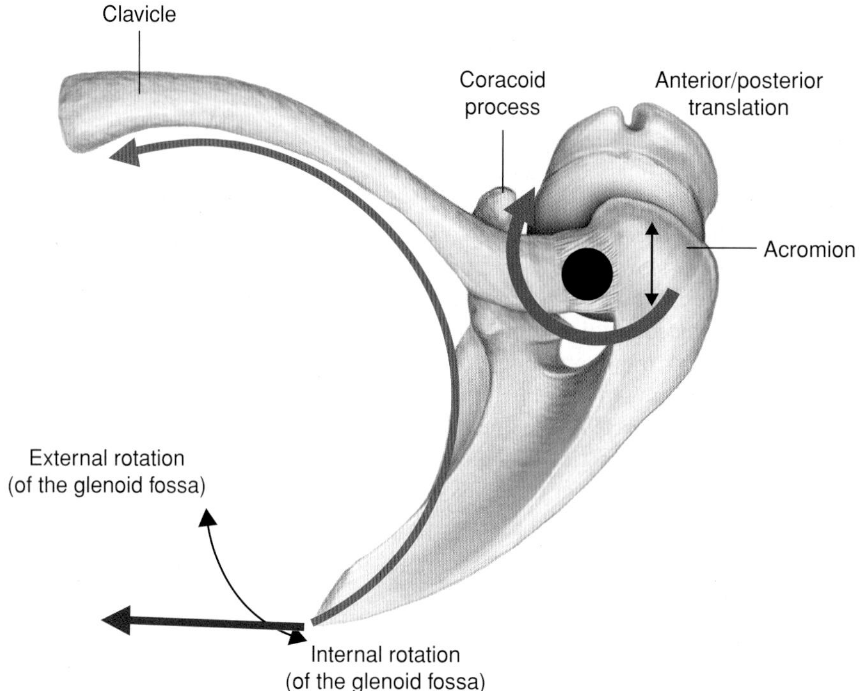

Figure 1.8 Muscles responsible for producing scapular external rotation. Black dot = axis of rotation; blue arrow = external rotation motion; red arrow = serratus anterior muscle; purple arrow = rhomboids. (From Oatis, Carol A. *Kinesiology: The Mechanics & Pathomechanics of Human Movement,* 3e. Philadelphia: Wolters Kluwer, 2016.)

© 2018 American Academy of Orthopaedic Surgeons

BIBLIOGRAPHY

Borich MR, Bright JM, Lorello DJ, Cieminski CJ, Buisman T, Ludewig PM: Scapular angular positioning at end range internal rotation in cases of glenohumeral internal rotation deficit. *J Orthop Sports Phys Ther* 2006;36(12):926–934.

Braman JP, Engel SC, Laprade RF, Ludewig PM: In vivo assessment of scapulohumeral rhythm during unconstrained overhead reaching in asymptomatic subjects. *J Shoulder Elbow Surg* 2009;18(6):960–967.

Culham E, Peat M: Functional anatomy of the shoulder complex. *J Orthop Sports Phys Ther* 1993;18(1):342–350.

Ebaugh DD, McClure PW, Karduna AR: Three-dimensional scapulothoracic motion during active and passive arm elevation. *Clin Biomech (Bristol, Avon)* 2005;20(7):700–709.

Johnson G, Bogduk N, Nowitzke A, House D: Anatomy and actions of the trapezius muscle. *Clin Biomech (Bristol, Avon)* 1994;9(1):44–50.

Kibler WB, Ludewig PM, McClure PW, Michener LA, Bak K, Sciascia AA: Clinical implications of scapular dyskinesis in shoulder injury: The 2013 consensus statement from the 'scapular summit'. *Br J Sports Med* 2013;47(14): 877–885.

Ludewig PM, Cook TM: Alterations in shoulder kinematics and associated muscle activity in people with symptoms of shoulder impingement. *Phys Ther* 2000;80(3):276–291.

Ludewig PM, Phadke V, Braman JP, Hassett DR, Cieminski CJ, LaPrade RF: Motion of the shoulder complex during multiplanar humeral elevation. *J Bone Joint Surg Am* 2009;91(2): 378–389.

McClure P, Tate AR, Kareha S, Irwin D, Zlupko E: A clinical method for identifying scapular dyskinesis, part 1: reliability. *J Athl Train* 2009;44(2):160–164.

Ozaki J: Glenohumeral movements of the involuntary inferior and multidirectional instability. *Clin Orthop Relat Res* 1989; 238:107–111.

Paine RM, Voight M: The role of the scapula. *J Orthop Sports Phys Ther* 1993;18(1):386–391.

Perry J: Normal upper extremity kinesiology. *Phys Ther* 1978; 58(3):265–278.

Roren A, Fayad F, Poiraudeau S, et al: Specific scapular kinematic patterns to differentiate two forms of dynamic scapular winging. *Clin Biomech (Bristol, Avon)* 2013;28(8):941–947.

Sheikhzadeh A, Yoon J, Pinto VJ, Kwon YW: Three-dimensional motion of the scapula and shoulder during activities of daily living. *J Should Elbow Surg* 2008;17(6):936–942.

Teece RM, Lunden JB, Lloyd AS, Kaiser AP, Cieminski CJ, Ludewig PM: Three-dimensional acromioclavicular joint motions during elevation of the arm.*J Orthop Sports Phys Ther* 2008;38(4):181–190.

Triffitt PD: The relationship between motion of the shoulder and the stated ability to perform activities of daily living. *J Bone Joint Surg Am* 1998;80(1):41–46.

Weiser WM, Lee TQ, McMaster WC, McMahon PJ: Effects of simulated scapular protraction on anterior glenohumeral stability. *Am J Sports Med* 1999;27(6):801–805.

Yanagawa T, Goodwin CJ, Shelburne KB, Giphart JE, Torry MR, Pandy MG: Contributions of the individual muscles of the shoulder to glenohumeral joint stability during abduction. *J Biomech Eng* 2008;130(2):021024.

© 2018 American Academy of Orthopaedic Surgeons

2 Patient-Related Outcome Measures for Shoulder Surgery and Rehabilitation

Lori A. Michener, PhD, PT, ATC, and Phillip W. McClure, PT, PhD

INTRODUCTION

Outcome measures can be used to systematically assess the effects of surgical interventions and rehabilitation for musculoskeletal shoulder disorders. Ernest Codman, MD, was the first to describe this "end result idea" in 1905. He subsequently was also the first physician to describe the outcomes of the patients he treated in order to improve quality of care. To systematically assess the outcomes of care, outcome measures should be selected that can be simply and routinely performed, with adequate psychometric properties, and that are relevant to the patient. Patient-rated outcome (PRO) measures can fit these requirements to assess the effects of care for both individuals and groups of patients, as well as to guide treatment decision-making in daily clinical practice for individual patients. By providing the patient perspective, PROs can assess the direct impact of a shoulder disorder and its treatment on the patient's daily activities and participation in work and recreational pursuits, which facilitates the assessment of the effectiveness and efficacy of treatment interventions. Moreover, PROs aid in the assessment of cost-effectiveness and value.

Clinician-rated impairment measures, such as shoulder range of motion (ROM) and strength, assess muscle and joint capacity in isolation, thus do not specifically determine the ability of the patient to use the upper extremity during required daily activities. These assessments of tissue or joint impairments are inadequate to comprehensively assess outcomes of care. PROs assess the patient perspective, which is frequently more reflective of the desired functional status, and is ultimately the most important aspect of outcome of care. Moreover, most PROs meet the requirements of simple routine use. Why are they not being used by clinicians consistently? Reported reasons for the lack of PRO use are unfamiliarity with the measures, time considerations for the patient and clinician, and lack of knowledge to interpret and use the final scores. This chapter will provide an overview of PROs for shoulder disorders—how to interpret and use the scores for treatment decision-making and quality improvement.

PSYCHOMETRIC MEASUREMENT PROPERTIES OF PATIENT-RATED OUTCOMES

PRO measures should have established measurement properties of reliability, validity, error estimates, and responsiveness. In Table 2.1, these psychometric properties and common terms are defined. The properties of a PRO should be evaluated in a sample group of patients in whom the PRO is intended to be used. A PRO score should be reliable and reproducible over time in patients whose shoulder symptoms and function/disability are not changing. Items used to generate the total score or subscales scores should demonstrate internal consistency, which is the similarity of the items used to form the score. Types of validity of a scale include: (1) concurrent validity—correlated with other similar scales or measures of shoulder disability, (2) convergent validity—not related to scales that are not measures of shoulder disability, and (3) discriminate validity—ability to discriminate between patients with different levels of disability.

For daily clinical use and interpretation of a scale, the most helpful metrics are the error and responsiveness values. Error estimates are used to interpret the scale's single score or a changed score. The standard error of the measure (SEM) is an estimate of error of a score when a patient completes a score just one time; SEM = standard deviation × [(1 − internal consistency coefficient or reliability coefficient)$^{1/2}$]. The minimal detectable change (MDC), also known as the smallest detectable difference (SDD), is the error associated with change scores (e.g., before and after treatment); MDC = SEM × [(2)$^{1/2}$]. The SEM and MDC both have a 68% confidence interval (CI).

Dr. McClure or an immediate family member serves as a board member, owner, officer, or committee member of the Journal of Orthopaedic and Sports Physical Therapy. *Dr. Michener or an immediate family member has received nonincome support (such as equipment or services), commercially derived honoraria, or other non-research–related funding (such as paid travel) from the* Journal of Orthopaedic and Sports Physical Therapy; *and serves as a board member, owner, officer, or committee member of the ACOEM–American College of Occupational and Environmental Medicine, the American Physical Therapy Association–Orthopaedic Section, the ASSET–American Society of Shoulder and Elbow Therapists, the* Journal of Orthopaedic and Sports Physical Therapy, *and the Shoulder and Elbow–British Elbow and Shoulder Society.*

© 2018 American Academy of Orthopaedic Surgeons

Table 2.1 PSYCHOMETRIC MEASUREMENT PROPERTIES OF PATIENT-RATED OUTCOMES

Property	Definition
Test-retest reliability; Interclass correlation coefficient (ICC)	Consistency of scale scores in a stable population
Internal consistency, Cronbach's alpha	Homogeneity of the items (questions) of the scale
Error Estimates	Error in the scale score based on reliability of the scale
Standard Error of the Measure (SEM)	Error value associated with a change score (e.g., change in score between pretreatment and posttreatment) with 68% confidence bounds unless otherwise stated; distribution-based error value
Minimal Detectable Change (MDC) Smallest Detectable Difference (SDD)	Error value associated with a single score with 68% confidence bounds unless otherwise stated; distribution-based error value
Responsiveness	Ability of a scale to measure clinical change
Standardized Response Mean (SRM)	Mean change scores/standard deviation of changes scores
Effect Size (ES)	Mean change scores/standard deviation of baseline scores
Minimally Clinically Important Difference (MCID)	The minimal/smallest amount of change in the score associated with patient-rated improvement; anchor-based method for calculating change that is clinically meaningful minimal or small amount of change
Substantial Clinical Benefit (SCB)/Major Clinically Important Improvement (MCII)	The amount of change in the score associated with substantial or major patient-rated improvement; anchor-based method for calculating change that is a large clinically meaningful change
Validity	Degree by which a scale measures what it intends to measure. Variety of types, which include: construct, convergent, divergent, factorial, discriminant

To determine the 90% CI, the SEM and MDC are multiplied by the corresponding z-score of 1.64 for the SEM_{90} and MDC_{90}, respectively. A critical feature of these error estimates is that they are in the same units or points as the scale itself; therefore, they allow a direct interpretation of error rather than a standardized reliability coefficient.

Responsiveness, as an aspect of validity, is the ability of a scale to measure clinical change when it has occurred. Two established metrics, effect size (ES) and standardized response mean (SRM), are used to assess the size of treatment effect over time by calculating the magnitude of the change that has occurred and taking into account the variability (standard deviation) of the scores. To determine if the change is clinically meaningful, an external criterion of improvement is used as an anchor to establish meaningful clinical change. The minimally clinically important difference (MCID), also known as the minimal important change (MIC) value, is the PRO change value that indicates the *minimally* clinically important change in the PRO score. A more recent term—the substantial clinical benefit (SCB), also known as major clinically important improvement (MCII)—is the PRO change value of *substantial* or large change that may be expected over a longer period of treatment or as a long-term outcome. The MCID and SCB are both anchor-based metrics that can be used to determine if change in a PRO score is clinically meaningful.

PATIENT-RATED OUTCOMES FOR MUSCULOSKELETAL SHOULDER DISORDERS

Shoulder pain and symptoms, difficulty with activities and participation, and patient satisfaction with shoulder use are the major elements assessed in PRO measures for shoulder disorders. PROs that are commonly used to assess outcomes of surgery and rehabilitation and have established measurement properties are presented in Table 2.2. These measures include two PROs, the Disabilities of the Arm, Shoulder, and Hand (DASH) and the Quick-DASH, which consider both upper extremities as a single unit when assessing symptoms and disability. This is accomplished by asking the patient to answer based on ability to perform the tasks "regardless of how you perform the task," stating that "it doesn't matter which hand or arm you use to perform the activity." Thus, the DASH and Quick-DASH do not allow for the specific assessment of only the involved shoulder. Three other PROs assess function/disability, two including symptoms of pain of the involved shoulder specifically. The American Shoulder and Elbow Surgeon's (ASES) Patient Self-Report, developed by the American Shoulder and Elbow Surgeons, assesses pain and function/disability considering the right or left shoulder individually with respect to the level of difficulty with daily tasks. The ASES function subscale has 10 questions, with ratings of difficulty using a 4-point Likert scale. The Simple

© 2018 American Academy of Orthopaedic Surgeons

Table 2.2 SCALE MEASUREMENT PROPERTIES PATIENT-RELATED OUTCOMES

Outcome	Scale Dimensions Scoring	Test-retest Reliability Internal Consistency	Error Estimate (SEM, MDC)	Validity	Responsiveness (SRM, ES, MCID)
ASES: American Shoulder & Elbow Standardized Form	Pain: 1 item, 10 pts/50% of total Function: 10 items 30 pts/50% of total Scoring: 0–100 pts, 100 = no disability	Test-retest reliability ICC: Range = 0.84–0.96; Average = 0.91 Internal consistency α: Range = 0.61–0.96	SEM = 6.7 MDC 90% CI = 9.4	Content Construct	SRM: Range = 0.5–1.6 Average = 1.1 ES: Range = 0.9–3.5 Average = 1.3 MCID = 6.4, 12–17
Constant Shoulder Score	Pain: 1 item,10 pts/15% of total Function: 4 items, 20 pts/20% of total Clinician measure: Range of Motion: 4 items 40 pts/40% of total Strength: 1 item, 25 pts/25% of total Scoring: 0–100 pts, 100 = no disability	Test-retest reliability ICC: Range = 0.80– 0.96 Internal consistency α: Range = 0.61–0.96	SEM = 4.5 Error estimate: SD = 8.86 (95% CI = 15, 20 pts)	Content Construct	SRM: Range = 0.59–2.16 ES: Range = 0.20–2.72 MCID = 5.4
DASH: Disabilities of the Arm, Shoulder, and Hand	Symptoms: 5 items, 30 pts/16.7% of total Disability: 25 items, 125 pts/83.3% of total Scoring: 0–100%; 0 = no disability	Test-retest reliability ICC: Range = 0.77–0.98 Average = 0.90 Internal consistency α: Range = 0.92–0.98	SEM: Range = 2.8–5.2; Average = 4.5 MDC 90% CI: Range = 6.6–12.2; Average = 10.5	Content Construct	SRM: Range = 0.5–2.2 Average = 1.1 ES: Range = 0.4–1.4 Average = 1.1 MCID = Range 10.2–10.8
Quick DASH	Symptoms: 3 items, 15 pts/37.5% of total Disability: 8 items, 40 pts/62.5% of total Scoring: 0–100% 0 = no disability	Test-retest reliability ICC: Range = 0.90–0.94 Internal consistency α: Range = 0.92–0.95	SEM: Range = 3.3–10.2 MDC 95% CI = Range = 11–13.3	Content Construct	SRM: Range = 0.63–1.1 ES = 1.02 and 1.26 MCID = 8.0, 15.9
Penn: University of Pennsylvania Shoulder Score	Pain: 3 items, 30 pts/30% of total Satisfaction: 1 item 10 pts/10% of total Function: 20 items 60 pts/60% of total Scoring: 0–100 pts 100 = no disability	Test-retest reliability ICC: 0.94 Internal consistency α = 0.93	SEM 90% CI = 8.5 MDC 90% CI = 12.1	Content Construct	SRM = 1.27 ES = 1.01 MCID = 11.4 (SD 9.5)
SST: Simple Shoulder Test	Function: 12 items,12 pts/100% of total Scoring: 0–12 pts 12 = full function	Test-retest reliability ICC: Range = 0.97–0.99 Average = 0.98 Internal consistency α = 0.85	SEM = 11.65 MDC 95% CI = 32.3	Content Construct	SRM: Range = 0.8–1.8 Average = 0.9 ES = 0.8 MCID = 2.33 points

© 2018 American Academy of Orthopaedic Surgeons

Table 2.2 SCALE MEASUREMENT PROPERTIES PATIENT-RELATED OUTCOMES *(Continued)*

Outcome	Scale Dimensions Scoring	Test-retest Reliability Internal Consistency	Error Estimate (SEM, MDC)	Validity	Responsiveness (SRM, ES, MCID)
WORC: Western Ontario Rotator-Cuff Index	Physical Symptoms: 6 items; 100 pts/28.7% of total Sports/Rec: 4 items, 100 pts/19% of total Work: 4 items, 100 pts/19% of total Lifestyle: 4 items, 100 pts/19% of total Emotional: 3 items, 100 pts/14.3% of total Scoring: 0–100% 0 = no disability	Test-retest reliability ICC: Range = 0.84–0.89 Internal Consistency α: Range = 0.91–0.95	SEM = 6.9 MDC 95% CI = 19.1	Construct	SRM = 0.91–2.1 ES = 0.96–1.37 MCID = 11.7–13.1
PSFS: Patient Specific Functional Scale	Function: 3–5 items, 10 pts each, average of item total Scoring: 0–10 10 = no disability	Test-retest reliability ICC = 0.71 Internal Consistency: none	SEM = 1.1 MDC = 3.0 (90% CI = 1.7, 4.2)	Construct	MCID = 1.2

CI = confidence interval, ES = effect size, ICC = interclass correlation coefficient, MDC = minimal detectable change, MCID = minimally clinically important difference, SEM = standard error of the measure, SRM = standardized response mean

Shoulder Test (SST) epitomizes its name. It contains 12 simple items of daily function with dichotomous (yes/no) response options. The University of Pennsylvania Shoulder Score (Penn) assesses function and pain as well as patient satisfaction with shoulder use for the involved shoulder. The Penn uses an 11-point numeric rating for pain and satisfaction, and a 5-point Likert scale for the functional items.

Other measurement tools are also used. The Constant shoulder score is a widely used shoulder scale. It contains two sections, one patient self-report and a clinician report. The patient-report section contains five questions regarding pain and daily functional activities, which contributes 35% of the total score. These few items may not adequately sample and assess shoulder disability. The clinician-based measures are ROM weighted 40% and strength weighted 25% of the total score. The Constant score is a combined measure of body structure and function, activities, and participation; the score is weighted toward the objective measures of body structure and function components. The Western Ontario Rotator Cuff Index (WORC) is a disease-specific scale, used to assess outcome in those with rotator cuff disease. The WORC assesses symptoms and function across multiple domains. It was originally described using a visual analog scale for each of the 21 items, but has been translated to an 11-point numeric rating scale that is easier to use and score in daily clinical practice. The last PRO is an individual patient function-specific scale, the patient-specific functional scale (PSFS). The PSFS asks patients to select three to five items that are important to them with which they have difficulty performing because of their injury. The difficulty level is rated for each of the items on an 11-point numeric rating scale (0 = unable to perform, 10 = able to perform the activity at preinjury level), then summed and divided by the number of items for an average score (interclass correlation coefficient [ICC] = 0.71, MDC 95% CI = 3.0, MCID = 1.2). The PSFS is quick and efficient to use, can be used for any part of the body, but may not adequately sample all activities that the patient is having difficulty with on a daily basis.

USE AND INTERPRETATION OF PATIENT-RATED OUTCOMES

Error estimates and responsiveness values can be used directly to interpret scores. For example, a patient completes the DASH at pretreatment and scores a 30/100 (0 = no disability). Using the average SEM_{90} of 7.4, the clinician can be 90% confident that the patient's score is 30 ± 7.4 points on the DASH. To judge change over time, the MDC, MCID, and SCB metrics can be used. The patient with a 30/100 DASH score on day 1 is reassessed 2 weeks later and scores a 15/100 on the DASH, which equates to a 15-point change in the DASH score. The DASH average MDC_{90} of 10.5 points indicates that there is 90% confidence that true change has occurred, and is not

© 2018 American Academy of Orthopaedic Surgeons

change due to error. A change of 15 points is greater than the MDC_{90} of 10.5 points; however, is this 15 points change clinically meaningful? The MCID can be used to determine if the amount of change is associated with clinically meaningful change—change that is deemed important to the patient. The range for the MCID for the DASH is 10.2 to 10.8 points. This indicates that the change of 15 points on the DASH, which is greater than the MCID 10.2 to 10.8, indicates meaningful change for the patient. There is a range of values for error and responsiveness metrics because they vary based on things such as the sample of patients studied, treatment delivered, patient characteristics, interval of change, and acuity.

A systematic search of the literature was performed to identify patient-rated outcomes of selected shoulder surgical procedures for rotator cuff disease. PUBMED, CINAHL, and Web of Science databases were searched for English-language only studies using free text and MeSh terms. For the purpose of this chapter, to illustrate reporting of PROs, studies of surgical interventions with follow-up rehabilitation for rotator cuff tears were retrieved. The most common PROs used to evaluate outcomes at both pre- and postsurgery in studies with at least 30 subjects were the ASES, Constant score, SST, DASH, QuickDASH, Penn shoulder score, and WORC. All these scales have established reliability and validity (including responsiveness to change) for assessing patient-rated shoulder function and disability.

It is not unusual for studies to report more than one PRO. Interestingly, there is also overlap in the assessment of symptoms and disability among most PROs. Clinically, it is reasonable to choose the PRO that is most suitable for the patient or patient population under study. Decisions regarding which PRO is most appropriate for a particular patient or patient population can be determined simply by reviewing the questions on the scales to determine their applicability. For example, both the ASES and the Quick-DASH ask about sports and recreational activity. However, the ASES specifically also asks about throwing a ball overhand and lifting 10 pounds overhead. While these questions may be critical for an athlete, they may be irrelevant for a relatively inactive elderly person who is simply concerned about difficulties performing activities of daily living (ACLs) such as grooming and toileting. PROs provide the clinician with a functional and quantitative means of determining patient progress for activities that are important to the patient.

To best determine if a patient is satisfied with the outcome of rehabilitation or surgery, we need to correlate information obtained from PROs along with key information from the rest of the process of care. A single PRO does not likely provide enough information for a comprehensive judgment of the patient's level of disability and symptoms. A suggested complement of patient-report information could include a PRO score, a report of patient satisfaction with use of the shoulder, and assessment of difficulty with patient-specific tasks that can be assessed with the PSFS. Patient satisfaction with shoulder use can be measured using the single question from the Penn score, which has demonstrated adequate measurement properties (ICC = 0.93, SEM = 1.3, MDC = 1.8) in patients with shoulder pain. Satisfaction can also be assessed by asking, "If your shoulder remained the same as it was today, would you be satisfied?" The patient-specific functional scale (PSFS) which asks patients to select and rate the level of difficulty with three to five daily tasks, can assist in most directly assessing individual patient needs. Using the PRO score, patient satisfaction with shoulder use, and the PSFS score can help the clinician judge if the patient is able to perform general daily activities, the specific activities the patient needs to do, and the patient's overall satisfaction with use of the shoulder.

Process-of-care variables are those aspects of care that potentially influence outcome, and therefore should be accounted for when interpreting patient outcomes. For surgery, these would include surgical approach and components performed (e.g., arthroscopic, tendon rotator cuff repair, and biceps tenodesis), patient characteristics (e.g., age, gender, comorbidities, and other prior surgeries) and patient–provider interaction. Process-of-care variables for rehabilitation should include patient characteristics (e.g., prior treatment, history of exercise, other areas of pain, age, gender, and comorbidities), patient–provider interaction, the type of treatment intervention performed, as well as the number of rehabilitation visits. These are variables that may influence outcome, thus may be important in interpreting PRO scores to judge quality of care. The process-of-care variables will allow the physician and therapist to better interpret outcomes of care, thus determine how to improve quality of care.

SUMMARY

PRO measures obtain information directly from a patient and provide a means to measure the effects of the disorder on the patient with respect to functional limitations and restrictions in daily work, social, and home tasks. PRO measures can be used to assess the impact of the disease or injury on the patient, to assist in treatment decision-making, and to assess the effect of treatment, be it nonoperative or surgical. Consideration of key error and responsiveness metrics facilitates use and provides a basis for interpretation of the PRO scores in daily clinical practice with a goal to improve patient care.

BIBLIOGRAPHY

Angst F, Schwyzer HK, Aeschlimann A, Simmen BR, Goldhahn J: Measures of adult shoulder function: Disabilities of the Arm, Shoulder, and Hand Questionnaire (DASH) and its short version (QuickDASH), Shoulder Pain and Disability Index (SPADI), American Shoulder and Elbow Surgeons (ASES) Society standardized shoulder assessment form, Constant (Murley) Score (CS), Simple Shoulder Test (SST), Oxford Shoulder Score (OSS), Shoulder Disability Questionnaire (SDQ), and Western Ontario Shoulder Instability Index (WOSI). *Arthritis Care Res (Hoboken)* 2011;63(Suppl 11): S174–S188.

© 2018 American Academy of Orthopaedic Surgeons

Beaton DE, Bombardier C, Katz JN et al: Looking for important change/differences in studies of responsiveness. OMERACT MCID Working Group. Outcome Measures in Rheumatology. Minimal Clinically Important Difference. *J Rheumatol* 2001;28(2):400–405.

Beaton DE, Katz JN, Fossel AH, Wright JG, Tarasuk V, Bombardier C: Measuring the whole or the parts? Validity, reliability and responsiveness of the DASH Outcome Measure in different regions of the upper extremity. *J Hand Ther* 2001;14(2):128–146.

Beaton DE, Wright JG, Katz JN: Development of the QuickDASH: comparison of three item-reduction approaches. *J Bone Joint Surg Am* 2005;87(5):1038–1046.

Conboy VB, Morris RW, Kiss J, Carr AJ: An evaluation of the Constant-Murley shoulder assessment. *J Bone Joint Surg Br* 1996;78(2):229–232.

Constant CR, Murley AHG: A clinical method of functional assessment of the shoulder. *Clin Orthop* 1987;214:160–164.

de Witte PB, Henseler JF, Nagels J, Vliet Vlieland TP, Nelissen RG: The Western Ontario Rotator Cuff index in rotator cuff disease patients: a comprehensive reliability and responsiveness validation study. *Am J Sports Med* 2012;40(7):1611–1619.

Dogu B, Sahin F, Ozmaden A, Yilmaz F, Kuran B: Which questionnaire is more effective for follow-up diagnosed subacromial impingement syndrome? A comparison of the responsiveness of SDQ, SPADI and WORC index. *J Back Musculoskelet Rehabil* 2013;26(1):1–7.

Ekeberg OM, Bautz-Holter E, Keller A, Tveita EK, Juel NG, Brox JI: A questionnaire found disease-specific WORC index is not more responsive than SPADI and OSS in rotator cuff disease. *J Clin Epidemiol* 2010;63(5):575–584.

Ekeberg OM, Bautz-Holter E, Tveita EK, Keller A, Juel NG, Brox JI: Agreement, reliability and validity in 3 shoulder questionnaires in patients with rotator cuff disease. *BMC Musculoskelet Disord* 2008;9:68.

Franchignoni F, Vercelli S, Giordano A, Sartorio F, Bravini E, Ferriero G: Minimal Clinically Important Difference of the Disabilities of the Arm, Shoulder, and Hand Outcome Measure (DASH) and Its Shortened Version (QuickDASH). *J Orthop Sports Phys Ther* 2013;41:30–39.

Gabel CP, Michener LA, Burkett B, Neller A: The Upper Limb Functional Index: development and determination of reliability, validity, and responsiveness. *J Hand Ther* 2006;19(3): 328–348.

Glassman SD, Copay AG, Berven SH, Polly DW, Subach BR, Carreon LY: Defining substantial clinical benefit following lumbar spine arthrodesis. *J Bone Joint Surg Am* 2008; 90(9):1839–1847.

Hefford C, Abbott JH, Arnold R, Baxter GD. The patient-specific functional scale: validity, reliability, and responsiveness in patients with upper extremity musculoskeletal problems. *J Orthop Sports Phys Ther* 2012;42(2):56–65.

Hudak PL, Amadio PC, Bombardier C: Development of an upper extremity outcome measure: the DASH (disabilities of the arm, shoulder and hand) [corrected]. The Upper Extremity Collaborative Group (UECG). *Am J Ind Med* 1996;29(6):602–608.

Kirkley A, Alvarez C, Griffin S: The development and evaluation of a disease-specific quality-of-life questionnaire for disorders of the rotator cuff: The Western Ontario Rotator Cuff Index. *Clin J Sport Med* 2003;13(2):84–92.

Kirkley A, Griffin S: Development of disease-specific quality of life measurement tools. *Arthroscopy* 2003;19(10):1121–1128.

Leggin BG, Michener LA, Shaffer MA, Brenneman SK, Iannotti JP, Williams GR, Jr: The Penn shoulder score: reliability and validity. *J Orthop Sports Phys Ther* 2006;36(3): 138–151.

Lippitt SB, Harryman DTI, Matsen FA: A practical tool for evaluation of function: the simple shoulder test, in Matsen FA, Fu FH, Hawkins RJ, eds: *The Shoulder: A Balance of Mobility and Stability.* Rosemont, IL, American Academy of Orthopaedic Surgery, 1993, pp 501–518.

MacDermid JC, Drosdowech D, Faber K: Responsiveness of self-report scales in patients recovering from rotator cuff surgery. *J Shoulder Elbow Surg* 2006;15(4):407–414.

Michener LA, Snyder Valier AR, McClure PW: Defining substantial clinical benefit for patient-rated outcome tools for shoulder impingement syndrome. *Arch Phys Med Rehabil* 2013;94(4):725–730.

Mintken PE, Glynn P, Cleland JA: Psychometric properties of the shortened disabilities of the Arm, Shoulder, and Hand Questionnaire (QuickDASH) and Numeric Pain Rating Scale in patients with shoulder pain. *J Shoulder Elbow Surg* 2009;18(6):920–926.

Polson K, Reid D, McNair PJ, Larmer P: Responsiveness, minimal importance difference and minimal detectable change scores of the shortened disability arm shoulder hand (QuickDASH) questionnaire. *Man Ther* 2010;15(4):404–407.

Razmjou H, Bean A, van Osnabrugge V, MacDermid JC, Holtby R: Cross-sectional and longitudinal construct validity of two rotator cuff disease-specific outcome measures. *BMC Musculoskelet Disord* 2006;7:26.

Richards RR, An KN, Bigliani LU et al: A standardized method for the assessment of shoulder function. *J Shoulder Elbow Surg* 1994;3(6):347–352.

Roddey TS, Olson SL, Cook KF, Gartsman GM, Hanten W: Comparison of the University of California–Los Angeles Shoulder Scale and the Simple Shoulder Test with the shoulder pain and disability index: single-administration reliability and validity. *Phys Ther* 2000;80(8):759–768.

Roy JS, MacDermid JC, Woodhouse LJ: Measuring shoulder function: a systematic review of four questionnaires. *Arthritis Rheum* 2009;61(5):623–632.

Roy JS, MacDermid JC, Woodhouse LJ: A systematic review of the psychometric properties of the Constant-Murley score. *J Shoulder Elbow Surg* 2009;19(1):157–164.

Schmitt JS, Di Fabio RP: Reliable change and minimum important difference (MID) proportions facilitated group responsiveness comparisons using individual threshold criteria. *J Clin Epidemiol* 2004;57(10):1008–1018.

© 2018 American Academy of Orthopaedic Surgeons

Tashjian RZ, Deloach J, Green A, Porucznik CA, Powell AP: Minimal clinically important differences in ASES and simple shoulder test scores after nonoperative treatment of rotator cuff disease. *J Bone Joint Surg Am* 2010;92(2):296–303.

Terwee CB, Roorda LD, Dekker J et al: Mind the MIC: large variation among populations and methods. *J Clin Epidemiol* 2009;63(5):524–534.

van de Water AT, Shields N, Davidson M, Evans M, Taylor NF: Reliability and validity of shoulder function outcome measures in people with a proximal humeral fracture. *Disabil Rehabil* 2014;36(13):1072–1079.

Wessel J, Razmjou H, Mewa Y, Holtby R: The factor validity of the Western Ontario Rotator Cuff Index. *BMC Musculoskelet Disord* 2005;6:22.

© 2018 American Academy of Orthopaedic Surgeons

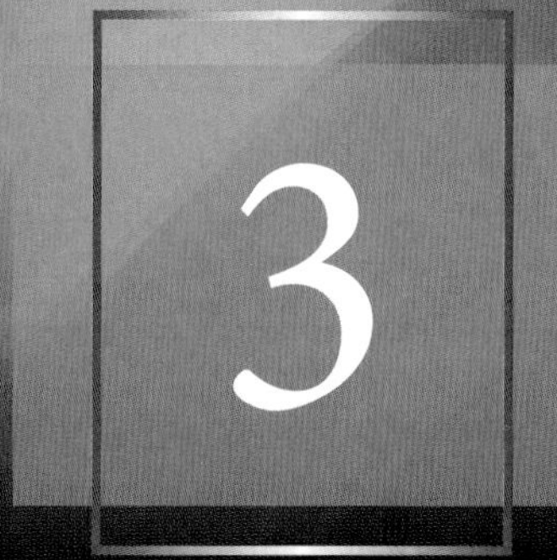

3 Acromioclavicular Separations

Mandeep Singh Virk, MD, MBBS, Mark P. Cote, PT, DPT, MSCTR, and Augustus D. Mazzocca, MS, MD

INTRODUCTION

Acromioclavicular (AC) joint separations commonly occur in contact sports (rugby, wrestling, ice hockey, and football). The usual mechanism of injury involves a fall with direct trauma to the posterosuperior part of the shoulder. Less commonly, injury occurs by an indirect mechanism, with a fall on an outstretched adducted arm or elbow driving the humeral head into the AC joint. AC joint separations involve varying degrees of injury to the AC ligaments, coracoclavicular ligaments, and deltotrapezial fascia. They are classified according to the severity of injury, radiographic findings, and position of the clavicle relative to the acromion (Table 3.1). Higher-grade separation results in AC joint instability, and can lead to shoulder girdle dysfunction. Less severe types I and II as well as many type III injuries are routinely treated nonoperatively (Figure 3.1).

Surgical treatment is pursued for more severe acute injuries, types IV to VI and selected type III injuries, as well as symptomatic chronic AC separations. Numerous surgical procedures, open and arthroscopic, have been described, but the ideal surgical procedure is not known. Reconstruction of the AC joint and the coracoclavicular (CC) space requires a thorough understanding of the relevant anatomy, biomechanics, and stabilizers of the AC joint. The AC and CC ligaments are primary stabilizers of the AC joint; the deltoid and trapezius muscles and fascia are the secondary dynamic stabilizers. The AC joint capsular ligaments, specifically the superior and posterior AC capsular ligaments, are the primary restraints to anterior-to-posterior translation and confer horizontal stability. The CC ligaments (trapezoid and conoid) contribute to the vertical stability. The trapezoid ligament attaches on the undersurface of the clavicle at an anterolateral position. The conoid is a broad, stout ligament located in a posterior and medial position (conoid tubercle) relative to the trapezoid ligament (Figure 3.2). Both the trapezoid and conoid ligaments are attached distally to the base of the coracoid posterior to the pectoralis minor insertion on the coracoid. Anatomical Coracoclavicular Ligament Reconstruction (ACCR) attempts to restore stability to the AC joint and shoulder girdle.

Postoperative rehabilitation plays a critical role in the success of surgical management both by protecting the repair to ensure appropriate healing and by leading a patient through a progressive program of exercise that results in anatomic restoration and functional recovery. Early on, postoperative immobilization is an integral part of the rehabilitation to protect the construct during the initial phases of healing. During this period of immobilization, restoring scapular control and shoulder range of motion (ROM) through gradual low-load exercises allows an effective transition into the strengthening phase of rehabilitation. During the strengthening phase, it is important to appreciate that patient-specific goals are met prior to advancing the intensity of the strengthening program. Thus, a guided postoperative rehabilitation program plays a critical role in the surgical management. In this chapter, we describe the indications and surgical techniques for treatment of AC joint separations, and detail the postoperative rehabilitation.

SURGICAL TREATMENT

The main goals of surgical treatment of AC joint separations are to achieve a pain-free shoulder with full ROM and strength. Treatment of acute type III AC separations is controversial and a matter of ongoing debate. Although many patients can be treated without surgery, there are cases such as higher-demand athletes and laborers who may benefit from acute repair. Higher-grade AC joint separations (types IV, V, and VI) are best managed surgically.

Multiple operative procedures have been described for treating AC joint separation, but there is a lack of consensus regarding the ideal procedure. These procedures can be broadly categorized into the following:

- *Acromioclavicular joint stabilization,* using hook plates, pins, or Kirschner wires (K-wires)

Dr. Mazzocca or an immediate family member serves as a paid consultant to Arthrex, and has received research or institutional support from Arthrex. Dr. Virk or an immediate family member serves as a board member, owner, officer, or committee member of the American Journal of Orthopedics *and* Techniques in Orthopaedics. *Neither Dr. Cote nor any immediate family member has received anything of value from or has stock or stock options held in a commercial company or institution related directly or indirectly to the subject of this article.*

© 2018 American Academy of Orthopaedic Surgeons

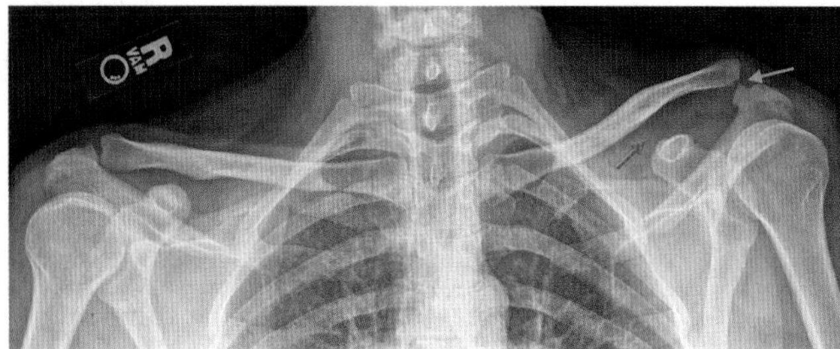

Figure 3.1 Radiograph of bilateral Zanca view demonstrating increased coracoclavicular distance (*red arrow*) and complete acromioclavicular joint separation (*blue arrow*) on the left.

- *Coracoclavicular space stabilization,* using suture loop, screw, endobutton, suture anchor
- *Ligament reconstruction:* CC ligament and/or AC ligament reconstruction with autograft or allograft and CC augmentation
- *Dynamic muscle transfer:* Proximally based conjoint tendon transfer

Open ACCR is our surgical procedure of choice for the treatment of complete AC joint separation. The postoperative rehabilitation described here is specific for the ACCR procedure, but can be modified to be adapted to other methods of surgical reconstruction of the AC joint.

Indications

- Types IV, V, and VI AC joint separations
- Type III AC joint separation in high-demand individuals, for example, athletes or failed conservative management

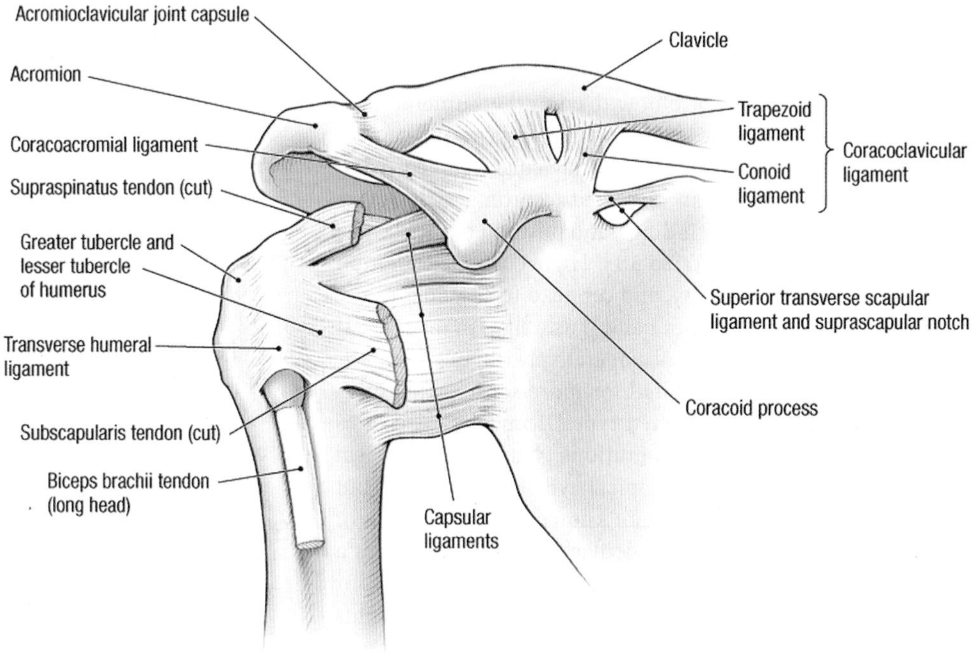

Figure 3.2 Illustration of the anatomy of the coracoclavicular ligaments and acromioclavicular ligaments. The conoid is a broad, stout ligament that fans out from the base of the coracoid and attaches to the conoid tubercle on the undersurface of the coracoid. The trapezoid ligament is a more anterolateral structure compared to the conoid ligament. (Reproduced with permission from Detton AJ: *Grant's Dissector,* ed 16. Philadelphia, PA, Wolters Kluwer Health, 2016.)

Table 3.1 ROCKWOOD CLASSIFICATION FOR ACROMIOCLAVICULAR INJURIES

Type	AC Ligaments	CC Ligaments	Deltopectoral Fascia	Radiographic CC Distance Increase	Radiographic AC Appearance	AC Joint Reducible
I	Sprained	Intact	Intact	Normal (1.1–1.3 cm)	Normal	N/A
II	Disrupted	Sprained	Intact	<25%	Widened	Yes
III	Disrupted	Disrupted	Disrupted	25%–100%	Widened	Yes
IV	Disrupted	Disrupted	Disrupted	Increased	Posterior clavicle displacement	No
V	Disrupted	Disrupted	Disrupted	100%–300%	N/A	No
VI	Disrupted	Intact	Disrupted	Decreased	N/A	No

AC = acromioclavicular, CC = coracoclavicular.

© 2018 American Academy of Orthopaedic Surgeons

Contraindications

- Types I and II AC joint separations

Anatomic Coracoclavicular Ligament Reconstruction

In ACCR (Figure 3.3, A–K), the conoid and trapezoid ligaments are reconstructed using autograft or allograft tendon tissue. The capsular ligaments of the AC joint are also reinforced posteriorly and superiorly with the same graft tissue. The fixation of the graft on the clavicle is performed using interference screws through the drill holes. The fixation of the graft on the coracoid can be performed by looping the graft around the coracoid base (loop technique, our preferred method) or by using

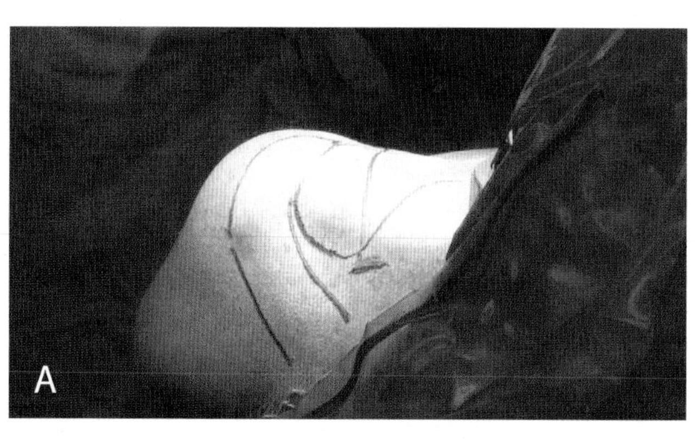

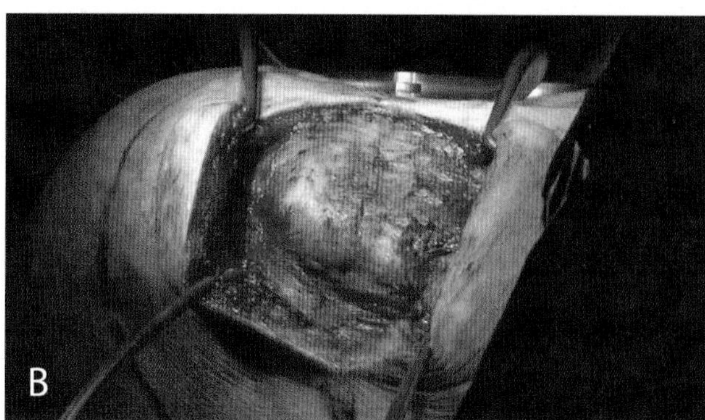

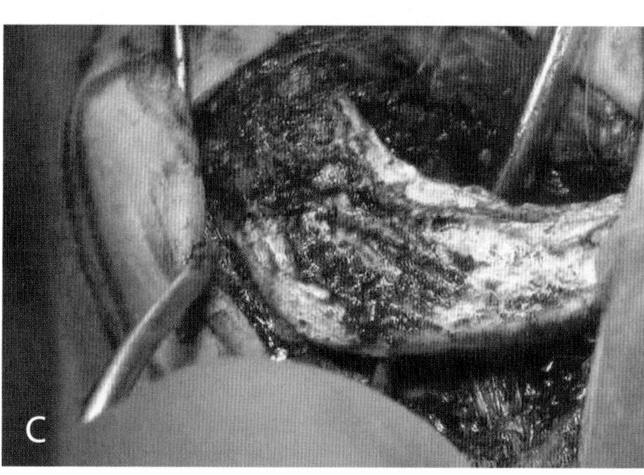

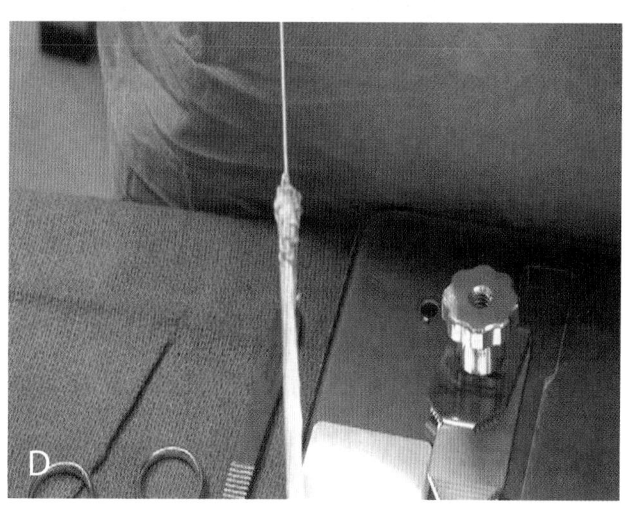

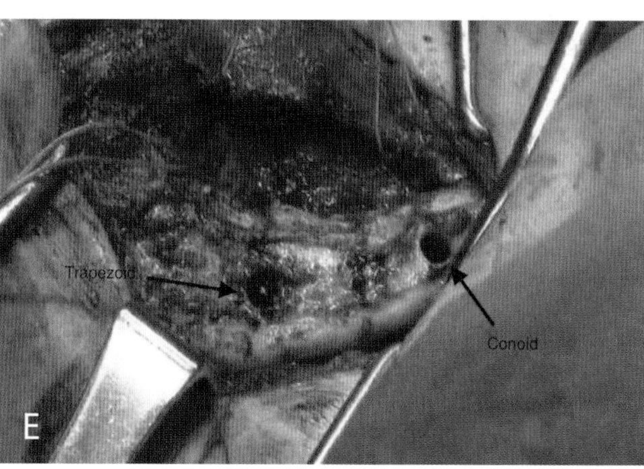

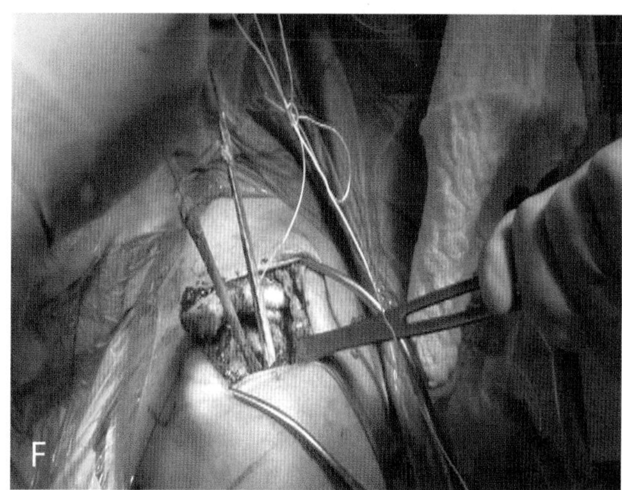

Figure 3.3 Clinical photographs of open anatomic coracoclavicular ligament reconstruction (ACCR). **A**, The saber skin incision is approximately an inch medial to the acromioclavicular joint. **B**, Full-thickness skin flaps are created to expose the deltotrapezial fascia. **C**, Periosteomuscular flaps are elevated to skeletonize the distal end of clavicle. **D**, The allograft (peroneus longus) is prepared and tendon ends are bulleted for easy passage through tunnels. **E**, The conoid (medial) and trapezoid tunnels (lateral) are created using a 5-mm reamer. **F**, The autograft or allograft tissue is looped around the coracoid along with a collagen-coated FiberWire. (*continued*)

© 2018 American Academy of Orthopaedic Surgeons

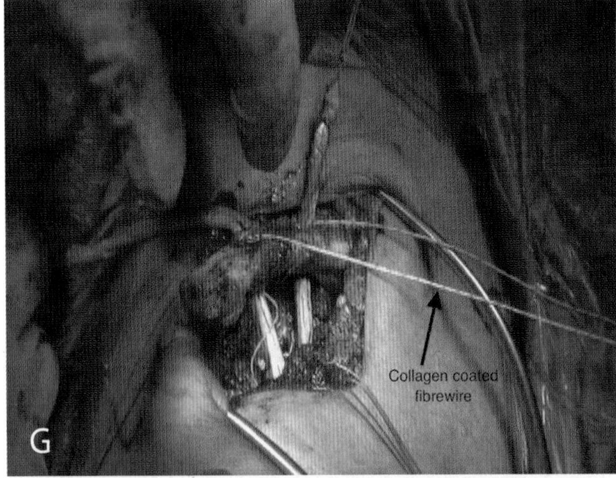

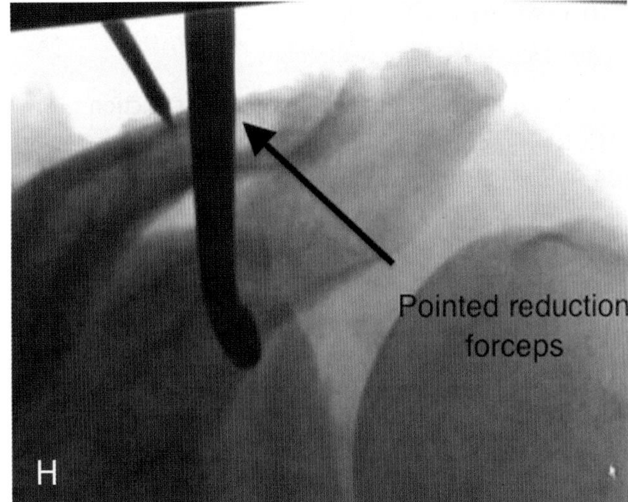

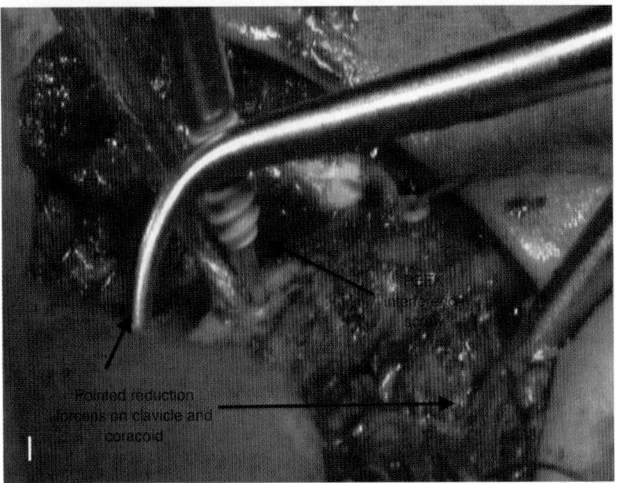

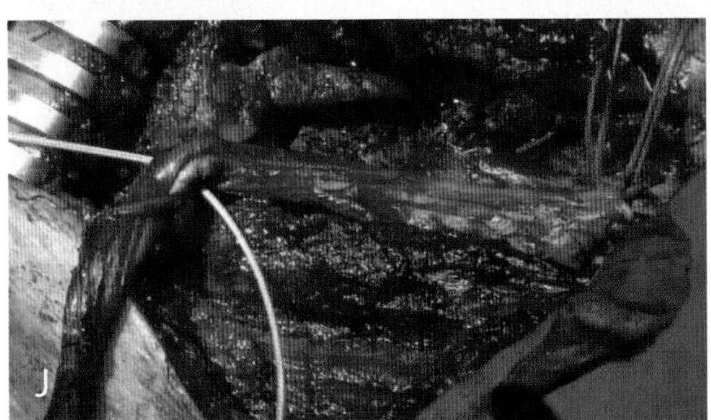

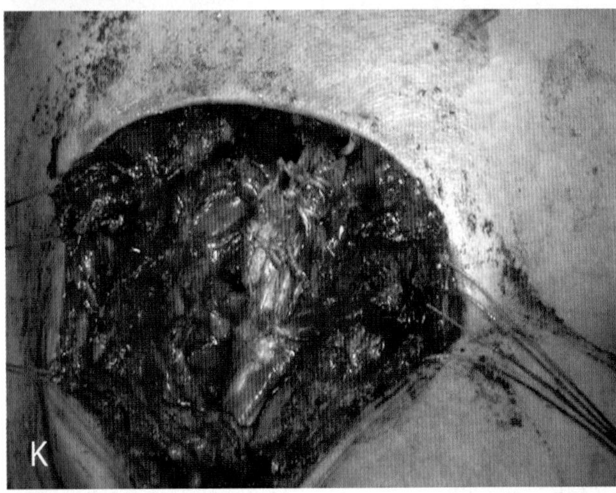

Figure 3.3 *(Continued)* **G**, The graft and collagen coated FiberWire is passed through both the tunnels in the clavicle and reduction of the acromioclavicular joint is performed by passively shrugging the shoulder. **H**, A large pointed reduction forceps with its tines on the coracoid and clavicle is used to further achieve and maintain reduction till final reconstruction is achieved and is held by a pointed reduction forceps. **I**, The conoid ligament is anchored into the tunnel using a 5.5 PEEK interference screw followed by securing the trapezoid ligament with a 5.5 PEEK interference screw. The collagen-coated FiberWire is then tied to itself to give nonbiologic support. **J**, Excess graft is used to reconstruct or reinforce the acromioclavicular ligaments. **K**, After the final ligament reconstruction is performed, the deltotrapezial fascia is then closed in layer and is an important component of ACCR.

an interference screw (tenodesis technique) in the coracoid. We incorporate a collagen-coated, braided, nonabsorbable suture along with the graft in our reconstruction. We believe that the graft provides the biologic form of fixation, while the collagen-coated suture provides the nonbiologic form of fixation.

The patient is placed in the beachchair close to the edge of the table with a small bump under the medial scapular edge to stabilize it and elevate the coracoid anteriorly. The arm is draped free so that maneuvers to reduce the AC joint can be performed. Prior to prepping and draping of the surgical field, fluoroscopy is used to ensure that appropriate imaging can be obtained during surgery.

A skin incision is centered approximately 1 inch medial to the AC joint starting at the posterior clavicle directed toward the

© 2018 American Academy of Orthopaedic Surgeons

coracoid process along Langer's lines (Figure 3.3, A). The deltotrapezial fascia is defined in the depth of the incision (Figure 3.3, B) and full-thickness fascio-periosteal flaps are elevated from the midline of the clavicle both posteriorly and anteriorly to expose the lateral end of the clavicle and AC joint (Figure 3.3, C).

An allograft (peroneus longus) or autograft (semitendinosus) tendon can be used for this procedure. The tendon is sized using a standard tendon sizer (usually 5 mm) and tendon ends are bulleted for easy passage through bone tunnels. A whipstitch or grasping suture is placed in the two free ends of the tendon for passage through the bone tunnels (Figure 3.3, D).

Two bone tunnels are drilled in the clavicle for the reconstruction of the conoid and trapezoid ligament attachment (Figure 3.3, E). To recreate the conoid ligament attachment on the clavicle, a cannulated guide pin is placed approximately 45 mm medial to the most distal end of the clavicle. The drill hole should be made as posterior as possible, taking into account the space needed to prevent a "blowout" of the posterior cortical rim during subsequent reaming. A 5-mm cannulated reamer is used to drill over the pin to create the tunnel. The depth of the tunnel is measured for appropriate interference screw length placement. The same procedure is repeated for the trapezoid ligament, which is a more anterior and lateral structure than the conoid ligament. This tunnel is centered on the clavicle, approximately 15 mm lateral to the center portion of the previous tunnel, approximately 25 mm to 30 mm medial to the distal end of the clavicle (Figure 3.3, E).

In the loop technique, the graft is passed under the coracoid. Soft-tissue dissection is performed to expose the base of the coracoid process and its medial and lateral margins. A Stanitsky clamp, or suture-passing device, is passed in a medial to lateral direction around the coracoid to shuttle a suture. A loop is created at the one end of this suture and is used to pass the graft and no. 2 high-strength suture around the coracoid (Figure 3.3, F).

The limbs of the graft can be passed through the bone tunnels in a crossed (figure-of-eight) or a noncrossed fashion ("U loop," Figure 3.3, G). If there is predominant posterior displacement, we prefer a noncrossed graft through the tunnels and if there is superior displacement, a figure-of-eight configuration is used. Each limb of the graft is accompanied by one of the two ends of a no. 2 suture (Figure 3.3, G). After the grafts and suture are passed through the bone tunnels, the AC joint is reduced by applying an upwards-directed force to the elbow or arm and a large pointed reduction forceps placed on the coracoid process and the clavicle to hold the reduction. Fluoroscopy is used to confirm adequate reduction of the AC joint (Figure 3.3, H).

The medial (conoid) limb of the tendon graft is secured first. The graft is positioned so that the graft tail representing the conoid ligament is left 2 cm proud from the superior margin of the clavicle. The long tail of the graft exits the trapezoid tunnel and will later be used to augment the AC joint repair. With traction placed on the graft, ensuring tension, a nonabsorbable radiolucent interference screw of appropriate size and length is placed in the conoid tunnel. While holding reduction and tension on the ligament, another nonabsorbable radiolucent screw (5.5 size PEEK screw) is placed in the lateral trapezoid tunnel anterior to the trapezoid ligament graft (Figure 3.3, I). With both grafts secured, the no. 2 collagen coated FiberWire is tied over the top of the clavicle. The pointed reduction forceps is removed and fluoroscopic images obtained to demonstrate anatomic reduction of the AC joint.

For acute AC joint separations, our preferred approach is to also repair the AC joint capsule and ligaments with no. 0 nonabsorbable suture. The long limb of the graft exiting the lateral (trapezoid) tunnel is taken laterally and looped on top of the AC joint, and used for augmentation of the AC joint capsule repair superiorly and posteriorly (Figure 3.3, J and H). Lastly, the deltoid and trapezius are repaired over the distal clavicle and AC joint (Figure 3.3, K). In chronic dislocations, two options exist. One approach is to repair the AC joint, as described earlier. An alternative approach is to perform a distal clavicle excision, especially if AC joint arthritis is a concern. An oscillating saw is used to remove enough bone from the distal end of the clavicle (<1 cm) to prevent any mechanical contact with the acromion.

POSTOPERATIVE REHABILITATION

Postoperative rehabilitation is an essential component of the AC joint reconstructive process. The goal of anatomic reconstruction of the CC ligaments is to restore stability to the AC joint by reconstructing the CC ligaments and AC ligaments. In concept, this process has two primary steps: (1) the surgery itself, which recreates the anatomy that was damaged as a result of injury; and (2) the incorporation of the tendon graft within the tunnel to establish permanent stability of the AC joint. In this regard, guidelines for postoperative rehabilitation are based on tissue healing time frames for tendon healing in a bone tunnel, the biomechanical properties of the surgical construct, and potential joint forces associated with rehabilitative exercises and activities.

It is estimated that a tendon graft in a bone tunnel requires up to 12 weeks before achieving a resilient union at the bone–tendon interface. Thus, for the first 12 weeks following reconstruction, the surgical construct progressively gains stability as healing occurs. Initially, the stability of the construct is largely dependent on the biomechanical properties of the repair, as little in the way of biologic healing has occurred. After 8 weeks, the stability of the reconstruction has likely improved as a result of partial incorporation of the graft in the bone tunnel through the development of scar tissue. This process is far from complete, however, as the construct is still susceptible to failure from excessive force. From 12 weeks and beyond, the bone–tendon interface is far more resilient, and while healing will continue to occur over the ensuing months and weeks, the construct is considered stable. This serves as the biologic basis underlying our rehabilitative protocol for postoperative rehabilitation of AC joint separations.

It is important to distinguish rehabilitation of nonoperatively managed AC joint injury versus rehabilitation after AC joint reconstruction. In a nonoperative setting, early intervention is focused on reducing pain and inflammation associated with the injury to allow ROM and strengthening exercise to begin as soon as possible. This differs from postoperative

© 2018 American Academy of Orthopaedic Surgeons

rehabilitation, in which the repair is protected for a period of time before initiating strength-based and functional exercise.

A home exercise should be initiated early on, coordinated with the formal therapist-directed rehabilitation, and continued throughout the entire rehabilitation process. This program is designed to mirror the exercises performed during each phase of rehabilitation. Early in the postoperative period, this program is focused on maintaining and improving ROM and scapular control, which optimizes transition into the next phase of rehabilitation. During the strengthening phase, the home exercise program is modified to allow a safe but progressive advancement of strength-based exercises. Patients are encouraged to continue a home exercise program following discharge from supervised rehabilitation.

Author's Preferred Postoperative Protocol for Open ACCR

Phase I (6–8 Weeks Postoperative): Immobilization to Protect the Repair

- Postoperative immobilization in a platform brace (Donjoy Lerman shoulder orthosis, Gunslinger shoulder orthosis) for 6 to 8 weeks. The platform brace minimizes the stress on the AC joint reconstruction by preventing the gravity-dependent downward pull on the scapulohumeral complex.
- Remain in the brace at all times other than during self-care and prescribed therapeutic activities.

Phase II (6 to 12 Weeks Postoperative): Rehabilitation Focused on Restoring Shoulder Range of Motion and Scapular Control

- Begin ROM exercise emphasizing closed-chain exercises in which the hand is fixed to allow the limb to be supported, and progress toward open-chain exercises as mobility improves.
- Closed-chain exercises are ideal for initiating ROM as they unweight the limb and elicit low amounts of shoulder muscle activity, allowing the patient to move the arm within the patient's comfort range with little stress on the AC joint. These exercises can be started on a flat surface (Figure 3.4, A and B) and gradually progressed to inclined surfaces, and finally a vertical surface (Figure 3.4, C and D).

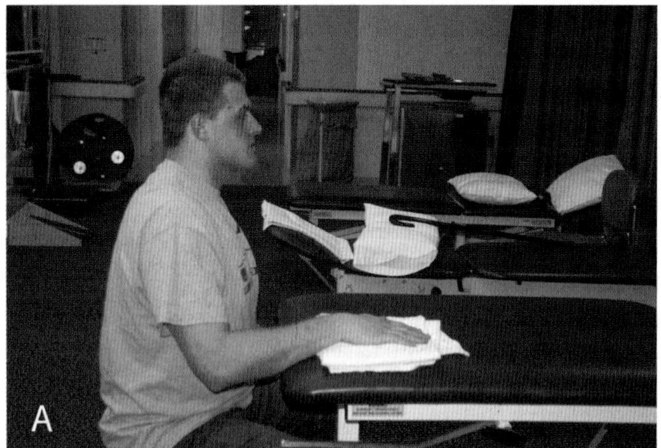

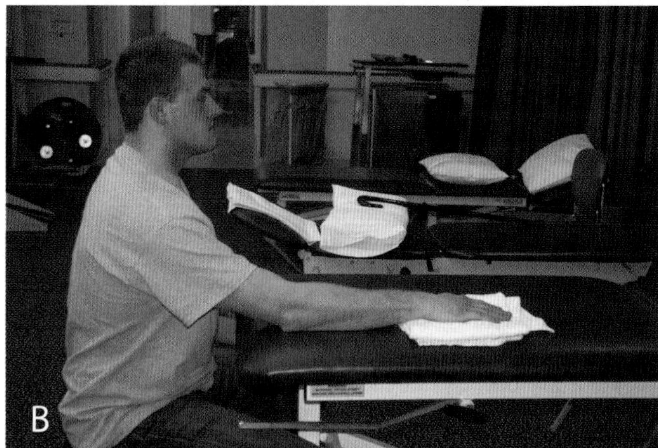

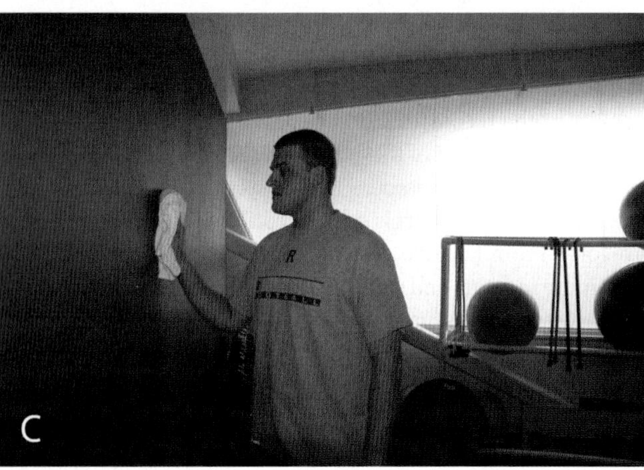

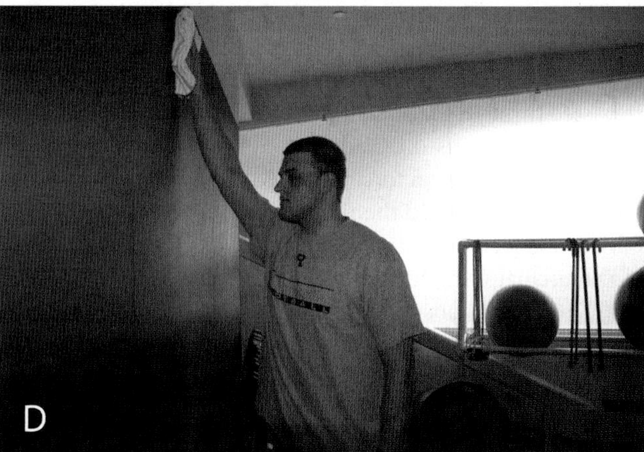

Figure 3.4 Photographs of closed-chain progression of active assistive range of motion. **A**, The patient is instructed to keep the hand fixed to the table while sliding the arm forward. **B**, A towel or pillowcase is positioned between the patient's hand and the surface of the table or wall to reduce friction, allowing the exercise to be performed smoothly with minimal resistance. **C**, **D**, This exercise is initially performed on a flat surface and gradually progresses to a vertical surface as pain decreases and motion improves.

 © 2018 American Academy of Orthopaedic Surgeons

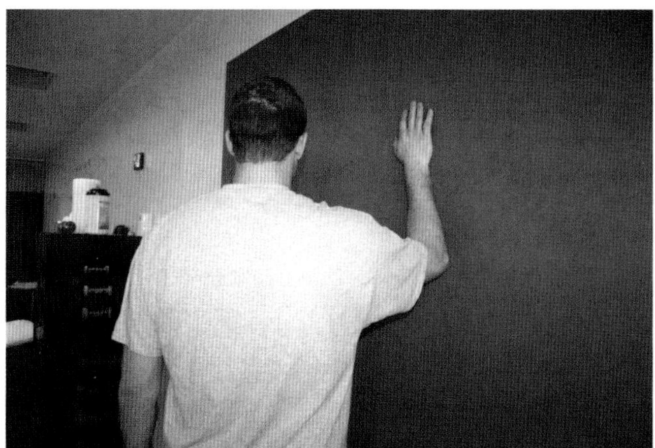

Figure 3.5 Photograph of scapular clocks to facilitate muscle activity of the parascapular muscles and motion and control of the scapula. The patient is positioned with the shoulder in the plane of the scapula with the hand on the wall. The patient is then instructed to try to depress and retract the scapula. The image of the scapula as a clock can be useful to assist the patient in understanding the direction of scapular motion. For the right shoulder, the patient is instructed to move the scapula toward 8:00 (4:00 for the left). As the patient demonstrates the ability to retract and depress the scapula, isometric holds are introduced, with the patient maintaining a position of a retracted scapula for 10 seconds.

- While not expressly limited, motions that may increase stress on the AC joint—specifically, internal rotation (IR) behind the back, cross-body adduction, and end-range forward elevation—are approached cautiously and within a patient's own pain threshold.
- Supine flexion and pulley exercises also assist in increasing forward elevation and facilitate the transition to open-chain exercise.
- Scapular muscle–strengthening exercises to facilitate motion of the scapula and muscle recruitment. Closed-chain scapular exercises, such as the scapular clock, allow patients to focus on scapular control and establish movement patterns without creating excessive loads about the shoulder (Figure 3.5).
- It is important to note that, while fixing the hand to the wall is advantageous for unweighting the limb, weight bearing on the operative side is not permitted.
- Early integration of kinetic-chain exercises that incorporate movement of the legs, trunk, and scapula is also recommended to facilitate recovery of shoulder function.
- Activities in single-leg stance as well as exercises such as shoulder dumps and trunk bends are ideal initial exercises, as they can be performed without movement of the upper extremity.
- As ROM improves, exercises combining leg and trunk activity with shoulder motions can be incorporated to reinforce normally occurring movement patterns of the upper extremity.

At 10 weeks postoperatively, patients typically present with near full-shoulder mobility, lacking only the ability to perform IR behind the back. This limitation is often associated with restrictions in posterior shoulder mobility, which may prompt the prescription of exercises to isolate posterior shoulder tissues. Horizontal adduction and behind-the-back exercises are typically prescribed to patients to improve IR of the shoulder. It is important to be mindful when considering these activities prior to 12 weeks as these motions produce motion and potentially pathologic forces at the AC joint. In our experience, this limitation in motion seems to be related to the mechanics of the AC joint rather than restrictions in glenohumeral joint mobility. If a patient presents with restriction in IR, behind-the-back stretching is allowed if the patient can maintain scapular retraction while performing the exercise. Gradual progression of this exercise is often sufficient to restore ROM.

Phase III (12 to 18 Weeks): Focus is on Strengthening

- Begin isotonic strength activities after 12th week.
- Scapular strengthening exercises
  - Isometric exercises, such as low row, involving no motion of the upper extremity
  - Horizontal abduction with external rotation
  - Prone horizontal extension with the arm at 100° of shoulder abduction
  - Multilevel rowing exercises focusing on combined motions with resistance band tubing or cable resistance (Figure 3.6)
  - These exercises can be modified to allow continued integration of the legs and trunk to help facilitate scapular control (Figure 3.7, A and B)
  - "Ts" and "Ys" are prescribed when the patient is able to demonstrate minimal to no scapular substitution with active forward elevation, with the medial border of the scapula appearing symmetrical and remaining protracted to the rib cage during shoulder flexion and retracted and upwardly rotated during abduction (Figure 3.8A–D)

Phase IV (4–6 Months Postoperative): Functional Restoration

- Isotonic shoulder and scapula strengthening
- Initiate sports-related rehabilitation with returning to throwing, swimming, tennis, and golf at 4 to 5 months postoperative
- Return to contact sports after 6 months

OUTCOMES

There is a general consensus that types I and II AC injuries should be managed nonoperatively with limited immobilization and early return to function. Treatment of type III AC injuries is controversial, and there is fair evidence that favors initial nonoperative management. General consensus exists that high-grade AC injuries (types IV, V, and VI) should be managed operatively. There is insufficient evidence to recommend for the optimum timing of operative repair (early vs. delayed), the ideal type of surgical repair (anatomic vs. nonanatomic), the type of graft for surgical repair (allograft

© 2018 American Academy of Orthopaedic Surgeons

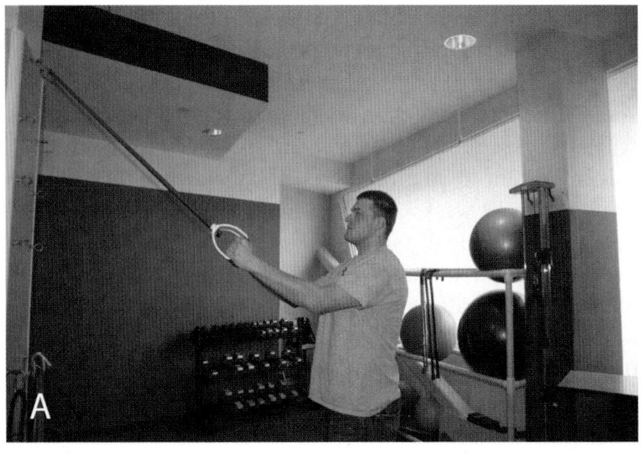

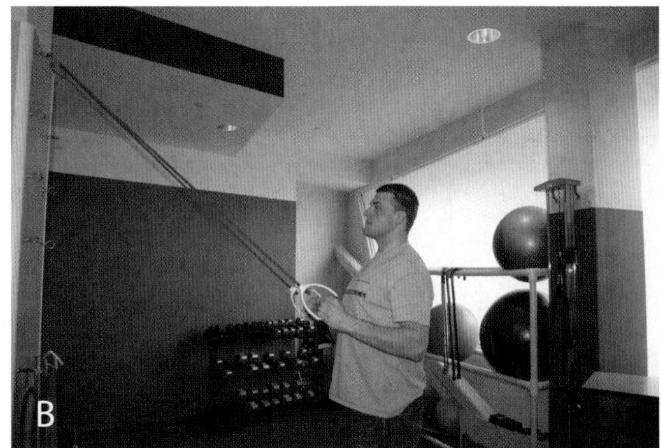

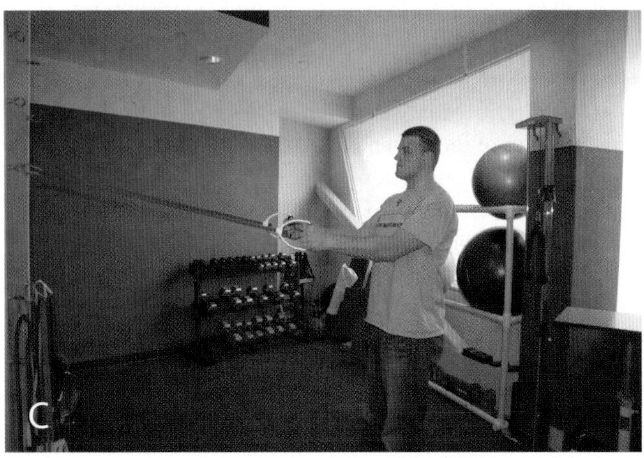

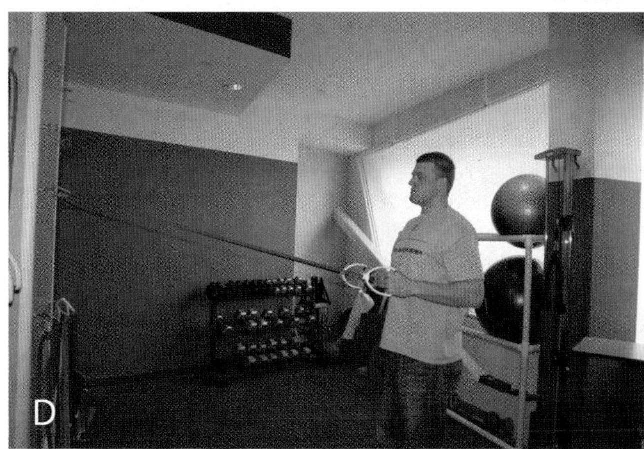

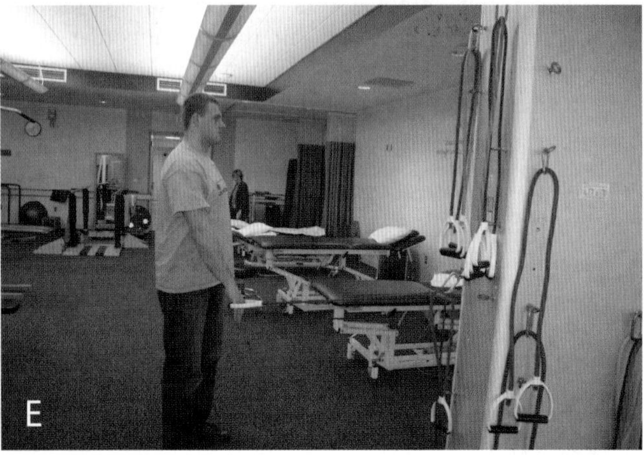

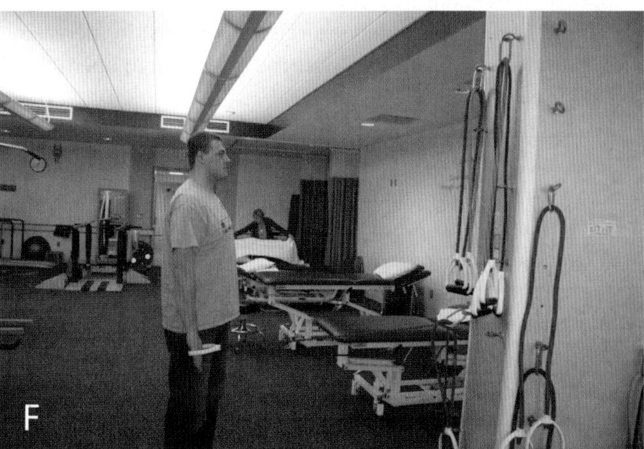

Figure 3.6 Photographs of multilevel rows performed with resistive tubing. These exercises combine upper extremity and scapular motion to facilitate the transition between closed- and open-chain exercises. **A**, **C**, **E**, Starting with the arm out in front of the body, the patient is instructed to pull the arms back (**B**, **D**, **F**) by focusing on retracting and depressing the scapula.

vs. autograft), and open versus arthroscopic repair for chronic AC joint dislocations.

Anatomic CC ligament reconstruction and the Weaver-Dunn procedure are the two most common open techniques for AC joint reconstruction. The short-term data demonstrates that the majority of patients report a significant relief of pain, return of normal strength and function, and negligible loss of motion. Some loss of radiographic reduction (<5 mm change in CC distance) is common, but not reported to be clinically significant. Subjective and standardized outcome measures show high satisfaction rates. Complications reported with ACCR include loss of reduction and recurrence of deformity, coracoid fracture, clavicle fracture, infection, adhesive capsulitis, graft failure, clavicular or coracoid osteolysis, hypertrophic

 © 2018 American Academy of Orthopaedic Surgeons

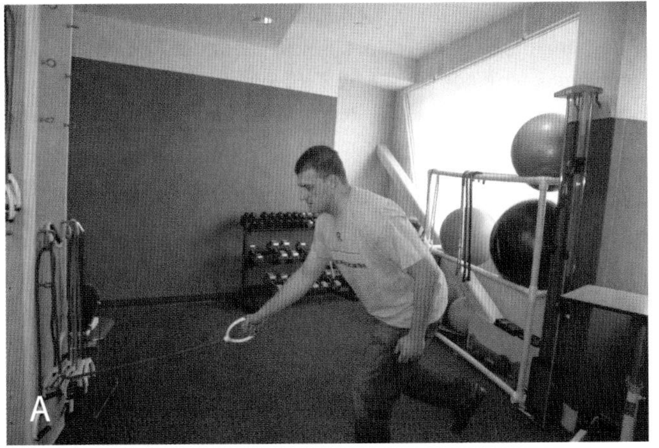

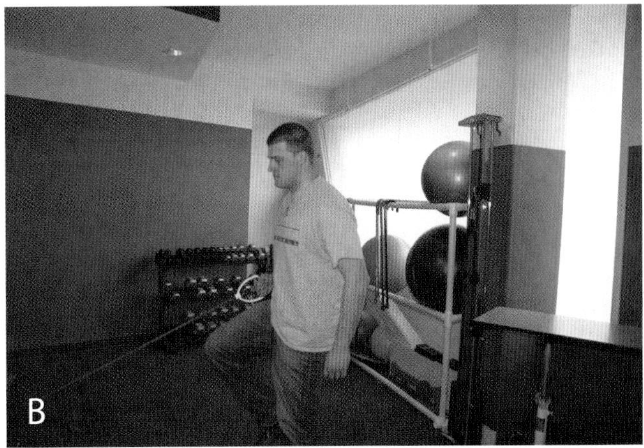

Figure 3.7 Photographs of rowing exercise with integration of the legs and trunk. The patient starts in a single leg stance on the opposite side of the affected shoulder. The exercise is performed by initiating a controlled bend at the trunk with reaching forward with the hand (**A**), then returning to an upright position while retracting and depressing the scapula (**B**).

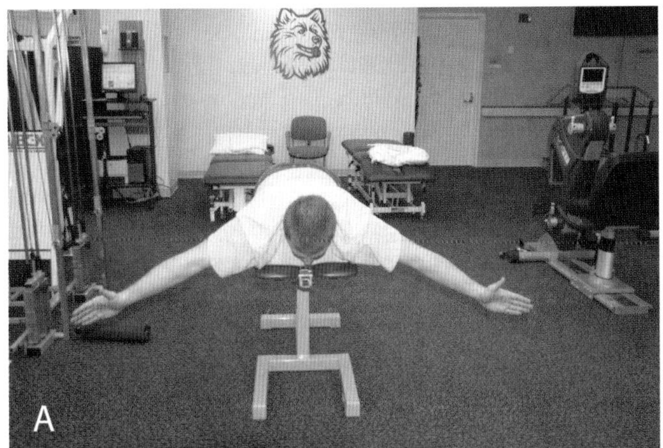

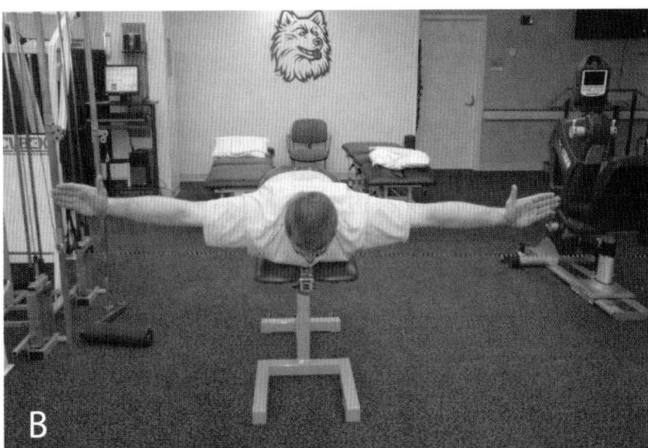

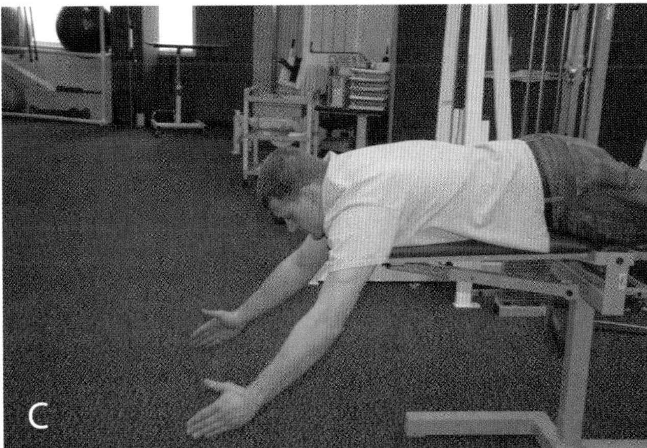

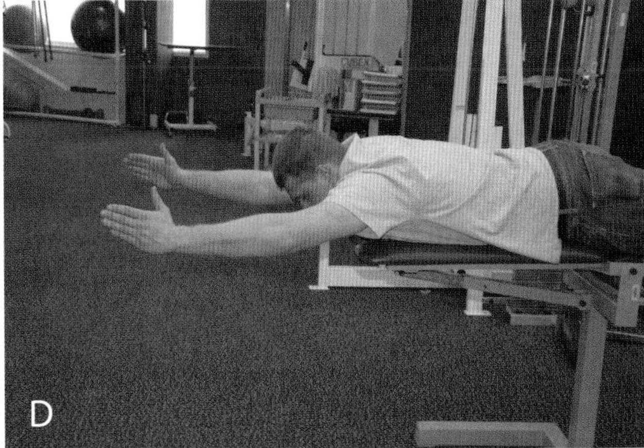

Figure 3.8 Photographs of prone horizontal extension with the arm at 100° and horizontal abduction with external rotation. These exercises are often referred to as "Ts" (**A**, **B**) and "Ys" (**C**, **D**) and involve the patient moving the limb in an open-chain fashion to produce muscle activity of the parascapular muscles. For both exercises, the patient is instructed to lift the arms up while maintaining extension through the elbows. When introducing these exercises it is important to closely monitor the patient to ensure that the motion is performed in a controlled and form-appropriate manner. These exercises are initially performed using only the weight of the limb and can be progressed to include a handheld weight as strength improves.

© 2018 American Academy of Orthopaedic Surgeons

distal clavicle, brachial plexopathy, hardware complications (broken hardware, symptomatic hardware), and osteoarthritis of AC joint.

PEARLS

Surgical Pearls

- Chronic AC dislocations require ligament reconstruction.
- The patient's head position needs to be considered in order to facilitate drilling of the more medial conoid tunnel.
- Smaller clavicle drill holes (5 mm), sufficient distance between the two tunnels, avoiding drill holes in the lateral 15 mm of the distal clavicle, and using the loop technique for coracoid fixation can minimize the risk of postoperative coracoid and clavicle fracture.
- The graft ends should be narrow (like the nose of a bullet) for easy graft passage through tunnels and to prevent graft laceration.
- The deltotrapezial fascia should be meticulously repaired as it provides additional stability to the reconstructed ligaments.

Rehabilitation Pearls

- Shoulder stiffness is relatively uncommon despite prolonged shoulder immobilization of up to 8 weeks following reconstruction.
- Low-load active assistive exercises are often sufficient to restore ROM after bracing is discontinued.
- Scapular mobility and control is important throughout the entire postoperative period.

SUMMARY

In the ACCR procedure, autograft or allograft tendon tissue is used to reconstruct the conoid and trapezoid ligaments with or without reinforcement of the AC joint capsular ligament. Postoperative immobilization is an important component of rehabilitation following ACCR to protect the surgical reconstruction during the initial phases of healing. The goal during the initial phase of rehabilitation is to restore scapular control and shoulder ROM through gradual low-load exercises. During the strengthening phase, it is important to appreciate that patient-specific goals are met prior to advancing the intensity of the strengthening program. A home exercise program plays an important role in accelerating restoration of strength and ROM.

BIBLIOGRAPHY

Beitzel K, Cote MP, Apostolakos J, et al: Current concepts in the treatment of acromioclavicular joint dislocations. *Arthroscopy* 2013;29(2):387–397.

Bradley JP, Elkousy H: Decision making: operative versus nonoperative treatment of acromioclavicular joint injuries. *Clin Sports Med* 2003;22:277–290.

Carofino BC, Mazzocca AD: The anatomic coracoclavicular ligament reconstruction: surgical technique and indications. *J Shoulder Elbow Surg* 2010;19(2 Suppl):37–46.

Cools AM, Dewitte V, Lanszweert F, Notebaert D, Roets A, Soetens B, Cagnie B, Witvrouw EE: Rehabilitation of scapular muscle balance: which exercises to prescribe? *Am J Sports Med* 2007;35(10):1744–1751.

Cote MP, Wojcik KE, Gomlinski G, Mazzocca AD: Rehabilitation of acromioclavicular joint separations: operative and nonoperative considerations. *Clin Sports Med* 2010;29(2): 213–228, vii.

Debski RE, Parsons IM 4th, Woo SL, Fu FH: Effect of capsular injury on acromioclavicular joint mechanics. *J Bone Joint Surg Am* 2001;83A:1344–1351.

Ekstrom RA, Donatelli RA,Soderberg GL: Surface electromyographic analysis of exercises for the trapezius and serratus anterior muscles. *J Orthop Sports Phys Ther* 2003;33(5): 247–258.

Geaney LE, Beitzel K, Chowaniec DM, Cote MP, Apostolakos J, Arciero RA, Mazzocca AD: Graft fixation is highest with anatomic tunnel positioning in acromioclavicular reconstruction. *Arthroscopy* 2013;29(3):434–439.

Kibler WB, Sciascia A, Wilkes T: Scapular dyskinesis and its relation to shoulder injury. *J Am Acad Orthop Surg* 2012; 20(6):364–372.

Lynch TS, Saltzman MD, Ghodasra JH, Bilimoria KY, Bowen MK, Nuber GW: Acromioclavicular joint injuries in the National Football League: epidemiology and management. *Am J Sports Med* 2013;41(12):2904–2908.

Phillips AM, Smart C, Groom AF: Acromioclavicular dislocation. Conservative or surgical therapy. *Clin Orthop Relat Res* 1998; (353):10–17.

Renfree KJ, Wright TW: Anatomy and biomechanics of the acromioclavicular and sternoclavicular joints. *Clin Sports Med* 2003;22(2):219–237.

Rios CG, Arciero RA, Mazzocca AD: Anatomy of the clavicle and coracoid process for reconstruction of the coracoclavicular ligaments. *Am J Sports Med* 2007;35:811–817.

Rockwood CA, Williams GR, Young DC: Disorders of the acromioclavicular joint, in Rockwood CA, Matsen F, eds: *The Shoulder*, ed 2. Philadelphia, PA, WB Saunders, 1990, pp 495–554.

Rodeo SA, Arnoczky SP, Torzilli PA, Hidaka C, Warren RF: Tendon-healing in a bone tunnel. A biomechanical and histological study in the dog. *J Bone Joint Surg Am* 1993; 75(12):1795–1803.

Schlegel TF, Burks RT, Marcus RL, Dunn HK: A prospective evaluation of untreated acute grade III acromioclavicular separations. *Am J Sports Med* 2001;29:699–703.

Takase K: The coracoclavicular ligaments: an anatomic study. *Surg Radiol Anat* 2010;32(7):683–688.

Walton J, Mahajan S, Paxinos A, et al: Diagnostic values of tests for acromioclavicular joint pain. *J Bone Joint Surg Am* 2004; 86A(4):807–812.

Wise MB, Uhl TL, Mattacola CG, Nitz AJ, Kibler WB: The effect of limb support on muscle activation during shoulder exercises. *J Shoulder Elbow Surg* 2004;13(6):614–620.

© 2018 American Academy of Orthopaedic Surgeons

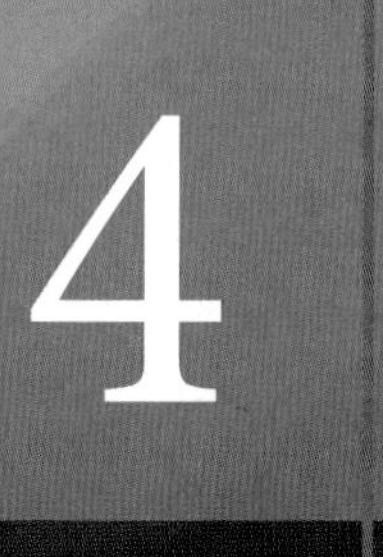

Capsular Releases for Shoulder Stiffness: Considerations for Treatment and Rehabilitation

Jacqueline Munch, MD, Andrea Tychanski, PT, DPT, ATC, CSCS, Sarah E. McLean, PT, MSPT, Samuel Arthur Taylor, MD, and Scott Alan Rodeo, MD

INTRODUCTION

Frozen shoulder, or adhesive capsulitis, is a common cause of loss of both active and passive shoulder motion. Originally described by Duplay in 1872, Codman and Neviaser lent the terms "frozen shoulder" and then "adhesive capsulitis" to this condition. Idiopathic adhesive capsulitis presents in the absence of any underlying shoulder pathology, trauma, or systemic condition. Risk factors for idiopathic adhesive capsulitis include female sex, diabetes, thyroid disease, or other autoimmune disease, age over 40 years, stroke, and cardiopulmonary disease. Frozen shoulder can also be a significant cause of delay and difficulty in reestablishing shoulder range of motion (ROM) in the postoperative or posttraumatic setting. The precise cause of this condition remains unknown, but our understanding of the pathologic process has improved substantially.

In the absence of any surgery or known trauma, idiopathic adhesive capsulitis generally manifests as a gradual onset of global shoulder pain and stiffness. This global loss of motion is in contrast to directional capsular tightness, as in the case of the throwing shoulder (in which the posterior capsule is typically tight, due to adaptive changes secondary to repetitive high-velocity external rotation [ER]) or an iatrogenic motion loss such as that seen in the setting of an overly tight anterior instability repair, such as the now-defunct Putti Platt procedure.

Pain associated with adhesive capsulitis is typically constant in the early period. Patients have trouble sleeping, and find particular difficulty with activities involving reaching to the extremes of their motion, including overhead or behind the back. Rapid shoulder movement—a vigorous handshake or unexpected "bump," for instance—often causes particularly severe pain. In the early presentation, before there is severe loss of motion, the condition is often confused with rotator cuff or impingement syndromes. Patients can avoid pain by minimizing or avoiding movements that cause pain.

As our understanding of the pathogenesis of adhesive capsulitis has improved, the process has been divided into four typical stages. In stage 1, adhesive capsulitis, which typically lasts for about 3 months, patients note pain with active and passive motion, and progressive limitation of shoulder motion in all directions. If pain is controlled or eliminated (such as by injection or nerve block), examination will demonstrate minimal loss of passive motion. The glenohumeral joint has diffuse synovitis on arthroscopic examination, and microscopic examination demonstrates a normal capsule, with a hypertrophic synovium.

In stage 2, or "freezing" adhesive capsulitis, from 3 to 9 months from the onset of symptoms, patients continue to suffer from pain with active and passive motion, but experience true loss of passive range of motion (PROM) as well as limited glenohumeral translation that can be demonstrated on physical examination. Pathologic evaluation reveals synovitis as in stage 1, but with additional scarring and changes in the glenohumeral capsule.

Patients in stage 3, or "frozen" adhesive capsulitis, from 9 to 15 months from the onset of symptoms, have relief of pain except at the extremes of motion, but continue to suffer from significant limitation of active range of motion (AROM) and PROM. The capsule is dense and shows global volume loss. Histologic evaluation demonstrates a synovium that is no longer hypervascular, but the capsule has fibroblastic scarring (Figure 4.1).

Stage 4 adhesive capsulitis is called the "thawing" phase, which can last from 15 to 24 months after the onset of symptoms. During this time, patients have diminishing pain, and gradually regain their ROM.

The diagnosis of adhesive capsulitis is made primarily based on history and physical examination, with imaging studies utilized mainly to rule out other known causes of shoulder pain and stiffness, such as rotator cuff disease, osteoarthritis, or

Dr. Munch or an immediate family member has received nonincome support (such as equipment or services), commercially derived honoraria, or other non-research–related funding (such as paid travel) from Acumed and Arthrex. Dr. Rodeo or an immediate family member has stock or stock options in Rotation Medical and Ortho RTI (not paid consultant to Ortho RTI). Also—consultant to Joint Restoration Foundation. None of the following authors or any immediate family member has received anything of value from or has stock or stock options held in a commercial company or institution related directly or indirectly to the subject of this article: Dr. Taylor and Dr. Tychanski.

© 2018 American Academy of Orthopaedic Surgeons

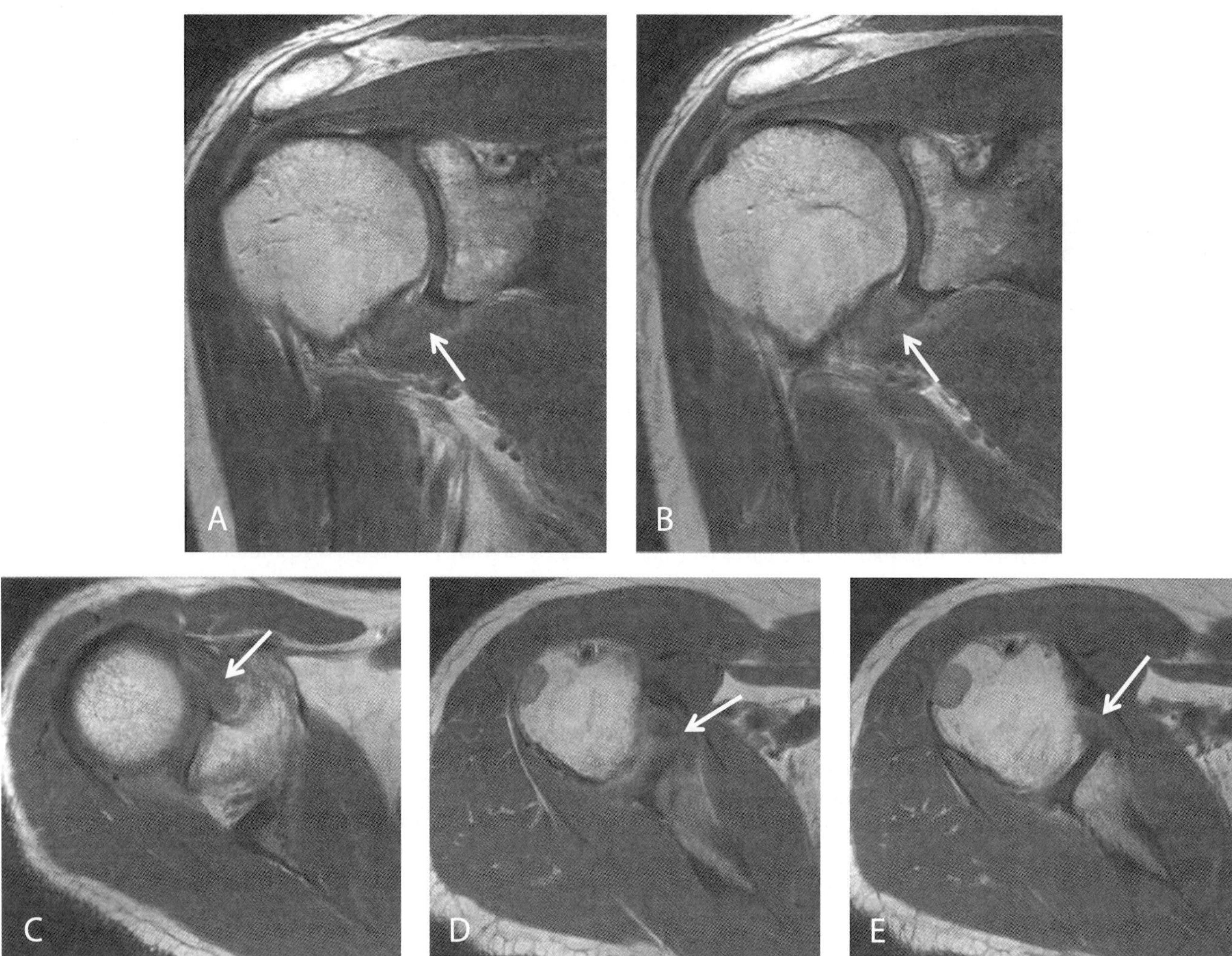

Figure 4.1 MRIs demonstrating global contraction of the axillary pouch with scarring of the glenohumeral ligaments, consistent with stage 3 adhesive capsulitis. Arrows indicate the thickened and scarred glenohumeral ligaments/capsule.

calcific tendinitis. Plain radiographs may demonstrate disuse osteopenia, and depending on the stage in which the imaging is obtained, MRI may show a thickened capsule with loss of overall intra-articular volume.

TREATMENT

Treatment of adhesive capsulitis is individualized. Underlying risk factors should be addressed, such as optimizing glucose control or thyroid balance. Patients are treated with oral nonsteroidal anti-inflammatory drugs (NSAIDs), activity modifications, and PT aimed at preserving and restoring ROM while avoiding pain. Intra-articular corticosteroid injection can be a useful adjunct if patients are diagnosed within 3 months of symptom onset. The therapeutic effects of corticosteroids are lessened in chronic cases. Injections can be both diagnostic and therapeutic in stage 1. If a patient regains full active shoulder motion following intra-articular injection of local anesthetic, the diagnosis of early stage adhesive capsulitis is confirmed.

SURGICAL PROCEDURE: ARTHROSCOPIC CAPSULAR RELEASE WITH MANIPULATION UNDER ANESTHESIA

Indications

As mentioned earlier, the natural history of adhesive capsulitis involves a prolonged course of pain followed by progressive stiffness for up to 2 years, which eventually resolves in the vast majority of cases. Many patients are dependent on their shoulder ROM for their livelihood; thus, if no progress is being made after 6 months of conservative treatment, more aggressive intervention may be considered.

Contraindications

Patients who are deemed too high risk for surgery for medical reasons are counseled to continue PT until their stiffness improves, rather than attempt to accelerate their course by undergoing capsular release. Many arthroscopic shoulder surgeries are performed in a "beach chair" position, which

 © 2018 American Academy of Orthopaedic Surgeons

involves sitting relatively upright. This positioning, combined with general anesthesia, can result in intraoperative hypotension that is dangerous for patients with heart disease, hypertension, a history of stroke, and so on. If a patient is cleared for surgery from a medical standpoint, however, the procedure is generally straightforward.

Procedure

Closed manipulation under anesthesia can result in improvements in ROM, but risks involved in exertion of significant force against relatively thickened and rigid tissues include fracture, dislocation, rotator cuff or labral tears, or possible neurovascular injury. As a result, the surgeon may recommend arthroscopic capsular release prior to manipulation. Arthroscopy allows synovectomy to be performed, and any coexisting shoulder pathology can be documented and treated. After direct arthroscopic capsular release, a controlled manipulation is carried out, allowing predictable improvement in ROM while minimizing the risk of bone or soft-tissue injury.

Arthroscopic capsular release is accomplished in a stepwise fashion. Preoperative ROM and stability under anesthesia are carefully documented prior to introducing the arthroscope into the glenohumeral joint. Given the thickness of the joint capsule, a blunt trocar is essential to avoid injury to articular structures as the capsule is penetrated. Distension of the joint with an intra-articular injection may aid insertion of the arthroscope into the joint. The global capsular volume loss is documented on diagnostic arthroscopy, and the capsule is released in a systematic fashion. It is important for the arthroscopic capsular release to be carried out expediently, under low fluid distension pressures when possible, since fluid will quickly extravasate from the joint after the capsule is incised. The rotator interval is released first, typically using an intra-articular cautery device. Once the rotator interval has been addressed, the instruments are removed from the joint, and ROM and joint stability are assessed again. If the ROM has not normalized, the anterior capsule is released next: the plane between the subscapularis and the middle glenohumeral ligament (MGHL) is developed in order to protect the subscapularis tendon while releasing the MGHL. The anterior portion of the inferior glenohumeral ligament (IGHL) is also released (Figure 4.2). Again, the instruments are removed and the ROM and stability are evaluated. In some cases, the stiffness is sufficiently profound as to require release of the inferior glenohumeral capsule. This anatomic location is perilous due to the proximity of the axillary nerve. As a result, care is taken to release the inferior capsule, and consideration is given to keeping the inferior capsule intact to be released with the manipulation. The arthroscope is switched to an anterior viewing position to allow the posteroinferior capsule to be released. Once the capsule is completely released, the shoulder is manipulated to release any remaining capsular scaring and assess the shoulder ROM.

Once the glenohumeral portion of the procedure is complete, some surgeons will also perform a subacromial bursectomy in order to completely release any remaining adhesions, and treat any symptoms of impingement that may arise as patients work to improve their ROM. A final assessment of ROM and stability is performed and documented. When the bursectomy is complete, the subacromial space may be injected with corticosteroid. The glenohumeral joint is generally not injected in the perioperative setting, because the capsular releases will allow extravasation of the corticosteroid into the surrounding tissues. Some surgeons elect to treat patients with systemic steroids to prevent recurrence of synovitis and subsequent adhesive capsulitis.

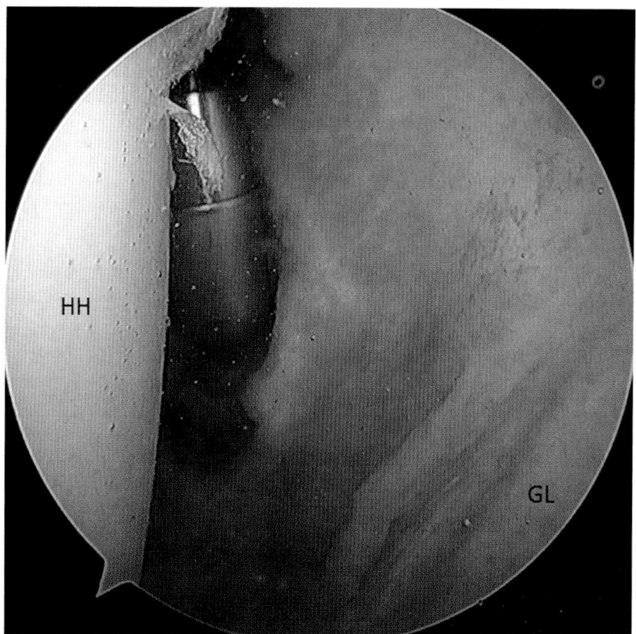

Figure 4.2 Arthroscopic anterior capsule release of the left shoulder using an electrocautery device, as viewed from a standard posterior viewing portal. GL = glenoid labrum, HH = humeral head.

Interscalene regional anesthesia may be used as a perioperative adjunct for assistance with intraoperative pain control. In addition, an indwelling interscalene catheter can be used to administer long-acting anesthetic to help the patient regain ROM before early postoperative pain might become prohibitive.

POSTOPERATIVE REHABILITATION

Patients are referred immediately to PT, in order to maintain the ROM that was obtained intraoperatively. Focused rehabilitation after capsular release is essential to restore function and achieve patient goals. As this surgical procedure is indicated and performed on patients who have failed conservative measures, it is important to consider that a patient may be frustrated with the process and the prospect of more PT. Patient education on the importance of regaining ROM in a timely manner is critical to the success of this procedure.

Communication among the physician, physical therapist, and patient is extremely important. The ROM that was

© 2018 American Academy of Orthopaedic Surgeons

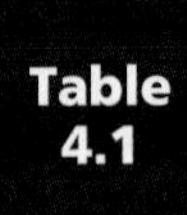

Table 4.1 EXAMPLE OF A HOME EXERCISE PROGRAM FOLLOWING ARTHROSCOPIC CAPSULAR RELEASE FOR ADHESIVE CAPSULITIS

Home Exercise Plan

Perform the following >5 times per day:

- Pendulums
- AAROM forward flexion with the contralateral arm
- AAROM external rotation with a cane
- Towel pass for internal rotation
- Cryotherapy

AAROM = active assisted range of motion.

achieved intraoperatively should be conveyed to the physical therapist following capsular release in order to set realistic goals. The initial PT evaluation should take place in the recovery room on the day of surgery, prior to discharge from the hospital. During this session, the physical therapist will perform PROM of the shoulder into end-range forward flexion, ER, and internal rotation (IR). In addition, the patient and family are educated on home ROM exercises, with appropriate information regarding frequency and duration of each maneuver clearly outlined in a written home exercise program (HEP; Table 4.1). The patient is scheduled to begin formal outpatient PT as early as postoperative day one. The importance of pain management, especially during the early postoperative phase, cannot be overestimated. Adequate analgesia and cryotherapy are critical to the success of a rehabilitation protocol.

The postoperative rehabilitation following arthroscopic capsular release can be divided into four phases (Table 4.2). In the initial phase, PT visits following capsular release for adhesive capsulitis should be very frequent, up to 4 to 5 times per week for the first 1 to 2 weeks with a primary focus on maximizing ROM in all planes during the first 2 weeks. Appropriate interventions depend on the available motion and the patient's pain level. It is particularly important to set proper expectations; the patient should anticipate some degree of pain and discomfort throughout the process, especially during end-range stretching.

Beginning the treatment session with modalities, such as a moist heat pack, will decrease muscle spasm and maximize

Table 4.2 THE FOUR PHASES OF POSTOPERATIVE REHABILITATION FOLLOWING ARTHROSCOPIC CAPSULAR RELEASE

Phase I (Days 0–14): Control pain and inflammation while regaining motion

- Frequent PT visits up to 4–5 times per week for the first 1–2 weeks
- Primary focus on maximizing ROM in all planes during the first 2 weeks
- Moist heat to relax and decrease spasm
- Manual therapy with PROM, grades I–IV joint mobilization and soft-tissue manipulation
- Pendulum, supine AAROM FE, supine AAROM ER, supine AAROM IR, supine AAROM horizontal adduction

Phase II (Weeks 2–6): Normalize ROM and scapular kinematics

- Progress ROM: Once AAROM supine FE to 100°, begin with a cane in both hands.
- Pulleys in the scapular plane may be initiated when the patient achieves at least 130° of AAROM FE.
- Incorporate higher degrees of abduction with ER
- Posterior capsular stretch: cross-chest adduction, side-lying IR
- Aqua therapy
- Scapular mobility and stability exercises

Phase III (Weeks 6–10): Improve strength while avoiding impingement/overuse

- Progress ROM
- Deltoid isometrics: short-lever arm progressed to long-lever arm
- IR and ER strengthening: Submaximal IR and ER isometrics against manual resistance to submaximal isometrics against a wall, to side-lying ER in a modified neutral position
  - Standing ER and IR with elastic tubing is initiated once the patient is able to perform side-lying ER with light resistance and without compensation
- Progress scapular mobility exercises: Closed-chain scapular stability exercise on a ball below 90° of elevation

Phase IV (Weeks 10–14): Prepare for return to work and sporting activities

- Continue exercises to achieve maximal ROM
- Progressive strengthening
- Functional exercises based on patient goals

AAROM = active assisted range of motion, ER = external rotation, FE = forward elevation, IR = internal rotation, PROM = passive range of motion, PT = physical therapy, ROM = range of motion.

© 2018 American Academy of Orthopaedic Surgeons

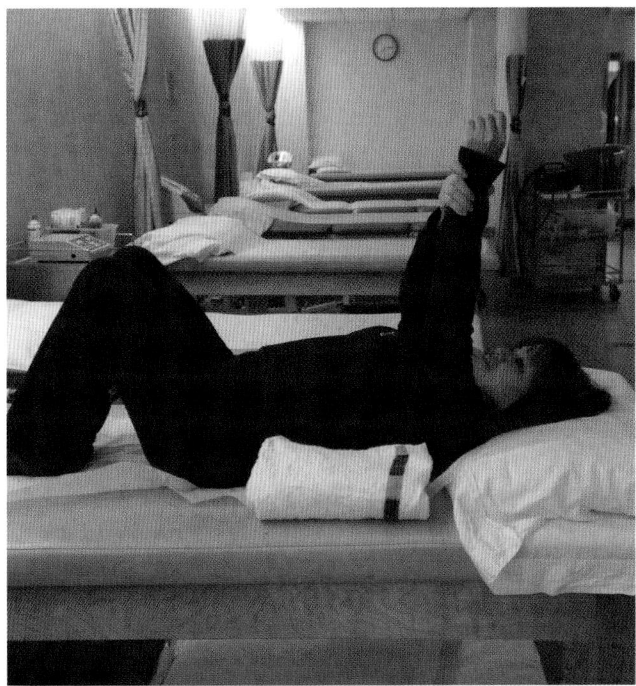

Figure 4.3 Photograph of supine active assisted forward flexion range of motion, with the contralateral upper extremity in the scapular plane.

relaxation. Next, pendulums are performed to provide gentle joint distraction and capsular stretching, and to increase blood flow to the tissues. Manual treatments—including PROM, grades I–IV joint mobilization and soft-tissue manipulation—should be incorporated into each PT session in order to maximize potential ROM gains. This is particularly true with regard to inferior and posterior glenohumeral joint mobilizations, which have been shown to be helpful for improving glenohumeral ROM.

Active assisted range of motion (AAROM) for forward elevation (FE) in the scapular plane is first performed in a supine position with assistance from the contralateral arm (Figure 4.3). Once FE reaches 100° and the patient demonstrates adequate humeral head control, the patient may progress to supine FE with a cane in both hands (Figure 4.4). Pulleys in the scapular plane may be initiated when the patient achieves at least 130° of AAROM FE (Figure 4.5). The physical therapist must be sure to monitor the patient to prevent compensatory motor patterns such as superior migration of the shoulder girdle (i.e., "shrug") during elevation with pulleys. Ultimately, elevating the arm up along a doorway and leaning the trunk forward until a stretch is felt may help achieve terminal FE (Figure 4.6).

AAROM ER is first performed supine with the aid of a cane or wand. The affected arm is positioned in the scapular plane at 30° to 45° of abduction and 90° of elbow flexion, with the humerus resting on a towel roll (Figure 4.7). With the cane in both hands, gradually increasing ER force is applied by the unaffected arm to move the affected arm into ER. Care is taken to avoid substituting elbow extension for shoulder ER. As ROM improves, the patient advances by incorporating higher

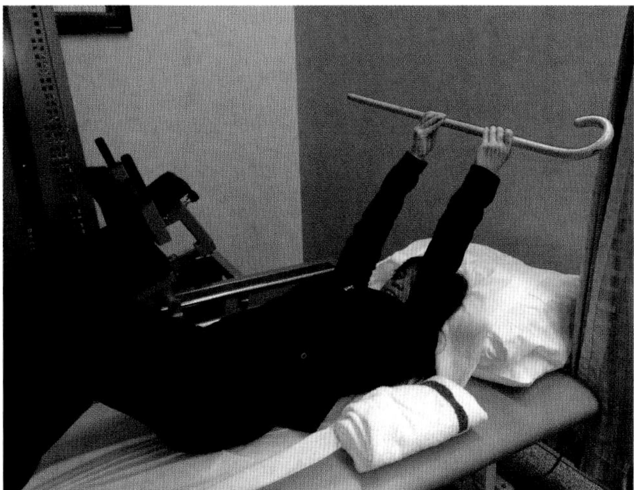

Figure 4.4 Photograph of supine active assisted forward flexion range of motion in the scapular plane, utilizing a cane.

degrees of abduction with ER. Terminal ER may be achieved by utilizing a doorway to stretch: the elbow is flexed to 90° at the patient's side, and the hand is firmly planted on the wall of the doorway. The patient rotates the body away from the hand, externally rotating the shoulder until a stretch is felt.

Manual techniques, including soft-tissue and glenohumeral joint mobilizations, are performed by the physical therapist to stretch the posterior capsule and restore IR. To stretch the posterior capsule, the body is supine and the arm is positioned

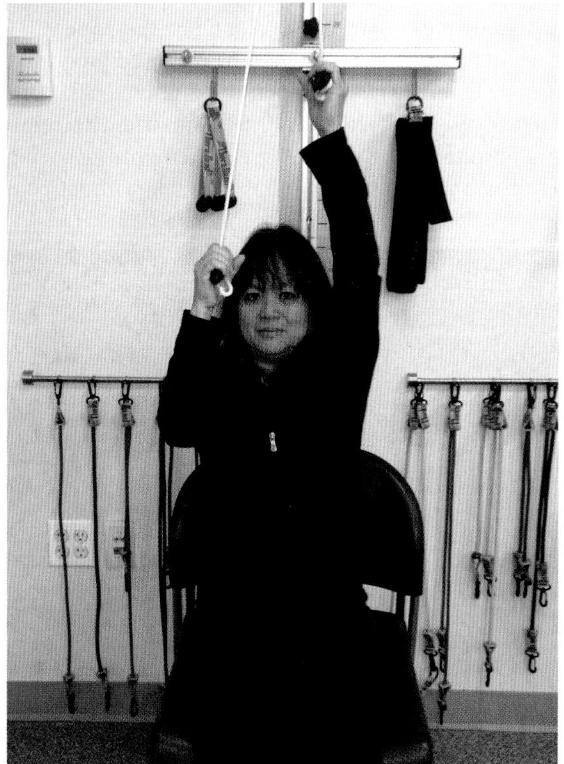

Figure 4.5 Photograph of active assisted forward flexion with pulleys in the scapular plane.

© 2018 American Academy of Orthopaedic Surgeons

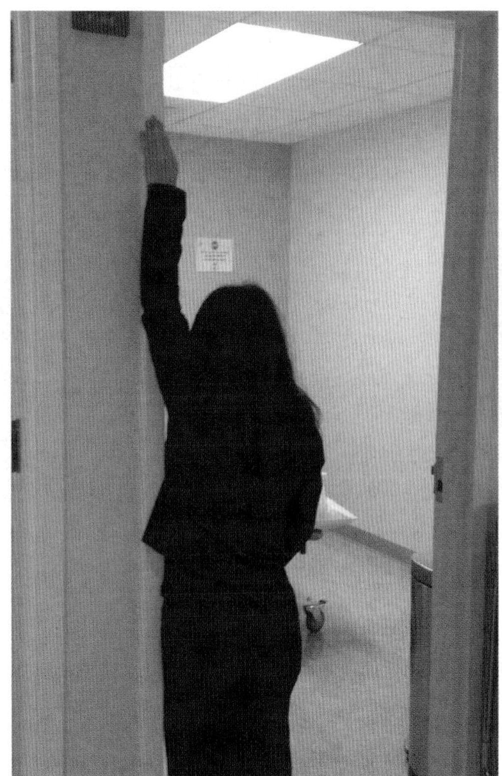

Figure 4.6 Photograph of end-range forward flexion stretch against a wall.

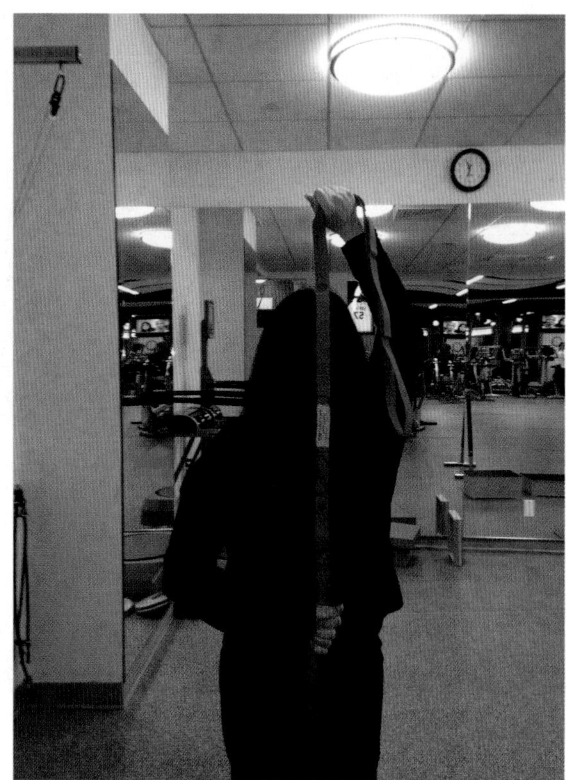

Figure 4.8 Photograph of active assisted internal rotation with a strap.

in horizontal adduction across the chest to stabilize the scapula, which minimizes compensatory motion and maximizes stretching of the posterior capsule. Once the patient is able to reach behind the back, IR stretching can be progressed by passing an object (e.g., towel, pen) behind the back from the affected to the unaffected arm. It is important to reinforce patient posture during this exercise and emphasize having the patient reach as far up the back as tolerable without pain. IR

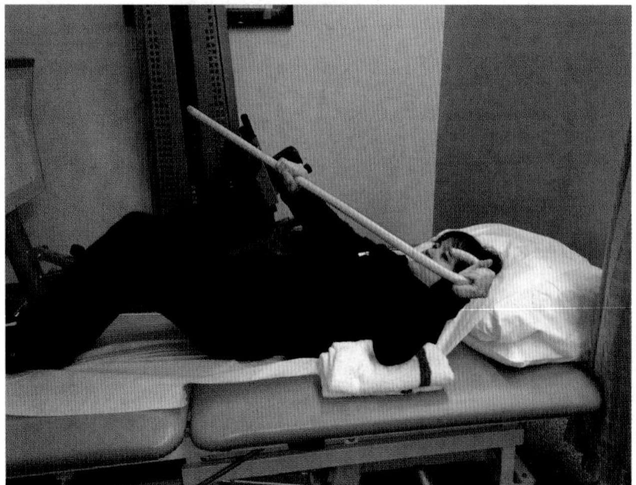

Figure 4.7 Photograph of supine active assisted external rotation in the neutral position with a cane. The humerus is resting on a towel roll.

can be progressed further by performing an IR stretch with a strap (Figure 4.8). Posterior capsule stretching can be more aggressive as IR ROM improves. Side-lying IR is performed with the patient in a lateral decubitus position with the affected arm down, the shoulder flexed to 90° and the elbow flexed to 90°. The contralateral hand is then used to push the affected wrist down toward the table, internally rotating the affected shoulder (Figure 4.9).

Hydrotherapy is a useful adjunct to land-based therapy in the early period following capsular release. Several authors have advocated the incorporation of aqua therapy into the postoperative rehabilitation. Occlusive dressings should be applied when wounds are not yet fully healed to help prevent contamination and potential infection. It is reported that aqua therapy is as effective as land-based therapy with regard to pain, edema, strength, and ROM in the early postoperative period without increased risk of wound-related complications. Patients are often more relaxed, thus less guarded while performing exercises in the pool. Furthermore, the buoyancy of the water supports the arm, allowing the patient to move with less pain than on the land. Gentle ROM exercises in a pool include scapular retraction, underwater arm circles, ER ROM with assistance from a paddle, stretching into FE and abduction with assistance from a noodle, small buoy passes behind the back, and supine stretches into abduction (Figure 4.10). Early strengthening may also begin in the water, focusing on the scapula and deltoid without pain, and progress to the use of fins, paddles, and resistance from a current, if available.

© 2018 American Academy of Orthopaedic Surgeons

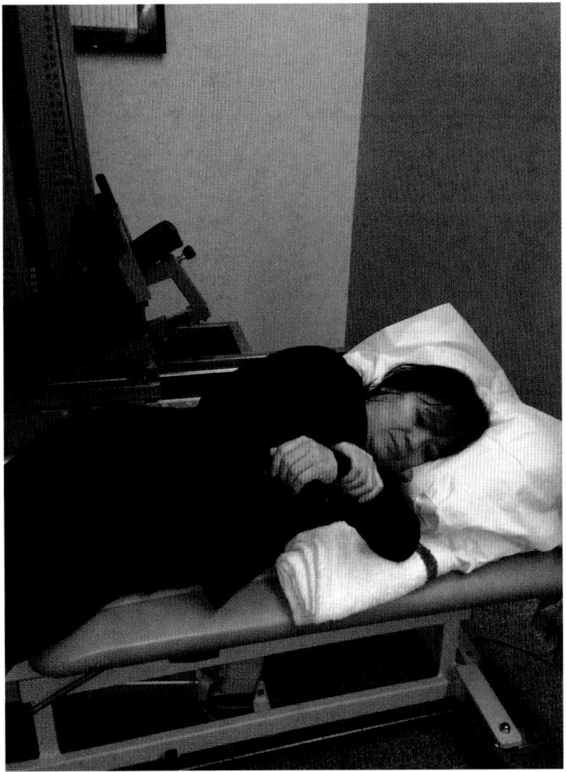

Figure 4.9 a Photograph of side-lying internal rotation stretch with the scapula stabilized ("sleeper stretch").

Once 90° of forward elevation AAROM is achieved, deltoid isometrics for strengthening may be initiated. Deltoid isometrics in the anterior, posterior, and abducted positions are performed with a short-lever arm at first, and progressed to a long-lever arm. Isometrics should be pain-free and submaximal at approximately 20% to 30% maximum contraction. Activation of the rotator cuff musculature is important for neuromuscular reeducation in order to restore humeral head control. When the patient displays at least 30° of ER and IR, submaximal IR and ER isometrics against manual resistance from the physical therapist may be initiated. If manual resistance is well tolerated, submaximal IR and ER isometrics against a wall are introduced. A towel roll is placed between the trunk and upper arm to position the arm in slight abduction (modified neutral). This position will decrease tension on the supraspinatus and may enhance vascular flow to the rotator cuff. As ROM and rotator cuff activation continues to improve, side-lying ER in a modified neutral position is initiated. Once the patient is able to perform side-lying ER with light resistance and without compensation, standing ER and IR with elastic tubing is initiated.

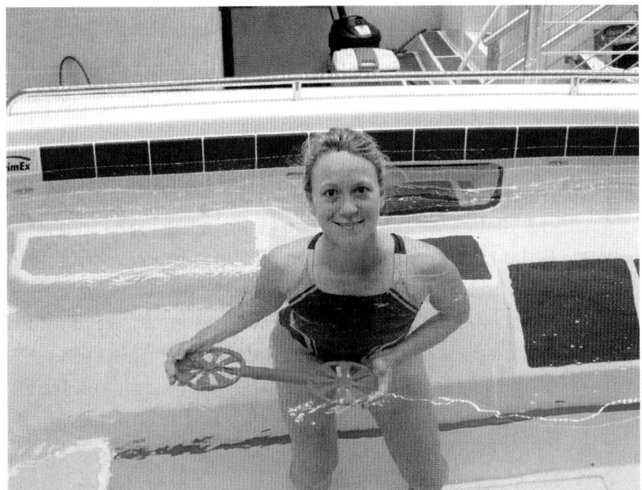

Figure 4.10 Photograph of aquatic active assisted external rotation range of motion with a paddle.

Scapular mobility and stability exercises are essential, and should be introduced according to patient tolerance. Scapular mobilizations by the physical therapist in a lateral decubitus position will help encourage early scapular mobility. The patient will also perform side-lying scapular retraction/protraction and elevation/depression independently as part of the HEP. As the patient's symptoms improve, these scapular mobility exercises are progressed to a seated position. Closed-chain scapular stability exercise on a ball below 90° of elevation is often well tolerated early in rehabilitation and helps to reinforce proper scapulothoracic kinetics and proprioception. Resisted scapular exercises are introduced once the patient demonstrates improved scapular control. For postural reeducation and scapular strengthening, supine scapular protraction, scapular retraction, and shoulder extension with elastic tubing are performed. Once the patient displays adequate scapular stability and glenohumeral control (absence of a shrug), FE in the scapular plane is introduced in the supine position and gradually progressed to a standing position. Continuous monitoring by the rehabilitation specialist for scapular dyskinesias—notably a scapular shrug as the arm elevates—is essential. Focused rotator cuff strengthening can progress as well at this time. As the patient continues to develop scapular stability, glenohumeral control and strength, additional closed-chain exercises and proprioceptive neuromuscular facilitation patterns are included to reeducate functional movements.

OUTCOMES

Grant and coworkers reported on a systematic review that compared arthroscopic capsular release and manipulation under anesthesia for frozen shoulder, and found no difference to suggest an advantage of capsular release over manipulation alone. We would argue that the quality of studies available is poor, however, and that addition of a capsular release improves the safety of the manipulation by mitigating risk of iatrogenic fracture. Arthroscopic capsular release and manipulation under anesthesia have demonstrated excellent functional and clinical results in early and midterm studies. Barnes et al found that the procedure demonstrated immediate improvements in pain and ROM. ROM improvements noted at 1 week declined slightly by 6 weeks, but continued to improve thereafter. Other authors have found the procedure

© 2018 American Academy of Orthopaedic Surgeons

to be safe and effective for improving ROM and patient-reported outcomes. Hagiwara et al found that preoperative injection of steroid improved ROM and pain outcomes following capsular release. Several authors have demonstrated durability of improvements in ROM and functional outcomes scores in studies with 3- to 7-year follow-up.

More recently, some authors have stratified results of arthroscopic capsular release and manipulation under anesthesia for those with and without diabetes, and found slower recovery among diabetic patients. Cho et al found that while diabetics and nondiabetics demonstrated similar final results for American Shoulder and Elbow Surgeons (ASES) score and ROM, the diabetic group exhibited lower scores at the 3, 6, and 12 months. Mehta et al also compared outcomes for patients with and without diabetes treated surgically for adhesive capsulitis and found that while both groups demonstrated significant improvements in Constant scores, the improvements were less in the diabetic group. Furthermore, only 70% of diabetic patients ultimately regained full ROM, while 90% of the nondiabetics reached normal motion. Others have found similarly inferior results for diabetic patients with adhesive capsulitis who underwent capsular release.

Other authors have reported that the results of arthroscopic capsular release for posttraumatic and postoperative stiffness are inferior to the results of treatment of idiopathic adhesive capsulitis.

No surgical procedure is without complications. While the complication rate is exceedingly low among many reported studies, some authors have reported iatrogenic instability and dislocation, glenohumeral chondrolysis, and possibly fracture or axillary nerve injury. Patients must be counseled accordingly, and the decision for surgical intervention made after careful consideration.

PEARLS

- Most patients recover from adhesive capsulitis without requiring manipulation under anesthesia or arthroscopic capsular release.
- Restoring and retaining ROM early after capsular release is of upmost importance.
- Patient education on a home exercise program, activity modification, and cryotherapy is crucial in the early phase after capsular release surgery.
- Communication between the physician and physical therapist is essential for successful rehabilitation.
- Manual PT—including PROM, soft-tissue manipulation, scapular and glenohumeral joint mobilizations, manual resistance, and rhythmic stabilization—has an important role in recovery.
- Strengthening is initiated and progressed once ROM is restored.
- Once the patient reports pain-free ADLs with normalized scapulohumeral rhythm throughout ROM, and manual muscle testing strength is 5/5 for the shoulder and scapular musculature, the patient may prepare for discharge with a HEP.

BIBLIOGRAPHY

Barnes CP, Lam PH, Murrell GA: Short-term outcomes after arthroscopic capsular release for adhesive capsulitis. *J Shoulder Elbow Surg* 2016;25(9):e256–e264.

Berghs BM, Sole-Molins X, Bunker TD: Arthroscopic release of adhesive capsulitis. *J Shoulder Elbow Surg* 2004;13(2):180–185.

Cho CH, Kim DH, Lee YK: Serial comparison of clinical outcomes after arthroscopic capsular release for refractory frozen shoulder with and without diabetes. *Arthroscopy* 2016;32(8): 1515–1520.

Ellsworth AA, Mullaney M, Tyler TF, McHugh M, Nicholas S: Electromyography of selected shoulder musculature during un-weighted and weighted pendulum. *N Am J Sports Phys Ther* 2006;1(2):73–79.

Grant JA, Schroeder N, Miller BS, Carpenter JE: Comparison of manipulation and arthroscopic capsular release for adhesive capsulitis: a systematic review. *J Shoulder Elbow Surg* 2013; 22(8):1135–1145.

Hagiwara Y, Sugaya H, Takahashi N, Kawai N, Ando A, Hamada J, Itoi E: Effects of intra-articular steroid injection before pancapsular release in patients with refractory frozen shoulder. *Knee Surg Sports Traumatol Arthrosc* 2015;23(5):1536–1541.

Hannafin JA, Chiaia TA: Adhesive capsulitis: a treatment approach. *Clin Orthop Relat Res* 2000;(372):95–109.

Holloway GB, Schenk T, Williams GR, Ramsey ML, Iannotti JP: Arthroscopic capsular release for the treatment of refractory postoperative or post-fracture shoulder stiffness. *J Bone Joint Surg Am* 2001;83-A(11):1682–1687.

Jerosch J, Nasef NM, Peters O, Mansour AM: Mid-term results following arthroscopic capsular release in patients with primary and secondary adhesive shoulder capsulitis. *Knee Surg Sports Traumatol Arthrosc* 2013;21(5):1195–1202.

Le Lievre HM, Murrell GA: Long-term outcomes after arthroscopic capsular release for idiopathic adhesive capsulitis. *J Bone Joint Surg Am* 2012;94(13):1208–1216.

Mehta SS, Singh HP, Pandey R: Comparative outcome of arthroscopic release for frozen shoulder in patients with and without diabetes. *Bone Joint J* 2014;96-B(10):1355–1358.

Villalta, E, Peiris CL: Early aquatic therapy improves function and does not increase risk of wound-related adverse events for adults after orthopaedic surgery: a systematic review and meta-analysis. *Arch Phys Med Rehabil* 2013;94:138–148.

Warner JJ, Allen A, Marks PH, Wong P J: Arthroscopic release for chronic, refractory adhesive capsulitis of the shoulder. *Bone Joint Surg Am* 1996;78(12):1808–1816.

© 2018 American Academy of Orthopaedic Surgeons

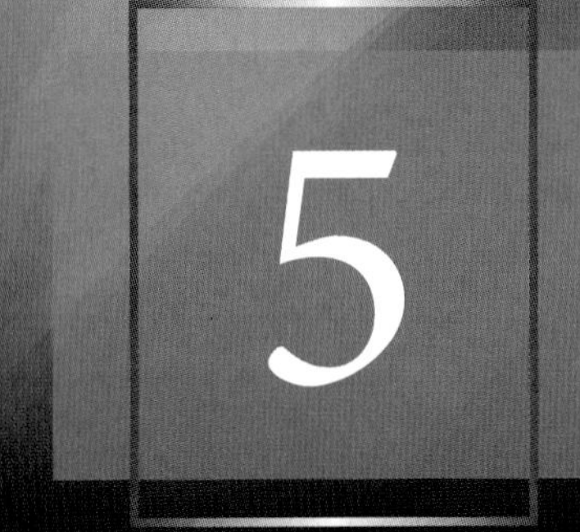

Shoulder Instability Repairs

Marc S. Haro, MD, MSPT, Todd R. Hooks, PT, ATC, Kevin E. Wilk, DPT, FAPTA, Lucy Oliver-Welsh, MBChB, and Brian J. Cole, MD, MBA

INTRODUCTION

Shoulder instability is common in young individuals. Whether it is a relatively straightforward acute anterior traumatic dislocation, posterior instability, or a more subtle multidirectional instability, it is important to ascertain the type of shoulder instability in order to correctly guide treatment. Shoulder instability can be unidirectional or multidirectional, as well as both traumatic and atraumatic in nature. The classical acronyms TUBS (Traumatic Unidirectional Bankart Surgery) and AMBRI (Atraumatic Multidirectional Bilateral Rehabilitation Inferior capsular shift) have long been used to help the clinician guide treatment based on the type of instability. While these simple acronyms have been used for years and may not cover all types of shoulder instability, they are still helpful in drawing attention to the mechanism of instability and the nature of treatment often recommended.

When evaluating a patient with possible shoulder instability, several critical factors must be assessed. First is the patient's age. Younger individuals with anterior shoulder dislocations are at a significantly higher risk to have recurrent instability compared to older individuals. Among 15 to 35 year olds, about 50% will have a subsequent instability in the first 2 years following primary dislocation, and about two-thirds within 5 years. Due to the high recurrence rate, and the significant impact that shoulder instability can have on an individual, surgical stabilization is often recommended to treat young active patients. In contrast, older patients are much less likely to have recurrent instability, and those over age 40 years are far more likely to sustain a rotator cuff injury at the time of an initial anterior dislocation.

Most unidirectional shoulder instability is anterior and traumatic. Anterior instability usually manifests as a dislocation event and often requires a closed reduction. Typically, the mechanism of injury is an abduction and external rotation (ER) force on the arm. The anterior inferior glenohumeral ligaments (AIGHL) and the posterior inferior glenohumeral ligaments (PIGHL) are the primary restraints to anteroposterior translation with the arm abducted. The Bankart lesion, considered the "essential" lesion, is an avulsion injury of the anterior labrum that typically extends from the 2 o'clock position to the 6 o'clock position (in a right shoulder) (Figure 5.1) and disrupts the AIGHLs and has variable healing. There are several varieties of anterior labral injuries, including glenoid labral articular defect (GLAD) lesions and anterior labral periosteal sleeve avulsion (ALPSA) lesions. If these lesions are not treated surgically, patients may suffer from recurrent instability. Anterior glenohumeral instability without labral injury and atraumatic anterior instability is relatively uncommon.

Several other lesions are also associated with acute shoulder dislocation, including humeral avulsions of the glenohumeral ligament (HAGL) lesions and glenoid rim fractures. Also seen,

Dr. Cole or an immediate family member has received royalties from Arthrex, DJ Orthopaedics, and Elsevier Publishing; serves as a paid consultant to Arthrex, Regentis, and Zimmer; has stock or stock options held in Carticept and Regentis; has received research or institutional support from Aesculap/B.Braun, Arthrex, Cytori, Medipost, National Institutes of Health (NIAMS and NICHD), and Zimmer; has received nonincome support (such as equipment or services), commercially derived honoraria, or other non-research–related funding (such as paid travel) from Athletico, Ossur, Saunders/Mosby-Elsevier, SLACK Incorporated, Smith & Nephew, and Tornier; and serves as a board member, owner, officer, or committee member of the American Journal of Orthopedics, *the American Orthopaedic Society for Sports Medicine, the American Shoulder and Elbow Surgeons, the journal* Arthroscopy, *the Arthroscopy Association of North America, the International Cartilage Repair Society, the* Journal of Bone and Joint Surgery–*American, the* Journal of Shoulder and Elbow Surgery, *and the* Journal of the American Academy of Orthopaedic Surgeons. *Dr. Wilk or an immediate family member serves as a paid consultant to LiteCure Laser Company Intelliskin Zetroz and Performance Health; serves as an unpaid consultant to AlterG; has received research or institutional support from Intelliskin; and has received nonincome support (such as equipment or services), commercially derived honoraria, or other non-research–related funding (such as paid travel) from Churchill Livingstone CV, Mosby Slack Publishing, and Dynasplint Bauerfeind ERMI Device. Neither of the following authors nor any immediate family member has received anything of value from or has stock or stock options held in a commercial company or institution related directly or indirectly to the subject of this article: Dr. Haro and Dr. Hooks.*

© 2018 American Academy of Orthopaedic Surgeons

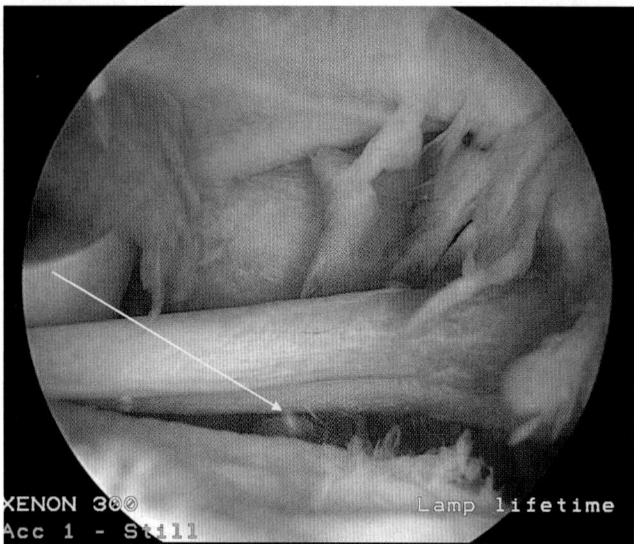

Figure 5.1 Arthroscopic image of a Bankart lesion (*yellow arrow*).

especially after repeated anterior shoulder dislocation, are Hill Sachs lesions, or osteochondral impaction injuries to the posterosuperior humeral head. These are caused by impaction of the posterosuperior humeral head on the anterior glenoid rim with a dislocation event. Recurrent glenohumeral instability often leads to glenoid bone loss and can affect the decision regarding the surgical technique and the outcome of repair (Figure 5.2).

Traumatic posterior instability is much less common, involving the posterior labrum and PIGHLs and a reverse Bankart lesion. Posterior instability can be either traumatic dislocation or atraumatic repetitive microtrauma to the posterior capsule and labrum. Traumatic posterior instability is often seen with a posterior directed force on a shoulder that is flexed, adducted, and internally rotated, or it may be associated with a seizure or electric shock when a forceful tetanic muscle contracture causes the stronger posterior shoulder muscle to dislocate the humeral head posteriorly. Atraumatic posterior instability is more common; it is seen in individuals who perform activities with repetitive posterior-directed forces, such as football offensive linemen, weight lifters, and overhead athletes.

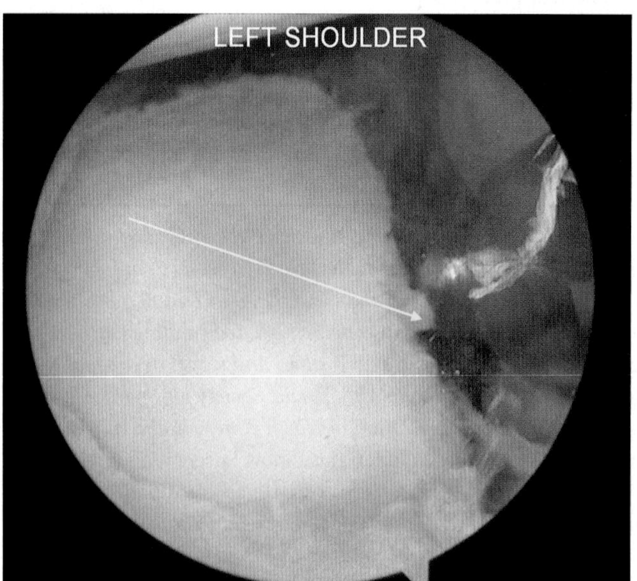

Figure 5.2 Arthroscopic image showing anteroinferior glenoid bone loss (*yellow arrow*).

Multidirectional instability (MDI) is typically defined as instability in two or more directions. While MDI is generally thought of as being atraumatic in nature, and associated with repetitive microtrauma or congenital laxity, it can also be due to extensive labral tears. Those with MDI coupled with large labral tears are probably an extension of traumatic unilateral instability. Patients with atraumatic MDI usually complain of pain or subjective instability with particular activities or arm positions. Often, MDI is seen in overhead athletes, especially those who participate in swimming, volleyball, and gymnastics. They may have associated hyperlaxity and collagen disorders, such as Marfan's disease and Ehler's Danlos. These associated collagen disorders decrease the likelihood of a successful surgical outcome.

PREOPERATIVE EVALUATION

A thorough history and physical examination should be performed to ascertain the nature of the instability. Both shoulders are examined to assess range of motion (ROM), strength, direction of shoulder instability, as well as signs of generalized ligamentous laxity.

Plain radiographs, including true anteroposterior, axillary lateral, and West Point views, should be obtained to evaluate for humeral and glenoid bone loss. A computed tomography (CT) scan with three-dimensional reconstructions should be considered for any patient who demonstrates instability at low angles of abduction, planned revision surgery, or presence of bone loss on plain radiographs. Bone loss greater than 20% may result in failed isolated arthroscopic soft-tissue repair (Figure 5.3). An MR arthrogram is commonly used to assess for the extent of capsulolabral injury, a HAGL lesion, rotator cuff integrity, or posterior pathology.

SURGICAL MANAGEMENT

When patients have failed conservative measures and continue to have pain and recurrent instability, surgical intervention is often warranted. The nature of the surgery is dependent on the patient's age, mechanism of injury, and type of instability present. Regardless of the surgical procedure, the patient must be mentally prepared for the surgery, which frequently requires a long rehabilitation period.

Unidirectional Anterior Glenohumeral Instability

The goal of surgical intervention is to restore the attachment of the labrum and AIGHL. Open repair was traditionally achieved with the Bankart procedure. While these procedures are very effective, over the past 10 to 20 years, the advances in shoulder arthroscopy have allowed us to perform these

© 2018 American Academy of Orthopaedic Surgeons

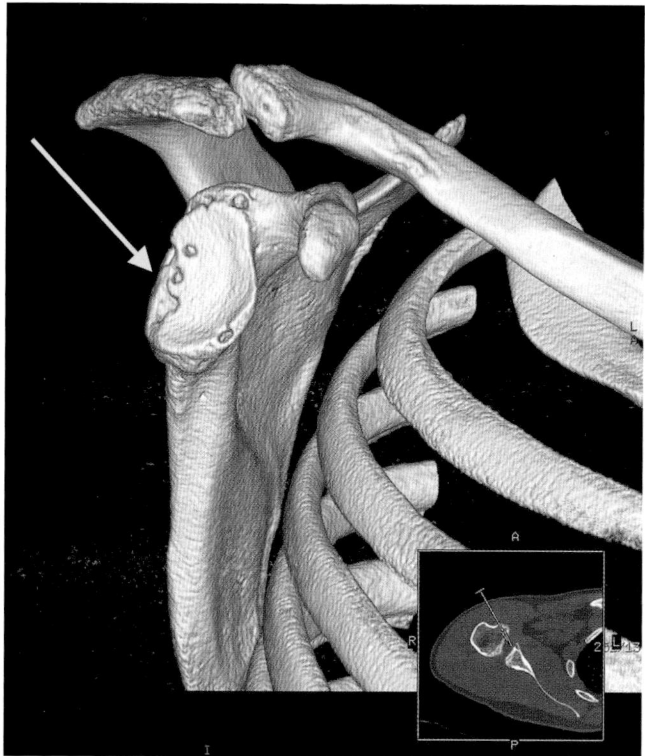

Figure 5.3 A three-dimensional CT scan showing significant posterior bone loss after 2 failed posterior instability repairs (*yellow arrow*).

procedures minimally invasively with comparable results. Additionally, arthroscopic repairs have advantages over open surgery, including lower complication rates (fewer infections and nerve injuries) as well as avoiding surgical disruption of the subscapularis anteriorly and the infraspinatus posteriorly.

Arthroscopic Repair

The patient can be placed in a beach chair or lateral decubitus position depending on the surgeon's preference. Our preference is to perform all instability procedures in the lateral decubitus position. Accurate portal placement is the key to visualization, tissue mobilization, and accurate hardware placement. A standard posterior viewing portal is placed 1 cm medial and 2 cm inferior to the posterolateral acromion. A standard anterior midglenoid (AMG) portal low in the rotator interval, just above the subscapularis tendon, is also established and used for suture management and the easy passage of arthroscopic tools. A posteroinferior (PI) portal, or a 7 o'clock portal (left shoulder), can be placed 3 cm distal and 1 cm lateral to the posterolateral acromion. It gives excellent access to the inferior glenoid and is useful for glenoid preparation, posterior anchor placement, and suture management. The portal also provides access to the posterior glenoid should the lesion extend more posteriorly. Other commonly used portals include an anterior superior portal through the rotator interval and an accessory lateral (Wilmington) portal 1 cm lateral to the acromion.

A standard diagnostic arthroscopy is performed to evaluate the labrum, rotator cuff, and biceps tendon. The humeral head is evaluated for the presence and size of a Hill Sachs lesion (Figure 5.4). Specific attention must be paid to the integrity of the labrum to evaluate for any sign of a Bankart lesion or associated fracture. Glenoid bone loss is assessed, as this may alter the surgical procedure. An ALPSA is found when the disrupted labroligamentous heals medially along the glenoid. This lesion is often found in recurrent dislocators and can be best seen from the anterior superior viewing portal. Special attention is also paid to the anterior capsule to evaluate for the presence of a HAGL. Visualization of the subscapularis muscle fibers through the capsule suggests the presence of this lesion. The arthroscope should also be placed through the anterior portal to fully evaluate the posterior structures. Failure to recognize and address all associated pathology will likely result in an unsatisfactory outcome.

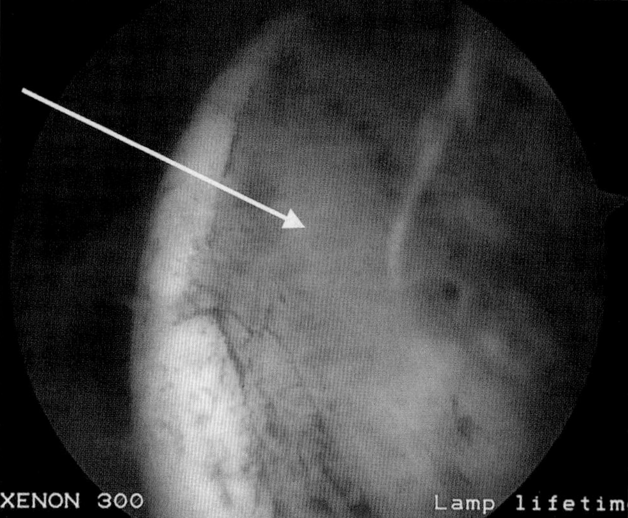

Figure 5.4 Arthroscopic image of a Hill Sachs lesion of the humeral head (*yellow arrow*).

Once a thorough diagnostic arthroscopy is completed, an arthroscopic elevator is used to develop a plane between the glenoid and capsulolabral complex (Figure 5.5, A) in order to fully release the capsule and labrum so that they can be mobilized onto the glenoid rim (Figure 5.5, B). The glenoid rim is then carefully prepared using an arthroscopic burr or rasp. The bony surface should be decorticated to remove any overlying fibrous tissue and to achieve a bleeding surface, but excessive bone should not be removed.

Once the glenoid rim has been prepared, suture anchors are placed into the glenoid rim to repair the labral tissue back to the glenoid. Regardless of the type of suture anchor used, the key maneuver of the shoulder stabilization procedure is to reestablish the tension of the AIGHL. The most inferior anchor is placed first as a drill guide is introduced into the posterior inferior portal, from which both limbs of the suture pass. The tip of the drill guide is placed between the 5:30 to 6:00 position on the glenoid (right shoulder). This will allow the tissue captured with the suture to be brought anteriorly and superiorly (Figure 5.5, C).

© 2018 American Academy of Orthopaedic Surgeons

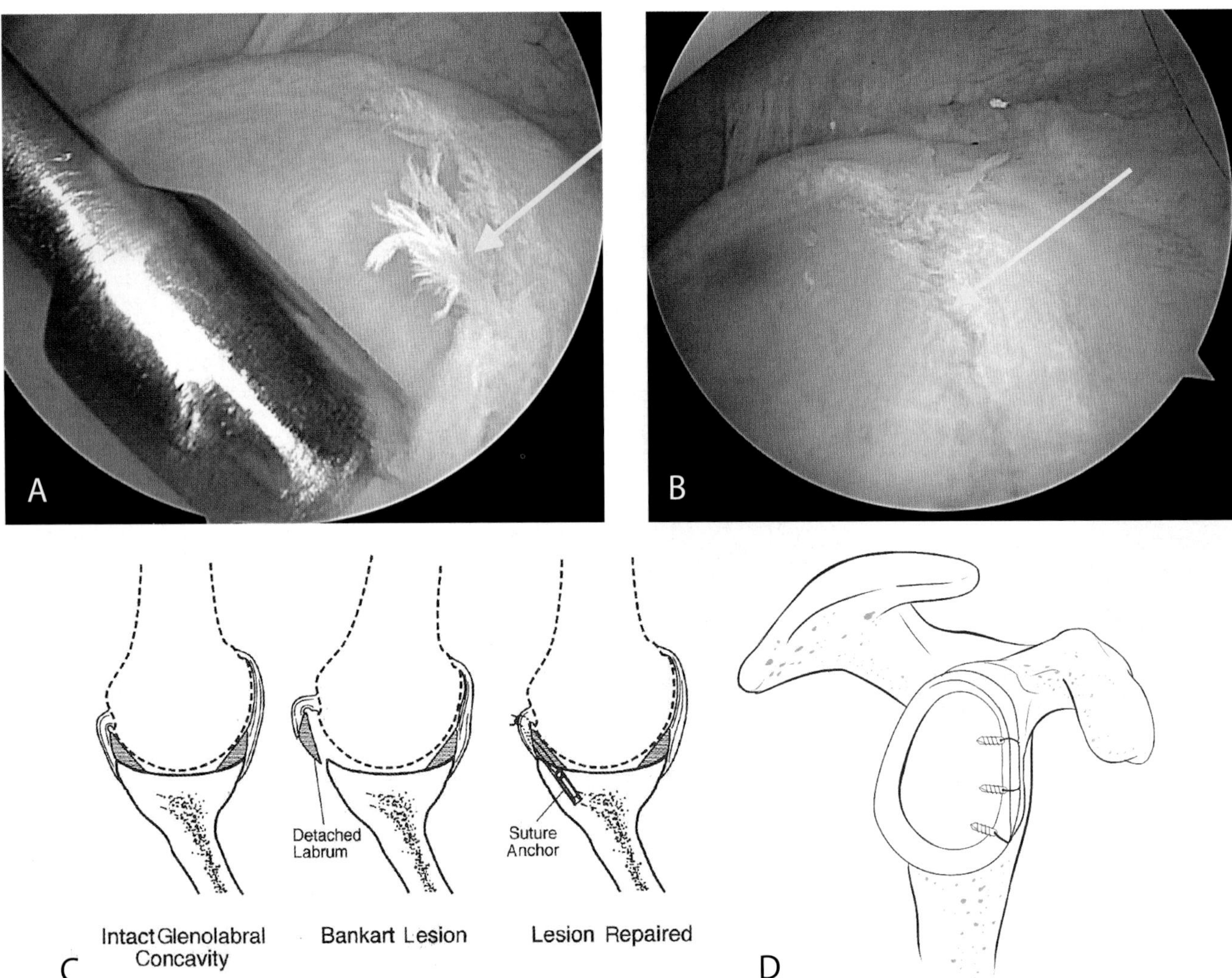

Figure 5.5 Arthroscopic images showing development of a plane between the glenoid and capsulolabral complex. **A**, The labrum should be thoroughly elevated with an arthroscopic elevator (*yellow arrow*). **B**, An adequate release has been achieved when the labrum rests without tension at the level of the glenoid (*yellow arrow*). **C**, Illustration of an axial image of an arthroscopic Bankart repair for anterior glenohumeral instability of a right shoulder. **D**, Illustration of a sagittal image of an arthroscopic Bankart repair for anterior glenohumeral instability of a right shoulder. (**C** reproduced with permission from Trumble TE, Budoff JE, Cornwall R: *Hand, Elbow, & Shoulder: Core Knowledge in Orthopaedics.* Philadelphia, PA, Elsevier, 2006.)

We prefer to work from a posterior to anterior direction. In order to restore the disrupted labral tissue back to the glenoid rim and reestablish the appropriate tension, the suture-passing instrument should enter the capsule approximately 1 cm posterior and inferior to the planned anchor site. In the inferior capsule, one needs to be careful to avoid passing the device too deeply into the soft tissue to avoid injury to the axillary nerve. Once this anchor has been placed, the surgeon should note the reduction of the inferior capsular redundancy. The suture can then be cut with an arthroscopic suture cutter. It is important to cut the suture without tails to prevent mechanical irritation and damage to the articular surface. This process is then repeated from an inferior to superior direction in order to elevate the labral tissue back to the glenoid and to restore tension. For typical Bankart lesions, we use three anchors; however, this is ultimately dictated by the size of the labral tear.

Posterior Glenohumeral Instability

Many of the technical aspects of arthroscopic posterior instability repairs are similar to anterior repairs. A complete diagnostic arthroscopy should be performed with careful inspection of the posterior labrum and capsule. With careful inspection, one may encounter a reverse Bankart lesion or a reverse Hill Sachs lesion. Injuries to the posterior capsule, a posterior HAGL, or a Kim lesion (incomplete avulsion of the posterior labrum) may also be present. As with anterior instability, the labrum is elevated to an anatomic position and the associated capsulolabral tears are repaired with the use of

© 2018 American Academy of Orthopaedic Surgeons

suture anchors. However, in these procedures, the process of placing anchors begins anteriorly and progresses posteriorly to recreate the sling effect of the PIGHL and to decrease the posterior capsular volume.

Multidirectional Instability

The surgical repair for multidirectional instability involves capsular plication. It requires the same basic setup and portal placement as is noted with the anterior instability repair. However, in this procedure, the main focus is addressing the generalized capsular laxity. To do this, anchors are placed along the glenoid rim with the focus on trying to remove the capsular redundancy that leads to multidirectional instability. In what is called a pinch-tuck technique, anchors are placed and then a "pinch" of capsular tissue is obtained with an arthroscopic suture passer; the capsular tissue is then tied down to the anchor. This decreases the capsular volume and stabilizes the shoulder. As with anterior or posterior instability, stabilization proceeds from inferior to superior. To encourage the redundant capsular tissue to scar to itself and permanently decrease the capsular volume, the surface of the capsule is abraded with a rasp prior to suture plication. If additional capsular plication is desired to further decrease the capsular volume, plication stitches without anchors can be placed around the intact labrum in areas between the previously placed suture anchors.

POSTOPERATIVE REHABILITATION

Rehabilitation plays a vital role in the functional outcome following shoulder stabilization surgery. The goal of the postoperative treatment is to ensure a balance between mobility and stability. We utilize a criteria-based approach to rehabilitation that divides the rehabilitation into 4 progressive phases, each tailored to the specific surgical procedure. Each phase consists of specific goals and exercises that are designed to systematically introduce forces and loads to the healing tissues while avoiding overstressing them. It is the intent of these programs to serve as a guideline. therefore, based on the patient and surgical intervention, the clinician will be able to make appropriate adjustments to each program. Although there are many common principles that can be applied to the rehabilitation of all instability repairs, there are also specific differences that relate to the direction of instability as well as to the repair.

When designing a shoulder instability rehabilitation program, the therapist must take into account several patient-related (Table 5.1) and surgery-related (Table 5.2) variables that may impact the rehabilitation. First, healing tissues should never be overstressed; therefore, the program must be progressive and sequential, with each phase building from the prior phase. Based on our experience of poorer outcomes following prolonged immobilization followed by a rapid progression of ROM, we implement the restoration of ROM in a gradual, systemic format with stretching precautions for the first 8 to 10 weeks following surgery. Second, the effects of immobilization must be minimized, especially in the overhead athlete.

Table 5.1 PATIENT FACTORS AFFECTING THE REHABILITATION PROGRAM

- Patient's tissue status
- Hyperelasticity ↔ hypermobility
- Dynamic stabilizers status
- Muscle–bone
- Muscular strength and balance
- Proprioceptive ability
- Classification of instability
- Previous activity level
- Desired activity level (expectations)
- Healing abilities (rapid healers, slow healers)

After shoulder stabilization surgery, a short period of immobilization may be indicated to allow initial healing. During this phase, however, the clinician can incorporate mild dynamic stabilization drills, gentle restricted passive motions, and submaximal isometrics to enhance dynamic stability, assist in collagen organization, and prevent loss of motion. In addition, the quality of end feel should be continually monitored throughout the rehabilitation by applying a slight overpressure at the end range of passive ROM (PROM). If a firm or hard end feel is noted, the clinician may accelerate the rate of ROM progression; with a soft or empty end feel, the patient's stretching program will be slowed. Third, the patient must fulfill specific criteria to progress from one phase to the next, thus allowing the rehabilitation program to be individualized based on the patient's unique healing rate and constraints. Finally, a successful outcome is related to a team effort, with the physician, therapist, and patient all working together toward a common goal.

Phases of Rehabilitation After Surgery

Phase I

In the immediate postoperative period, ROM is restricted. The primary goal of this phase is to prevent excessive scarring by allowing movement, but avoiding overaggressive motion that may compromise the surgical repair. For example, after an

Table 5.2 SURGICAL FACTORS AFFECTING THE REHABILITATION PROGRAM

- Type of surgical procedure (exposure, specific procedure, tissue used)
- Method of fixation
- Type of instability (instability classification)
- Patient's tissue status (hyperelasticity, normal, hypoelasticity)
- Patient's response to surgery
- Patient's dynamic stabilization (muscle strength, dynamic stability, proprioception)
- Patient's activity level (past, present, desired goals)
- Physician's philosophical approach

© 2018 American Academy of Orthopaedic Surgeons

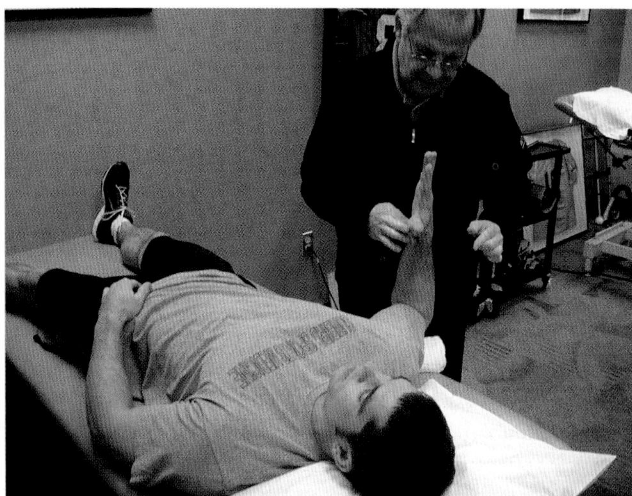

Figure 5.6 Photograph of rhythmic stabilization drills performed in the plane of the scapula to facilitate rotator cuff activation and neuromuscular control.

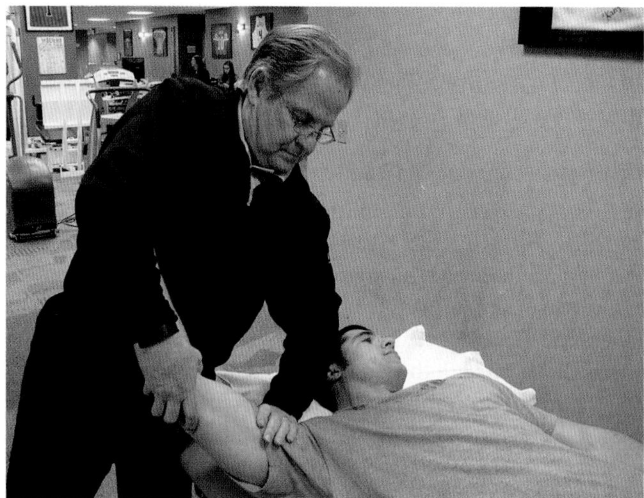

Figure 5.7 Photograph of joint mobilization performed in a posterolateral direction to improve posterior capsular mobility.

anterior stabilization procedure, external rotation is restricted, as this may overstress the capsulolabral repair. Submaximal and subpainful isometric contractions are also initiated during phase 1 to stimulate muscle training, neuromodulate pain, and prevent muscle atrophy that occurs as a result of immobilization (Figure 5.6).

Phase II

During this intermediate phase, the emphasis is on advancing shoulder mobility. Active assistive range of motion (AAROM) and PROM exercises are incorporated into the treatment program. The patient's ROM and capsular end feel will be used to determine the rate of progression. Patients with sufficient ROM and a soft end feel will be progressed slower than a patient with restricted ROM and a hard end feel. Joint-mobilization techniques are used to restore normal motion and to correct asymmetric capsular tightness. If one side of the capsule is excessively tight, the humeral head may translate in the opposite direction away from the tightness (Figure 5.7). In an overhead athlete, the clinician will progress the stretching exercises to allow the athlete to obtain "thrower's motion" of approximately 115° ± 5° ER to allow the athlete to return to throwing. Strengthening exercises can be progressed to include isolated rotator cuff and scapular exercises. Performing dynamic stabilization drills, manual resistance training, and proprioceptive neuromuscular facilitation (PNF) drills with rhythmic stabilizations can enhance neuromuscular control and reestablish muscular balance (Figure 5.8). During this phase, we usually initiate the "thrower's ten exercise" program.

Phase III

Phase III is designed to maintain shoulder ROM while improving strength, power, and endurance. Strengthening exercises are progressed to restore optimal sufficient muscle ratios (Table 5.3). Muscular balance and dynamic joint stability should be achieved before initiating aggressive strengthening exercises, such as plyometrics or functional activities. During this phase, eccentric muscle training and proprioceptive training are emphasized. Muscular endurance training also is performed to enhance dynamic functional joint stability and to prevent fatigue-induced subluxation. Plyometric training drills are utilized to increase the athlete's functional mobility and to gradually increase the functional stresses onto the shoulder joint. Overhead athletes are also progressed to the thrower's ten program to improve strength, endurance, and posture during this period.

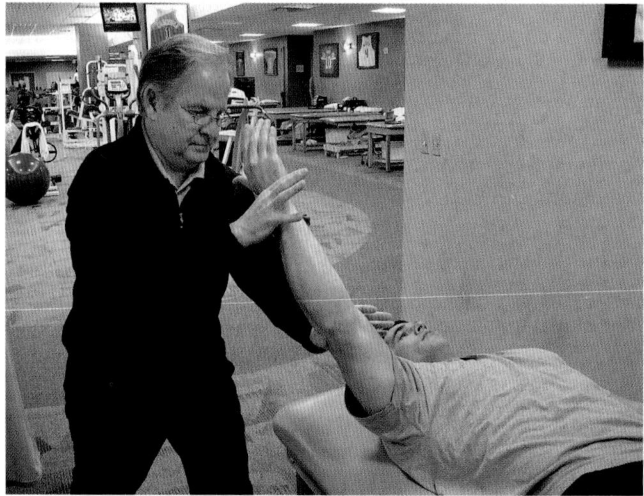

Figure 5.8 Photograph of manual resistance proprioceptive neuromuscular facilitation drills incorporating rhythmic stabilizations to facilitate dynamic joint stability.

© 2018 American Academy of Orthopaedic Surgeons

Table 5.3 ISOKINETIC SHOULDER STRENGTH CRITERIA FOR OVERHEAD ATHLETES

Bilateral Comparison (Dominant Arm vs. Nondominant Arm)

Velocity[a]	ER	IR	Abduction	Adduction
180	98%–105%	110%–120%	98%–105%	110%–128%
300	85%–95%	105%–115%	96%–102%	111%–129%

Peak Torque (ft-lb) to Body Weight (lb) Ratios

Velocity[a]	ER	IR	Abduction	Adduction
180	18%–23%	28%–33%	26%–33%	32%–38%
300	12%–20%	25%–30%	20%–25%	28%–34%

Unilateral Muscle Ratios

Velocity[a]	ER/IR	Abduction/Adduction	ER[2]/Abduction
180	66–76%	78%–84%	67%–75%
300	61%–71%	88%–94%	60%–70%

[a]Degrees per second.
ER = external rotation, IR = internal rotation.

Phase IV

During this phase, the goal is to increase the functional demands on the shoulder and return the patient to unrestricted sport or daily activities. Upon successful completion of the rehabilitation program and achieving the desired goals, the patient may initiate a gradual return to sport activity in a controlled manner. Other goals of this phase are to maintain the patient's muscular strength, dynamic stability, and functional motion established in the previous phase. Therefore, the patient is encouraged to maintain a stretching and strengthening program on an ongoing basis to maintain optimal shoulder function.

Arthroscopic Anterior Instability Repair Rehabilitation Protocol

Phase I: Immediate Postoperative Phase (Weeks 0–6)

Goals

- Protect the anatomic repair
- Prevent negative effects of immobilization
- Promote dynamic stability and proprioception
- Diminish pain and inflammation

Weeks 0 to 2

- Sling at all times during THE day for 3 to 4 weeks and sleep in an immobilizer for 4 weeks
- Elbow/hand ROM, hand-gripping exercises
- PROM and gentle AAROM exercise
  - Flexion to 70° week 1, 90° by week 2
  - ER/internal rotation (IR) performed with the arm in 30° abduction
    - ER to 5° to 10°
    - IR to 45°

Note: No active ER, extension, abduction

- Submaximal isometrics for shoulder musculature
- Rhythmic stabilization drills ER/IR
- Proprioception drills
- Cryotherapy, modalities as indicated

Weeks 3 and 4

- Discontinue use of the sling during the day but continue the immobilizer during sleep

Note: To be discontinued at 4 weeks unless otherwise directed by physician

- Continue gentle ROM exercises (PROM and AAROM)
  - Flexion to 90°
  - Abduction to 90°
- ER/IR at 45° abduction in the scapular plane
  - ER in the scapular plane to 15° to 20°
  - IR in the scapular plane to 55° to 60°

Note: The rate of progression is based on evaluation of the patient. No excessive ER, extension, or elevation.

- Continue isometrics and rhythmic stabilization (submaximal)
- Core stabilization program
- Initiate scapular strengthening program
- Continue use of cryotherapy

Weeks 5 and 6

- Gradually improve ROM
  - Flexion to 145°
  - ER at 45° of abduction: 55° to 50°
  - IR at 45° of abduction: 55° to 60°
- May initiate stretching exercises

© 2018 American Academy of Orthopaedic Surgeons

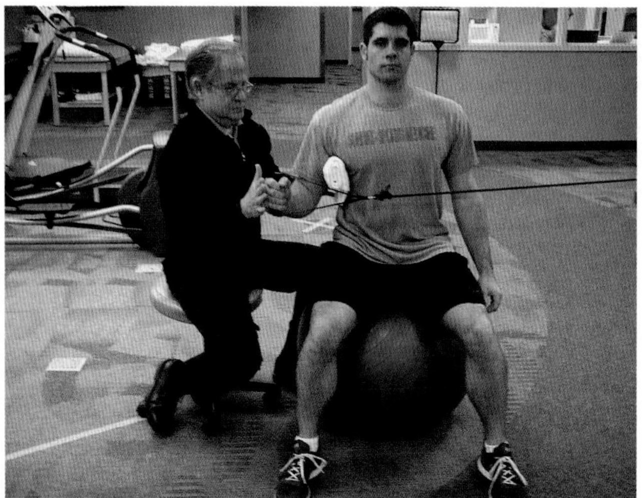

Figure 5.9 Photograph of external rotation tubing performed with concomitant rhythmic stabilizations to promote dynamic stability, neuromuscular control, and core stability.

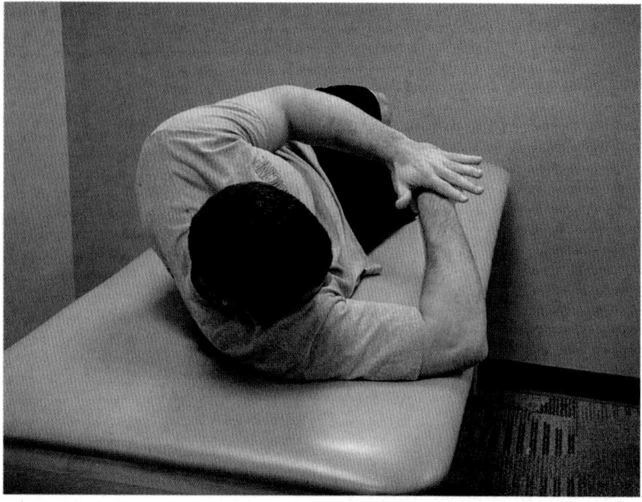

Figure 5.10 Photograph of modified sleeper stretch performed in the scapular plane to decrease stress on the subacromial structures.

- Initiate exercise tubing ER/IR (arm at side; Figure 5.9)
- Scapular strengthening
- PNF manual resistance

Note: In general, all exercises begin with 1 set of 10 repetitions and should increase by 1 set of 10 repetitions daily, as tolerated, to 3 sets of 10 repetitions.

Phase II: Intermediate Phase (Weeks 7–14)

Goals

- Gradually restore full ROM (week 10)
- Preserve the integrity of the surgical repair
- Restore muscular strength and balance
- Enhance neuromuscular control

Weeks 7 to 9

- Gradually progress ROM
  - Flexion to 160°
  - Initiate ER/IR at 90° of abduction
  - ER at 90° of abduction: 70° to 80° at week 7
  - ER to 90° at weeks 8 to 9
  - IR at 90° of abduction: 70° to 75°
- Continue to progress isotonic strengthening program
- Continue PNF strengthening

Weeks 10 to 14

- May initiate slightly more aggressive strengthening
- Progress isotonic strengthening exercises
- Continue all stretching exercises
- Progress ROM to functional demands (i.e., overhead athlete)
  - Progress to isotonic strengthening (light and restricted ROM)

Phase III: Minimal Protection Phase (Weeks 15–20)

Goals

- Maintain full ROM
- Improve muscular strength, power, and endurance
- Gradually initiate functional activities

Criteria to Enter Phase III

- Full nonpainful ROM
- Satisfactory stability
- Muscular strength (good grade or better)
- No pain or tenderness

Weeks 15 to 18

- Continue all stretching exercises (capsular stretches, including the sleeper stretch) (Figure 5.10)
- Continue strengthening exercises
  - Throwers ten program or fundamental exercises
  - PNF manual resistance
  - Endurance training
  - Restricted sport activities (light swimming, half golf swings)
- Initiate interval sport program weeks 16 to 18

Weeks 18 to 20

- Continue all exercise listed earlier
- Process interval sport program (throwing, and so on)

Phase IV: Advanced Strengthening Phase (21 Weeks and Beyond)

Goals

- Enhance muscular strength, power, and endurance
- Progress functional activities
- Maintain shoulder mobility
- Gradual return to sports at 7 to 9 months

Criteria to Enter Phase IV

- Full nonpainful ROM
- Satisfactory static stability
- Muscular strength 75% to 80% of contralateral side
- No pain or tenderness

© 2018 American Academy of Orthopaedic Surgeons

Weeks 21 to 24

- Continue flexibility exercises
- Continue isotonic strengthening program
- Neuromuscular control drills
- Plyometric strengthening
- Progress interval sport programs
- Continue stretching and strengthening program
- Gradually progress sport activities to unrestrictive participation when full functional ROM and satisfactory strength and stability are achieved

Arthroscopic Posterior Instability Repair Rehabilitation Protocol

Phase I: Immediate Postoperative Phase (Weeks 0–6)

Precautions

- Postoperative brace in 20° of abduction, and approximately 30° of ER for 4 weeks (physician will determine length of time and position)
- Brace must be worn at all times, with the exception of exercise activity and bathing
- No activities above the head or across the body
- Precautions: No IR motions, horizontal adduction, or pushing motions for 4 to 6 weeks
- Must sleep in brace for 4 to 6 weeks

Goals

- Allow healing of repaired capsule
- Initiate early protected and restricted ROM
- Minimize muscular atrophy
- Decrease pain/inflammation

Weeks 0 to 4

- Cryotherapy
  - Ice before and after exercises for 20 minutes and up to 20 minutes per hour to control pain and swelling

Exercises

- Gripping exercises with putty
- Active elbow flexion/extension, wrist flexion/extension and pronation/supination
- Passive shoulder ROM only for the first 2 to 3 weeks. May begin to initiate AAROM at 4 weeks.
  - Flexion to 90° for 2 to 4 weeks
  - ER at 45° abduction to 0° to 10° (first 2 weeks)
  - ER at 45° abduction to 15° to 20° (weeks 3–4)
  - No IR for 6 to 8 weeks (unless specified by physician)
  - No cross-body motion for 6 weeks
- Submaximal shoulder isometrics: Flexion, abduction, extension, ER, IR
- Scapular manual resistance
- Rhythmic stabilization drills ER/IR in scapular plane at 45° abduction
- Scapular neuromuscular control drills, manual resistance in sling
- Avoid closed kinetic-chain exercises, pushing motion, and crossed body activities

Weeks 4 to 6

Goals

- Gradual increase in ROM
  - Flexion to increase 125° to 145°
  - Begin light easy increase in ER at 45° of abduction
- Normalize arthrokinematics
- Improve strength
- Decrease pain/inflammation
- May discontinue brace 4 to 6 weeks postsurgery (per physician discretion)

Range of Motion Exercises

- L-Bar active-assisted exercises
- Initiate ER at 90° of abduction to tolerance
- Shoulder flexion to tolerance to 90° at week 4, then 125° at week 6
- No IR for 6 to 8 weeks (unless physician specifies)
- Rope and pulley (flexion only)
  - Shoulder scaption to 90° at week 4, 125° to 145° at week 6
- All exercises should be performed to tolerance
- Do not push or aggressively stretch into IR, or horizontal adduction

Strengthening Exercises

- Exercise tubing ER/IR at 45° of abduction (IR to neutral rotation only)
- Active shoulder flexion (full can) to 90° elevation
- Active shoulder abduction to 90° elevation
- Isotonic biceps and triceps
- Scapular strengthening with arm at 0° or 30° of abduction
  - Prone horizontal abduction and horizontal abduction with ER
  - Prone rowing and prone extensions
- Sidelying ER with dumbbell
- Rhythmic stabilization ER/IR and flexion/extension
- Avoid closed-chain kinetic exercises
- Proprioception and kinesthesia training
  - Initiate joint reposition training

Phase II: Intermediate Phase (Weeks 7–15)

Goals

- Gradually reestablish ROM
- Normalize arthrokinematics
- Increase strength
- Improve neuromuscular control
- Enhance proprioception and kinesthesia

Weeks 7 to 10

Range of Motion Exercises

- L-Bar active-assisted exercises
  - ER at 90° of abduction to tolerance (should be 80°–85° by week 8)
  - ER at 90° of abduction to 115° (if patient is a thrower) by week 10 to 12

© 2018 American Academy of Orthopaedic Surgeons

- Shoulder flexion to tolerance (180° by week 8)
- IR at 90° of abduction to 30° to 45° by week 10
- Rope and pulley: elevation in scapular plane

Strengthening Exercises

- Tubing for IR/ER at 0° of abduction
- Initiate isotonic dumbbell program
  - Shoulder abduction, shoulder scaption with ER (full can), seated rowing
- Horizontal abduction
  - Horizontal abduction full can
  - Prone rowing
- Biceps curls and triceps pushdowns
- Scapular muscle training (sidelying)
- No push-ups or pushing movements (until 12 weeks)
- Prone dumbbell rows, horizontal abduction, and horizontal abduction ER
- Sidelying ER dumbbell
- Initiate Neuromuscular Control Exercises for Scapulothoracic Joint

Weeks 11 to 15

Continue all exercises listed earlier. Initiate the following:

- Progress ER/IR at 90° abduction
- ER to 90° or 115° for overhead athletes
- IR to 45° to 50°
- Full elevation
- Progress strengthening program
- Initiate push-ups into wall at week 12
- Initiate plank (bilateral) against wall and onto floor
- Emphasize muscle strength of ER, scapular region

Phase III: Minimal Protection Phase (Weeks 16–21)

Goals

- Maintain/progress to full ROM
- Improve strength/power/endurance
- Emphasize posterior shoulder muscles and scapular muscles
- Improve neuromuscular control
- Enhance dynamic stability
- Improve scapular muscular strength

Weeks 13 to 20

Exercises

- Continue isotonic program (emphasize posterior glenohumeral joint and scapular retraction)
- Continue trunk/lower extremity (LE) strengthening and conditioning exercises
- Continue neuromuscular control exercises
- Machine resistance (limited ROM)
  - Latissimus dorsi pulldowns
  - Seated row
  - Seated bench press (week 14)
- May progress closed kinetic chain program
  - Ball on wall
  - Push-up with rhythmic stabilization on unstable surface (if appropriate)

Week 16 to 20

- Continue all exercises as listed before
- Emphasis on gradual return to recreational activities
- Progress plyometrics—2-hand drills

Criteria to Progress to Phase IV

- Full ROM
- No pain/tenderness
- Satisfactory clinical exam
- Satisfactory isokinetic test

Phase IV: Return to Activity Phase (Weeks 21–32)

Goals

- Progressively increase activities to prepare the patient for unrestricted functional return

Exercises

- Continue isotonic strengthening exercises outlined in Phase III
- Clearance for bench press, pushups, football blocking drills, and so forth (determined by physician)
- Continue ROM exercises—light stretching
- Initiate interval programs between 22 to 26 weeks (if the patient is an athlete), (physician determines)
- Gradual return to sports but continue scapular and glenohumeral joint muscle training

Arthroscopic Multidirectional Instability Repair Rehabilitation Protocol

Phase I: Immediate Postoperative Phase (Weeks 0–6)

Goals

- Reduce postoperative pain and inflammation
- Promote capsular healing
- Slow muscular atrophy
- Controlled motion to shoulder

Weeks 0 to 2

- Sling and swathe for 4 weeks at all times, except for exercises
- Pendulum exercises
- AAROM with L-bar and PROM
  - Flexion to 70° by week 1, and 90° by week 2
  - ER in scapular plane 30° of abduction to 5° to 10°
  - IR in scapular plane 30° of abduction to 15° to 20°
- Rope and pulley to 70° and 90°
- Isometrics for shoulder flexion, abduction, and scapular retraction
  - Rhythmic stabilization IR/ER
  - Biceps isometrics (if SLAP repair not for 6 weeks)

Modalities

- Cryotherapy for first 7–10 days

© 2018 American Academy of Orthopaedic Surgeons

Weeks 3 and 4

- Continue use of sling and swathe
- AAROM and PROM exercises
  - Flexion to 90° to 100°
  - ER at 45° of abduction, scapular plane to 30°
  - IR at 45° of abduction, scapular plane to 45°
- Continue pendulum and rope/pulley
- Muscular strengthening exercises
  - Tubing ER/IR at 0° of abduction
  - Continue isometrics
  - Prone rowing
  - Prone horizontal abduction (limited ROM)
  - Lower trapezius table lifts
  - Continue manual resistance rhythmic stabilization for IR/ER
- Initiate proprioception drills

Weeks 5 and 6

- Discontinue sling and swathe (week 4)
- Progress ROM overhead (above 90° of abduction)
- AAROM and PROM
  - Flexion to 145° (week 5)
  - Flexion to 160° (week 6)
  - ER at 90° of abduction to 70° at week 6
  - IR at 90° of abduction to 65° at week 6
- Initiate light isotonics (week 5)
  - Full can (begin with 1 Ib)
  - Shoulder abduction (begin with 1 Ib)
  - Sidelying ER
  - Scapular strengthening
  - Continue manual resistance
  - Initiate light resistance closed kinetic chain wall drills (Figure 5.11)

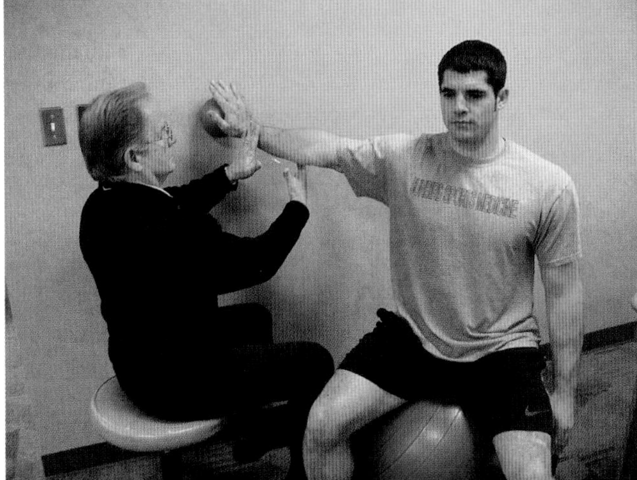

Figure 5.11 Photograph of stabilization exercise performed with the arm in the scapular plane, with the hand placed on a ball on a wall to facilitate dynamic stabilization and providing compressive forces into the glenohumeral joint.

- Continue proprioception drills
- Initiate core stabilization drills

Phase II: Intermediate Phase (Weeks 7–16)

Goals

- Gradually increase ROM and flexibility
- Enhance dynamic stabilization
- Improve muscle strength and endurance
- Gradually increase applied loads

Weeks 7 to 9

- Flexibility and ROM exercises
  - ER at 90° of abduction to 90° (week 8)
  - IR at 90° of abduction to 65° (week 8)
  - Full flexion at 180°

Muscle Training

- Continue rhythmic stabilization drills
- Proprioceptive neuromuscular facilitation D2 flexion/extension with rhythmic stabilization
- Begin "throwers ten program"
  - Progress 1 Ib/week if nonpainful
- Progress scapular strengthening program
- Push-ups on ball on table with rhythmic stabilization
- Wall stabilization onto ball into wall
- Tubing ER strengthening
- Closed kinetic chain drills
- Proprioception drills

Weeks 10 to 12

- Continue all exercises listed earlier
- Progress ER at 90° of abduction to 110° to 115° at week 12
- Initiate self-capsular stretches
- Initiate 2-hand plyometrics (weeks 10–11)

Weeks 13 to 16

- Continue all exercises listed earlier
- Initiate progressive resistance exercises
  - Bench press (narrow grip)
  - Pull-downs (in front of body)
  - Push-ups
  - Seated rowing
  - Pectoralis flies
- Plyometrics 1-hand drills/throws (week 14)
- Wall dribble with 2-Ib plyoball

Phase III: Minimal Protection Phase (Weeks 16–23)

Goals

- Progress strengthening, power, and endurance
- Enhance dynamic stabilization
- Initiate overhead throwing program

Weeks 16 to 20

- Continue all flexibility and ROM exercises
- Continue self-capsular stretches

© 2018 American Academy of Orthopaedic Surgeons

- Continue ER/IR stretch at 90° of abduction
- Throwers ten program
- Plyometrics 2-hand and 1-hand drills
- Endurance drills
- Core stabilization drills
- Initiate interval throwing program (Phase I)

Weeks 21 to 23

- Continue all of the previously listed exercises
- Initiate interval throwing program (Phase II) at weeks 21 to 22

Phase IV: Return to Activity Phase (Weeks 24–32)

Goals

- Progress to unrestricted full activity
- Continue/progress strengthening exercise

Weeks 26 to 30

- Stretch and improve ROM and flexibility
- Throwers ten program
- Plyometrics 2-hand and 1-hand drills
- Progress throwing program

Criteria for Return to Play

- Full nonpainful ROM
- Satisfactory isokinetic test
- Satisfactory clinical exam
- Completion of interval throwing program
- Physician approval

OUTCOMES

Mazzocca et al reported on an average 37-month (range 24–66 months) follow-up following arthroscopic anterior Bankart repair in collision athletes. The authors found an 11% overall recurrent dislocation rate that was isolated to football players. A recent meta-analysis by Harris and colleagues comparing the rate of return to sport for open anterior Bankart repair to arthroscopic suture anchor repair found similar results (89% vs. 87%) for both procedures. Bradley et al published successful results in 200 athletes following arthroscopic posterior capsulolabral reconstruction, with 90% overall returning to full sport. In addition, 91% of the contact athletes were able to return to sport without recurrence of instability. Similarly, Provencher et al published a series of 33 patients, in which 88% remained stable at a mean follow-up of 39 months after a posterior labral repair. The return-to-sport rate has been reported following capsular plication for multidirectional instability to be 86% in the cohorts of Baker et al and Treacy et al. Similarly, Jones et al reported at a mean follow-up of 3.6 years (range, 2.0–5.5 years) following capsular plication for MDI; 18 (90%) patients returned to overhead sports, with 17 (85%) at their preinjury level.

PEARLS

- Imaging should be carefully scrutinized for associated lesions. If there is concern for bone loss, a CT scan should be performed.
- Accurate portal placement is key for proper placement of suture anchors.
- Capsulolabral repair should start far inferior to recreate the sling effect to the inferior glenohumeral ligament complex.
- During rehabilitation, never overstress healing tissue. The rehabilitation program must match the surgical procedure, the patient's tissue quality, and the patient's desired functional goals.
- ROM is progressed based on the clinical assessment of quality of end feel. A firm end feel necessitates acceleration in restoration of motion; a softer end feel should alert the therapist to slow the restoration of motion.
- The systematic implementation of incorporating stresses and forces via functional and sport-specific drills is imperative to allow a return to activity.

BIBLIOGRAPHY

Baker CL 3rd, Mascarenhas R, Kline AJ, Chhabra A, Pombo MW, Bradley JP: Arthroscopic treatment of multidirectional shoulder instability in athletes: A retrospective analysis of 2- to 5-year clinical outcomes. *Am J Sports Med* 2009;37:1712–1720.

Bradley JP, McClincy MP, Arner JW, Tejwani SG: Arthroscopic capsulolabral reconstruction for posterior instability of the shoulder: A prospective study of 200 shoulders. *Am J Sports Med* 2013;41(9):2005–2014.

Harris JD, Gupta AK, Mall NA, Abrams GD, McCormick FM, Cole BJ, Bach BR Jr, Romeo AA, Verma NN: Long-term outcomes after Bankart shoulder stabilization. *Arthroscopy* 2013;29(5):920–933.

Jones KJ, Kahlenberg CA, Dodson CC, Nam D, Williams RJ, Altchek DW: Arthroscopic capsular plication for microtraumatic anterior shoulder instability in overhead athletes. *Am J Sports Med* 2012;40(9):2009–2014.

Mazzocca AD, Brown FM, Carreira DS, Hayden J, Romeo AA: Arthroscopic anterior shoulder stabilization of collision and contact athletes. *Am J Sports Med* 2005;33(1):52–60.

Provencher MT, LeClere LE, King S, McDonald LS, Frank RM, Mologne TS, Ghodadra NS, Romeo AA: Posterior instability of the shoulder: Diagnosis and management. *Am J Sports Med* 2011;39(4):874–886.

Reinold MM, Wilk KE, Reed J, Crenshaw K, Andrews JR: Interval sport programs: guidelines for baseball, tennis, and golf. *J Orthop Sports Phys Ther* 2002;32(6):293–298.

Treacy SH, Savoie FH 3rd, Field LD: Arthroscopic treatment of multidirectional instability. *J Shoulder Elbow Surg* 1999;8:345–350.

© 2018 American Academy of Orthopaedic Surgeons

Wilk KE, Andrews JR, Arrigo CA, Keirns MA, Erber DJ: The strength characteristics of internal and external rotator muscles in professional baseball pitchers. *Am J Sports Med* 1993;21:61–66.

Wilk KE, Andrews JR: Rehabilitation following arthroscopic subacromial decompression. *Orthopaedics* 1993;16:349–358.

Wilk KE, Andrews JR, Arrigo CA: The abductor and adductor strength characteristics of professional baseball pitchers. *Am J Sports Med* 1995;23:307–311.

Wilk KE, Yenchak AJ, Arrigo CA, Andrews JR: The advanced throwers ten exercise program: a new exercise series for enhanced dynamic shoulder control in the overhead throwing athlete. *Phys Sportsmed* 2011;39(4):90–97.

© 2018 American Academy of Orthopaedic Surgeons

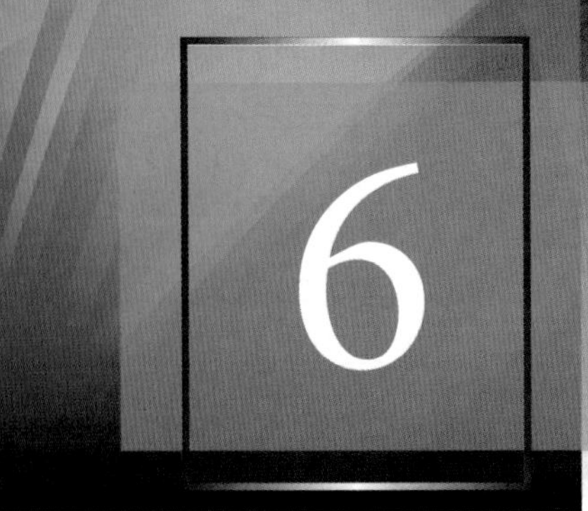

Open Anterior Glenohumeral Instability Repair

E. Scott Paxton, MD, and Brett D. Owens, MD

INTRODUCTION

Open anterior shoulder stabilization remains an essential procedure for the orthopaedic surgeon. Historically, a number of procedures, anatomic and nonanatomic, have been described. The open Bankart procedure, which involves anterior capsulolabral repair, was described initially by Sir Blundell Bankart in 1923 and later popularized by Carter Rowe. Variations of this procedure are used to treat traumatic recurrent anterior dislocations with anterior labral injury. The Latarjet procedure, coracoid transfer, was described in 1953 by Michel Latarjet. The mechanism of stability of the Latarjet procedure includes the elongation of the anterior bony glenoid, anterior capsular reconstruction, and the inferior sling effect of the conjoined tendon. In the last two decades, open stabilization surgery was supplanted by arthroscopic stabilization procedures. However, reported failures of arthroscopic instability repairs, as well as a greater understanding of the implications of glenoid and humeral bone loss, have resulted in a renewed appreciation and study of both the open Bankart repair and Latarjet coracoid transfer.

The rehabilitation of all anterior shoulder stabilization procedures share some common aspects. The goal is to allow the capsulolabral tissues to heal without undue tension while allowing return of motion by 12 weeks and the initiation of strengthening with return to sport at approximately 24 weeks. The major differences in the rehabilitation after open Bankart repair stabilization and Latarjet procedures stem from the surgical management of the subscapularis tendon and the goal of osseous healing of the coracoid bone block. These differences direct the alterations in the approaches to rehabilitation; therefore, the chapter will differentiate between the open Bankart and Latarjet procedures.

SURGICAL PROCEDURE

Open Bankart Procedure

Indications

The indications for open Bankart repair are first-time anterior dislocation in a young athlete or recurrent anterior instability. This procedure is a great option for the surgical treatment of patients who are at high risk for recurrence, including young contact athletes and military personnel. The open Bankart repair is also a great option for shoulder instability with "subcritical" bone loss or for revision anterior stabilization in shoulders without significant glenoid bone loss.

Contraindications

A relative contraindication for open Bankart repair is glenoid bone loss greater than 20%, for which many surgeons would recommend a bone augmentation procedure, such as the Latarjet procedure, autogenous glenoid bone graft (iliac crest), or osteochondral allograft. Another relative contraindication for open Bankart repair is poor-quality capsular tissue, as can be encountered following thermal modification or cases of multiple failed stabilization procedures.

Voluntary shoulder instability is a contraindication to surgical reconstruction in general. Additionally, uncontrolled epilepsy, instability associated with significant permanent

---

Dr. Owens or an immediate family member serves as a paid consultant to CONMED Linvatec, Mitek, Musculoskeletal Transplant Foundation, and Rotation Medical; has received research or institutional support from Hisogenics; has received nonincome support (such as equipment or services), commercially derived honoraria, or other non-research–related funding (such as paid travel) from the American Journal of Sports Medicine, *Saunders/Mosby-Elsevier, SLACK Incorporated, and Springer; and serves as a board member, owner, officer, or committee member of American Academy of Orthopaedic Surgeons, the* American Journal of Sports Medicine, *the American Orthopaedic Association, the American Orthopaedic Society for Sports Medicine, the Arthroscopy Association of North America, the journal* Orthopedics, *and* Orthopedics Today. *Dr. Paxton or an immediate family member serves as a paid consultant to Tornier; has received nonincome support (such as equipment or services), commercially derived honoraria, or other non-research–related funding (such as paid travel) from Arthrex, Smith & Nephew, and Tornier; and serves as a board member, owner, officer, or committee member of the* Journal of Bone and Joint Surgery–American.

© 2018 American Academy of Orthopaedic Surgeons

nerve injury, and multidirectional instability are thought to be contraindications.

Procedure

Relevant Anatomy

The open Bankart repair is performed through a true internervous plane, the deltopectoral interval. Deep to this interval is the conjoint tendon. A critical decision in performing this procedure is how to approach the subscapularis tendon. The stabilization can be performed through a horizontal subscapularis split or by a vertical tenotomy and retraction of the subscapularis tendon with subsequent repair. The axillary nerve located along the lower border of the subscapularis and inferior to the capsule is at risk of injury. The musculocutaneous nerve, which enters the deep aspect of the coracobrachialis and short head of the biceps, is at risk for injury as well.

Technique

A several-centimeter anterior skin incision is made following Langer's lines and extending superiorly from the anterior axillary fold. The cephalic vein is identified deep to the subcutaneous tissue and dissected to be retracted laterally with the deltoid muscle while the pectoralis muscle is retracted medially. Once the deltoid and pectoralis major muscles are retracted, the clavipectoral fascia is incised and the conjoint tendon retracted medially, exposing the subscapularis tendon and muscle. We describe a subscapularis tenotomy in this chapter with relevant rehabilitation protocols. However, a subscapularis split may also be performed, thus avoiding the risk of failed healing of the subscapularis tendon.

We prefer to enter the glenohumeral joint through a vertical tenotomy of the upper two-thirds of the subscapularis tendon approximately 1 cm medial to the insertion on the lesser tuberosity. This leaves good tendon tissue laterally for repair at the end of the procedure. The subscapularis tendon and anterior capsule can either be left together as a single layer or separated in order to perform a capsular shift. The subscapularis tendon and capsular tissues are controlled with traction sutures.

A humeral head retractor (Fukuda) is placed into the glenohumeral joint and behind the posterior glenoid to expose the anterior glenoid and the Bankart lesion. The labrum is mobilized from the anterior glenoid neck with an elevator so that it can be repaired. The anteroinferior glenoid rim and neck are abraded with a burr or rasp in preparation for the repair. The capsule and labrum can be repaired with sutures placed through bone tunnels on the glenoid rim or with suture anchors. Sutures are passed around the avulsed labrum and medial capsule in a mattress fashion, and knots are tied in succession from inferior to superior on the anterior capsule (Figure 6.1).

The humeral head retractor is removed if needed and a laterally based capsular shift can be performed. We prefer to use suture anchors in the anatomic neck of the humeral head to facilitate the capsular shift repair and perform a pants-over-vest

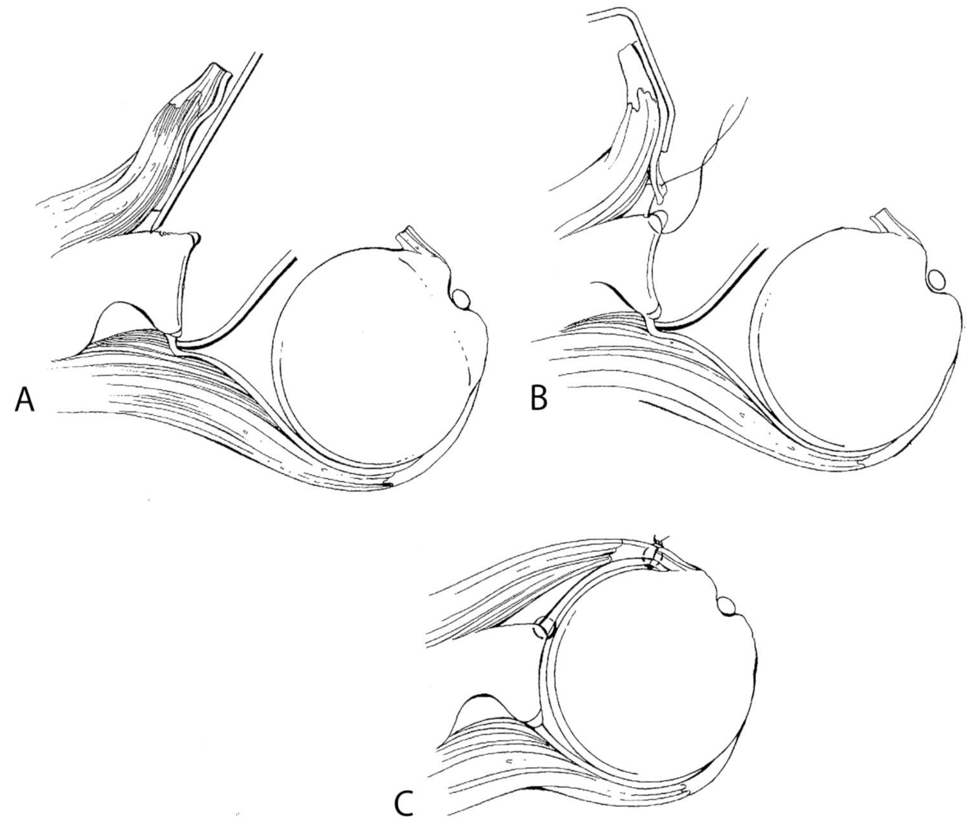

Figure 6.1 Radiographs of Bankart lesion with anterior inferior labral detachment: sagittal view (**A**) and axial view (**B**). Bankart anterior inferior capsulolabral repair: sagittal view (**C**).

© 2018 American Academy of Orthopaedic Surgeons

closure. Last, the subscapularis tendon is securely repaired with nonabsorbable sutures, and the wound is closed.

Complications

The most serious complication is injury to the axillary nerve, which can be palpated as it traverses posteriorly deep to the subscapularis and capsule. It is critical to gently place retractors superior to the nerve to protect it and to avoid injury while passing sutures during Bankart repair. Failure of the subscapularis repair is also a substantial concern and can result from inadequate repair, early postoperative injury, patient noncompliance, or overly aggressive rehabilitation.

Postoperative Rehabilitation

In general, the rehabilitation protocol for an open Bankart repair follows a course of initial immobilization and protection of the subscapularis repair, early protected range of motion (ROM) exercises, progressive strengthening after early soft-tissue healing, and eventual return to premorbid activities. A more conservative approach may be warranted for high-risk patients or revision cases. Our rehabilitation protocol is guided by the need to protect the healing of the subscapularis tendon repair along with healing of the capsulolabral repair. One area of debate is the length of sling immobilization. While there is no consensus, most surgeons recommend a sling for at least 4 weeks and at most 6 weeks. Protection of the subscapularis repair is critically important, as failure can lead to disastrous results.

As the restrictions are released, the ROM is advanced and early strengthening is begun. The focus shifts to progressive strengthening and work on proprioception. The final phase involves sport-specific training and preparation for return to play. Another point of debate is the return-to-play timing. There are few reports on return-to-play criteria, in contrast to return following anterior cruciate ligament (ACL) reconstruction.

Authors' Preferred Protocol

Week 1

- Sling for 6 weeks, even while sleeping
- Hand-squeezing exercises
- Elbow and wrist active range of motion (AROM) with shoulder in neutral position at side
- Supported pendulum exercises
- Shoulder shrugs/scapular retraction without resistance
- Cryotherapy

Goals

- Pain control
  - Protection

Week 2

- Continue sling for 6 weeks
- Continue appropriate previous exercises
- Active assisted range of motion (AAROM) supine with wand
- Flexion and abduction motion to 90°
- Gentle AAROM external rotation (ER; elbow at side) to neutral position
- *No Active Internal Rotation (IR)*
- Resisted elbow/wrist exercises (light dumbbell)
- Stationary bike (must wear sling)

Goal

- AAROM flexion and abduction to 90°

Weeks 3 to 4

- Continue sling for 6 weeks
- Continue appropriate previous exercises
- AAROM supine with wand
- Elevation motion to 120°
- Abduction motion to 110°
- Gentle ER motion (elbow at side) to within 50% of opposite shoulder
- *No Active IR*

Goal

- AAROM flexion to 120°, abduction to 110°

Weeks 5 to 6

- Continue sling for 6 weeks
- Continue appropriate previous exercises
- Full pendulum exercises
- AAROM: Flexion (supine wand, pulleys) >120°, as tolerated
- Abduction motion (supine wand, pulleys) to 120°
- Gentle ER motion (elbow at side) to within 75% of opposite shoulder
- *No Active IR*
- Push-up plus against wall—no elbow flexion >90°
- Prone scapular retraction exercises (without weights)
- Treadmill—walking progression program

Goal

- AAROM flexion >120°, abduction to 120°

Weeks 7 to 9

- Discontinue sling
- Continue appropriate previous exercises
- AAROM (pulleys, wall climbs, doorway stretches) through full range
- AROM through full range, as tolerated
- Rotator cuff strengthening with light resistance band
- ER and IR with arm at side and pillow or towel roll under arm (Figure 6.2)
- Active flexion to 60°
- Active abduction to 60°
- Active scaption to 60°
- Active extension to 30°
- Standing rows with resistance band
- Prone scapular retraction exercises (with light weight; Figure 6.3)
- Ball on wall (arcs, alphabet)
- BAPS/BOSU board on hands (Figure 6.4)

© 2018 American Academy of Orthopaedic Surgeons

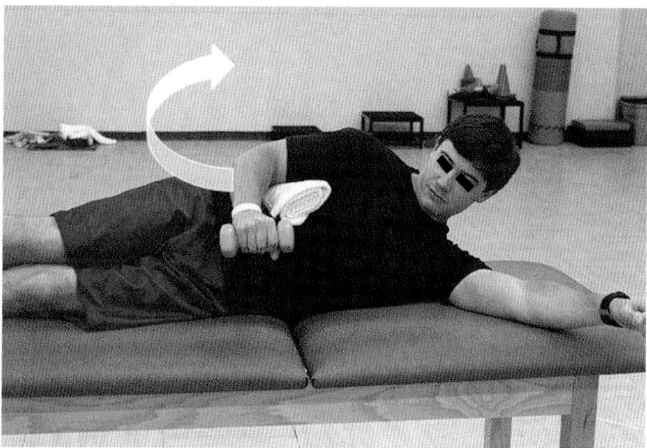

Figure 6.2 Photograph of external rotation strengthening.

- Push-up progression: Wall to table (no elbow flexion >90°)
- Bodyblade (Mad Dogg Athletics, Venice, CA)
- Upper body exercise (UBE) forward and backward at low resistance
- Stair training/elliptical trainer
- Pool walking/running—No upper extremity (UE) resistive exercises

Goals

- Full AROM
  - 30 wall push-ups

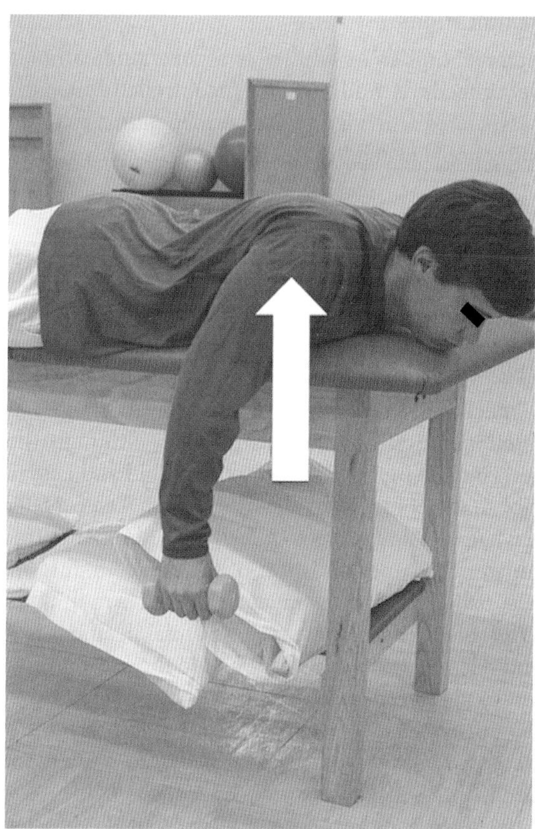

Figure 6.3 Photograph of prone scapular retraction exercises.

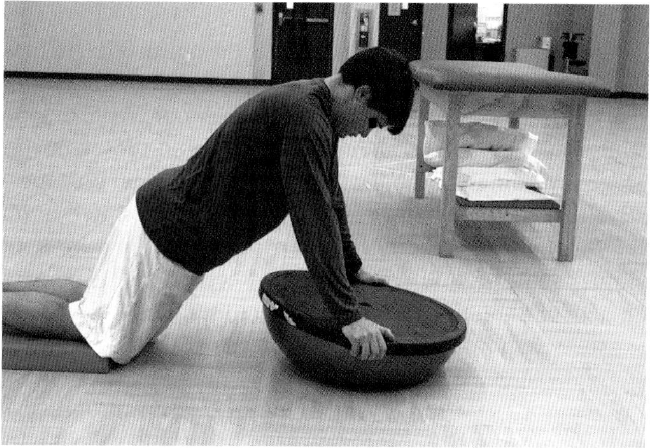

Figure 6.4 Photograph of BAPS/BOSU on hands.

Weeks 10 to 12

- Continue appropriate previous exercises with increased resistance, as tolerated
- PROM/mobilization as needed to regain full ROM
- Push-up progression: Table to chair (no elbow flexion >90°)
- Ball toss with arm at side using light ball
- Running progression program
- Pool walking/running, with UE resistance (no swimming)

Goal

- Normal rotator cuff strength

Months 3 to 4

- Continue appropriate previous exercises
- Ball toss overhead
- Push-ups, regular: No elbow flexion >90°
- Weight training with light resistance
- No overhead press or pull-downs behind head
- No elbow flexion >90° with bench, dips, and so on
- Pool therapy

Goals

- Run at easy pace
- Able to perform regular push-ups

Months 5 to 6

- Continue appropriate previous exercises
- Push-ups: No elbow flexion >90°
- Core strengthening
- Swimming
- Running progression to track
- Progressive weight training
- No elbow flexion >90° with bench, dips, and so on
- Transition to home/gym program
- Sport-specific training

Goals

- Resume all activities
- *No contact sports until 6 months postoperatively*
- Motion-limiting brace recommended for collision athletes during first season back, if possible

© 2018 American Academy of Orthopaedic Surgeons

Outcomes

There is no known level 1 evidence of the optimal rehabilitation following open Bankart repair. However, there are studies that evaluated rehabilitation after arthroscopic repairs. One study compared an accelerated rehabilitation protocol with 3 weeks of sling immobilization to a conventional postoperative rehabilitation. The accelerated protocol resulted in no increase in recurrence, less pain, earlier return of motion, and similar subjective outcomes scores. Recently, the American Society of Shoulder and Elbow Therapists published a consensus rehabilitation guideline for arthroscopic stabilization procedures, including 4 weeks of sling immobilization, progressive ROM improvement over 12 weeks, progressive strengthening starting at 6 weeks, and return to full activity between months 4 and 6. However, Dampkjaer and colleagues compared patients treated under this guideline to a cohort of arthroscopic stabilization patients treated with "standard care" protocol (which they describe briefly as a protocol of progressive motion and strengthening), and no differences were noted.

It is also important to note that randomized controlled trials of open versus arthroscopic Bankart repair using the same rehabilitation protocol among groups have failed to show significant differences in outcome or ROM.

Pearls

- Like all surgical procedures, patient selection is key.
- Preoperative generalized ligamentous laxity should be evaluated and may suggest the need for adjunctive anterior inferior capsular shift with open Bankart repair.
- Meticulous repair of the subscapularis tendon is essential.
- Avoidance of excessive or unsupervised passive ER and active IR during the first 6 weeks is critical to avoid excessive stress on the subscapularis repair.
- The procedure can also be performed through a subscapularis splitting approach, which should be considered in selected patients.

Latarjet Procedure

Indications

The principle indication for the Latarjet procedure is anterior glenohumeral instability in the presence of glenoid bone loss. Glenoid bone loss greater than 20% is considered the threshold for bony reconstruction (Figure 6.5). Soft-tissue repairs, such as arthroscopic and open Bankart repairs, have higher failure rates in the presence of substantial glenoid bone loss. Some surgeons also prefer to use the Latarjet procedure to treat anterior instability without glenoid bone loss, especially for treating younger, highly active male patients who participate in contact sports. Failed anterior instability repair is also an indication for the Latarjet procedure, even without glenoid bone loss, as these patients often have deficient labral tissue and poor-quality capsular tissue. In a revision setting, this procedure may be indicated in patients with less bone loss who have already failed a soft-tissue repair.

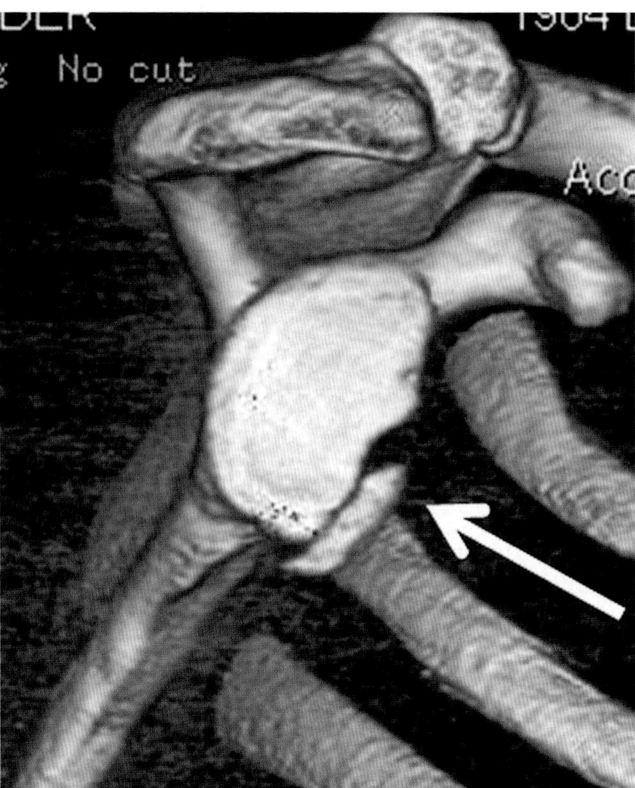

Figure 6.5 A 3-D CT scan of a right shoulder with >20% anterior glenoid bone loss (*arrow*).

Contraindications

Voluntary shoulder instability is a contraindication to the Latarjet procedure. Additionally, uncontrolled epilepsy, instability associated with significant permanent nerve injury and multidirectional instability are thought to be contraindications.

Procedure (Figure 6.6)

An interscalene nerve block is typically performed preoperatively along with a general anesthetic. The patient is placed in the beach chair position and examination under anesthesia is performed to confirm the diagnosis and to rule out co-existing posterior instability. The operative arm is draped free and a sterile mechanical arm holder is used for assistance. A standard deltopectoral approach is utilized, although the skin incision is made in line with the axillary fold and extends just superior to the coracoid (typically 4–5 cm). The cephalic vein is taken laterally and protected. A sharp Hohmann retractor is placed over the superior aspect of the coracoid, just anterior to the coracoclavicular ligaments, with the arm in abduction and external rotation. The coracoacromial ligament is identified and released from its insertion onto the acromion, leaving enough tissue to repair to the anterior capsule after the coracoid is transferred. Medially, care is taken to protect the adjacent neurovascular structures as the pectoralis minor tendon is released from its insertion on the medial coracoid.

With the coracoid exposed, a 90° saw blade or osteotome is used to cut the coracoid just anterior to the coracoclavicular

 © 2018 American Academy of Orthopaedic Surgeons

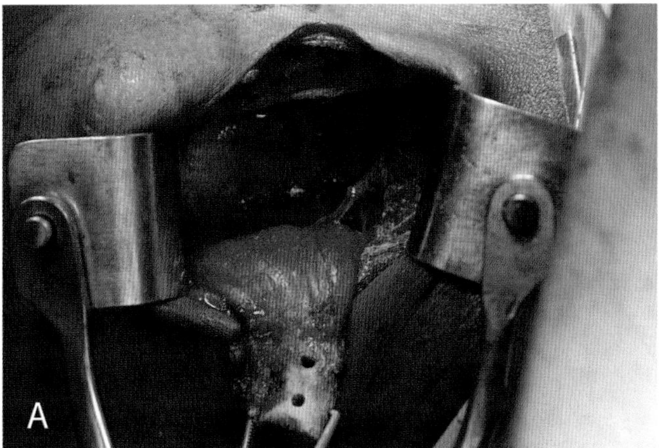

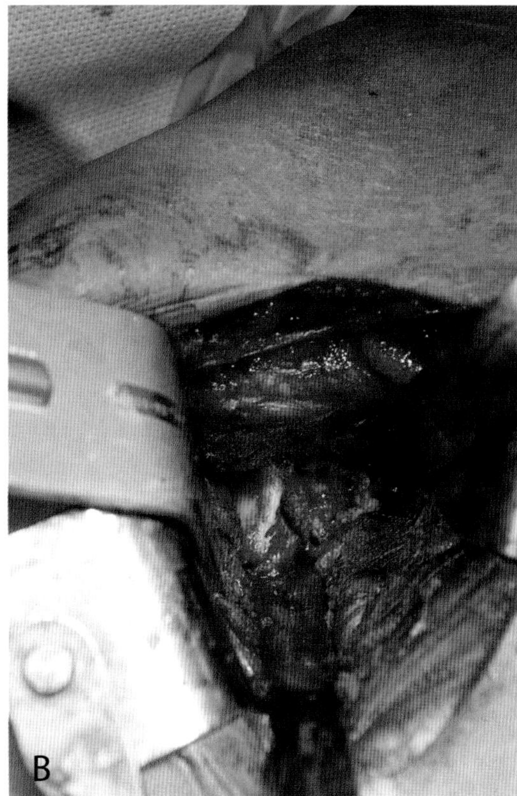

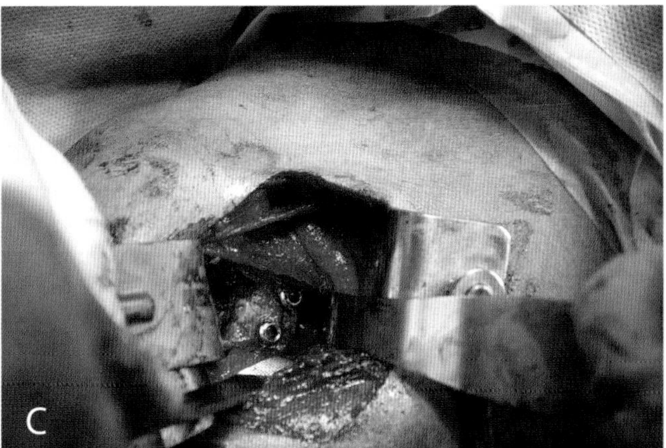

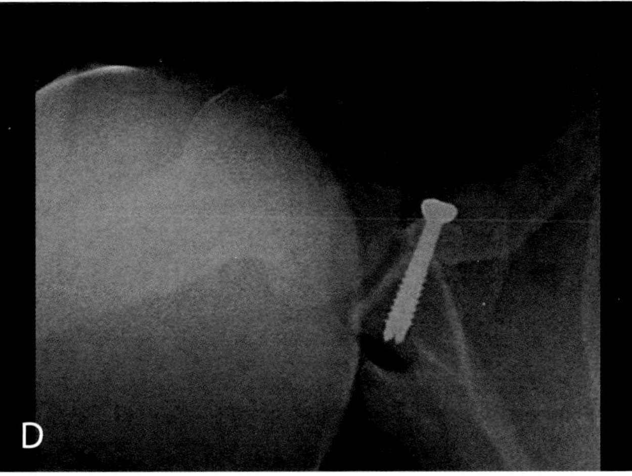

Figure 6.6 **A**, Clinical photograph of coracoid graft after harvest and preparation with drill holes. **B**, Clinical photograph of glenoid exposure through a subscapularis split. **C**, Clinical photograph of solid screw fixation of the coracoid on the anterior glenoid. **D**, Postoperative axillary lateral plain radiograph demonstrating the transferred coracoid and the fixation screws.

ligaments, with care taken to avoid violating the glenoid. This should produce a graft of 2.5 cm to 3 cm in length. The coracoid is then gently delivered from the wound, and adhesions and tissue connections laterally and inferiorly are released. Care is taken not to pull the coracoid excessively, as this can cause a traction injury to the musculocutaneous nerve. The musculocutaneous nerve is identified as it enters the strap muscles distal to the coracoid tip. The coracoid is then prepared by flattening the side that will contact the glenoid. We typically position the inferior surface of the coracoid on the anterior inferior glenoid and scapular neck. Others perform a "congruent arc" technique, placing what was the original medial side of the coracoid against the glenoid. Two holes are drilled in the coracoid, and attention is turned to the glenoid.

The arm is placed at the side and in ER. The subscapularis is split in line with its muscle fibers at the interval between the superior two-thirds and the inferior one-third. The plane between the subscapularis and underlying anterior capsule is

© 2018 American Academy of Orthopaedic Surgeons

developed with an elevator. It is useful to pack a sponge in this space to help separate the tissue planes. The anterior capsule is incised vertically at the joint line and a humeral head retractor is placed within the joint. A double-pronged Bankart retractor is placed on the anterior glenoid after the anterior capsule and labrum have been elevated using the Cobb elevator. Then, 2.0-mm Kirschner wires (K-wires) are placed as retractors: one at the coracoid base and bent superiorly and one at the inferior-most aspect of the glenoid. This decreases the number of assistants needed to hold retractors in a somewhat crowded space. The anterior glenoid is examined and a burr is used to prepare the surface to fit with the coracoid graft (Figure 6.5, B).

The coracoid is then placed in position and held flush with the native glenoid articular surface and guidewires for the screws are placed to hold it in position. The holes are sequentially drilled and measured, and the coracoid is secured with two screws (3.5–4.5 mm diameter, 30–35 mm length; Figure 6.5, C and D). If there is any overhang of the coracoid beyond the face of the glenoid, the burr is used to remove any overhang. It is extremely important for the coracoid to be flush with the glenoid, with no lateral overhang and only 1 mm to 2 mm of medialization. The anterior capsule is repaired to the coracoacromial ligament remaining on the coracoid. This is done with the arm in 45° of ER, to not overtighten the anterior tissues. A final examination is performed to ensure stability and assess ROM. The wound is routinely closed.

Complications

The majority of complications resulting from this procedure are related to graft harvest and intraoperative exposure and fixation. The suprascapular nerve can be injured as a result of an improperly placed screw that enters the spinoglenoid notch posteriorly. This typically requires hardware removal. Hematoma formation and infection are reported, but are relatively uncommon. Violent trauma postoperatively can result in graft displacement, fracture, and/or recurrent dislocation. Fibrous union or nonunion is not uncommon and can occur if the graft is not secured sufficiently or if the patient is noncompliant with postoperative restrictions. Joint mobilizations should be avoided postoperatively, as they put pressure on the bone graft and increase the chance for failure. Mild loss of ER is common after this procedure (10°–15°). Overzealous passive stretching can disrupt the anterior capsular repair or the subscapularis repair if it was tenotomized.

Postoperative Rehabilitation

It should be noted that rehabilitation after this procedure may vary depending on the surgeon. Some surgeons, more commonly in Europe, discontinue the sling at 2 weeks and allow full return to sport at 3 months. Others are more conservative, recommending a period of 9 to 12 months prior to contact sports or heavy labor. We believe that once the coracoid bone has solidly healed and strength and motion have returned, these patients can return to full activity, generally by 4 to 5 months after surgery.

Weeks 0 to 6

- A sling is used for 6 weeks.
- PROM in all planes
- Patients should perform sets of 10, 5 times a day of passive:
  - Supine forward flexion
  - Supine ER at the side
  - Cross-body adduction
  - Standing extension and IR behind the back
- ER should not extend beyond what was found intraoperatively. If there is a question, the operative note or the surgeon should be consulted for the safe limitations to motion.
- Isometric scapular stabilization exercises are begun immediately.
- Prone or upright scapular retraction exercises may be employed as well as isometric strengthening of the trapezius, rhomboids, serratus anterior, and deltoid.
- Radiographs are taken periodically to evaluate for bony healing, which typically occurs by 4 to 6 weeks.
- We do not recommend joint mobilizations until there is clear bony healing, as these exercises may displace the coracoid fragment if done too aggressively and too early.
- If the subscapularis tendon is detached and repaired during the surgery, active IR is not performed.

Weeks 6 to 10

- Patients may discontinue the sling and use the arm for light activities.
- AROM is begun once bony healing occurs, with attention paid particularly to forward elevation and ER.
- Wall walks
- Table slides
- Pulley exercises
- Continue PROM stretching regiment of 5 times per day.
- Initiate isometric IR and ER strengthening.
- Rhythmic stabilization and proprioceptive exercises with therapist
- Standing rows and prone scapular retraction exercises
- Ball on wall alphabet exercises

Week 10+

- When AROM has plateaued and is near full, resistive strengthening is begun, typically at 10 weeks. Resistive strengthening should not be instituted if correctable stiffness remains.
- It is not uncommon for patients to lose some ER with this procedure, but this is usually no more than 10° to 15° compared to preoperatively.
- Initiate closed- and open-chain strengthening exercises.
- Home resistance band exercises daily for rotator cuff strengthening
- Full push-ups
- Vibration training
- Patients are typically released to full activity without restriction in around 4 months if motion is near full, strength is full, and there is radiographic evidence of graft healing.

© 2018 American Academy of Orthopaedic Surgeons

Outcome

Outcomes after the Latarjet procedure are generally expected to be good. Reported failure due to recurrent instability rates are generally less than 5%, and often associated with early violent postoperative trauma. Return to play in collision athletes has been reported to be greater than 70%, with almost 90% of the patients feeling that their shoulder is stable enough to return to premorbid collision sports. Patients generally regain near full motion, with the exception of ER, which can be limited by 5° to 10°, on average, when the subscapularis is split. With subscapularis tenotomy and repair, ER loss can be more severe and has been reported to be about 30°.

Glenohumeral arthritis can be a late finding after this procedure, especially if there is overhang of the graft on the glenoid, making correct initial graft placement critically important. It should be noted, however, that rates of glenohumeral arthritis reported after the Latarjet procedure in general are lower than rates of glenohumeral arthritis seen in patients with nonoperatively treated recurrent shoulder instability.

Pearls

- Laterjet reconstruction is usually indicated for treatment of anterior glenohumeral instability associated with glenoid bone loss.
- Coracoid transfer can be performed without subscapularis tenotomy, eliminating the risk of subscapularis failure.
- Neurologic complications involving the axillary and musculocutaneous nerves can occur.

SUMMARY

Open shoulder stabilization involves either soft-tissue repair in isolation (open Bankart repair) or bony reconstruction through coracoid transfer (Latarjet procedure). These procedures rely on adequate tissue healing for stabilization, but also need return of ROM to maximize outcome. Rehabilitation after these procedures requires a thorough knowledge of the procedure performed in order to ensure adequate protection of the repair while maximizing functional outcome.

BIBLIOGRAPHY

Allain J, Goutallier D, Glorion C: Long-term results of the Latarjet procedure for the treatment of anterior instability of the shoulder. *J Bone Joint Surg Am* 1998;80(6):841–852.

Balg F, Boileau P: The instability severity index score. A simple pre-operative score to select patients for arthroscopic or open shoulder stabilisation. *J Bone Joint Surg Br* 2007;89-B(11): 1470–1477.

Bessière C, Trojani C, Carles M, Mehta SS, Boileau P: The open Latarjet procedure is more reliable in terms of shoulder stability than arthroscopic Bankart repair. *Clin Orthop Relat Res* 2014;472(8):2345–2351.

Bottoni CR, Smith EL, Berkowitz MJ, Towle RB, Moore JH: Arthroscopic versus open shoulder stabilization for recurrent anterior instability: a prospective randomized clinical trial. *Am J Sports Med* 2006;34(11):1730–1737.

Burkhart SS, de Beer JF: Traumatic glenohumeral bone defects and their relationship to failure of arthroscopic Bankart repairs: significance of the inverted-pear glenoid and the humeral engaging Hill-Sachs lesion. *Arthroscopy* 2000;16(7):677–694.

Delaney RA, Freehill MT, Janfaza DR, Vlassakov KV, Higgins LD, Warner JJ: 2014 Neer Award Paper: neuromonitoring the Latarjet procedure. *J Shoulder Elbow Surg* 2014;23(10): 1473–1480.

Gaunt BW, Shaffer MA, Sauers EL, Michener LA, McCluskey GM III, Thigpen CA: The American Society of Shoulder and Elbow Therapists' consensus rehabilitation guideline for arthroscopic anterior capsulolabral repair of the shoulder. *J Orthop Sports Phys Ther* 2010;40(3):155–168.

Griesser MJ, Harris JD, McCoy BW, Hussain WM, Jones MH, Bishop JY, Miniaci A: Complications and re-operations after Bristow-Latarjet shoulder stabilization: a systematic review. *J Shoulder Elbow Surg* 2013;22(2):286–292.

Kim SH, Ha KI, Jung MW, Lim MS, Kim YM, Park JH: Accelerated rehabilitation after arthroscopic Bankart repair for selected cases: a prospective randomized clinical study. *Arthroscopy* 2003;19(7):722–731.

Mizuno N, Denard PJ, Raiss P, Melis B, Walch G: Long-term results of the Latarjet procedure for anterior instability of the shoulder. *J Shoulder Elbow Surg* 2014;23(11):1691–1699.

Mohtadi NG, Chan DS, Hollinshead RM, et al: A randomized clinical trial comparing open and arthroscopic stabilization for recurrent traumatic anterior shoulder instability. *J Bone Joint Surg Am* 2014;96(5):353–360.

Moroder P, Odorizzi M, Pizzinini S, Demetz E, Resch H, Moroder P: Open Bankart repair for the treatment of anterior shoulder instability without substantial osseous glenoid defects: results after a minimum follow-up of twenty years. *J Bone Joint Surg Am* 2015;97(17):1398–1405.

Owens BD: Been around the block before. *Am J Sports Med* 2014;42(11):2557–2559.

Owens BD, Harrast JJ, Hurwitz SR, Thompson TL, Wolf JM: Surgical trends in Bankart repair: an analysis of data from the American Board of Orthopaedic Surgery certification examination. *Am J Sports Med* 2011;39(9):1865–1869.

Rowe CR, Patel D, Southmayd WW: The Bankart procedure: a long-term end-result study. *J Bone Joint Surg Am* 1978; 60(1):1–16.

Shah AA, Butler RB, Romanowski J, Goel D, Karadagli D, Wanner JJ: Short-term complications of the Latarjet procedure. *J Bone Joint Surg Am* 2012;94(6):495–501.

Shaha JS, Cook JB, Song DJ, Rowles DJ, Bottoni CR, Shaha SH, Tokish JM: Redefining "critical" bone loss in shoulder instability: functional outcomes worsen with "subcritical" bone loss. *Am J Sports Med* 2015;43(7):1719–1725.

Tjong VK, Devitt BM, Murnaghan ML, Ogilvie-Harris DJ, Theodoropoulos JS: A qualitative investigation of return to sport after arthroscopic Bankart repair: beyond stability. *Am J Sports Med* 2015;43(8):2005–2011.

© 2018 American Academy of Orthopaedic Surgeons

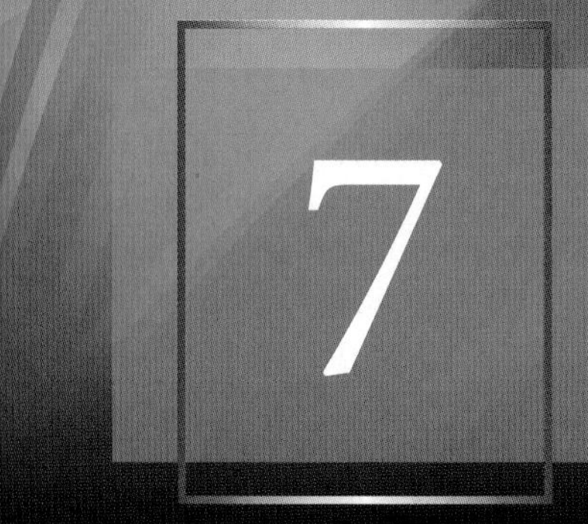

7 SLAP Repairs

W. Ben Kibler, MD

INTRODUCTION

Rehabilitation following superior labral anterior posterior (SLAP) repair is a key component to returning the patient to functional status. Since SLAP injuries are most frequently associated with multiple functional deficits in many areas of the kinetic chain, a comprehensive approach to evaluation and functional rehabilitation is needed. Although much of the focus of this chapter is directed to the treatment of the overhead throwing athlete, many of the principles of surgical repair and postoperative rehabilitation can be applied to other patients who undergo SLAP repair.

RELEVANT ANATOMY AND PATIENT EVALUATION

The clinically significant SLAP injury is one in which the anatomic alteration in the labrum results in elements of the clinical history of the dysfunction that can be attributed to the loss of labral roles; the injury can be highlighted by specific physical examination tests that are clinically useful for detection of the injured labrum. It is a positive diagnosis, not a catch-all term in the presence of shoulder pain of unknown etiology in which the diagnosis is uncertain.

The history findings suggestive of loss of labral roles include pain upon external rotation/cocking, weakness in clinical or functional arm strength, symptoms of internal derangement (clicking, popping, catching, sliding), or decreased capsular tension, and a feeling of a "dead arm." These are not exclusively seen in a labral injury, but point toward the loss of labral roles.

Kinetic chain deficits are discovered on examination in a majority of patients with SLAP injuries. Deficits in hip abductor or extensor strength, hip rotation flexibility, or core strength weakness have been identified in 50% of SLAP injuries, while scapular dyskinesis is seen in around 90% of patients with labral injuries. These alterations can be identified by specific screening examinations.

Labral examination tests can provide intra-articular clues to the presence of a labral injury. Of the labral examination tests, the modified dynamic labral shear (M-DLS) test has been shown to be of high clinical utility in the evaluation of labral injuries when the test is performed in the manner described. Other labral examination tests advocated include O'Brien's active compression test; the relocation test, with pain as the indicator; and an anterior levering maneuver to place a posterior load and shear.

The labral injury can be confirmed by MRI, MRI arthrography, or CT arthrogram, but should not be defined by imaging. Specific criteria have been developed to distinguish a labral alteration, but MRI is best viewed as a static estimation of labral status with inconsistent relation to the dynamic roles. A percentage of patients will demonstrate "labral tears" without symptoms relating to loss of the labral roles. There is some evidence that rehabilitation can decrease symptoms and provide functional control in 40% to 50% of patients with SLAP injuries.

SURGICAL PROCEDURES

Indications and Contraindications

There is continuing debate regarding which characteristics of the lesion and the patient should be considered as helpful criteria for surgical indications. Most papers suggest that SLAP tears classified as type I should not be repaired, and that types 2, 3, and 4 should be surgically addressed. However, there is a wide variability in the accuracy, reliability, and consistency of making the determination of the specific lesion type. Also, many papers recommend an upper age limitation, usually 40 years, for surgical repair, based on rates of stiffness and less successful outcomes, although no anatomic evidence supports this recommendation. Finally, most papers recommend that anticipated physical demands be considered since the importance of an intact labral complex to maximize joint concavity-compression is greater in patients with higher-demand activities such as overhead athletes or overhead workers. All of these factors should be considered in the

Dr. Kibler or an immediate family member serves as an unpaid consultant to Alignmed; has stock or stock options held in Alignmed; and serves as a board member, owner, officer, or committee member of the Arthroscopy Association of North America and the British Journal of Sports Medicine.

© 2018 American Academy of Orthopaedic Surgeons

evaluation of the patient with a suspected clinically significant labral injury, but they should be evaluated with the rest of the clinical presentation.

Given these parameters, the indications for surgical repair of SLAP injuries include the proper history, a positive clinical examination for findings associated with a labral injury, and failure to respond to a rehabilitation program that addresses the deficits found on the examination. The findings of arthroscopic examination have a critically important role in the management of superior labral tears. The arthroscopic findings most frequently associated with a clinically significant labral injury include (1) a type II or higher lesion; (2) a peel-back phenomenon indicating labral detachment and increased compliance; (3) glenoid articular cartilage damage or chondromalacia; (4) loss of capsular tension indicated by a drive-through sign or loss of tension in the posterior band of the inferior glenohumeral ligament (PIGHL); (5) increased posterior labral thickness, indicating increased translation and shear with compression on the labrum; and/or (6) excessive posterior inferior capsular thickness and scar indicating end-stage capsular damage that helps create glenohumeral internal rotation deficit.

Contraindications for a SLAP repair include (1) lack of demonstrated clinical significance, by history and physical exam, in a patient with an MRI finding of labral injury; (2) repair at the same time as a capsular release for adhesive capsulitis; and (3) repair in the face of advanced arthrosis. In these cases, the symptoms and dysfunction are not due to the loss of labral roles and may lead to more dysfunction. Relative contraindications to SLAP repair are those that are associated with rotator cuff injury. SLAP injuries can be frequently seen in patients undergoing rotator cuff repair—the majority of these do not need to be treated, as they are usually degenerative. However, if the patients exhibit a positive M-DLS on preoperative examination, the SLAP injury probably does play a role in the clinical picture, and needs to be treated in conjunction with the rotator cuff injury.

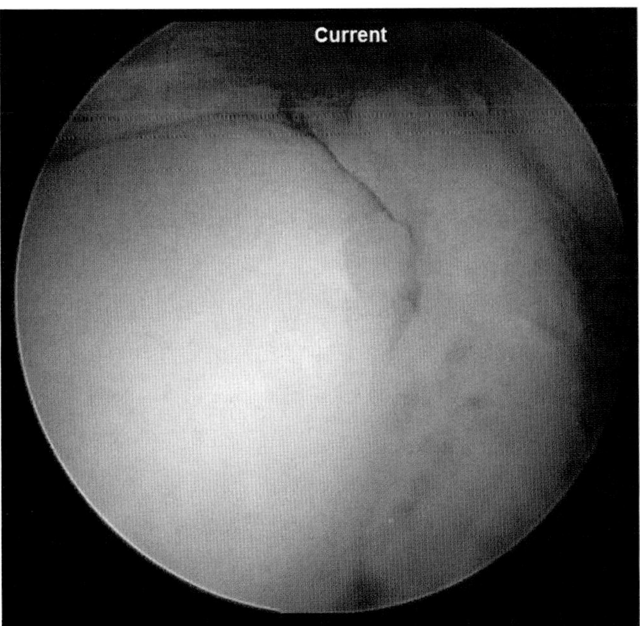

Figure 7.1 Arthroscopic view of left shoulder posterior superior labral injury.

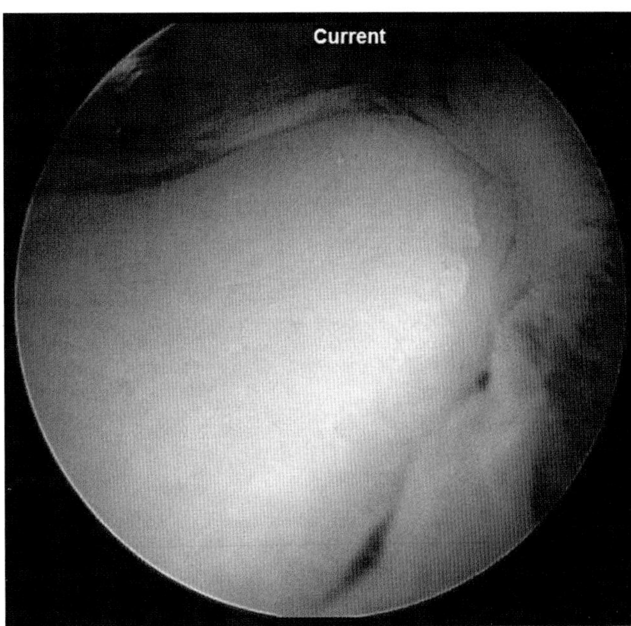

Figure 7.2 Arthroscopic view of example of peel-back lesion with external rotation.

Procedure

The arthroscopic evaluation of the suspected labral injury must be specific in order to understand and treat the labral injury properly. Arthroscopic treatment guidelines for labral injury include (1) evaluation of the labral injury and mobility (Figure 7.1), peel-back (Figure 7.2), glenoid surface, and capsular tension (Figure 7.3) by direct visualization;

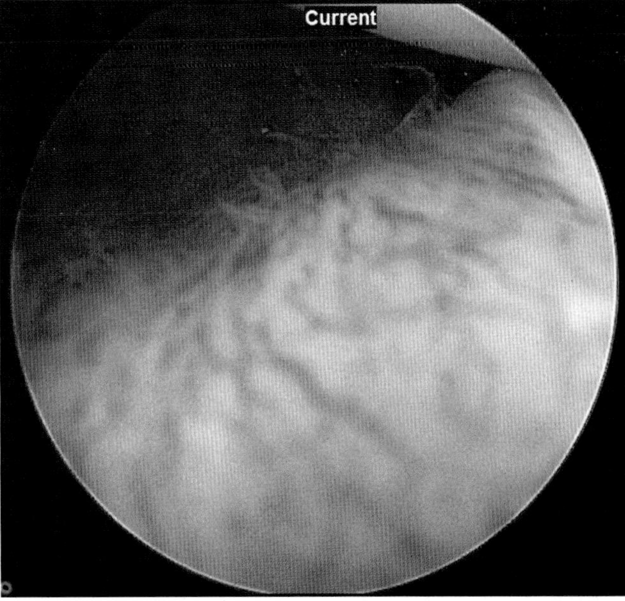

Figure 7.3 Arthroscopic visualization of lack of PIGHL tension.

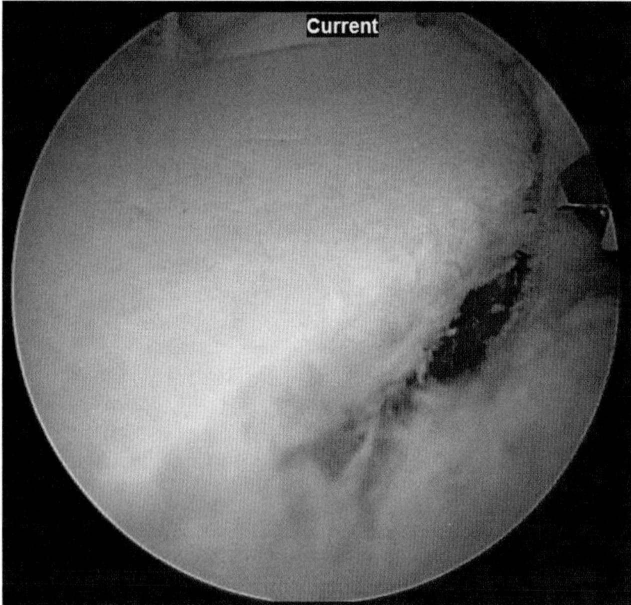

Figure 7.4 Arthroscopic view of bone preparation prior to labral repair.

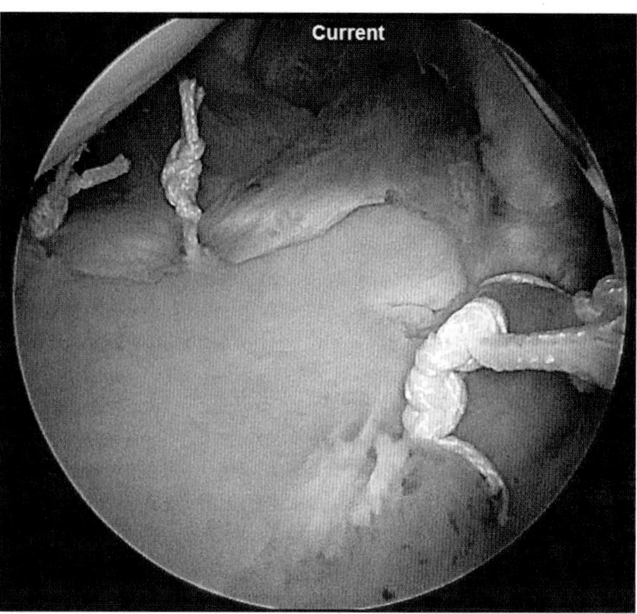

Figure 7.6 Arthroscopic view of completed superior labral repair. Note that anterior repair was also performed.

(2) preparation of the glenoid to maximize bone to labrum healing (Figure 7.4); (3) multiple anchor placement to secure at least 2-point fixation of the labrum on the posterior superior glenoid (12:30 and 1:30 on the left shoulder, a double-loaded single anchor is still only one point fixation; Figure 7.5); (4) placement of enough posterior superior anchors to eliminate the peel-back (Figure 7.6); (5) evaluation of biceps mobility after anchor and suture placement to make sure that there is adequate motion of the biceps in shoulder external rotation; (6) rare placement of anchors and sutures in the anterior superior glenoid (12:00–10:30 on the left shoulder) to reduce the chance of biceps tethering; (7) evaluating the effect of the labral repair on capsular tension by evaluation in the PIGHL tautness and elimination of the drive-through (Figure 7.7); (8) assessing total glenohumeral rotation to ensure that no external rotation has been lost; and (9) treatment of the associated pathology in the glenohumeral joint.

POSTOPERATIVE REHABILITATION

The goals of postoperative therapy are to facilitate healing of the SLAP repair, while restoring shoulder and upper

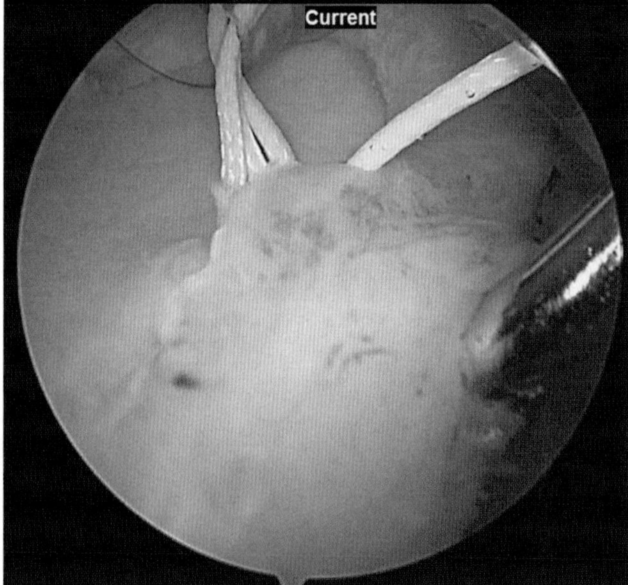

Figure 7.5 Labral mobilization and suture passage

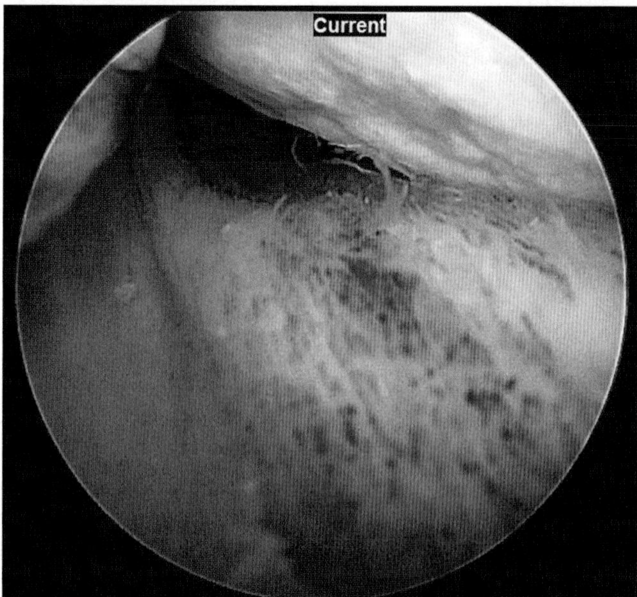

Figure 7.7 Establishment of tension in the PIGHL as a result of the labral repair

© 2018 American Academy of Orthopaedic Surgeons

Table 7.1	FUNCTIONAL REHABILITATION PARAMETERS

1. Kinetic Chain
   a. Leg drive and lower extremity strength
   b. Hip mobility
   c. Proximal core stability
   d. Dynamic core strength/power
   e. Scapular stabilization
2. Shoulder Mobility
   a. Restoring internal and external rotation deficits to achieve safe total ROM
   b. Addressing joint restrictions in the spine and shoulder complex
   c. Addressing muscular flexibility imbalances in the spine and scapula
3. Arm Strength and Endurance
   a. Restoring scapular motor control for functional and pain-free motion
   b. Facilitating inhibited or weak scapular musculature
   c. Integrating scapular exercises with functional tasks
   d. Facilitating endurance and eccentric control by advanced shoulder and scapular exercises
   e. Strengthening forearm, wrist, and hand

extremity function through optimizing glenohumeral rotation, scapular stability and motion, local muscle strength and balance, and kinetic chain strength and flexibility (Table 7.1). Functional restoration may be initiated even while the repair is protected, starting with kinetic chain activation, progressing to scapular control, and then involving the glenohumeral rotation and strength.

The exercise program is progressive and sequential, and is divided into 3 phases based on the level of disability and tissue irritability. Movement through the phases is variable and based on achieving functional capabilities rather than adhering to specific time frames. Phase 1, the acute phase, should minimize loads on the injured tissues, and should focus on scapular and glenohumeral muscular activation, particularly in correcting timing of muscular activation to ensure that they are working synchronously. Phase 2, the recovery phase, should focus on strengthening and restoring core, kinetic chain, and progressive isotonic strengthening. Phase 3, the functional phase, should focus on sport-specific actions, and include endurance and ballistic exercises. Strengthening exercises are oriented toward endurance, emphasizing higher repetitions and lower resistance. An athlete should demonstrate the ability to perform 3 to 4 sets of 15 to 20 repetitions with correct form prior to progressing to a greater resistance.

Kinetic Chain

During the initial evaluation of the athlete's kinetic chain, deficits in hip mobility or single leg stability are likely to be identified. Strengthening and stability of the core and lower extremity musculature is critical due to their contributions to the throwing motion. During pitching, the stance or back leg balances the body weight during the wind up and drives the body forward during the push off, but the lead or front leg requires sufficient leg and hip strength to control the landing force of body weight. One exercise does not target all the abdominal muscles; therefore, a program that addresses anterior, lateral, and posterior sides of the torso should be undertaken. Mat exercises emphasizing endurance are good starting points, with consideration given to positions that limit stress to the shoulder. The athlete should be engaged in lower extremity and core exercises that simulate the demands of throwing. The use of unstable surfaces, such as stability balls or foam mats, has demonstrated increased core activation and improvement in core strength, but has not necessarily demonstrated carryover into functional tasks. Lunges can be performed in multiple planes (Figure 7.8). They should start and end in the "ideal position" of hip extension and trunk extension. All of these core and hip exercises can be implemented early, even while the shoulder repair is protected.

Restoration of scapular stability is covered in the chapter on scapular dyskinesis (Chapter 10). The patient with a SLAP injury and repair will frequently exhibit scapular dyskinesis from muscle activation inhibition and/or inflexibilities. Many types of exercises for scapular rehabilitation can also be implemented while the repair is protected, especially scapular pinches and maneuvers that facilitate scapular retraction, such as the lawnmower exercise (Figure 7.9).

Shoulder Mobility

Exercises to restore shoulder mobility can be instituted before surgery to maximize preoperative motion and make postoperative motion easier to obtain. The goal of the intervention program is restoration of range of motion (ROM) to acceptable values. Deficits in glenohumeral internal rotation (GIR) and total range of motion (TROM) should be addressed to restore safe ROM values. However, it is important to remember that ROM values are affected by previous throwing activities for at least 24 hours. GIR of the throwing shoulder should be within 18° (range 13°–20°) of the nondominant shoulder, TROM in the throwing shoulder should be within 5° of the nondominant shoulder, and TROM should not exceed 186° to avoid an increased risk of injury. The cross-body stretch and sleeper stretch target the posterior shoulder musculature and capsule to effectively improve GIR and glenohumeral abduction (Figures 7.10 and 7.11). Additional beneficial treatment techniques include joint mobilizations, muscle energy techniques, and soft-tissue mobilization. Loss of glenohumeral adduction is becoming more frequently identified as a possible limiting factor in shoulder function. A multimodal treatment approach that included posterior shoulder stretching and joint mobilization demonstrated that change in adduction is as important as change in GIR in reduction of symptoms.

© 2018 American Academy of Orthopaedic Surgeons

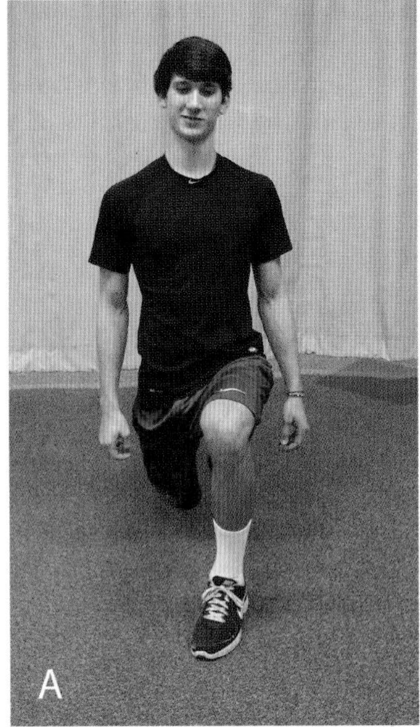

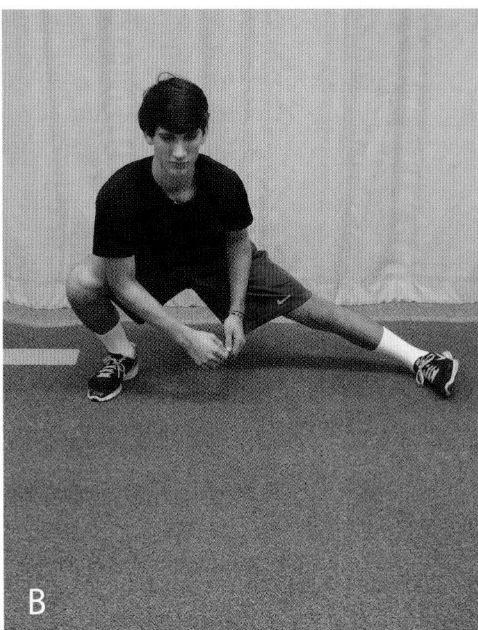

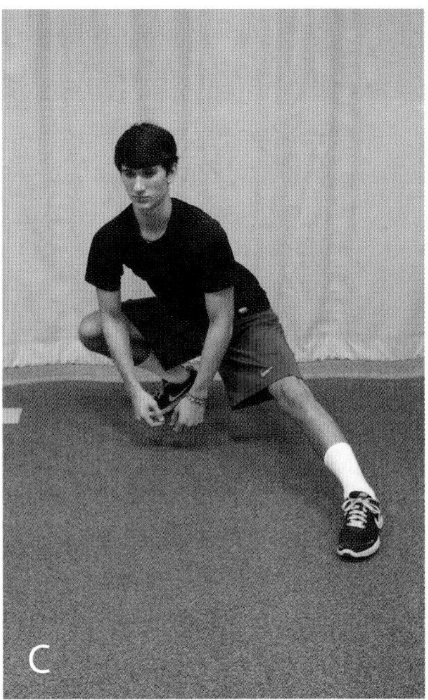

Figure 7.8 Multidirectional lunges can be performed for comprehensive lower extremity strengthening and stability, which include the following: **A,** forward, **B,** lateral, and **C,** diagonal directions.

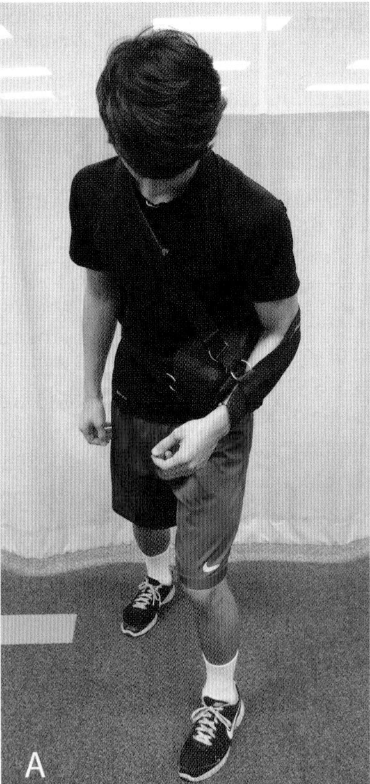

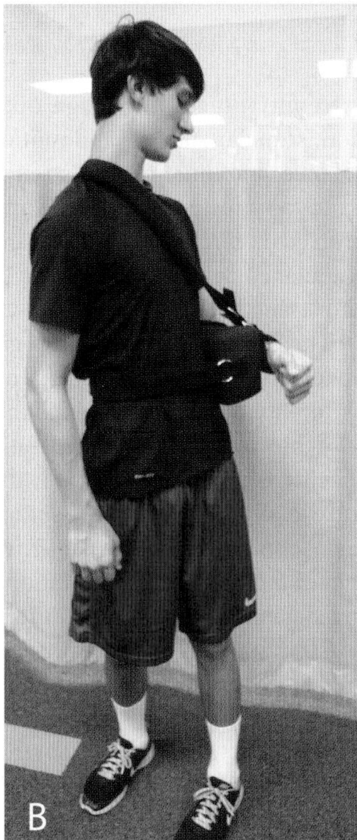

Figure 7.9 The lawnmower exercise can be modified for post-operative use by allowing the patient to perform the maneuver in the post-operative immobilizer.

© 2018 American Academy of Orthopaedic Surgeons

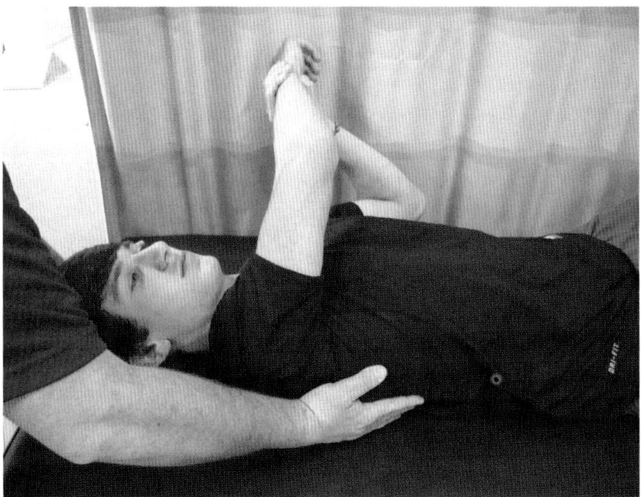

Figure 7.10 The cross-body stretch is more effective when stabilization is applied to the scapula.

Muscular adaptations that can alter scapular kinematics during elevation can occur due to tight anterior structures such as the pectoralis minor. Pectoralis minor tightness has been identified in the dominant side of tennis players, and is associated with increased scapular anterior tilt and scapular internal rotation. Pectoralis minor tightness can be effectively treated with corner stretching exercises (Figure 7.12).

The latissimus dorsi is also commonly found to be inflexible. Tightness in this large muscle will affect arm forward flexion and glenohumeral rotation, especially in abduction over 90°. Latissimus stretches and deep tissue mobilization can be employed to restore flexibility.

Arm Strength, Power, and Endurance

Prior to their injury, throwing athletes often demonstrate strength deficits and imbalances that will still be present after treatment. Deficits in shoulder strength are predictive of future injury, particularly in external rotation and supraspinatus activation. Athletes presenting with shoulder symptoms are typically found to have strength deficits of the rotator cuff and scapular musculature, which may present with various

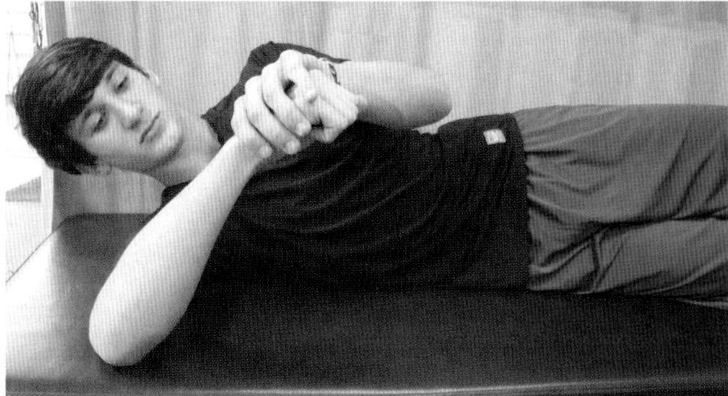

Figure 7.11 The sleeper stretch is a patient-performed stretch that helps combat posterior shoulder tightness.

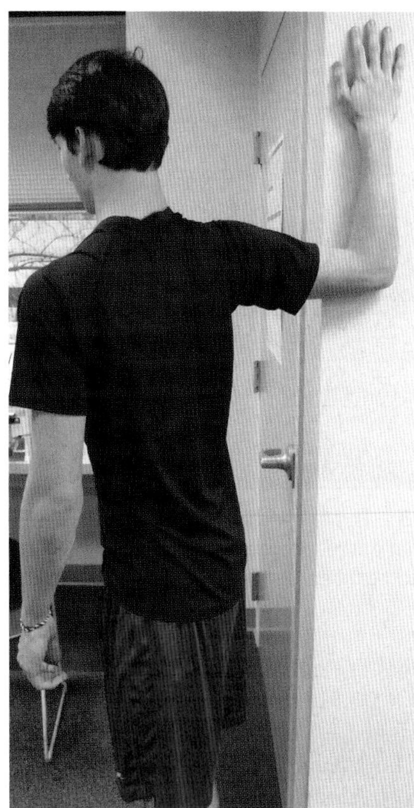

Figure 7.12 The patient is instructed to stand with the involved arm in a 90/90 position on a wall or other firm surface. The patient then rotates the body in the opposite direction to stretch the anterior musculature.

movement patterns. Treatment of these deficits has many common themes and treatment protocols. Initial management should focus on scapular musculature control, which facilitates stability in order to prepare the shoulder musculature for more dynamic and stressful exercises. Repeated emphasis on proper position and movement instructions are important, as many of the movement strategies learned are only temporary. Establishment of proximal stability, such as scapular orientation exercises, should precede longer lever arm activities (i.e., prone horizontal abduction exercises) in order to establish proximal functional control. Overactivation of the upper trapezius during elevation, indicating a muscular imbalance around the scapular force couple, has been found in injured shoulders. Scapular setting exercises have been shown to primarily activate trapezius musculature; they can facilitate muscular balance between the scapular force couple of the serratus anterior, and upper and lower trapezius. The focus of the scapular exercise program should be on the rhomboids, lower trapezius, and middle trapezius musculature. Facilitation of serratus anterior and lower trapezius musculature can be targeted with isometric adduction (Figure 7.13) and extension exercises (Figure 7.14) with continued focus on proper scapular orientation of posterior tilting and retraction.

Specific emphasis on rotator cuff strengthening should be done after initial scapular control as been reestablished.

© 2018 American Academy of Orthopaedic Surgeons

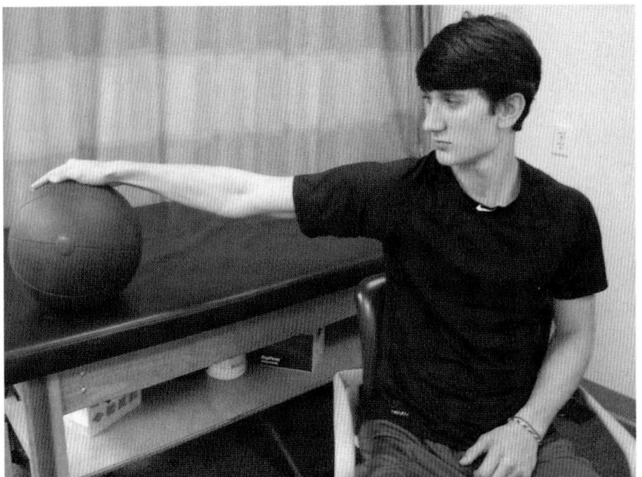

Figure 7.13 The active inferior glide exercise is an isometric maneuver that utilizes co-contraction of both shoulder and scapular muscles to help depress the humeral head and scapula.

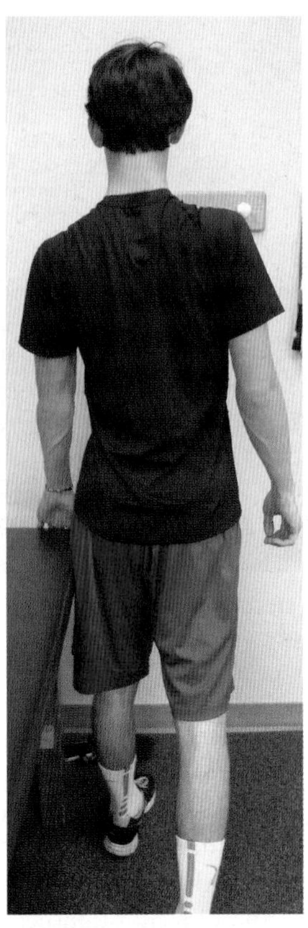

Figure 7.14 The low row exercise is performed with the patient standing and the hand of the involved arm against the side of a firm surface. The patient actively extends the hips and trunk to facilitate scapular retraction, holding the final position for approximately 5 to 10 seconds.

Multiple types of exercises may be employed. Exercises that conform to a graded increase in muscle activation and load have been shown to be effective. Progression from closed to open chain, horizontal to vertical to diagonal, and slow speed to fast speed creates graded activation. More difficult rotator cuff–strengthening exercises should be performed in functional positions and motions. Examples include humeral rotation tubing exercises at 90° abduction (Figure 7.15), punches (Figure 7.16), and wall washes (Figure 7.17).

Plyometric and eccentric exercises are important in developing power. They are high-load exercises, using high

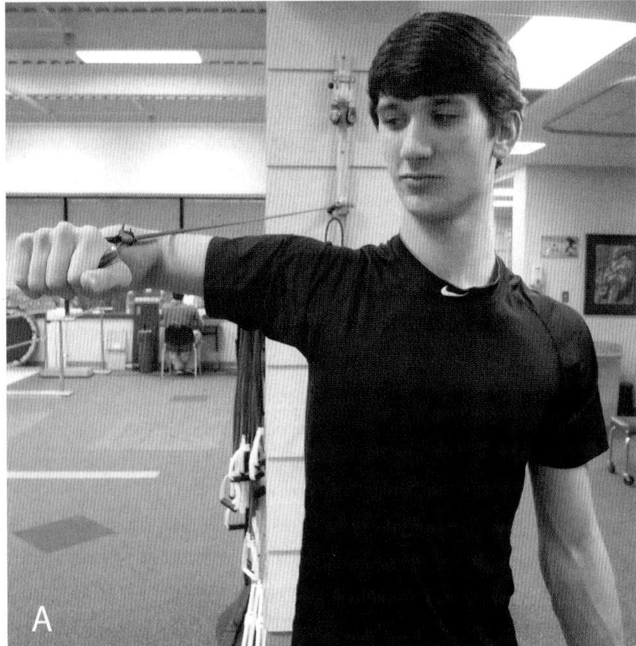

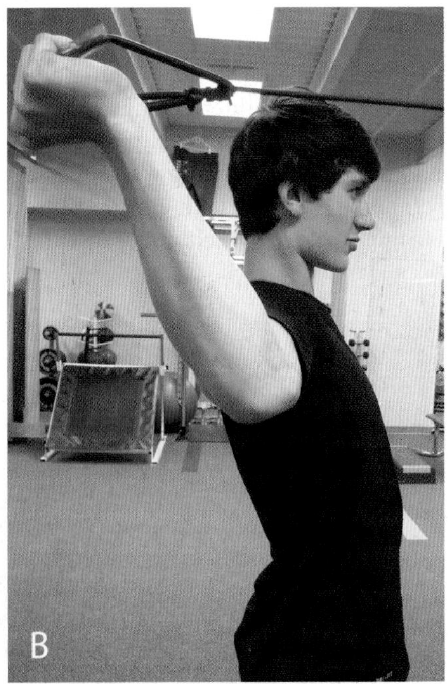

Figure 7.15 Humeral rotation exercises—**A**, internal and **B**, external rotation—performed at 90° of abduction, aid in creating strength and endurance in the rotator cuff musculature.

 © 2018 American Academy of Orthopaedic Surgeons

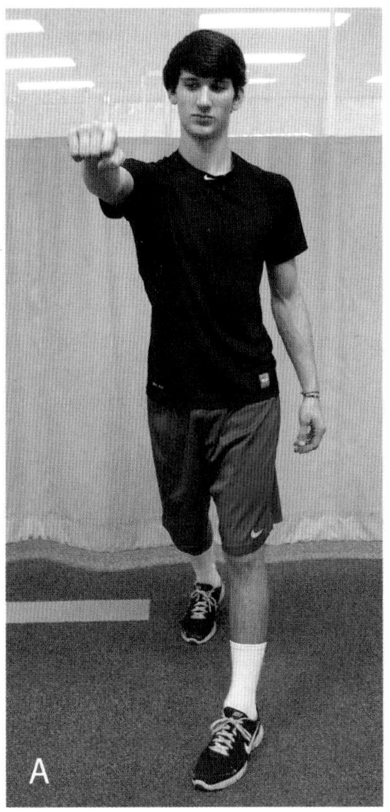

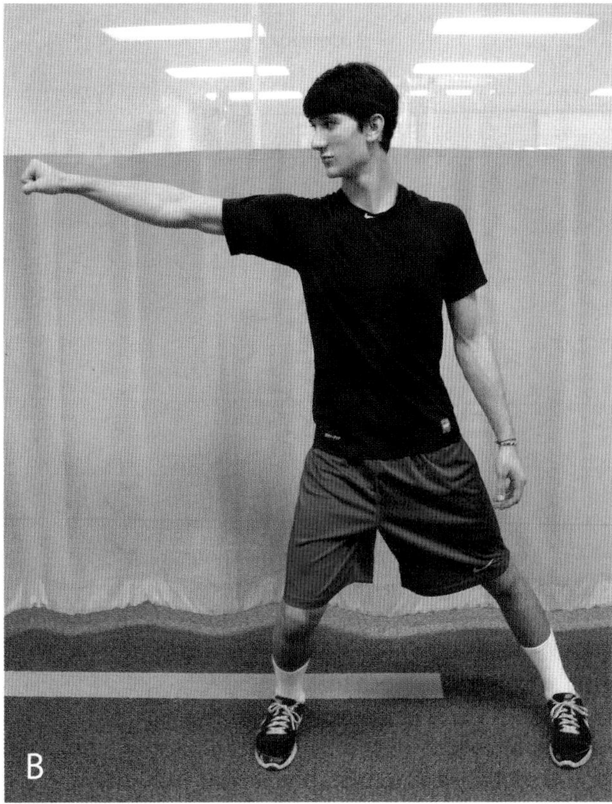

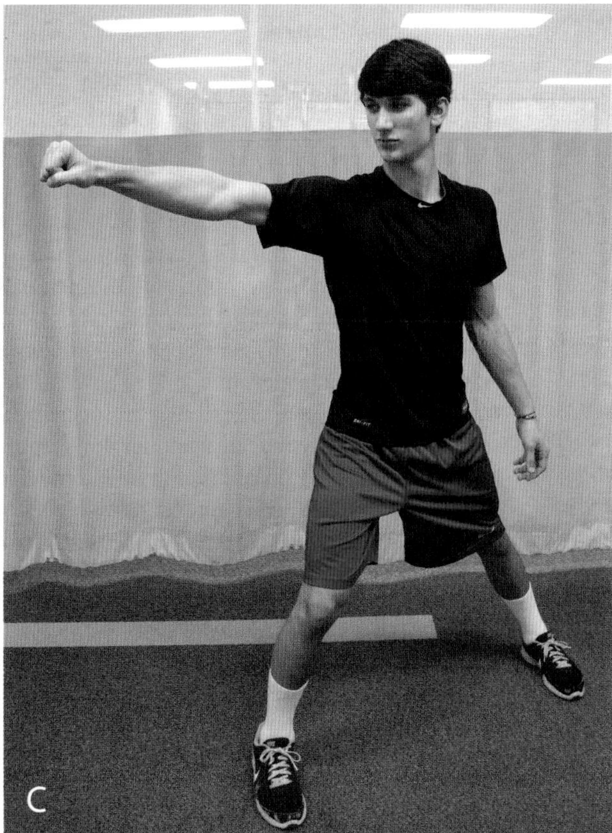

Figure 7.16 Open-chain, multidirectional punches can be performed for increasing strength and stability of the arm, which include the forward (**A**), lateral (**B**), and diagonal (**C**) directions.

© 2018 American Academy of Orthopaedic Surgeons

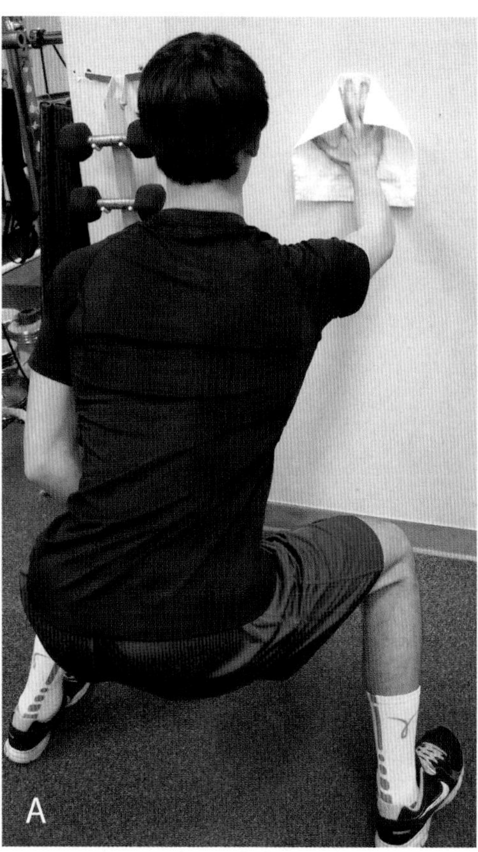

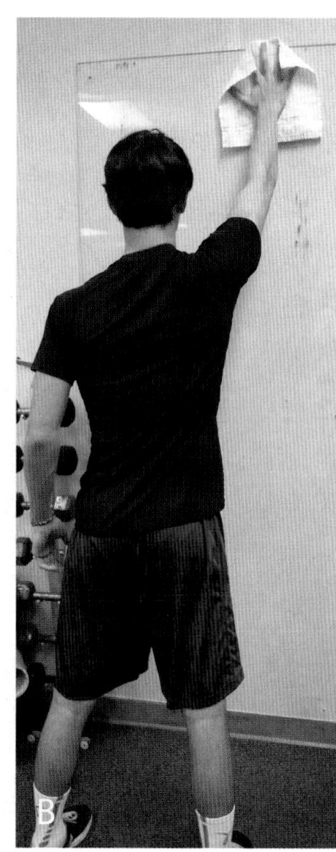

Figure 7.17 Wall washing is an integrated exercise which allows the larger muscles of the lower extremity and core to drive the arm in a vertical direction (**A, B**).

repetition and long lever arms, and should be employed in the functional phase of rehabilitation. Effective exercises include device-assisted maneuvers such as rebounding drills with weighted balls and rhythmic devices.

Rehabilitation after SLAP repair should shade into prehabilitation for returning to throwing or working. A maintenance core stability program should be established. Scapular stabilization exercises should be performed on a regular basis. Daily stretching exercises should be completed either statically or dynamically. Static stretches are to be held for 30 seconds and repeated 4 times. Dynamic stretches are to be performed for 12 repetitions with a minimal hold time of no longer than 2 seconds. All stretching should be performed until a strong pull is experienced, but without pain or neurologic symptoms. The actual throwing capability can be helped by the advanced throwers ten program. This program challenges the endurance of the athlete with the application of sustained holds and alternating arm motions, and can be incorporated in the functional rehabilitation phase.

Author's Preferred Protocol

Therapeutic exercise for superior labral repairs begins 5 to 7 days after surgery. Exercises can be fairly aggressive below and up to 90° of glenohumeral elevation. If after approximately 3 weeks, there are no ROM limitations and rehabilitation can progress as tolerated. Pain should guide all active range of motion (AROM).

Early Phase: Acute (Usually 1–3 Weeks)

- Sling for the first 10 to 14 days with progression out of sling by 2 to 3 weeks.
- Begin by establishing quality scapular motion, using complementary trunk motion, hip activation, and scapular kinematic patterns, without concern for glenohumeral motion.
- Promote scapular retraction with thoracic extension.
- Use the hips to position the spine.
- De-emphasize the upper trapezius—emphasize medial and inferior scapular motion.
- Address soft-tissue inflexibilities, especially in the pectoralis minor, upper trapezius, and levator scapulae.
- During this early phase, glenohumeral movement includes:
  - Closed-chain pendulum exercises on ball or table
  - AROM exercises up to 90° of elevation, provided there is good scapular motion with this elevation
  - Axially loaded AROM exercises, which facilitate glenohumeral congruency and effectively decrease the intrinsic weight of the upper limb
  - Short lever closed kinetic chain exercises such as weight shifts, low row, and inferior glide maneuvers to promote force couple contractions
  - ROM goals include achievement of 90° abduction and flexion
  - Avoid external rotation beyond neutral with posterior superior labral repairs.
- In conjunction with biceps tenodesis, avoid biceps loading.

© 2018 American Academy of Orthopaedic Surgeons

Intermediate Phase: Recovery (Usually Week 4–8)

- Move toward full AROM with quality scapulo-thoraco-humeral rhythm.
- "Open the upper extremity chain," continuing to use functional movement patterns and complementary motion in the proximal segments.
- Address all planes of motion.
- Load the rotator cuff using punches, with complementary hip and trunk movement, in various planes and angles. (Begin in downward angles and progress to horizontal for maximal load. Overhead punches and presses require normal scapular kinetics.)
- Address internal rotation deficit—muscular and capsular.
- Avoid external rotation/horizontal abduction posterior to the plane of the body.
- May begin introducing plyometrics at weeks 6 to 8 provided there is full AROM, good scapular control, and good rotator cuff strength.
- ROM goals include 120° to 140° of abduction and forward flexion as well as 40° of external rotation.

Later Phase: Functional (Beyond Week 8)

- Begin to integrate larger kinetic chain movements to re-educate the patient on using the lower extremity to drive the upper extremity.
  - Employ synchronous single-leg and transverse-plane exercises, which aid in improving proprioception as well as muscle education.
- Focus on muscle endurance and proprioception with high-repetition, low-load exercises.
  - High-repetition exercises designed to increase lower extremity muscle endurance should be employed with focus on the major muscle groups (gastrocnemius/soleus, quadriceps, hamstrings, and hip abductor muscles).
- Upper extremity power and endurance should be addressed only after the lower extremity segments are optimized.
  - High-repetition, long-lever exercises performed in standing and prone positions are recommended after week 12.

OUTCOMES

A number of outcomes studies have suggested that return to athletic participation is possible following injury and/or surgery. However, full return to preinjury level of activity has been shown to be elusive for some individuals. The orthopaedic literature has reported an inconsistent rate of return to preinjured level of activity (8%–94%) in overhead athletes with isolated SLAP repairs, and those who are not baseball pitchers have higher rates of return. Those with concomitant surgery for other shoulder lesions have lower rates of return. Non-overhead athletes have at least two times greater chances to return to full levels of activity.

Multiple factors probably affect the return to activity rate. They include lack of a consistent diagnosis, differences in specific surgical technique, type and number of suture anchors and sutures, and variable rehabilitation programs. Improvement in knowledge and skills in each of these areas would be expected to result in more consistency and increase in the rate of return to activity.

PEARLS

Surgical Pearls

- Develop diagnostic techniques to reliably identify the clinically significant SLAP injury.
- Correlate arthroscopic findings with the clinical presentation.
- Use enough anchors to adequately repair the entire extent of the labral injury.
- Avoid anchors and sutures that limit normal biceps excursion.
- Avoid high-strength, stiff, suture material.
- Develop specific criteria to determine adequacy of the repair: elimination of the peel-back, no loss of biceps motion, PIGHL tension, addressing all other intra-articular pathology.

Rehabilitation Pearls

- Develop a function-based rehabilitation protocol.
  - Kinetic chain restoration
  - Scapular control
  - Glenohumeral ROM
  - Rotator cuff co-contraction and eccentric strength

CONCLUSIONS

Rehabilitation of postoperative SLAP repairs focuses on restoring deficits identified before surgery that contributed to the clinical injury, overall kinetic chain functionality, local joint rotation, effective rotator cuff strength, and prehabilitation to minimize future injury risk.

BIBLIOGRAPHY

Borstad JD, Ludewig PM: Comparison of three stretches for the pectoralis minor muscle. *J Shoulder Elbow Surg* 2006; 15(3):324–330.

Byram IR, et al.: Preseason shoulder strength measurements in professional baseball pitchers: Identifying players at risk for injury. *Am J Sports Med* 2010;38(7):1375–1382.

Cools AM, et al.: Evaluation of isokinetic force production and associated muscle activity in the scapular rotators during a protraction-retraction movement in overhead athletes with impingement symptoms. *Br J Sports Med* 2004;38:64–68.

Edwards SL, et al.: Nonoperative treatment of superior labrum anterior posterior tears: Improvements in pain, function, and quality of life. *Am J Sports Med* 2010;38(7):1456–1461.

© 2018 American Academy of Orthopaedic Surgeons

Ellenbecker TS, Cools A: Rehabilitation of shoulder impingement syndrome and rotator cuff injuries: An evidence-based review. *Br J Sports Med* 2010;44:319–327.

Escamilla R, et al.: Core muscle activation during swiss ball and traditional abdominal exercises. *J Orthop Sports Phys Ther* 2010;40(5):265–276.

Imai A, et al.: Trunk muscle activity during lumbar stabilization exercises on both a stable and unstable surface. *J Orthop Sports Phys Ther* 2010;40(6):369–375.

Kibler WB, McMullen J, Uhl TL: Shoulder rehabilitation strategies, guidelines, and practice. *Oper Tech Sports Med* 2000;8(4): 258–267.

Kibler WB, et al.: Electromyographic analysis of specific exercises for scapular control in early phases of shoulder rehabilitation. *Am J Sports Med* 2008;36(9):1789–1798.

Kibler WB, et al.: The disabled throwing shoulder—Spectrum of pathology: 10 year update. *Arthroscopy* 2013;29(1):141–161.

Lin JJ, et al.: Adaptive patterns of movement during arm elevation test in patients with shoulder impingement syndrome. *J Orthop Res* 2010;29(5):653–657.

Ludewig PM, Reynolds JF: The association of scapular kinematics and glenohumeral joint pathologies. *J Orthop Sports Phys Ther* 2009;39(2)90–104.

MacWilliams BA, et al.: Characteristic ground-reaction forces in baseball pitching. *Am J Sports Med* 1998;26:66–71.

McClure P, et al.: A randomized controlled comparison of stretching procedures for posterior shoulder tightness. *J Orthop Sports Phys Ther* 2007;37(3):108–114.

McMullen J, Uhl TL: A kinetic chain approach for shoulder rehabilitation. *J Athl Train* 2000;35(3):329–337.

Moore SD, et al.: The immediate effects of muscle energy technique on posterior shoulder tightness: A randomized controlled trial. *J Orthop Sports Phys Ther* 2011;41:400–407.

Sciascia AD, et al.: Return to pre-injury levels of play following superior labral repair in overhead athletes: a systematic review. *J Athl Train* 2015;50(7):767–777.

Uhl TL, et al.: Shoulder musculature activation during upper extremity weight-bearing exercise. *J Orthop Sports Phys Ther* 2003;33(3):109–117.

Voight M, Hoogenboom BJ, Cook G: The chop and lift reconsidered: integrating neuromuscular principles into orthopedic and sports rehabilitation. *N Am J Sports Phys Ther* 2008;3:151–159.

Wilk KE, et al.: Loss of internal rotation and the correlation to shoulder injuries in professional baseball pitchers. *Am J Sports Med* 2011;39(2):329–335.

© 2018 American Academy of Orthopaedic Surgeons

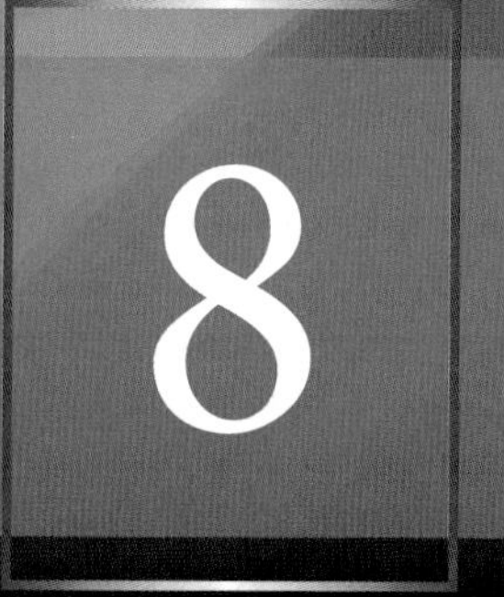

8 Rotator Cuff Repairs

Brian E. Richardson, PT, MS, SCS, CSCS, and Charles L. Cox, MD, MPH

INTRODUCTION

Rotator cuff disease is a common cause of pain and dysfunction, as approximately one in three individuals over the age of 65 years reports shoulder pain with some degree of disability. Approximately 5 million physician visits were due to rotator cuff–related issues from 1998 to 2004, which represents a 40% increase during this time period. Most rotator cuff repairs are performed in an outpatient setting, and although accurate numbers are not available, estimates for outpatient rotator cuff repair surgery range up to 250,000 per year. As rotator cuff disease is a condition that primarily affects individuals from middle age and beyond, the impact will only increase as the population in the United States ages.

Patients present to clinicians with a history of shoulder pain and dysfunction and a physical examination with varying degrees of limitation of motion and weakness. It is important to determine whether there was an acute injury or a more chronic evolution of symptoms. Magnetic resonance imaging, ultrasound, or CT arthrogram is frequently performed to confirm the diagnosis and quantify the size of the tear (number of tendons involved, amount of retraction, and so on) and muscle quality (muscular atrophy and fatty infiltration). Muscular atrophy generally increases with the chronicity of the tear and is associated with decreased healing rates following repair.

The indications for surgery vary from surgeon to surgeon and case to case, with wide variation across geographical areas.

Rotator cuff repair surgery continues to evolve with the advent of arthroscopic techniques and various implants. In general, the basic premise of the technique involves repairing the detached tendon(s) to the footprint of the insertion(s) on the proximal humerus. As with any tendon repair surgery, the postoperative focus relies heavily on protecting the site of repair while trying to simultaneously restore function in a protected and graduated fashion. The primary goal of surgery is to alleviate pain and to restore function. Postoperative rehabilitation plays a critically important role in the success of surgery.

Relevant Anatomy

The rotator cuff consists of four muscles that originate on the scapula and insert onto the proximal humerus. The site of origin and insertion determines the biomechanical function of the muscle. The subscapularis inserts onto the lesser tuberosity and assists in internal rotation (IR) of the humerus. The supraspinatus inserts onto the greater tuberosity and assists in overhead elevation of the humerus. The teres minor and infraspinatus insert more posteriorly and assist with external rotation (ER) of the humerus. The four-tendon complex assists in providing compressive forces to the glenohumeral joint and maintaining the humeral head in a centered position relative to the glenoid. Injury to the rotator cuff usually involves the tendinous attachments and ranges from partial tearing to full detachment of the tendon from the bone. Often, the tendon ends retract from the insertion point after a tear. As time passes following detachment, atrophy coupled with fatty infiltration of the muscles can occur from relative disuse.

SURGICAL TREATMENT

Indications and Contraindications

It is important to recognize that there are both clinical and anatomic indications for rotator cuff repair. The primary clinical indications for rotator cuff repair surgery are shoulder pain and/or dysfunction. In the setting of chronic atraumatic rotator cuff tear, surgical treatment is usually considered after failed nonoperative treatment. In contrast, in cases of acute traumatic tears, especially larger tears in active individuals, early surgery is considered. Due to the known natural history of rotator cuff tears, clinicians more often consider earlier surgical repair for younger patients. When considering the anatomy of the rotator cuff, repair is indicated if there is a reparable tear, as not all rotator cuff tears are reparable. This may be the case in the presence of a chronic large or massive tear, especially if there is severe muscle atrophy and fatty infiltration.

Dr. Cox or an immediate family member is an employee of Smith & Nephew; and serves as a board member, owner, officer, or committee member of the American Orthopaedic Society for Sports Medicine. Neither Dr. Richardson nor any immediate family member has received anything of value from or has stock or stock options held in a commercial company or institution related directly or indirectly to the subject of this article.

© 2018 American Academy of Orthopaedic Surgeons

Rotator cuff repair is contraindicated in the presence of severe adhesive capsulitis, glenohumeral arthritis, and chronic massive irreparable rotator cuff tear.

Rotator Cuff Repair

Traditionally, rotator cuff repairs were performed with open techniques or mini-open techniques. In the former, the anterior deltoid is detached to gain exposure; in the latter, the deltoid muscle is split after arthroscopic evaluation, preparation, and acromioplasty. Currently, most rotator cuff repairs are performed with a variety of arthroscopic techniques. Open repairs are now more typically reserved for revision surgery or procedures that augment the repair site with a soft-tissue graft. Arthroscopic techniques provide a less invasive means to evaluate and manage concomitant pathology, such as labral tears and intra-articular long-head biceps pathology. A variety of suture anchor techniques are available, including single-row, double-row, and transosseous equivalent suture bridge techniques with various suture techniques including simple, mattress, or knotless constructs. Less commonly, arthroscopic repairs are performed with transosseous sutures in the humerus (Figure 8.1).

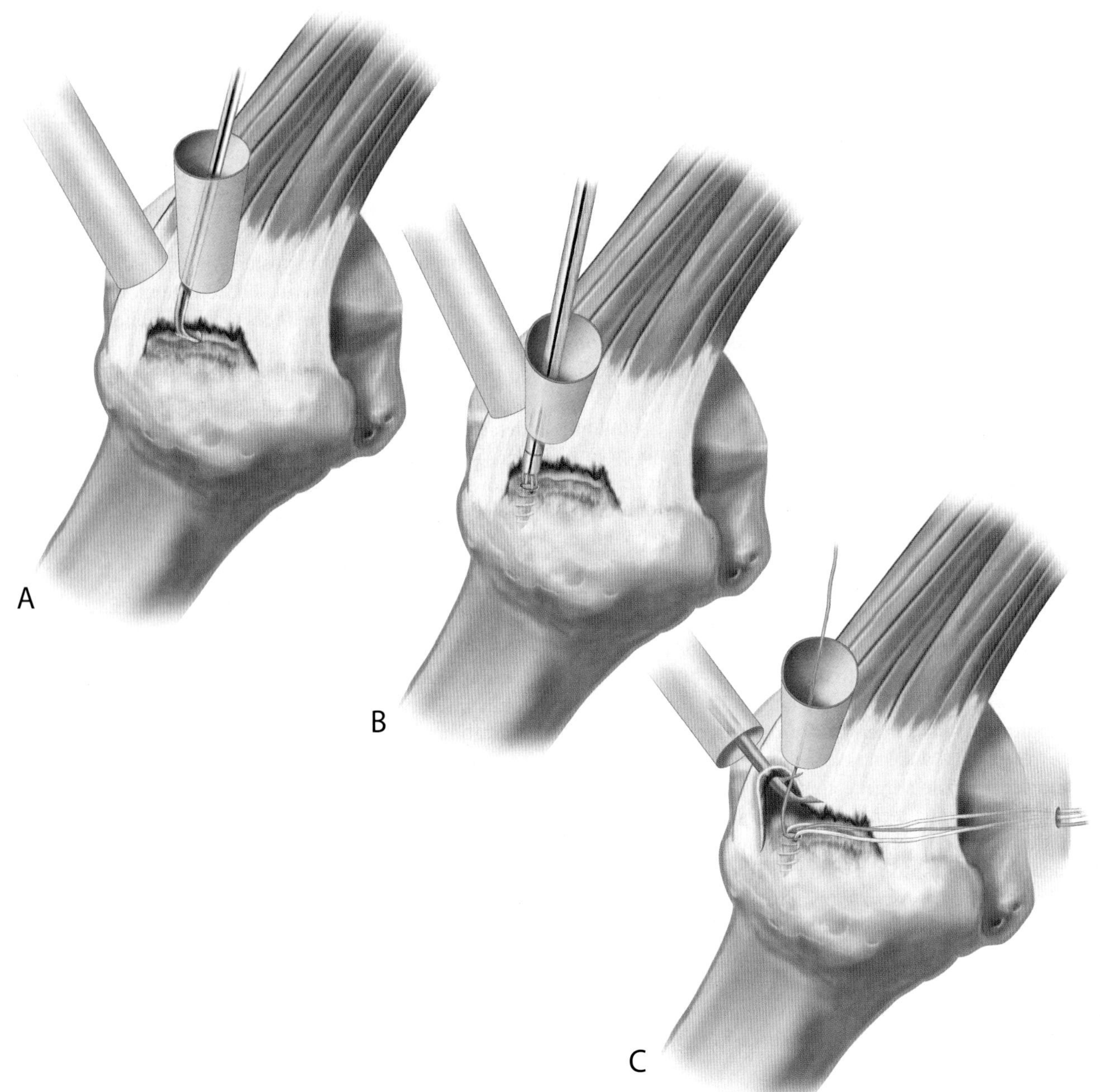

Figure 8.1 **A–H**, Diagram of transosseous equivalent suture bridge technique for arthroscopic rotator cuff repair. (Reproduced with permission from Miller MD, Chhabra AB, Konin J, Mistry D: *Sports Medicine Conditions: Return To Play: Recognition, Treatment, Planning.* Philadelphia, PA, Wolters Kluwer, 2014.)

© 2018 American Academy of Orthopaedic Surgeons

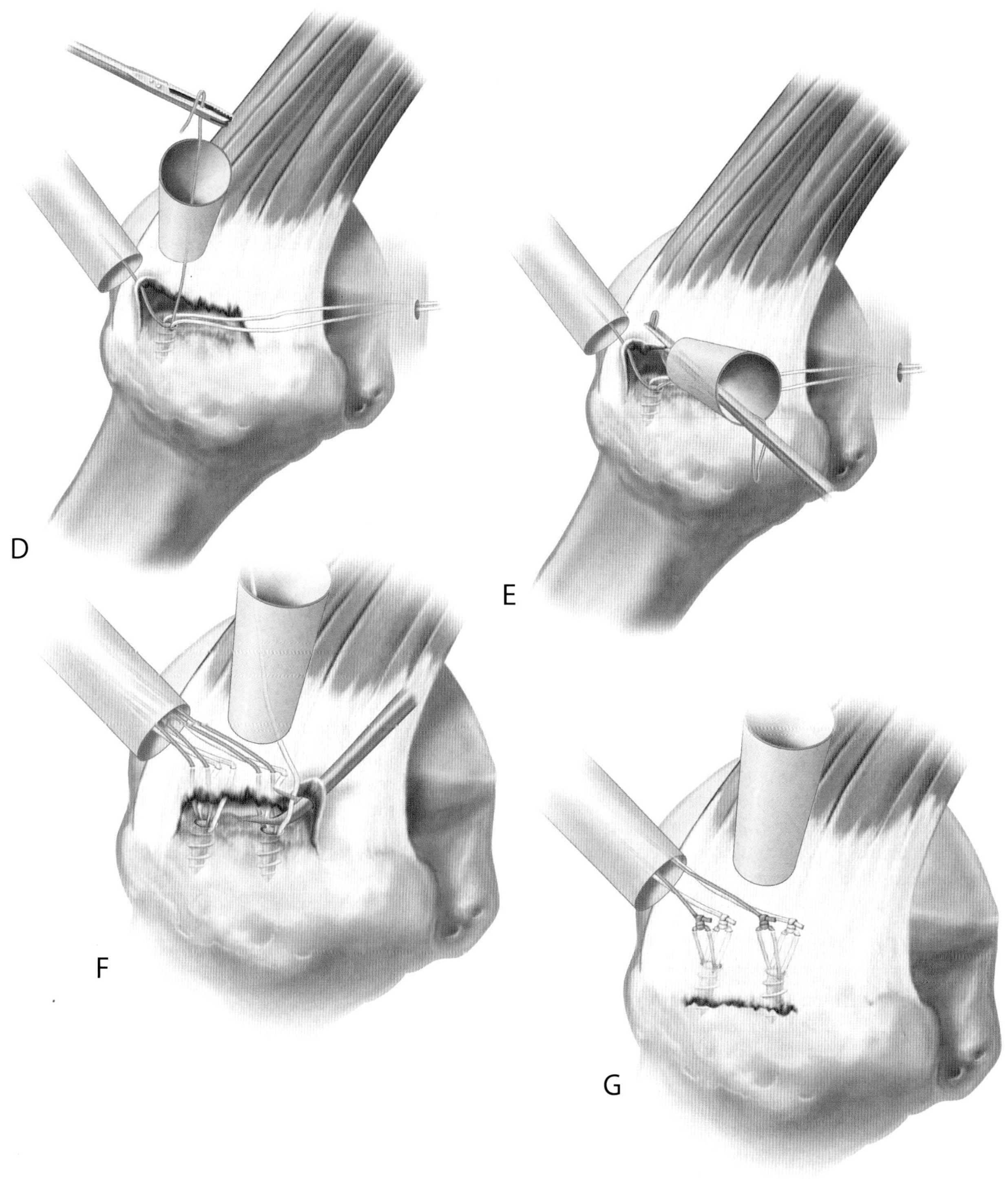

Figure 8.1 *(Continued)*

© 2018 American Academy of Orthopaedic Surgeons

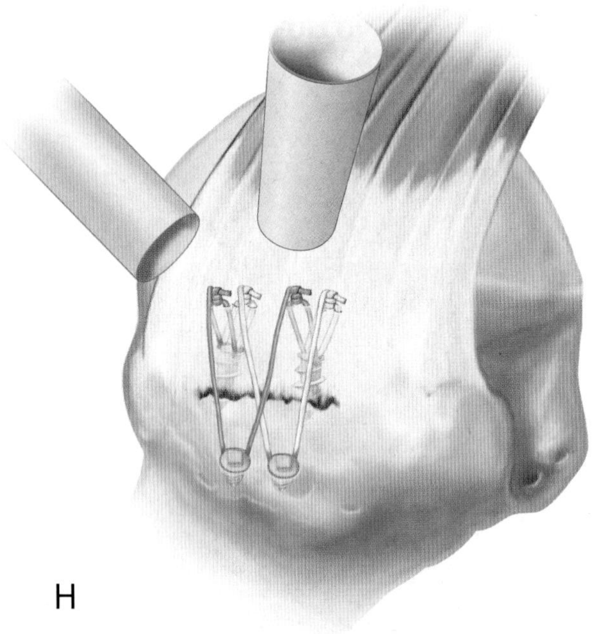

Figure 8.1 *(Continued)*

Traditionally, acromioplasty was recommended in conjunction with rotator cuff repair. However, recent clinical trials have shown little short-term benefit in healing rates or patient-reported outcomes when comparing patients who underwent simultaneous acromioplasty at the time of rotator cuff repair versus patients in whom the acromial morphology was left alone. Similarly, there is no evidence to suggest that a careful and appropriately performed acromioplasty is detrimental to the outcome. This remains a controversial topic, and long-term outcome studies are needed.

POSTOPERATIVE REHABILITATION

In discussing rehabilitation following arthroscopic rotator cuff repair, one must realize that each tear and repair is different and that a specific protocol should be used as a guide for treatment that is coordinated with the individual patient's response to treatment. Communication between the orthopaedic surgeon and rehabilitation provider is critical for the success of the rehabilitation. The surgeon should discuss with the physical therapist the surgical technique, location of the repair, severity and shape of the tear, and the tissue quality in addition to any adjunctive procedures. All of these factors are important in the success of the rehabilitation.

The guidelines outlined in this chapter describe an arthroscopic rotator cuff repair; special consideration should be made if the procedure was performed as an open repair. It should be noted that with an open repair, the deltoid is usually detached from the anterior acromion in order to improve visualization. The rehabilitation following an open repair will need to be modified in order to limit stress across the reattached deltoid. Communication with the physician is important to determine any additional precautions that need to be taken in the rehabilitation process.

Regardless of the technique utilized, the postoperative protocol hinges on protecting the repaired tendons to facilitate tendon-to-bone healing. The most common reported anatomic complication in rotator cuff surgery involves re-tearing of the tendons, and most rehabilitation protocols try to progress slowly, initially limiting active range of motion (AROM) while healing takes place. Patient-reported outcomes do not always correlate with integrity of the repaired tendons, and it is possible to achieve good results even if re-tear (partial or complete) occurs. In contrast, postoperative stiffness has a tremendous impact on the progress of recovery even though most patients eventually recover range of motion (ROM).

Authors' Preferred Protocol

These guidelines are designed for rehabilitation after arthroscopic rotator cuff repair of small to medium cuff tears (<5 cm) with good tissue quality. Patients who have poor tissue quality, tears of multiple tendons, and larger tears (>5 cm) will need to be progressed slower. The rehabilitation program for patients who have massive rotator cuff tears should focus on regaining motion, controlling pain, and regaining periscapular strength, and should emphasize deltoid strengthening.

Phase I (0–4 Weeks)

Goals

- Protect the repair
- Control pain and inflammation
- Allow for wound healing
- Prevent the development of adhesions

Precautions

- No active shoulder motion for 6 weeks
- Wear a sling at all times for 6 weeks
- Avoid heavy lifting using the involved upper extremity (UE)
- No quick sudden movements with the involved UE

Exercises (Table 8.1)

- Elbow/wrist ROM exercises/gripping
- Pendulum exercises (Figure 8.2)
- Pain-free PROM shoulder (Figure 8.3)
  - Elevation to tolerance
  - ER and IR in scapular plane
- Grade I/II joint mobilizations
- Manual scapular resistance
- Scapular retraction
- Ice to control pain and inflammation for 15 minutes

Phase II (4–6 Weeks)

Goals

- Protect the repair
- Control pain and inflammation
- Attain full PROM

 © 2018 American Academy of Orthopaedic Surgeons

Table 8.1 PHASE I EXERCISES AFTER ROTATOR CUFF REPAIR

Exercise	Week Initiated	Number of Sets/Reps	Frequency
Therapist-assisted PROM	1		2–3 d/wk
Therapist-assisted manual scapular resistance	2	1 set of 10 reps	2–3 d/wk
Elbow/wrist/gripping	1	3 sets of 10 reps	3–5 times/d
Pendulum	1	3 sets of 10 reps	3–5 times/d
Scapular retraction	1	3 sets of 10 reps	3–5 times/d

PROM = passive range of motion, reps = repetitions.

Exercises (Table 8.2)

- Pain-free PROM shoulder
  - Elevation
  - ER and IR at 90° of abduction
- Grades I to IV joint mobilizations
- Manual scapular resistance/proprioceptive neuromuscular facilitation (PNF)
- Active assistive ROM (AAROM, flexion, abduction, ER, IR), table slides, wand, pulleys (Figure 8.4)

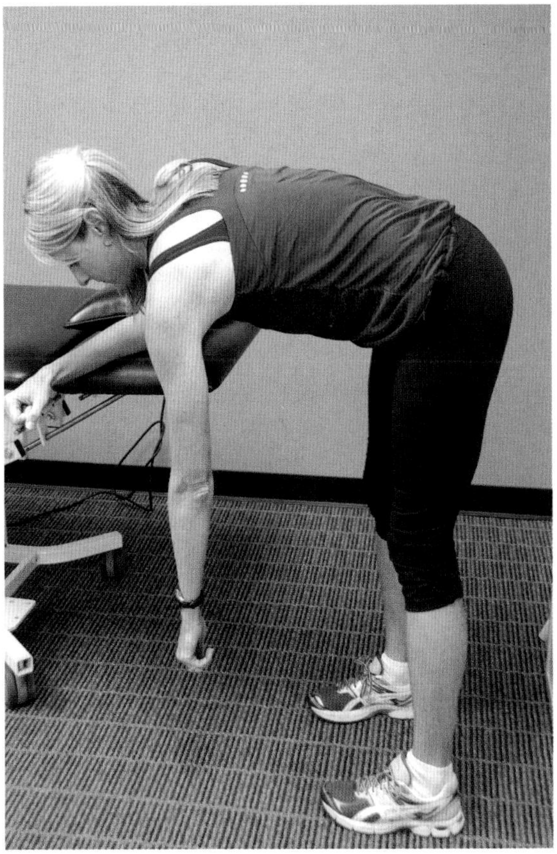

Figure 8.2 Photograph of pendulum exercises. Let the involved arm dangle. Make clockwise and counterclockwise circles. Make forward and backward motions, followed by side-to-side motions. Perform 3 sets of 10 repetitions.

- Submaximal isometrics in neutral position with elbow flexed to 90° (Figure 8.5)
  - ER/IR
  - Flexion
  - Extension
- Dynamic stabilization activities (Figure 8.6)
  - Flexion
  - ER/IR in scapular plane
- Ice to control pain and inflammation for 15 minutes

Phase III (6–12 Weeks)

Goals

- Maintain full PROM
- Attain full pain-free AROM
- Initiate strengthening program

Exercises (Table 8.3)

- Continue PROM, as needed
- Continue AAROM activities, as needed
- Dynamic stabilization techniques
- Scapular stabilization
  - Prone rows (Figure 8.7)
  - Prone shoulder extension (Figure 8.8)
  - Serratus punch (Figure 8.9)
- Ice PRN

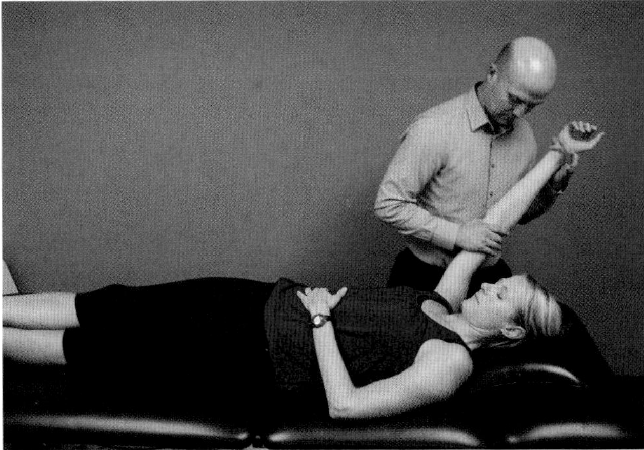

Figure 8.3 Photograph of physical therapist performing passive range of motion.

Table 8.2 PHASE II EXERCISES FOLLOWING ROTATOR CUFF REPAIR

Exercise	Week Initiated	Number of Sets/Reps	Frequency
Therapist-assisted PROM	1		2–3 d/wk
Therapist-assisted manual scapular resistance	2	1 set of 10 reps	2–3 d/wk with therapist
Therapist-assisted dynamic stabilization	4	3 sets of 10 s, hold	2–3 d/wk with therapist
Submaximal isometrics	6	1 set of 10 reps	3–5 times/d
AAROM (table slides, wand, pulleys)	4	1 set of 15 reps	3–5 times/d

AAROM = active-assistive range of motion, PROM = range of motion, reps = repetitions.

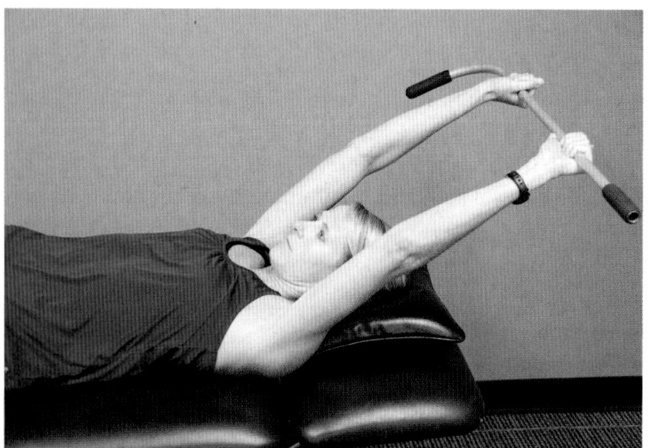

Figure 8.4 Photograph of active-assistive range of motion. While lying supine, elevate the cane overhead using both arms. Allow the uninvolved arm to guide the involved arm. Increase the elevation of the involved arm according to patient tolerance and comfort.

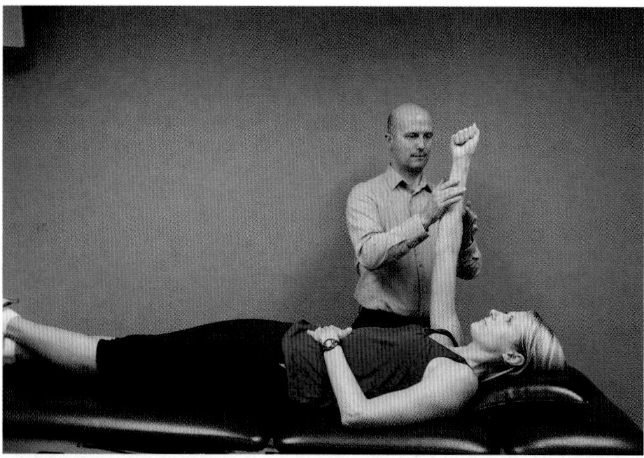

Figure 8.6 Photograph of therapist-guided dynamic stabilization. While the patient is lying supine, place the involved arm at 90° of elevation. Instruct the patient to hold the arm in place while the physical therapist provides light manual resistance.

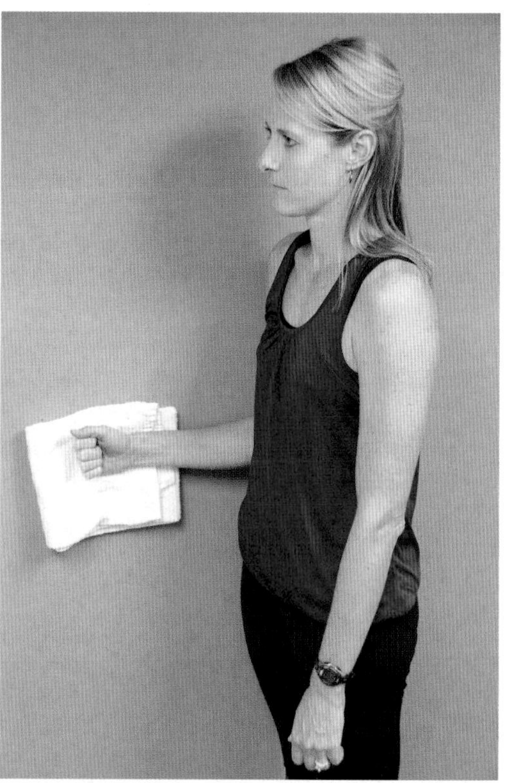

Figure 8.5 Photograph of submaximal isometrics. While standing with elbow flexed at 90°, push the involved hand out against the wall (external rotation). Perform facing the wall and pushing inward (internal rotation), in front of the wall pushing forward (flexion), back against the wall and pushing backward (extension).

Phase IV (12–16 Weeks)

Goals

- Maintain full pain-free AROM
- Restore strength in involved UE
- Increase functional activities

Exercises (Table 8.4)

- Isotonics
  - Prone rows
  - Prone shoulder extension
  - Prone horizontal abduction
  - Serratus punch

© 2018 American Academy of Orthopaedic Surgeons

Table 8.3 PHASE III EXERCISES FOLLOWING ROTATOR CUFF REPAIR

Exercise	Week Initiated	Number of Sets/Reps	Frequency
Therapist-assisted PROM	1		2–3 d/wk
AAROM (table slides, wand, pulleys, internal and external rotation)	4	1 set of 15 reps	3–5 times/d
Therapist-assisted dynamic stabilization	4	3 sets of 20 sec holds	2–3 d/wk
Prone rows	10	3 sets of 10 reps	2–3 d/wk for strengthening
Prone shoulder extension	10	3 sets of 10 reps	2–3 d/wk for strengthening
Serratus punch	10	3 sets of 10 reps	2–3 d/wk for strengthening
Submaximal isometrics	6	1 set of 10 reps	Daily

AAROM = active-assistive range of motion.

  - Dynamic bear hugs
  - Scapular retraction with ER combo
  - ER (Figure 8.10)
  - IR
- Dynamic stabilization techniques
- Ice PRN

Phase V (16–24 Weeks)

Goals

- Gradual return-to-work activities
- Gradual return to sport

Exercises

- Progress strengthening program.
- Initiate sport-specific program and return-to-work program, as indicated by the physician.
- A gradual return-to-sport program should be initiated once the patient has been cleared by the physician and the patient exhibits full ROM and strength as well as normal scapular kinematics.
- Return to competitive sports may range from 8 to 12 months from surgery and will depend on the type of sport,

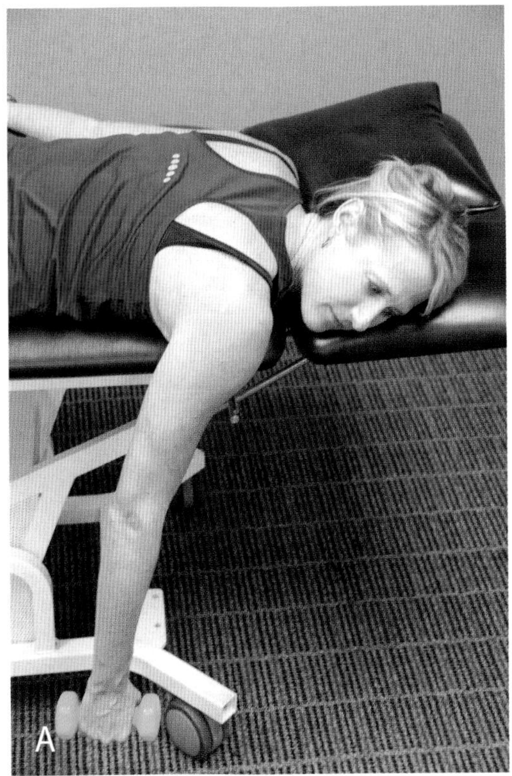

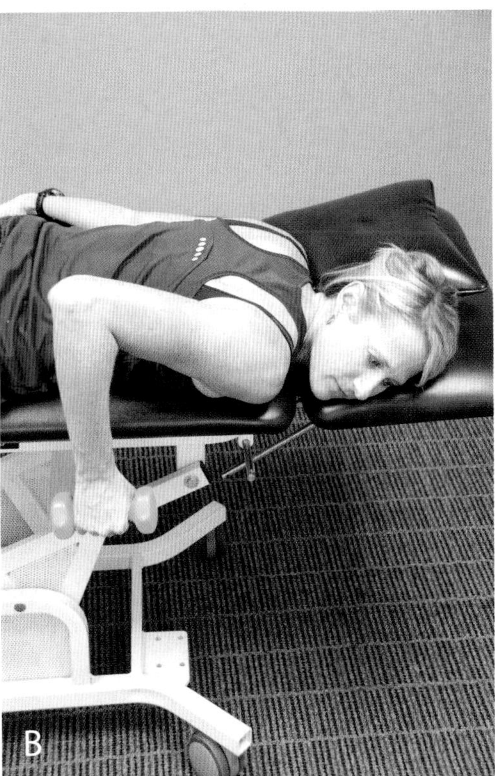

Figure 8.7 **A, B,** Photographs of prone rows. While the patient is lying prone, instruct the patient to lift the arm and raise the elbow to shoulder height while performing scapular retraction.

© 2018 American Academy of Orthopaedic Surgeons

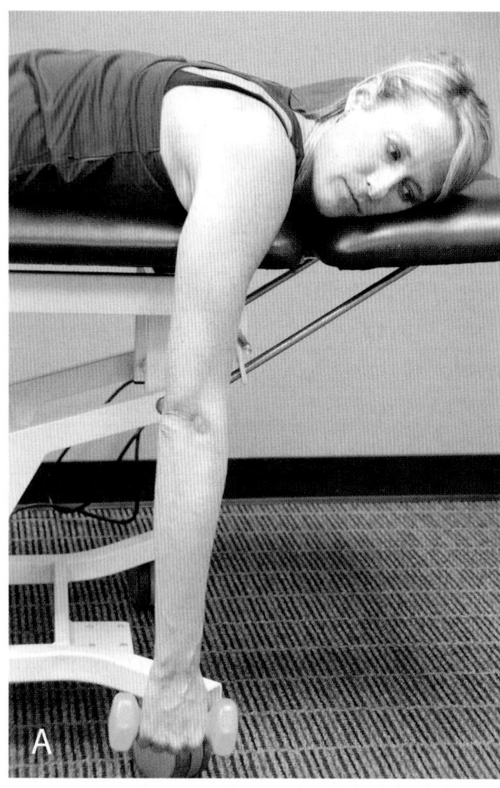

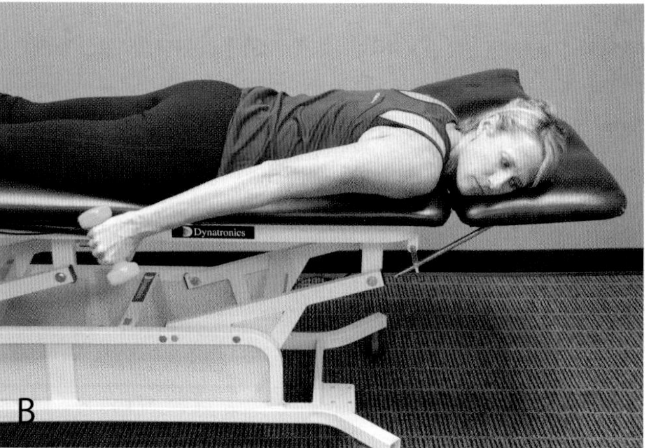

Figure 8.8 **A**, **B**, Photographs of prone shoulder extension. While the patient is lying prone, instruct the patient to lift the arm in line with the body while performing scapular retraction.

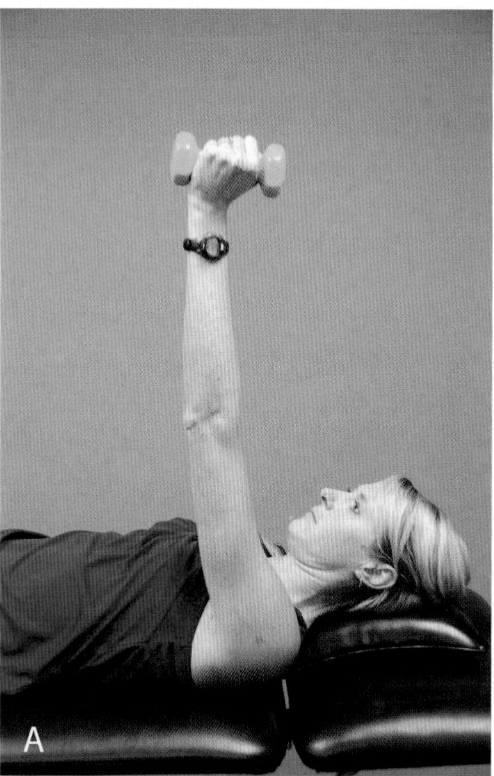

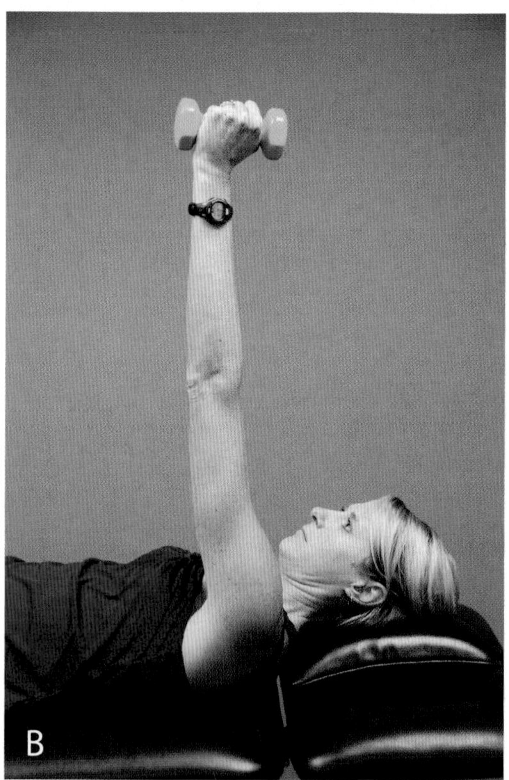

Figure 8.9 **A**, **B**, Photographs of serratus punch. While the patient is lying supine, instruct the patient to keep the elbow straight and move the arm toward the ceiling.

© 2018 American Academy of Orthopaedic Surgeons

Table 8.4 PHASE IV STRENGTHENING EXERCISES FOLLOWING ROTATOR CUFF REPAIR

Exercise	Week Initiated	Number of Sets/Reps	Frequency
Prone rows	10	3 sets of 10 reps	2–3 d/wk
Prone shoulder extension	10	3 sets of 10 reps	2–3 d/wk
Serratus punch	10	3 sets of 10 reps	2–3 d/wk
Scapular retraction with external rotation combo	12	3 sets of 10 reps	2–3 d/wk
External rotation	12	3 sets of 10 reps	2–3 d/wk
Internal rotation	12	3 sets of 10 reps	2–3 d/wk
Dynamic bear hugs	12	3 sets of 10 reps	2–3 d/wk
Prone horizontal abduction	12	3 sets of 10 reps	2–3 d/wk

size of the tear, tissue quality, associated labral pathologies, and the physician's preferences.

Outcomes

A recent meta-analysis reported that early ROM after arthroscopic rotator cuff repair resulted in a greater recovery of IR and shoulder flexion motion when compared to delayed ROM. Nevertheless, the study reported that delayed motion was associated with higher American Shoulder and Elbow Surgeons (ASES) scores at 12 months postoperatively as well as higher healing rates. When delaying ROM, one must consider the implications of postoperative stiffness. Patients with calcific tendinitis, adhesive capsulitis, PASTA repair, a concomitant labral repair, or a single-tendon rotator cuff repair appear to be at greater risk of postoperative stiffness. These groups of patients may benefit from starting ROM earlier to prevent stiffness.

The primary goals of rotator cuff repair are to improve patient pain and function. Repair healing is considered to be an important component of outcome. Studies have shown that small to medium tears (1–3 cm) have a higher healing rate of 79% when compared to large tears (57%) and massive tears (40%). Iannotti et al reported that the mean time to re-tear after arthroscopic rotator cuff repair of 1-cm to 4-cm tears was 19.2 weeks, with a linear increase in re-tears over the first 26 weeks after surgery. Several factors—including patient age, tear size, tear retraction, and rotator cuff muscle degeneration—affect repair healing. Harryman et al were the first to study the relationship between rotator cuff healing and functional outcome. They reported re-tear in 20% of supraspinatus repairs and 50% of larger tears. Although patients with larger tears at follow-up had inferior function, 87% of the patients with a recurrent tear were satisfied with the results. Russell et al reported the findings of a systematic review and meta-analysis of 14 rotator cuff repair studies. Patients with intact repairs had better, but not clinically relevant, outcomes; patients with intact repairs had significantly greater strength than those with re-tears. Last, Salbaugh and coworkers performed a systematic review and reported that patients with intact rotator cuffs had statistically better improvement in objective outcome measures (Constant, UCLA scores) and that there was no correlation between healing and patient-reported outcome (ASES, Simple Shoulder Test [SST]).

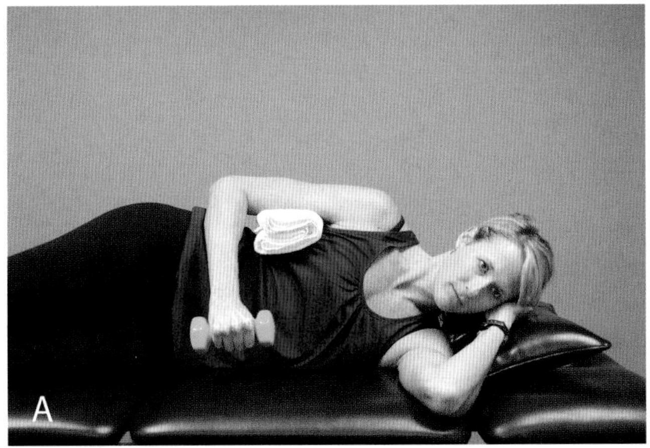

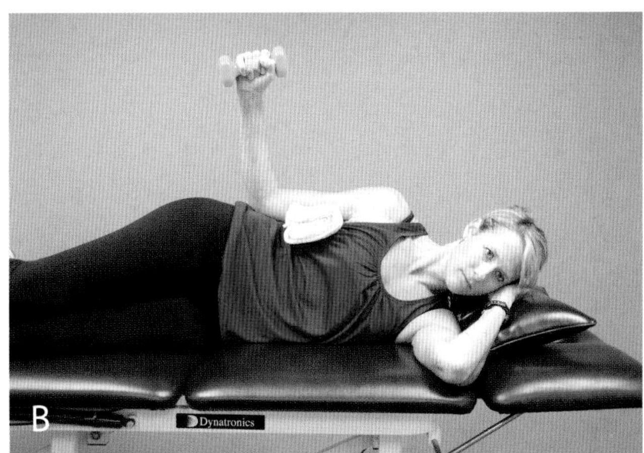

Figure 8.10 **A**, **B**, Photographs of external rotation. While the patient is lying on the uninvolved side with the involved arm bent, instruct the patient to lift the bent arm up.

© 2018 American Academy of Orthopaedic Surgeons

PEARLS

- It is important to discuss patient expectations prior to initiating treatment, as these may vary considerably.
- Communication between the treating therapist and surgeon is critical. Each tear configuration is unique, and intraoperative findings may affect the postoperative plan.
- Most therapy protocols progress through a graduated plan from PROM to AROM, followed by strengthening.
- Tear size and tissue quality should dictate the rate of progression of postoperative rehabilitation, with larger tears dictating a slower and less aggressive protocol.
- Patient-reported outcomes do not always correlate with integrity of the repaired tendons, and it is possible to achieve good results even if re-tear (partial or complete) occurs.

SUMMARY

Rotator cuff tears are quite common and surgical management has high reported success rates. The postoperative rehabilitation is as important as the surgical repair. Repair healing is a major concern and is related to several factors, including patient age, the original tear size, rotator cuff muscle degeneration, repair technique, and the postoperative management. Rotator cuff repair rehabilitation should be individualized based on patient goals and expectations, the anatomic pathology, and the quality of the repair. Communication between the surgeon and the rehabilitation provider to coordinate postoperative care is very important in order to optimize the outcome.

BIBLIOGRAPHY

American Academy of Orthopaedic Surgeons, Research Statistics on Rotator Cuff Repairs, National Ambulatory Medical Care Survey, 1998–2004. Data obtained from: U.S. Department of Health and Human Services; Centers for Disease Control and Prevention; National Center for Health Statistics; Retrieved on May 9, 2007 from http://www.aaos.org/Research/stats/patientstats.asp

Bishop J, Klepps S, Lo IK, Bird J, Gladstone JN, Flatow EL: Cuff integrity after arthroscopic versus open rotator cuff repair: a prospective study. *J Shoulder Elbow Surg* 2006;15(3):290–299.

Chakravarty K, Webley M: Shoulder joint movement and its relationship to disability in the elderly. *J Rheumatol* 1993; 20:1359–1361.

Chard MD, Hazleman R, Hazleman BL, King RH, Reiss BB: Shoulder disorders in the elderly: a community survey. *Arthritis Rheum* 1991;34:766–769.

Chen L, Peng K, Zhang D, Peng J, Xing F, Xiang Z: Rehabilitation protocol after arthroscopic rotator cuff repair: early versus delayed motion. *Int J Clin Exp Med* 2015;8(6):8329–8338.

Harryman DT 2nd, Mack LA, Wang KY, Jackins SE, Richardson ML, Matsen FA 3rd: Repairs of the rotator cuff. Correlation of functional results with integrity of the cuff. *J Bone Joint Surg Am* 1991;73(7):982–989.

Iannotti JP, Deutsch A, Green A, Rudicel S, Christensen J, Marraffino S, Rodeo S: Time to failure after rotator cuff repair: a prospective imaging study. *J Bone Joint Surg Am* 2013;95:965–971.

Koo SS, Parsley BK, Burkhart SS, Schoolfield JD: Reduction of postoperative stiffness after arthroscopic rotator cuff repair: results of a customized physical therapy regimen based on risk factors for stiffness. *Arthroscopy* 2011;27:(2):155–160.

Russell RD, Knight JR, Mulligan E, Khazzam MS: Structural integrity after rotator cuff repair does not correlate with patient function and pain a meta-analysis. *J Bone Joint Surg Am* 2014; 96:265–271.

Slabaugh MA, Nho SJ, Grumet RC, Wilson JB, Seroyer ST, Frank RM, Romeo AA, Provencher MT, Verma NN: Does the literature confirm superior clinical results in radiographically healed rotator cuffs after rotator cuff repair? *Arthroscopy* 2010;26(3): 393–403.

Vitale MA, Vitale MG, Zivin JG, Braman JP, Bigliani LU, Flatow EL: Rotator cuff repair: an analysis of utility scores and cost-effectiveness. *J Shoulder Elbow Surg* 2006;16:181–187.

© 2018 American Academy of Orthopaedic Surgeons

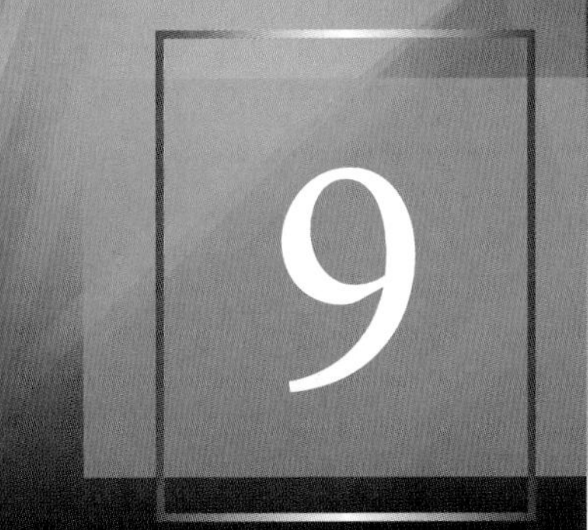

9 Shoulder Arthroplasty

Andrew Green, MD, Daniel DeBottis, MD, and David Pezzullo, MS, PT, SCS, ATC

INTRODUCTION

The modern era of shoulder arthroplasty was championed by Dr. Charles Neer, who pioneered the use of an anatomically conceived implant for treatment of proximal humerus fractures and later developed a polyethylene glenoid component to perform total shoulder arthroplasty to treat glenohumeral arthritis. After only a slight increase in the incidence of shoulder arthroplasty between 1990 and 2000, there has been a subsequent rapid increase in the number of shoulder arthroplasties performed in the United States. The introduction of reverse shoulder arthroplasty to the United States in 2004 was accompanied by an even greater increase in shoulder arthroplasty, with a projection of greater than 80,000 procedures by 2015.

The evolution of anatomic shoulder prosthesis design led to humeral implants that have modular humeral heads with various sizes and offsets to facilitate accurate anatomic reconstruction of the articular segment. In addition, variable neck-shaft angles further provide the surgeon the ability to closely recreate the anatomy of the patient. More recently, humeral head resurfacing and stemless humeral implants have been introduced. The importance of recreating the native anatomy has been demonstrated by multiple studies (Figure 9.1).

The modern reverse shoulder arthroplasty was initially developed by Grammont in France to treat rotator cuff–deficient shoulders. The major design features that allow this are the inverted constrained ball-and-socket orientation with a scapula-based glenosphere and a humeral-based socket that provide a stable fulcrum. The relative lengthening and tensioning of the deltoid muscle provide dynamic stability, as well as the strength and power for shoulder function (Figure 9.2).

Beyond specific design characteristics and surgical technique, numerous authors have emphasized the importance of postoperative rehabilitation in achieving successful outcomes. Although rehabilitation is considered a critically important factor in the outcome of shoulder arthroplasty, there has been little reported investigation of specific rehabilitation protocols. Most references to postoperative rehabilitation are sections on the postoperative management included in reports on the technique and outcome of shoulder arthroplasty. Nevertheless, there are principles of implant design and surgical technique that must be considered in order to ensure a successful outcome.

SURGICAL INDICATIONS AND CONTRAINDICATIONS

The primary indications for prosthetic shoulder arthroplasty are shoulder pain and dysfunction in the presence of advanced glenohumeral arthritis that cannot be managed with appropriate nonoperative treatments and modalities. Anatomic total shoulder arthroplasty requires an intact and functioning rotator cuff as well as sufficient glenoid bone for implant fixation, and is most commonly performed for primary glenohumeral osteoarthritis. A number of other less common conditions—including inflammatory arthropathy, posttraumatic arthritis, osteonecrosis, and capsulorraphy arthropathy—can also be treated with anatomic arthroplasty. Humeral head replacement with or without biologic glenoid preparation (soft-tissue resurfacing and "ream and run") is indicated for some younger patients and patients who desire a very active and physical lifestyle.

In contrast, reverse total shoulder replacement was specifically developed for the treatment of shoulders with rotator cuff

Dr. Green or an immediate family member has received royalties from Tornier and Wright Medical Technology; is a member of a speakers' bureau or has made paid presentations on behalf of DJ Orthopaedics; serves as a paid consultant to Tornier and Wright Medical Technology; has stock or stock options held in IlluminOss Medical and Pfizer; has received research or institutional support from DJ Orthopaedics and Tornier; has received nonincome support (such as equipment or services), commercially derived honoraria, or other non-research–related funding (such as paid travel) from Arthrex, Journal of Bone and Joint Surgery–American, *and Smith & Nephew; and serves as a board member, owner, officer, or committee member of the American Academy of Orthopaedic Surgeons, the American Shoulder and Elbow Surgeons, the* Journal of Bone and Joint Surgery–*American, and* Techniques in Shoulder and Elbow Surgery.

© 2018 American Academy of Orthopaedic Surgeons

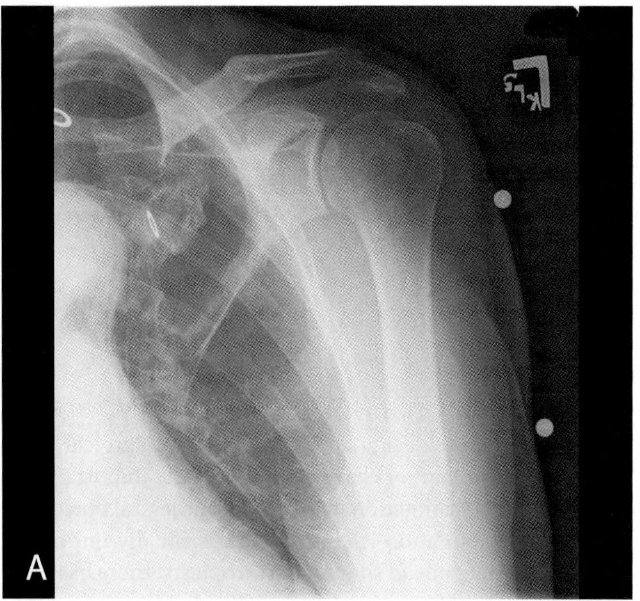

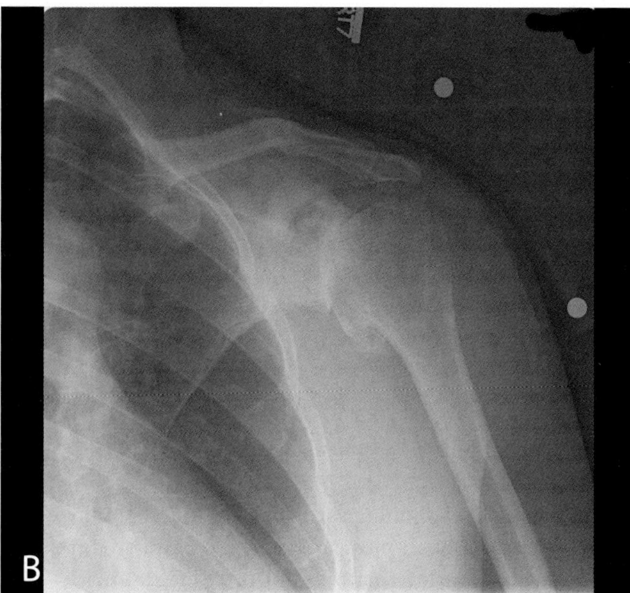

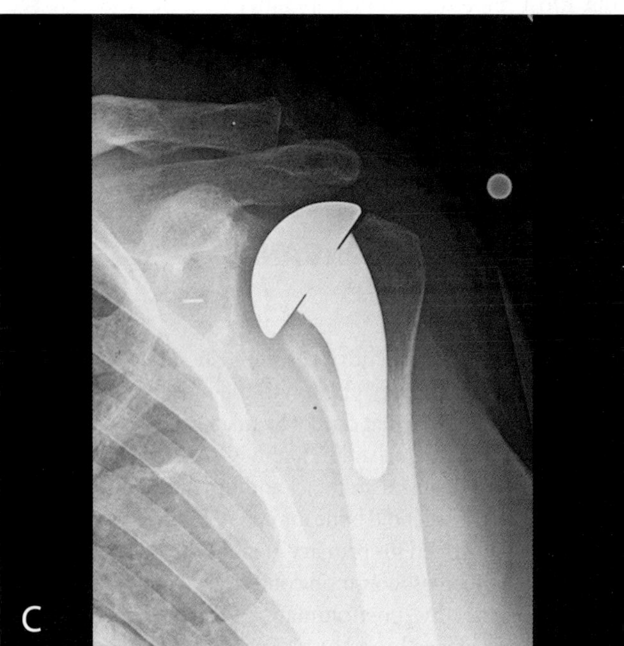

Figure 9.1 **A**, True anterior posterior plain radiograph of a normal proximal humerus. **B**, Anterior posterior plain radiograph of a shoulder with advanced osteoarthritis. **C**, True anterior posterior plain radiograph of an anatomic total shoulder arthroplasty. The humeral head implant conforms to the anatomy of the native proximal humerus.

deficiency. In a rotator cuff–deficient shoulder, deltoid contraction causes the proximal humerus to migrate superiorly and the glenohumeral joint does not provide a stable fulcrum for the deltoid. Mechanical advantage is thus lost, which can lead to the inability to elevate the arm above 90°, often referred to as pseudoparalysis. The results of anatomic total shoulder surgery in patients with combined glenohumeral arthritis and rotator cuff deficiency are usually poor. The indications for reverse total shoulder arthroplasty are expanding and generally apply to patients with rotator cuff deficiency, including patients with rotator cuff tear arthropathy, irreparable rotator cuff tears, posttraumatic arthropathy, and failed primary arthroplasty. More recently, reverse shoulder arthroplasty has been used in cases of primary glenohumeral osteoarthritis with glenoid deficiency or soft-tissue severe contracture.

Contraindications to anatomic and reverse shoulder arthroplasty include infection, deltoid paralysis, deficient deltoid musculature, unreconstructable bone loss, as well as patient comorbidities and noncompliance.

SURGICAL PROCEDURE

The preoperative evaluation includes assessment of active range of motion (AROM) and passive range of motion (PROM) as well as shoulder strength. The postoperative range of motion (ROM)

© 2018 American Academy of Orthopaedic Surgeons

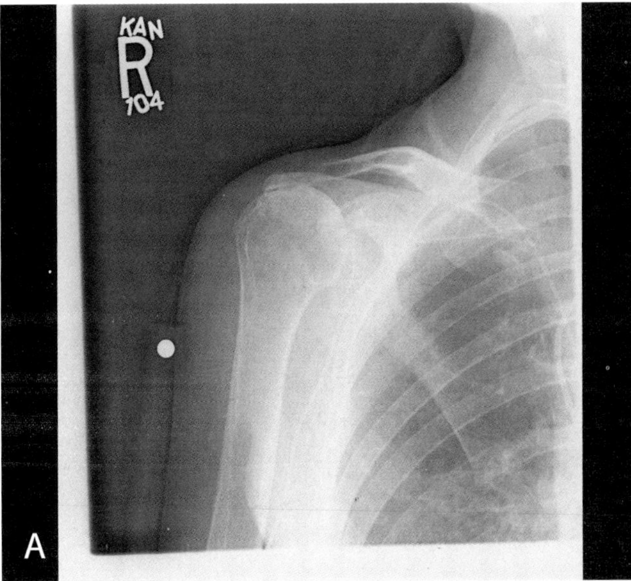

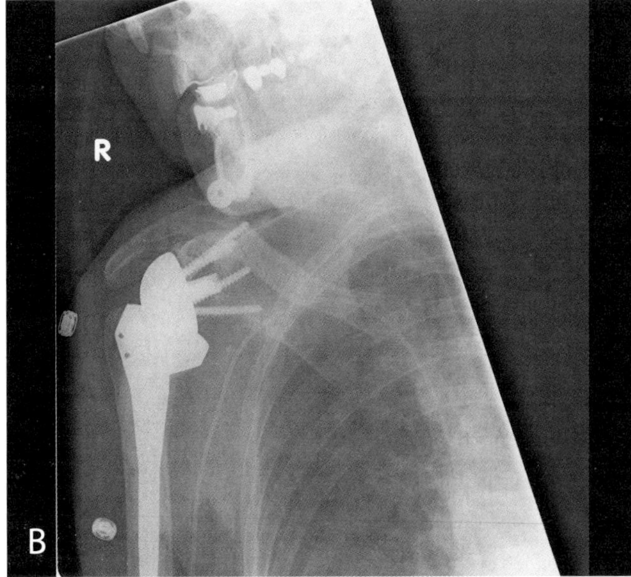

Figure 9.2 **A**, Preoperative true anterior posterior plain radiograph of a patient with rotator cuff tear arthropathy demonstrating elevation of the humeral head, narrowing of the acromial humeral space, and glenohumeral arthritis. **B**, Postoperative anterior posterior plain radiograph after reverse shoulder arthroplasty demonstrating inferior/distal positioning of the humerus with lengthening of the deltoid muscle.

achieved after shoulder arthroplasty is related to the preoperative motion, as patients with more severe contracture may not regain as much motion. Shoulder strength is related to the integrity and function of the rotator cuff and deltoid muscles. External rotation (ER) and internal rotation (IR) weakness due to rotator cuff tearing or dysfunction is not restored with anatomic shoulder arthroplasty. Consequently, patients with substantial rotator cuff weakness and dysfunction are preferentially treated with reverse shoulder arthroplasty.

Shoulder arthroplasty surgery can be performed with interscalene nerve block, with or without general anesthesia. Nerve block provides the advantage of better perioperative pain, control with reduced narcotic and general anesthetic requirement.

Anatomic Shoulder Arthroplasty

Anatomic shoulder arthroplasty is performed through a deltopectoral approach, which is an extensile approach that takes advantage of the internervous plane between the deltoid (axillary nerve) and pectoralis major (lateral and medial pectoral nerves) muscles (Figure 9.3). The skin incision is made on the anterior shoulder over the deltopectoral interval. Shorter incisions can be used in smaller and thinner patients. The subcutaneous tissue overlying the deltopectoral interval is incised and the cephalic vein is identified between the deltoid laterally and pectoralis major medially. The cephalic vein is retracted either medially or laterally. Lateral retraction preserves the often numerous branches from the deltoid muscle.

After developing the deltopectoral interval, the clavipectoral fascia is incised, exposing the underlying subscapularis muscle and tendon, lesser tuberosity, biceps tendon and groove, and the anterior circumflex humeral artery and its venae comitantes (see Figure 9.3). These vessels can be suture ligated or coagulated. The pectoralis major insertion on the humerus is identified and the superior 1 cm can be released to allow better exposure. The axillary nerve is palpated under the conjoined tendon by sweeping a finger from superior to inferior along the anterior aspect of the subscapularis muscle. Identification of the axillary nerve is essential in order to protect it from injury. The subacromial and subdeltoid planes are freed of any scarring to improve deeper exposure and postoperative shoulder motion. The long head of the biceps tendon is identified within the bicipital groove, routinely tenodesed to the pectoralis major insertion, and released proximally.

The glenohumeral joint can be entered via subscapularis tenotomy, subscapularis peel, or lesser tuberosity osteotomy. Subscapularis management in shoulder arthroplasty is an extremely important and somewhat controversial issue. Regardless of the technique, a strong anatomic repair is required to avoid subscapularis failure. The subscapularis originates on the anterior aspect of the scapula, is innervated by the upper and lower subscapular nerves, and is the largest of the rotator cuff muscles. The major function of this muscle is to internally rotate the shoulder and counterbalance the posterior aspect of the rotator cuff. At the least, subscapularis failure can result in internal rotation weakness. At the worst, it can result in glenohumeral instability and pseudoparalysis.

Subscapularis tenotomy is performed by vertically incising the tendon, leaving a cuff of tendon laterally to allow for secure repair (Figure 9.4, A). The technique relies on tendon-to-tendon healing. The subscapularis peel involves elevating the subscapularis insertion and underlying capsuloligamentous structures off of the lesser tuberosity and proximal humerus metaphysis, and relies on tendon-to-bone

© 2018 American Academy of Orthopaedic Surgeons

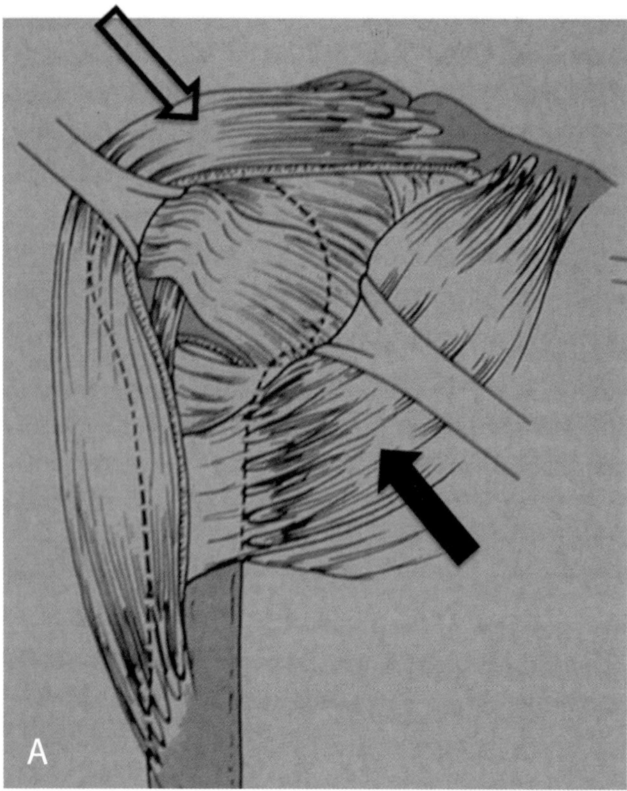

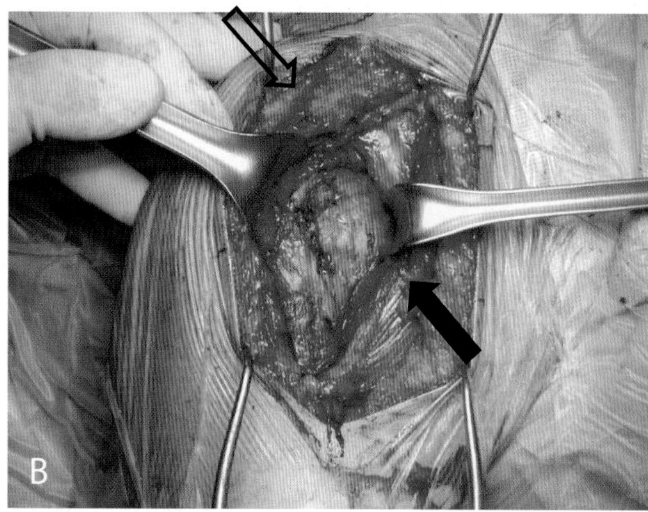

Figure 9.3 **A**, Illustration of the deltopectoral interval (*white arrow* = deltoid muscle; *black arrow* = pectoralis major muscle). **B**, Intraoperative photograph of the deltopectoral exposure. (**A** reproduced with permission from Browner BD, Jupiter JB, Levine AM, Trafton PG, Krettek C, eds: *Skeletal Trauma: Basic Science, Management, and Reconstruction,* ed. 4. Philadelphia, PA, Elsevier, 2009.)

healing (Figure 9.4, B and C). Lesser tuberosity osteotomy was developed in response to the observation that some patients have IR weakness after subscapularis tenotomy. The thought is that bone-to-bone healing is more predictable than tendon-to-tendon healing, and that lesser tuberosity osteotomy reduces the rate of subscapularis failure. The osteotomy is performed using either an osteotome or oscillating saw. A wafer of bone from the lesser tuberosity is elevated in continuity with the subscapularis tendon and muscle (Figure 9.4, D and E). Recent studies comparing lesser tuberosity osteotomy to the subscapularis peel technique demonstrate equivalent outcomes both with regard to healing and functional outcome. Regardless of the subscapularis technique, a complete release of the capsular contracture is carried out to mobilize the tendon and muscle, and restore soft-tissue balance.

The humeral head is dislocated to expose the articular segment of the humerus as well as the posterior insertion of the rotator cuff. After humeral osteophytes are removed, the humeral head articular segment is removed by cutting along the anatomic neck with a saw, and the medullary canal is prepared (Figure 9.5). The anatomic neck cut determines the retroversion of the humeral component. In anatomic arthroplasty, the patient's natural version is usually followed.

Soft-tissue releases are performed to adequately mobilize the subscapularis, as well as to release the anterior, inferior, and posterior capsular contractures and facilitate exposure of the glenoid as well as to restore glenohumeral motion. The glenoid is prepared with concentric reaming in order to optimize the seating of the glenoid component (Figure 9.6). Once the glenoid implant is placed, attention is returned to the humerus.

The humeral head component is then sized, and a trial reduction is done in order to assess glenohumeral stability, ROM, and soft-tissue balance (Figure 9.7). Different implant systems have different humeral head size options. In general, there are two philosophies in approaching this surgery; anatomic humeral head replacement and soft-tissue balancing replacement. The goal of both is to restore the center of rotation of the humerus to an anatomic position as well as to restore appropriate soft-tissue balance to achieve ROM, stability, and strength. The final humeral component is implanted with or without cement depending on the specific implant design and surgeon preference, and the glenohumeral joint is reduced.

Regardless of the technique used for subscapularis management, the repair must be strong in order to allow early shoulder motion. Subscapularis tenotomy is repaired by suturing the subscapularis tendon to the cuff of tissue remaining on the lesser tuberosity with heavy, nonabsorbable sutures. In addition, the repair can be reinforced by incorporating transosseous sutures. Subscapularis tendon peel is repaired anatomically to the lesser tuberosity using transosseous, heavy, nonabsorbable sutures. The suture limb passing through the medullary canal is passed through the tendon in Mason-Allen locking fashion and tied to the limb exiting the lateral bone tunnel. Several techniques for repair of the lesser tuberosity osteotomy are described. The authors prefer a transosseous repair with heavy nonabsorbable sutures that are passed into

© 2018 American Academy of Orthopaedic Surgeons

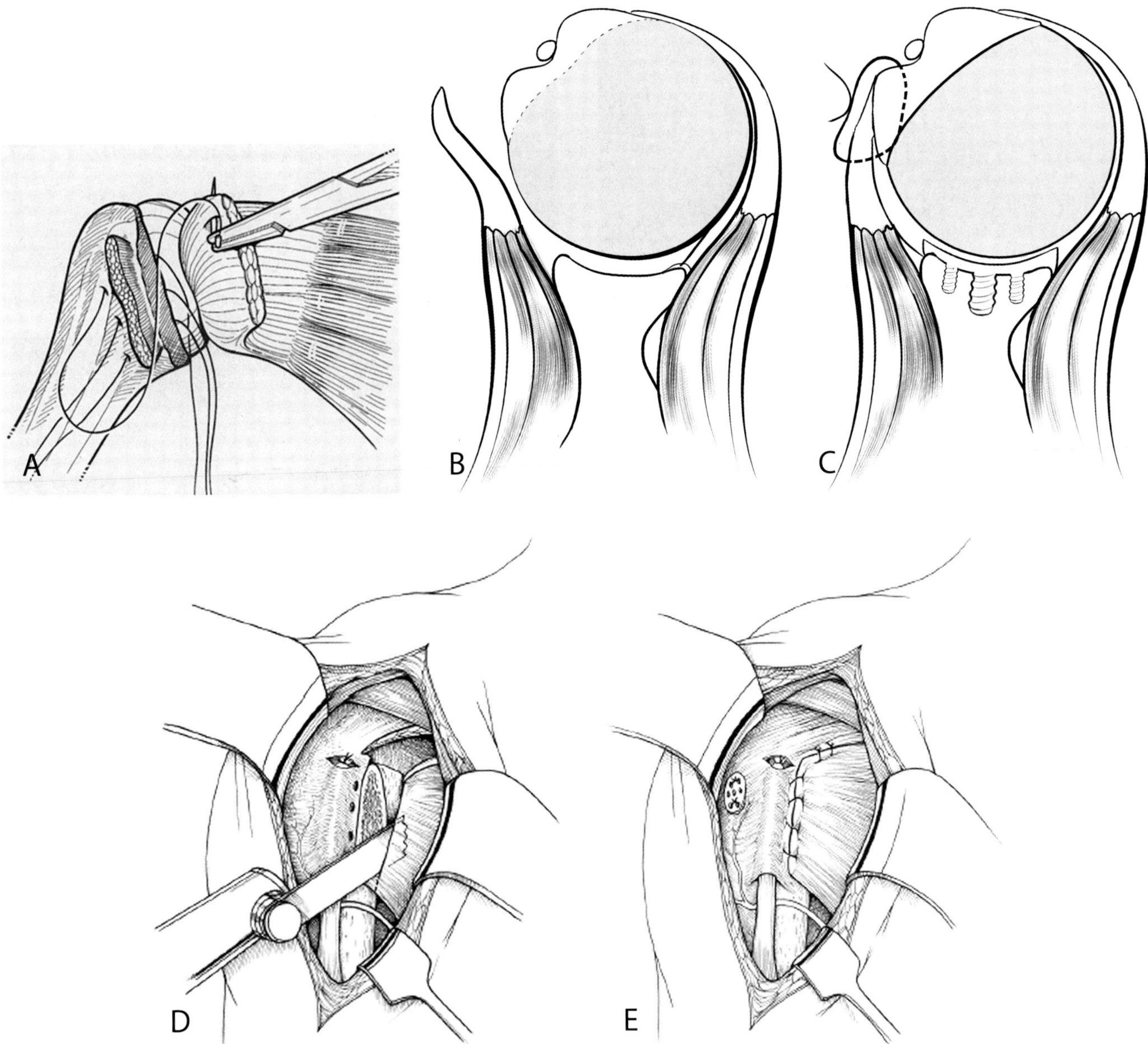

Figure 9.4 Illustrations of surgical management of the subscapularis tendon and muscle. **A**, Subscapularis tenotomy with tendon-to-tendon suture repair. **B**, **C**, Axial view of subscapularis peel with tendon-to-bone transosseous suture repair (*solid arrows* indicate subscapularis peel and repair). **D**, **E**, Lesser tuberosity osteotomy with bone-to-bone suture repair. (**A** reproduced with permission from Gartsman GM, Edwards TB, eds: *Shoulder Arthroplasty.* Philadelphia, PA, Elsevier, 2008; **D**, **E** reproduced with permission from DeFranco MJ, Higgins LD, Warner JJP: Subscapularis management in open shoulder surgery. *J Am Acad Orthop Surg* 2010;18(12):707–717.)

the intramedullary canal and around the humeral implant. The bone is then reduced anatomically, and the sutures are tied over top, allowing for bone-to-bone contact.

Once the subscapularis is securely repaired, ROM and stability are assessed. In most cases, near full shoulder motion is possible. Glenohumeral translation should permit the humeral head to easily move to the posterior glenoid rim. If there is a question about stability, this should be addressed surgically. Shoulders with posterior instability can be treated with posterior capsular plication. ROM and the effect on the subscapularis repair and shoulder stability are noted to guide the early rehabilitation. Communication with the physical therapist regarding the integrity of the subscapularis will assist in the education of the patient and progression of the rehabilitation. The remainder of the wound is then closed, and the arm is placed in a sling.

Reverse Shoulder Arthroplasty

Reverse total shoulder arthroplasty is performed through either a standard deltopectoral or a superior deltoid splitting

© 2018 American Academy of Orthopaedic Surgeons

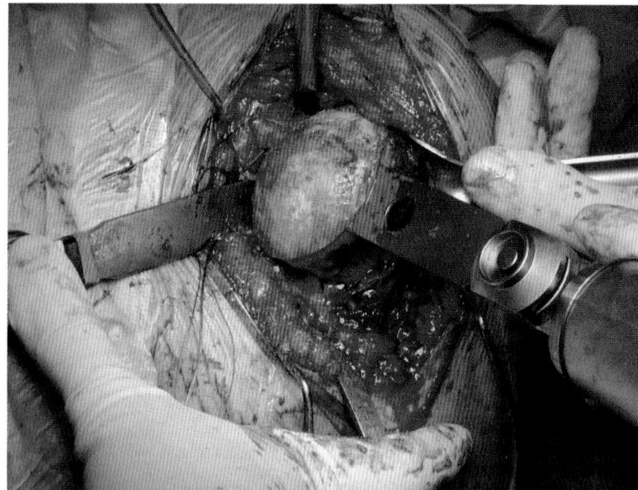

Figure 9.5 Intraoperative photograph of exposure of a left shoulder with saw blade used to perform anatomic neck osteotomy to remove the arthritic articular segment.

approach. The deltopectoral approach is the same as it is for an anatomic shoulder arthroplasty. Management of the subscapularis is somewhat controversial. Although absence of the subscapularis has been associated with instability, there is no strong evidence to support this concern. The reality of the situation is that, in many cases, the subscapularis is either deficient or very degenerative and not likely to be functional even if it is repaired. Additionally, if repairing the subscapularis would limit ER, then it can be left unrepaired. The inherent stability of the constrained reverse ball and

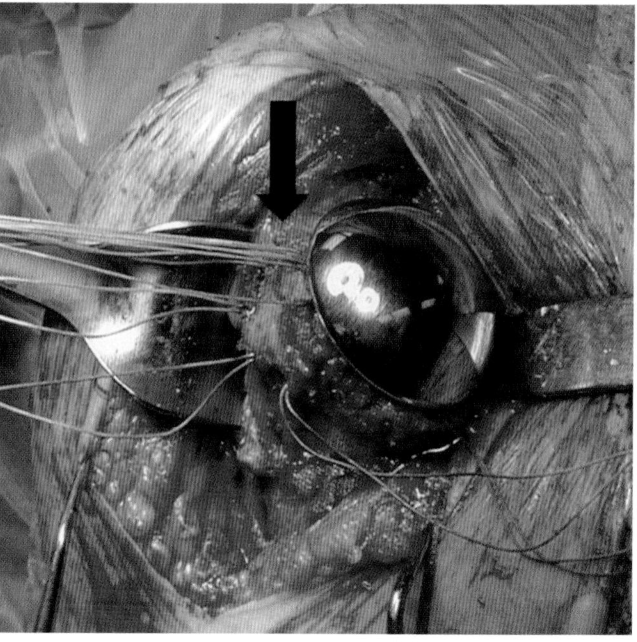

Figure 9.7 Intraoperative photograph of a humeral head component in position. Solid arrow points to transosseous sutures that will be used to repair the subscapularis.

socket likely obviates the need for intact anterior soft tissues. The decision to repair the subscapularis should consider these factors.

The humerus is dislocated and exposed to allow the humeral osteotomy. The angle of the osteotomy cut follows

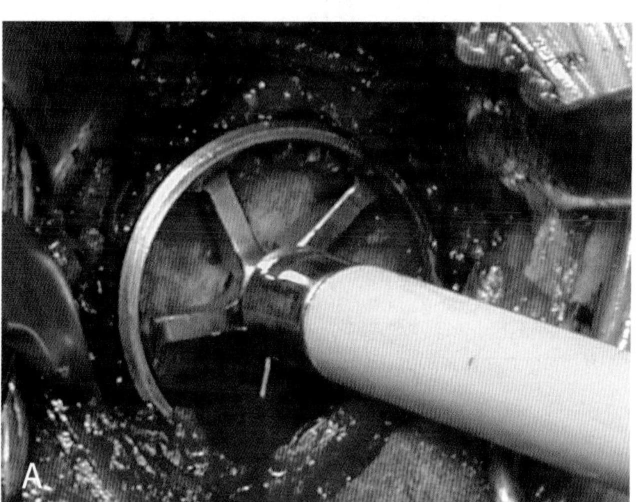

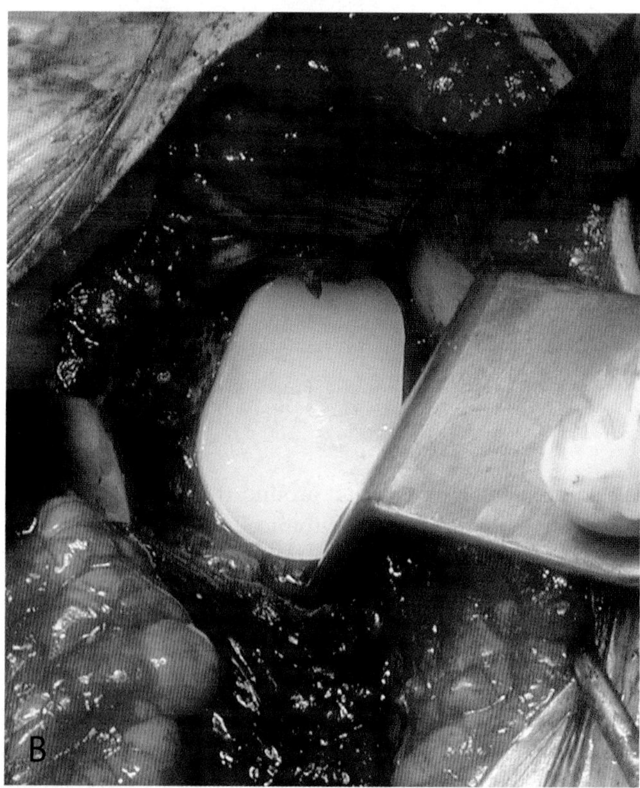

Figure 9.6 Intraoperative photographs of a right shoulder. **A**, Glenoid reamer preparing the bone surface. **B**, Polyethylene glenoid implant in place.

© 2018 American Academy of Orthopaedic Surgeons

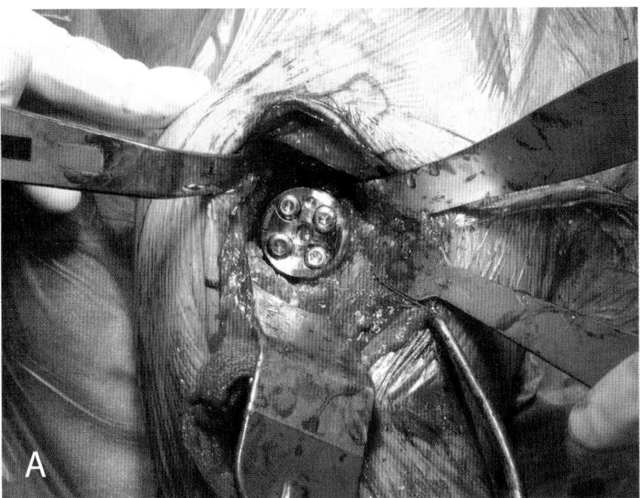

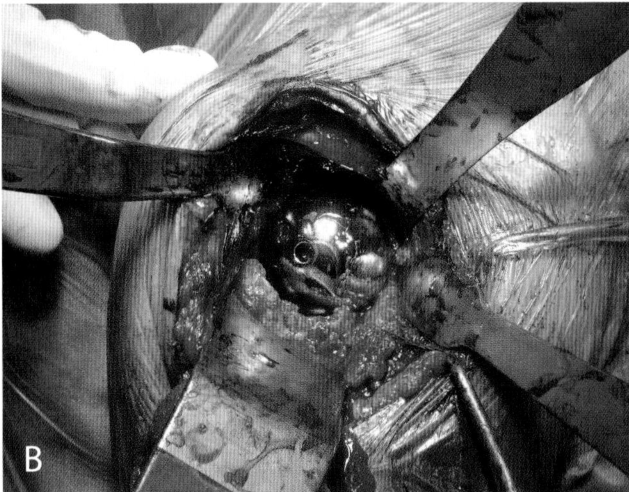

Figure 9.8 Intraoperative photographs of a right shoulder. **A**, Glenoid baseplate in position. **B**, Glenosphere implanted onto the baseplate.

the design of the specific implant. The degree of retroversion appears to be related to the implant design as well as surgeon preference, and the degree of retroversion affects the rotation that can be achieved. Greater retroversion may permit greater ER motion with diminished IR. In contrast, less retroversion has the opposite effect, with less ER but more IR. The position of the baseplate and glenosphere (Figure 9.8) is an important factor in the stability of fixation and the potential for scapular notching. The baseplate is usually positioned inferiorly on the glenoid, with a neutral or slight inferior tilt (Figure 9.9). The humeral component has a polyethylene socket and can be either cemented or press fit, depending on the specific implant design and the surgeon's preference (Figure 9.10). The shoulder is then reduced and ROM and stability are assessed.

The anterior superior deltoid splitting approach is preferred by some surgeons for reverse shoulder arthroplasty. The anterior deltoid is released from the anterior acromion

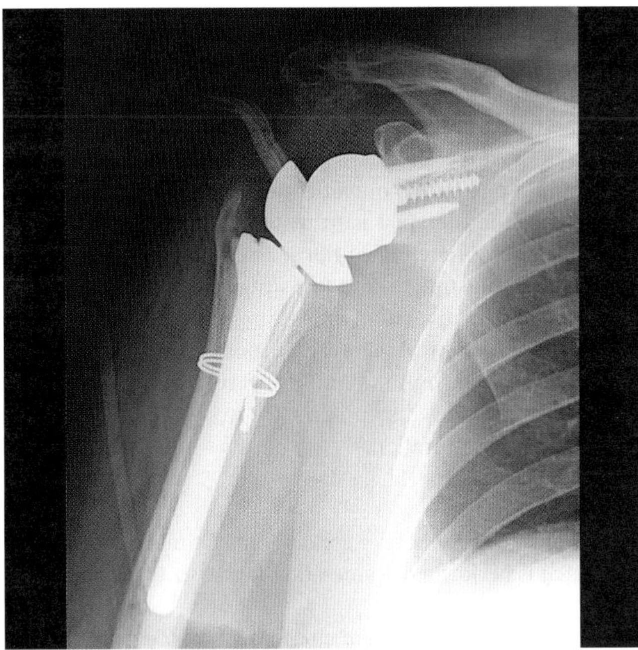

Figure 9.9 Postoperative true anterior posterior plain radiograph demonstrating positioning of the glenosphere at the inferior aspect of the native glenoid.

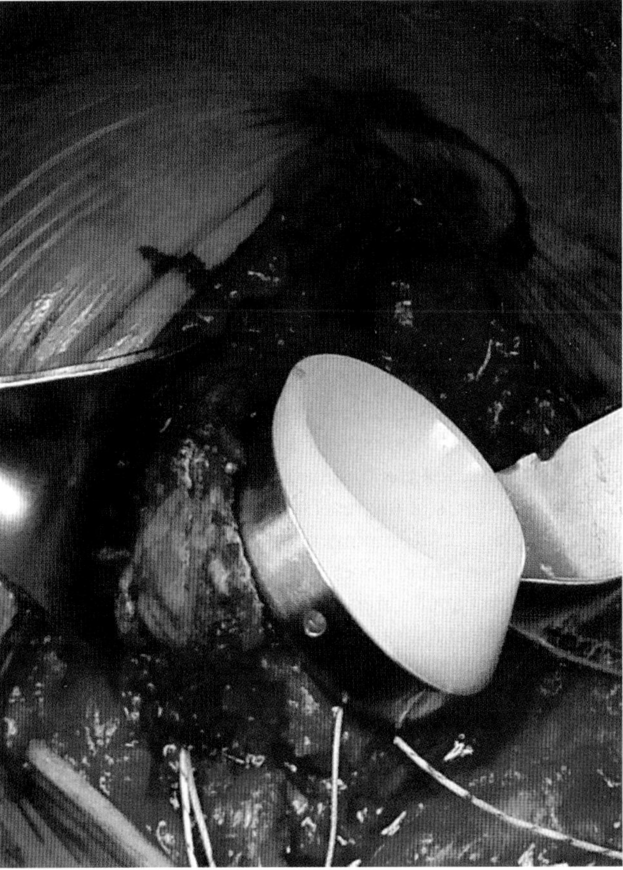

Figure 9.10 Intraoperative image of a press fit humeral component of a right reverse shoulder arthroplasty.

© 2018 American Academy of Orthopaedic Surgeons

and split laterally. Care must be taken to avoid injuring the axillary nerve when splitting the deltoid. Most surgeons are more familiar with the deltopectoral approach. In the superior approach, the deltoid must be securely repaired and the postoperative rehabilitation correspondingly modified to protect the deltoid repair.

The surgical wound is closed in layers and the arm is immobilized in a sling with an abduction cushion. The abducted position is used to direct the humeral socket against the glenosphere.

POSTOPERATIVE REHABILITATION

General Considerations

Postoperative rehabilitation is a critically important determinant of the outcome of shoulder arthroplasty. Despite this belief, there are few published references that specifically evaluate protocols and the results. Many protocols are based on Neer's original total shoulder protocol, which was published in 1975. These protocols commonly include phases that begin with early PROM exercises, a progression to AROM exercises, and later strengthening exercises and functional restoration. Considerations of tissue healing and implant stability are important in focusing the early postoperative stages.

It is important to highlight the major distinctions between anatomic and reverse shoulder arthroplasty. The most obvious is the presence or absence of a functioning rotator cuff. Rehabilitation of the rotator cuff is a critical aspect of early recovery after anatomic shoulder arthroplasty, as well as long-term functional outcome. In contrast, most shoulders that are treated with reverse arthroplasty have a deficient or poorly functioning rotator cuff; thus, rehabilitation should focus on deltoid muscle rehabilitation as well as the remaining rotator cuff. The next important difference is the effect of the implant design on stability and shoulder motion. Anatomic arthroplasty designs provide the potential for a greater arc of motion in all directions and are unconstrained, thus requiring a balanced capsule and rotator cuff for glenohumeral stability. The nature of the ball-and-socket constraint and design of the reverse arthroplasty potentially limits shoulder motion while providing increased glenohumeral stability.

Various aspects of the reverse implant design and position of the implant limit impingement-free ROM. Lateral offset glenosphere implants, lower glenosphere position, and lower humeral socket angles are associated with less scapular notching. Lateral offset may also allow greater rotational motion.

As noted earlier, healing of the subscapularis is a very important consideration in the early rehabilitation after anatomic shoulder arthroplasty. Subscapularis failure following anatomic shoulder arthroplasty is a major complication that can lead to weakness, glenohumeral instability, and poor functional outcome. A clear distinction needs to be made between acute traumatic tear and attritional failure. The former is almost always associated with poor outcome and should be repaired on an urgent basis. The latter has a more variable effect on outcome, often resulting in IR weakness, but does not preclude an overall successful outcome. Subscapularis integrity is assessed functionally by testing IR strength, and performing the belly press and the lift-off tests. Any concern for early failure should prompt evaluation with advanced imaging such as ultrasound, CT scan, or MRI.

Early implant fixation is not a major issue of concern after anatomic shoulder arthroplasty and usually does not factor into the rehabilitation. Posterior instability may be encountered in anatomic total shoulder arthroplasty; if identified intraoperatively, the early rehabilitation is directed to avoid aggravating the situation. In rare cases, a posterior capsulorraphy is performed at the time of the arthroplasty. If posterior instability is an issue, the shoulder should initially be immobilized and braced in a position of neutral or slight ER and early shoulder elevation motion should be posterior to the scapular plane to avoid overstretching the posterior capsule and rotator cuff. In addition, IR and horizontal adduction should be avoided for the first 4 weeks.

Although reverse shoulder arthroplasty is a more constrained construct than anatomic shoulder arthroplasty, glenohumeral joint stability is an important consideration in the early rehabilitation. Postoperative instability is one of the more commonly reported complications of reverse total arthroplasty. In the early postoperative course, positions that cause implant impingement, such as adduction-IR-extension are avoided. Glenohumeral instability of reverse total shoulder is more common in revision cases with scarred and stiff periarticular soft tissue, cases with complete absence of a rotator cuff, or cases with preoperative dislocation.

Authors' Preferred Protocol

Anatomic Shoulder Arthroplasty

The postoperative rehabilitation protocol begins on the morning after surgery while the patient is in the hospital. The patient is instructed by a therapist in a home exercise program that focuses on appropriate precautions and passive shoulder ROM. Most patients are discharged directly home the day after surgery. A physical or occupational therapist is also engaged in the outpatient postoperative care and rehabilitation. Patients typically attend one or two outpatient therapy sessions per week. The role of the therapist is to instruct in proper technique, reinforce appropriate precautions, assess progress, and make appropriate adjustments and transitions in the rehabilitation program. Adjunctive modalities, including analgesics and ice, are used to control pain. The major early emphasis is on regaining shoulder motion and protecting the subscapularis repair. This is followed by progressive strengthening exercises and functional restoration.

Phase I (0–6 Weeks)

- Self-assisted PROM exercises at home 5 times per day. Each stretch is performed 5 times, holding 10 to 15 seconds each repetition.
    - Unweighted pendulum circumduction (Figure 9.11)
    - Supine passive self-assisted forward elevation in the scapular plane (Figure 9.12)
    - Supine passive self-assisted ER (Figure 9.13)

 © 2018 American Academy of Orthopaedic Surgeons

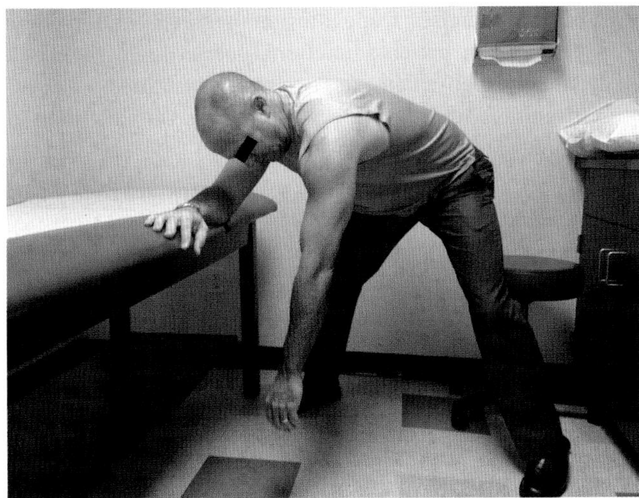

Figure 9.11 Photograph of pendulum circumduction of the left shoulder. The shoulder girdle muscles are relaxed and the arm is moved clockwise and counterclockwise with minimal muscle activity.

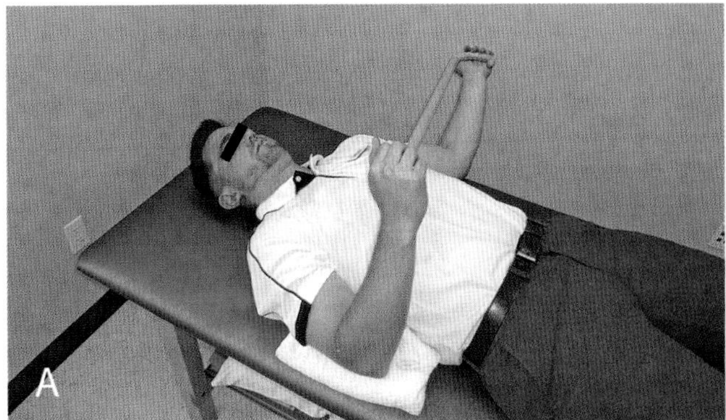

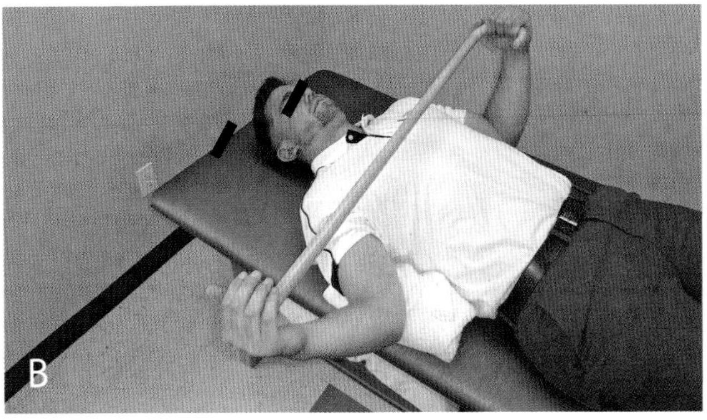

Figure 9.13 Photographs of right shoulder supine passive self-assisted external rotation. **A** is the initiation of the motion and **B** is the completion.

- Supine passive self-assisted cross-body adduction (Figure 9.14)
- Standing IR reaching behind the back assisted with a rod, unaffected upper extremity, or over the shoulder strap (Figure 9.15)
- Active-assisted elbow, forearm, wrist, and hand motion exercises are performed.
- Sling worn at all times, except during exercises. Assistance with dressing and hygiene.
- Postoperative distal extremity swelling control with elastic stockinette and arm elevation, as needed
- Cervical spine motion: AROM in flexion, extension, and rotation to maintain normal cervical mobility during the immobilization phase of recovery.
- Scapular muscle-stretching exercises for the levator scapulae and upper trapezius muscles to prevent cervical/scapular pain associated with use of the sling.
- Scapular stabilization: Active recruitment of the scapular stabilizers, including retraction and protraction, elevation, and depression to maintain neuromuscular control of the scapulothoracic muscles.

Most patients are very comfortable at 4 to 6 weeks after surgery. ROM goals for week 6 include passive forward elevation to 140°, active forward elevation above shoulder level, passive ER to 40°, and passive IR to the lower lumbar level.

Phase II (7–12 Weeks)

- Sling is discontinued; begin light activities of daily living (ADLs)

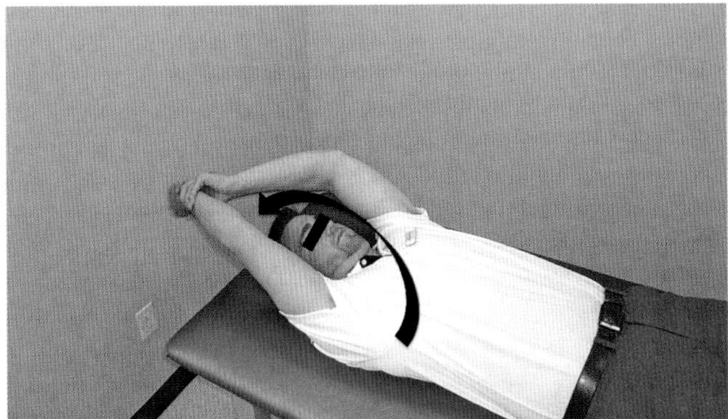

Figure 9.12 Photograph of right shoulder supine passive self-assisted forward elevation in the scapular plane (*black arrow* indicates direction and arc of motion).

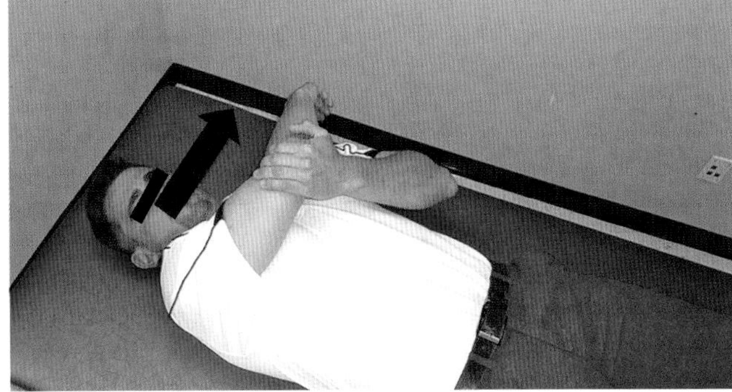

Figure 9.14 Photograph of right shoulder supine passive self-assisted cross-body adduction (*black arrow* indicates the direction of motion).

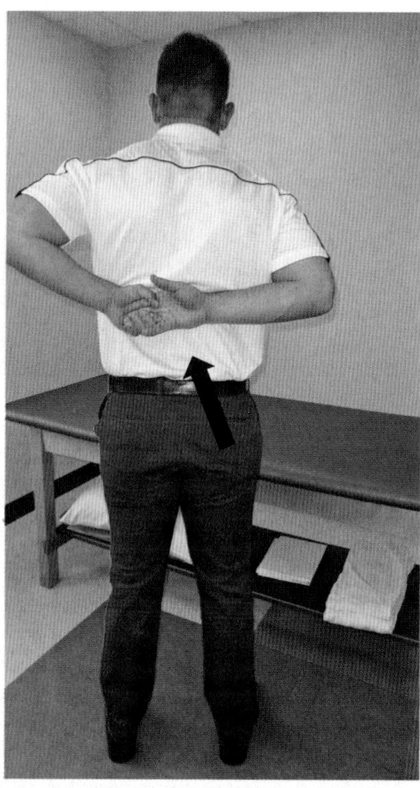

Figure 9.15 Photograph of right shoulder standing self-assisted internal rotation reaching behind the back (*black arrow* indicates the right arm being pushed upward by the left hand).

- Continue self-assisted passive shoulder motion exercises to improve and maintain shoulder motion.
- Supine active shoulder elevation initiated—reduces effect of gravity
- Overhead pulley to facilitate active elevation in the upright position
- Gentle strengthening initiated with isometric deltoid (anterior, middle, and posterior), IR and ER
- Supine deltoid exercises adapted from the Reading protocol (Figure 9.16)
- Scapular stabilization exercises. Rhythmic stabilization exercises can be performed in side-lying position once the patient demonstrates good neuromuscular control actively.
- Advanced exercises: Depending on the sophistication of the patient and the patient's functional goals. Closed-chain and eventually open-chain exercises can be instituted.
- Active use is advanced during this phase, with attention to avoiding excessive resistance.

The goals for ROM after 12 weeks are active elevation above 140°, active ER greater than 45°, and IR to upper lumbar level. Although there is clearly variation in the final ROM, these are very reasonable goals for the majority of patients with primary glenohumeral osteoarthritis.

Phase III (After 12 Weeks)

- Stretching exercises continued to optimize shoulder motion
- Isotonic strengthening with elastic resistance bands and light weights

The overall goal is for the patient to be very comfortable and functional after 3 months. The maximal outcome after anatomic shoulder arthroplasty can take up to 1 year to achieve (Figure 9.17).

Phase IV: Advanced Function and Recreational Activities

- Exercises tailored to specific functional demands and expectations

Many patients have goals and expectations that include physical, recreational, and athletic activities. McCarty and coworkers reported that 64% of patients who participated in sports or recreation before arthroplasty had surgery to be able to participate in sports or recreation. Similarly, Zarkadas and coworkers reported that 89% of total shoulder arthroplasty patients and 77% of humeral head replacement (HHR) patients participated in medium and high-demand activities and sports after arthroplasty. Advancing patients to more demanding or complex activities requires satisfactory ROM and restoration of strength. The subscapularis repair should have sufficient healing at 3 to 4 months after surgery to allow functional progression with minimal risk of failure. Because glenoid failure is the primary long-term concern of anatomic total shoulder arthroplasty, we recommend refraining from heavy lifting and impact activities. Activities such as golf, tennis, swimming, bowling, and moderate yard work are considered acceptable.

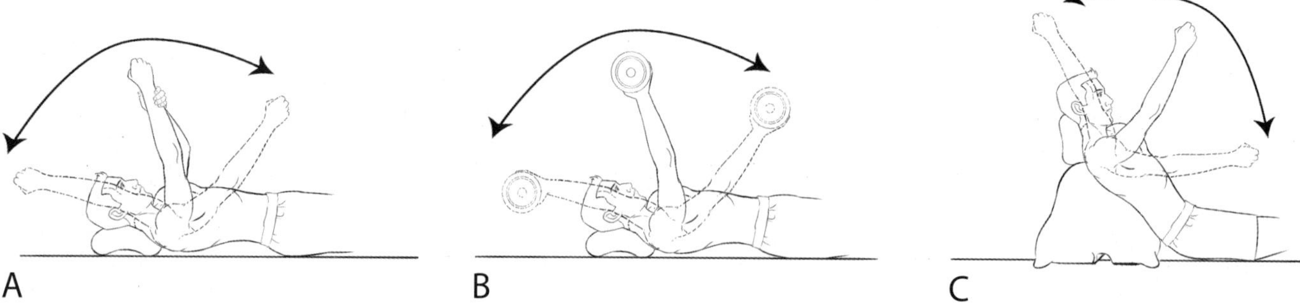

Figure 9.16 Illustrations of shoulder exercises that emphasize anterior deltoid strengthening. **A**, The exercises are initiated in the supine position without weights. **B**, With improvement in comfort and strength, a hand-held weight is added. **C**, With further improvements, the exercise is progressed from flat supine to inclined to a fully upright position.

© 2018 American Academy of Orthopaedic Surgeons

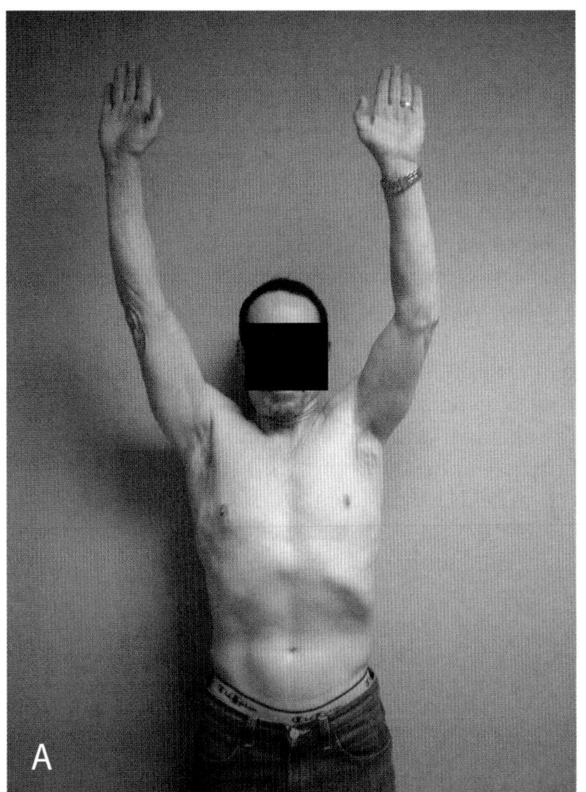

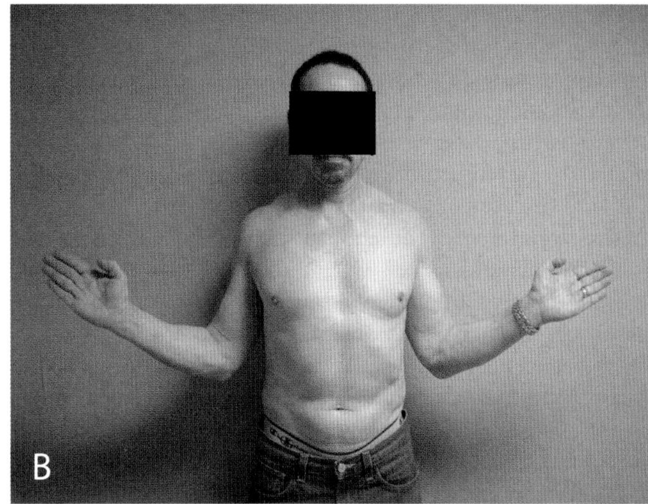

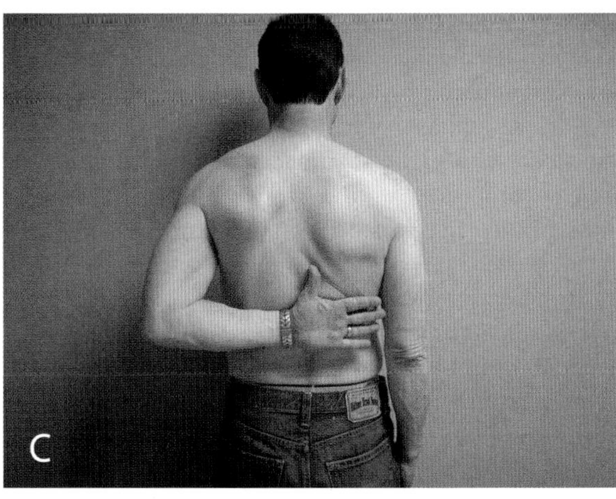

Figure 9.17 Postoperative photographs of a patient who had a left anatomic total shoulder to treat glenohumeral osteoarthritis. **A**, Active forward elevation. **B**, Active external rotation. **C**, Internal rotation.

Reverse Total Shoulder Arthroplasty

Postoperative rehabilitation begins in the hospital prior to discharge. As with anatomic total shoulder replacement, there are few published references that address specific rehabilitation protocols and the effect on outcome of reverse total shoulder arthroplasty. Factors that can affect postoperative outcome include quality and functional status of the remaining rotator cuff, the type of prosthesis design (lateral vs. medial center of rotation; low- vs. high-angle humeral socket), and preoperative functional status. The key concepts when formulating a postoperative rehabilitation course for reverse total shoulder arthroplasty include protecting the joint from dislocation, improving deltoid function, and managing patient expectations. The potential ROM, especially IR and ER, after reverse shoulder arthroplasty is less than anatomic arthroplasty. Implants with built-in lateral offset of the center of rotation, or reverse shoulder arthroplasty performed with glenoid interposition bone graft, have the potential for greater rotational motion. Patients with remaining functioning posterior cuff, including the teres minor, will have better active ER motion as well as ER strength. Patients with weak or absent ER strength may have substantial functional limitations.

Phase I (0–6 Weeks)

- Sling with small abduction cushion worn at all times, except during therapy exercises
- Assistance with dressing and hygiene activities
- Unweighted pendulum circumduction exercises

© 2018 American Academy of Orthopaedic Surgeons

- Passive self-assisted scapular plane elevation and ER with elbow at the side if there is repaired subscapularis and good posterior rotator cuff
- Active shoulder motion is not permitted
- Active-assisted elbow, forearm, wrist, hand, and finger motion to prevent stiffness
- Cervical spine (same as anatomic total shoulder)
- Active recruitment of the scapular stabilizers (same as anatomic total shoulder)
- Dislocation precautions: Avoid using the arm to assist in getting up from a seated position, and avoid adduction-IR-extension positions
- Week 5: Begin passive self-assisted ROM exercises in supine scapular plane forward elevation, supine ER, supine horizontal adduction, and standing IR reaching behind the back.
- If a deltoid-splitting approach is used, greater care and attention is directed at protecting the deltoid repair. Delay active deltoid exercises.
- Most patients are very comfortable at 4 to 6 weeks after surgery.
- Passive forward elevation should be greater than 90° and ER beyond neutral.
- Patients are often able to actively elevate above shoulder level.

Phase II (Weeks 7–12)

- Discontinue sling and begin light active use.
- Initiate active shoulder elevation in the supine position to reduce the effect of gravity.
- Progress ROM in all directions.
- Overhead pulleys to facilitate active elevation
- Isometric exercises for the deltoid, IR and ER
- Supine deltoid strengthening
- Scapular stabilization exercises

Phase III (Beyond Week 12)

- Stretching exercises are continued to maximize shoulder motion. Do not force IR stretching.
- Progress resistance exercises with elastic bands and light weights
- Open chain strengthening of the deltoid, IR and ER.

Most patients are comfortable and functional after 3 months, with the final results being achieved around 12 months (Figure 9.18). The ROM goals remain variable and relate to the implant and underlying pathology. Patients with cuff tear arthropathy or massive cuff tear without arthritis can expect active elevation of 120° or greater and active ER of 20°. Patients with reverse shoulder arthroplasty for fracture sequelae or revision shoulder arthroplasty may have more limited motion.

Phase IV: Advanced Function and Recreational Activities

- Exercises tailored to specific functional demands and expectations.

Most of the early experience with reverse shoulder arthroplasty has been with elderly individuals with somewhat limited functional goals and expectations. More recent expansion of the indications for reverse shoulder arthroplasty will lead to the same questions about advanced functions that are addressed regarding anatomic arthroplasty. Golant and coworkers surveyed shoulder surgeons about recommendations for return to athletic activity and found that while 59% percent of the respondents would allow low-impact sports without limitations after anatomic arthroplasty, only 26% would allow low-impact sports without limitations after reverse shoulder arthroplasty. Magnussen and co-workers also surveyed shoulder specialists about activity restrictions and similarly reported greater restrictions after reverse shoulder arthroplasty. In contrast, Lawrence and coworkers surveyed patients after reverse shoulder arthroplasty and reported that 80% percent participated in medium- or high-demand activities, similar to what patients with anatomic total shoulder reported.

Because the nature of the design of reverse total shoulder limits the amount of rotational motion that can be achieved, there may be some limitations of advanced functions. The constrained design most probably results in different stress transfer to the implants, which may have significant implications for long-term durability of the glenosphere and glenoid baseplate, as well as polyethylene wear.

Complications of Shoulder Arthoplasty

Although a variety of complications are reported after total shoulder arthroplasty, they are relatively uncommon. While some are easily managed and have little effect on outcome, others are more serious and may necessitate altering the postoperative management. Reverse shoulder arthroplasty is associated with higher complication rates than anatomic shoulder arthroplasty.

Intraoperative periprosthetic humeral fractures are rare and reported to occur in 1.5% of shoulder arthroplasty. Although many are nondisplaced or minimally displaced, some—especially humeral shaft fractures—may require supplemental internal fixation. In the ideal situation, the fracture is either stable or is rendered stable. The stability of the fracture may warrant adjustment in the postoperative rehabilitation to ensure uneventful healing of the fracture.

Upper trunk brachial plexopathy is the most common postoperative nerve injury associated with shoulder arthroplasty. In the majority of cases, there is complete or near-complete recovery. Axillary nerve injury is less common but has a poorer prognosis. Aside from requiring prolonged sling support in cases with delayed recovery, the initial postoperative rehabilitation should not be modified in the presence of nerve injury. ROM exercises are maintained to regain motion and prevent stiffness. Persistent weakness can delay later phases of recovery.

Although early postoperative infection is relatively uncommon after shoulder arthroplasty, it is important to recognize the early signs of infection. Beyond the obvious local signs of swelling, erythema, and drainage, persistent pain and stiffness are more subtle signs of periprosthetic infection and should be noted.

Although rotator cuff failure is a potential late problem after anatomic total shoulder arthroplasty, early subscapularis

 © 2018 American Academy of Orthopaedic Surgeons

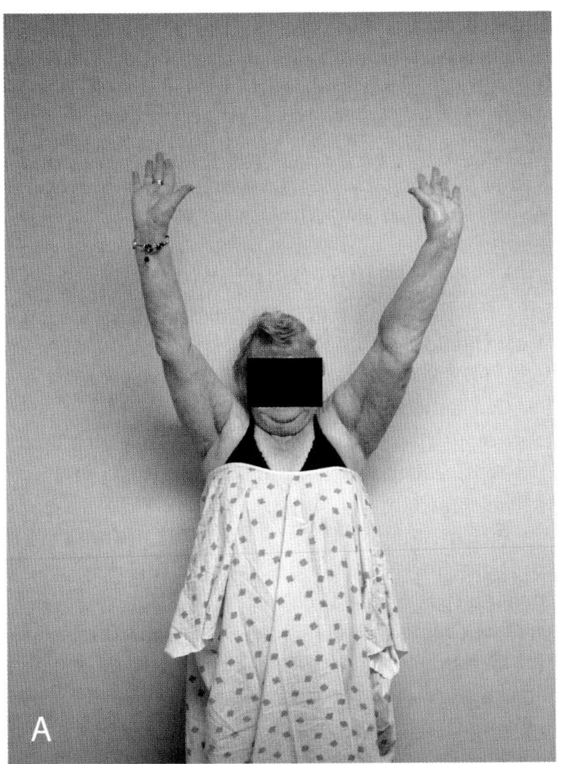

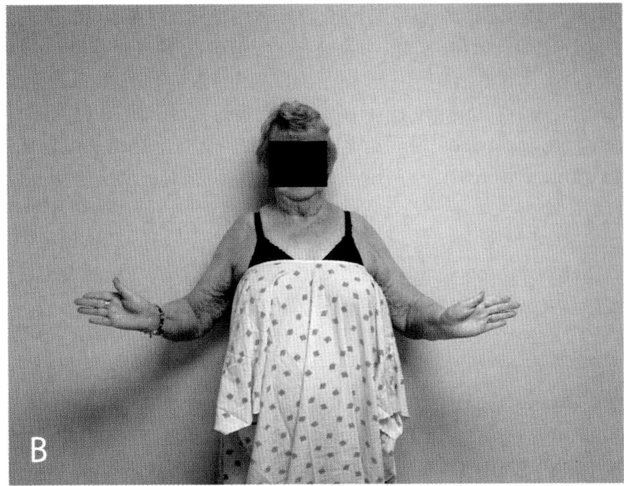

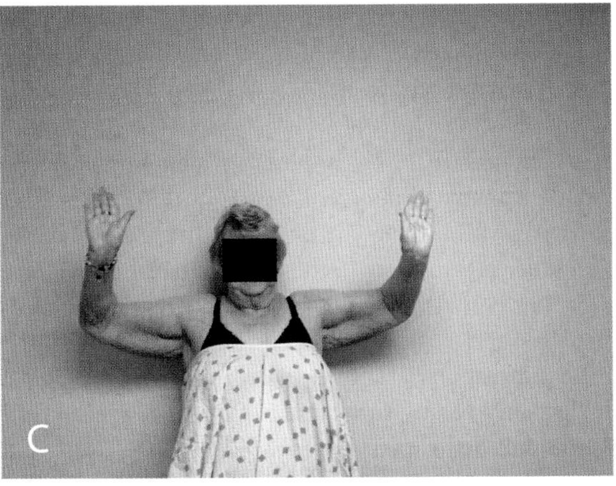

Figure 9.18 Postoperative clinical images of a patient who had rotator cuff tear arthropathy treated with bilateral reverse shoulder arthroplasty. **A**, Active forward elevation. **B**, Active external rotation. **C**, Active abduction and external rotation.

failure should not be overlooked or ignored. Early subscapularis failure is usually the result of a traumatic injury or a noncompliant patient. Postoperative trauma should be evaluated with advanced imaging (ultrasound, CT scan, or MRI) to rule out subscapsularis disruption. Avoidance of early active use of the extremity is essential to protect the subscapularis repair.

Postoperative dislocation is relatively uncommon after anatomic shoulder arthroplasty. If it occurs, evaluation for rotator cuff tear is mandatory. Instability is more commonly reported after reverse shoulder arthroplasty, which appears to be more common after revision cases and primary cases performed for posttraumatic sequelae. Substantial changes in function and ROM after reverse shoulder arthroplasty should be investigated with plain radiographs. Although the majority of cases of dislocation after reverse shoulder arthroplasty can be treated with closed reduction, some will require revision surgery.

Acromial fracture is unique to reverse shoulder arthroplasty, and can occur spontaneously as well as with trauma. Patients with prior acromioplasty or preexisting acromial erosion are at increased risk for acromial fracture. Patients usually report new-onset pain at rest and with attempted shoulder elevation. Treatment is difficult, and there can be a substantial effect on functional outcome.

Evidence and Outcomes

Numerous studies report high success rates for both anatomic and reverse total shoulder arthroplasty, with substantial and significant improvements in pain, shoulder motion, and functional outcomes. The effects of specific aspects of postoperative rehabilitation have not been well studied. Although the importance of rehabilitation after shoulder arthroplasty is universally acknowledged, the role of formal supervised physical

© 2018 American Academy of Orthopaedic Surgeons

therapy remains controversial. Most published rehabilitation protocols are structured and require supervision of a physical therapist. Boardman et al evaluated the 2-year outcome of a home-based therapy program. The patients had several sessions with a physical therapist prior to discharge from the hospital, and a follow-up session at 5 weeks postoperatively to get instructions for new exercises. They reported that 70% of all patients (85% with osteoarthritis) achieved elevation within 20° of that obtained intraoperatively, whereas 90% achieved final ER within 20° of the intraoperative motion. Mulieri and coworkers compared the effectiveness of a standard formal physical therapy program to a home-based, physician-guided program after anatomic total shoulder arthroplasty, and did not find any statistically significant differences in final outcome.

The recent focus on the concepts of cost-effectiveness and value in musculoskeletal care will likely lead to further assessment of the role of rehabilitation in the outcome of shoulder arthroplasty. Limitations on available financial resources will also promote utilization of alternative methods to instruct patients and monitor their progress. Regardless of future changes, the outcome of shoulder arthroplasty is highly dependent on the postoperative rehabilitation.

PEARLS

- Differentiate between anatomic and reverse shoulder arthroplasty.
- Subscapularis repair is protected during early rehabilitation.
- ROM gains are achieved with passive stretching exercises.
- Delay active use and shoulder strengthening until early soft-tissue healing to prevent subscapularis disruption.
- Patient participation and independence are critically important to outcome.
- Identify signs of complications, including nerve injury, subscapularis failure, and infection.

SUMMARY

Regardless of the indications for surgery, shoulder arthroplasty consistently provides patients with pain relief and functional improvement. The importance of postoperative rehabilitation is universally recognized. It is critically important that the surgeon, therapist, and patient understand the rational for treatment, surgical procedure, and the principles of postoperative rehabilitation in order to ensure the optimal outcome of treatment.

BIBLIOGRAPHY

Boardman ND 3rd, Cofield RH, Bengston KA, Little R, Jones MC, Rowland CM: Rehabilitation after total shoulder arthroplasty. *J Arthroplasty* 2001;16:483–486.

Boileau P, Sinnerton RJ, Chuinard C, Walch G: Arthroplasty of the shoulder: Review article. *Bone Joint Surg Br* 2006;88-B:562–575.

Boileau P, Watkinson D, Hatzidakis AM, Hovorka I: Neer Award 2005. The Grammont reverse shoulder prosthesis: Results in cuff tear arthritis, fracture sequelae, and revision arthroplasty. *J Shoulder Elbow Surg* 2006;15:527–540.

Boudreau S, Boudreau E, Higgins LD, Wilcox RB 3rd: Rehabilitation following reverse total shoulder arthroplasty. *J Orthop Sports Phys Ther* 2007:37:734–743.

Brems JJ: Rehabilitation following total shoulder arthroplasty. *Clin Orthop Relat Res* 1994;(307):70–85.

Brown DD, Friedman RJ: Postoperative rehabilitation following total shoulder arthroplasty. *Orthop Clin North Am* 1998;29:535–547.

Gerber C, Yian EH, Pfirrmann CA, Zumstein MA, Werner CM: Subscapularis muscle function and structure after total shoulder replacement with lesser tuberosity osteotomy and repair. *J Bone Joint Surg Am* 2005;87-A:1739–1745.

Golant A, Christoforou D, Zuckerman JD, Kwon YW: Return to sports after shoulder arthroplasty: a survey of surgeons' preferences. *J Shoulder Elbow Surg* 2012;21:554–560.

Gutierrez S, Comiskey CA 4th, Luo ZP, Pupello DR, Frankle MA: Range of impingement-free abduction and adduction deficit after reverse shoulder arthroplasty hierarchy of surgical and implant-design-related factors. *J Bone Joint Surg Am* 2008;90:2606–2615.

Harryman DT, Sidles JA, Harris SL, Lippitt SB, Matsen FA 3rd: The effect of articular conformity and the size of the humeral head component on laxity and motion after glenohumeral arthroplasty: a study in cadavers. *J Bone Joint Surg Am* 1995;77-A:555–563.

Jobe CM, Iannotti JP: Limits imposed on glenohumeral motion by joint geometry. *J Shoulder Elbow Surg* 1995;4:281–285.

Kim SH,Wise BL, Zhang Y, Szabo RM: Increasing incidence of shoulder arthroplasty in the United States. *J Bone Joint Surg Am* 2011;93(24):2249–2254.

Lapner PL, Sabri E, Rakhra K, Bell K, Athwal GS: Healing rates and subscapularis fatty infiltration after lesser tuberosity osteotomy versus subscapularis peel for exposure during shoulder arthroplasty. *J Shoulder Elbow Surg* 2013;22:396–402.

Lawrence TM, Ahmadi S, Sanchez-Sotelo J, Sperling JW, Cofield RH: Patient reported activities after reverse shoulder arthroplasty: Part II. *J Shoulder Elbow Surg* 2012;21:1464–1469.

Magnussen RA, Mallon WJ, Willems WJ, Moorman CT 3rd: Long-term activity restrictions after shoulder arthroplasty: an international survey of experienced shoulder surgeons. *J Shoulder Elbow Surg* 2011;20:281–289.

McCarty EC, Marx RG, Maerz D, Altchek D, Warren RF: Sports participation after shoulder replacement surgery. *Am J Sports Med* 2008;36:1577–1581.

Miller SL, Hazrati Y, Klepps S, Chiang A, Flatow EL: Loss of subscapularis function after total shoulder replacement: a seldom recognized problem. *J Shoulder Elbow Surg* 2003;12(1):29–34.

Mulieri PJ, Holcomb JO, Dunning P, Pliner M, Bogle RK, Pupello D, Frankle MA: Is a formal physical therapy program necessary after total shoulder arthroplasty for osteoarthritis? *J Shoulder Elbow Surg* 2010;19:570–579.

© 2018 American Academy of Orthopaedic Surgeons

Neer CS 2nd: Replacement arthroplasty for glenohumeral arthritis. *J Bone Joint Surg Am* 1974;56:1–13.

Saltzman MD, Chamberlain AM, Mercer DM, Warme WJ, Bertelsen AL, Matsen FA 3rd: Shoulder hemiarthroplasty with concentric glenoid reaming in patients 55 years old or less. *J Shoulder Elbow Surg* 2011;20:609–615.

Werner CM, Steinmann PA, Gilbart M, Gerber C: Treatment of painful pseudoparesis due to irreparable rotator cuff dysfunction with Delta III reverse-ball-and-socket total shoulder prosthesis. *J Bone and Joint Surg Am* 2005;87-A:1476–1486.

Wilcox RB, Arslanian LE, Millett PJ: Rehabilitation following total shoulder arthroplasty. *J Orthop Sports Phys Ther* 2005; 35:821–836.

Wirth MA: Humeral head arthroplasty and meniscal allograft resurfacing of the glenoid. *J Bone Joint Surg Am* 2009; 91:1109–1119.

Zarkadas PC, Throckmorton TQ, Dahm DL, Sperling J, Schleck CD, Cofield R: Patient reported activities after shoulder replacement: total and hemiarthroplasty. *J Shoulder Elbow Surg* 2011;20:273–280.

© 2018 American Academy of Orthopaedic Surgeons

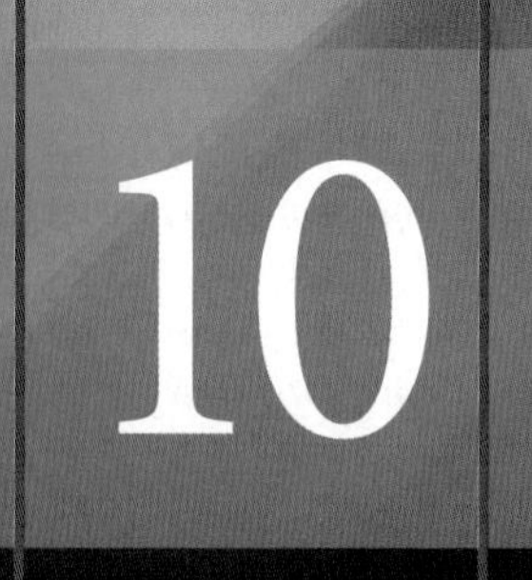

10 Proximal Humerus Fractures

Surena Namdari, MD, MSc, and Gerald R. Williams, Jr, MD

INTRODUCTION

Fractures of the proximal humerus are relatively common injuries, accounting for 5% of all fractures. The incidence increases rapidly with age, with more than 70% of proximal humerus fractures occurring in patients older than 60 years of age. Upper extremity fractures can considerably limit independence and function in an elderly individual, and may lead to a permanent move to a nursing home in 6% of patients. The male-to-female gender ratio for proximal humerus fractures has been estimated at 3:7. Approximately 20% to 50% of proximal humerus fractures are displaced or unstable. Given the risks of malunion and nonunion, the preference in unstable fracture patterns is for surgical intervention to reduce fracture fragments and generate the stability necessary for early motion. Despite this, nonoperative treatment for displaced fractures may be indicated for low-demand or medically debilitated patients. Some patients who undergo nonoperative treatment of a displaced proximal humerus fracture can achieve satisfactory pain relief and very functional results; however, the results may be less predictable than anatomic reconstruction.

While many options for fixation exist, the selected treatment must be able to withstand the loads placed on the proximal humerus while motion is initiated and fracture healing is taking place. The rotator cuff, deltoid, pectoralis major, latissimus, and teres major muscles invoke substantial deforming forces on the fracture fragments of the proximal humerus. The combination of multiple deforming forces and poor bone quality can lead to complications, including fracture malunion, hardware failure, and a poor clinical result. Possible fixation techniques include locked plating, percutaneous fixation with screws and pins, intramedullary nailing, and external fixation. Hemiarthroplasty and reverse arthroplasty are both used as treatment options for proximal humerus fractures that are not amenable to nonoperative treatment or surgical fixation. Arthroplasty can be technically challenging, requiring anatomic placement of the prosthesis and anatomic healing of the tuberosities to achieve an optimal functional result. Rehabilitation following surgical management of the proximal humerus is similar, regardless of the type of surgical procedure, and is dependent on achieving stable fixation. In this chapter, we will discuss the surgical treatment of proximal humerus fractures with an emphasis on surgical details that facilitate rehabilitation.

SURGICAL PROCEDURES

Locked Plate Fixation

Indications

Locked plating can be utilized for all fractures that meet the indications for operative treatment as outlined by Neer (angulation of the articular surface of >45° or displacement of >1 cm between the major fracture segments) or are unstable. Locked plating provides for enhanced axial stability of the fracture fixation. The determination of whether a fracture is amenable to surgical fixation or is better suited for arthroplasty is controversial and based on multiple variables, including age, activity level, bone quality, comminution, and

Dr. Namdari or an immediate family member has received royalties from DJ Orthopaedics and Miami Device Solutions; is a member of a speakers' bureau or has made paid presentations on behalf of DJ Orthopaedics; serves as a paid consultant to DJ Orthopaedics, Integra Life Sciences, and Miami Device Solutions; has received research or institutional support from Arthrex, Integra, and Zimmer; has received nonincome support (such as equipment or services), commercially derived honoraria, or other non-research–related funding (such as paid travel) from Saunders/Mosby-Elsevier; and serves as a board member, owner, officer, or committee member of the American Journal of Orthopedics and the Bone & Joint 360. *Dr. Williams or an immediate family member has received royalties from DePuy, A Johnson & Johnson Company, DJ Orthopaedics, and IMDS; has stock or stock options held in CrossCurrent Business Analytics, Force Therapeutics, ForMD, In Vivo Therapeutics, and OBERD; has received research or institutional support from DePuy, A Johnson & Johnson Company, Synthasome, and Tornier; and has received nonincome support (such as equipment or services), commercially derived honoraria, or other non-research–related funding (such as paid travel) from Wolters Kluwer Health–Lippincott Williams & Wilkins.*

© 2018 American Academy of Orthopaedic Surgeons

fracture displacement. In general, locked plating is indicated in two-part surgical neck fractures (especially those with medial comminution), three-part fractures, and selected four-part fractures (patients under the age of 50). Minimally invasive osteosynthesis techniques, such as percutaneous pin or screw fixation, are less rigid forms of fixation and are not generally performed in cases of substantial calcar comminution or fracture displacement.

Contraindications

Contraindications to locked plating include active infection, irreducible fractures, and medically unstable patients. Elderly patients with severe comminution of the humeral head or tuberosities and poor bone quality are often better treated with arthroplasty.

Procedure

A deltopectoral or anterolateral (deltoid-split) exposure can be used to expose the proximal humerus. In both procedures, we routinely identify and protect the axillary nerve. Rehabilitation protocol is not affected by the approach utilized. We prefer a deltopectoral approach. After development of the deltopectoral interval, the biceps is routinely tenodesed to the upper border of the pectoralis major and is resected proximal to this tenodesis site. Heavy nonabsorbable sutures are placed in the subscapularis, supraspinatus, and infraspinatus tendons at the myotendinous junction to control fracture fragments. Sutures are placed in the stronger rotator cuff tendons rather than through the soft bone of the tuberosities to improve fixation strength. Secure tuberosity fixation is among the most important factors that allow early rehabilitation. A low-profile proximal humeral locking plate with angular stable locking screws and suture eyelets is selected to provide fracture fixation (Figure 10.1). A provisional reduction of the surgical neck and humeral head fragment can be obtained using blunt elevators or joysticks and held with Kirschner wires. The tuberosities are reduced via the traction sutures with minimal manipulation and impaction of the cancellous bone underlying the tuberosities. The plate is secured to the humeral head and/or the shaft using Kirschner wires. The initial screw

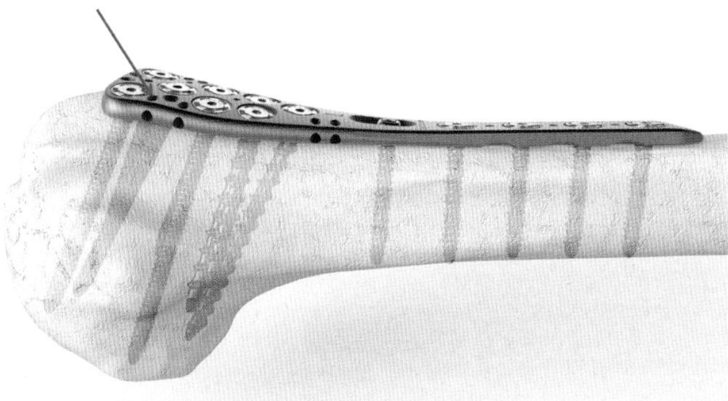

Figure 10.1 Illustration of low-profile proximal humeral locking plate (Miami Device Solutions, Miami, FL) with angular stable locking screws and suture eyelets (red arrow).

should be diaphyseal, bicortical, and nonlocking. This allows compression of the plate against the humeral shaft and allows subsequent reduction of the tuberosities to the shaft via the plate. It is critical not to reduce a fracture in internal rotation, as this will limit the patient's ability to regain functional external rotation postoperatively. To ensure that this does not occur, reduction and plating are performed with the arm in 30° of external rotation. In addition, the biceps groove can be identified in the proximal fragment and in the distal shaft, and can be used as a guide to reduction alignment. Plate height should be confirmed fluoroscopically so that the plate is not too proximal to impinge with shoulder abduction. Similarly, if using a plate with fixed-angled locking screws, accurate plate position ensures the correct location and trajectory for the inferior humeral head screw(s), which is critical to the stability of the construct. Once plate position is confirmed, fixation into the head is performed with five or more locking screws. Care is taken to avoid intra-articular screw penetration. In general, three nonlocking, bicortical screws are placed in the humeral shaft. Finally, separate tuberosity sutures are passed through the plate eyelets and tied. Ideally, a superior suture is placed for the supraspinatus tendon, an anterior suture for the subscapularis, and a posterior suture for the infraspinatus tendon. The augmentation of fixation constructs with intramedullary fibular grafts, calcium phosphate or sulfate cement, and/or cancellous bone chips is determined subjectively at the time of the procedure and is dictated primarily by the bone quality. Multiple fluoroscopic views are utilized to ensure that screws have not violated the glenohumeral joint.

Complications

Complications of proximal humeral locking plate fixation include malreduction, intra-articular screw penetration, primary screw cutout and loss of reduction, malunion, nonunion, avascular necrosis, and infection. A typical failure mode involves loss of fixation in the humeral head, varus collapse of the head fragment, and screw cutout (Figure 10.2). Screw cutout and intra-articular screw penetration can result in rapid glenoid destruction and need for arthroplasty. Excessive superior plate placement can result in pain and motion limitation from acromial impingement. Alternatively, excessively inferior plate placement can result in inadequate fixation in the humeral head and/or ineffective buttress fixation of the greater tuberosity fragment. Overly aggressive rehabilitation may result in fixation failure. Therefore, the timing and intensity of rehabilitation should be adjusted based on bone quality and stability of fixation.

Arthroplasty

Indications

Arthroplasty is indicated in proximal humerus fractures that are not amenable to surgical fixation. This includes certain three-part and four-part fractures, fracture-dislocations, and head-splitting fractures. The decision to proceed with arthroplasty is dependent on multiple patient-specific and

© 2018 American Academy of Orthopaedic Surgeons

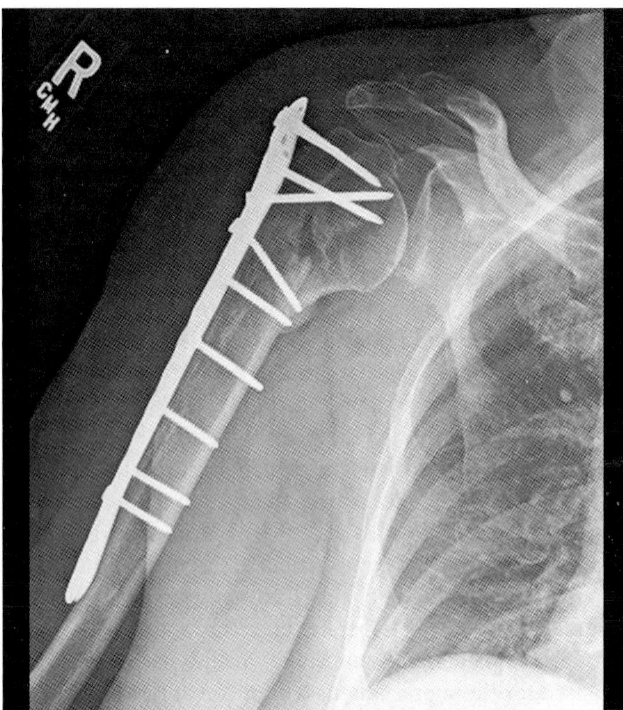

Figure 10.2 Plain radiograph of example of a failed proximal humerus ORIF with varus collapse of the head segment and screw cutout.

fracture-specific factors, including patient age, activity level, medical comorbidities, expectations of treatment, fracture pattern, displacement, bone quality, comminution, and chronicity of the injury. Indications for reverse arthroplasty versus hemiarthroplasty are controversial. In general, reverse arthroplasty is indicated in selected patients over the age of 70 or in patients younger than 70 with pre-existing rotator cuff tears, extreme tuberosity comminution, or poor bone quality. Although the popularity of hemiarthroplasty has decreased as the use of reverse arthroplasty has increased, there remains a role for hemiarthroplasty in younger patients (over 50 and under 70 years of age) whose fractures cannot be reduced and fixed adequately (Figure 10.3).

Contraindications

Contraindications to arthroplasty include active infection, medically unstable patients, and those with neurologic deficits that would preclude shoulder function and/or implant stability.

Procedure

The surgical techniques for hemiarthroplasty (humeral head replacement) and reverse arthroplasty are similar, especially regarding management of the tuberosities.

The procedure is performed via a standard deltopectoral approach. The pectoralis major insertion is identified so that it can be used to confirm accurate head placement. The long head of the biceps tendon is identified in its sheath and traced proximal through the rotator interval, and released from its intra-articular origin. It is tenodesed routinely to the upper border of the pectoralis major, and is resected proximal to this tenodesis site. A heavy, nonabsorbable suture is placed through the bone–tendon junction of each of the greater and lesser tuberosity fracture fragments. Care is taken to preserve as much of the periosteal connection between the fragments and the shaft as possible. Next, the humeral head is excised. Any

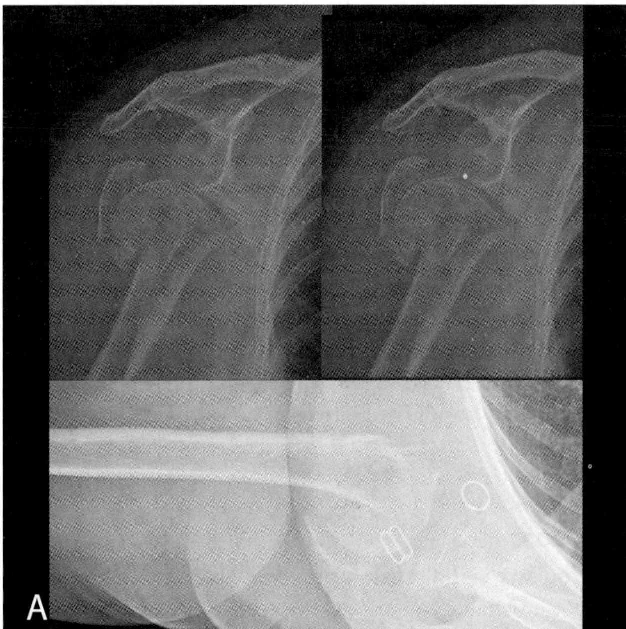

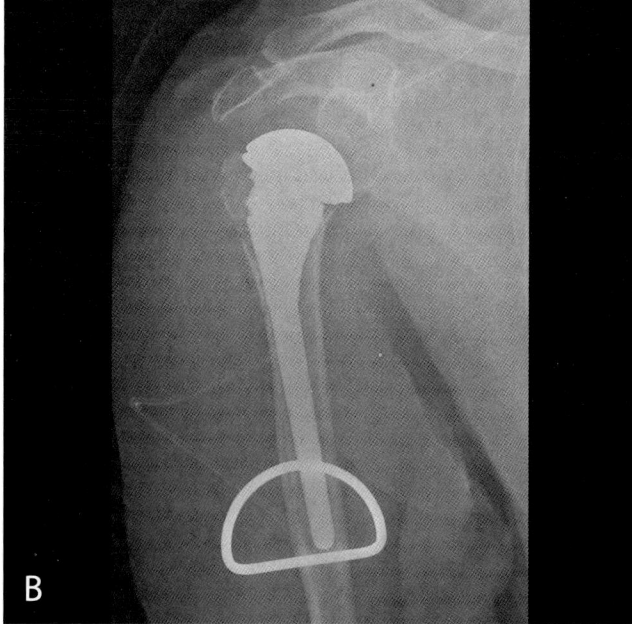

Figure 10.3 **A**, Plain radiograph of proximal humerus fracture with displacement of the greater tuberosity, lesser tuberosity, and impaction of the humeral head. **B**, Plain radiograph of hemiarthroplasty with anatomic reduction of the greater tuberosity fragment.

© 2018 American Academy of Orthopaedic Surgeons

remaining head, often attached to the tuberosities, is resected so that the residual head does not interfere with tuberosity reduction. Cancellous bone from the humeral head is used for bone grafting of the tuberosities. Prior to preparing the humerus for implant placement, the glenoid is visualized to determine if any concomitant pathology exists. The baseplate and glenosphere are placed at this time when reverse arthroplasty is indicated.

The specific steps for humeral bone preparation, prosthetic placement, and tuberosity reduction and fixation are dependent on the prosthetic design used. Once the humerus is prepared, a trial stem is placed in the proper version and height. Cementless fixation may be possible in the absence of substantial calcar comminution, but cement is often required to provide component stability. The head size is determined by measuring the excised head. The humerus is reduced and the tuberosities are reduced to the implant using the previously placed traction sutures. Fluoroscopy is then used to evaluate stem height, tuberosity-to-head distance, and reduction of the greater tuberosity to the shaft. Ideally, the greater tuberosity is either reduced anatomically to the shaft or overlaps it slightly, and the head-to-tuberosity distance is approximately 1 cm. When implant position is confirmed, trial components are removed and the final components are impacted into position. Cement is utilized in cases in which there is medial calcar comminution or adequate stability for cementless fixation is not present.

Anatomic and secure tuberosity fixation is a critical part of the procedure. In general, heavy, nonabsorbable sutures are passed in horizontal cerclage configurations around and/or through holes in the prosthesis and from the greater to the lesser tuberosity at the bone–tendon junction. Similarly, heavy, nonabsorbable sutures are passed in vertical tension-band configurations from the bone–tendon junction of the tuberosities and through drill holes in the humeral shaft. Cancellous bone from the excised humeral head is placed under the tuberosity repair. Sutures are tied securely; however, overtightening should be avoided so that the tuberosities are not overreduced. Final tuberosity position is confirmed on fluoroscopy. The shoulder is taken through a gentle range of motion (ROM) to ensure that the tuberosities and prosthesis move as a single unit and to determine limits of early motion for postoperative rehabilitation. A deep surgical drain is placed and a layered closure is undertaken.

Complications

Aside from typical postoperative complications, hemiarthroplasty can be affected by technical and biologic failures. Technical failures involve tuberosity malreduction, oversized or undersized humeral head, and improper stem version. These technical failures impact the soft-tissue tension and configuration of the rotator cuff tendons, and can have a significant impact on the potential for functional gains during rehabilitation. For example, if a stem is placed in excessive retroversion, internal rotation will be limited and increased traction forces will be placed on the tuberosity repair. Biologic failures include tuberosity nonunion and painful glenoid wear. Tuberosity healing can be improved with use of fracture-specific stems with ingrowth surfaces and windows for bone grafting. Additional complications include stiffness, infection, nerve injury, and dislocation. Complications following reverse arthroplasty are similar, but also include dislocation and acromial stress fracture.

POSTOPERATIVE REHABILITATION

The postoperative rehabilitation process requires a team-based approach that involves the patient, the therapist, and the surgeon. The aim of rehabilitation should be to reestablish shoulder function while taking care to protect the fixation and avoid creating complications. This is accomplished by recognizing the functional interdependence of joints and soft tissues in the upper quadrant when treating dysfunction of the shoulder. After a proximal humerus fracture and surgery, there are alterations in the neuromuscular patterns of the shoulder. Postoperative glenohumeral joint stiffness can result in compensatory movements in the shoulder girdle, including excessive scapular vertical movement. Restoring normal neuromuscular patterns, glenohumeral motion, and scapular kinematics is essential to proper kinetic chain function, as deficits can negatively impact the desired function of the shoulder girdle.

The primary goal of fixation of a displaced/unstable proximal humerus fracture is to create a stable construct that will allow for early rehabilitation. The fracture pattern, amount of medial calcar comminution, bone quality, and surgical technique play a substantial role in determining the quality of the fixation. Early complications of locking plates, related to poor initial fixation, are not uncommon and include screw perforations and loss of fixation. Because of this, rehabilitation is meant to be a gentle process and should not involve encouraging patients to push through pain early on in the process at the risk of fixation failure. For this reason, motion exercises initiated during the first 6 postoperative weeks, when bone healing is most critical, are passive, self-directed by the patient, and initially performed in the supine position. In the case of arthroplasty, tuberosity healing is less reliable than after locking plate fixation; thus, rehabilitation is a slower process as compared to locked plate fixation.

Authors' Preferred Protocol

Our rehabilitation protocols for both locked plate fixation and hemiarthroplasty are significantly influenced by quality of fracture reduction/tuberosity fixation. Assuming anatomic fracture reduction and secure fixation, the authors' preferred protocols are as follows.

Locked Plate Fixation

- Postoperatively, the arm is placed in a sling for comfort.
    - We attempt to discontinue sling use at home as quickly as possible provided that fixation is felt to be adequate.

© 2018 American Academy of Orthopaedic Surgeons

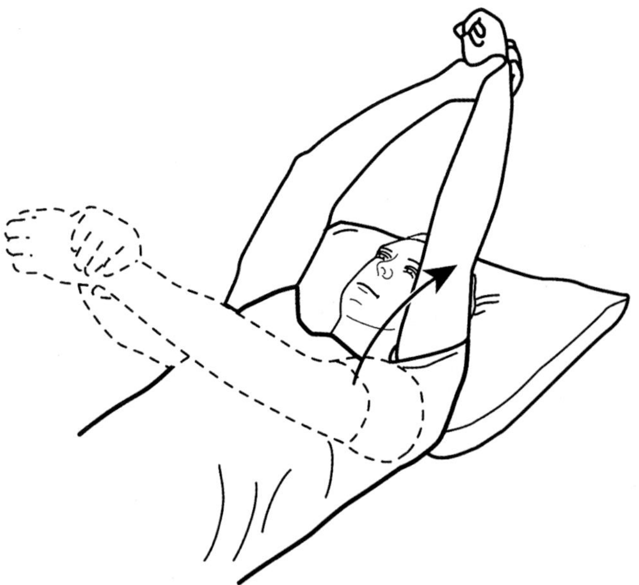

Figure 10.4 Illustration demonstrating supine passive forward elevation utilizing the contralateral limb. (Reproduced with permission from Burkhart S, Lo IK, Brady PC, Denard PJ: *Cowboy's Companion: A Trail Guide for the Arthroscopic Shoulder Surgeon*. Philadelphia, PA: Wolters Kluwer; 2012.)

However, the sling is used intermittently for protection in crowds and public places for 4 to 6 weeks.

- Padding may be placed in the axilla and around the elbow in the sling to prevent skin maceration.

- Patients are encouraged to perform active and passive ROM exercises of the elbow, wrist, and hand immediately after surgery.
- Gentle, patient-directed, passive ROM exercises within the safe ranges determined on the operating table (passive supine forward elevation, external rotation and internal rotation to the chest/abdomen) and pendulum exercises of the shoulder are initiated on the first postoperative day and continued until the first postoperative visit (Figures 10.4 and 10.5). For routine cases, safe ranges include 140° of elevation and 40° of external rotation. If there is concern about fixation, a safe range is usually 90° of elevation and 0° of external rotation.
- Suture removal typically occurs at 10 to 14 days. If radiographs reveal no loss of reduction, passive elevation is advanced to 160° and external rotation is advanced to 40°. This can usually be accomplished through a home exercise program with one or two initial visits to a physical or occupational therapist. If the patient is having difficulty performing the exercises, additional formal therapy can be instituted.
- Active-assisted mobilization with abduction and flexion is started at 4 to 6 weeks postoperatively, depending on maintenance of fracture reduction. During active-assisted motion, the patient actively uses the muscles surrounding the shoulder to perform the exercise but requires some help from the therapist, equipment, or the patient's contralateral arm.
  - Therapy can be supervised in one or three weekly sessions and performed three to five times daily at home by the patient.
  - Exercises are initially performed in the supine position and progressed to the sitting position.
  - An overhead pulley is added at approximately 6 weeks (Figure 10.6). Overhead pulleys are used by placing the pulley over the top of a door. The patient places the back of an armless chair against the door and positions the pulley handles at eye level. The handle of the pulley is placed in the hand of the operative limb first. The patient then reaches up with the other hand and grasps the

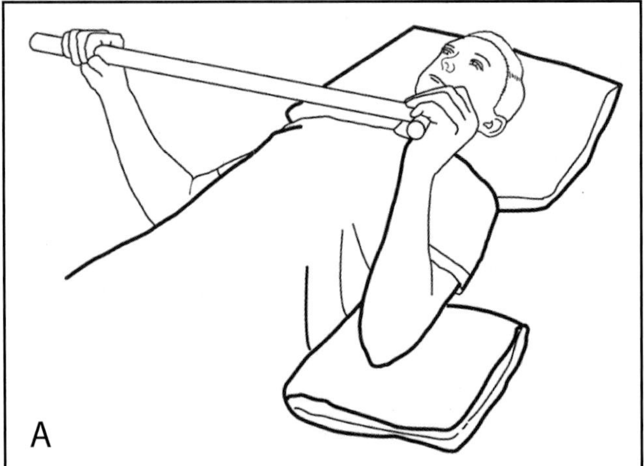

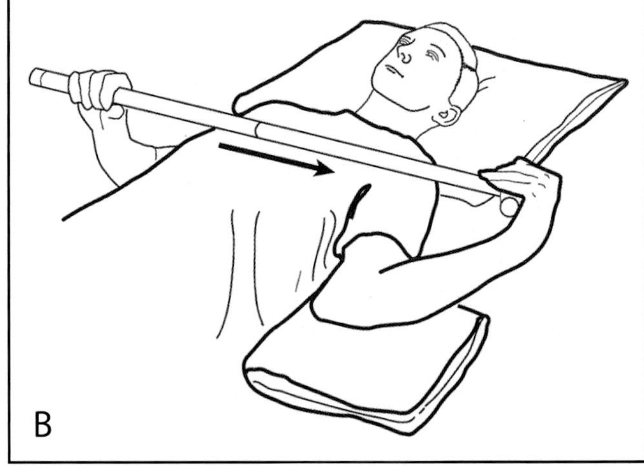

Figure 10.5 **A**, **B**, Illustrations demonstrating cane-assisted, passive external rotation utilizing the contralateral limb. (Reproduced with permission from Burkhart S, Lo IK, Brady PC, Denard PJ: *Cowboy's Companion: A Trail Guide for the Arthroscopic Shoulder Surgeon*. Philadelphia, PA: Wolters Kluwer; 2012.)

© 2018 American Academy of Orthopaedic Surgeons

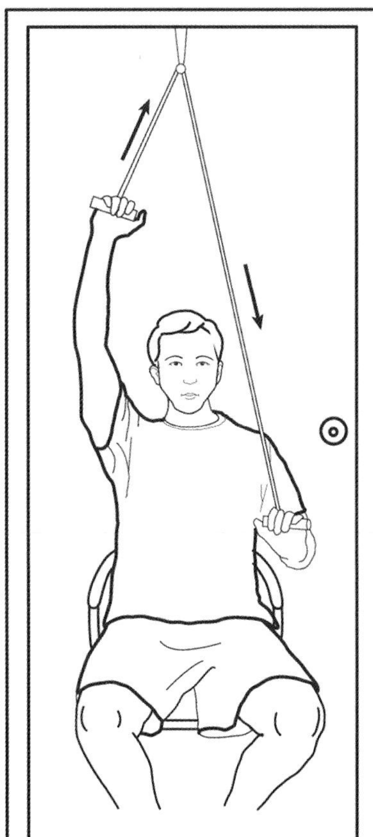

Figure 10.6 Illustration demonstrating passive forward elevation using a pulley system. (Reproduced with permission from Burkhart S, Lo IK, Brady PC, Denard PJ: *Cowboy's Companion: A Trail Guide for the Arthroscopic Shoulder Surgeon*. Philadelphia, PA: Wolters Kluwer; 2012.)

second pulley hand. With a slow and steady downward pull, the operative limb goes upward.

- One should be cautious of overly aggressive formal physical therapy during this early postoperative period, as this may lead to construct failure.

- If there are no signs of reduction loss, patients are progressed to full active motion at between 8 to 10 weeks. However, they will not achieve maximum active ROM until about 1 year postoperatively.
- Isometric deltoid and rotator cuff strengthening exercises are added to the therapy regimen at approximately 8 to 10 weeks after surgery and resistive deltoid. Rotator cuff strengthening exercises are added at 10 to 12 weeks.
    - Strengthening is initiated when active ROM is at least 130° of elevation and 30° to 40° of external rotation, significant bony consolidation is confirmed on plain radiographs, and adequate coordination of the extremity has been achieved. Higher-level activities, such as manual labor and heavy lifting, can be slowly added once strength and motion are optimized, but generally are not initiated before 6 months have passed.

Arthroplasty

The rehabilitation for arthroplasty is similar to the rehabilitation for osteosynthesis, except that safe ranges are initially smaller and transitions are slower. Reverse arthroplasty patients seem to progress more easily than hemiarthroplasty patients. However, they are typically older with poorer bone quality. As a result, the timing and intensity of rehabilitation should more closely resemble hemiarthroplasty than osteosynthesis.

- Postoperatively, the arm is placed in a sling for comfort. Range of motion for the elbow, wrist, and hand should be performed daily. No active or active-assisted ROM of the shoulder is performed for 6 to 8 weeks postoperatively. The sling may be discontinued around the house at 2 to 4 weeks, but should be used in public for 6 to 8 weeks. These time frames may be adjusted and extended based on the tuberosity fixation stability obtained in the operating room.
- Patients perform pendulum exercises, passive supine forward elevation, passive external rotation, and internal rotation to the chest/abdomen for the first 6 to 8 weeks. Safe ranges of motion are determined by fracture stability determined in the operating room.
- The amount of motion is individualized for each patient depending on the safe ROM attained on the operating table. For routine cases, safe ranges include 130° of elevation and 30° of external rotation. If there is concern about fixation, a safe range is usually 90° of elevation and 0° of external rotation.
- Sutures are removed at 10 to 14 days, and passive ROM exercises are maintained at their current levels.
- At 4 to 6 weeks postoperatively, assuming no loss of reduction, passive ROM is advanced as tolerated in both forward elevation and external rotation.
- At 8 weeks postoperatively, again assuming no loss of reduction, active assisted ROM with an overhead pulley, and passive stretching is initiated.
- Full active motion is initiated at approximately 10 to 12 weeks, but will improve for up to 1 year postoperatively.
- Strengthening is added at 12 to 14 weeks postoperatively (Table 10.1).

Functional Goals and Restrictions

While restoration of normal motion and strength is the goal of physical therapy, it is important to realize that normal ROM is not necessary to comfortably and effectively perform activities of daily living. Based on electromagnetic tracking system data from asymptomatic shoulders, the average shoulder motions required to perform the functional tasks are as follows: flexion, 121°; extension, 46°; abduction, 128°; cross-body adduction, 116°; external rotation with the arm 90° abducted, 59°; and internal rotation with the arm at the side, 102°.

On average, patients achieve reliable pain relief and active forward elevation between 100° and 130° and active external rotation between 30° and 50° with either hemiarthroplasty or plate fixation.

© 2018 American Academy of Orthopaedic Surgeons

Table 10.1 **AUTHOR'S PREFERRED REHABILITATION PROTOCOLS FOR LOCKED PLATING AND HEMIARTHROPLASTY**

Postop Weeks	Goals	Sling Wear	Motion	Strengthening	Schedule
Weeks 0–4 **Weeks 0–6**	• Pain/Edema Control • Main ROM of adjacent joints • Protect fracture • Prevent shoulder capsular contracture	For comfort and sleeping	• AROM/AAROM/PROM neck, elbow, wrist, hand • Pendulums, supine passive forward elevation, external rotation, and internal rotation to abdomen (not behind back)	• None	• Home-based
Weeks 4–6 **Weeks 6–8**	• Same as above • Minimize deconditioning • Maintain muscle flexibility and neuromuscular pattern • Normalize scapulohumeral kinematics	For comfort and sleeping	• Same as above • Passive motion in all planes • Active-assisted motion in all planes • Begin scapular retraction and depression	• Instruct in program of postural correction • Lower extremity aerobic conditioning	• 2 visits per week, everyday home program
Weeks 6–8 **Weeks 8–10**	• Same as above • Prevent muscle atrophy • Regain normal motion	For comfort and sleeping	• Same as above • Add overhead pulley	• Same as above	• 2 visits per week, everyday home program
Weeks 8–10 **Weeks 10–12**	• Same as above • Initiate strengthening	Discontinued	• Same as above • Active motion in all planes • Posterior capsular stretching program	• Same as above • Isometric rotator cuff/ deltoid strengthening • Periscapular strengthening	• 2 visits per week, everyday home program
Weeks 10–12 **Weeks 12–14**	• Same as above • Progress stretching • Increase rotator cuff/deltoid strength • Strengthen scapular rotators • Improve scapulohumeral rhythm	Discontinued	• Same as above • AROM/AAROM/PROM of shoulder in all planes • Self-stretching in all planes, bilateral hanging stretches	• Same as above • Resistive exercises: standing forward press, Theraband exercises, rowing	• Progress to home exercise program when: - Maximized ROM - Full independent ADLs - Normal scapulohumeral rhythm >100° elevation

AAROM, active assisted range of motion; ADLs, activities of daily living; AROM, active range of motion; PROM, passive range of motion; ROM, range of motion.
Black = locked plate fixation.
Red = hemiarthroplasty.

PEARLS

Pearls	Description
Medial Calcar Restoration	• Reduction of the medial calcar is critical for stability and allowance of early ROM. • In cases of medial comminution, proper placement of medial calcar screw(s) is important. • If using fixed-angle locking screws, plate position will dictate position of the medial calcar screw(s). Thus, it is important to confirm calcar screw position before placing multiple screws into the humeral head or shaft.
Arm Position	• Reducing and fixating the fracture in internal rotation will limit postoperative external rotation. • Perform reduction and fixation with the arm in 30° of external rotation.
Early Protected Motion	• Initiating early motion is important; however, motion should be passive and self-directed by the patient utilizing the contralateral limb when possible while fracture healing is taking place.
Fracture Pattern Considerations in Rehab	• Rotator cuff tendons can place significant force on greater tuberosity and lesser tuberosity fracture fragments. • Knowledge of the specific fracture fragments and the quality of the fixation is important when creating a rehabilitation protocol. • When greater tuberosity fixation is a concern, abduction and external rotation exercises should be limited or delayed. • When lesser tuberosity fixation is a concern, active internal rotation and passive external rotation should be limited or delayed.

BIBLIOGRAPHY

Brorson S, Rasmussen JV, Frich LH, Olsen BS, Hrobjartsson A: Benefits and harms of locking plate osteosynthesis in intraarticular (OTA Type C) fractures of the proximal humerus: a systematic review. *Injury* 2012;43:999–1005.

Court-Brown CM, Caesar B: Epidemiology of adult fractures: A review. *Injury* 2006;37:691–697.

Court-Brown CM, Garg A, McQueen MM. The epidemiology of proximal humeral fractures. *Acta Orthop Scand* 2001;72: 365–371.

Fankhauser F, Schippinger G, Weber K, et al.: Cadaveric-biomechanical evaluation of bone-implant construct of proximal humerus fractures (Neer type 3). *J Trauma* 2003; 55:345–349.

Helmy N, Hintermann B: New trends in the treatment of proximal humerus fractures. *Clin Orthop Related Res* 2006;442: 100–108.

Hodgson S: Proximal humerus fracture rehabilitation. *Clin Orthop Related Res* 2006;442:131–138.

Koval KJ, Gallagher MA, Marsicano JG, Cuomo F, McShinawy A, Zuckerman JD: Functional outcome after minimally displaced fractures of the proximal part of the humerus. *Journal Bone Joint Surg Am* 1997;79:203–207.

Kristiansen B, Barfod G, Bredesen J, et al.: Epidemiology of proximal humeral fractures. *Acta Orthop Scand* 1987;58: 75–77.

Lanting B, MacDermid J, Drosdowech D, Faber KJ.: Proximal humeral fractures: a systematic review of treatment modalities. *J Shoulder Elbow Surg* 2008;17:42–54.

Lubbeke A, Stern R, Grab B, Herrmann F, Michel JP, Hoffmeyer P: Upper extremity fractures in the elderly: consequences on utilization of rehabilitation care. *Aging Clin Exp Res* 2005; 17:276–280.

Maldonado ZM, Seebeck J, Heller MO, et al.: Straining of the intact and fractured proximal humerus under physiological-like loading. *J Biomech* 2003;36:1865–1873.

Mills HJ, Horne G: Fractures of the proximal humerus in adults. *J Trauma* 1985;25:801–805.

Namdari S, Voleti PB, Mehta S: Evaluation of the osteoporotic proximal humeral fracture and strategies for structural augmentation during surgical treatment. *J Shoulder Elbow Surg* 2012;21:1787–1795.

Namdari S, Yagnik G, Ebaugh DD, et al.: Defining functional shoulder range of motion for activities of daily living. *J Shoulder Elbow Surg* 2012;21:1177–1183.

Neer CS, 2nd: Displaced proximal humeral fractures. I. Classification and evaluation. *J Bone Joint Surg Am* 1970;52:1077–1089.

Seebeck J, Goldhahn J, Stadele H, Messmer P, Morlock MM, Schneider E: Effect of cortical thickness and cancellous bone density on the holding strength of internal fixator screws. *J Orthop Res* 2004;22:1237–1242.

Sudkamp N, Bayer J, Hepp P, et al.: Open reduction and internal fixation of proximal humeral fractures with use of the locking proximal humerus plate. Results of a prospective, multicenter, observational study. *J Bone Joint Surg Am* 2009;91: 1320–1328.

Thanasas C, Kontakis G, Angoules A, Limb D, Giannoudis P. Treatment of proximal humerus fractures with locking plates: a systematic review. *J Shoulder Elbow Surgery* 2009;18: 837–844.

© 2018 American Academy of Orthopaedic Surgeons

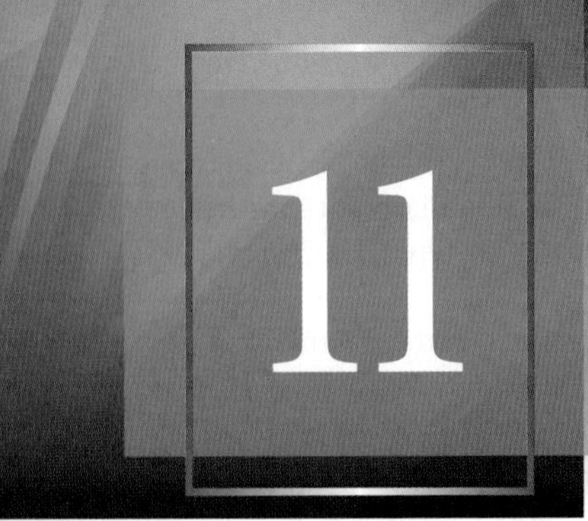

Scapular Dyskinesis

W. Ben Kibler, MD

INTRODUCTION

Alterations of scapular motion are frequently seen in association with shoulder injury. Restoration of scapular motion and strength should be a part of any comprehensive shoulder rehabilitation protocol to restore normal scapulohumeral rhythm and shoulder function. These exercises can be instituted in conjunction with shoulder rehabilitation; the extent of the exercise will be determined by the extent of shoulder healing.

Postoperative restoration of optimal scapular function is more commonly implemented after surgery for glenohumeral or acromioclavicular problems rather than for the relatively rare surgical procedures relating directly to the scapula. Scapular dyskinesis is frequently associated with all types of shoulder pathology, and should be addressed as part of the comprehensive rehabilitation protocol following shoulder surgery. Scapular rehabilitation can often be implemented early in the rehabilitation sequence, even while the shoulder repair is being protected.

PROCEDURES

Scapular dyskinesis has been associated with almost every type of shoulder pathology. Its presence or absence should be evaluated preoperatively as part of the comprehensive examination for the specific pathology. The specific operations, their indications, contraindications, and techniques are all described in the specific chapters on those pathologies. Rehabilitation of scapular dyskinesis should be included when scapular dyskinesis is observed on clinical examination.

REHABILITATION

The goal of rehabilitation of the dyskinetic or winged scapula is to recreate the normal kinematics of the scapula, allowing it to participate in the normal scapulohumeral rhythm (SHR). Restoration of SHR requires the restoration of stability and strength in the legs and core, the motion of the scapula, and the flexibility, strength, and muscle activation patterns of the periscapular structures. The basic program, discussed later, may be implemented during the rehabilitation of most shoulder pathologies, with variations depending on tissue healing and range-of-motion (ROM) restrictions.

Proximal Kinetic Chain Exercises

Maximal scapular muscle strength results from a stabilized platform comprised of leg strength combined with hip and trunk (commonly referred to as "core") strength and stability. Early emphasis on core strength and stability, even while the scapula and shoulder are protected, provides this proximal base for distal mobility and maximal activation. Strengthening exercises for the trunk and hip start from and end at the position of hip extension and trunk extension. These exercises include trunk and hip flexion and extension, rotation, and diagonal motions. Emphasis also should be placed on flexibility of the hips, lumbar spine, and thoracic spine, because these areas are frequently tight. The exercises should be done first to restore the base; then, they can be integrated with the scapular exercises.

To create a stable base, the rehabilitation protocols start with the primary stabilizing musculature, such as the transverse abdominis and multifidi. These groups are responsible for segmental spinal stability and provide the foundation for adequate trunk stability because of their direct attachment to the spine and pelvis; they are responsible for the most central portion of core stability. The internal and external oblique, erector spinae, rectus abdominis, and quadratus lumborum muscles then should be incorporated for trunk stability. Together, these local and global stabilizers provide ultimate core stability. The larger global muscles, including the abdominal muscles, erector spinae, and hip abductors, are vital for power generation and stability in upper extremity function. The incorporation of core strengthening into rehabilitation regimens

Dr. Kibler or an immediate family member serves as an unpaid consultant to Alignmed; has stock or stock options held in Alignmed; and serves as a board member, owner, officer, or committee member of the Arthroscopy Association of North America and the British Journal of Sports Medicine.

© 2018 American Academy of Orthopaedic Surgeons

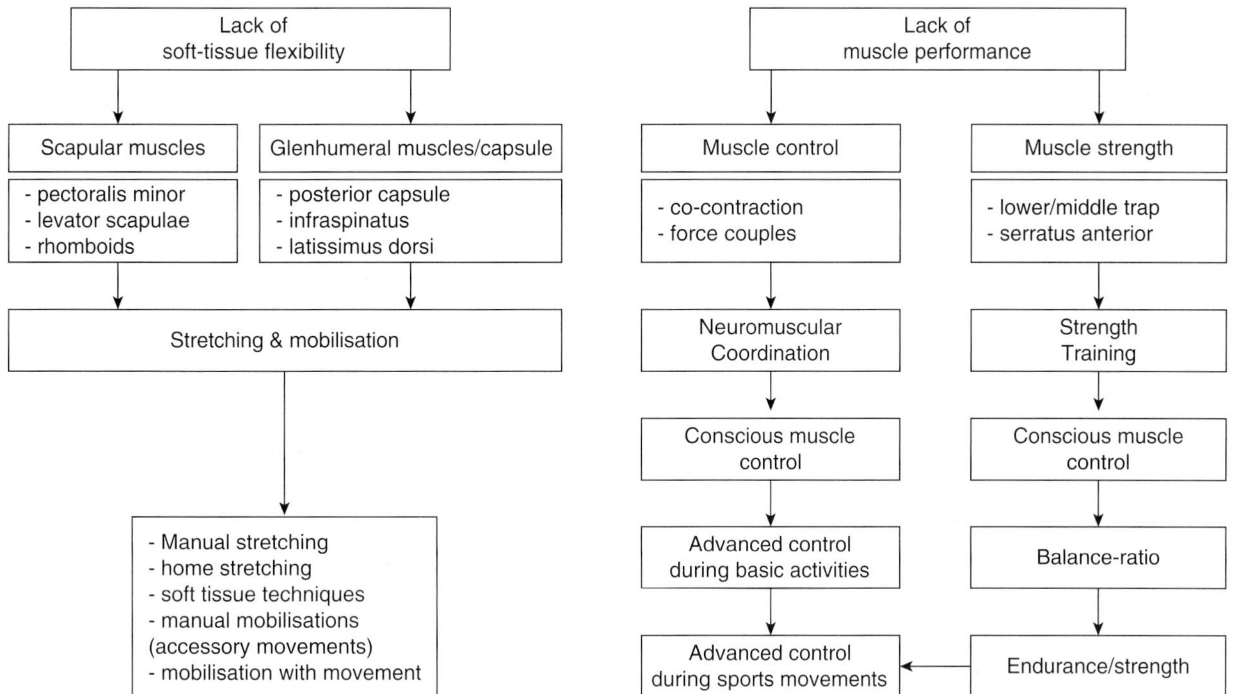

Figure 11.1 Algorithm developed by Cools and Ellenbecker. (Reproduced with permission from Ellenbecker TS, Cools A: Rehabilitation of shoulder impingement syndrome and rotator cuff injuries: an evidence-based review. *Br J Sports Med* 2010;44:319–327.)

has been shown to increase hip extensor muscle strength and balance. Core strengthening programs also have been shown to reduce pain and increase the strength of the core musculature in patients with low back pain. This stage of rehabilitation is undertaken to restore core function but also is the first stage of extremity rehabilitation, because the core is the critical base for development and transfer of energy.

Periscapular Rehabilitation

Ellenbecker and Cools have published a very useful rehabilitation algorithm to guide the implementation of scapular rehabilitation (Figure 11.1). The goals are restoration of scapular motion and periscapular muscle strength. Altered scapular motion can result from a lack of soft-tissue flexibility in the periscapular muscles or the glenohumeral muscles and capsule. The most commonly affected periscapular muscles include the pectoralis minor, short head of the biceps, upper trapezius, and latissimus dorsi. These combined inflexibilities create a forwardly tilted posture of scapular protraction. It is this alteration that frequently must be addressed at the beginning of the scapular rehabilitation program. The glenohumeral structures most commonly involved include the posterior rotator cuff musculature and the glenohumeral capsule. They affect scapular posture by increasing the tightness of the internal glenohumeral rotation so that forward arm motion or rotation "winds up" the scapula into protraction.

Stretching and mobilization techniques may be used for both types of alterations. Flexibility exercises focusing on the anterior coracoid (pectoralis minor and short head of the biceps) and shoulder rotation include the open book (Figure 11.2) and corner stretches (Figure 11.3) for the

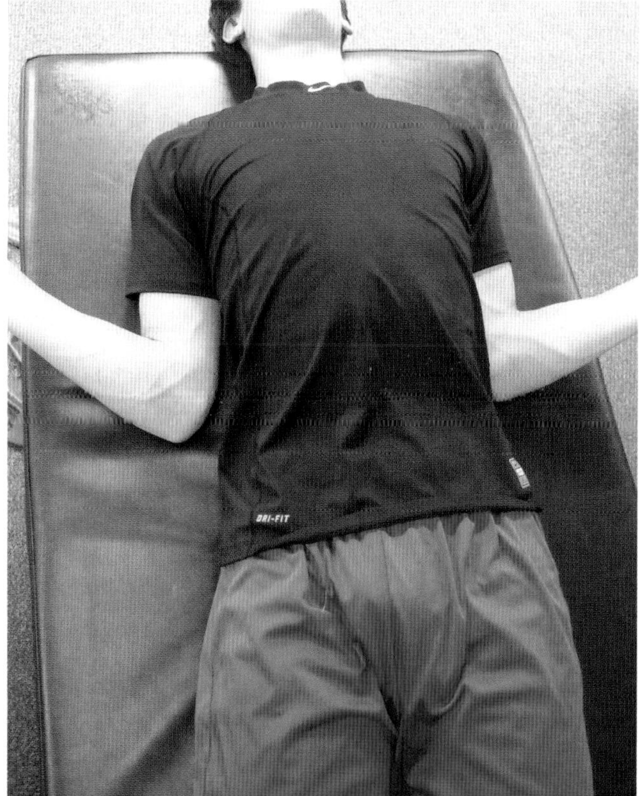

Figure 11.2 Photograph showing the open book stretch. This maneuver is performed by having the patient lie supine on a bolster with the elbows of both arms positioned against the body. The patient is instructed to externally rotate both arms, stretching the anterior musculature.

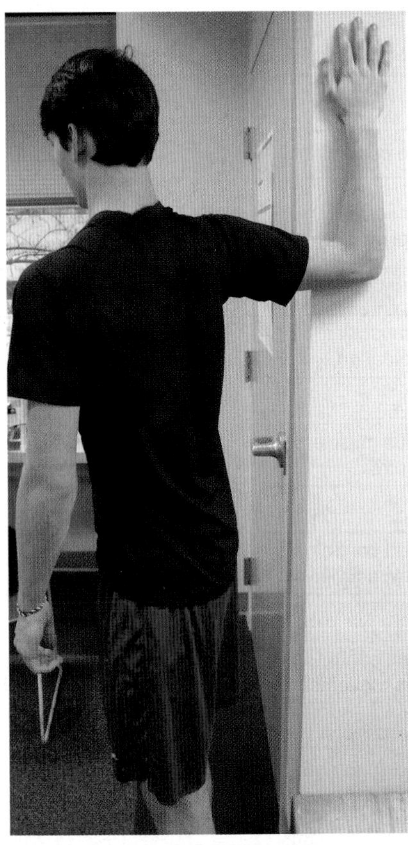

Figure 11.3 Photograph showing the corner stretch. The patient is instructed to stand with the involved arm in a 90° position on a wall or other firm surface. The patient then rotates the body in the opposite direction to stretch the anterior musculature.

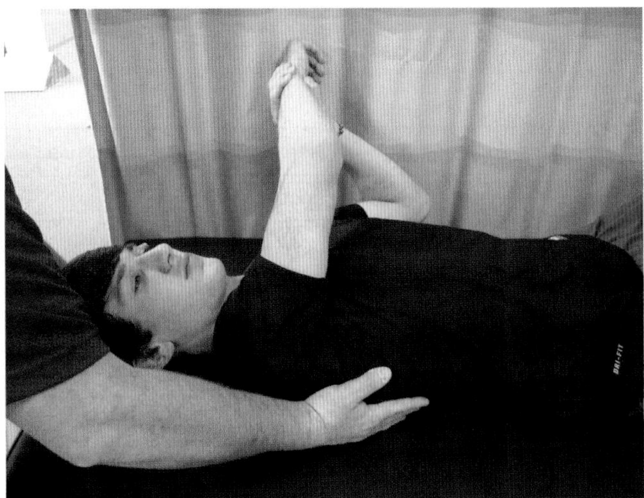

Figure 11.5 Photograph demonstrating the cross-body adduction stretch. This stretch also combats posterior shoulder tightness. It is more effective to stabilize the scapula when performing this maneuver.

coracoid muscles and the sleeper (Figure 11.4) and cross-body stretches (Figure 11.5) for shoulder rotation. Manual stretching and mobilization also can improve the flexibility of the periscapular muscles. Mobilization also can be effective in altering poor posture, especially thoracic kyphosis. Addressing the thoracic spine and the posterior and inferior soft-tissue components of the shoulder have been shown to be effective in correcting posture.

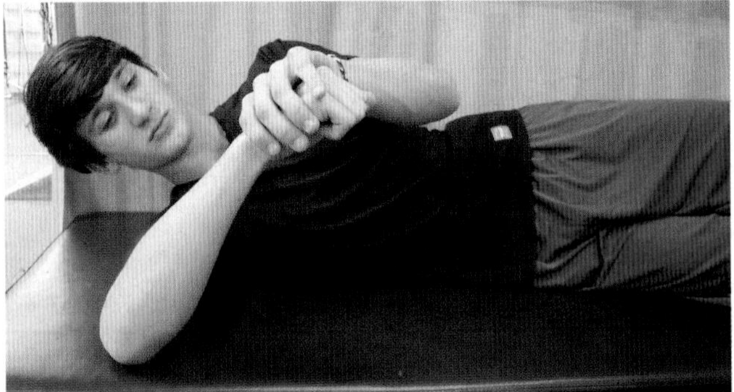

Figure 11.4 Photograph depicting the sleeper stretch. This stretch is helpful in addressing tight posterior rotator cuff muscles and allows the arm position to be varied based on need.

Taping and bracing can help to maintain increased motion, especially in patients who have improved their symptoms with postural correction or manual scapular repositioning. Several taping techniques have been used and several brands of lightweight scapular braces are available. They can be used between treatment sessions in patients who have difficulty maintaining the optimal scapular position.

Lack of muscle performance affecting scapular position and motion may derive from not only the loss of muscle strength, but also alterations in muscle activation. Periscapular strengthening should emphasize achieving a position of scapular retraction, which is the most effective position to maximize scapular roles. Scapular retraction exercises may be done in a standing position to simulate normal activation sequences and allow proximal to distal sequencing. Scapular pinch and trunk extension/scapular retraction exercises may be started early in rehabilitation, even when the shoulder is being protected, because minimal tensile load or shear is exerted on the glenohumeral joint in these exercises. The muscles most commonly found to be weak include the serratus anterior and lower trapezius. Several specific exercises have been shown to be very effective in activating the key scapular stabilizers—the lower trapezius and serratus anterior muscles—and in minimizing upper trapezius activation. They are the low row (Figure 11.6), inferior glide (Figure 11.7), fencing (Figure 11.8), lawnmower (Figure 11.9), and robbery (Figure 11.10) exercises. These are collectively called the scapular stability series. They have been shown to activate the target muscles at 18% to 30% of maximal activation. This activation, combined with the performance of these exercises at arm angles below 90° of abduction, make these exercises particularly effective in the early stages of rehabilitation, after injury or surgery.

© 2018 American Academy of Orthopaedic Surgeons

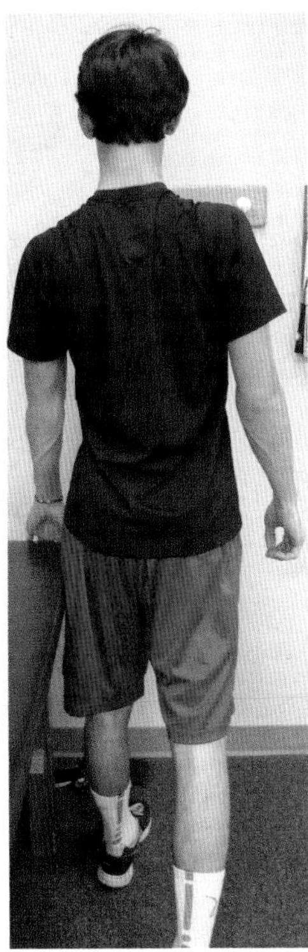

Figure 11.6 Photograph showing the low row exercise. The patient is positioned standing with the hand of the involved arm against the side of a firm surface. The patient is instructed to extend the hips and trunk to facilitate scapular retraction and hold the contraction for 5 seconds.

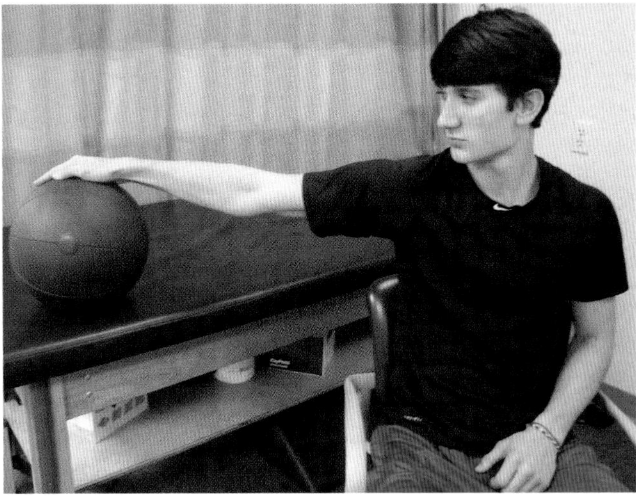

Figure 11.7 Photograph depicting the inferior glide exercise. The active inferior glide exercise uses co-contraction of both the shoulder and scapular muscles to help depress the humeral head and scapula.

After this early phase, in which moderate levels of strength are obtained, exercise can shift to higher loads, performed prone or standing. Exercises that emphasize lower trapezius and serratus anterior muscle activation, while limiting upper trapezius activation, include side-lying external rotation and prone arm extension exercises. High-load scapular

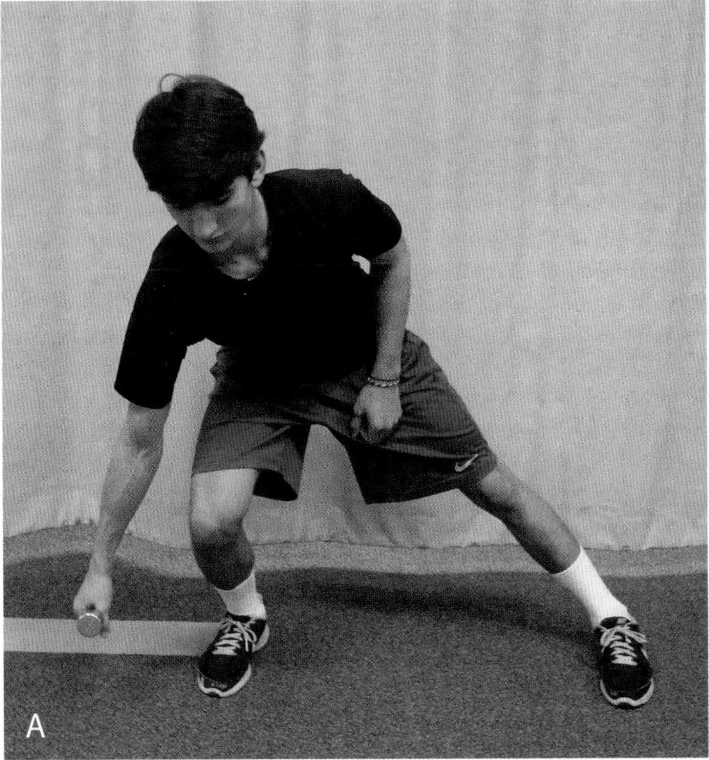

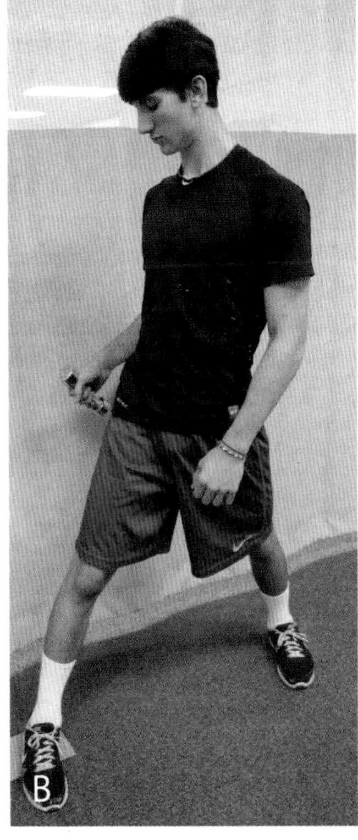

Figure 11.8 Photograph demonstrating the fencing exercise. **A**, The patient begins with the trunk flexed and arm abducted to approximately 45°. **B**, The patient then extends and rotates the trunk with simultaneous arm adduction to encourage scapular retraction.

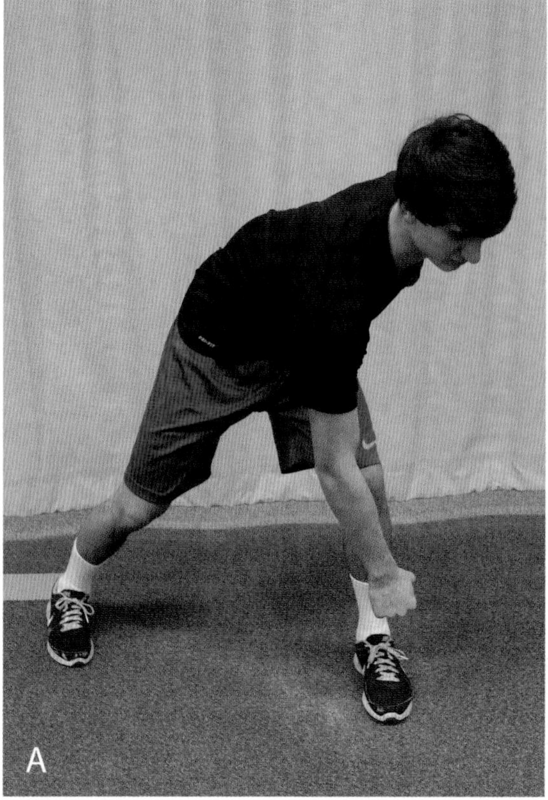

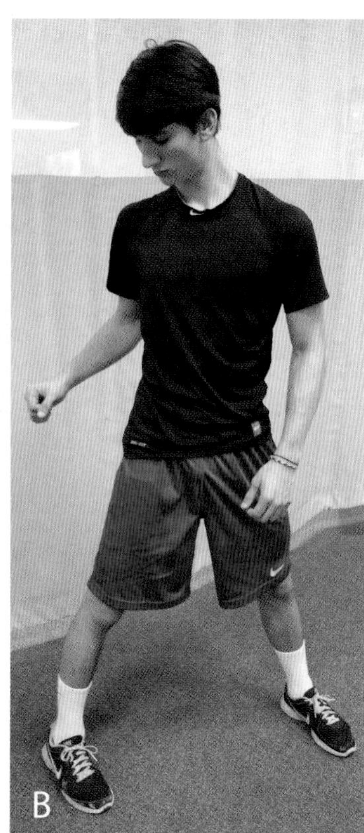

Figure 11.9 Photograph showing the lawnmower exercise. **A**, The exercise begins with the hips and trunk flexed and the arm slightly elevated forward. **B**, The patient is instructed to extend the hips and trunk, then rotate the trunk to facilitate scapular retraction.

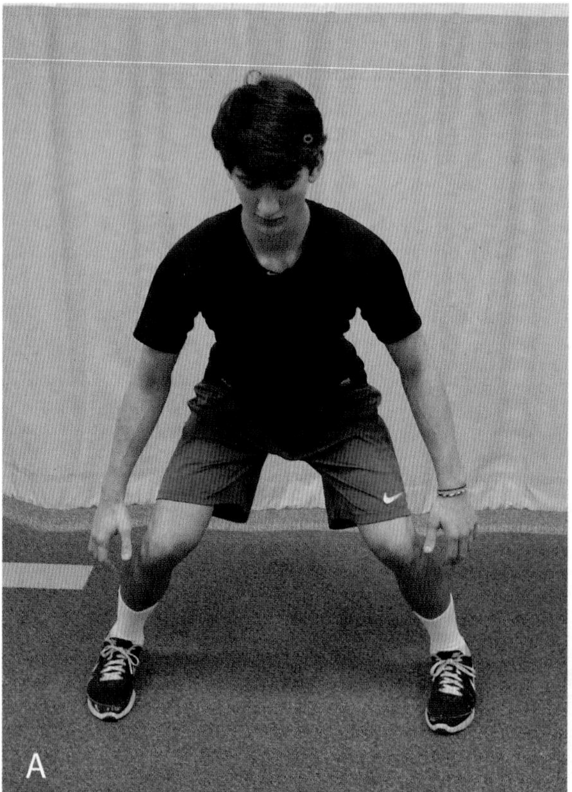

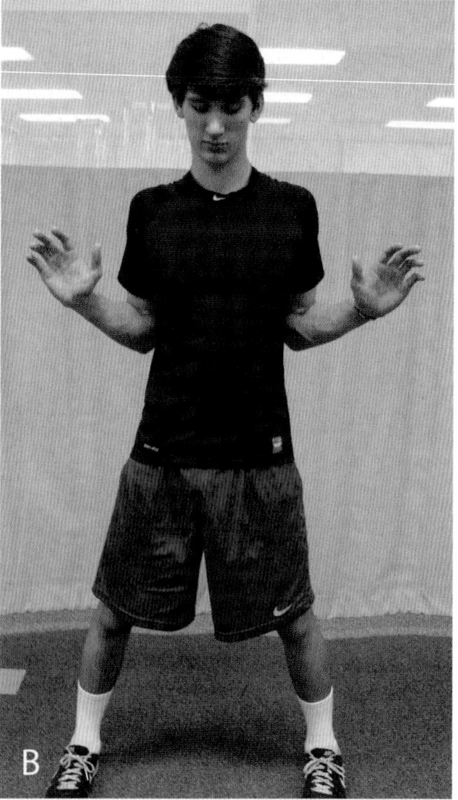

Figure 11.10 Photograph demonstrating the robbery exercise. **A**, The maneuver begins with the knees and trunk flexed and the arms held away from the body. **B**, The patient is instructed to extend the hips and trunk and to try to place the elbows in the back pockets, holding this final position for 5 seconds.

© 2018 American Academy of Orthopaedic Surgeons

strengthening exercises include the push-up plus (activating the serratus anterior muscle), low row with tubing or weight, horizontal abduction with external rotation (activating the lower trapezius and rhomboid), and press up (activating the serratus anterior and lower trapezius) exercises.

A loss of coordinated muscle activation patterns, along with inhibition of activation or delay in onset of activation, are frequently found. These deficits require reestablishment of the normal kinetic chain activations starting from the core. Early training should incorporate the trunk and hip to facilitate the kinetic chain proximal-to-distal sequence of muscle activation. Little stress is placed on the shoulder during the movements of hip and trunk extension combined with scapular retraction. All exercises are started with the feet on the ground, and involve hip extension and pelvic control. The patterns of activation are both ipsilateral and contralateral. Diagonal motions involving trunk rotation around a stable leg simulate the normal pattern of throwing. As the shoulder heals and becomes ready for motion and loading in the intermediate or recovery stage of rehabilitation, the patterns can include arm motion as the final part of the exercise.

Occasionally, the dynamic activation patterns are so inhibited that isometric, short lever arm positioning is necessary to restore neural activation at specific points of arm elevation before activation throughout the arc of motion. This series of exercises is called "Connect the Dots" (Figure 11.11). After the pattern of isolated control has been reestablished, more advanced exercises may be implemented.

Author's Preferred Protocol

For postoperative rehabilitation of scapular dyskinesis, this protocol may be used in conjunction with the postoperative rehabilitation of specific shoulder pathology. The early phase, which emphasizes core and scapular retraction, may be undertaken while the specific shoulder pathology is perfected and healing. The more advanced phases can be undertaken when healing is complete.

Phase I: Acute Phase (Weeks 1–3)

- Use hips to position trunk and spine.
- Glenohumeral motion has lower priority than scapular motion.
- Promote scapular retraction and depression with thoracic extension.
- De-emphasize the upper trapezius.
- Address soft-tissue inflexibilities of the pectoralis minor, upper trapezius, and levator scapulae (Figures 11.2–11.5). If addressing inflexibilities as part of postoperative rehabilitation, these maneuvers should be utilized in phase II after adequate tissue healing has occurred.
- Closed-chain exercise for glenohumeral joint is a must; emphasize glenohumeral depression (Figures 11.6 and 11.7).

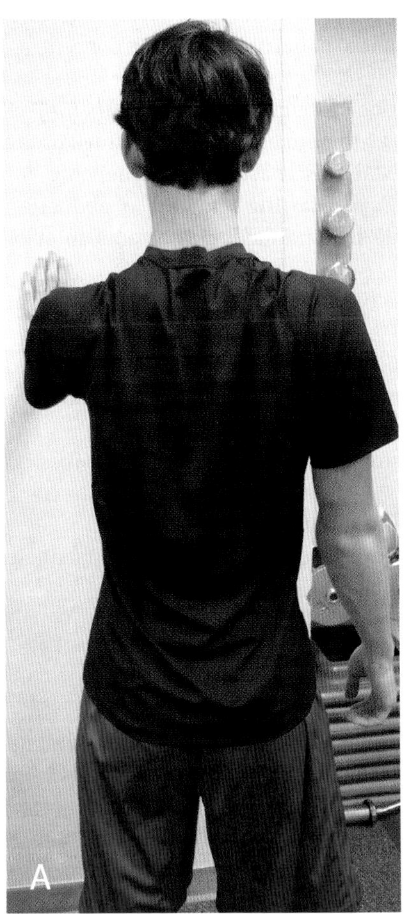

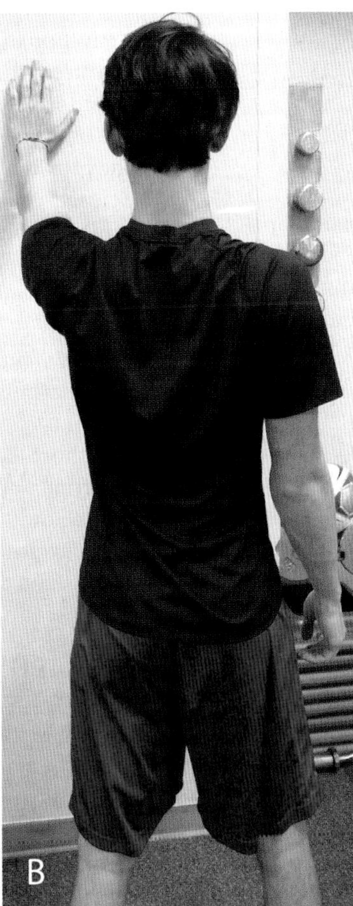

Figure 11.11 Photograph depicting the "Connect the Dots" exercise. **A**, The patient begins with the involved hand on a wall, with the arm extended. The patient is instructed to retract the scapula and hold the position for 5 to 10 seconds. **B**, After performing 2 to 3 sets of 10 repetitions, the patient can then move the arm to higher ROMs to repeat the exercise.

© 2018 American Academy of Orthopaedic Surgeons

Goals

- Achieve 90° abduction and flexion by end of phase I.
- Establish normal scapular motion using complementary trunk and hip motion (Figures 11.8–11.10).

Phase II: Recovery Phase (Weeks 4–8)

- Increase the difficulty of scapular strengthening exercises (Figures 11.8–11.10). Difficulty can be increased through the change in arm position, adding resistance tubing or bands, or the addition of light free weights (1–3 pounds).
- Open the upper extremity chain.
- Address all planes of motion.
- Promote glenohumeral depression.
- Progress from below 90° to above 90° of abduction and flexion.
- Begin to load the rotator cuff in various planes and angles, with caution.
- Address the glenohumeral internal rotation deficit, if present.
- Avoid external rotation and horizontal abduction posterior to the plane of the body.
- Address soft-tissue tightness and inflexibilities more aggressively.

Goals

- Good scapular control and rotator cuff strength
- Full active ROM
- Minimal pain

Phase III: Functional Activity Phase (Weeks 8+)

- Fine tune scapular motion to alleviate all dyskinesis (Figure 11.11).
- Increase the strength and endurance of the rotator cuff and scapular stabilizing muscles.

Multiple studies have identified methods to activate scapular muscles that control scapular motion, and have identified effective body and scapular positions that allow optimal activation. Scapular muscle performance is improved and clinical symptoms are decreased with use of these exercises, but there are equivocal results regarding a change in scapular motion, position, or dyskinesis in patients with shoulder pain. Only two randomized clinical trials have examined the effects of a scapular focused program by comparing it to a general shoulder rehabilitation. The findings indicate that the use of scapular exercises result in higher patient-rated outcomes.

Multiple clinical trials have incorporated scapular exercises within their rehabilitation programs, and have found positive patient-rated outcomes in patients with impingement syndrome. Studies in other populations are also starting to indicate positive outcomes. A multicenter study of patients with chronic full-thickness rotator cuff tears showed that an exercise program that included scapular exercises reduced symptoms and 80% of patients opted for no surgery. Three studies documented that a rehabilitation program that included scapular exercises improved symptoms and function and avoided surgery in up to 50% of patients with superior labral tears.

It appears that it is not the scapular exercises alone, but the inclusion of the scapular exercises as part of a rehabilitation program that may include the use of the kinetic chain that achieves positive outcomes. When the scapular exercises are prescribed, multiple components must be emphasized, including activation sequencing, force couple activation, concentric/eccentric emphasis, strength, endurance, and avoidance of unwanted patterns.

PEARLS

Several key principles have been found to facilitate the often difficult scapular rehabilitation, especially in the beginning phases.

1. The hip, trunk, and core are the base for scapular muscle attachment and activation.
   a. The core muscles must be strong to serve as the base for proximal to distal activation.
   b. Drive the rehabilitation exercises with coordinated core and scapula activations. These start with ipsilateral activation and progress to contralateral activation.
   c. Use trunk rotation to facilitate lower trapezius and rhomboid activation.
2. Restore muscle flexibility prior to muscle strengthening. The most commonly affected muscles are the pectoralis minor, short head of the biceps brachii, upper trapezius, scalene, and latissimus dorsi.
3. The focus of scapular rehabilitation is on coordinated muscle activation in sequential patterns, rather than concentrating on strength.
   a. Avoid isolated prone scapular muscle strengthening as the only exercises as these maneuvers discourage use of the proximal to distal muscle activation sequencing
4. Use closed-chain exercises starting below 90° of abduction to inhibit upper trapezius and facilitate serratus anterior activation.
5. Use manual cues (tactile or taping) to facilitate scapular tracking.
6. Alteration of muscle activation patterns is especially noticed when the arm is away from the body in forward flexion or abduction.
   a. Use short lever arm exercises to decrease the forces on the arm.
   b. Stay below 90° abduction in the early phases.
7. Use arm external rotation and trunk extension to facilitate scapular retraction.

BIBLIOGRAPHY

Blackburn TA, McLeod WD, White B, Wofford L: EMG analysis of posterior rotator cuff exercises. *J Athl Train* 1990;25(1):40–45.

Brudvig TJ, Kulkarni H, Shah S: The effect of therapeutic exercise and mobilization on patients with shoulder dysfunction: A systematic review with meta-analysis. *J Orthop Sports Phys Ther* 2011;41(10):734–748.

© 2018 American Academy of Orthopaedic Surgeons

Cools AM, Dewitte V, Lanszweert F, et al.: Rehabilitation of scapular muscle balance: Which exercises to prescribe? *Am J Sports Med* 2007;35(10):1744–1751.

Decker MJ, Hintermeister RA, Faber KJ, Hawkins RJ: Serratus anterior muscle activity during selected rehabilitation exercises. *Am J Sports Med* 1999;27(6):784–791.

De Mey K, Danneels L, Cagnie B, Cools A: Are kinetic chain rowing exercises relevant in shoulder and trunk injury prevention training? *Br J Sports Med* 2011;45(4):320.

De May K, Danneels L, Cagnie B, Cools AM: Scapular muscle rehabilitation exercises in overhead athletes with impingement symptoms: effect of a 6-week training program on muscle recruitment and functional outcome. *Am J Sports Med* 2012;40(8):1906–1915.

De Mey K, Danneels LA, Cagnie B, Huyghe L, Seyns E, Cools AM: Conscious correction of scapular orientation in overhead athletes performing selected shoulder rehabilitation exercises: The effect on trapezius muscle activation measured by surface electromyography. *J Orthop Sports Phys Ther* 2013;43(1):3–10.

Edwards SL, Lee JA, Bell JE, et al: Nonoperative treatment of superior labrum anterior posterior tears: Improvements in pain, function, and quality of life. *Am J Sports Med* 2010;38(7):1456–1461.

Ellenbecker TS, Cools A: Rehabilitation of shoulder impingement syndrome and rotator cuff injuries: An evidence-based review. *Br J Sports Med* 2010;44(5):319–327.

Johnson AJ, Godges JJ, Zimmerman GJ, Ounanian LL: The effect of anterior versus posterior glide joint mobilization on external rotation range of motion in patients with shoulder adhesive capsulitis. *J Orthop Sports Phys Ther* 2007;37(3):88–99.

Kibler WB, Sciascia A: Current concepts: Scapular dyskinesis. *Br J Sports Med* 2010;44(5):300–305.

Kibler WB, Sciascia A, Thomas SJ: Glenohumeral internal rotation deficit: Pathogenesis and response to acute throwing. *Sports Med Arthrosc* 2012;20(1):34–38.

Kibler WB, Sciascia AD, Uhl TL, Tambay N, Cunningham T: Electromyographic analysis of specific exercises for scapular control in early phases of shoulder rehabilitation. *Am J Sports Med* 2008;36(9):1789–1798.

Kromer TO, Tautenhahn UG, de Bie RA, Staal JB, Bastiaenen CH; Effects of physiotherapy in patients with shoulder impingement syndrome: a systematic review of the literature. *J Rehabil Med* 2009;41(11):870–880.

Laudner KG, Moline MT, Meister K: The relationship between forward scapular posture and posterior shoulder tightness among baseball players. *Am J Sports Med* 2010;38(10):2106–2112.

Manske RC, Meschke M, Porter A, Smith B, Reiman M: A randomized controlled single-blinded comparison of stretching versus stretching and joint mobilization for posterior shoulder tightness measured by internal rotation motion loss. *Sports Health* 2010;2(2):94–100.

McClure PW, Bialker J, Neff N, Williams GN, Karduna A: Shoulder function and 3-dimensional kinematics in people with shoulder impingement syndrome before and after a 6-week exercise program. *Phys Ther* 2004;84(9):832–848.

McMullen J, Uhl TL: A kinetic chain approach for shoulder rehabilitation. *J Athl Train* 2000;35(3):329–337.

Michener LA, Walsworth MK, Burnet EN: Effectiveness of rehabilitation for patients with subacromial impingement syndrome. *J Hand Ther* 2004;17:152–164.

Moseley JB Jr, Jobe FW, Pink M, Perry J, Tibone J: EMG analysis of the scapular muscles during a shoulder rehabilitation program. *Am J Sports Med* 1992;20(2):128–134.

Myers JB, Laudner KG, Pasquale MR, Bradley JP, Lephart SM: Glenohumeral range of motion deficits and posterior shoulder tightness in throwers with pathologic internal impingement. *Am J Sports Med* 2006;34(3):385–391.

Nadler SF, Malanga GA, Bartoli LA, Feinberg JH, Prybicien M, Deprince M: Hip muscle imbalance and low back pain in athletes: Influence of core strengthening. *Med Sci Sports Exerc* 2002;34(1):9–16.

Network MOO. Effectiveness of Physical Therapy in Treating Atraumatic Full Thickness Rotator Cuff Tears. A Multi-Center Prospective Cohort Study. *The American Shoulder and Elbow Surgeons Open Meeting.* San Diego, CA, 2011.

Petrofsky JS, Batt J, Brown J: Improving the outcomes after back injury by a core muscle strengthening program. *Journal of Applied Research* 2008;8(1):62–75.

Roy JS, Moffet H, Hebert LJ, Lirette R: Effect of motor control and strengthening exercises on shoulder function in persons with impingement syndrome: A single-subject study design. *Man Ther* 2009;14:180–188.

Sciascia A, Cromwell R: Kinetic chain rehabilitation: A theoretical framework. *Rehabil Res Pract* 2012;2012:853037.

Sciascia A, Kuschinsky N, Nitz AJ, Mair SD, Uhl TL: Electromyographical comparison of four common shoulder exercises in unstable and stable shoulders. *Rehabil Res Pract* 2012; 2012:783824.

Struyf F, Nijs J, Baeyens JP, Mottram SL, Meeusen R: Scapular positioning and movement in unimpaired shoulders, shoulder impingement syndrome, and glenohumeral instability. *Scand J Med Sci Sports* 2011;21(3):352–358.

Struyf F, Nijs J, Mollekens S, et al.: Scapular-focused treatment in patients with shoulder impingement syndrome: a randomized clinical trial. *Clin Rheumatol* 2013;32(1):73–85.

Tate AR, McClure PW, Young IA, Salvatori R, Michener LA: Comprehensive impairment-based exercise and manual therapy intervention for patients with subacromial impingement syndrome: A case series. *J Orthop Sports Phys Ther* 2010;40(8):474–493.

Townsend H, Jobe FW, Pink M, Perry J: Electromyographic analysis of the glenohumeral muscles during a baseball rehabilitation program. *Am J Sports Med* 1991;19(3):264–272.

Tyler TF, Nicholas SJ, Lee SJ, Mullaney M, McHugh MP: Correction of posterior shoulder tightness is associated with symptom resolution in patients with internal impingement. *Am J Sports Med* 2010;38(1):114–119.

Tyler TF, Nicholas SJ, Roy T, Gleim GW: Quantification of posterior capsule tightness and motion loss in patients with shoulder impingement. *Am J Sports Med* 2000;28(5):668–673.

Worsley P, Warner M, Mottram S, et al.: Motor control retraining exercises for shoulder impingement: effects on function, muscle activation, and biomechanics in young adults. *J Shoulder Elbow Surg* 2013;22(4):e11–e19.

© 2018 American Academy of Orthopaedic Surgeons

SECTION 2

Elbow

12 Elbow Anatomy

H. Mike Kim, MD

INTRODUCTION

Together with the shoulder, the elbow enables us to move and position the hand to a desired location to perform functions that are fundamental to our daily living activities. The elbow is also the intermediate of the upper extremity kinetic chain and provides a foundation for powerful upper extremity motions in various physical occupational and recreational activities. The elbow is a highly complex trocho-ginglymoid joint composed of the ulnohumeral, radiocapitellar, and proximal radioulnar joints. The capsuloligamentous and muscular structures that act across the elbow are responsible for controlled range of motion (ROM) as well as static and dynamic stability of the elbow and forearm. A thorough understanding of elbow anatomy and biomechanics is a key to accurate assessment and treatment of various elbow conditions.

OSSEOUS ANATOMY

The distal humerus, proximal ulna, and proximal radius form a highly congruent skeletal articulation that contributes to joint stability and determines ROM. The bony anatomy provides approximately 50% of elbow joint stability. The distal humerus articular surface is comprised of two components that articulate with the proximal end of the radius and ulna (Figure 12.1, A and B). The spool-shaped trochlea is the medial articular aspect, and articulates with the greater sigmoid notch of the proximal ulna. The medial ridge of the trochlea projects more distally than the lateral ridge, which results in 6° to 8° of valgus tilt at the ulnohumeral articulation. The hemispherical capitellum is the lateral articular component, and articulates with the radial head. In the sagittal plane, the orientation of the articular surface of the distal humerus is positioned approximately 30° anterior to the long axis of the humerus, which facilitates flexion while limiting the maximum extension of the elbow (Figure 12.2). The center of the rotation of the arc formed by the trochlea and capitellum is in line with the anterior cortex of the distal humerus.

The proximal ulna has two articular components—the greater sigmoid notch and lesser sigmoid (radial) notch—which form highly congruent articulations with the trochlea and radial head (Figure 12.3). The guiding ridge of the greater sigmoid notch articulates with the apex of the trochlea groove. In the sagittal plane, the greater sigmoid notch opens posteriorly by 30° with respect to the long axis of the ulna shaft (Figure 12.4). In flexion, the coronoid process of the proximal ulna locks into the coronoid fossa of the distal humerus, while the radial head fits into the radial fossa. In extension, the tip of the olecranon is engaged in the olecranon fossa increasing the osseous stability of the joint.

The radial head has a concave proximal end, which articulates with the capitellum, and an articular rim, which articulates with the lesser sigmoid notch of the proximal ulna (Figure 12.5). The shape of the radial head is elliptical and is highly variable among individuals. The radial tuberosity marks the distal margin of the radial neck; it is the site of attachment of the distal end of the biceps tendon.

CAPSULOLIGAMENTOUS ANATOMY

In addition to the highly congruent bony articulations, the capsuloligamentous structures are primary static stabilizers of the elbow. The static soft-tissue stabilizers include the anterior and posterior joint capsule, and the medial and lateral collateral ligament complexes.

The medial collateral ligament (MCL) complex consists of three parts: anterior, posterior, and transverse components

Neither Dr. Kim nor any immediate family member has received anything of value from or has stock or stock options held in a commercial company or institution related directly or indirectly to the subject of this article.

 © 2018 American Academy of Orthopaedic Surgeons

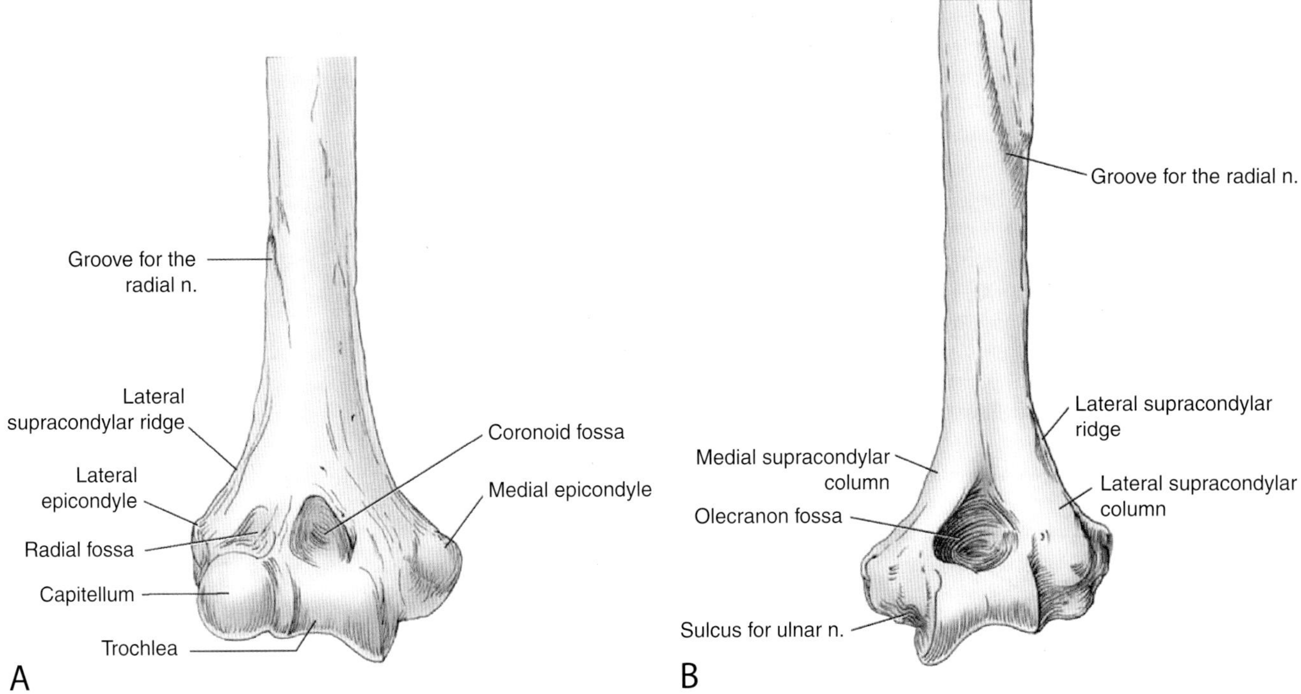

Figure 12.1 Illustrations of the bony landmarks of the anterior aspect (**A**) and of the posterior aspect (**B**) of the distal humerus. (Reproduced with permission from Morrey BF: Anatomy of the elbow joint, in Morrey BF, ed: *The Elbow and Its Disorders*, ed 4. Philadelphia, Saunders Elsevier, 2009, p 14.)

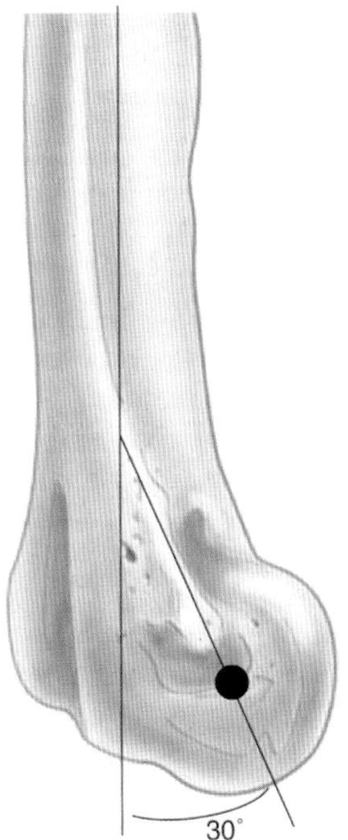

Figure 12.2 In the sagittal plane, the orientation of the articular surface of the distal humerus is rotated anteriorly approximately 30° with respect to the long axis of the humerus. This illustration shows that the center of the rotation of the arc formed by the trochlea and capitellum (black dot) is in line with the anterior cortex of the distal humerus. (Reproduced with permission from Morrey BF: Anatomy of the elbow joint, in Morrey BF, ed: *The Elbow and Its Disorders*, ed 4. Philadelphia, Saunders Elsevier, 2009, p 17.)

(Figure 12.6). The origin of the complex is at the anteroinferior aspect of the medial epicondyle. The anterior bundle is the most discrete component, and inserts on the sublime tubercle on the anteromedial aspect of the coronoid process. Numerous studies have demonstrated increased valgus joint laxity after sectioning of the anterior bundle of the MCL even with an intact radial head. Clinically, the functional importance of the anterior bundle has been confirmed, and various ligament reconstructions have been developed. The posterior bundle is a thickening of the posterior capsule forming the floor of the cubital tunnel, and is well defined at about 90° of flexion. Although the posterior bundle contributes little to the static stability of the elbow, it does provide a moderate contribution to rotational stability. In addition, contracture of the posterior bundle can limit elbow flexion. The transverse ligament runs between the coronoid and the tip of the olecranon, and consists of horizontally oriented fibers that often cannot be separated from the capsule. The transverse ligament appears to contribute little or nothing to elbow stability.

The lateral collateral ligament (LCL) complex is less discrete than the medial complex, and there is often individual variance. The LCL complex consists of four components: the lateral ulnar collateral ligament (LUCL), the annular ligament, the radial collateral ligament, and the variably present accessory LCL (Figure 12.7). The LUCL originates from the lateral epicondyle, and blends with the fibers of the annular ligament inserting on the tubercle of the supinator crest of the ulna. This ligament is considered to be one of the primary elbow constraints, and provides varus and posterolateral

© 2018 American Academy of Orthopaedic Surgeons

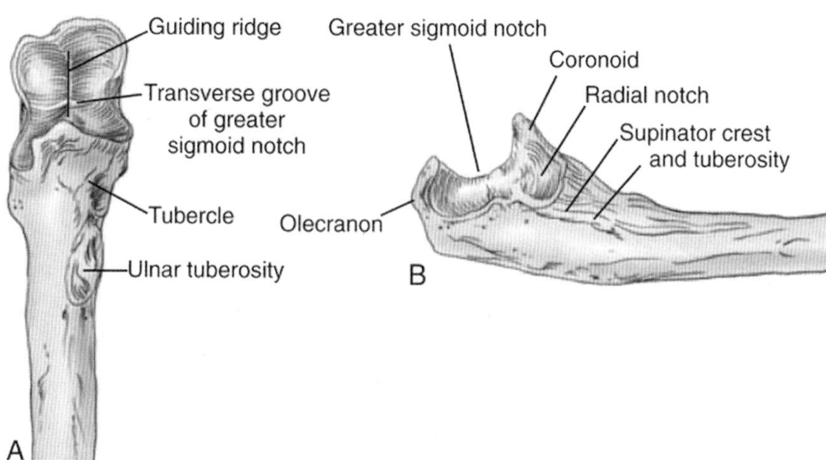

Figure 12.3 Illustrations of the bony landmarks of the anterior aspect (**A**) and lateral aspect (**B**) of the proximal ulna. (Reproduced with permission from Morrey BF: Anatomy of the elbow joint, in Morrey BF, ed: *The Elbow and Its Disorders*, ed 4. Philadelphia, Saunders Elsevier, 2009, p 16.)

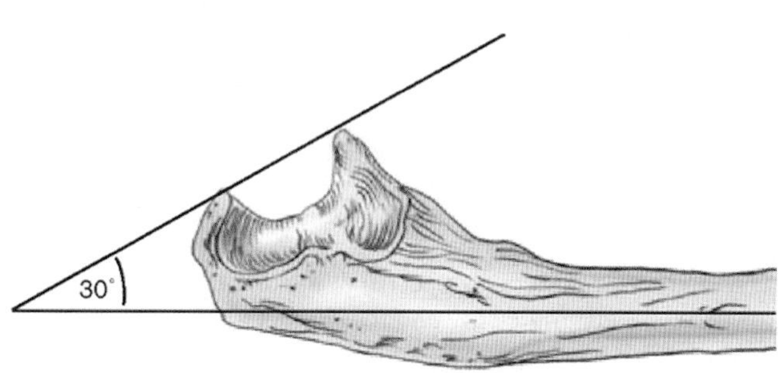

Figure 12.4 Illustration of the line connecting the olecranon tip with the coronoid process tip, which has approximately 30° of angulation with the long axis of the ulnar shaft. This matches the 30° anterior rotation of the distal humerus articular surface shown in Figure 12.2. (Reproduced with permission from Morrey BF: Anatomy of the elbow joint, in Morrey BF, ed: *The Elbow and Its Disorders*, ed 4. Philadelphia, Saunders Elsevier, 2009, p 19.)

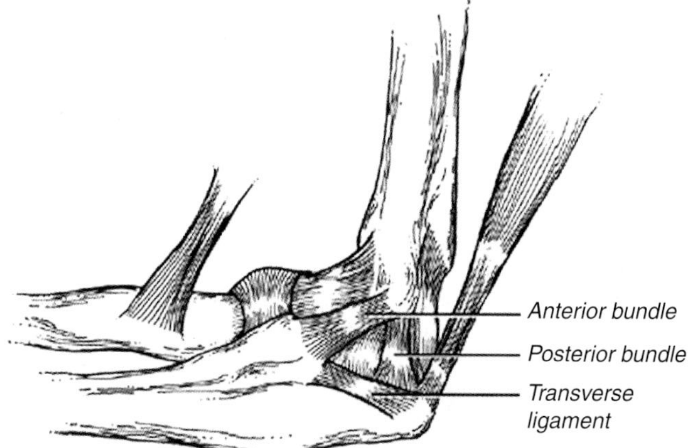

Figure 12.6 Illustration of the medial collateral ligament complex. (Reproduced with permission from Armstrong AD, King GJ, Yamaguchi K: Total elbow arthroplasty design, in Williams GR, Yamaguchi K, Ramsey ML, et al., ed: *Shoulder and Elbow Arthroplasty*. Philadelphia, Lippincott Williams & Wilkins, 2005, p 303.)

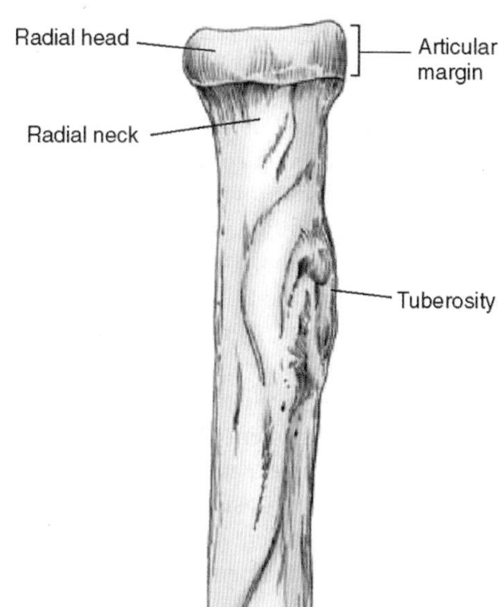

Figure 12.5 Illustration of the bony landmarks of the proximal radius. (Reproduced with permission from Morrey BF: Anatomy of the elbow joint, in Morrey BF, ed: *The Elbow and Its Disorders*, ed 4. Philadelphia, Saunders Elsevier, 2009, p 15.)

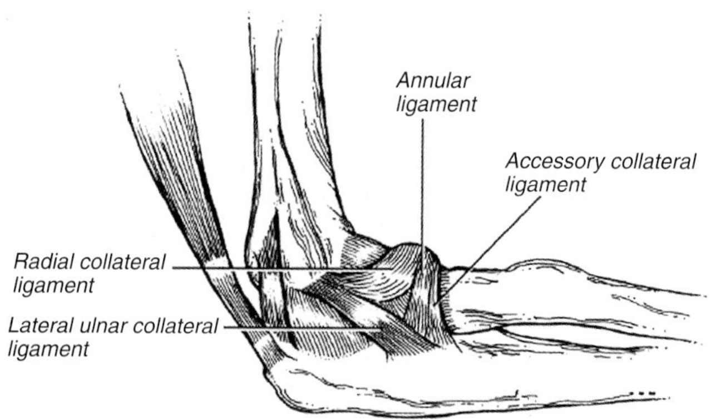

Figure 12.7 Illustration of the lateral collateral ligament complex. (Reproduced with permission from Armstrong AD, King GJ, Yamaguchi K: Total elbow arthroplasty design, in Williams GR, Yamaguchi K, Ramsey ML, et al., ed: *Shoulder and Elbow Arthroplasty*. Philadelphia, Lippincott Williams & Wilkins, 2005, p 303.)

© 2018 American Academy of Orthopaedic Surgeons

stability. Disruption of the LUCL has been demonstrated to be an important cause of both acute and recurrent dislocation of the elbow. The annular ligament is a strong band of tissue that wraps around the radial neck, originating and inserting on the anterior and posterior margins of the lesser sigmoid notch. This funnel-shaped ligament stabilizes the proximal radius throughout the range of pronation and supination. The radial collateral ligament originates from the lateral epicondyle and inserts into the annular ligament. This ligament contributes to the stability of the radial head. The accessory LCL originates from the supinator crest and inserts into the annular ligament. It is believed that this ligament contributes to the stability of the annular ligament during varus stress.

MUSCULAR ANATOMY

The muscles around the elbow joint provide the motor for motions for the elbow, forearm, wrist, and fingers, as well as contributing to the dynamic stability of the elbow joint. There are four groups of muscles that are primarily related to the elbow joint: elbow flexors, elbow extensors, forearm flexor-pronators, and forearm extensors.

The elbow flexors are the biceps, brachialis, and brachioradialis (Figure 12.8, A). The biceps has a smaller cross-sectional area as an elbow flexor than the brachialis, but it has a better mechanical moment arm. When the forearm is pronated, the biceps acts as a strong supinator. Its distal insertion on the radial tuberosity can be disrupted by forceful resisted elbow flexion, which requires a surgical repair depending on the activity and symptom severity of the patient. The biceps is innervated by the musculocutaneous nerve. The biceps aponeurosis, lacertus fibrosus, is a strong fibrous band that arises from the distal biceps tendon and blends into the deep fascia of the flexor-pronator muscle and reinforces the antecubital fossa, helping to protect the brachial artery and median nerve running underneath it (Figure 12.8, B). The lacertus fibrosus can be a source of median nerve compression. The brachialis has the largest cross-sectional area among the elbow flexors, but has a poor mechanical moment arm being so close to the axis of the rotation. It inserts on the coronoid process approximately 2 mm distal to the articular margin. It is well known that the brachialis is often injured during elbow trauma including elbow dislocations, which can lead to the development of heterotopic ossification. The brachialis is innervated mainly by the musculocutaneous nerve while a variable amount of its lateral portion is innervated by the radial nerve. The internervous plane along the midline of the muscle provides an access to the anterior aspect of the distal humerus during surgical procedures. The brachioradialis originates from the lateral supracondylar ridge of the humerus and inserts into the radial styloid. It protects the radial nerve and is innervated by the nerve. The brachioradialis is a weak elbow flexor but can provide elbow flexion function in cases of musculocutaneous nerve palsy.

Elbow extension is almost solely attributed to the triceps. The triceps has three components—the long, lateral, and medial heads—and inserts onto the tip of the olecranon. The long and lateral heads originate more proximally and are more superficial than the medial head. The three heads become confluent in the midline of the humerus to form a common muscle, that tapers into the triceps tendon. The radial nerve innervates all three heads. The medial head is innervated distal to the spiral or radial groove of the humerus, whereas the lateral and long heads are innervated proximal to the spiral groove. Therefore, a lesion of the nerve at the mid-portion of the humerus usually spares the triceps function as the lateral and long heads are innervated more proximally.

The flexor-pronator group arises from the medial epicondyle of the distal humerus and consists of the pronator teres, flexor carpi radialis (FCR), palmaris longus, flexor digitorum superficialis (FDS), and flexor carpi ulnaris (FCU) (Figure 12.8, A and B). The median nerve innervates all of the flexor-pronator muscles except for the FCU, which is innervated by the ulnar nerve. The pronator teres has two origins; the larger humeral head arises from the medial epicondyle, and the smaller ulnar head from the medial aspect of the coronoid process. The space between the two heads can be a source of median nerve compression in so-called "pronator syndrome." The pronator is a strong pronator of the forearm. The FCU is the most posterior of the common flexor tendons originating from the medial epicondyle. It has two origins: one from the medial epicondyle (the humeral head) and the other from the medial aspect of the proximal ulna (the ulnar head). The palmaris longus shares its origin from the medial epicondyle with the flexor carpi radialis and ulnaris. The palmaris longus becomes tendinous at the proximal forearm level and inserts into the palmar aponeurosis. It is absent in approximately 10% of extremities. The FCR inserts into the base of the second, and occasionally third, metacarpal, functioning as a wrist flexor. The FDS has two origins: one from the medial epicondyle and the other from the proximal two-thirds of the radius. This unique origin of the muscle forms a fibrous margin, which occasionally causes compression of the median nerve as the nerve passes under the muscle. It inserts into the base of the middle phalanges of the four fingers and functions as the flexor of the proximal interphalangeal joints.

The forearm extensors include the extensor carpi radialis longus (ECRL), the extensor carpi radialis brevis (ECRB), the extensor digitorum communis (EDC), and the extensor carpi ulnaris (ECU); all innervated by the radial nerve (Figure 12.9, A). The ECRL originates from the lateral supracondylar ridge of the distal humerus; its origin consists of largely fleshy fibers. It inserts into the dorsum of the second metacarpal base and functions as a wrist extensor. Unlike the ECRL, the ECRB has a tendinous origin. Its origin is more distal and deeper than that of the longus and is located on the lateral and superior aspect of the lateral epicondyle. The ECRB origin is covered by the ECRL origin. The common extensor origin of the EDC is located just distal to the origin of the ECRB. This relationship is important to recognize, as the ECRB is most commonly

© 2018 American Academy of Orthopaedic Surgeons

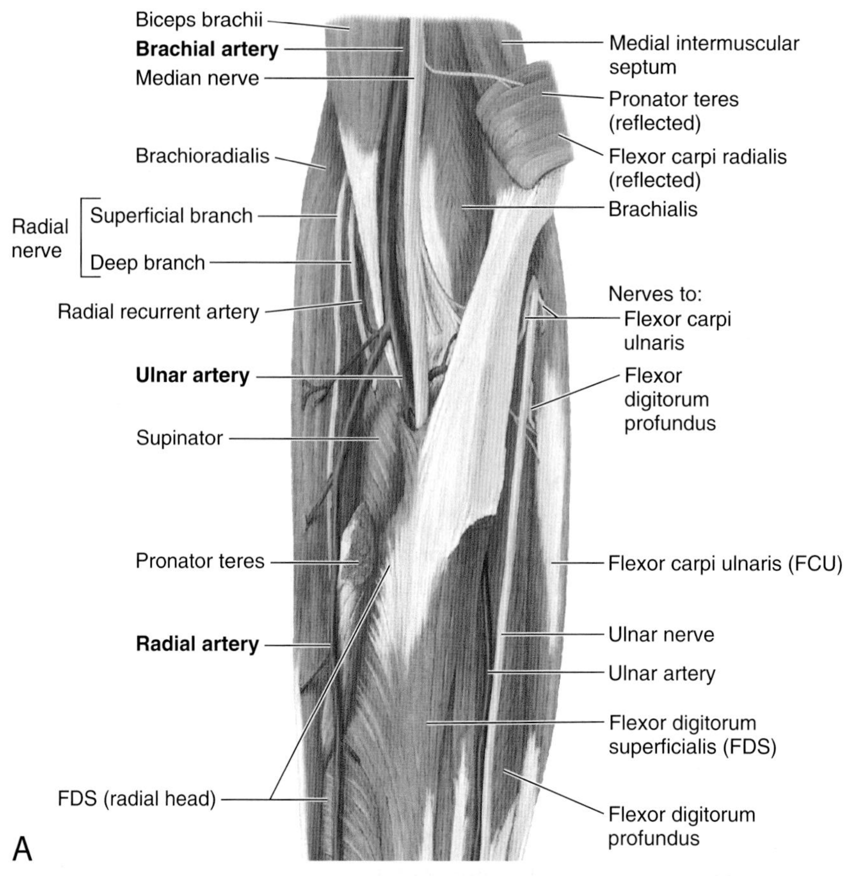

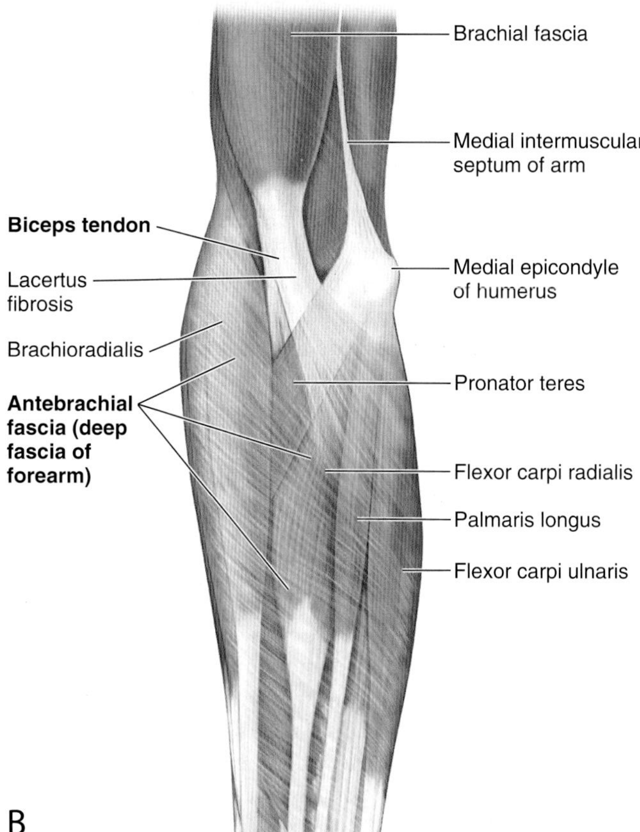

Figure 12.8 Illustration of the muscles and nerves of the anterior aspect of the elbow and forearm. The biceps brachii, brachialis, and brachioradialis are the elbow flexors. The bicipital aponeurosis or lacertus fibrosus blends into the deep fascia of the flexor-pronator muscle. The flexor-pronator muscle group arises from the medial epicondyle of the distal humerus and includes pronator teres, flexor carpi radialis, flexor carpi ulnaris, palmaris longus, and flexor digitorum superficialis. (Reproduced with permission from Moore KL, Agur AMR, Dalley AF, eds: *Clinically Oriented Anatomy*, 7th edition. Baltimore, Wolters Kluwer, 2014.)

© 2018 American Academy of Orthopaedic Surgeons

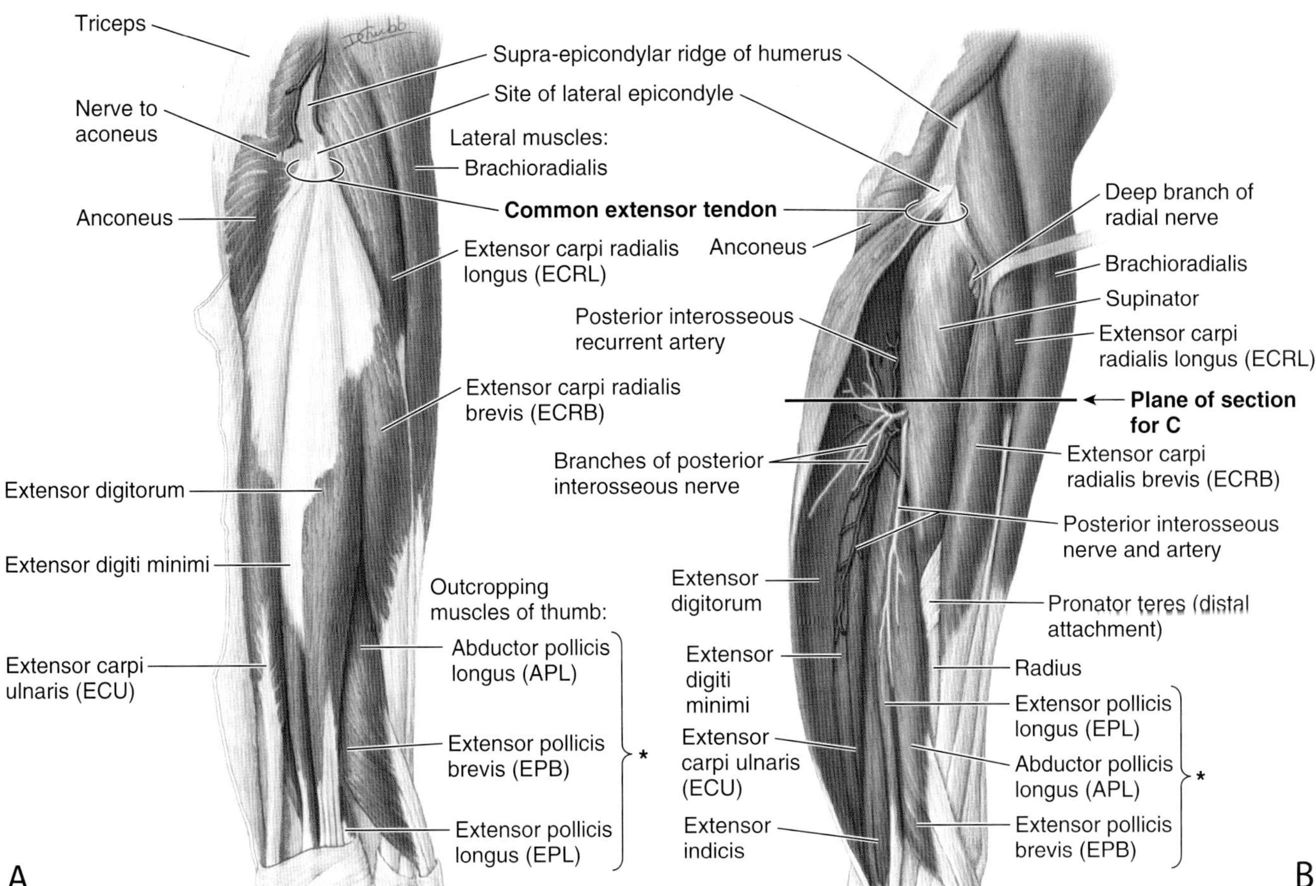

Figure 12.9 Illustration of muscles and nerves of the posterior aspect of the elbow and forearm. The triceps is the sole extensor of the elbow and inserts onto the olecranon tip. The forearm extensors originate from the lateral epicondyle of the distal humerus and include the extensor carpi radialis longus, extensor carpi radialis brevis, extensor digitorum communis, and extensor carpi ulnaris. The anconeus originates from the posterior aspect of the lateral epicondyle and lateral triceps fascia. (Reproduced with permission from Moore KL, Agur AMR, Dalley AF, eds: *Clinically Oriented Anatomy*, 7th edition. Baltimore, Wolters Kluwer, 2014.)

implicated as the site of lateral epicondylitis. The ECRB inserts into the dorsum of the third metacarpal base and functions as a wrist extensor. The humeral origin of the ECU is the most medial of the common extensor group. The interval between the ECU and the anconeus is commonly utilized for the approach to the lateral elbow structures during various surgical procedures.

Although the anconeus and the supinator are not part of the extensor group, they are in close proximity to the region on the lateral side of the elbow. The anconeus originates from the posterior aspect of the lateral epicondyle and lateral triceps fascia (Figure 12.9, B). It inserts on the lateral dorsal surface of the proximal ulna and covers the annular ligament and radial head. It is innervated by a terminal branch of the radial nerve. The exact function of the anconeus is unknown, but one possible suggestion is that it acts as an elbow joint stabilizer. The supinator is a flat muscle that has a complex origin consisting of three sites: the lateral epicondyle, the LCL, and the proximal lateral aspect of the ulnar along the supinator crest. It inserts diffusely on the proximal radius starting proximal to the radial tuberosity and continuing distal to the insertion of the pronator teres at the junction of the proximal and middle one-third of the radius. It functions as a supinator of the forearm, but is weaker than the biceps. Unlike the biceps, however, the effectiveness of the supinator is not affected by the degree of the elbow flexion. The supinator is innervated by the deep radial nerve as the nerve travels through the muscle.

BIOMECHANICS OF THE ELBOW

Stability

The stability of the elbow is provided by static and dynamic constraints (Figure 12.10). The three primary static constraints include the ulnohumeral articulation, anterior bundle of the MCL, and LCL complex. The elbow remains stable as long as these three primary constraints are intact. The secondary static constraints include the radiocapitellar articulation, the common flexor tendon, the common extensor tendon, and the joint capsule. The muscles crossing the elbow joint are dynamic constraints and augment the static constraints.

© 2018 American Academy of Orthopaedic Surgeons

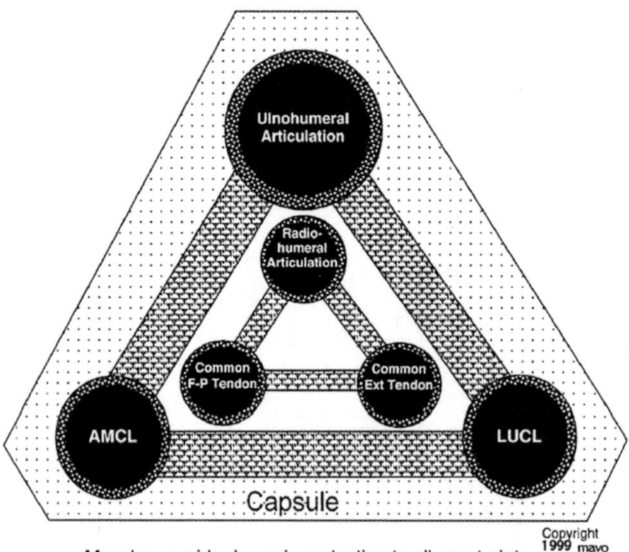

Figure 12.10 Illustration of stability of the elbow, maintained by the primary static constraints (the outer triangle) and the secondary static constraints (the inner triangle). The primary static constraints are the ulnohumeral articulation, the anterior bundle of the medial collateral ligament (AMCL), and the lateral ulnar collateral ligament (LUCL). The secondary static constraints are the radiocapitellar articulation, the common extensor tendon, the flexor-pronator tendon, and the joint capsule. The muscles crossing the elbow are the dynamic stabilizers of the elbow. (Reproduced with permission from O'Driscoll SW, Jupiter JB, King GJ, Hotchkiss RN, Morrey BF: The unstable elbow. *Instr Course Lect* 2001;50:91.)

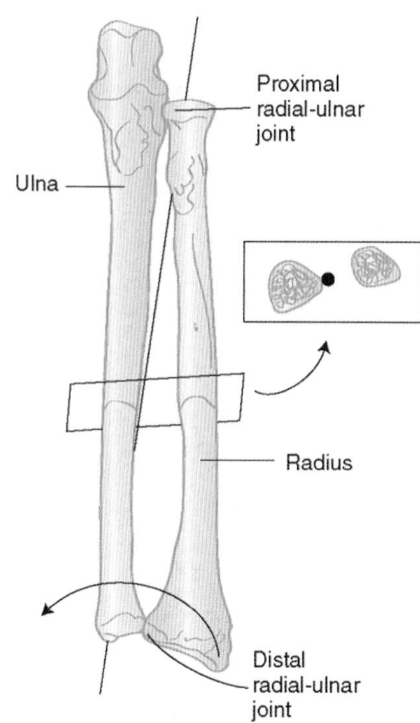

Figure 12.11 Illustration of the axis of forearm supination and pronation, which runs from the center of the radial head to the fovea near to the base of the ulnar styloid process. The axis is at the ulnar cortex in the distal one-third of the forearm. (Reproduced with permission from An KN, Zobitz ME, Morrey BF. Biomechanics of the elbow. In: Morrey BF, ed: *The Elbow and Its Disorders*, ed 4. Philadelphia, Saunders Elsevier, 2009, p 42.)

Flexion and Extension

The elbow joint normally has a ROM of approximately 0° to 140°. Of this total arc, only approximately 30° to 130° is necessary for most activities of daily living (ADLs). Because of the highly congruent ulnohumeral joint and soft-tissue constraints, the elbow joint motion is primarily a hinge type. It has been reported by many investigators that the center of rotation does not follow a perfect hinge, but rather follows an irregular course. Despite different findings from various studies, the deviation of the center of rotation is relatively minimal. Therefore, the ulnohumeral joint can be regarded as a uniaxial joint except at the extremes of flexion and extension. The radiocapitellar joint, which is the lateral half of the elbow joint, has a common transverse axis with the ulnohumeral joint. The axis of the rotation passes through the center of the arc formed by the trochlear groove and capitellum. The axis of rotation is internally rotated 3° to 8° relative to the plane of the epicondyles. In the coronal plane, the axis forms a valgus angle of 4° to 8° with the long axis of the humerus.

Pronation and Supination

Pronation and supination occurs at the radiocapitellar and proximal radioulnar joints. The normal range of forearm rotation is approximately 180° with pronation of 80° to 90° and supination of approximately 90°. Most ADLs can be achieved with 100° of forearm rotation (50° of pronation and 50° of supination). Loss of pronation can be compensated to a certain extent by shoulder abduction, but loss of supination can hardly be compensated. The axis of forearm rotation passes through the center of the radial head and the fovea near the base of the ulnar styloid (Figure 12.11). It has been reported clinically and experimentally that an angular deformity of less than 10° of either the radius or ulna causes no functionally significant loss of forearm rotation. The radius migrates proximally 1 mm to 2 mm with pronation. It has been shown that the ulna rotates with forearm rotation; it rotates externally with forearm supination and rotates internally with pronation. Thus, forearm rotation plays an important role in elbow stability, especially when the elbow is moved passively. With passive flexion, the elbow with a deficient MCL is more stable in supination while the elbow with a deficient LCL is more stable in pronation. This provides the basis of the forearm positioning for immobilization following elbow dislocations.

NERVES CROSSING THE ELBOW

Musculocutaneous Nerve (C5–C8)

The musculocutaneous nerve is a terminal branch of the lateral cord of the brachial plexus. It innervates the main elbow flexors, the biceps, and the brachialis at the level of the proximal

© 2018 American Academy of Orthopaedic Surgeons

arm. It continues through the brachial fascia and passes lateral to the biceps tendon. It becomes as superficial as the antecubital veins in the antecubital fossa, and terminates as the lateral antebrachial cutaneous nerve. A lesion of the lateral antebrachial cutaneous nerve causes paresthesia and anesthesia of the lateral proximal forearm area.

Median Nerve (C5–T1)

The median nerve arises from contributions from the medial and lateral cords of the brachial plexus and travels along with the brachial artery on the medial side of the arm between the brachialis and biceps brachii muscles. It courses straight distally into the medial aspect of the antecubital fossa, travelling medial to the biceps tendon and the brachial artery. At the elbow level, it passes under the bicipital aponeurosis or lacertus fibrosus, then between the ulnar and humeral heads of the pronator teres. Both locations under the lacertus fibrosus and between two heads of the pronator teres can be a source of median nerve compression. It continues distally to enter the forearm travelling between the FDS and flexor digitorum profundus (FDP). The median nerve innervates the pronator teres, FCR, palmaris longus, and FDS. It gives off two branches as it travels further distally in the forearm: the anterior interosseous nerve (AIN) and the palmar cutaneous nerve. The AIN arises near the inferior border of the pronator teres and travels distally along the anterior aspect of the interosseous membrane parallel to the anterior interosseous artery. The AIN innervates the lateral half of the FDP and the flexor pollicis longus. The palmar cutaneous branch arises from the lateral aspect of the median nerve at the distal forearm level and supplies the skin sensation at the lateral palmar aspect of the hand. The median nerve proper continues distally into the hand, giving off motor branches (recurrent branch) to the muscles of the thenar eminence and the two lateral lumbricals and sensory branches (digital cutaneous branches) to the palm and the lateral 3.5 digits.

Radial Nerve (C5–T1)

The radial nerve arises from the posterior cord of the brachial plexus and enters the posterior compartment of the upper arm. It travels distally in a medial-to-lateral direction, innervating the three heads of the triceps. It lies deep to the lateral head of the triceps and runs along the origin of the medial head of the triceps. It penetrates the lateral intermuscular septum just distal to the deltoid insertion along the spiral groove. The nerve is at risk for injury from fractures or surgery involving this site. As it approaches the elbow, it stays in the anterior compartment anterior to the lateral epicondyle, but deep to the brachioradialis. It innervates the brachioradialis, a variable amount of the lateral portion of the brachialis, ECRL, and anconeus. The nerve, then, divides into the deep and superficial branches in the antecubital fossa. The superficial radial nerve is the direct extension of the radial nerve, and travels distally in the anterior compartment of the forearm to innervate the mid-dorsal aspect of the forearm. The deep radial nerve innervates the ECRB and the supinator. The deep radial nerve becomes the posterior interosseous nerve (PIN) as it exits the distal margin of the supinator and travels in the posterior compartment of the forearm. The tendinous proximal border of the supinator or Arcade of Frohse can be a site of radial nerve compression. The PIN innervates the EDC, extensor pollicis longus, extensor pollicis brevis, ECU, abductor pollicis longus, extensor digiti minimi, and extensor indicis.

Ulnar Nerve (C8–T1)

The ulnar nerve arises from the medial cord of the brachial plexus. It penetrates the medial intermuscular septum at the mid-arm level, then travels intimately anterior to the intermuscular septum. The Arcade of Struthers refers to a fibrous canal formed by the medial intermuscular septum and the deep fascia of the triceps at the medial upper arm. The ulnar nerve is vulnerable to compression as it travels in this fibrous canal. As it approaches the elbow, it enters the cubital tunnel, which is formed by the medial epicondyle, the ligament of Osborne, and the posterior bundle of the MCL. The posterior bundle of the MCL becomes taut as the elbow flexes, which reduces the volume of the cubital tunnel. This explains the worsening of ulnar nerve symptoms with elbow flexion in patients with cubital tunnel syndrome. The ulnar nerve does not give off any branch in the upper arm except variable tributaries to the triceps. At the elbow, it gives off a few articular branches. It then passes between the two heads of the FCU, giving off a few branches to this muscle. The ulnar half of the FDP is innervated by the ulnar nerve. The dorsal and palmar cutaneous branches arise at the distal forearm level and supply the skin sensation of the dorsal and palmar sides of the hand, respectively.

BIBLIOGRAPHY

An KN, Zobitz ME, Morrey BF: Biomechanics of the elbow, in Morrey BF, ed: *The Elbow and its Disorders,* ed. 4. Philadelphia, Saunders Elsevier, 2009, pp 39–63.

Boone DC, Azen SP: Normal range of motion of joints in male subjects. *J Bone Joint Surg Am* 1979;61(5):756–759.

Bryce CD, Armstrong AD: Anatomy and biomechanics of the elbow. *Orthop Clin North Am* 2008;39(2):141–154, v.

Floris S, Olsen BS, Dalstra M, et al.: The medial collateral ligament of the elbow joint: anatomy and kinematics. *J Shoulder Elbow Surg* 1998;7(4):345–351.

Johnson JA, King GJ. 2005. Anatomy and biomechanics of the elbow, in Williams GR, Yamaguchi K, Ramsey ML, Galatz LM, eds: *Shoulder and Elbow Arthroplasty.* Philadelphia, Lippincott Williams and Wilkins, 2005, pp. 279–296.

Morrey BF, An KN: Articular and ligamentous contributions to the stability of the elbow joint. *Am J Sports Med* 1983;11(5):315–319.

Morrey BF: Anatomy of the elbow joint, in: Morrey BF, ed. *The Elbow and Its Disorders*, ed. 4. Philadelphia, Saunders Elsevier, 2009, pp 11–38.

Morrey BF, Chao EY: Passive motion of the elbow joint. *J Bone Joint Surg Am* 1976;58(4):501–508.

O'Driscoll SW, Bell DF, Morrey BF: Posterolateral rotatory instability of the elbow. *J Bone Joint Surg Am* 1991;73(3): 440–446.

© 2018 American Academy of Orthopaedic Surgeons

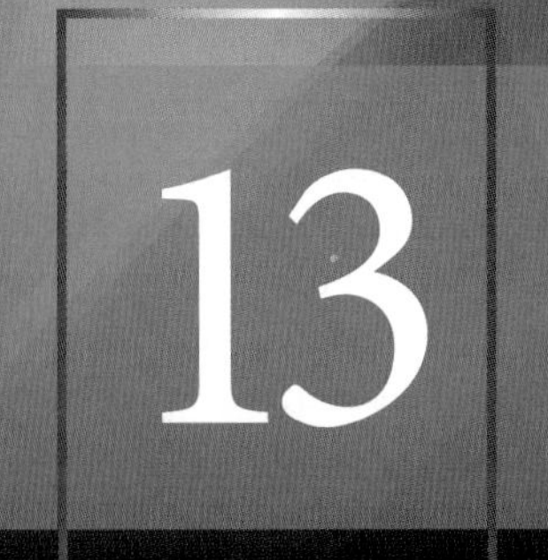

13 Elbow Contracture Release

Joaquin Sanchez-Sotelo, MD, PhD

INTRODUCTION

Among the major joints, the elbow is especially prone to stiffness and contracture. This is due, in part, to the constrained articular anatomy as well as the surrounding capsular and ligamentous structures. Contracture of varying degrees is very common after elbow trauma. Loss of motion and contracture also occurs in the setting of hypertrophic osteoarthritis, inflammatory arthritis, postoperative contracture, neuromuscular disease, and burns.

Although capsular fibrosis contributes to contracture in most elbows, motion may also be limited by bony impingement, heterotopic ossification, malunion, cartilage adhesions, prominent hardware, nonisometric ligaments, and other abnormalities of the articular surface. The term *intrinsic stiffness* refers involvement of the articular surfaces to such extent that motion cannot be reliably restored without addressing the articular surfaces surgically, whereas *extrinsic stiffness* refers to involvement of the periarticular soft tissues. In many cases, elbow stiffness is the result of combined involvement.

The normal elbow flexion arc is about 0° to 140°, and normal pronation and supination is about 80°. The majority of activities of daily living (ADLs) require a flexion arc of 30° to 130° and 50° of pronation and supination. A flexion arc of 30° to 130° reduces the space reached by the hand by about 20%. More recent work suggests that a greater range is required for certain activities, such as cell phone use.

Refractory elbow stiffness and contracture can be overcome by surgical removal of the contracted capsule and all sources of bony impingement, including areas of heterotopic ossification. Various surgical approaches have been described to remove a contracted capsule, loose bodies, osteophytes, and ectopic bone from the elbow joint. Arthroscopic contracture release, also known as arthroscopic osteocapsular arthroplasty, has gained popularity over the last few years, but open contracture release is also commonly performed.

Intraoperative restoration of a functional arc of motion can be achieved in the majority of elbows with extrinsic stiffness. However, maintenance of the range of motion (ROM) achieved in surgery is difficult, and the rehabilitation program after contracture release is paramount for the final outcome of any of these procedures. In general, improvements in flexion and extension are easier to obtain and maintain than improvements in pronation and supination.

This chapter reviews the surgical management and postoperative rehabilitation program typically recommended after surgical treatment of extrinsic stiffness.

SURGICAL PROCEDURE

Indications and Contraindications

Release of elbow joints with extrinsic contracture is indicated when the degree of stiffness interferes with the patient's function. Patients' expectations vary based on their occupation and interests. Although it is traditionally accepted that most activities of daily living (ADLs) are possible when the elbow can be flexed from 30° to 130° degrees, and the arc of pronation and supination is of 50° in each direction, some patients may require greater mobility to perform their ADLs or more demanding athletic or artistic activities.

The main absolute contraindication for contracture release in our practice is active infection. Compromised skin and surrounding soft-tissue envelope is a relative contraindication, as these conditions can be managed in some cases with the incorporation of plastic surgical interventions. In addition, inability to comply with the postoperative rehabilitation program and severe neuromuscular dysfunction or paralysis are relative contraindications, although release of the hyperflexed elbow may be required in these circumstances to facilitate skin hygiene in the elbow flexion crease. In patients with intrinsic contracture, surgical release needs to be combined with other

Dr. Sanchez-Sotelo or an immediate family member has received royalties from Stryker; is a member of a speakers' bureau or has made paid presentations on behalf of Merck and Stryker; serves as a paid consultant to Tornier; has received research or institutional support from Stryker; has received nonincome support (such as equipment or services), commercially derived honoraria, or other non-research–related funding (such as paid travel) from Elsevier and the Journal of Shoulder and Elbow Surgery; *and serves as a board member, owner, officer, or committee member of the American Shoulder and Elbow Surgeons and the* Journal of Shoulder and Elbow Surgery.

© 2018 American Academy of Orthopaedic Surgeons

procedures, such is interposition arthroplasty or total elbow arthroplasty.

Careful consideration should be given when considering arthroscopic capsular release in posttraumatic cases after open reduction and internal fixation. These cases may have extensive scarring related to the surgical procedure as well as the original injury, which may substantially increase the risk of the nerve injury.

The timing of contracture release needs to be carefully considered in some circumstances. Stiffness after fracture fixation is best addressed once fracture healing is confirmed. Resection of heterotopic ossification is considered typically 3 to 6 months after injury, substantially earlier than in the past. Controversy remains about the timing of contracture release for children and adolescents as well as patients with chronic regional pain syndrome (CRPS). Contracture release may be less reliable in older children and adolescents, attributed partly to increased fibrotic activity around growth spurts and partly to compliance issues. Early surgery may be considered in type II CRPS when ulnar neurolysis or release is considered, especially if a brachial plexus block will be used postoperatively.

Finally, the condition of the soft tissues needs to be assessed carefully to determine the need for soft-tissue coverage at the time of contracture release, especially in patients with previous open fractures, skin grafting, and/or soft-tissue flaps.

Surgical Technique

Preoperative evaluation is paramount for the success of surgical release of elbow contracture. Prior skin incisions and the condition of the elbow soft-tissue envelope should be noted. Motion should be accurately measured and recorded in flexion, extension, pronation, and supination. Neurovascular examination of the involved upper extremity is directed to identification of associated nerve deficits and is particularly directed to the ulnar nerve. Plain radiographs and computed tomography with three-dimensional reconstruction are the imaging modalities of choice to assess articular and bony anatomy, as well as ectopic ossification.

The principles of contracture release are the same for open and arthroscopic procedures and include (1) the removal of fibrotic anterior and posterior capsule, including the posterior band of the medial collateral ligament (MCL); and (2) elimination of bony impingement by removing osteophytes and bone from the olecranon, coronoid, radial head, and their respective fossae in the distal humerus.

The surgical procedure is typically performed with general anesthesia. A brachial plexus nerve block is performed once the neurovascular status of the affected extremity has been confirmed to be normal right after surgery, and provided there are no contraindications. An indwelling axillary catheter can be placed to provide pain relief for the first 2 to 3 days after surgery.

Open Contracture Release

In open contracture release, the capsule is first dissected free from the overlying muscle fibers and resected, and followed by bone removal. An effort is made to preserve the integrity of the collateral ligaments (lateral collateral ligament complex) and anterior band of the MCL. Table 13.1 lists the most common surgical exposures described for open contracture release. The decision to use the lateral or medial column approaches is based on the location of the associated pathology. In both approaches, the collateral ligaments are preserved whenever possible in order to avoid iatrogenic instability.

Table 13.1 COMMON PROCEDURES DESCRIBED FOR OPEN ELBOW CONTRACTURE RELEASE

Procedure	Posterior Compartment	Anterior Compartment
Lateral column	Raising triceps-anconeus laterally	ECRB–ECRL interval
Medial column	Raising triceps medially	Flexor–pronator interval
Ulnohumeral arthroplasty	Triceps split followed by oval fenestration at olecranon fossa	Through humeral oval fenestration

ECRB = extensor carpi radialis brevis, ECRL = Extensor carpi radialis longus.

In the lateral column procedure, a lateral incision is made and the interval between the extensor carpi radialis longus and brevis is developed to access the anterior compartment. The more anterior extensor muscles are detached and elevated with the brachialis muscle off of the anterior capsule, which is then resected across the anterior compartment of the elbow. The lateral approach is preferred if there is lateral pathology such as following a radial head fracture or if there is heterotopic bone more laterally based. The posterior compartment is accessed by elevating the anconeus and triceps off of the posterior capsule and posterior humerus (Figure 13.1).

In the medial column approach, a medial incision is made and the deeper dissection is carried through the common flexor pronator interval. These muscles are elevated with the brachialis muscle off of the anterior capsule, which is resected. The ulnar nerve can be exposed in the posterior compartment, and is accessed by elevating the triceps off of the posterior capsule and distal humerus. The medial approach is preferred if there is ulnar nerve involvement, after open reduction and internal fixation of distal humerus fractures that may have involved dissection of the ulnar nerve or heterotopic bone that is more medially located.

Open ulnohumeral arthroplasty, the Outerbridge-Kashiwagi procedure, is performed through a posterior incision and triceps-splitting approach to access the posterior compartment. The posterior capsule is released and excised, then the posterior osteophytes and spurring are removed. A complete fenestration of the distal humerus through the olecranon fossa is created to access the anterior compartment. This procedure is most commonly used to treat primary degenerative arthritis of the elbow.

© 2018 American Academy of Orthopaedic Surgeons

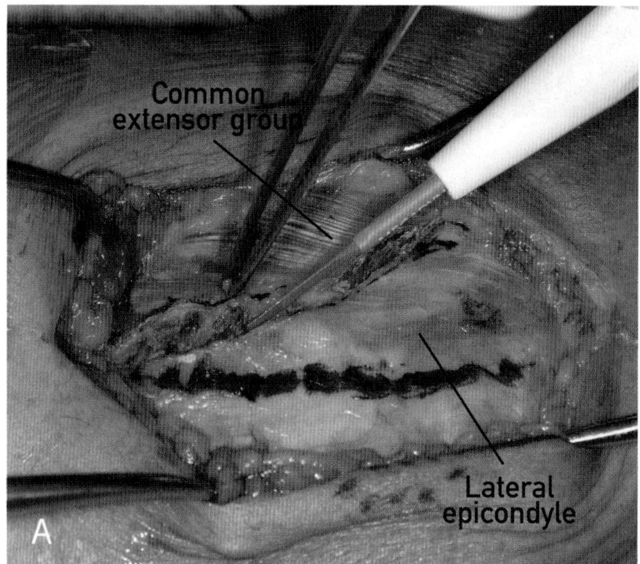

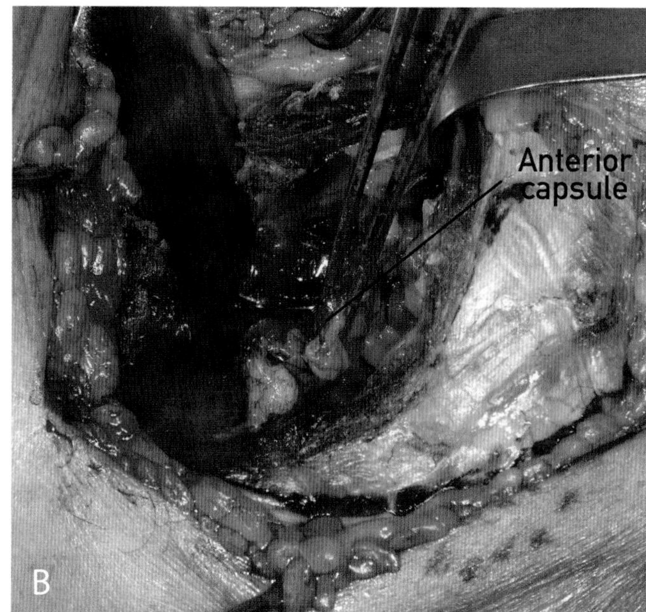

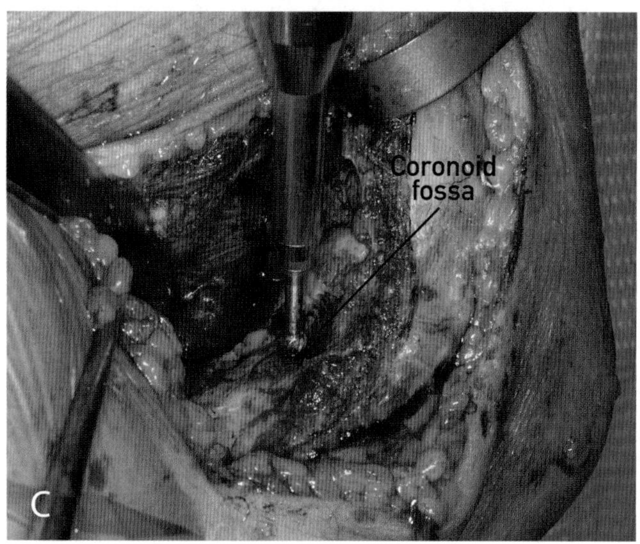

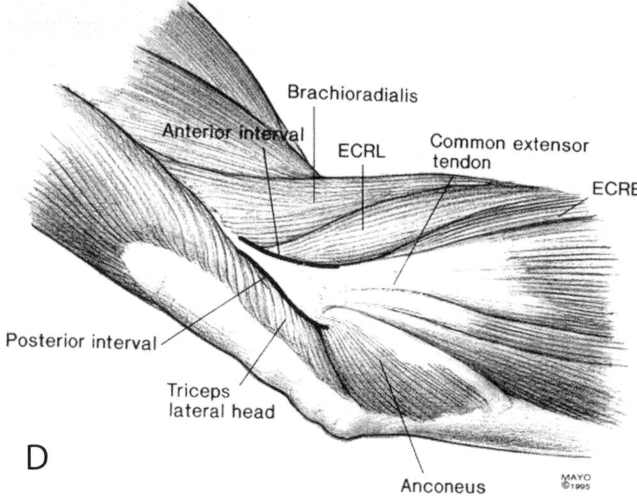

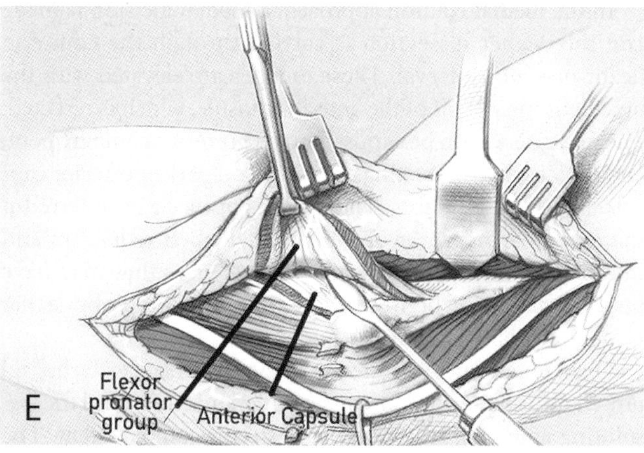

Figure 13.1 Clinical photographs of open contracture release. **A**, The anterior and posterior compartment of the elbows can be exposed using ligament-preserving intervals. Restoration of motion usually requires capsulectomy (**B**) and bone removal (**C**). Illustrations of the lateral (**D**) and medial (**E**) column procedures. (Part D reproduced with permission from the Mayo Foundation for Medical Education and Research, Rochester, MN.)

© 2018 American Academy of Orthopaedic Surgeons

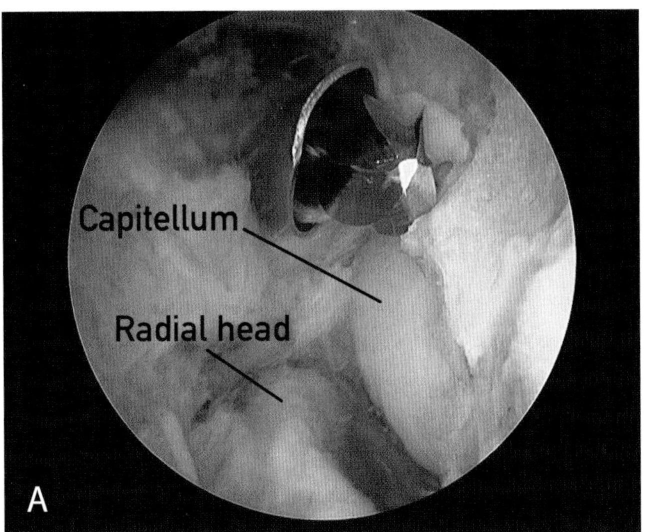

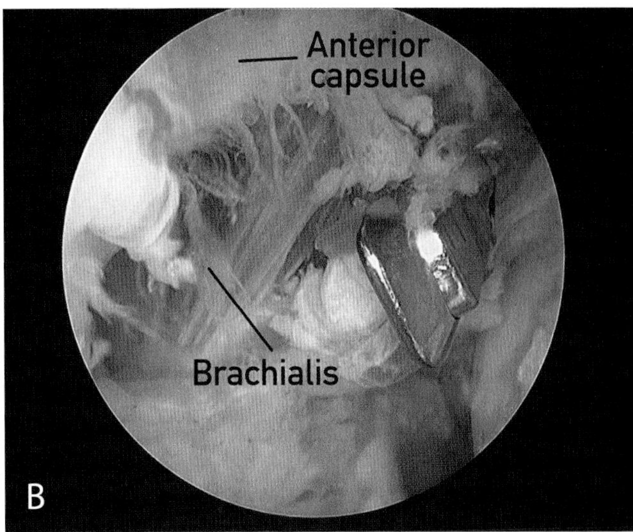

Figure 13.2 Photographs of arthroscopic osteocapsular arthroplasty. Bone removal (**A**) and capsulectomy (**B**) may also be completed arthroscopically.

Arthroscopic Contracture Release

Advances in arthroscopy have led to the use for elbow contracture release. Arthroscopic capsular release is technically demanding, but has the advantage of being minimally invasive. In arthroscopic contracture release, the bony work is performed first, followed by capsulectomy (Figure 13.2). The anterior or posterior compartment may be addressed first based on surgeon's preference. Bone removal is performed with arthroscopic burrs, whereas capsule resection is completed with a combination of arthroscopic bitters, shavers, and radiofrequency devices. Arthroscopic contracture release is thought to be more technically demanding and risky, especially as it relates to nerve injuries.

The Ulnar Nerve in Elbow Stiffness

The ulnar nerve is at risk of injury during elbow contracture release. Acute increases in elbow motion, especially flexion, may be poorly tolerated by the ulnar nerve secondary to perineural scarring and limited nerve mobility that results from previous injury and surgery, as well as a period of restricted elbow motion. In addition, the ulnar tunnel may be already compromised by bone spurs. In rare cases, heterotopic ossification can encase and surround the ulnar nerve.

Some patients may present with a subclinical or clinical ulnar neuropathy. Failure to address the ulnar nerve at the time of contracture release may lead to severe postoperative neuropathy or inability to maintain flexion motion secondary to pain on the medial side.

Controversy remains regarding the indications of in situ ulnar nerve release or subcutaneous transposition at the time of contracture release. In our practice, the ulnar nerve is addressed surgically in patients with preoperative symptoms of ulnar neuropathy, a positive Tinel sign at the ulnar tunnel, or flexion less than 90°. Some recommend routine in situ release in all elbows undergoing contracture release, and transposition for those with established motor neuropathy or a subluxating ulnar nerve.

The need to address the ulnar nerve is considered by some an indication to proceed to open surgery using the medial column procedure. However, in situ decompression of the ulnar nerve may be performed through a small incision and combined with either a lateral column procedure or arthroscopic contracture release (Figure 13.3). In situ decompression of the ulnar nerve also provides excellent exposure for resection of the posterior band of the MCL.

Surgical Restoration of Pronation and Supination

Forearm rotation may be compromised by pathology at the distal radioulnar joint, interosseous membrane, shapes of the radius and ulna, ectopic bone, and proximal radioulnar joint. Procedures designed to eliminate the contribution of the proximal radioulnar joint to limited pronation and supination include periarticular soft-tissue release around the radial head, radial head resection with or without replacement or soft-tissue interposition, removal of heterotopic ossification, and intercalary resection of the proximal radius (reverse Sauve-Kapandji). These may need to be combined with other procedures for the forearm and wrist. Restoration of both flexion and extension as well as pronation and supination can be extremely challenging in terms of both the surgical procedure and rehabilitation program. In general, restoration of flexion arc motion takes precedence over restoration of forearm rotation.

Complications

The main complications of elbow contracture release include nerve injury and wound complications, including infection. Incomplete restoration of motion or recurrence of contracture or heterotopic ossification may also adversely affect the outcome of these procedures. Rarely, an overzealous soft-tissue release may lead to instability. Patients with primary, posttraumatic or

© 2018 American Academy of Orthopaedic Surgeons

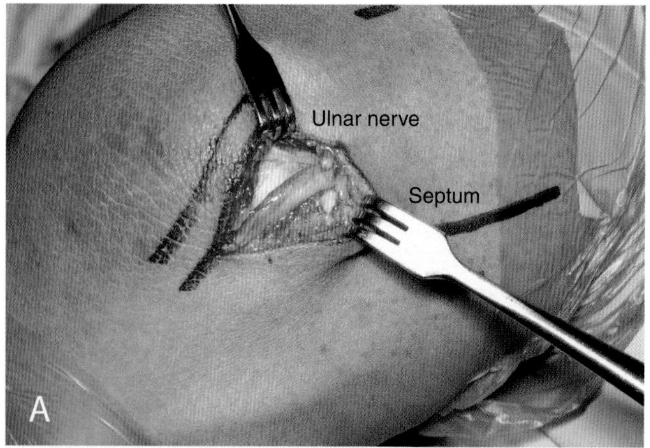

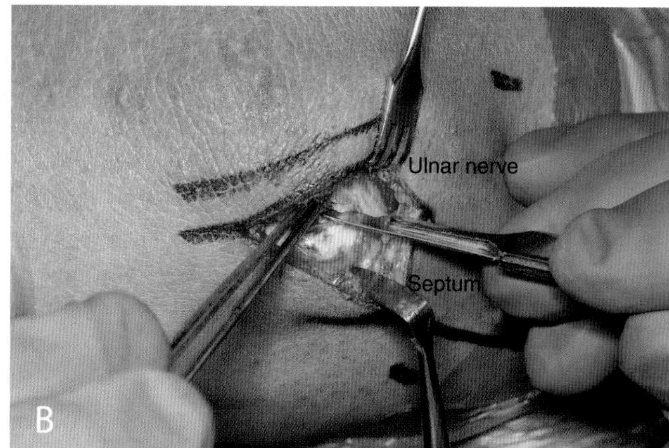

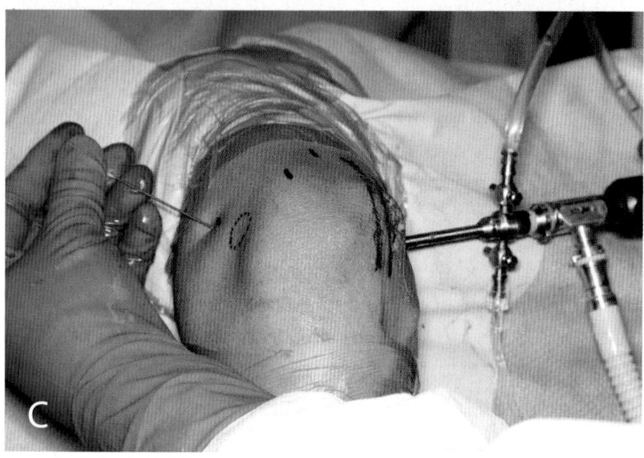

Figure 13.3 **A**, Clinical photograph of the ulnar nerve being decompressed though a small incision. **B**, Clinical photograph of the posterior band of the MCL being resected by retracting the nerve. **C**, Clinical photograph of contracture release then completed arthroscopically.

inflammatory arthritis may experience progression of their disease over time, with increased pain and stiffness.

POSTOPERATIVE REHABILITATION

General Principles

Rehabilitation after elbow contracture release is aimed at maintaining the ROM obtained intraoperatively. Stretching of the elbow joint in flexion and extension, as well as the forearm in pronation and supination, is the mainstay of postoperative treatment. This is accomplished with a combination of formal physical therapy, continuous passive motion (CPM), dynamic orthosis, or static adjustable orthosis. Our preference is to use a combination of CPM and static adjustable orthosis in addition to ROM exercises. Modulation of the inflammatory response is extremely important in the early phases of rehabilitation. Adjunctive radiation therapy, pharmacologic treatments, and manipulation under anesthesia are used for selective indications. Progression from the immediate postoperative period to the end result can follow a specific protocol that focuses on reducing the effects of the surgical trauma and maintains ROM (Table 13.2).

In the earliest phase, there is a focus on modulating the postoperative inflammatory response including pain and swelling. Elevation and compression help to minimize early postoperative swelling (Figure 13.4). Early ROM exercises and CPM can be extremely painful after surgery, especially in patients who undergo extensive open dissections or major bone work. Pain management with indwelling analgesic catheters and local

Table 13.2 OVERVIEW OF POSTOPERATIVE REHABILITATION AFTER ELBOW CONTRACTURE RELEASE

Postoperative Period	Stages of Rehabilitation
Up to first 24 postoperative hours	Modulate inflammatory response (RICE)
Weeks 1 to 4	Continuous passive motion
Up to Month 3	Physical therapy or orthosis
Adjunctive modalities	Manual stretching Radiation therapy Indomethacin Manipulation under anesthesia Neuropathic agents Botulinum toxin

RICE = Rest, Ice, Compression and Elevation.

© 2018 American Academy of Orthopaedic Surgeons

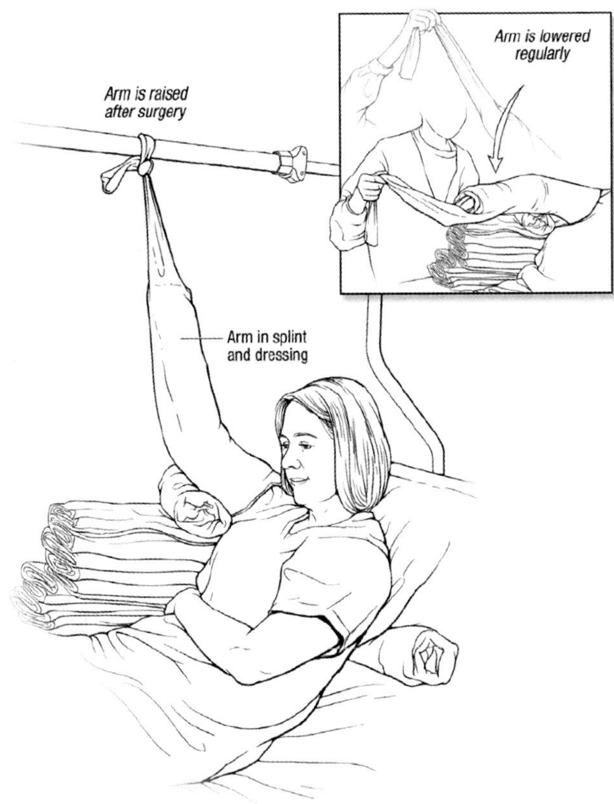

Figure 13.4 Immediately after surgery, edema is controlled by keeping the elbow in extension and elevated, as shown in this illustration.

anesthetic can provide early pain relief, while subsequent use of oral narcotics, analgesics, and anti-inflammatory medications can be helpful.

Formal physical therapy provides guidance and assistance as a patient progresses after surgery. Static and dynamic orthoses provide additional passive stretching and are used as adjuncts to restore and maintain motion after CPM is discontinued.

Author's Preferred Protocol

- *Immediate Postoperative Period (Up to 24 Hours):* Modulation of the inflammatory response
  - Compressive dressing to minimize swelling
  - Immobilize the elbow in extension (plaster or thermoplastic splint).
  - Elevation of the elbow (hang the arm or use pillows or blankets; Figure 13.4)
  - Apply ice frequently.
  - Active wrist and finger flexion and extension
  - Brachial plexus block with indwelling axillary catheter and local anesthetic pump for the first 2 to 3 days after surgery; after the first 2 to 3 days, most patients tolerate CPM using oral pain medication.
  - Oral narcotics, analgesics, and anti-inflammatory medications as needed
- *Weeks 1 to 4*
  - Continue compression, elevation, icing, and oral analgesics
  - CPM with extension and flexion end-range stretching
  - Daily wound check to assess healing and breakdown
- *Weeks 5 to 12*
  - Passive and active assisted elbow and forearm ROM
  - Dynamic or static progressive orthoses
- *Weeks 12+*
  - Continue stretching to avoid loss of motion.
  - Initiate progressive strengthening: elbow flexion/extension; forearm pronation/supination; wrist flexion/extension; hand

Continuous Passive Motion

CPM is instituted immediately after surgery. Although the protocol for usage may vary depending on the patient's response, it is critically important that the patient be an active participant in the management of his or her postoperative rehabilitation. CPM has several purposes. Initiation of early motion helps to avoid stiffness, and CPM requires less effort from the patient. Early on, CPM physically squeezes surgical hematoma and soft-tissue edema outside of the elbow joint. With continuous motion, CPM is also thought to be helpful in maintaining healthy cartilage and preventing intra-articular adhesions. The benefit of CPM is best obtained by moving the elbow joint through a full ROM. CPM is most effective for maintaining elbow flexion and extension motion. Some CPM machines provide pronation and supination motion, but this is usually less effective. When restoration of pronation and supination is a major goal, the patients may be better off coming out of the CPM machine to perform manual stretches of forearm rotation.

Careful attention to details is required when using elbow CPM. The CPM machine is set up so that the arm is comfortable positioned by the bedside or a chair, with the height adjusted so that the elbow rests above the level of the heart to minimize swelling. The CPM machine is set to move through a full flexion arc with the speed at the maximum setting to minimize the time spent in the mid-range of the flexion arc.

Circumferential dressings are removed and replaced with a lightweight elastic compression sleeve. Failure to do so may cause soft-tissue injury secondary to shear stresses. The elbow flexion crease should be directed upward and centered over the hinge of the CPM machine. The arm is then secured with wide soft bands around the forearm and arm. The patient can use the machine to provide end-range stretching (Figure 13.5). The patient stops the CPM machine when extension becomes uncomfortable. After 1 to 2 minutes of rest, blood and fluid have been squeezed out of the soft tissues, and patients are typically able to get a few more degrees of extension. This process of gaining progressive extension is continued until maximum extension is achieved. The patients can best understand the rationale of this process by thinking that they are "milking" their elbow. In order to stretch in flexion, the patient stops the CPM machine when flexion becomes uncomfortable. After 1 to 2 minutes of rest in the flexed position, the patient tries to gain a few more degrees by "milking" the elbow. Achieving

© 2018 American Academy of Orthopaedic Surgeons

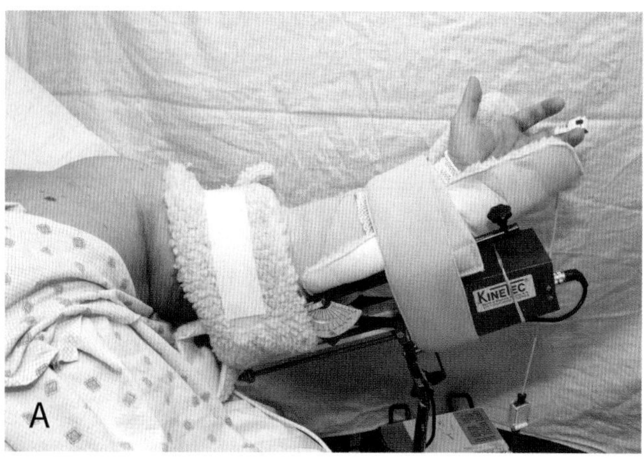

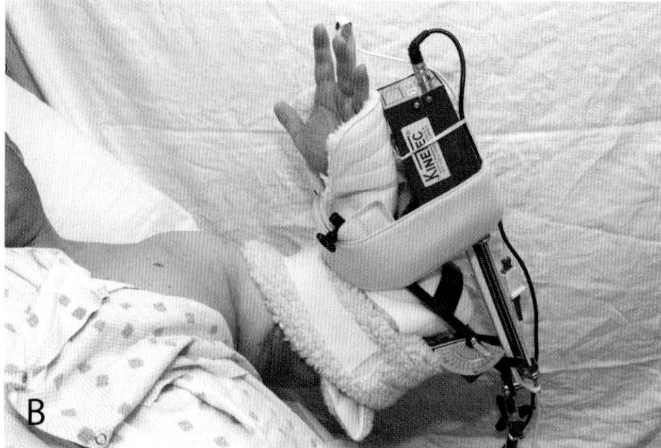

Figure 13.5 Photographs of continuous passive motion machine to work on terminal extension (**A**) and flexion (**B**).

maximum flexion is often more difficult that achieving maximum extension. Once the patient has worked on the ends of ROM, the CPM machine is run continuously. The amount of flexion provided by the CPM machine may be increased by using folded towels underneath the forearm, while using folded towels underneath the arm may increase extension.

The number of hours of CPM machine used each day and the overall duration vary according to the response of the elbow. Some patients are able to maintain their motion on their own with limited use of the CPM machine, whereas others require more CPM machine use to prevent loss of motion. The CPM machine is used as much as possible for the first few days after surgery, with breaks only for meals and bathroom use.

CPM machine use is not without risks. Unsupervised use may lead to serious complications, especially early after surgery in patients with a dense brachial plexus block when pain cannot be relied on as a sign of problems. Peripheral neuropathy may involve the ulnar, radial, and median nerves secondary to shearing of nerves, extreme stretching, or prolonged compression. The ulnar nerve is at risk if it was not decompressed or transposed. The radial nerve is at risk for compression resting against the CPM machine. The median and radial nerves are at risk in patients with high-degree flexion contractures, as the acute stretching of the nerves may lead neuropathies. Last, compartment syndrome due to postoperative swelling may go undetected in patients with dense blocks.

Static Adjustable Orthosis

These orthoses allow passive stretching of the elbow to a position that may be maintained over time to assist in maintaining the motion gained from elbow contracture release (Figure 13.6). Separate orthoses are required for flexion–extension and

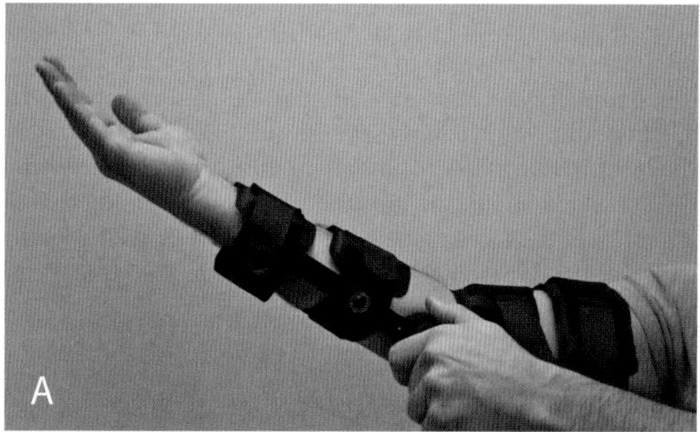

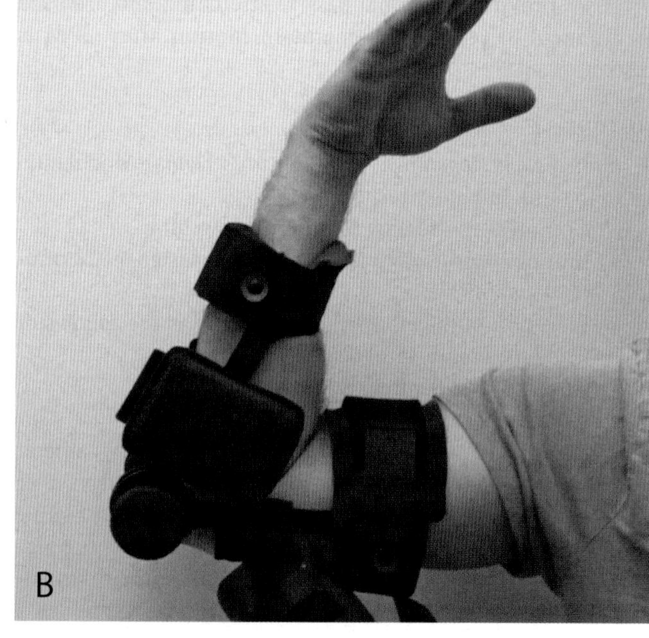

Figure 13.6 Photographs of static adjustable orthosis that may be used to stretch the elbow in extension (**A**) and flexion (**B**).

© 2018 American Academy of Orthopaedic Surgeons

pronation–supination. Maintained stretching is believed to lead to (1) plastic elongation of the soft tissues secondary to their viscoelastic nature, and (2) remodeling of the extracellular matrix. Most patients benefit from use of a static adjustable orthosis for 3 to 4 months after surgery, but the duration of use of the orthosis may need to be adjusted according to the response of the elbow. The typical program recommended to most patients is summarized in Table 13.3.

The amount of time spent stretching the elbow in flexion and extension should be proportional to the severity of stiffness in each direction; patients with a severe flexion contracture prior to surgery should spend more time stretching the elbow in extension, and vice versa.

Manual Stretching

In addition to a CPM machine and elbow orthoses, active assisted and passive stretching ROM exercises may be performed by the patient, a family member, or a physical therapist for selected patients when a CPM machine and orthosis are impractical or not available. The elbow may be stretched in extension by laying the posterior aspect of the arm on a flat surface (e.g., table) and using the opposite arm, the help of a physical therapist, a stick, or a free weight in an attempt to lie the forearm flat on the surface (Figure 13.7, A). The elbow may be stretched in flexion by forcing the forearm close to the arm with the opposite arm (Figure 13.7, B), the help of a physical therapist, or a flat static surface, such as a wall. Stretching of forearm rotation is best performed grabbing the forearm proximal to the wrist. Stretching by grasping the hand is less effective due to the flexibility of the carpus, and can also cause wrist pain. Maintaining the elbow in 90° of flexion with the arm at the side of the trunk blocks shoulder internal and external rotation to avoid the impression of false gains in forearm rotation.

Table 13.3 TYPICAL PROGRAM FOR STATIC ADJUSTABLE ORTHOSIS USE

Period	Program
Dinner time	Break—Do not use the orthosis.
Prior to bedtime **(extension)**	Apply the orthosis, extend the elbow to a point where there is some discomfort, but not severe pain; after 15 min, extend the elbow a little further.
Overnight	Sleep with the orthosis on, keeping the elbow in the extension position achieved prior to bedtime.
Early morning—Breakfast time **(break)**	Break—Do not use the brace, warm up the elbow with a hot shower, slowly work the elbow into flexion.
After breakfast **(flexion)**	Apply the orthosis, flex the elbow to a point where there is some discomfort, but not severe pain; after 15 min, flex the elbow a little further—leave the orthosis on for 2 hr.
Mid morning	Break—Do not use the brace, gently use the elbow as needed.
Rest of the day	Alternate periods of **extension, break,** and **flexion** throughout the day as detailed before.

Radiation Therapy

A single dose of radiation can be used after surgical removal of heterotopic ossification. In addition, it is used selectively for patients with severe or refractory arthrofibrosis. The rationale for using radiation therapy at the elbow is extrapolated

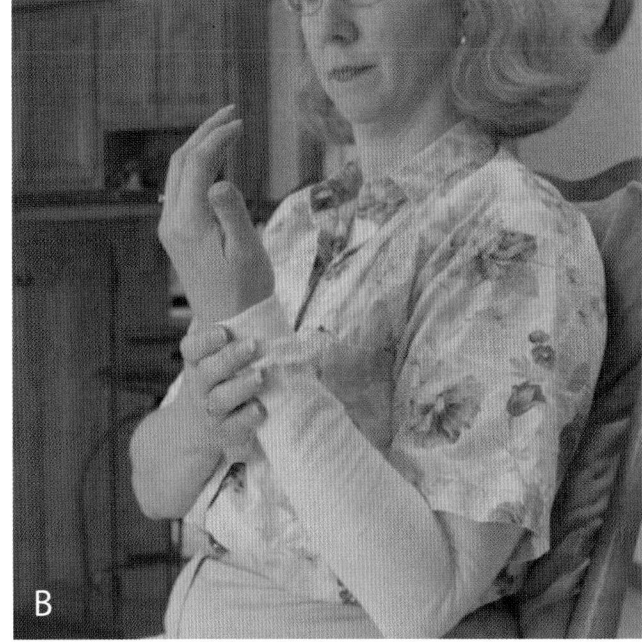

Figure 13.7 Exercises to work on elbow extension (**A**) and flexion (**B**).

© 2018 American Academy of Orthopaedic Surgeons

from the hip literature on heterotopic ossification complicating arthroplasty or acetabular fractures. A single low dose of 700 cGy should be delivered between 24 hours prior to the procedure and 72 hours after surgery. Potential complications of radiation therapy include bone nonunion, wound healing problems, and postradiation sarcoma.

Pharmacologic Agents

Nonsteroidal Anti-inflammatory Drugs (NSAIDs)

Indomethacin is also used as part of the postoperative program after contracture release based on the proven reduction of heterotopic bone formation around the hip joint. We typically recommend oral indomethacin for 6 weeks after surgery for all patients undergoing contracture release; however, we do not have a scientific basis for this practice. Indomethacin and other NSAIDs do not carry the risk of complications outlined for radiation therapy, and their analgesic and anti-inflammatory properties make them attractive. However, they do carry some risk of adverse effects, such as gastrointestinal ulcers, as well as hepatic and renal dysfunction. The recommended dose of indomethacin after contracture release is a single dose of 75 mg sustained daily.

GABA-Analogues (Anti-Epileptics)

Clinical or subclinical neuropathies, such as ulnar neuritis and chronic regional pain syndrome, may play a role in some patients with elbow contracture. Pharmacologic agents such as gabapentin (Neurontin) or pregabalin (Lyrica) may be considered in patients with persistent dysesthesias or suspected neuropathy.

Botulinum Toxin

Refractory muscle contracture may also play an adverse role in the rehabilitation program of some patients after contracture release, including individuals with spasticity or Parkinson disease. Botulinum toxins A and B may be considered as adjunctive modalities in these circumstances to temporarily paralyze the involved muscles. Injections are best performed under EMG guidance targeting the biceps, brachialis, and brachioradialis for flexion spasm and contracture, and the triceps for extension spasm and contracture. The effect of botulinum toxin is slowly lost over time, and most patients need a single treatment to correct muscle contracture over the first few weeks after surgery.

Manipulation Under Anesthesia

Manipulation under anesthesia of the elbow may be considered for patients with substantial difficulties in maintaining the ROM obtained in surgery. We typically consider manipulation under anesthesia approximately 6 weeks after contracture release when motion gains are suboptimal and have clearly reached a plateau. General anesthesia with pharmacologic paralysis is followed by gentle progressive flexion and extension; the elbow joint may be injected with a local anesthetic and corticosteroids after manipulation. Manipulation is followed by intensive CPM, orthosis, or manual stretching protocols that are instituted immediately after manipulation.

Functional Goals and Restrictions

The goal of elbow contracture release is restoration of a pain-free and complete, or at least functional, arc of motion. Most patients benefit from approximately 3 months of postoperative rehabilitation. At the end of their program, many patients are able to achieve a functional arc of motion, but only a few regain complete motion. The best results are achieved in patients with primary osteoarthritis (as opposed to posttraumatic), as well as those requiring removal of heterotopic ossification after a neurologic injury or burn injury (as opposed to posttraumatic ectopic bone formation). Once the rehabilitation program is completed and motion is restored, activity restrictions are dictated by the underlying pathology. Most patients resume their activities with no restrictions. Heavy weight lifting may aggravate symptoms in patients with arthritis.

OUTCOMES

Surgical release of stiff elbows with extrinsic contracture has been shown to reliably improve ROM. Most studies have reported improved motion in approximately 85% of the patients and restoration of a functional arc in most of the patients that improve their motion. Mansat and Morrey reported mean gains of 45° degrees of motion in 38 elbows treated with open contracture release. Similar gains were reported in a systematic review by Kodde et al., with average motion gains of 40° to 51° for arthroscopic and open contracture release, respectively. There is published evidence on the beneficial effects of various types of orthosis in maintaining elbow motion. Muller et al. performed a systematic review on the effectiveness of bracing and found mean improvements of 38.4° ± 8.9° during the course of treatment.

The benefits of CPM after elbow contracture release have been difficult to prove scientifically. The evidence in favor of postoperative manipulation under anesthesia is limited but strong. Araghi et al. reported on 51 patients treated with manipulation under anesthesia. The mean premanipulation arc of 40° increased to 78° at most recent follow-up. Heterotopic ossification usually does not recur after resection. Radiation therapy and indomethacin are used based on evidence published in the hip literature. Ploumis et al. reviewed all available literature and found only weak evidence supporting the use of radiation therapy for prevention of heterotopic ossification of the elbow. Most other adjuvant modalities lack strong scientific supportive basis.

PEARLS

Surgical Procedure

- Use advanced imaging studies to plan bone removal.
- Identify and address clinical and subclinical ulnar neuropathy as well as other elbows at risk for postoperative neuropathy.
- Plan your open or arthroscopic surgery to maximize efficacy and minimize complications, especially iatrogenic nerve injuries.

© 2018 American Academy of Orthopaedic Surgeons

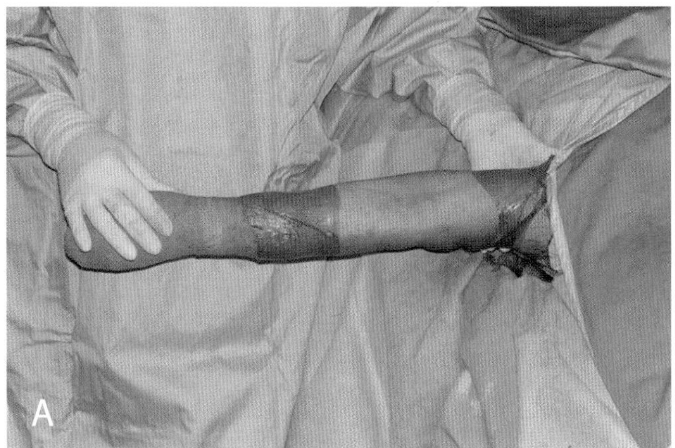

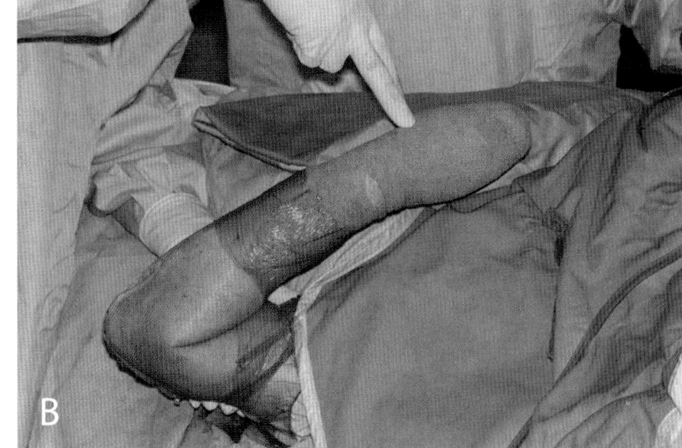

Figure 13.8 **A**, Clinical photograph of intraoperative extension after contracture release. **B**, Clinical photograph of intraoperative flexion after contracture release.

- Try to restore complete ROM at the end of the procedure whenever possible; most elbows are at risk of losing some motion during postoperative recovery (Figure 13.8).
- Do not remove hardware prior to complete restoration of elbow motion to prevent iatrogenic intraoperative fractures through stress risers.

Postoperative Rehabilitation

- Patient education and compliance are paramount for the success of the procedure and the rehabilitation program.
- Concentrate efforts on modulating the postoperative inflammatory response, introducing early ROM exercises throughout the whole range, and continued stretching though CPM, orthosis, and/or manual stretching exercises.
- Pay specific attention to restoration of pronation and supination.
- Add adjunctive treatment modalities selectively as needed.

CONCLUSION/SUMMARY

Rehabilitation is extremely important after elbow contracture release. The most critical elements include measures to control inflammation in the first postoperative days, use of CPM devices, and use of braces. Manual manipulation may be very effective, but may also become detrimental if it leads to increased inflammation. Adjuvant pharmacologic treatment in the form of NSAIDs is commonly used as well, sometimes for several weeks, to prevent the formation of heterotopic bone. Radiation therapy is also selectively considered, specifically after excision of heterotopic ossification. Manipulation under anesthesia may have a role in patients unable to make much progress over the first few weeks after surgery. In most cases, the combination of technically well-performed surgery and appropriately applied rehabilitation results in restoration of functional elbow motion.

BIBLIOGRAPHY

Araghi A, Celli A, Adams R, Morrey B: The outcome of examination (manipulation) under anesthesia on the stiff elbow after surgical contracture release. *J Shoulder Elbow Surg* 2010; 19(2):202–208.

Kodde IF, van Rijn J, van den Bekerom MP, Eygendaal D: Surgical treatment of post-traumatic elbow stiffness: a systematic review. *J Shoulder Elbow Surg* 2013;22(4):574–580.

Mansat P, Morrey BF: The column procedure: a limited lateral approach for extrinsic contracture of the elbow. *J Bone Joint Surg Am* 1998;80(11):1603–1615.

Muller AM, Sadoghi P, Lucas R, et al.: Effectiveness of bracing in the treatment of nonosseous restriction of elbow mobility: a systematic review and meta-analysis of 13 studies. *J Shoulder Elbow Surg* 2013;22(8):1146–1152.

Ploumis A, Belbasis L, Ntzani E, Tsekeris P, Xenakis T: Radiotherapy for prevention of heterotopic ossification of the elbow: a systematic review of the literature. *J Shoulder Elbow Surg* 2013;22(11):1580–1588.

© 2018 American Academy of Orthopaedic Surgeons

14 Lateral and Medial Epicondylitis

Eugene W. Brabston III, MD, James J. Perry, OT/L, OTR, CHT, RNCST, and John-Erik Bell, MD, MS

INTRODUCTION

Lateral and medial epicondylitis are common causes of elbow pain and dysfunction. The appropriate management of epicondylitis is based on an understanding of the natural history as well as the anatomic, biochemical, and biomechanical principles underlying the condition. Management should always start with nonsurgical treatment, which is typically successful. Surgical treatment is reserved for recalcitrant and chronic cases that have exhausted nonoperative measures over a prolonged period of time. Treatment options are tailored to individual patients depending on professional and recreational demands and activities.

Lateral epicondylitis is the most common cause of elbow pain, and is noted to occur up to 10 times more commonly than medial epicondylitis, with an equal prevalence among male and female patients. Risk factors for developing lateral epicondylitis include advancing age, smoking, obesity, heavy lifting, and repetitive motion use. Although the diagnosis carries the eponym "tennis elbow," tennis itself is actually the cause in very few cases of lateral epicondylitis. Nevertheless, it is common among tennis and other racquet sport players and affects 20% to 50%, with increased frequency noted among amateur or recreational players. The pathology predominantly involves the extensor carpi radialis brevis (ECRB) origin and occasionally the extensor digitorum communis (EDC).

Medial epicondylitis tends to affect patients in the fourth and fifth decades of life, usually affecting the dominant extremity, with an equal prevalence in males and females. Similar to lateral epicondylitis, medial epicondylitis results from repetitive stress in the setting of chronic inflammation. The pathology is found in the flexor pronator mass, particularly the pronator teres, flexor carpi radialis, palmaris longus, and sometimes the flexor carpi ulnaris (FCU) and flexor digitorum superficialis. Medial epicondylitis has earned the eponym "golfer's elbow," but can be seen in athletes and nonathletes alike.

Since epicondylitis was first described in the late 19th century, multiple theories have been proposed to explain the pathologic process. The current understanding is that epicondylitis represents microtearing of the medial or lateral tendons at their origin. A subsequent healing response is marred by vascular infiltration and changes in the normal structure of the musculotendinous junction. Nirschl and Pettrone (1979) described both the gross and histologic appearance of the pathologic process. They described the gross appearance of the tissue as a grayish amorphous substance. On a histologic level, the normal collagen architecture of the tissue is disrupted, with immature vascular invasion noted with a background surprisingly bereft of chronic and acute inflammatory cells. In the chronic setting, this leads to tendon degeneration that is described as "angiofibroblastic hyperplasia." Stage 1 represents the early portion of the process, with acute inflammation and no architectural changes. Stage 2 has pathologic changes, with angiofibroblastic invasion, but integrity of the tendon is maintained. In stage 3, the structure of the tendon becomes altered; stage 4 marks the addition of fibrosis or calcification, as in a chronic setting. The term "tendonitis" is a confusing term that can be a misnomer in describing the pathologic process, especially in the chronic setting. Although inflammatory cells can be present, the pathologic specimen is not marked by a typical inflammatory presentation, but rather by an abundance of fibroblasts, vascular hyperplasia, and collagen lacking normal structure.

RELEVANT ANATOMY

Lateral Epicondyle

The lateral epicondyle is the site of origin of the extensors of the fingers and wrist as well as the lateral ulnar collateral ligament (LUCL). The extensor carpi radialis longus (ECRL) originates from the supracondylar ridge in close proximity to the origin of the brachioradialis. The ECRB origin is deep, lateral, and inferior to the origin of the longus tendon. The EDC is noted to arise just posterior and distal to the ECRL. The origin of the ECRB is most often the site of pathology, although approximately one-third of patients also have involvement

None of the following authors or any immediate family member has received anything of value from or has stock or stock options held in a commercial company or institution related directly or indirectly to the subject of this article: Dr. Bell, Dr. Brabston, and Dr. Perry.

© 2018 American Academy of Orthopaedic Surgeons

of the EDC. The lateral ligament complex, which is deep to the ECRB, ECRL, and EDC tendons, is composed of four major components: the lateral ulnar collateral ligament, the radial collateral ligament, the annular ligament, and the accessory collateral ligament. Due to the close proximity of the ligament, it has been implicated in the clinical picture of the lateral epicondylitis as MRI findings have noted ligament tendon tears and thickening. The LUCL is also at risk for iatrogenic injury during lateral epicondylitis surgery.

Medial Epicondyle

The medial epicondyle is the site of origin for the flexor pronator mass, which is composed of the pronator teres, flexor carpi radialis, palmaris longus, flexor digitorum superficialis, and the FCU in a radial to ulnar direction. The medial collateral ligament (MCL) is noted to be in close proximity to the flexor pronator mass, and may be involved in the pathologic process. The MCL is composed of three distinct bands—the anterior, posterior, and transverse bands—with the anterior band being the most important in stabilizing the elbow against valgus stress. Ulnar nerve symptoms may also be clinically apparent due to the close proximity of the ulnar nerve to the origin of the flexors. When ulnar nerve symptoms present in the setting of medial epicondylitis, the most common site of ulnar nerve compression is between the two heads of the FCU.

PATIENT EVALUATION

The accurate diagnosis of medial and lateral epicondylitis depends on a thorough, but focused, history and physical. Chronicity of symptoms, location of symptoms, type of pain, exacerbating activities, associated paresthesias, and muscle weakness must be addressed. History of sports or other resisted and repetitive activities that could explain the inciting event should be noted.

Medial epicondylitis is associated with pain along the medial epicondyle made worse with resisted forearm pronation or wrist flexion. Placing the elbow in an extended position provides maximal physiologic stretch to the tendons being assessed. Tenderness is more pronounced just distal and anterior to the medial epicondyle over the attachment of the flexor carpi radialis and pronator teres.

The ulnar nerve should be assessed both for subluxation and reproducible symptoms of paresthesia. A Tinel's test or elbow flexion test may also be used to assess for ulnar nerve compression or irritation. The medial ulnar collateral ligament is evaluated with the moving valgus stress test and milking maneuver to rule it out as a source of medial-sided elbow pain.

Examination of the lateral elbow may elicit pain with palpation directly distal and slightly anterior to the epicondyle. Specific examination maneuvers include resisted wrist extension and resisted long finger extension. These maneuvers are typically more painful with the elbow extended than flexed. To rule out other causes of lateral elbow pain, the radiocapitellar joint should be palpated for arthritic pain and crepitus or snapping plica syndrome. The radial tunnel should also be palpated for tenderness.

In most cases of epicondylitis, plain radiographs are normal. Some patients have lateral epicondylar spurring or calcification. MRI scans are not necessary for diagnosis or treatment of epicondylitis. An MRI, however, may be used to rule out other pathology such as collateral ligament injury or plica if the diagnosis is unclear. Diagnostic ultrasound can show thickening and hypoechoic tendon origin or even small fluid collections.

NONSURGICAL TREATMENT AND REHABILITATION

Nonsurgical treatment is the mainstay of management of lateral and medial epicondylitis. A thorough review of randomized controlled trials regarding nonsurgical treatment of lateral epicondylitis demonstrates a high rate of long term success with nonsurgical treatment. Surgical treatment of medial and lateral epicondylitis is often reserved for recalcitrant cases, typically after 6 to 12 months of nonsurgical treatment. Less than 10% of patients with epicondylitis fail to improve with nonsurgical treatment and ultimately require surgical intervention.

SURGICAL TREATMENT

Indications and Contraindications

Although nonoperative management is the mainstay of treatment for both medial and lateral epicondylitis, surgical treatment is usually considered if a patient has failed 6 to 12 months of treatment. Contraindications to surgical intervention include elbow pain unrelated to epicondylitis such as elbow instability, radial tunnel and posterior interosseous nerve syndromes, ulnar neuropathy, and advanced elbow arthritis. Other contraindications are inability to comply with a postoperative treatment regimen and comorbidities that preclude safe use of surgical anesthesia.

Surgical Treatment of Lateral Epicondylitis

Surgical treatment includes both excision of inflammatory tissue and postoperative modification of the mechanical factors that predispose microinjury at the tendon origin. Surgical procedures to treat epicondylitis can be open, arthroscopic, or percutaneous; there is no clear advantage of one technique over the others regarding postoperative outcomes. Prior to the definitive surgical procedure, the elbow is examined under anesthesia to assess range of motion (ROM) and stability. Epicondylitis is rarely associated with loss of passive motion. In rare cases, lateral elbow pain can be a manifestation of posterolateral rotatory instability.

Open Lateral Epicondylitis Surgery (Figure 14.1)

An oblique skin incision over the lateral elbow is made to expose the common extensor origin. The common extensor origin and ECRL are identified with the ECRB deep and

© 2018 American Academy of Orthopaedic Surgeons

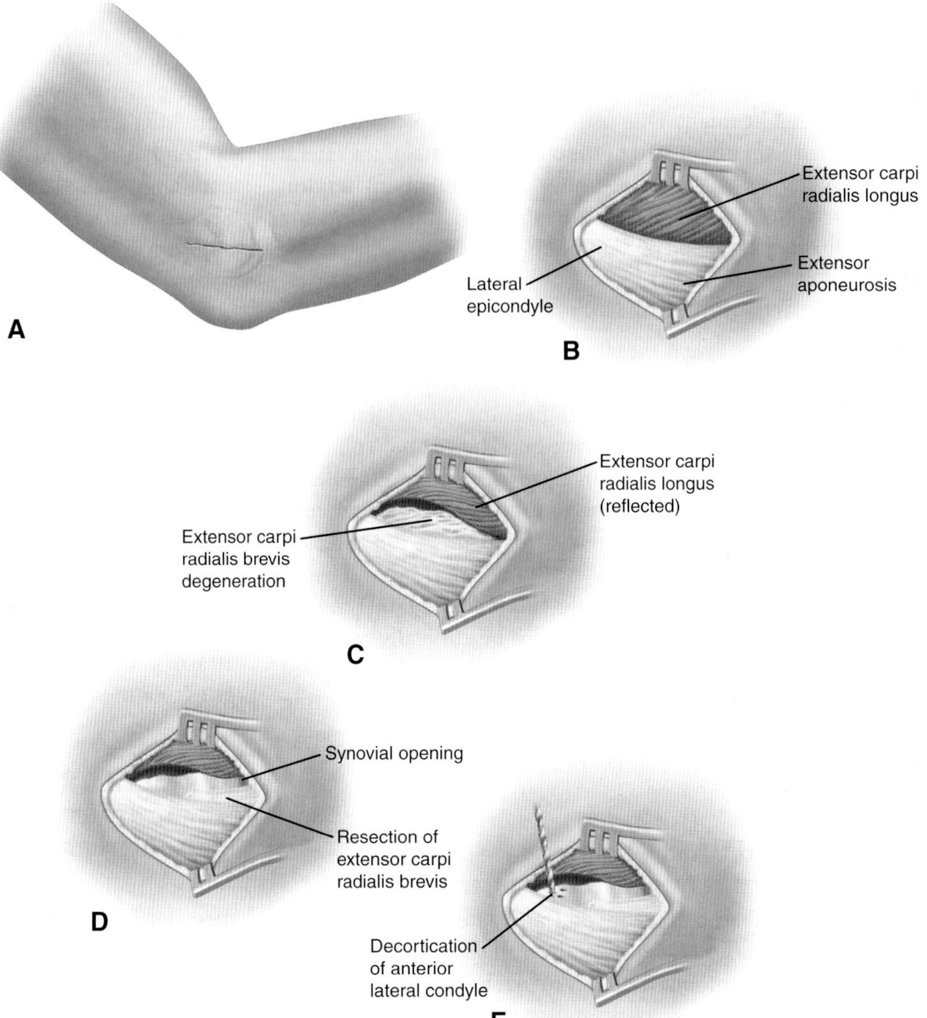

Figure 14.1 Illustration of open debridement for lateral epicondylitis. **A**, Incision is based over the extensor origin and lateral epicondyle. **B**, **C**, The pathologic tissue is primarily within the tendon origin of the extensor carpi radialis brevis (ECRB), which is deep to the extensor carpi radialis longus (ECRL). The longus is incised in line with the fibers to gain access. **D**, The pathologic tissue is excised from the origin. **E**, The exposed lateral epicondyle is decorticated to encourage neovascularization and healing of the ECRB. A suture anchor may also be used at this site to repair the longitudinal incision of the ECRL. (Reproduced with permission from Miller MD, Chhabra AB, Konin J, Mistry D: *Sports Medicine Conditions: Return To Play: Recognition, Treatment, Planning.* Philadelphia, PA, Lippincott Williams & Wilkins, 2014.)

posterior. Degenerative tissue often having a grayish appearance within the substance of the ECRB is debrided. The lateral epicondyle may be decorticated as well, but care should be taken to avoid damage to the LUCL. The overlying remaining tendon is then reapproximated. The subcutaneous tissues and skin are closed, a sterile dressing is applied to the wound, and the arm is immobilized in a sling.

Arthroscopic Lateral Epicondylitis Surgery

The arthroscopic surgical technique involves placement of arthroscopic portals, usually proximal anterior medial and anterior lateral, and an initial diagnostic evaluation of the joint (Figure 14.2). Using a shaver, the lateral capsule is debrided to be able to view the undersurface of the ECRB. The ECRB is then released from its origin at the lateral epicondyle and the release is extended from the anterior half of the radial head proximally to the point of the ECRL origin. The portion of the tendon overlying the posterior half of the radial head is used as a reference and is preserved in an effort to minimize damage to the lateral collateral ligament complex. The epicondyle may be decorticated to create a bleeding bed for healing. Some surgeons repair the reflected ECRB tendon, but many do not. The arthroscopic portals are closed, sterile dressings are applied to the wounds, and the arm is immobilized in a sling.

Surgical Treatment of Medial Epicondylitis

The surgical treatment of medial epicondylitis follows similar principles to those of lateral epicondylitis. Due to the close proximity of the ulnar nerve, most surgeons prefer an open surgical approach to treat medial epicondylitis. A medial skin incision is used over to the medial epicondyle and extending distally with careful subcutaneous dissection to protect the medial antebrachial cutaneous nerve. Both the ulnar nerve and the origin of the flexor pronator mass are noted, with the ulnar nerve being careful protected. An interval between the pronator teres and flexor carpi radialis is developed and any pathologic tissue is then removed. If deeper debridement is required, the MCL must be protected. Once the debridement is completed, the surrounding tissue is repaired. In the clinical

 © 2018 American Academy of Orthopaedic Surgeons

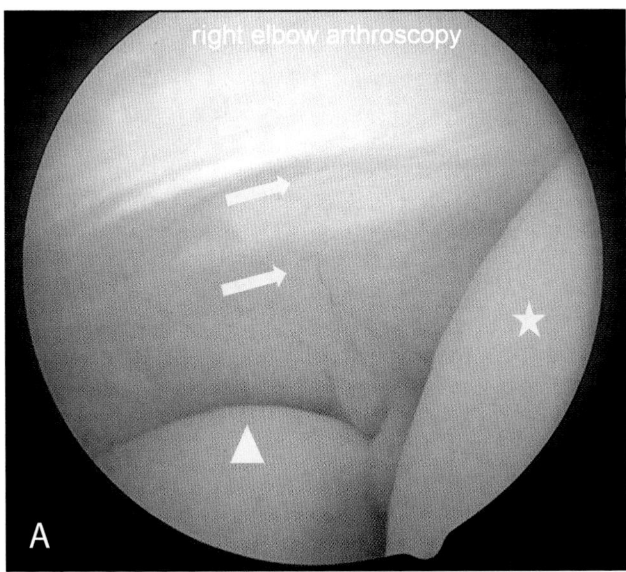

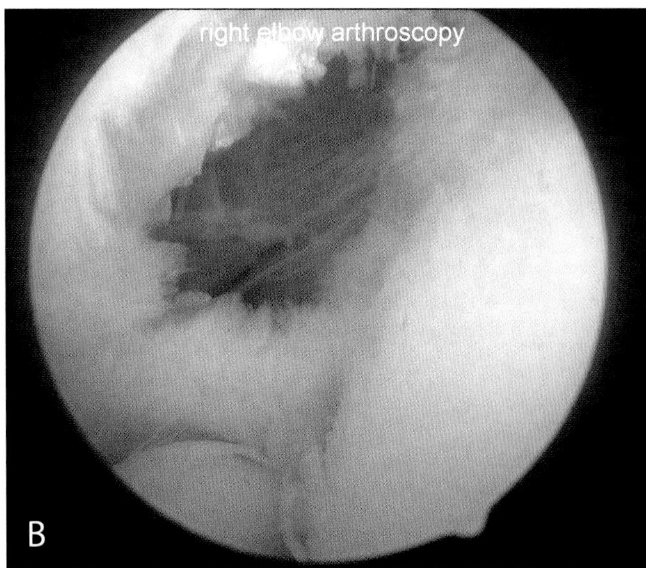

Figure 14.2 Clinical photographs of arthroscopic debridement for lateral epicondylitis. **A**, The lateral capsule (marked with arrows) overlies the ECRB. The capitellum is marked with a star and the radial head is marked with a triangle. **B**, The ECRB tendon is released and the surrounding degenerative tissue is debrided. (Courtesy of Andrew Green, MD)

setting of accompanying cubital tunnel symptoms, decompression or transposition of the ulnar nerve can be done. Decortication of the epicondyle may be performed taking care to avoid damage to the MCL. Repair of the flexor tendon origin to the medial epicondyle can be performed, but is usually not necessary. The subcutaneous tissues and skin are closed, the wound is dressed in a sterile fashion, and the arm is immobilized in a sling (Figure 14.3).

There has been some recent interest in arthroscopically assisted debridement as a surgical intervention for medial epicondylitis. This may require an additional medial anterior accessory portal in an effort to gain access to the degenerative medial epicondylitis tissue. Despite the possibility of addressing medial epicondylitis arthroscopically, no studies have shown patient outcomes, and the concern regarding iatrogenic injury to the ulnar nerve and underlying MCL has prevented many surgeons from undertaking this surgical technique.

POSTOPERATIVE REHABILITATION

The initial postoperative rehabilitation begins 3 to 5 days after surgery. Treatments are focused on reduction of swelling and edema with elevation, ice, and/or compression, and controlled mobilization. Active digit and shoulder motion should be emphasized to help with edema mobilization and prevention of joint stiffness. Often, a posterior splint or sling is utilized to prevent tissue irritation, minimize pain, and enable rest to the healing tissues. Immobilization in 90° of flexion relieves tension on the surgical site at the origin of the tendon and is typically used for the initial 1 to 2 weeks postoperatively.

The patient is seen for an initial postoperative visit at 10 to 14 days postsurgery for wound examination and suture removal, if necessary. Active assisted wrist and elbow motion is initiated within the patient's comfort range and in a gravity-eliminated or assisted plane if necessary. Splint use is continued between exercises as pain dictates. High-voltage galvanic stimulation can be utilized to promote edema reduction and healing. Scar therapy may be initiated after the wound has demonstrated initial phases of healing with resolution of any scab formation. Treatment options include massage, ultrasound, silicone sheets or elastomers, desensitization, and light compression. Taping can also be used for scar mobilization (Figure 14.4).

Early Postoperative Phase

General Goals

- Protect healing tissue.
- Decrease pain and inflammation.
- Prevent muscular atrophy.
- Avoid early strengthening of the extensor/flexor mass muscle groups to protect healing depending on diagnosis (medial vs. lateral epicondylitis).

Weeks 1 and 2

- Brace/splint/sling: 90° elbow flexion
- Cryotherapy: To elbow
- Active assisted elbow ROM
- Brace: Elbow ROM 0° to 120° (gradually increase ROM – 5° of extension/10° of flexion per week)
- Wrist ROM exercises
- Light scar mobilization incision

At 3 weeks postsurgery, full motion of the elbow in all planes against gravity is initiated. Stretching and counterforce bracing

© 2018 American Academy of Orthopaedic Surgeons

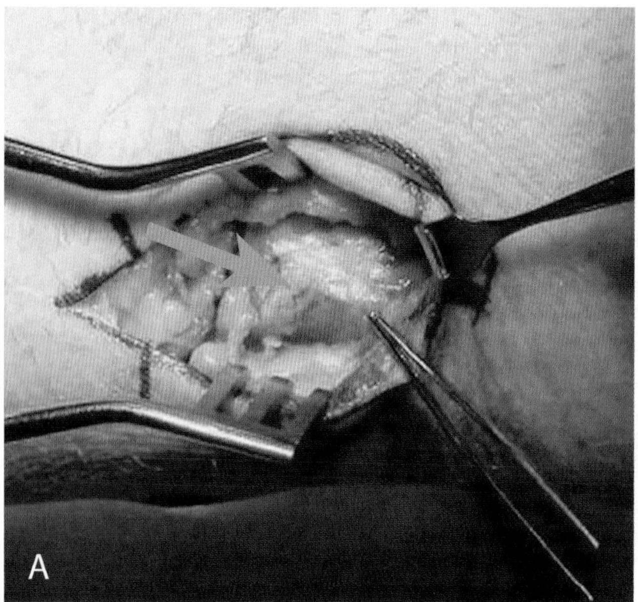

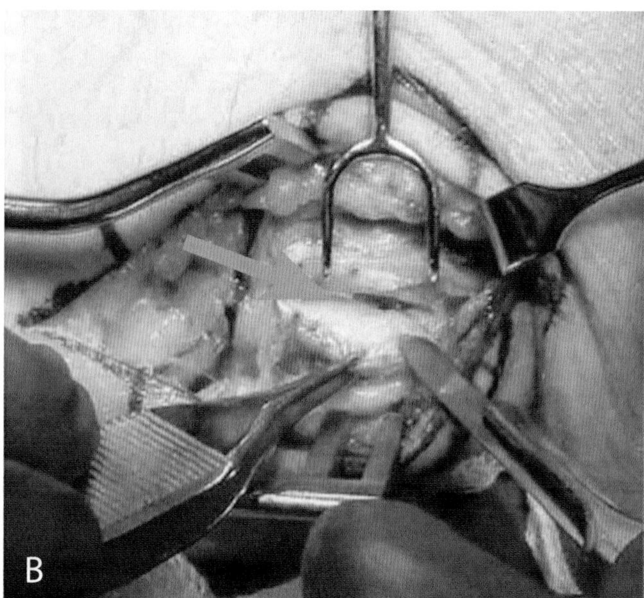

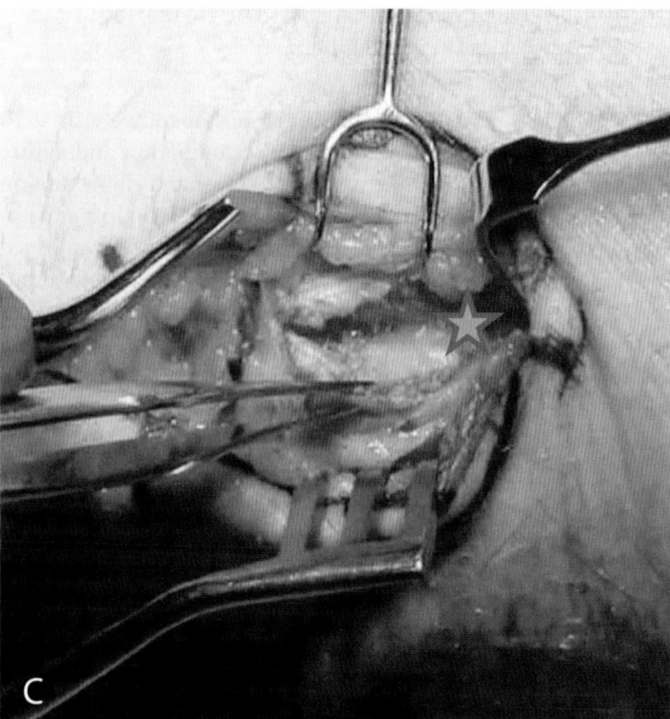

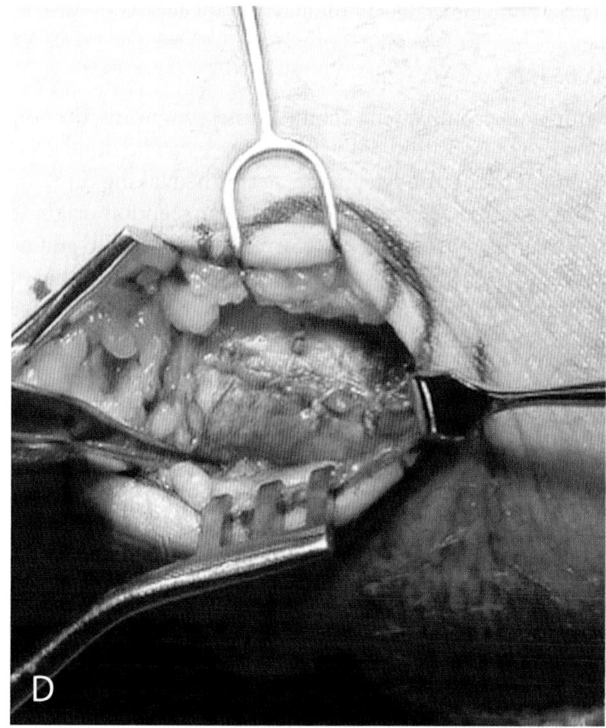

Figure 14.3 Clinical photographs of open debridement for medial epicondylitis. **A**, The pathologic changes within the tendon may be recognized (arrow). **B**, The medial epicondyle is exposed (star). **C**, The pathologic tissue is removed (arrow). **D**, Following removal of the tissue, the tendon is repaired in a side-to-side technique. (Reproduced with permission from Amin NH, Kumar NS, Schickendantz MS: Medial epicondylitis: Evaluation and management. *J Am Acad Orthop Surg* 2015;23(6):348–355.)

may be utilized to control pain if needed in an effort to advance motion. Once ROM is regained and pain is controlled, extensor wad mobilization begins with the elbow in 90° of flexion. Composite active and active assisted wrist ROM and digit flexion/extension stretching may be started in addition to soft massage and joint mobilizations about the elbow. The patient may return to aerobic exercise and light functional hand use with daily tasks. Due to an increased risk of impingement symptoms and scapular dyskinesia with immobilization, rotator cuff and scapular mobilization and stabilization training may be initiated with light resistance. Composite stretching should be progressed to gradually include elbow into full extension (Figure 14.5).

© 2018 American Academy of Orthopaedic Surgeons

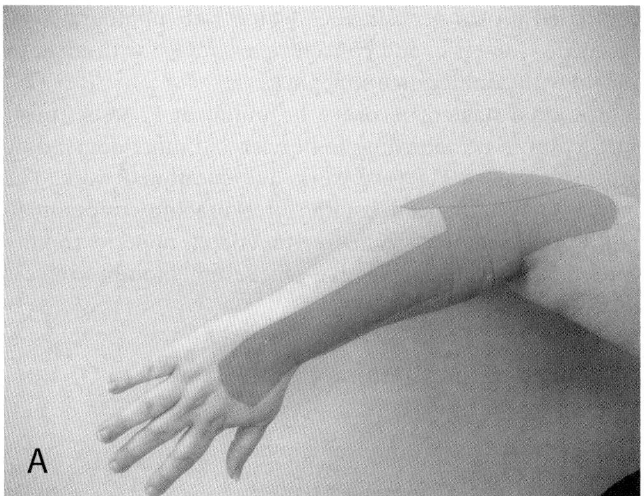

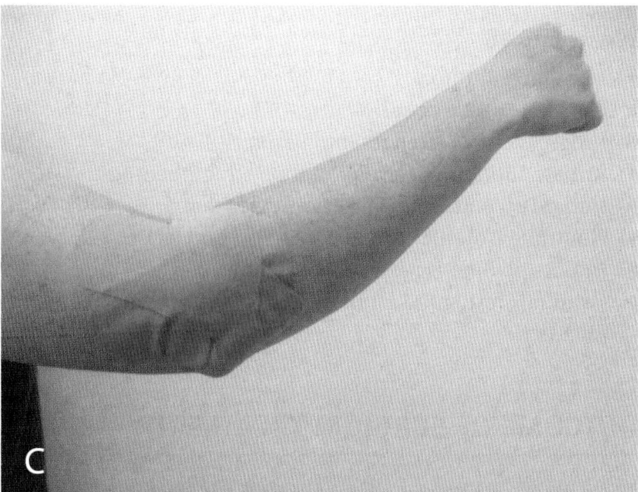

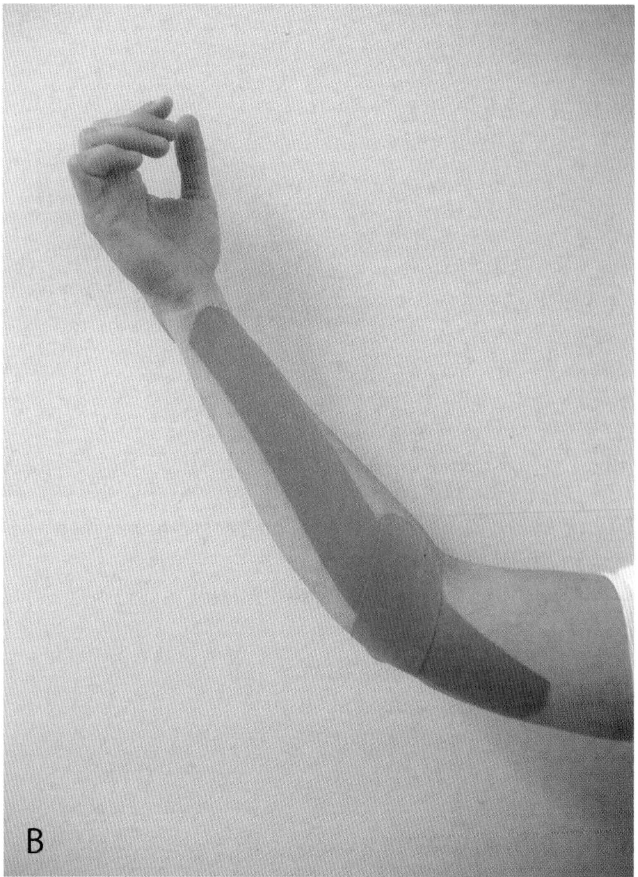

Figure 14.4 Clinical photographs of kinesiotape applied for conservative management of lateral epicondylitis (**A**) and medial epicondylitis (**B**). **C**, Kinesiotape can also be applied for scar correction status post lateral epicondylar surgery.

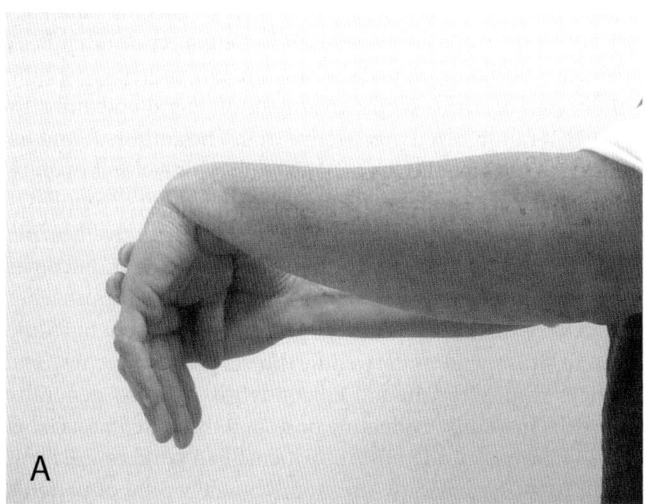

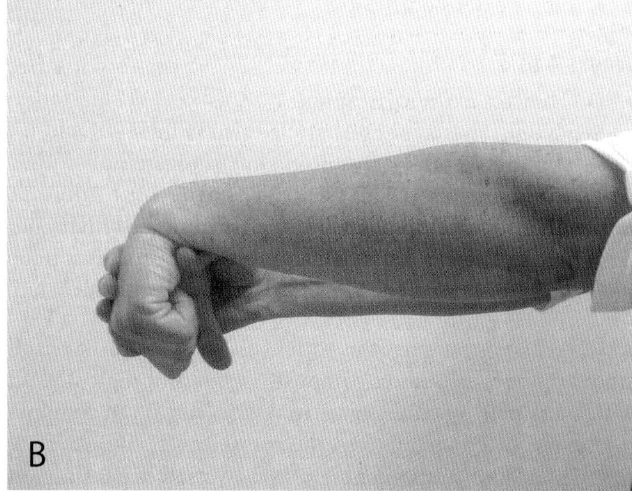

Figure 14.5 **A**, Photograph of wrist extensor stretch. **B**, Photograph of composite wrist and finger extensor stretch. *(continued)*

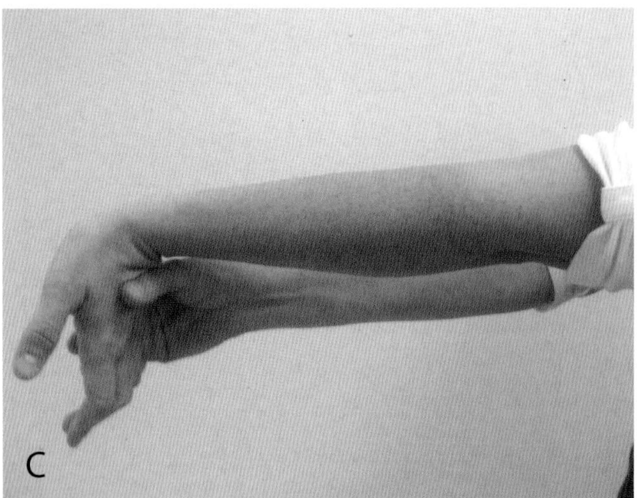

Figure 14.5 (*Continued*) **C**, Photograph of flexor wad stretching.

Intermediate Postoperative Phase

General Goals

- Gradual increase to full ROM
- Promote healing of repaired tissue.
- Regain and improve strength.

Weeks 3 and 4

- Eliminate all elbow immobilization.
- Continue all exercises listed earlier.
- Initiate active ROM wrist and elbow (no resistance).
- Initiate light wrist extension/flexion stretching.
- Initiate active ROM shoulder.
- Initiate light scapular strengthening exercises.
- Wrist splint
- Begin light resistance exercises (1 lb):
  - Wrist curls, extensions, pronation, supination
  - Elbow extension/flexion

Weeks 4 to 6

- D/C brace and use wrist splint
- Begin light resistance exercises for arm (1 lb):
  - Wrist curls, extensions, pronation, supination
  - Elbow extension/flexion
- Progress shoulder program, emphasizing rotator cuff and scapular strengthening.
- Initiate shoulder strengthening with light dumbbells.

At 6 weeks postsurgery, the patient is expected to have full elbow motion, including composite wrist and digit flexion with a less than 10° difference from wrist flexion to composite flexion or comparable to the nonsurgical side. Activity restrictions and strengthening may be varied depending on the surgical approach (arthroscopic vs. open) and surgical repair technique. Gradual strengthening of the wrist extensors should be initiated, progressing from isometric to eccentric to concentric. Use of a counterforce brace during exercise is continued if pain persists. (See Figure 14.6: photographs of eccentric isometric, and concentric exercises, with band or weight with counterforce strapping.)

The final stage of recovery, beginning at 12 weeks postsurgery, involves returning to heavier and more demanding tasks, such as sports, yard work, and vocational work. The patient may still need counterforce bracing/strapping to minimize discomfort. Pain-free functional upper extremity use independent of activity may take several months to a year to achieve.

Advanced Strengthening Phase

General Goals

- Increase strength, power, endurance
- Maintain full elbow ROM
- Gradually initiate sports/functional activities

Weeks 6 to 18

- Full elbow motion
- Continue all exercises.
- Progress elbow strengthening exercises.
- Initiate shoulder external rotation strengthening.
- Initiate eccentric elbow flexion/extension.
- Continue isotonic program: forearm and wrist.
- Initiate plyometric exercise program.
- Gradual return to sports/vocational requirements, as tolerated.

OUTCOME OF SURGICAL TREATMENT

The results of surgical treatment of both medial and lateral epicondylitis are generally favorable. However, persistent pain is noted after both open and arthroscopic release, with up to 40% of patients experiencing some level of chronic pain specifically with surgical intervention for lateral epicondylitis. A recent article has examined the outcomes of patients receiving either open or arthroscopic treatment of lateral epicondylitis through a randomized prospective trial. The authors found no difference in outcomes for patients undergoing either open or arthroscopic approaches with age, gender, worker's compensation status, and smoking status having no predictive bearing on outcomes. A similar study examining 3- to 6-year outcomes in patients having undergone arthroscopic or open approaches did reveal a small, but statistically significant, patient outcome score in those who underwent arthroscopic approaches. The surgical results for medial epicondylitis are also generally favorable. In a study evaluating postoperative outcomes, Gabel and Morrey noted that 87% of patients had good to excellent results at a 7-year follow-up. Approximately 50% of patients with surgically treated medial epicondylitis also had ulnar nerve symptoms. Those patients with more severe concomitant ulnar nerve symptoms have a less favorable outcome with surgical intervention.

© 2018 American Academy of Orthopaedic Surgeons

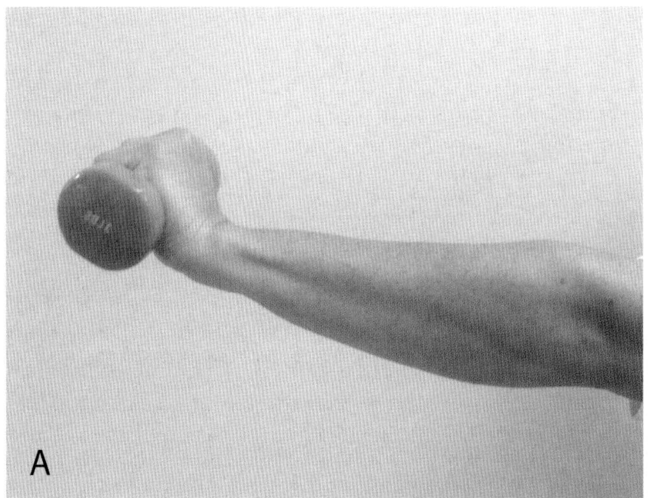

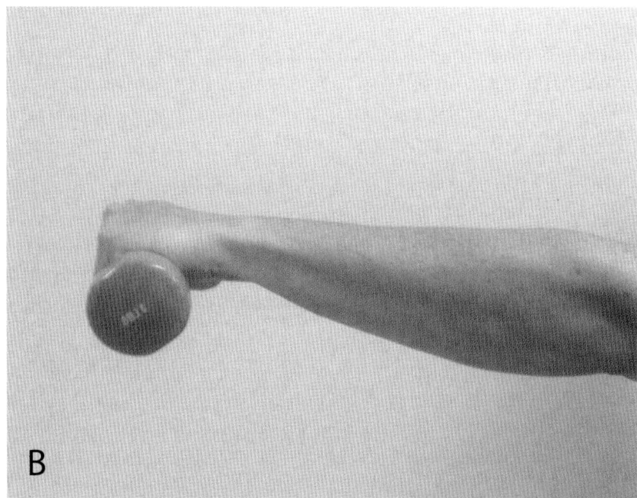

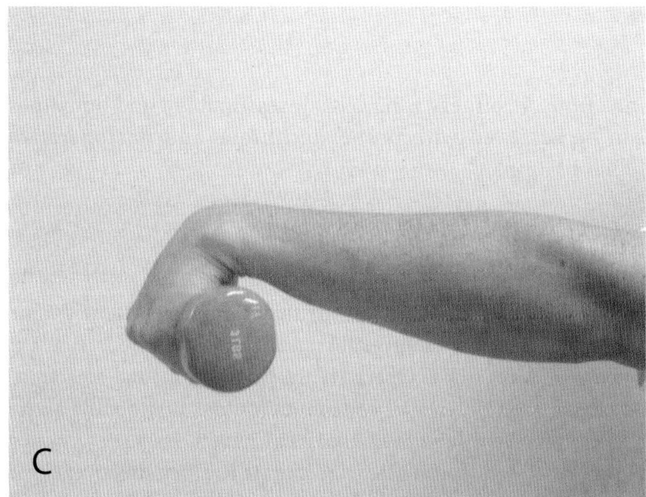

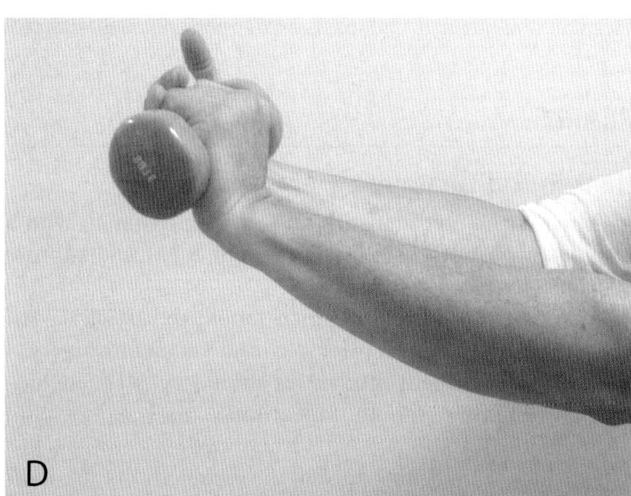

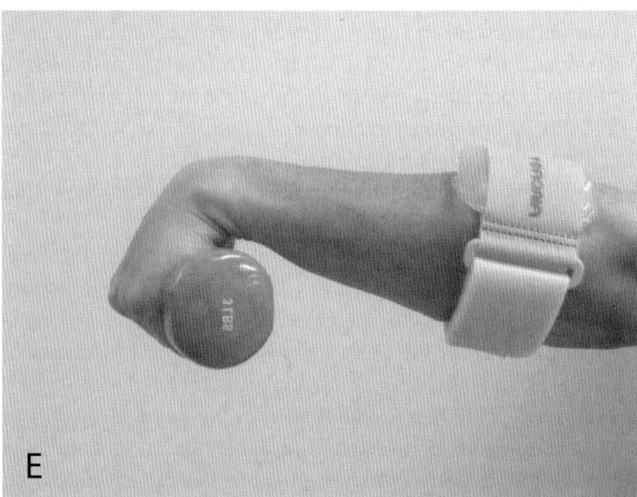

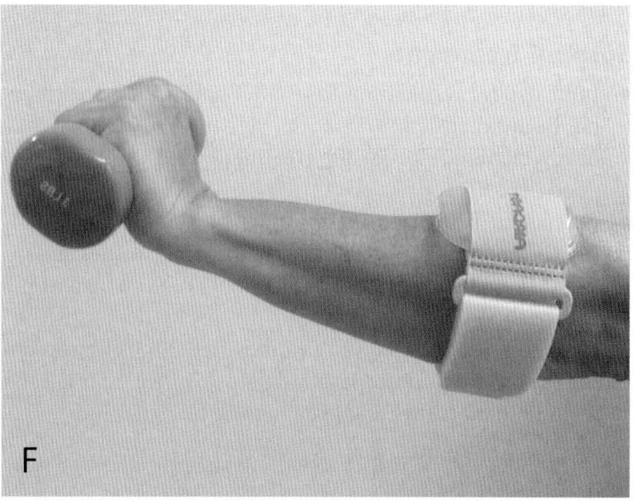

Figure 14.6 **A**, Photograph of eccentric strengthening for lateral epicondylitis starting position with tension through the wrist extensors. **B**, Photograph of eccentric strengthening controlled tension using 8-second count. **C**, Photograph of eccentric strengthening finish in composite flexion for full extensor wad mobility. **D**, Photograph of eccentric strengthening passive extension back to starting position to prevent concentric exercise in initial recovery. **E**, Photograph of eccentric strengthening in composite flexion with counterforce bracing. **F**, Photograph of eccentric strengthening in composite extension with counterforce bracing. (*continued*)

© 2018 American Academy of Orthopaedic Surgeons

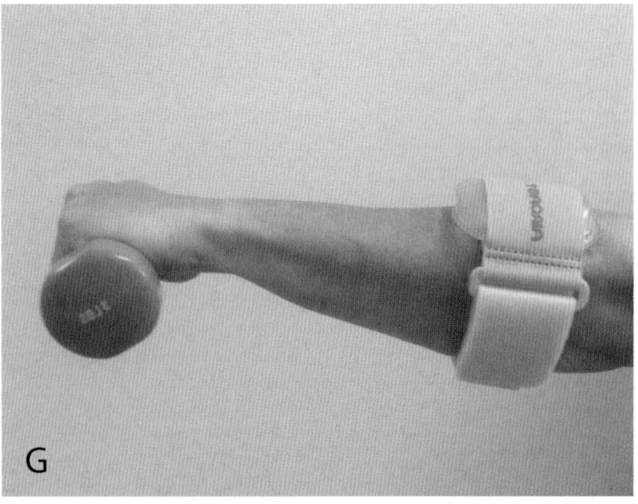

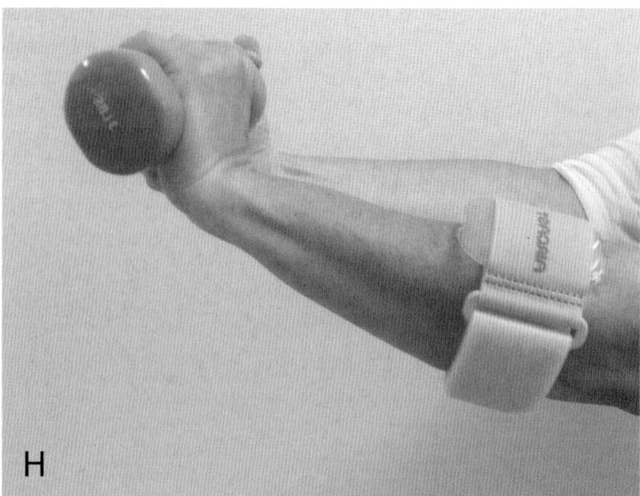

Figure 14.6 (*Continued*) **G**, Photograph of eccentric strengthening with 8 second count with counterforce bracing. **H**, Photograph of eccentric strengthening with passive extension and counterforce bracing.

PEARLS

Nonsurgical Treatment

- A well-structured nonsurgical treatment regimen with a progressive protocol to regain strength, ROM, and improve pain is often successful.
- A sustained treatment regimen should consist of at least 6 months of treatment prior to consideration for surgery.
- Multiple treatment modalities should be used, including stretching, taping, injections, and various pain modalities.
- Patients should be informed of the chronicity of the condition so that they understand that meaningful improvement and full return to function will take time.

Surgical Treatment

- Indicated for recalcitrant cases after appropriate treatment has been exhausted.
- Many techniques exist for treatment, and most do have good outcomes.
- Open and arthroscopic approaches for lateral epicondylitis have similar outcomes, with some studies potentially showing a small improvement in an arthroscopic approach.
- Structured therapy should resume after surgical intervention to improve postoperative pain, control edema, and regain function after adequate healing has occurred.

SUMMARY

The treatment of medial and lateral epicondylitis represents a spectrum of options from observation to surgical intervention. The majority of cases are successfully treated with nonsurgical options, including exercises, bracing, and injections. If surgery is necessary, reasonably good outcomes can be achieved with proper technique and postoperative rehabilitation.

BIBLIOGRAPHY

Cyriax JH: The pathology and treatment of tennis elbow. *J Bone Joint Surg* 1936;18:921–940.

Gabel GT, Morrey BT: Operative treatment of medial epicondylitis: The influence of concomitant ulnar neuropathy at the elbow. *J Bone Joint Surg Am* 1995;77:1065–1069.

Hoogvliet P, Randsdorp MS, Dingemanse R: Does effectiveness of exercise therapy and mobilisation techniques offer guidance for the treatment of lateral and medial epicondylitis? A systematic review. *Br J Sports Med* 2013;47:1112–1119.

MacDonald PB, Clark T, McRae S, Leiter J, Dubberley J: Arthroscopic versus open lateral release for the treatment of lateral epicondylitis: a prospective randomized controlled trial. *J Shoulder Elbow Surg* 2016 Jun 1;25(6):e176.

Morrey BF: Functional anatomy of the ligaments of the elbow. *Clin Orthop* 1985;201:84–90.

Mullett H, Sprague M, Brown G, Hausman M: Arthroscopic treatment of lateral epicondylitis: Clinical and cadaveric studies. *Clin Orthop Relat Res* 2005;439:123–128.

Nirschl RP, Pettrone FA: Tennis elbow: the surgical treatment of lateral epicondylitis. *J Bone Joint Surg Am* 1979;61:832–839.

Peerbooms JC, Sluimer J, Bruijn DJ, Gosens T: Positive effect of an autologous platelet concentrate in lateral epicondylitis in a double-blind randomized controlled trial platelet-rich plasma versus corticosteroid injection with a 1-year follow-up. *Am J Sports Med* 2010 Feb 1;38(2):255–262.

Roquelaure Y, Ha C, Goldberg M, Zins M, Descatha A: Work-related risk factors for incidence of lateral epicondylitis in a large working population. *Scand J Work Environ Health* 2013 Nov 1;39(6):578.

 © 2018 American Academy of Orthopaedic Surgeons

Shiri R, Viikari-Juntura E, Varonen H, Heliövaara M: Prevalence and determinants of lateral and medial epicondylitis: a population study. *Am J Epidemiol* 2006;164(11):1065–1074.

Smidt N, van der Windt DA WM, Assendelft WJJ, Deville WLJM, Korthals-deBos IBC, Bouter LM: Corticosteroid injections, physiotherapy, or a wait and see policy for lateral epicondylitis: a randomized controlled trial. *Lancet* 2002;359:657–662.

Solheim E, Hegna J, Øyen J. Arthroscopic versus open tennis elbow release: 3- to 6-year results of a case-control series of 305 elbows. *Arthroscopy* 2013 May 31;29(5):854–859.

Struijs PA, Kerkhoffs GM, Assendelft WJ, Van Dijk CN: Conservative treatment of lateral epicondylitis: brace versus physical therapy or a combination of both—a randomized clinical trial. *Am J Sports Med* 2004;32:462.

Szabo SJ, Savoie FH, Field LD, et al: Tendinosis of the extensor carpi radialis brevis: an evaluation of three methods of operative treatment. *J Shoulder Elbow Surg* 2006;15:721.

Tyler TF, Thomas GC, Nicholas SJ, McHugh MP: Addition of isolated wrist extensor eccentric exercise to standard treatment for chronic lateral epicondylitis: A prospective randomized trial. *J Shoulder Elbow Surg* 2010;19:917–922.

Zonno A, Manuel J, Merrell G, Ramos P, Akelman E, DaSilva MF: Arthroscopic technique for medial epicondylitis: Technique and safety analysis. *Arthroscopy* 2010;26(5): 610–616.

© 2018 American Academy of Orthopaedic Surgeons

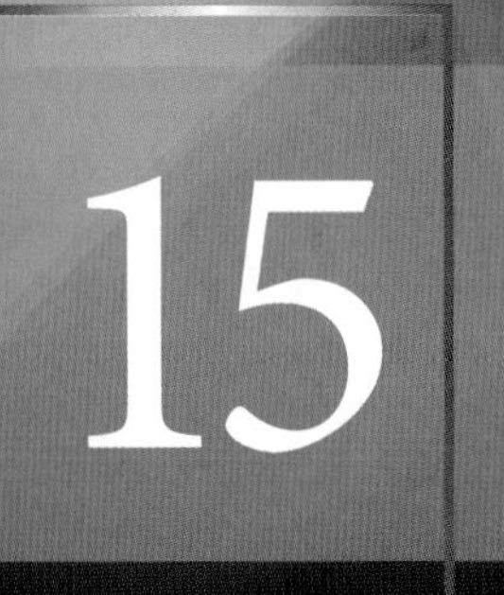

Current Concepts in Surgical Techniques and Postoperative Rehabilitation Strategies Following Ulnar Collateral Ligament Reconstruction of the Elbow

Christopher S. Ahmad, MD, Adrian James Yenchak, DPT, PT, and Joseph L. Ciccone, PT, DPT, SCS, CIMT, CSCS

INTRODUCTION

Injuries to the ulnar collateral ligament (UCL) of the elbow are well recognized in throwing athletes and cause significant absence from sporting activity. Although the first documented cases of UCL insufficiency were described in javelin throwers, baseball pitchers constitute the largest grouping of athletes. The act of throwing generates repetitive forces during the acceleration phase of the motion in which elbow varus torque reaches upwards of 120 Nm and extension velocity of 2300 deg/s. The repetitive valgus loading of the elbow during the transition from the throwers late cocking phase to the follow-through phase produce tensile forces at the medial elbow that challenge the ultimate strength of the ligament. These repetitive tensile forces can result in both acute and repetitive microtrauma to the elbow.

Patients that develop ligament insufficiency resulting from throwing can present with a multitude of impairments that may include medial elbow discomfort, instability, ulnar nerve paresthesia, loss of elbow/shoulder strength, loss of elbow motion, lack of shoulder musculature endurance, reduction in arm velocity, and compromise of controlling pitch location. These factors, coupled with physical changes in elbow chondral integrity and olecranon osteophytic formation, can jeopardize sporting careers and require the need for orthopaedic consultation, treatment, and possible operative intervention.

OPERATIVE TREATMENT

Indications

UCL reconstructions are indicated in patients with persistent medial elbow pain with throwing/overhead activities despite nonoperative treatments who are willing to participate in a postoperative rehabilitation program. Seasonal timing, competitive level, personal expectation, and concomitant pathology of the elbow can influence the indications for the surgery.

Although there is limited literature documenting the efficacy of nonoperative management of UCL tears in overhead throwing athletes, conservative management is the initial approach in most cases. There is uniform consensus that initial strategies for recovery include a 6- to 8-week period of cessation from sport that also incorporates principles of restoration of elbow and shoulder motion, shoulder rotator cuff endurance, scapular stability, and eventual introduction of a modified throwing program. Platelet-rich plasma (PRP) injections to the medial elbow have been advocated by some to enhance healing of the injured ligament before and/or during rehabilitation, but current supporting outcomes research is lacking to provide universal agreement regarding the efficacy of PRP treatments.

A successful rehabilitation program will address specific areas of the kinetic chain (lower extremity/core) with particular attention to restoration of shoulder motion/strength. Principles of total range of motion (TROM) and strength ratios of the rotator cuff are evaluated and treated to significantly decrease potential injury risk upon return to competitive sport. Once motion is restored, adequate shoulder strength ratios are achieved, and total glenohumeral ROM is within acceptable parameters, an athlete may begin a modified two-phase throwing program. This program encompasses flat ground throwing followed by mound throwing progressions designed to safely expose the elbow/shoulder to progressive stresses with gradual return to full competition.

UCL reconstruction is contraindicated if the tear is asymptomatic (no associated symptoms with throwing), the patient is unwilling or not able to participate in a postoperative rehabilitation program, or the patient has inappropriate expectations following surgical procedure despite counseling.

SURGICAL PROCEDURE/TECHNIQUE

Surgical reconstruction of the UCL restores stability to the medial elbow and eliminates symptoms. Concomitant

Dr. Ahmad or an immediate family member serves as a paid consultant to Arthrex; and has received research or institutional support from Arthrex, Major League Baseball, and Stryker. Neither of the following authors nor any immediate family member has received anything of value from or has stock or stock options held in a commercial company or institution related directly or indirectly to the subject of this article: Dr. Ciccone and Dr. Yenchak.

 © 2018 American Academy of Orthopaedic Surgeons

procedures, such as osteophyte débridement of the posteromedial ulna for valgus extension overload and ulnar nerve transposition, may also be performed based on the degree of coexisting pathology and their related symptoms and examination. Autogenous graft harvest options for reconstruction include the palmaris longus or gracilis tendons from the ipsilateral or contralateral limb. There are several different elbow ligament reconstructive procedures that differentiate themselves by surgical approach, bone tunnel placement, ulnar nerve repositioning, and graft fixation/strand number. The two most cited in the literature include the modified Jobe technique and the docking procedure.

Modified Jobe Technique

The ipsilateral palmaris longus or gracilis tendon is harvested. A curved 8-cm to 10-cm skin incision is centered over the medial epicondyle. The dissection protects the medial antebrachial cutaneous nerve branches. A muscle-splitting approach is then used, which incises the raphe of the flexor carpi ulnaris (FCU). The muscle fibers are bluntly separated from the UCL. The ulnar nerve traverses posterior to the border of the MCL and is retracted for its protection. Eventual transposition of the ulnar nerve is carried out following completion of the MCL reconstruction if indicated based on significant ulnar nerve symptoms or ulnar nerve subluxation. A longitudinal incision is made in the UCL (Figure 15.1). Gapping of the ulnohumeral articulation indicates UCL insufficiency. Pathology, such as ulnar or humeral detachment and midsubstance damage, is observed. Two converging tunnels are made with a drill in the ulna, one anterior and one posterior to the sublime tubercle. Tunnels are created on the inferior medial epicondyle at the anatomic origin of the anterior bundle without penetrating the posterior cortex. One 3.2-mm drill tunnel is placed just anterior to the attachment of the medial intermuscular septum and directed to communicate with the central drill hole.

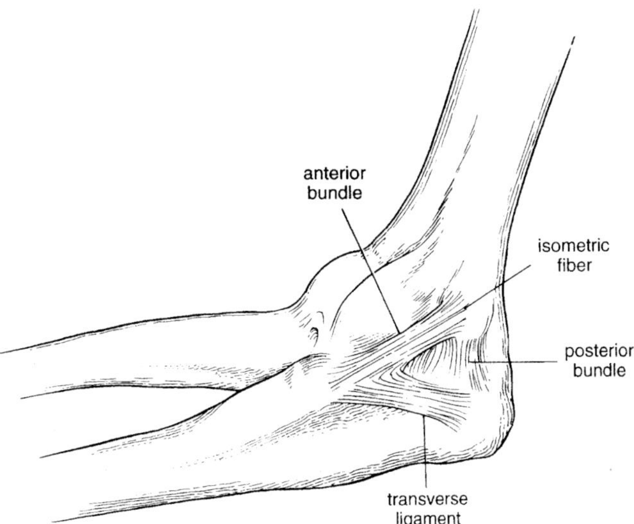

Figure 15.1 Anatomy of the UCL. The UCL is composed of three bundles, the anterior, posterior, and oblique. The anterior bundle is the primary restraint to valgus stress.

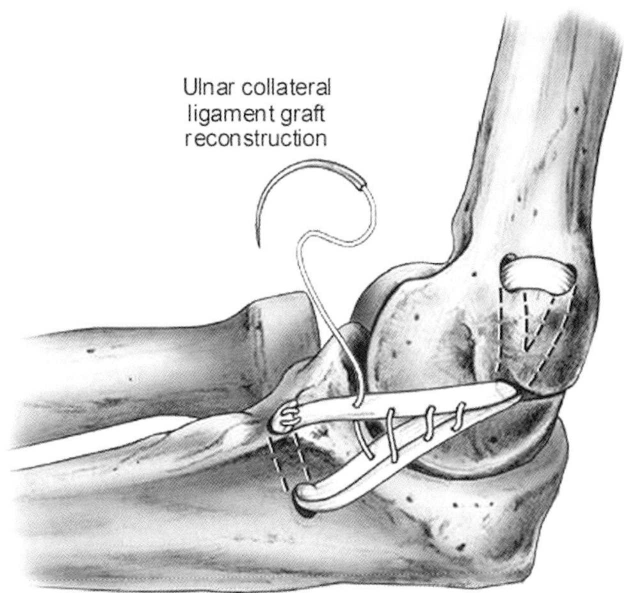

Figure 15.2 Modified Jobe surgical reconstruction. The surgical reconstruction places the graft in a figure-of-8 fashion through bone tunnels on the ulna and humeral epicondyle.

A second 3.2-mm drill tunnel is made, leaving at least a 1-cm bone bridge. The graft is passed through the ulna bone tunnels and through the medial epicondyle, creating a figure-eight configuration (Figure 15.2). Tension is applied to the graft and the ulnar side of the graft is sutured to the remnants of the UCL adjacent to the sublime tubercle. The proximal limb of the graft is sutured to the medial intermuscular septum. If possible, the native ligament is repaired over the graft. The muscle fascia and skin are closed.

Docking Technique

The docking technique is a modification to the Jobe method to ease graft passage, decrease epicondylar tunnel diameters, and improve graft tensioning. The docking technique uses the muscle-splitting approach with similar ulna tunnels as described for the modified Jobe technique. A central distal humeral tunnel is located in the medial epicondyle at the anatomic insertion of the native UCL. The upper border of the epicondyle is exposed, incising the overlying muscular fascia. Two 2-mm exit tunnels with a 5-mm to 1-cm bone bridge are drilled from superior to inferior, communicating with the central tunnel at its proximal apex. The graft is passed through the ulnar tunnels; then, the posterior limb of the graft is passed into the central humeral tunnel and tensioned on the far cortex by pulling its associated sutures through the posterior exit tunnel. The anterior limb of the graft is then estimated for proper length; sutures are placed in it and docked into the humeral tunnel (Figure 15.3). The sutures controlling the graft are then tied over the bony bridge on the humeral epicondyle with the elbow in 40 to 60 degrees of flexion, forearm supination, and varus stress. The fascia overlying the flexor pronator mass is repaired, and the skin is closed in standard fashion.

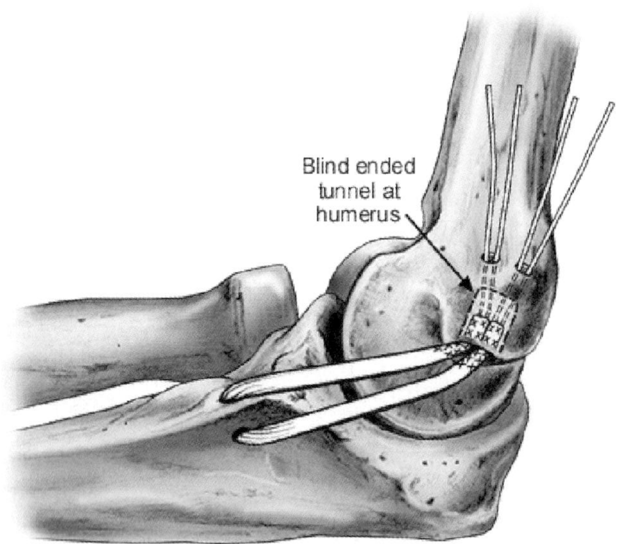

Figure 15.3 Docking procedure. The surgical reconstruction docks the two free limbs of the graft into the humeral epicondyle and sutures controlling the graft are tied over a bone bridge for graft fixation.

POSTOPERATIVE MANAGEMENT/ REHABILITATION

Postoperative rehabilitation of the elbow is tailored to the UCL reconstruction technique and any concomitant procedures performed. The rehabilitation follows a stepwise multiphase approach that minimizes immobilization, applies appropriate stress to healing tissue, and adapts to the individual needs of the patient. A holistic approach to the rehabilitation of the entire kinetic chain helps to ensure optimal restoration of function. The collaborative efforts of both physician and rehabilitation specialist are integral for proper progression through the rehabilitation process to achieve prior level of function in a safe and timely manner.

Immediate Postoperative Management (Weeks 0–3)

The rehabilitation specialist must consider the surgical technique utilized to properly design safe and progressive isotonic strengthening exercises for the patient. The modified Jobe technique will allow the rehabilitation specialist to perform ROM and resistive exercise earlier in the rehabilitation course secondary to a muscle-splitting/sparing visualization to the medial elbow when compared to previous techniques that utilized a complete detachment of the flexor/pronator complex. The modified Jobe technique will allow for earlier flexibility to the wrist and forearm. Scar tissue mobilization is utilized at the proximal wrist to limit a dimple effect (indentation resulting from palmaris longus graft harvesting). Palmar aponeurosis extensibility will also be promoted with early mobilization of the wrist and hand, which allows greater extensibility for wrist/hand motion and dexterity (Figure 15.4).

The rate of progression toward achieving full passive range of motion (PROM) and transitioning to the intermediate strengthening phase will be based on the surgical procedure performed, physiologic healing response of the patient (end feel), and patient subjective reports. The elbow is initially immobilized in a posterior splint in 90 degrees of elbow flexion and neutral forearm rotation for 5 to 7 days to protect the graft, flexor/pronator musculature, and skin incision. The elbow is then placed in a hinged brace to allow ROM while continuing to protect the reconstruction.

Postoperative complications can present in the early rehabilitation phase regarding elbow extension. Pain associated with arthroscopy/osteophytic débridement, elbow edema, and resultant spasmodic activity of the forearm flexors and extenders can cause limitation in elbow ROM. Prolonged pain and muscle spasm may produce elbow flexion soft-tissue contractures and elbow joint capsular stiffness secondary to anterior capsular adhesions. The rehabilitation specialist can minimize the propensity for elbow stiffness by consistently evaluating the end feel when performing ROM exercise during the early rehabilitation course. If the patient exhibits a loss of motion and a firm elbow capsular end feel with no pain, more

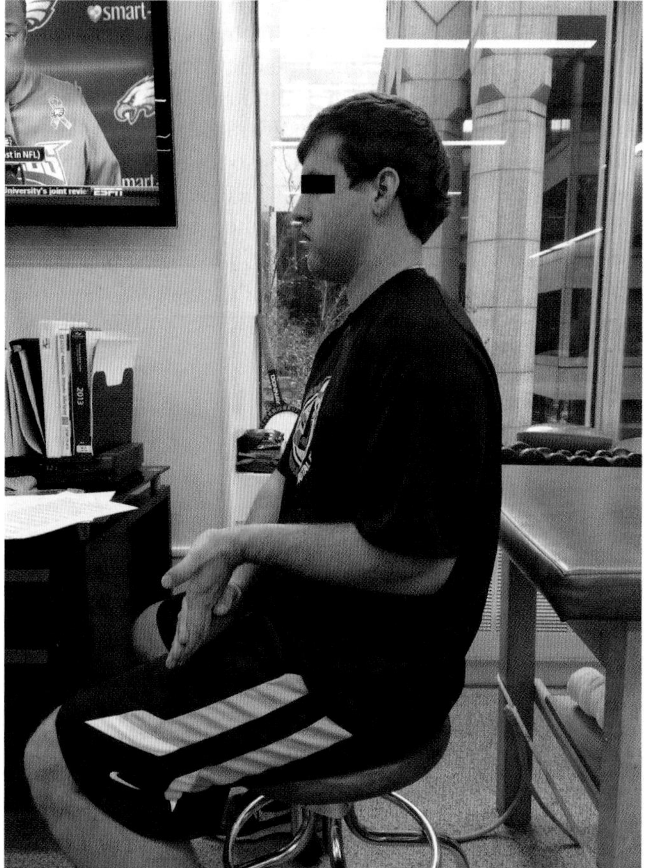

Figure 15.4 Forearm wrist extensor stretching (elbow bent). Exercise begins with elbow flexed at 90 degrees with palm facing up. The opposite hand grasps all four fingers and pulls the wrist and fingers into extension until a light stretch is felt.

© 2018 American Academy of Orthopaedic Surgeons

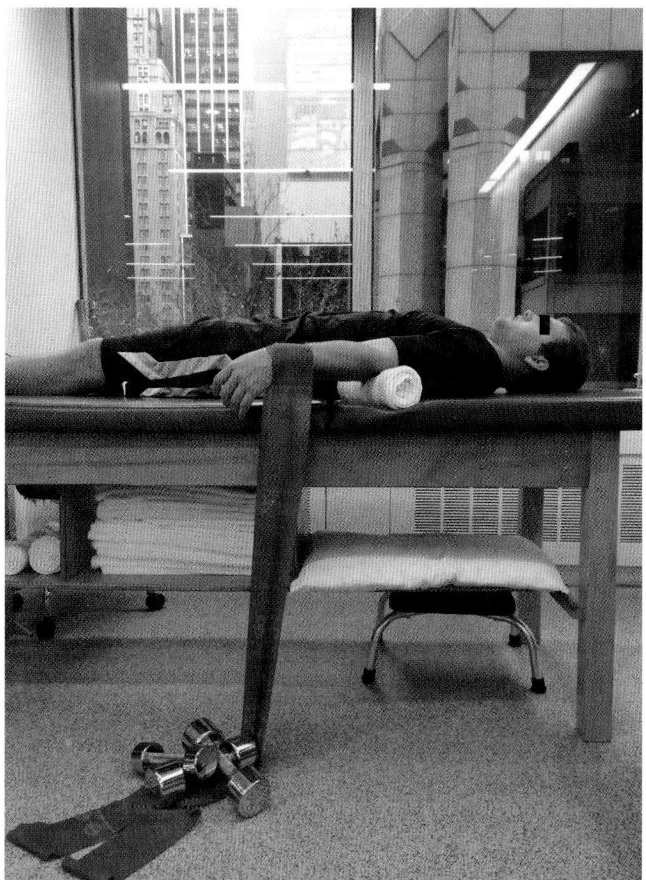

Figure 15.5 Static progressive range of motion. With the patient in supine position, a towel roll is placed under the distal humerus and a wide resistance band is placed on the distal forearm and secured with weights once desired tension is established by the therapist. The elbow and wrist should be in neutral position.

aggressive PROM techniques, such as grade 3 or grade 4 joint mobilization and static progressive stretching (Figure 15.5), can be employed. If pain is present with a loss of motion prior to an end feel being established, a more conservative approach utilizing soft-tissue massage, heat modalities, grade 1 or grade 2 ulnohumeral joint distraction, and low-amplitude stretching may be warranted.

Intermediate Strengthening Phase (Weeks 4–8)

The transition from the immediate postoperative phase to the intermediate strengthening phase begins at week 4 and progresses to week 8. There are specific clinical markers pertaining to motion and strength that must be addressed during this time interval. Full elbow motion should be achieved by week 6. Upper extremity strengthening is progressed with particular attention placed on glenohumeral rotator cuff strengthening, scapular stabilization, and core endurance. Upper extremity strengthening progresses with elbow forearm flexors/extensors achieving grade 4 on manual muscle testing.

Isotonic strengthening of the shoulder and elbow complex is initiated during this phase to promote rotator cuff co-contraction for glenohumeral stability, elbow proximal stability, and periscapular neuromuscular control. The principles of the "throwers 10 program" are utilized during postoperative weeks 5 to 6, which include shoulder internal and external rotation (limited external ROM to neutral to decrease valgus stress to elbow) using resistance bands. Standing shoulder abduction and standing scaption are incorporated initially using arm weight and then slowly progressed with weighted dumbbells. Side-lying external rotation, prone extension, prone scaption, and prone abduction with external rotation are performed to enhance proximal shoulder girdle strength. Isotonic elbow strengthening includes wrist flexion, extension, and forearm pronation/supination with progression based on patient symptoms and endurance. Resistance exercises are progressed from 3 sets of 10.

Neuromuscular control drills for the scapula are performed in a side-lying position (Figure 15.6) and progressed to a seated position to challenge core musculature. A stability ball is introduced during postoperative weeks 8 to 10 for higher-level neuromuscular control of the upper and lower extremities. The patient performs shoulder isotonic exercise in a seated and prone position on the stability ball to promote higher levels of glenohumeral/scapulothoracic stabilization while performing isotonic shoulder strengthening (Figure 15.7). Lower extremity and core stability exercises are incorporated for enhanced kinetic chain recruitment. Resistance exercise is generally alternated between stability ball shoulder isotonic strengthening and plinth exercises, with higher repetitions and lower resistance utilized for stability ball exercises for the promotion of muscular endurance. Arm ergometry (arm cycle) further promotes muscular endurance and upper extremity (shoulder and elbow) mobility; thus, it should be incorporated and continued throughout the remainder of the rehabilitation program. Manual resistance exercises of the elbow flexors are also introduced and have an important role in medial elbow stabilization during throwing (Figure 15.8). Two sets of 10 repetitions are prescribed for these exercises to enhance muscular strength and endurance development. Shoulder manual side-lying external rotation (Figure 15.9A) and manual prone rowing are promoted for posterior rotator cuff strengthening (Figure 15.9B).

Neuromuscular control drills emphasizing proprioceptive facilitation such as rhythmic stabilizations with medicine ball perturbations (Figure 15.10) aid in co-contraction of musculature at the elbow and shoulder joint necessary for stabilization and controlled motion during sport-related activity. The exercises are initiated with proximal perturbations close to the glenohumeral joint and progressed to the distal extremity for higher-level neuromuscular control.

The intensity, duration, and frequency of the exercises discussed in this phase prepare the patient for advanced rehabilitation principles that incorporate strength, power, and endurance in functional postures relevant to the overhead athlete. Stresses applied to the elbow and shoulder joint become more relevant to the throwing motion with stresses that mimic those encountered with repetitious overhead throwing. The advanced strengthening phase serves as a crucial intermediary

© 2018 American Academy of Orthopaedic Surgeons

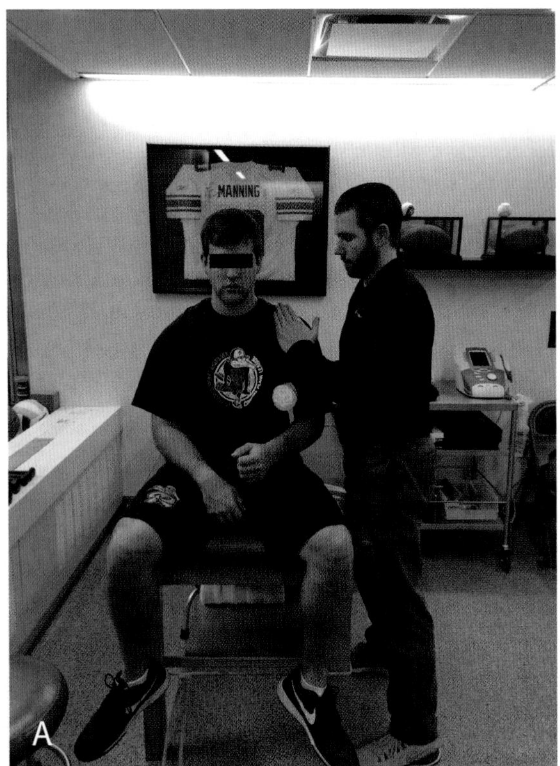
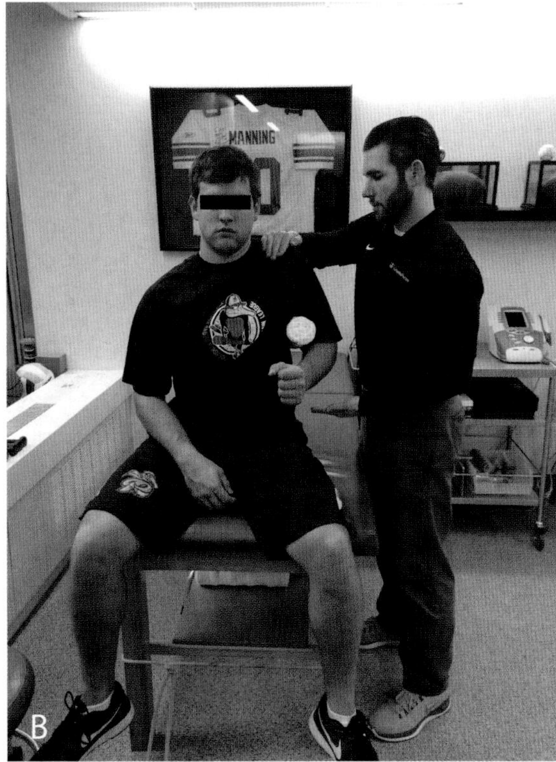

Figure 15.6 Neuromuscular control drills for scapula in seated position. The patient sits upright with a towel under arm while the therapist applies resistance to the scapula for protraction/retraction (**A**) and for elevation/depression (**B**).

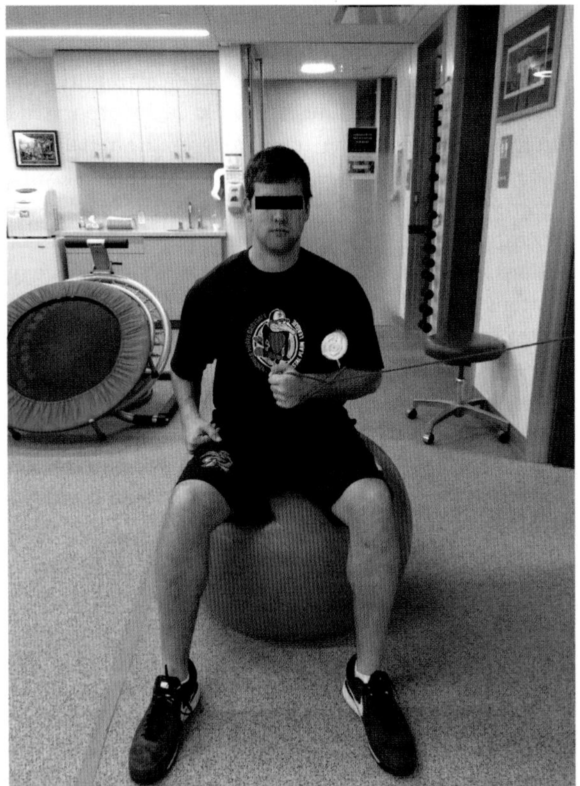

Figure 15.7 Stability ball isotonic strengthening. The patient sits with good posture on a stability ball with feet on the floor and performs external and internal rotation with a resistance band while maintaining a neutral spine position.

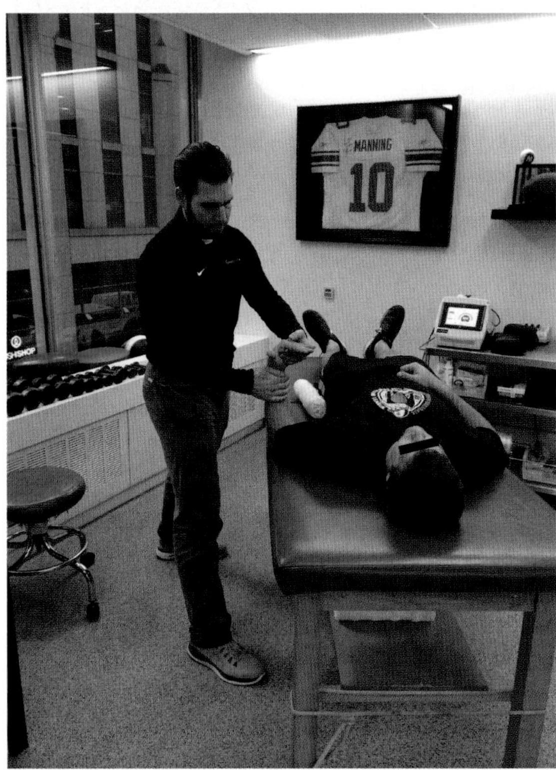

Figure 15.8 Resisted elbow flexor strengthening. The therapist places one hand on the patient's wrist and the other over the patient's fingers. The patient flexes the fingers, wrist, and elbow as the therapist provides resistance to strengthen the finger/wrist and elbow flexor complexes.

 © 2018 American Academy of Orthopaedic Surgeons

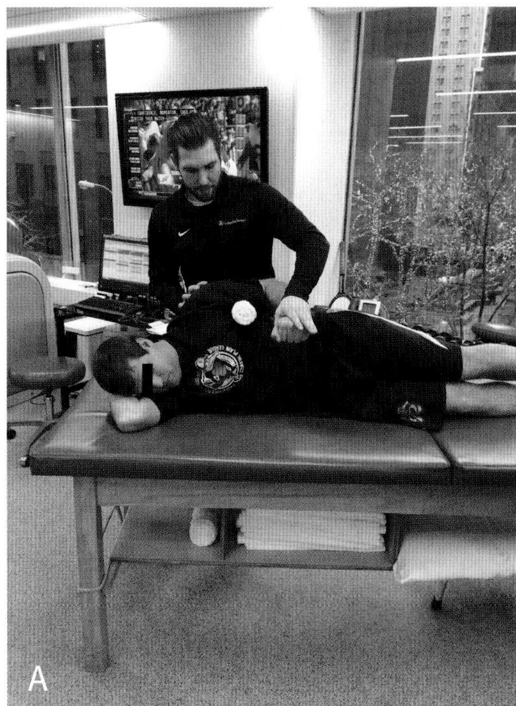

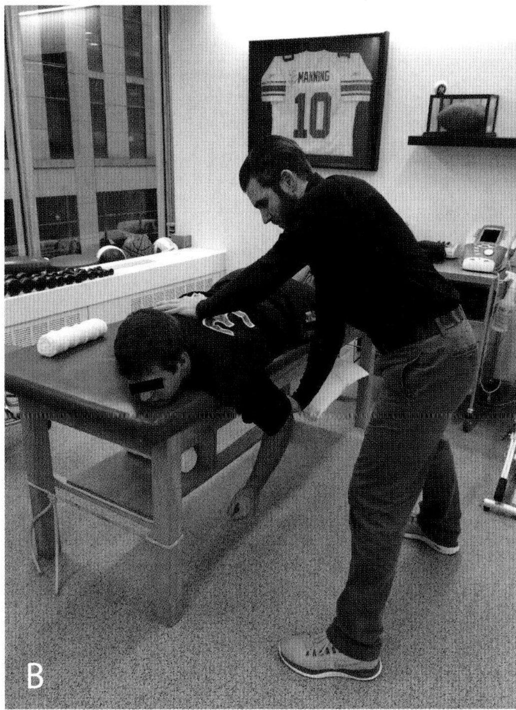

Figure 15.9 **A**, Side-lying manual external rotation. With the patient lying on the uninvolved side, a towel roll is placed under the arm and the therapist manually resists external rotation concentrically and eccentrically. As the program advances, the therapist imparts alternating isometrics of external rotation/internal rotation at the end range. **B**, Prone rowing manual resisted. The patient lies prone with affected arm hanging off the edge of the table. The therapist applies resistance to the distal humerus as the patient brings the humerus into the extended position. The therapist then applies pressure again as the patient resists eccentrically back to the starting position.

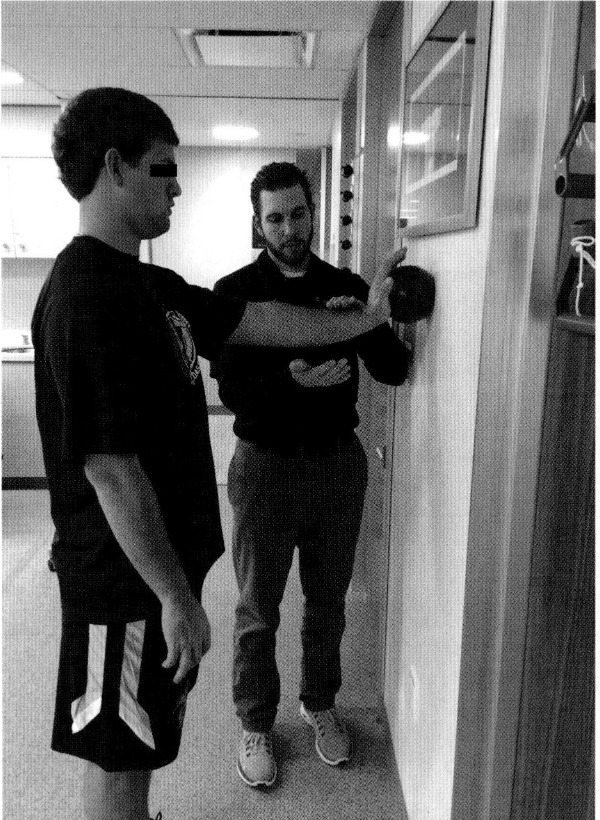

Figure 15.10 Ball on wall rhythmic stabilization. The patient places the palm on a small ball with the hand fully open against the wall. The therapist applies rhythmic stabilization drills while the patient maintains the starting position.

between progressive resistive exercise and the initiation of an athlete's return to sport.

Advanced Strengthening Phase (Weeks 8–16)

The advanced strengthening phase is characterized by a continuation of manual resistance exercise, shoulder and elbow isotonic strengthening, maintenance of elbow PROM, and the initiation of plyometric exercises for the elbow and shoulder complex. Plyometric exercise has been shown to excite muscle spindles with an eccentric prestretch that creates forceful muscle contractions. The exercises emphasize all aspects of strengthening about the elbow, glenohumeral joint, and scapula.

One-hand plyometric drills are initiated with the arm at 0 degrees of abduction for both internal and external rotation during postoperative weeks 12 to 14 (Figure 15.11). Chest passes, side passes, and overhead tossing using a weighted medicine ball are used to promote higher levels of stress to the medial elbow and prepare the soft tissue for more advanced stress with one-handed plyometric progressions. Drills performed in the thrower's position (90/90) are utilized for both internal and external rotation (Figure 15.12). One-handed drills are initiated at weeks 14 to 16 postoperatively. Wall dribbles, prone abduction wrist flips, and seated wrist flips are all incorporated for increased stress to the elbow and shoulder complex. Exercises are performed in 3 sets of 10 repetitions

© 2018 American Academy of Orthopaedic Surgeons

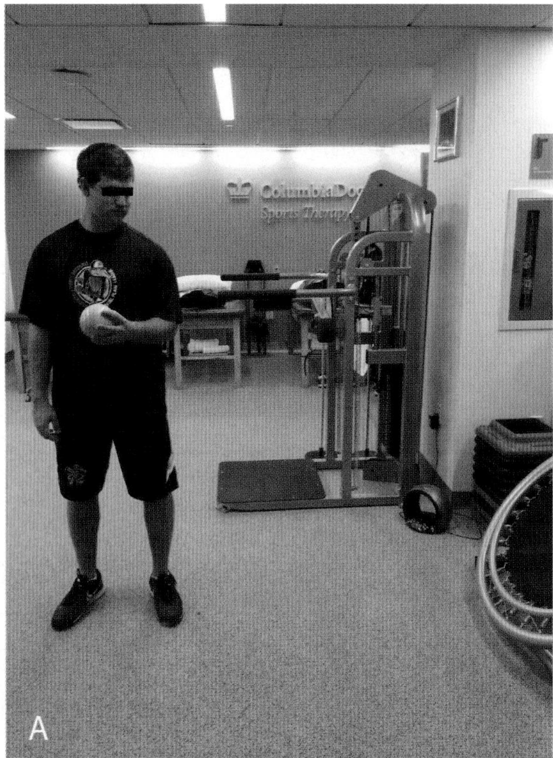

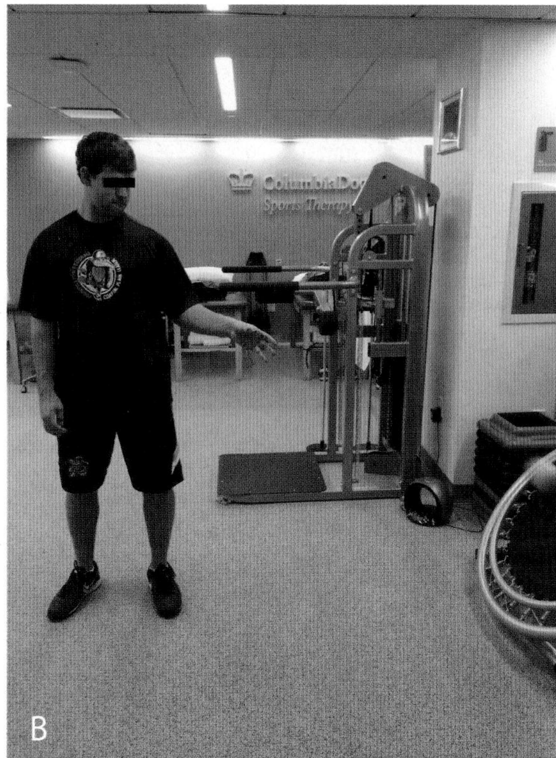

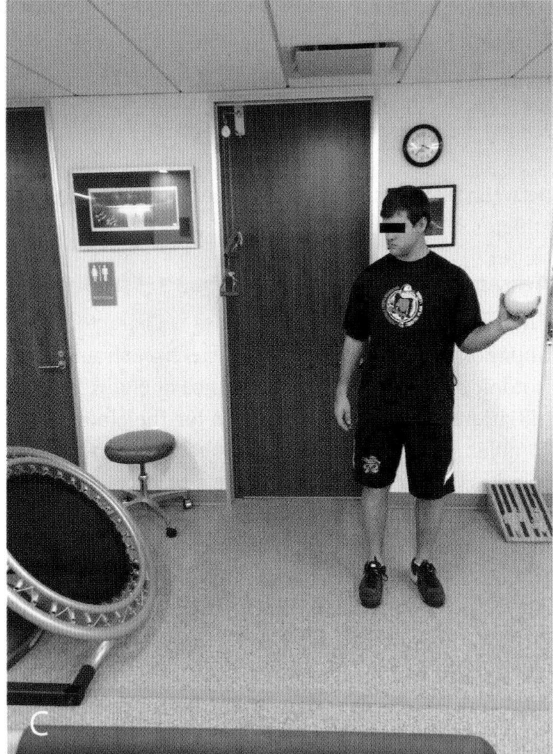

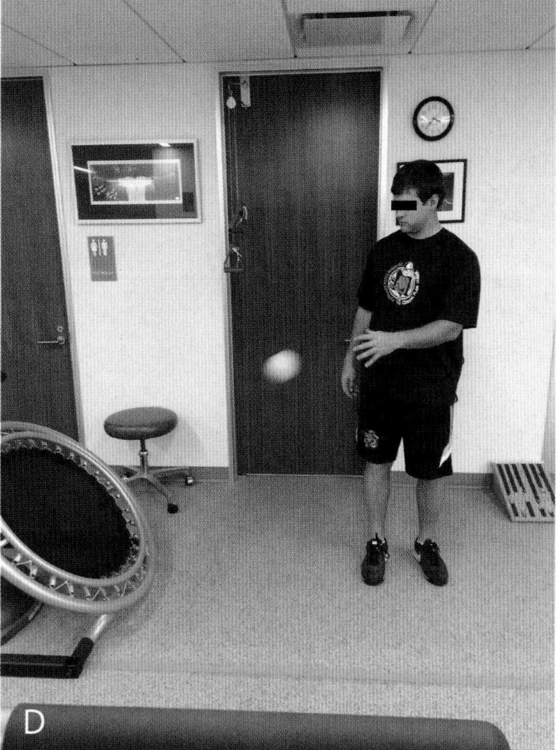

Figure 15.11 One-hand plyometric drills at 0 degrees of abduction external rotation (**A**) and internal rotation (**B**). The patient stands in front of a trampoline sideways with the surgical arm closest to the trampoline. With a small medicine ball, the patient keeps the shoulder at 0 degrees of abduction and rotates the arm to throw the ball out to the trampoline. As the ball is coming back, the athlete catches it while returning to starting position and immediately throws the ball out again (**A** and **B**). The patient stands sideways with surgical arm on far side and performs the same movement pattern for internal rotation. The ball is tossed out to the trampoline and then catching it as it returns to starting position and immediately throws the ball out again (**C** and **D**).

 © 2018 American Academy of Orthopaedic Surgeons

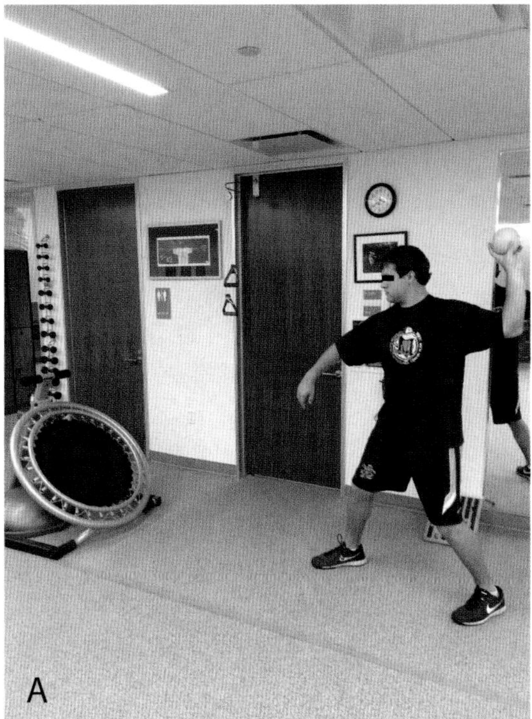

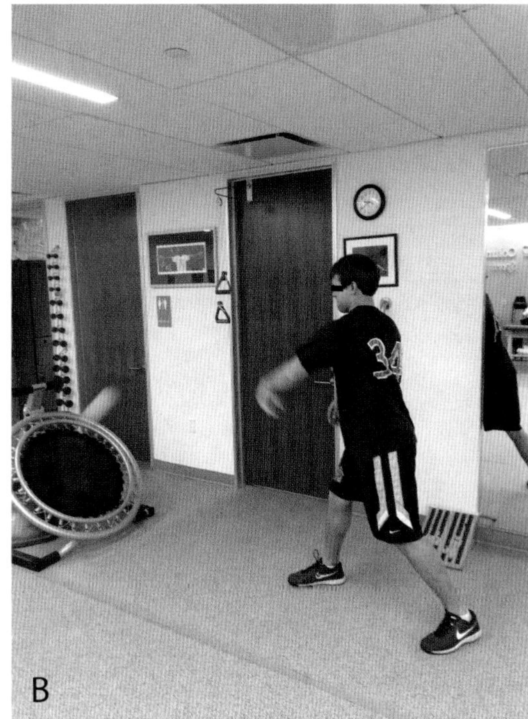

Figure 15.12 90/90 standing plyometric toss. With a small plyoball, the patient starts in a throwing position (**A**) and throws the ball into the trampoline (**B**). The patient then receives the ball back from the trampoline in the throwing position with a smooth movement pattern and immediately transitions to throwing the ball again.

while wall dribbles are performed for 30- to 60- to 90-second bouts. Strengthening exercises integrating higher-level neuromuscular control are included in our Advanced Throwers 10 program.

Elbow flexion exercises are altered to promote fast eccentric training secondary to the biceps role in eccentric deceleration of the arm through the follow-through phase of overhead motion. Fast bicep curls can be performed with exercise tubing or manual resistance (Figure 15.13). Triceps concentric exercise promotes its functional role in concentrically accelerating the arm during the acceleration phase of throwing.

End-range dynamic stabilization and advanced neuromuscular control drills—such as resistance bands in the 90/90 ER position with manual perturbations, manual concentric/eccentric external rotation on a stability ball with rhythmic stabilization (Figure 15.14), and stability ball wall dribble with perturbations at end-range external rotation—are employed to challenge the rotator cuff and promote proximal stability at the elbow joint. Side-lying scapular elevation, depression, protraction, and retraction are performed with manual resistance by the rehabilitation specialist to challenge the endurance of the periscapular musculature.

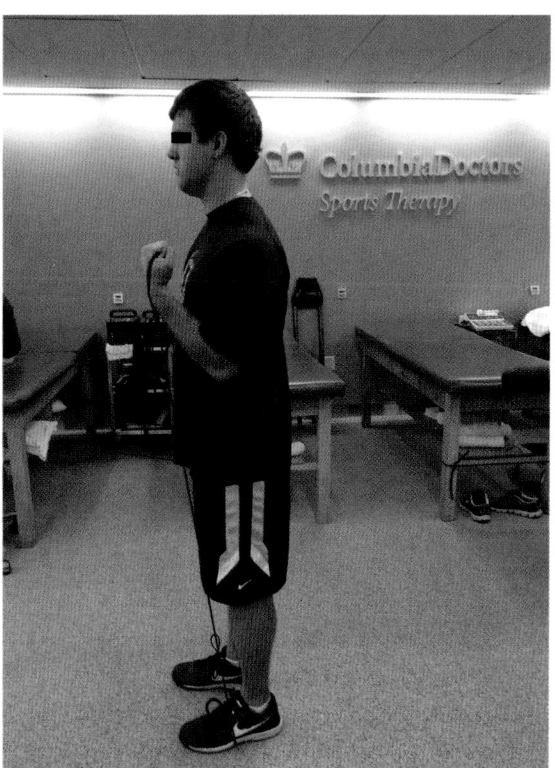

Figure 15.13 Biceps curls with exercise tubing. The patient stands upright on one end of a resistance band, holding the other end with the involved arm. The patient flexes the elbow to full flexion and then lowers to full extension. Speed is encouraged once the form is sound.

Return to Sport

An interval-throwing program is typically initiated at 16 weeks postoperatively following successful completion of a multiphased, progressive resistance and motion restoration rehabilitation program (Box 15.1). The patient begins throwing

© 2018 American Academy of Orthopaedic Surgeons

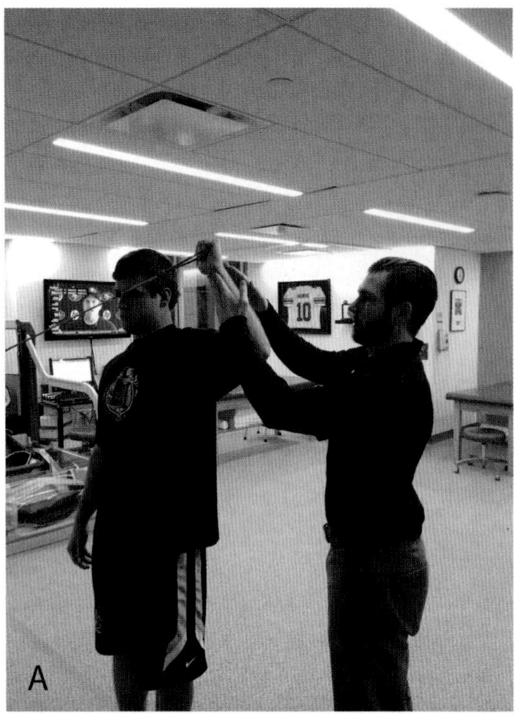

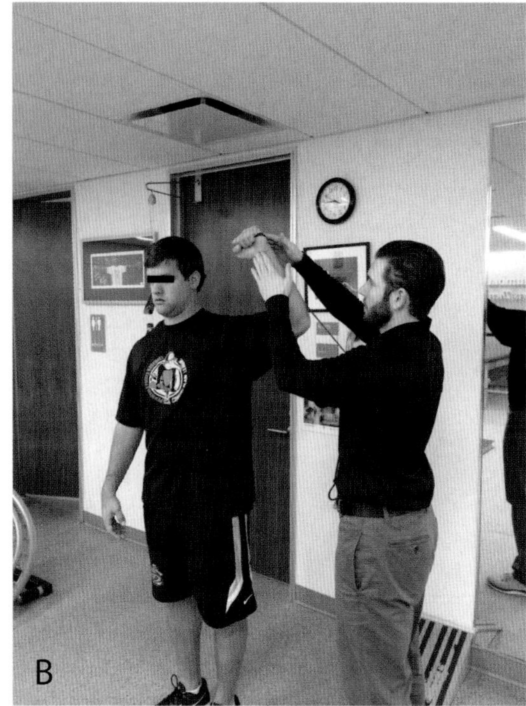

Figure 15.14 Resistance band 90/90 external rotation (**A**) and internal rotation (**B**) with perturbations. The patient stands in the throwing position performing resistance band external rotation while in 90 degrees of elbow flexion and 90 degrees of abduction. The patient remains in 90 degrees of abduction and elbow flexion while rotating the arm from 0 degrees to 90 degrees of external rotation with the therapist performing perturbations at the end range of external rotation (**A**). The patient then turns around and performs internal rotation from 90 degrees to 0 degrees of with the therapist performing perturbations at the 90 degrees position (**B**).

Box 15.1 RETURN TO SPORT AND INTERVAL THROWING PROGRAM

Phase 1

- Lob toss program is initiated at week 16 at distances no greater than 45 feet.
- Throwing activity is performed on an alternate day schedule with stretching, cardiovascular exercise, and core exercise performed on rest days.
- Proper warm-up is essential prior to beginning any throwing program.
- Isotonic shoulder exercises (Throwers 10) should be performed for 10 repetitions prior to throwing.
- An additional two sets of the isotonic strengthening program should be performed following successful completion of throwing.
- Phase 1 of the interval-throwing program will follow with progressions to 120 feet using a crow hop.
- Throwing on a line (flat ground) begins after successful completion of pain-free throwing at 120 feet.

Phase 2

- Mound progressions begin 4 to 6 weeks following the initiation of phase 1 depending on patient symptoms.
- Phase 2 mound progressions usually take 8 to 10 weeks to reestablish proper mechanics, confidence, and ball velocity.
- Competitive throwing will not commence until 9 to 12 months postoperatively.

based on stringent clinical criteria, including full PROM of the elbow, no pain or tenderness at the medial elbow, suitable isokinetic strength of the shoulder/elbow complex, and satisfactory thrower's PROM at the shoulder. It is not uncommon for an athlete to feel discomfort when progressing through the stages of the throwing program. This is usually addressed with rest (3–5 days) and restarting of the particular phase that created symptoms.

Postoperative Rehabilitation for Modified Jobe Technique Using Autograft

Phase 1: Postoperative Phase (Weeks 1–3)

Immediate Postoperative Goals

- Protect surgical procedure/healing tissue.
- Decrease postoperative discomfort/elbow edema.
- Limit elbow/shoulder muscle atrophy.

Week 1

- Posterior splint at 70 to 90 degrees of elbow flexion
- Cryotherapy hourly to decrease regional swelling, edema, and pain
- Compressive wrap worn for 1 to 2 weeks postoperatively
- Wrist PROM, gripping exercise with putty or foam ball
- Shoulder isometrics (no external rotation) preferably with electric stimulation to the posterior rotator cuff/biceps isometrics

 © 2018 American Academy of Orthopaedic Surgeons

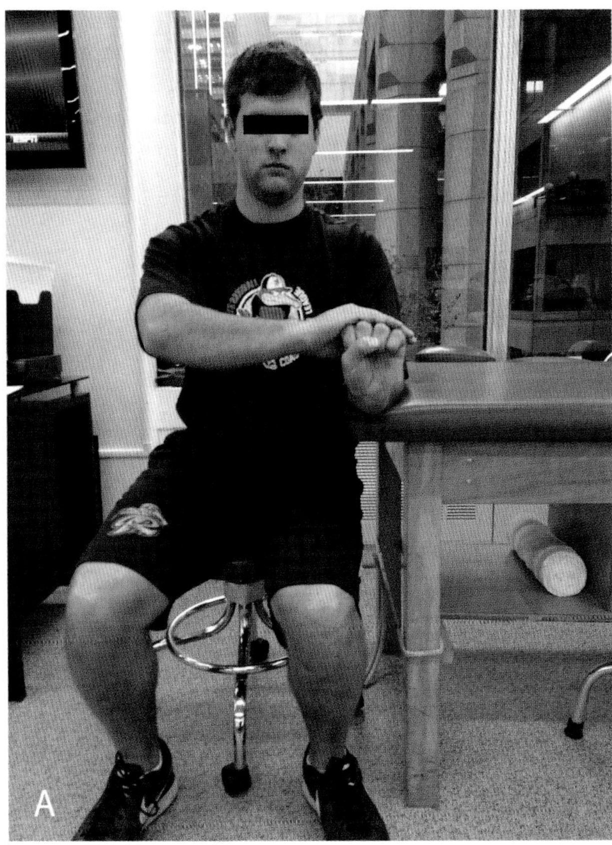

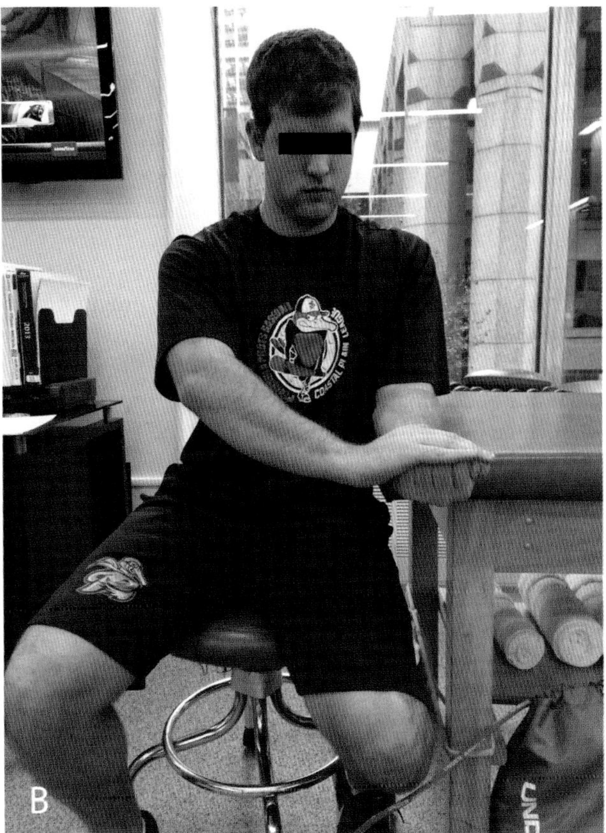

Figure 15.15 Isometric wrist exercises. The patient places the involved elbow on the table in 90 degrees of flexion. The uninvolved hand is placed on dorsal aspect of hand to resist active wrist extension (**A**). Next, the uninvolved hand is positioned on the volar aspect of fist to resist active wrist flexion (**B**).

Week 2

- Hinged elbow brace initiated 5 to 7 days postoperatively
- Hinged brace set at 30-degree to 100-degree arc of elbow motion
- Sleep in brace weeks 2 to 6
- Initiate wrist isometrics with gradual progression to wrist active range of motion (AROM) at week 3.
- Submaximal isometrics for the wrist and elbow (Figure 15.15) limit the effects of muscle atrophy to the forearm.
- Continue shoulder isometrics with initiation of shoulder external rotation to 50% to 75% maximum intensity.
- Begin PROM to elbow 15-degree to 110-degree arc with close supervision pertaining to end feel.
- Soft-tissue principles applied to elbow flexors/extensors to limit reflexive spasm
- Maintain PROM of the affected shoulder.

Week 3

- Continue shoulder isometrics, wrist AROM, and PROM of elbow.
- Hinged elbow brace settings 15 degrees to 110 degrees with gradual increase in extension by 5 degrees to 10 degrees per week/flexion 10 degrees to 15 degrees per week
- Continue soft tissue to forearm/brachium

Phase 2: Transitional Strengthening/Restoration of Elbow Joint Range of Motion (Weeks 4–8)

Goals for Phase 2

- Work toward restoration of elbow ROM.
- Protect the surgical repair site.
- Advance strengthening exercises to shoulder/scapula/elbow.
- Maintain muscle/soft-tissue flexibility.

Week 4

- Begin isotonic strengthening to wrist, shoulder with emphasis on internal rotation, external rotation (limit full arc of motion for 8 weeks), shoulder scaption, side-lying external rotation, and prone rowing.
- Brace specifications 10 degrees to 120 degrees of motion
- Continue to work toward restoration of full passive elbow extension (closely monitor end feel).
- Continue soft-tissue principles for elbow ROM/extensibility.
- Begin scapular neuromuscular control drills in seated position.
- Begin rhythmic stabilization drills to affected shoulder.

Weeks 5–6

- Brace set to 0 degrees to 130 degrees (week 5) with discontinuation at week 6

© 2018 American Academy of Orthopaedic Surgeons

- Continue isotonic strengthening exercise to shoulder (discontinue use of electrical stimulation).
- Patient should achieve full passive elbow extension by week 6.
- Continue scapular control drills.
- Initiate abdominal isometric/isotonic exercise.
- Patient may begin running program at week 6.
- Arm ergometry if applicable

Weeks 7–8

- Emphasize shoulder isotonic strengthening program with addition of prone extension, prone abduction, and prone scaption.
- Continue abdominal program and running program.
- Maintain elbow PROM (closely monitor end feel).
- May progress external rotation ROM with isotonic exercise through full arc of motion.
- Progress scapular control exercise.
- Maintain muscle length through soft-tissue techniques.
- Maintain shoulder PROM.

Phase 3: Progressive Strengthening Phase

Goals for Phase 3

- Advance strengthening, initiate power, and progress endurance exercise
- Maintain full passive/active range of motion of postoperative elbow
- Begin plyometric drills/interval sport programs

Weeks 9–12

- Continue isotonic shoulder, elbow, and abdominal exercises.
- Begin manual resistance exercise with emphasis on prone rowing and supine external rotation.
- Maintain thrower's motion in affected shoulder.
- Progress neuromuscular control drills to scapula.
- Progress abdominal program.
- Initiate Advanced Throwers 10 exercise program.
- May initiate interval hitting program (weeks 10–12).
- May initiate interval golf program (week 12).
- Initiate two-hand plyometric drills (chest, side throw, overhead throw).

Phase 4: Return to Sporting Activity Phase (Weeks 13–36; see Box 15.1)

Goals

- Continue to progress advanced strengthening exercises, neuromuscular control of the scapula, and upper extremity power/endurance.

Weeks 13–16

- Continue Advanced Throwers 10 program.
- Continue manual resistance exercise with emphasis on side-lying external rotation.
- Continue rhythmic stabilization exercise with emphasis on thrower's position.
- Initiate one-handed plyometric drills (internal/external rotation at side, wall dribble, week 14; see Figure 15.11).
- Initiate lob toss program (weeks 15–16).
- Initiate interval throwing programs (weeks 16–18).
- Initiate off-the-mound throwing programs (weeks 22–24).

Return to competitive sport (weeks 30–36)

Postoperative Rehabilitation for Autograft with Docking Procedure

Phase 1: Postoperative Phase (Weeks 1–3)

Immediate Postoperative Goals

- Protect surgical procedure/healing tissue.
  - Decrease postoperative discomfort/elbow edema.
  - Limit elbow/shoulder muscle atrophy.

Week 1

- Posterior splint at 90 degrees of elbow flexion
  - Cryotherapy hourly to decrease regional swelling, edema, and pain
  - Compressive wrap worn for 1 to 2 weeks postoperatively
  - Wrist PROM, gripping exercise
  - No shoulder isometrics until weeks 4 to 5

Week 2

- Hinged elbow brace initiated 5 to 7 days postoperatively
  - Hinged brace set at 30-degree to 90-degree arc of elbow motion
  - Sleep in brace weeks 2 to 6.
  - Initiate wrist isometrics with gradual progression to wrist AROM at week 3.
  - Submaximal isometrics for the wrist and elbow (see Figure 15.14) limit the effects of muscle atrophy to the forearm.
  - Soft-tissue principles applied to elbow flexors/extensors to limit reflexive spasm
  - Maintain PROM of the affected shoulder.

Week 3

- Continue wrist AROM, and PROM of postoperative elbow.
  - Hinged elbow brace settings 30 to 90 degrees
  - Continue soft tissue to forearm/brachium.

Phase 2: Transitional Strengthening/Restoration of Elbow Joint Range of Motion (Weeks 4–8)

Goals for Phase 2

- Begin elbow PROM.
  - Begin isometric strengthening exercises to shoulder.
  - Maintain muscle/soft-tissue flexibility.

Week 4

- Begin isometric strengthening to shoulder with emphasis on electrical stimulation to the posterior rotator cuff. No external rotation isometrics.
  - Brace specifications 15 degrees to 120 degrees of motion by week 6

© 2018 American Academy of Orthopaedic Surgeons

- Continue to work toward restoration of full passive elbow extension (closely monitor end feel).
- Continue soft-tissue principles for elbow ROM/extensibility.
- Begin scapular neuromuscular control drills in seated position.
- Begin rhythmic stabilization drills to affected shoulder.

Weeks 5–6

- Brace set to 10 degrees to 130 degrees (week 5) with discontinuation at week 8
  - Continue isometric strengthening exercise to shoulder (continue use of electrical stimulation).
  - Patient should achieve full passive elbow extension by week 6.
  - Continue scapular control drills.
  - Initiate abdominal isometric/isotonic exercise.
  - Patient may begin running program weeks 6–8.

Weeks 7–8

- Initiate and emphasize shoulder isotonic strengthening program. Continue abdominal program and running program.
  - Achieve full elbow PROM (closely monitor end feel).
  - Progress scapular control exercises.
  - Maintain muscle length through soft-tissue techniques.
  - Maintain shoulder PROM.

Phase 3: Progressive Strengthening Phase

Goals for Phase 3

- Advance strengthening, initiate power, and progress endurance exercise.
  - Maintain full PROM/AROM of postoperative elbow (closely monitor end feel).
  - Begin plyometric drills/interval sport programs.

Weeks 9–14

- Continue isotonic shoulder, elbow, abdominal exercise
  - Begin manual resistance exercise with emphasis on prone rowing and supine external rotation.
  - Maintain thrower's motion in affected shoulder.
  - Maintain full PROM of affected elbow.
  - Progress neuromuscular control drills to scapula.
  - Progress abdominal program.
  - May progress external rotation ROM with isotonic exercise through full arc of motion.
  - Initiate Advanced Throwers 10 program (weeks 10–12).
  - May initiate interval hitting program (week 12).
  - May initiate interval golf program (week 14).
  - Initiate two-hand plyometric drills (chest, side throw, overhead throw).

Phase 4: Return to Sporting Activity Phase (Week 14–Return to Sport; see Box 15.1)

Goals

- Continue to progress advanced strengthening exercises, neuromuscular control of the scapula, and upper extremity power/endurance.

Weeks 13–16

- Continue Advanced Throwers 10 program
  - Continue manual resistance exercise with emphasis on side-lying external rotation.
  - Continue rhythmic stabilization exercise with emphasis on thrower's position.
  - Initiate one-handed plyometric drills (internal/external rotation at side, wall dribble; week 14).
  - Initiate lob toss program (weeks 15–16).
  - Initiate interval throwing programs (weeks 16–18).
  - Initiate off-the-mound throwing programs (weeks 22–24).
  - Return to competitive sport 10 to 12 months.

OUTCOMES

In 2008, Vitale and Ahmad published a systematic review demonstrating excellent results among 83% of patients with only a 10% complication rate. This review highlighted the transition to a muscle-splitting approach instead of the conventional flexor pronator muscle detachment. Cain et al. reported that 83% of athletes returned to the same level of play with a relatively low complication rate. Makhni et al. evaluated the public records of 147 baseball pitchers returning from elbow UCL reconstruction to Major League Baseball. A total of 80% returned to pitch in at least one regular season game, while 67% of pitchers returned to their previous level of competition postoperatively. Of those established players returning, 57% returned to the disabled list as a result of injury to their throwing arm. Other factors, such as flexor pronator tear with UCL repair, substantially compromised success, with only 12.5% returning to previous level of competition. The presence of ulnohumeral chondromalacia, UCL calcification/bony deficiency noted at the time of repair has also demonstrated inferior results.

PEARLS

Surgical

- Exposure—Limited dissection of flexor-pronator mass is critical to optimize dynamic stability of elbow.
- Ulnar nerve—Less involvement/handling of nerve is associated with better outcome.
- Tunnel placement—Location of inferior humeral tunnel is imperative to isometric graft tensioning.
- Graft position—Extrasynovial to avoid delayed healing/tunnel expansion
- Bone deficiency—Hybrid interference screw fixation or cortical button fixation is preferred.

Rehabilitation

- Rehabilitation must be tailored to the specific procedure
  - Jobe technique earlier progression of elbow motion and shoulder strengthening
  - Docking technique: Allow more time for motion restoration, 8 to 10 weeks.

© 2018 American Academy of Orthopaedic Surgeons

- Put emphasis on wrist flexor/shoulder strengthening.
- Preparation for throwing involves longer plyometric duration.
- Long toss: Allow more time to develop during interval throwing program.
- Delay hard throwing 7 to 9 months.

SUMMARY

Optimizing clinical and functional outcomes following UCL injury or reconstruction is based on a sequential, progressive, multiphased rehabilitation approach. Clear understandings of the biomechanical and physiologic sequelae that lead to UCL disruption are necessary to properly treating this patient population. Clear knowledge of the surgical technique will help the rehabilitation specialist to guide the patient through a protective, comprehensive program with a particular focus on postsurgical factors within the rehabilitation process that appropriately stresses healing tissue, restores elbow ROM, enhances strength and endurance of the upper extremity musculature, and promotes a gradual return to sport based on interval sporting programs incorporating the entire kinetic chain. The collaborative efforts of the physician and the rehabilitation specialist are essential in the management and successful postoperative recovery.

BIBLIOGRAPHY

Bernas GA, Ruberte Thiele RA, Kinnaman KA, Hughes RE, Miller BS, Carpenter JE: Defining safe rehabilitation for ulnar collateral ligament reconstruction of the elbow: a biomechanical study. *Am J Sports Med* 2009;37(12):2392–2400.

Cain EL Jr, Andrews JR, Dugas JR, et al: Outcome of ulnar collateral ligament reconstruction of the elbow in 1281 athletes: Results in 743 athletes with minimum 2-year follow-up. *Am J Sports Med* 2010;38:2426–2434.

Dugas JR, Bilotta J, Watts CD, et al: Ulnar collateral ligament reconstruction with gracilis tendon in athletes with intraligamentous bony excision: technique and results. *Am J Sports Med* 2012;40:1578–1582.

Fleiseg GS, Escamilla RF: Biomechanics of the elbow in the throwing athlete. *Oper Tech Sports Med* 1996;4(2):62–68.

Makhni EC, Lee RW, Morrow ZS, Gualtieri AP, Gorroochurn P, Ahmad CS: Performance, Return to competition, and reinjury after Tommy John surgery in major league baseball players. A review of 147 cases. *Am J Sports Med* 2014;42(6): 1323–1332.

Osbahr DC, Dines JS, Rosenbaum AJ, Nguyen JT, Altchek DW: Does posteromedial chondromalacia reduce rate of return to play after ulnar collateral ligament reconstruction? *Clin Orthop Relat Res* 2012;470:1558–1564.

Osbahr DC, Swaminathan SS, Allen AA, Dines JS, Coleman SH, Altchek DW: Combined flexor-pronator mass and ulnar collateral ligament injuries in the elbows of older baseball players. *Am J Sports Med* 2010;38:733–739.

Reinold MM, Wilk KE, Reed J, Crenshaw K, Andrews JR: Interval sport programs: guidelines for baseball, tennis, and golf. *J Orthop Sports Phys Ther* 2002;32(6):293–298.

Rettig AC, Sherrill C, Snead DS, Mendler JC, Mieling P: Nonoperative treatment of ulnar collateral ligament injuries in throwing athletes. *Am J Sports Med* 2001;29(1):15–17.

Thomas SJ, Swanik KA, Swanik CB, Kelly JD 4th: Internal rotation deficits affect scapular positioning in baseball players. *Clin Orthop Relat Res* 2010;468(6):1551–1557.

Vitale MA, Ahmad CS: The outcome of elbow ulnar collateral ligament reconstruction in overhead athletes: a systematic review. *Am J Sports Med* 2008;36:1193–1205.

Werner SL, Fleisig GS, Dillman CJ, Andrews JR: Biomechanics of the elbow during baseball pitching. *J Orthop Sports Phys Ther* 1993;17:274–278.

Wilk KE, Macrina LC, Arrigo C: Passive range of motion characteristics in the overhead baseball pitcher and their implications for rehabilitation. *Clin Orthop Relat Res* 2012;470(6): 1586–1594.

Wilk KE, Obma P, Simpson CD, Cain EL, Dugas JR, Andrews JR: Shoulder injuries in the overhead athlete. *J Orthop Sports Phys Ther* 2009;39(2):38–54.

Wilk KE, Yenchak AJ, Arrigo CA, Andrews JR: The advanced throwers ten exercise program: a new exercise series for enhanced dynamic shoulder control in the overhead athlete. *Phys Sportsmed* 2011;39(4):90–97.

© 2018 American Academy of Orthopaedic Surgeons

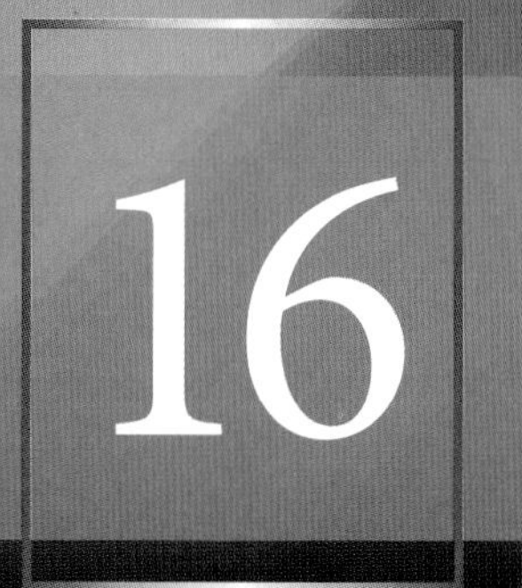

16 Elbow Rehabilitation After Lateral Collateral Ligament Reconstruction

Shannon R. Carpenter, MD, Vikram M. Sathyendra, MD, and Anand M. Murthi, MD

INTRODUCTION

The lateral ligament complex plays a critical role in stability of the elbow. All elbow dislocations and many elbow fracture dislocations include injury of the lateral ligament complex.

An incompetent lateral collateral ligament (LCL) complex may cause recurrent dislocations or posterior lateral rotatory instability (PLRI), the latter more commonly than the former. In addition, iatrogenic lateral ligament insufficiency is an uncommon complication of surgical treatment of lateral epicondylitis. Repair of the lateral capsule and ligamentous complex is recommended for adolescents and adults with symptomatic recurrent dislocation of the elbow to restore elbow stability and function.

RELEVANT ANATOMY

The LCL complex includes four components (Figure 16.1). The LCL originates from the lateral epicondyle of the humerus and attaches to the annular ligament. The lateral ulnar collateral ligament (LUCL) originates from the isometric point on the lateral epicondyle and attaches to the supinator crest on the ulna. The annular ligament originates from and inserts onto the anterior and posterior aspects of a sigmoid notch, respectively, and encircles the radial neck. The accessory LCL originates from the annular ligament and attaches onto the supinator crest of the ulna. The function of the LCL complex is to resist rotatory instability of the elbow. PLRI can occur after a simple elbow dislocation when the posterolateral capsular and ligamentous structures fail to reattach or from chronic attenuation of the LCL complex after multiple injuries. Incompetence of the lateral complex allows the forearm to rotate and translate in supination and posteriorly away from the distal humerus.

PATIENT EVALUATION

Patients with PLRI often have a history consistent with an ulnohumeral dislocation. In the acute injury setting, a thorough physical exam should be conducted, including neurovascular exam and range of motion (ROM) of the affected extremity. To perform a reduction of the elbow joint, an axial compressive and valgus force are applied to the elbow with the forearm in full supination. As the elbow is slowly brought from an extended position into a flexed position, the ulnohumeral joint would reduce from a subluxed or dislocated position. In the chronic setting, patients with PLRI present either later after a traumatic injury or after surgery with symptoms that range from mild mechanical clicking or vague elbow pain to frank subluxation or dislocation. Diagnosis of subtle PLRI can be very challenging, and because of guarding, it can be difficult to perform an adequate physical examination in the clinic on an awake patient. Examination under anesthesia with fluoroscopic imaging may be required to make a definitive diagnosis.

Two tests, in particular, are most helpful: the supine rotatory instability test (or pivot shift test) and the drawer test. In order to perform the supine lateral pivot shift test, the patient is placed supine on the examination table with the elbow in approximately 30° of flexion and full supination. This position causes the elbow to subluxate. The examiner then applies a valgus load to the elbow while continuing to flex the elbow fully. As this occurs, the subluxed radial head can be palpated as it relocates. A clunk may be elicited. This test may also be performed with the patient in the prone position. Patient

Dr. Murthi or an immediate family member has received royalties from Integra Orthopaedics; serves as a paid consultant to Arthrex, Integra Orthopaedics, and Zimmer; has received nonincome support (such as equipment or services), commercially derived honoraria, or other non-research–related funding (such as paid travel) from Current Opinion in Orthopaedics *and the* Journal of Bone and Joint Surgery–American; *and serves as a board member, owner, officer, or committee member of the American Academy of Orthopaedic Surgeons, the American Shoulder and Elbow Surgeons,* Current Orthopaedic Practice, *the* Journal of Bone and Joint Surgery–American, *and the* Journal of Shoulder and Elbow Surgery. *Neither Dr. Sathyendra nor any immediate family member has received anything of value from or has stock or stock options held in a commercial company or institution related directly or indirectly to the subject of this article.*

© 2018 American Academy of Orthopaedic Surgeons

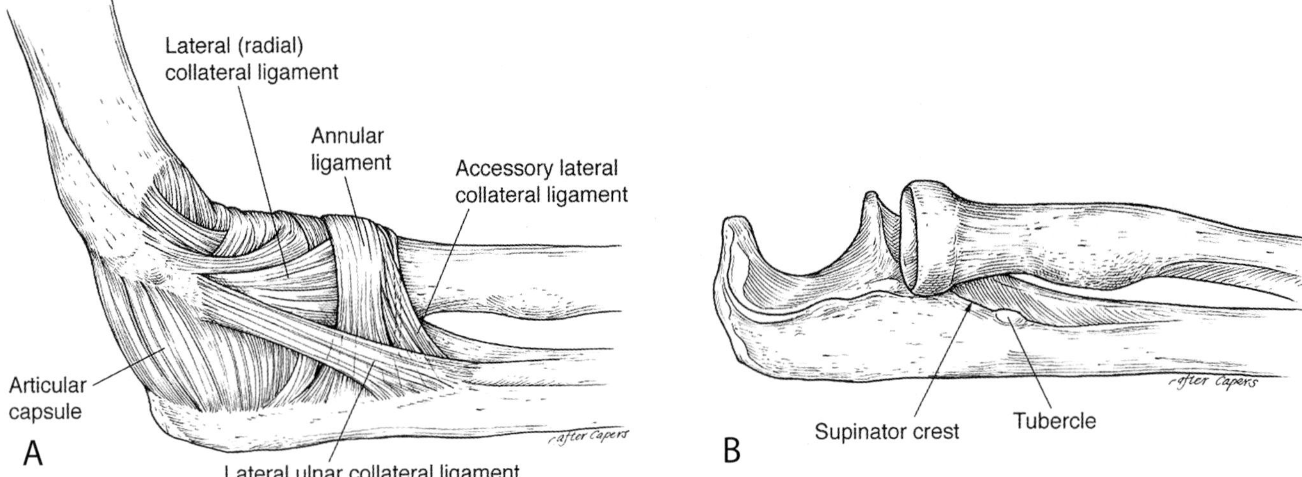

Figure 16.1 **A**, Illustration demonstrating the bony and ligamentous anatomy of the lateral elbow. **B**, Illustration of the bony anatomy of the lateral ulna and radius with the lateral collateral ligament complex stripped off. (**A** reproduced with permission from Mehta JA, Bain GI: Posterolateral rotatory instability of the elbow. *J Am Acad Orthop Surg* 2004;12:405–415. **B** adapted with permission from Bain GI, Mehta JA: Anatomy of the elbow joint and surgical approaches, in Baker CL Jr, Plancher KD [eds]: *Operative Treatment of Elbow Injuries.* New York, NY, Springer-Verlag, 2001, pp 1–27.)

guarding can make it difficult to elicit the diagnosis from this examination. The drawer sign can also be used to make the diagnosis of PLRI. With the patient supine on the table, the affected arm is brought over the patient's head, with the forearm fully supinated. The examiner then places the index finger posterior to the radial head and the thumb anterior. The examiner attempts to translate the radius posteriorly. The sign is considered positive if the radial head is felt to subluxate, in which case PLRI is likely present.

In addition, patients with PLRI can report pain and difficulty while rising from a chair using their arms or trying to perform push-ups. A chair push-up test may be performed in which patients are asked to push themselves up from a chair with the forearm in supination. The test is positive if there is pain with resisted elbow extension, which may be indicative of PLRI.

SURGICAL PROCEDURE

Indications

The indications for surgery include elbow pain, functional limitation, and instability. In the setting of chronic instability of the elbow in adolescents and adults, nonoperative treatment is attempted. Typically, in either acute or chronic dislocations, the lateral ligamentous complex is repaired first, then the MCL is examined for instability. In the absence of gross medial instability, the MCL is not repaired, even in complex elbow fractures such as a terrible triad.

Contraindications

The contraindications to LCL reconstruction include children with open physes and generalized ligamentous laxity. As children age, the capsule and ligaments around the elbow tend to become stiffer, and dislocations become less frequent and eventually stop occurring. When posterolateral rotatory instability occurs in children, the LUCL can be imbricated rather than formally reconstructed. Elbow arthritis is also a relative contraindication to LUCL reconstruction.

Procedure: Open Repair

The patient is given general anesthesia and a tourniquet is applied to the upper extremity. A lateral pivot shift test is performed to confirm posterolateral rotatory instability of the elbow joint. Next, a modified Kocher approach is made between the extensor carpi ulnaris and the anconeus muscles (Figure 16.2, A and B). In acute injuries, there is often a disruption of the extensor muscle and overlying fascia. This rent in the fascia and muscle can be extended proximally and distally. We extend it proximally to the lateral epicondyle. Once the lateral epicondyle is identified, the common extensor origin is elevated and the proximal stump of the LUCL is identified (Figure 16.2, C). The LCL complex typically avulses off of the humeral insertion, but can also avulse off of the ulna. The hematoma is removed and the forearm is pronated to reduce the ulnohumeral joint and, concomitantly, the radiocapitellar joint. Next, the isometric point of the elbow at the lateral epicondyle is identified and a suture anchor or transosseous drill holes are placed at the isometric point. A locking stitch is placed into the LUCL stump and reattached to the lateral epicondyle. The common extensor origin is also repaired to the lateral epicondyle. In the acute setting, associated bony injury that may contribute to instability must also be addressed and appropriately fixed and repaired.

Procedure: Open Reconstruction

The LUCL is reconstructed using tissue grafts fixed to the ulna and the isometric point of the lateral elbow (Figure 16.3). The

 © 2018 American Academy of Orthopaedic Surgeons

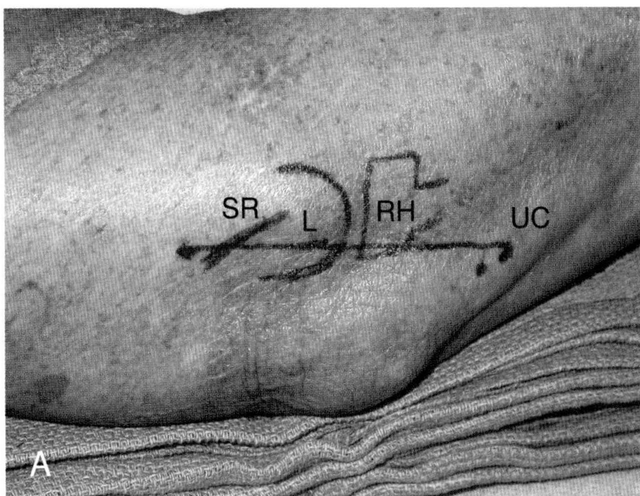

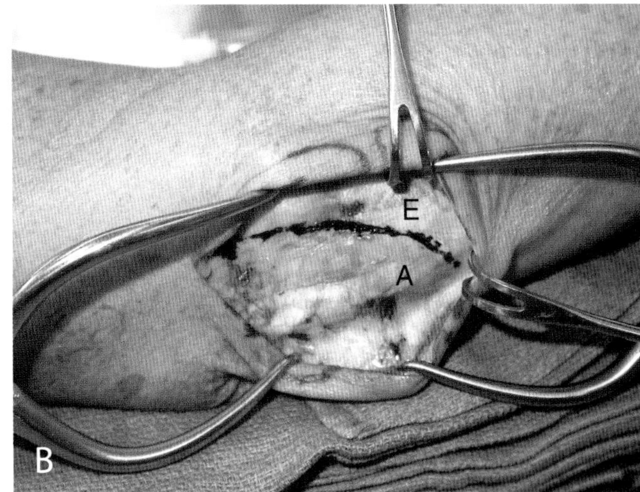

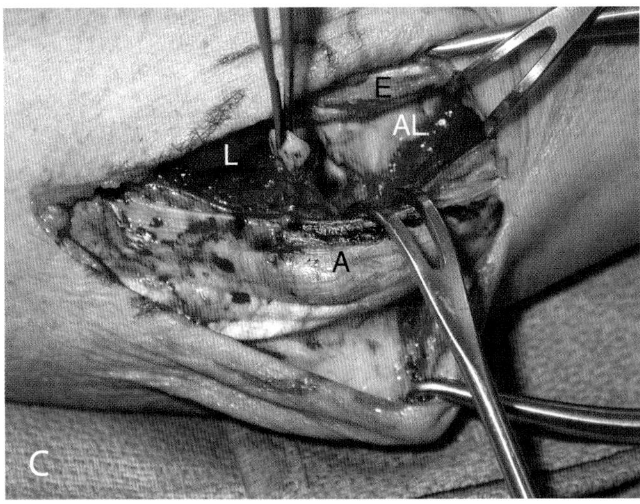

Figure 16.2 Standard Kocher approach to the elbow. **A**, Clinical photograph showing landmarks and incision. **B**, Clinical photograph showing interval between the anconeus (A) and extensor carpi ulnaris (E); supracondylar ridge (SR), lateral epicondyle (L), radial head (RH), ulnar crest (UC). **C**, This clinical photograph shows that after opening the interval, the torn LCL (L) and the annular ligament (AL) can be visualized.

set-up and approach for open reconstruction of the LUCL is very similar to that described earlier for the open-repair technique. A modified Kocher approach is used. The common extensors are reflected anteriorly and the anconeus is reflected posteriorly, revealing the disrupted and/or deficient ligaments. Both the lateral epicondyle and the supinator crest are exposed. A pivot shift test will reveal laxity of the capsule over the radiocapitellar joint. The joint is examined for any loose bodies or articular cartilage damage. If the ligament is lax but the tissue is of good quality, then both the radial and the ulnar portions of the LCL are imbricated. The anterior and posterior capsule surrounding the radiocapitellar joint is also imbricated. In cases of deficient or poor-quality tissue, a graft is used to reconstruct the ligament. A variety of grafts can be used. Most commonly, a palmaris longus autograft from the involved forearm is used. However, if the patient does not have a palmaris longus, a gracilis tendon autograft of allograft can be used.

The distal attachment site is prepared with two drill holes in the ulna. The first is drilled near the supinator crest and the second is approximately 1.25 cm proximal to that, near the insertion of the annular ligament. The drill holes are connected, being very careful to maintain the cortical bridge. The isometric insertion point on the lateral epicondyle is identified by passing a suture through the ulnar tunnels. The tails of the suture can then be held against the lateral epicondyle as the elbow is ranged through a flexion arc to find and mark the isometric point (Figure 16.4). A drill hole is made at the isometric point on the lateral epicondyle, and two additional drill holes, one anterior and one posterior on the supracondylar ridge, that connect to the isometric hole are made proximally on the lateral condyle. A bone bridge of at least 1 cm should be left intact between the two proximal holes. The tendon graft is placed through the ulnar tunnels. Next, the graft is passed through the isometric hole bony tunnel and fixed onto the isometric point (Figure 16.5). The suture tails are brought out through the two proximal holes in the humerus. The graft is tensioned with the forearm fully pronated and a valgus load applied to the elbow. Sutures are tied over the proximal bone bridge with the elbow flexed at 30° and the forearm in full pronation. The extensor carpi ulnaris–anconeus interval is closed with nonabsorbable sutures.

© 2018 American Academy of Orthopaedic Surgeons

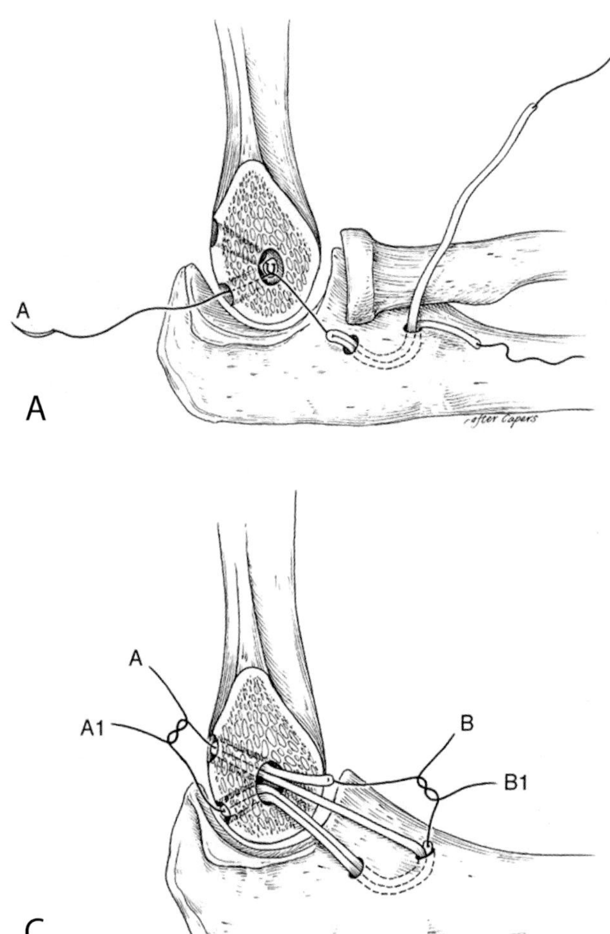

Figure 16.3 Illustration demonstrating reconstruction of the lateral collateral ligament using the open docking technique. **A**, The graft is passed through a tunnel created at the crista supinatoris. **B**, The posterior limb is passed through the isometric point at the lateral epicondyle. **C**, The anterior limb is passed through the isometric point and both limbs are tied together; then, the anterior limb is looped onto and tied to itself. (Reproduced with permission from Mehta JA, Bain GI: Posterolateral rotatory instability of the elbow. *J Am Acad Orthop Surg* 2004;12:405–415.)

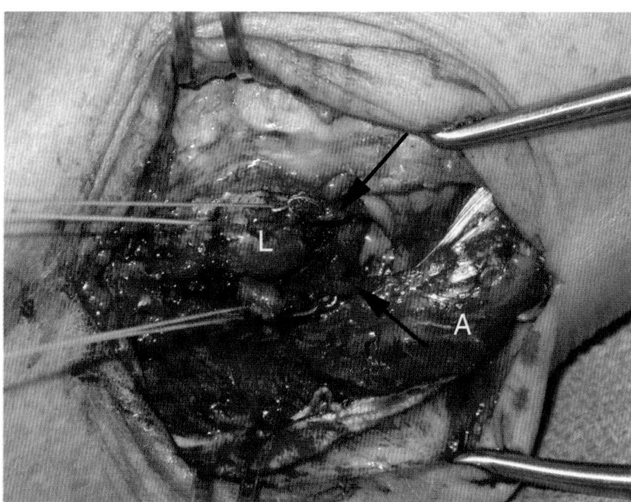

Figure 16.4 Photograph demonstrating the isometric point of the lateral elbow. Two arrows represent the limbs of the graft. (A) anconeus; (L) lateral epicondyle.

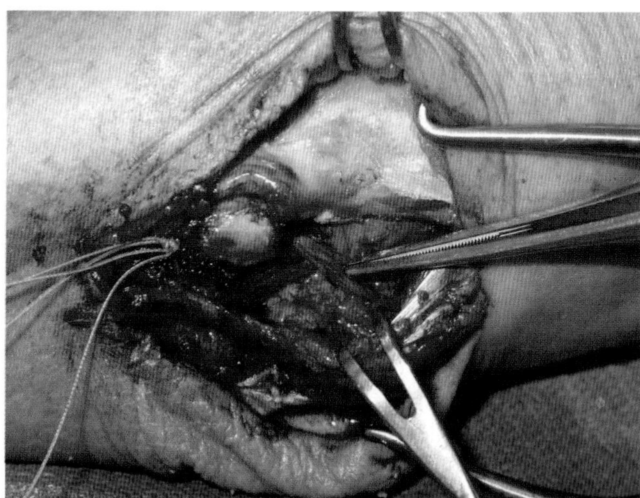

Figure 16.5 Photograph demonstrating fixation of the graft. The straight hemostat is pointing to the graft.

 © 2018 American Academy of Orthopaedic Surgeons

Procedure: Arthroscopic Repair and Reconstruction

The patient is positioned lateral on a beanbag with the use of an arm holder. A tourniquet is applied to the upper arm. Standard arthroscopic portals are used. Viewing from the anteromedial portal, we are able to identify subluxation of the radial head during the pivot shift maneuver. Viewing from the posterolateral portal, we are able to easily drive the arthroscope through the lateral gutter because of the laxity of the LUCL. This laxity can be treated with arthroscopic plication of the LUCL.

Plication is accomplished by placing six to seven sutures along the radial aspect of the ulna traveling proximally to the radial aspect of the humerus. Sutures are introduced into the elbow joint using a spinal needle, then are retrieved proximally using a retrograde retriever. During suture retrieval, one must be careful to position the retriever posterior along the lateral epicondyle to avoid injury to the radial nerve. Once sutures are retrieved, they are tied either superficial or deep to the anconeus tendon. These sutures are tied blindly arthroscopically through the medial portal and the tissue is monitored for imbrication. As sutures are tied from distal to proximal, the drive-through sign, in which the arthroscope can easily be moved from the posterolateral gutter through the ulnohumeral articulation into the medial gutter, will disappear. If there is any remaining residual laxity or an avulsion of the LUCL from the lateral epicondyle, this can be repaired using a suture anchor placed in the isometric point of the lateral epicondyle.

PITFALLS AND COMPLICATIONS

The main complications after ligament reconstruction of the elbow are persistent instability and stiffness. It is important to have clear communication between the surgeon and the physical therapist in terms of how much ROM is expected during the early phases of rehabilitation after surgery. Rehabilitation should establish a balance between protecting the ligament repair and establishing early ROM to prevent stiffness. In general, patient outcomes are similar with ligament repair, ligament reconstruction, or arthroscopic techniques. It is difficult to regain full ROM of the elbow after acute traumatic injuries, regardless of the technique used for treatment.

POSTOPERATIVE REHABILITATION

Communication between the treating surgeon and the therapist is critically important in the rehabilitation of the elbow after LUCL reconstruction or repair. The initial goal is to control pain and swelling while at the same time starting early active motion. Rehabilitation is progressed through stages that respect the healing of the repair and reconstruction in order to avoid injury. Icing, compression sleeves, and elevation of the extremity will help with edema and pain control. In addition, judicious use of narcotic as well as nonnarcotic pain relievers will help with pain control. For postoperative stiffness, a gentle passive stretching protocol should be utilized provided that it does not compromise the repair or reconstruction. Later, during rehabilitation, heat packs and whirlpools can help precondition tissues prior to stretching.

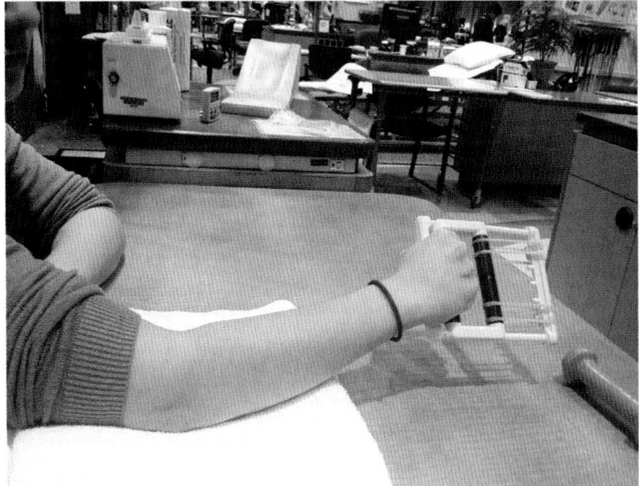

Figure 16.6 Photograph of patient demonstrating hand isometric exercises.

Patients are initially protected with a posterior elbow splint for 1 to 2 weeks. The elbow is flexed 90° and the forearm is usually kept in a pronated position to protect the repair. Pronation tensions the posterolateral soft tissues and helps to maintain the reduction of the radius and ulna on the distal humerus. Supination rotates the radius and ulna and relaxes the lateral soft tissues, which may lead to subluxation.

Initially, patients are immobilized for the first 3 weeks and are allowed to perform wrist and hand motion exercises as well as light gripping. The splint can be a removable thermoplastic splint or a commercial hinged brace that maintains the elbow at 90° of flexion and forearm pronation. Wrist and hand isometrics can be performed as tolerated, and shoulder active and passive ROM can be performed if necessary (Figure 16.6). We are careful to avoid shoulder abduction because this causes a varus moment at the elbow and can compromise the repair or reconstruction.

Subsequently, a hinged elbow brace is used to prevent varus and valgus forces and to allow protected elbow motion. During phase 2, elbow ROM is gradually increased and isometric strengthening of the flexor pronator muscle group is initiated. Flexor pronator isometric strengthening is incorporated to provide dynamic stability. Patients are usually kept in a hinged elbow brace, with limits set by the surgeon (Figure 16.7). Active assisted ROM of the elbow and active ROM of the elbow between 20° and 120° of flexion is permitted with the forearm kept in pronation to protect the lateral ligament repair or reconstruction (Figure 16.8, A and B). Forearm pronation tensions the common extensor group and reduces the stresses placed on the LCL complex repair, helping to maintain the reduction of the ulnohumeral joint. Shoulder, wrist, and hand exercises are continued as in phase 1. At this point, edema and swelling are usually less of a concern. Pain control is usually

© 2018 American Academy of Orthopaedic Surgeons

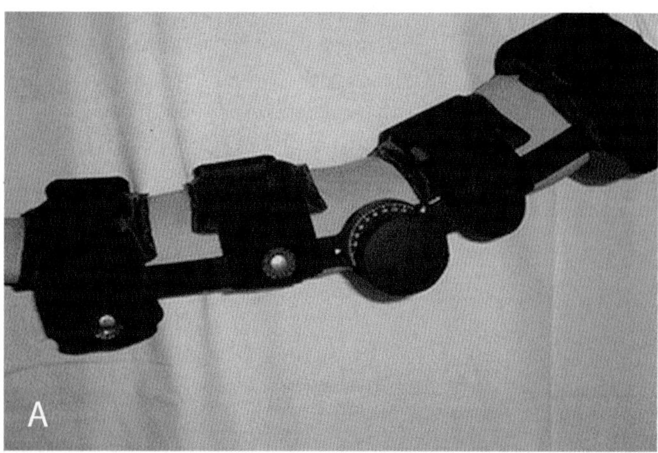

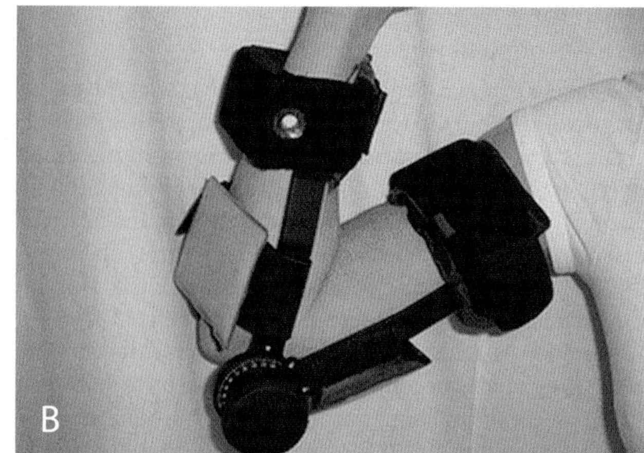

Figure 16.7 Photograph of patient demonstrating (**A**) elbow extension and (**B**) flexion ROM in a hinged elbow brace. (Reproduced with permission from Morrey BF: *Master Techniques in Orthopaedic Surgery: The Elbow,* ed. 3. Philadelphia, PA, Lippincott Williams & Williams, 2015.)

accomplished with a combination of narcotic and nonnarcotic pain medications. Wrist extensor strengthening is not permitted during the first 6 weeks after surgery.

Bracing and immobilization are discontinued after 6 weeks. Passive ROM and active assisted ROM of the elbow are continued to obtain full motion. The main goals during phase 3 include establishing full ROM of the elbow and strengthening of the wrist flexors and forearm pronators on the medial elbow forearm as well as the wrist extensors on the lateral side to provide dynamic stability. At the same time point, unrestricted strengthening of the flexors, pronators, and extensors and supination is allowed to tolerance. Elbow flexion and extension strengthening is also performed at this stage. Care must be taken to avoid shoulder abduction, which may place undue varus stress on the elbow and therefore stress the LCL complex. After 3 months, patients continue to work on strengthening and terminal elbow stretching, avoiding any varus stress to the elbow until 6 months postoperatively.

Stiffness is a major problem after lateral elbow ligament reconstruction. At this stage, heat packs and whirlpool massages may help precondition tissues before starting gentle passive stretching of the elbow. A nighttime elbow extension splint may be worn to help prevent flexion contracture of the elbow. If stiffness persists beyond 3 months, a static progressive stretching or dynamic brace can be used.

Beyond 3 months after surgery, progressive strengthening is continued. If ROM has been achieved, the focus of rehabilitation can shift to functional restoration. Heavier and more demanding activities, as well as activities that apply substantial varus stress to the elbow, are avoided for the first 6 months after surgery.

AUTHOR'S PREFERRED PROTOCOL

Phase 1: 0 to 3 Weeks

Allow elbow soft tissues to heal while maintaining motion in shoulder and wrist.

- Skin staples or sutures are removed at week 1.
- Compression sleeve to control edema and swelling.

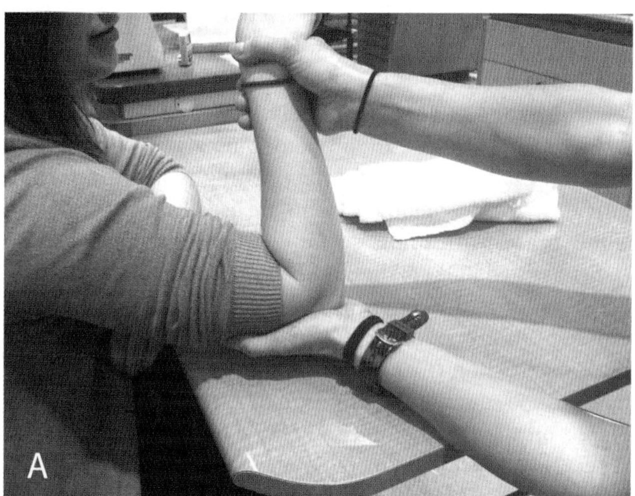

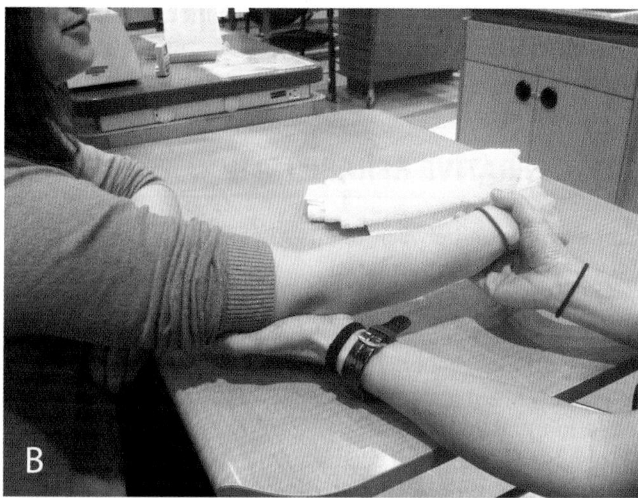

Figure 16.8 Photograph of patient performing elbow (**A**) flexion and (**B**) extension ROM exercises with the forearm in pronation.

© 2018 American Academy of Orthopaedic Surgeons

- Ice/cryotherapy.
- Elbow immobilization in posterior splint/brace.
- Wrist and hand isometrics as tolerated.
- Shoulder active and passive ROM (if necessary).
- Avoid varus elbow stress.

Phase 2: 4 to 6 Weeks

Start elbow motion, flexor pronator and wrist strengthening.

- Hinged elbow brace, with limits set by surgeon from 20° to 120°.
- Begin flexor/pronator isometrics.
- Continue with wrist/hand strengthening.
- Continue shoulder motion as above.
- Active assisted ROM elbow 20° to 120° of flexion, keeping forearm pronated at all times.

Phase 3: 6 to 12 Weeks

Regain full elbow ROM, strengthen forearm muscles.

- Discontinue immobilization.
- Passive ROM and active assisted elbow ROM to full motion.
- Begin unrestricted strengthening of flexors/pronators/extensors of forearm.
- Begin supination ROM to tolerance.

Phase 4: 3 to 6 Months

- Regain full strength in elbow, strengthen shoulder.
- Avoid varus stress to elbow and ballistic movement in terminal elbow ranges.
- Begin shoulder strengthening with light resistance (emphasis on rotator cuff).
- Start total body conditioning.
- Terminal elbow stretching in flexion and extension.
- Resistive elbow flexion and extension exercises as tolerated.

OUTCOMES

Overall, there are few large studies that evaluate the surgical outcomes of lateral elbow instability repair and reconstruction. Of those that are available, the results of lateral ligament surgery have shown good to excellent outcome scores with few complications.

The classic original article by O'Driscoll et al. in 1991 followed five patients, two who underwent a repair and three who underwent reconstruction with autograft. The patients were followed for 15 to 30 months and had full ROM with no recurrent episodes of instability or apprehension. Sanchez-Sotelo et al. subsequently reported the results of treatment of 44 patients with PLRI. A total of 86% of the patients were subjectively satisfied with their repairs; overall, the reconstruction patients did better than the repair patients.

A recent systematic review of eight studies that included a total of 130 patients who underwent surgery for posterolateral rotatory instability reported that among patients with reported Mayo elbow performance score and mean follow-up of 44.5 months, 91% had good or excellent results and improvement in ROM. Recurrent instability was noted in 8% of the 130 patients.

PEARLS

1. Posterolateral rotatory instability is relatively uncommon and difficult to diagnose.
2. Lateral pivot shift maneuver can confirm the diagnosis.
3. Surgical treatment of acute traumatic injury usually involves primary repair of the lateral ligament complex.
4. Surgical reconstruction is performed with tendon graft in chronic cases. Ensure appropriate graft tension.
5. Early phases of rehabilitation protect the ligament repair or reconstruction while initiating recovery of ROM.
6. Initiate elbow motion exercises with forearm pronated.
7. Avoid varus elbow stress. Shoulder abduction should be avoided during the first 3 months.
8. Mid-to-late phases of rehabilitation restore full elbow ROM and strengthen elbow extensors, flexors, and pronators.

CONCLUSION

The lateral ligament complex plays a critical role in elbow stability and is frequently injured in an elbow dislocation. The diagnosis of chronic lateral elbow instability can be very difficult. Acute lateral ligament insufficiency can be treated with open or arthroscopic repair, whereas a chronic injury usually requires ligament reconstruction. Rehabilitation after repair or reconstruction focuses on avoiding varus stress to the elbow for the first 3 months because it may compromise the surgical outcome. Typically, surgical outcomes for lateral ligament repair or reconstruction are favorable; most patients see functional improvement in pain, ROM, and elbow stability.

BIBLIOGRAPHY

Anakwenze OA, Kwon D, O'Donnell E, Levine WN, Ahmad CS: Surgical treatment of posterolateral rotatory instability of the elbow. *Arthrosc—J Arthrosc Relat Surg* 2014;30(7):866–71.

Clitherow HDS, McGuire DT, Bain, GI: Lateral elbow instability. *Sports Med Arthrosc Rehabil Ther Technol* 2014;1:11–18.

Fedorka CJ, Oh LS: Posterolateral rotatory instability of the elbow. *Curr Rev Musculoskelet Med* 2016;9:240–246.

Josefsson PO, Gentz CF, Johnell O, Wendeberg B: Surgical versus non-surgical treatment of ligamentous injuries following dislocation of the elbow joint. A prospective randomized study. *J Bone Joint Surg Am* 1987;69(4):605–608.

Mehta JA, Bain GI: Posterolateral rotatory instability of the elbow. *J Am Acad Orthop Surg* 2004;12(6):405–415.

Nestor BJ, O'Driscoll SW, Morrey BF: Ligamentous reconstruction for posterolateral rotatory instability of the elbow. *J Bone Joint Surg Am* 1992 Sep;74(8):1235–1241.

O'Driscoll SW, Bell DF, Morrey BF. Posterolateral rotatory instability of the elbow. *J Bone Joint Surg Am* 1991 Mar;73(3):440–446.

© 2018 American Academy of Orthopaedic Surgeons

Osborne G, Cotterill P: Recurrent dislocation of the elbow. *J Bone Joint Surg Br* 1966;48(2):340–346.

Safran MR, Baillargeon D: Soft-tissue stabilizers of the elbow. *J Shoulder Elbow Surg* 2005;14(1 Suppl S):179S–185S.

Sanchez-Sotelo J, Morrey BF, O'Driscoll SW: Ligamentous repair and reconstruction for posterolateral rotatory instability of the elbow. *J Bone Joint Surg Br* 2005;87-B:54–61.

Savoie FH, 3rd, Field LD, Gurley DJ: Arthroscopic and open radial ulnohumeral ligament reconstruction for posterolateral rotatory instability of the elbow. *Hand Clin.* 2009;25(3):323–329.

Savoie FH, 3rd, O'Brien MJ, Field LD, Gurley DJ: Arthroscopic and open radial ulnohumeral ligament reconstruction for posterolateral rotatory instability of the elbow. *Clin Sports Med* Oct;29(4):611–618.

Smith JP, 3rd, Savoie FH, 3rd, Field LD: Posterolateral rotatory instability of the elbow. *Clin Sports Med* 2001;20(1):47–58.

Stein JA, Murthi AM: Posterolateral rotatory instability of the elbow: our approach. *Oper Tech Orthop* 2009;19(4): 251–257.

Szekeres M, Chinchalkar SJ, King GJ: Optimizing elbow rehabilitation after instability. *Hand Clin* 2008;24(1):27–38.

Wolff AL, Hotchkiss RN: Lateral elbow instability: nonoperative, operative, and postoperative management. *J Hand Ther* 2006; 19(2):238–243.

© 2018 American Academy of Orthopaedic Surgeons

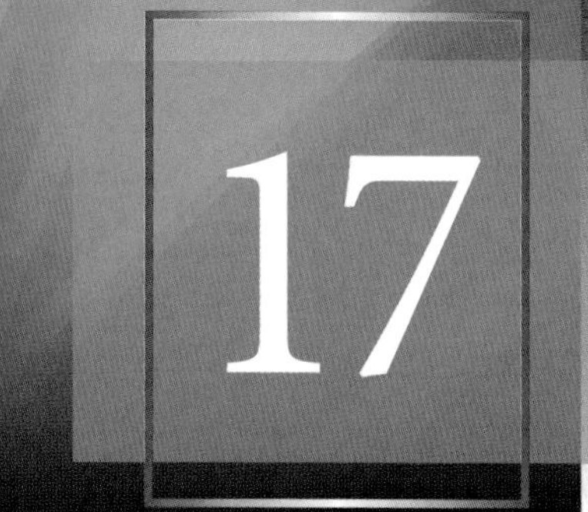

17 Rehabilitation Following Distal Biceps Tendon Repair

Jay D. Keener, MD

INTRODUCTION

The majority of distal biceps tendon injuries are treated operatively. The goal of surgery is to obtain successful tendon healing, thus maximizing the return of full elbow and forearm strength and function. A successful result is dependent not only on anatomic repair of the tendon but also on a comprehensive postoperative rehabilitation protocol and a compliant patient. Rehabilitation stages and return to activity timeline follow a progression based on the known stages of tendon healing. Recently, advances in surgical technique have provided improved tendon fixation strength in a minimally invasive fashion, and now permit earlier rehabilitation. This chapter will review the stages and principles of rehabilitation following distal biceps tendon repair.

SURGICAL PROCEDURE: DISTAL BICEPS TENDON REPAIR

Indications/Contraindications

Distal biceps tendon injuries are most common in middle-aged men and usually occur in the dominant arm as the result of a forceful eccentric load applied against active elbow flexion and forearm supination. Most injuries involve complete disruption of the tendon insertion, producing an obvious clinical deformity of the biceps muscle. Acute tears are usually accompanied by ecchymosis in the antecubital fossa and proximal volar forearm. Partial tendon injuries are less common but have a high failure rate with nonoperative treatment; therefore, they are often treated surgically. The primary goal of surgery is to maximize the return of elbow and forearm strength and function in contrast to the outcome of nonoperative treatment, which often results in normal range of motion (ROM) and resolution of pain. Injuries treated without surgery result in elbow flexion strength loss of 20% to 30% and forearm supination strength loss of 30% to 50%.

The optimal indication for surgery is acute injuries, defined as less than 4 to 6 weeks, in active patients medically fit for surgery. Delayed surgical repair is more difficult due to fixed retraction of the biceps tendon and shortening of the muscle. However, primary fixation can sometimes be performed in a delayed fashion if tendon and muscle retraction are minimized by attachment of an intact lacertus fibrosis. If a primary repair of a retracted tendon can be performed with the elbow at 90° of flexion, full ROM and good function can be reliably obtained. Delayed reconstruction often requires an interposition tendon graft. Partial distal biceps tendon injuries are treated with surgical repair after failure of conservative treatment for a period of 3 months.

Contraindications for surgery include low-demand patients, chronic tendon ruptures (>6 months) and patients with medical illnesses precluding surgery. Potential noncompliance must be factored into the decision-making process as well.

Surgical Technique

Distal biceps tendon repair is performed by reattachment of the tendon into the radial tuberosity of the radius. The surgery can be performed either through a single-incision (transverse or longitudinal) anterior approach or a dual-incision anterior and posterior approach. Care should be taken to reattach the tendon to the apex of the radial tuberosity, thus recreating the anatomic insertion and maximizing the supination function of the biceps muscle (Figure 17.1). Fixation of the tendon can be performed in a variety of ways, including the use of sutures through bone tunnels, suture anchors into bone, cortical button fixation, or tenodesis screw fixation into a bone tunnel (Figure 17.2). Current methods of fixation provide ample fixation strength to allow early passive and active ROM of the forearm and elbow. In some cases, the fixation strength rivals or exceeds the native strength of the biceps tendon.

Single-incision repairs are performed between muscular planes without violation of muscle or tendon tissue. Dissection is performed between the flexor/pronator mass and the brachioradialis muscle. Care is taken to protect the lateral antebrachial

Dr. Keener or an immediate family member has received royalties from Genesis, Shoulder Innovations; serves as a paid consultant to Arthrex; has received research or institutional support from the National Institutes of Health (NIAMS and NICHD) and Zimmer; and serves as a board member, owner, officer, or committee member of the Journal of Shoulder and Elbow Surgery.

© 2018 American Academy of Orthopaedic Surgeons

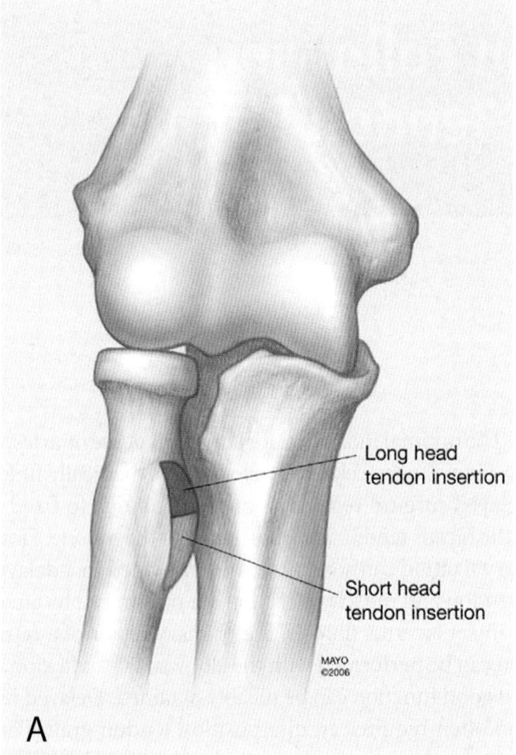

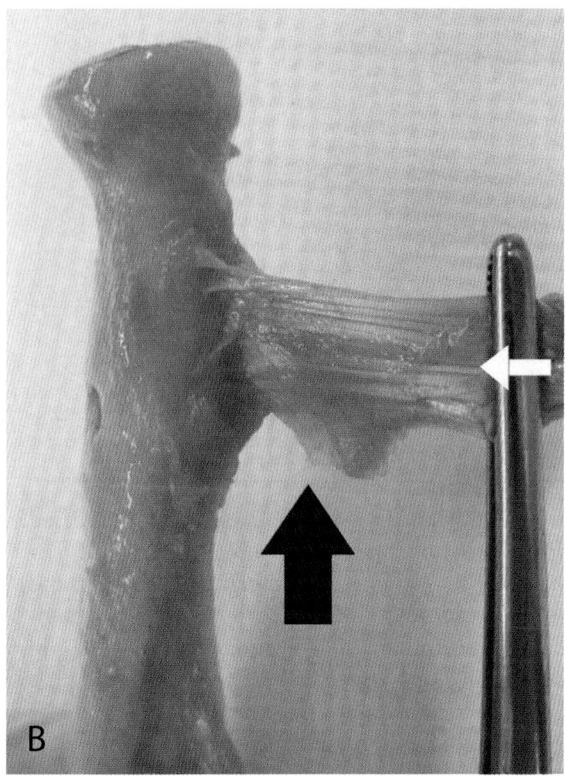

Figure 17.1 Biceps tendon insertion. **A**, Illustration of the long- and short-head biceps tendon insertions on the bicipital tuberosity. The mean average cadaver footprint area of the long head of the tendon is 48 mm^2 and of the short head of the tendon, 60 mm^2. **B**, Clinical photograph of a cadaver specimen demonstrates the separation between the short and long heads of the distal tendons (*white arrow*). *Black arrow* points to the short head of the biceps tendon. (**A** reproduced with permission from the Mayo Foundation of Medical Education and Research, Rochester, MN. **B** reproduced with permission from Athwal GS, Steinmann SP, Rispoli DM: The distal biceps tendon: Footprint and relevant clinical anatomy. *J Hand Surg Am* 2007;32:1225–1229.)

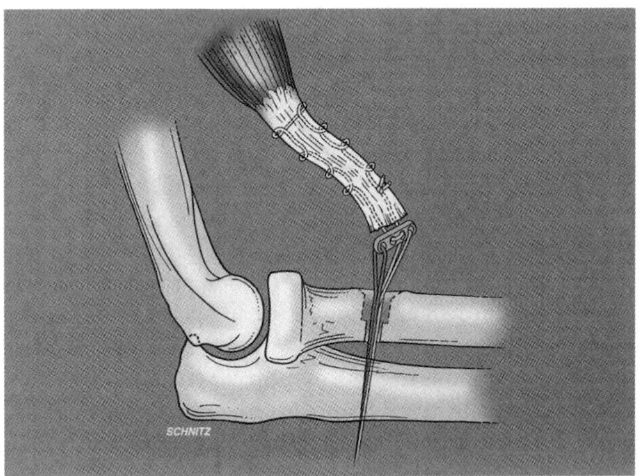

Figure 17.2 Illustration of the "loaded" ENDOBUTTON complex ready for vertical passage through the proximal radius. This technique is one of many utilized to achieve fixation of the biceps into the radial tuberosity. (Reproduced with permission from Greenberg JA, Fernandez JJ, Wang T, Turner C: Endobutton-assisted repair of distal biceps tendon ruptures. *J Should Elbow Surg* 2003;12: 484–490.)

cutaneous nerve, which lies adjacent to the cephalic vein superficial to the muscle fascia and the superficial radial nerve, which lies under the leading edge of the brachioradialis muscle. Deep dissection requires identification and control of crossing blood vessels superficial and distal to the biceps sheath. Medial to the biceps sheath are the brachial artery and the median nerve, which must be protected. The inflamed biceps sheath is incised superficially, often revealing the torn biceps tendon resting on the brachialis fascia. When the biceps is retracted, dissection proximal is performed to identify and retrieve the biceps tendon. Digital palpation of the supinated forearm within the biceps sheath allows exposure of the radial tuberosity. Careful placement of retractors around the exposed radial tuberosity aids visualization; however, care is taken not to trap the posterior interosseous nerve, and retraction force should be minimized to prevent compression of the nerve.

Dual-incision repairs require an anterior approach to retrieve the biceps tendon and a posterior approach to expose the radial tuberosity. Once the biceps is retrieved and secured with a running locked suture, a curved hemostat is passed ulnar to the radial tuberosity (with the elbow flexed) and pushed forward through the common extensor tendon on the posterior aspect of the forearm (Figure 17.3). This helps

 © 2018 American Academy of Orthopaedic Surgeons

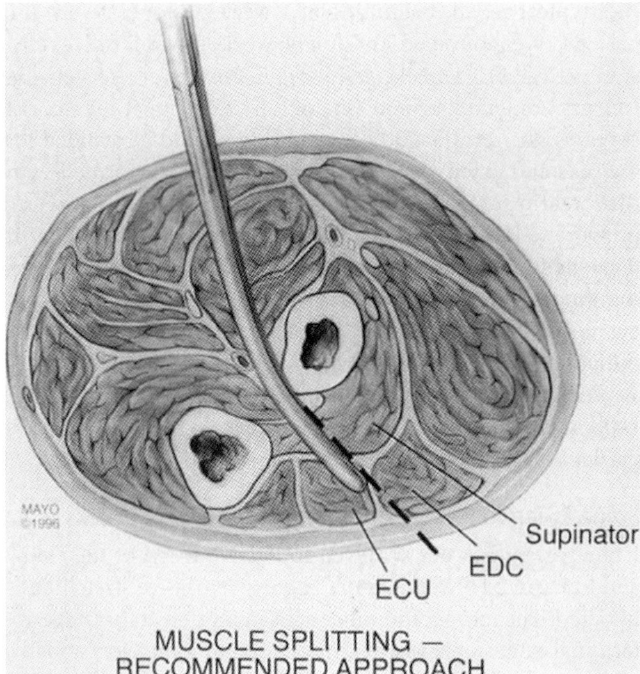

Figure 17.3 Diagram demonstrating the correct path for exposure of the radial tuberosity through a posterior incision. The preferred path utilizes a muscle-splitting approach through the extensor carpi ulnaris (ECU) and avoids exposure of the ulna. EDC – extensor digitorum communis. (Reproduced with permission from the Mayo Foundation for Medical Education and Research, Rochester, MN.)

to localize the posterior skin incision. The extensor tendons/muscle are split around the hemostat until the supinator muscle fibers are seen. Care is taken not to strip muscle tissue from the ulna to prevent heterotopic ossification. The supinator muscle is then split, with the forearm pronated to protect the posterior interosseous nerve and expose the radial tuberosity. The tuberosity is then prepared for tendon fixation, usually bone tunnels with a dual-incision approach.

Dual-incision repairs may lead to slightly increased early postoperative pain and stiffness compared to single-incision repairs. In addition, dual-incision repairs have historically been associated with higher rates of postoperative heterotopic bone formation and radioulnar synostosis, although these complications are much less common when the extensors are split and the ulna is not exposed. Both single- and dual-incision repairs have been associated with postoperative nerve palsies (10%–15% of cases). The most common nerves involved are the lateral antebrachial cutaneous nerve and, less commonly, the posterior interosseous nerve. Single-incision repairs may have a higher chance of nerve injuries given the retraction necessary to gain visualization of the radial tuberosity from the anterior approach.

In most instances, nerve injuries are transient and do not affect the final outcome. One recent series reported a 3.2% incidence of posterior interosseous nerve injury complicating a single-incision repair. All patients recovered nerve function, usually within 3 months of surgery.

POSTOPERATIVE REHABILITATION

Author's Preferred Protocol

Stage 1: Immediate Postoperative Period—Initial 7 Days

The elbow and forearm are typically splinted in a safe position dependent on the tension of the repair. Typically, the elbow is flexed 80° to 90° and the forearm is in neutral rotation or supinated if the repair is under tension. It is rarely necessary to splint the elbow in greater than 90° of flexion. A sling is used in the early postoperative period for additional support. Elevation of the extremity is recommended for the initial 72 hours. Finger motion is encouraged to decrease edema and stiffness. Ice is applied through the splint regularly for the first 72 hours and then as needed.

Stage 2: Subacute Period—1 to 6 Weeks

The goals of the initial stage of rehabilitation are to allow early elbow and forearm motion in a manner that protects the surgical repair. Conventional methods of tendon repair allow early, protected motion assuming adequate repair. At 1 week, a custom molded plastic splint is fashioned to splint the arm at 90° flexion and neutral forearm rotation (Figure 17.4), which is worn for 4 weeks. Alternatively, a hinged brace initially set with ROM from 30° to 120° with a sling strap can be used. The patient is instructed to remove the splint/brace 3 to 4 times per day to initiate gentle self-directed active assistive flexion and active or gravity-assisted extension ROM. Early active assisted forearm motion is critically important, given the intimate location of the proximal radius and ulna, to optimize recovery of forearm rotation motion and minimize the risk of synostosis formation.

- Elbow flexion active assistive motion is encouraged unrestricted as tolerated, with assist from the opposite extremity (Figure 17.5).
- Forearm rotation with the elbow flexed 90° is allowed unrestricted in both pronation and supination, as tolerated.

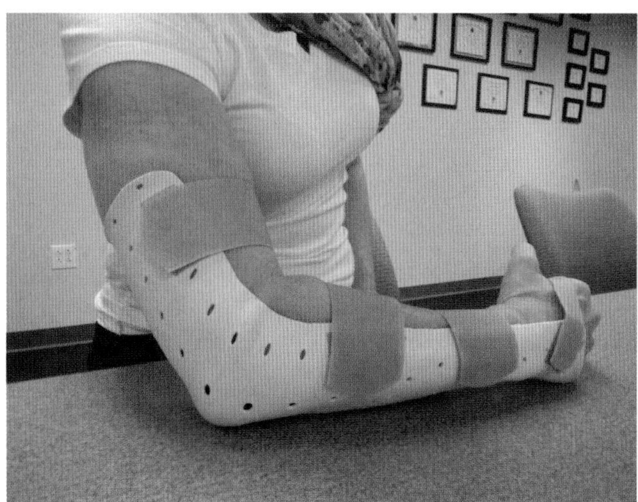

Figure 17.4 Photograph of custom-molded Orthoplast splint. Arm position is 80° to 90° of flexion and neutral forearm rotation.

© 2018 American Academy of Orthopaedic Surgeons

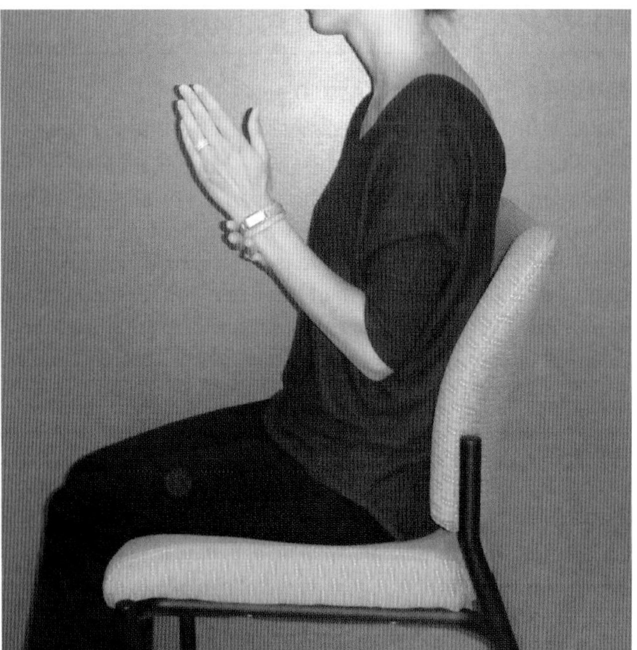

Figure 17.5 Photograph of active-assistive elbow flexion ROM. Forearm is in neutral rotation.

Assistance is provided by the opposite hand or a therapist or family member (Figure 17.6, A and B).

- Gravity-assisted elbow extension is permitted to a safe angle determined at the time of surgery (Figure 17.7, A). Repair tension can be minimized by stretching into elbow extension with the forearm in a supinated position.
- Gravity-assisted supine elbow extension stretching (Figure 17.7, B). Elbow muscles are relaxed and a static stretch is maintained for 3 to 4 minutes.

In a typical repair, beginning at 1 week postoperatively, the patient is encouraged to slowly work toward full extension within 3 to 4 weeks. With repairs under greater tension (repairs limited to 45°–60° shy of full extension at the time of surgery), the terminal 30° of extension should be avoided for 4 weeks and extension stretching should be performed with the forearm supinated during that time frame. After 4 weeks, unrestricted extension stretching is initiated. Even in the most tensioned repairs, it is unusual for a patient to develop a flexion contracture as long as early ROM is initiated. Physical/occupational therapy is prescribed selectively based on the individual needs or progress of each patient.

The skin is protected for the initial 3 weeks with a stockinette. Daily scar massage is initiated at 3 weeks postsurgery. This is particularly important for the anterior antecubitial incision.

Stage 3: Tendon Healing/Remodeling—6 to 12 Weeks

If the patient has not achieved full active ROM of the elbow and forearm by 6 weeks, more aggressive passive stretching is initiated. The most common deficits in motion at this stage are terminal extension and forearm rotation motion. Occasionally, nighttime static extension splinting (Figure 17.8) is needed as well as daytime static progressive splinting or dynamic splinting; however, the need for these is rare for distal biceps tendon repairs as joint contracture is uncommon.

- Passive terminal elbow flexion stretching (Figure 17.9). End-range stretch provided by therapist or family member.
- Passive terminal elbow extension stretching (Figure 17.10). End-range stretch provided by therapist or family member.
- Passive terminal forearm supination and pronation stretching.

Gentle isometric elbow, forearm, and grip strengthening are typically initiated 6 to 8 weeks postsurgery; however, a delay

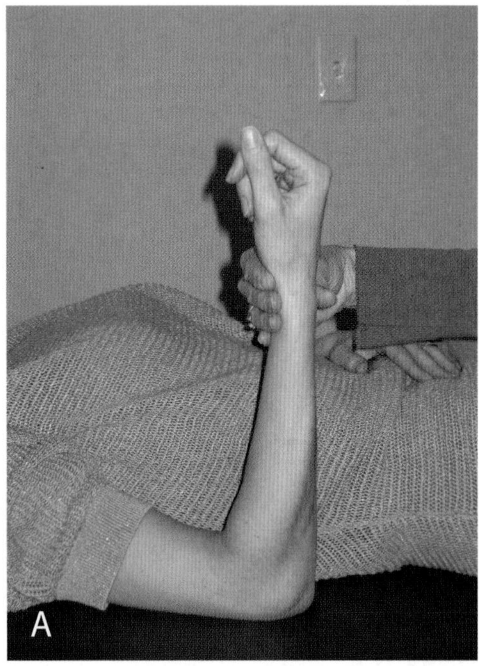

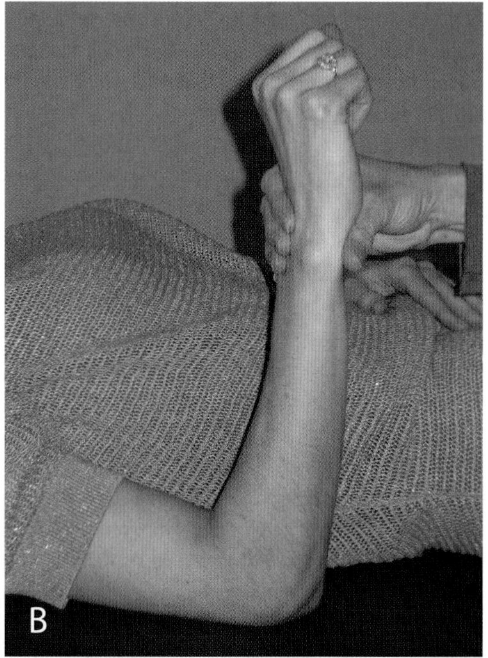

Figure 17.6 Photographs of passive forearm **A**, supination and **B**, pronation.

© 2018 American Academy of Orthopaedic Surgeons

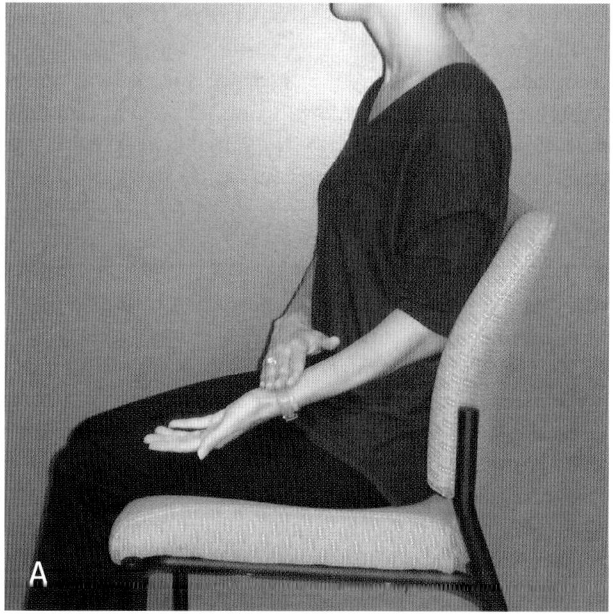

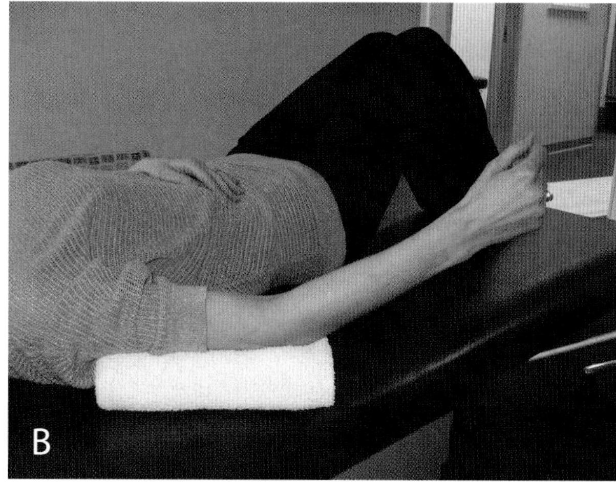

Figure 17.7 **A**, Photograph of gravity-assisted elbow extension: the forearm should initially be in a supinated position to minimize biceps tendon repair stretch. **B**, Photograph of gravity-assisted elbow extension performed supine.

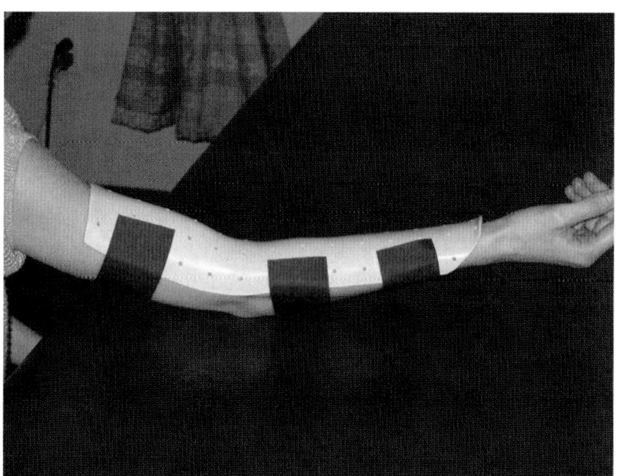

Figure 17.8 Photograph of static extension splint.

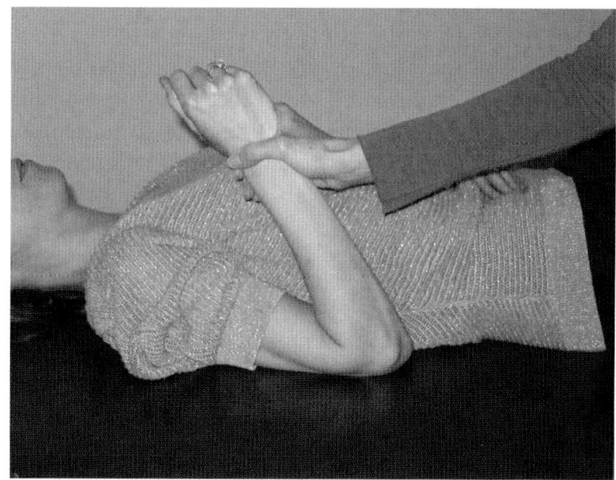

Figure 17.9 Photograph of passive terminal elbow flexion stretch.

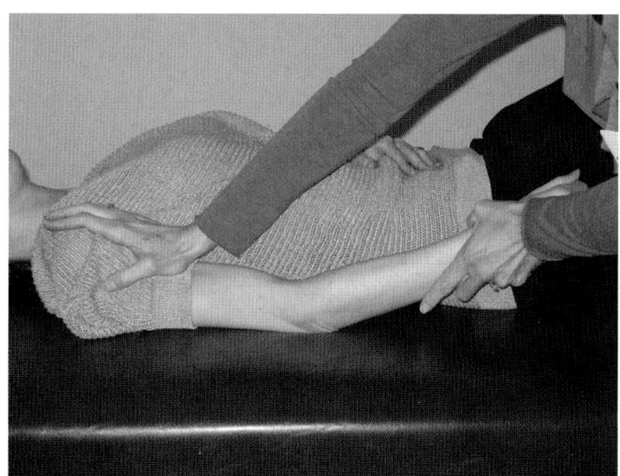

Figure 17.10 Photograph of passive terminal elbow extension stretch. Initially performed with the elbow supinated.

in strengthening until 12 weeks is acceptable. Strengthening of the biceps is allowed in pain-free arcs of motion emphasizing lighter weights and progressive increases in repetitions.

- Resisted elbow flexion (Figure 17.11). Lighter weights are used initially, emphasizing higher repetitions (2–5 lbs initially). Weight is progressed once 12 to 15 repetitions for 3 sets are well tolerated.
- Resisted forearm supination (Figure 17.12).

Lifting limits of 5 to 10 pounds are recommended for the first 4 weeks of strengthening. Resistance is progressed as tolerated from this point, emphasizing both strength and endurance (particularly with forearm supination). Full return to activity is based on the individual progress of each patient and specific functional demands, but is generally allowable by 6 months.

© 2018 American Academy of Orthopaedic Surgeons

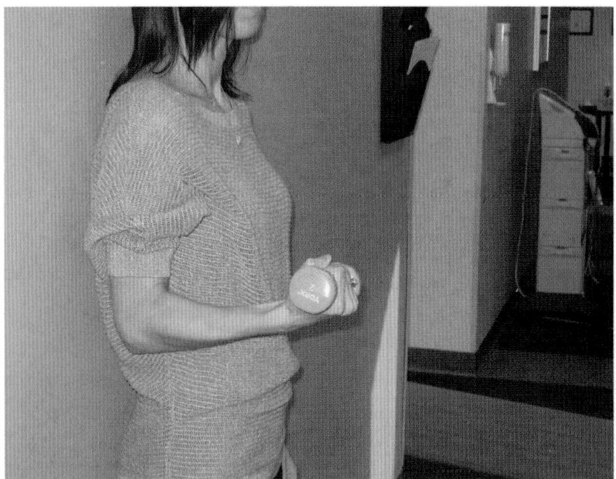

Figure 17.11 Photograph of resisted elbow flexion performed with the forearm supinated.

Functional Goals/Evidence Review

The functional goals following surgery are restoration of full elbow and forearm motion by 6 to 12 weeks and full strength by 6 to 9 months. Return to work is dictated by functional demands. The majority of outcome studies show excellent clinical results following distal biceps repair, with little residual disability. Multiple recent studies have advocated early, unprotected ROM allowing antigravity active flexion and extension stretching quickly after surgery without deleterious effects on tendon healing or outcomes. It is the preferred treatment of the author to allow early, unrestricted motion in compliant patients whose repairs are performed with minimal tension at 30° to 45° of elbow flexion. However, static immobilization is still advocated for the initial 4 weeks with several periods of exercise throughout the day.

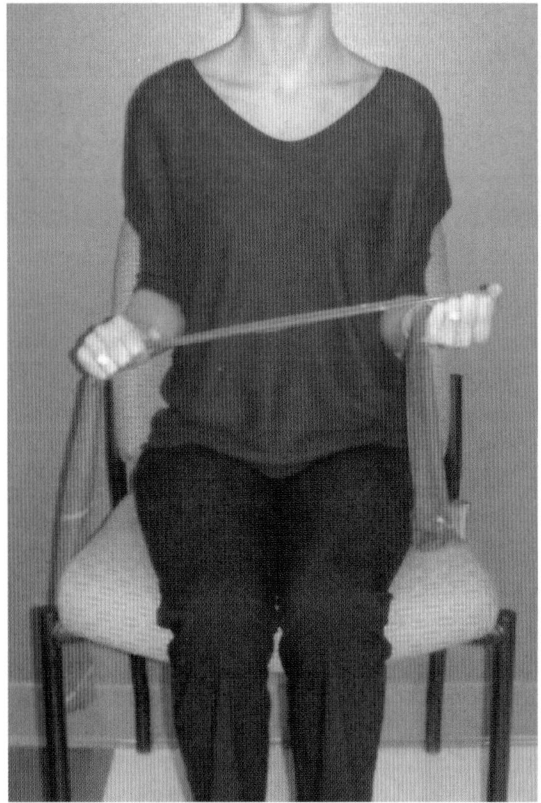

Figure 17.12 Photograph of Theraband-resisted forearm supination of the left upper extremity.

PEARLS

- Proper surgical technique is needed to optimize outcome and avoid complications.
- Judicious retractor placement and careful retraction can help avoid intraoperative nerve injuries. For dual-incision repairs, avoidance of violating the ulnar periosteum and careful irrigation of bone debris are important to prevent excessive heterotopic bone formation.
- Full mobilization of a retracted biceps tendon/muscle is necessary to avoid excessive repair tension.
- Anatomic reattachment of the distal biceps to the radial tuberosity probably optimizes strength recovery.
- In select cases, especially late or revision repairs, use of an interpositional graft is preferable to an excessively tensioned primary repair.
- The key to successful restoration of function is early mobilization. The arm should be immobilized for only a short period of time. Initial elbow extension ROM should be restricted based on intraoperative repair tension. Patients are instructed to perform light stretching and active assisted ROM several times per day.
- Close postoperative follow-up is needed to identify patients who are not progressing as expected with self-directed exercises where supervised rehabilitation can be prescribed.
- For patients with excessive elbow or forearm stiffness at 6 weeks, plain radiographs should be obtained to rule out heterotopic bone formation.

BIBLIOGRAPHY

Athwal GS, Steinmann SP, Rispoli DM: The distal biceps tendon: footprint and relevant clinical anatomy. *J Hand Surg Am* 2007;32(8):1225–1229.

Bain GI, Prem H, Heptinstall RJ, Verhellen R, Paix D: Repair of distal biceps tendon rupture: a new technique using the Endobutton. *J Shoulder Elbow Surg* 2000;9(2):120–126.

Baker BE, Bierwagen D: Rupture of the distal tendon of the biceps brachii. Operative versus non-operative treatment. *J Bone Joint Surg Am* 1985;67(3):414–417.

Cain RA, Nydick JA, Stein MI, Williams BD, Polikandriotis JA, Hess AV: Complications following distal biceps repair. *J Hand Surg Am* 2012;37(10):2112–2117.

Cheung EV, Lazarus M, Taranta M: Immediate range of motion after distal biceps tendon repair. *J Shoulder Elbow Surg* 2005; 14(5):516–518.

Greenberg JA, Fernandez JJ, Wang T, Turner C: EndoButton-assisted repair of distal biceps tendon ruptures. *J Shoulder Elbow Surg* 2003;12(5):484–490.

© 2018 American Academy of Orthopaedic Surgeons

Grewal R, Athwal GS, MacDermid JC, Faber KJ, Drosdowech DS, El-Hawary R, King GJ: Single versus double-incision technique for the repair of acute distal biceps tendon ruptures: a randomized clinical trial. *J Bone Joint Surg* 2012;94(13):1166–1174.

Hartman MW, Merten SM, Steinmann SP: Mini-open 2-incision technique for repair of distal biceps tendon ruptures. *J Shoulder Elbow Surg* 2007;16(5):616–620.

Idler CS, Montgomery WH 3rd, Lindsey DP, Badua PA, Wynne GF, Yerby SA: Distal biceps tendon repair: a biomechanical comparison of intact tendon and 2 repair techniques. *Am J Sports Med* 2006;34(6):968–974.

Kelly EW, Morrey BF, O'Driscoll SW: Complications of repair of the distal biceps tendon with the modified two-incision technique. *J Bone Joint Surg Am* 2000;82-A(11):1575–1581.

Kettler M, Lunger J, Kuhn V, Mutschler W, Tingart MJ: Failure strengths in distal biceps tendon repair. *Am J Sports Med* 2007;35(9):1544–1548.

Lemos SE, Ebramzedeh E, Kvitne RS: A new technique: in vitro suture anchor fixation has superior yield strength to bone tunnel fixation for distal biceps tendon repair. *Am J Sports Med* 2004;32(2):406–410.

Mazzocca AD, Burton KJ, Romeo AA, Santangelo S, Adams DA, Arciero RA: Biomechanical evaluation of 4 techniques of distal biceps brachii tendon repair. *Am J Sports Med* 2007; 35(2):252–258.

McKee MD, Hirji R, Schemitsch EH, Wild LM, Waddell JP: Patient-oriented functional outcome after repair of distal biceps tendon ruptures using a single-incision technique. *J Shoulder Elbow Surg* 2005;14(3):302–306.

Morrey ME, Abdel MP, Sanchez-Sotelo J, Morrey BF: Primary repair of retracted distal biceps tendon ruptures in extreme flexion. *J Shoulder Elbow Surg* 2014;23(5):679–685.

Nesterenko S, Domire ZJ, Morrey BF, Sanchez-Sotelo J: Elbow strength and endurance in patients with a ruptured distal biceps tendon. *J Shoulder Elbow Surg* 2010;19(2):184–189.

Nigro PT, Cain R, Mighell MA: Prognosis for recovery of posterior interosseous nerve palsy after distal biceps repair. *J Shoulder Elbow Surg* 2013;22(1):70–73.

Schmidt CC, Diaz VA, Weir DM, Latona CR, Miller MC: Repaired distal biceps magnetic resonance imaging anatomy compared with outcome. *J Shoulder Elbow Surg* 2012;21(12): 1623–1631.

© 2018 American Academy of Orthopaedic Surgeons

18 Evaluation and Treatment of Ulnar Neuropathy at the Elbow

Michael Darowish, MD, and Kathleen Beaulieu, OTR/L, CHT

INTRODUCTION

Cubital tunnel syndrome is the second most common compressive neuropathy of the upper extremity. Symptoms of cubital tunnel syndrome include numbness or tingling in the ring and small fingers, medial elbow pain, hand or grip weakness, dropping objects, or a generalized feeling of clumsiness of the hand. Numbness often occurs at night, waking patients from sleep, or is present upon awakening. Prolonged elbow flexion, as can occur when performing activities around one's face or head, talking on the telephone, or keyboard use, as well as repetitive elbow flexion and extension, can increase symptoms. External compression to the nerve, such as leaning one's elbow on a hard surface while driving, working on a table, or sitting on a chair with arms, can also increase numbness and pain in the hand.

Ulnar nerve compression from pressure and/or tension decreases blood flow to the ulnar nerve, resulting in demyelination. More severe nerve dysfunction eventually causes myopathic changes of the ulnar innervated muscles. The clinical manifestations of cubital tunnel syndrome are the result of nerve conduction abnormality as the ulnar nerve passes behind the medial epicondyle of the elbow. Nerve conduction can be affected by compression or traction across the ulnar nerve. Various anatomic structures, including the Arcade of Struthers (a fascial band from the medial triceps to the medial intramuscular septum), anconeus epitrochlearis muscle, Osborne's ligament, and the deep or superficial flexor carpi ulnaris fascia can cause compression. Space occupying lesions within the cubital tunnel, including ganglia, osteophytes, or loose bodies, are less common causes of increased pressure on the ulnar nerve. Last, external compression of the nerve, such as that which is caused by leaning on one's elbow, or positional factors, including prolonged elbow flexion, and ulnar nerve subluxation can cause symptoms.

In many cases, surgical treatment with ulnar nerve decompression with or without ulnar nerve transposition is required to relieve symptoms, as well as to prevent further neurologic deterioration. The postoperative treatment includes rehabilitation to ensure optimal recovery.

Relevant Anatomy

The ulnar nerve is the terminal branch of the medial cord of the brachial plexus, with contributions from the C8 and T1 cervical nerve roots. It traverses the thoracic inlet and outlet, entering the axilla. Proximally, the medial cord or ulnar nerve can be compressed by masses of the superior lung (Pancoast tumor), or at the thoracic outlet; these should be considered in the differential diagnosis. The nerve then pierces through the medial intermuscular septum, entering the posterior compartment at the level of the Arcade of Struthers, a band of fascia running from the medial intermuscular septum to the medial head of the triceps. The ulnar nerve then continues distally along the intermuscular septum, under the medial head of the triceps. At the elbow, the nerve lies in the condylar groove, then passes through the cubital tunnel, under the Osborne ligament. The nerve then enters the flexor carpi ulnaris (FCU), where it is covered both by the superficial fascia of the FCU as well as a deeper layer of fascia under the muscle fibers of the FCU. The ulnar nerve then begins branching, providing muscular branches to the FCU and the ulnar portion of the flexor digitorum profundus (FDP). The nerve continues distally, travelling deep and radial to the FCU tendon, entering the wrist. It then enters the hand at the Guyon canal, dividing into the superficial sensory branches (which provide sensation to the small finger and the ulnar ring finger) and the deep motor branch, which wraps around the hook of the hamate and traverses the palm, providing motor innervation to the hypothenar musculature, the interosseous muscles, the deep head of the flexor pollicis brevis, and the ulnar two lumbrical muscles.

At the level of the elbow, the ulnar nerve can be compressed by the Arcade of Struthers, the overlying triceps, the Osborne ligament, and the FCU. When the nerve is transposed, the medial intermuscular septum can become a compressive structure as the nerve travels from the posterior compartment

Dr. Darowish or an immediate family member serves as a board member, owner, officer, or committee member of the American Academy of Orthopaedic Surgeons. Neither Mrs. Beaulieu nor any immediate family member has received anything of value from or has stock or stock options held in a commercial company or institution related directly or indirectly to the subject of this article.

 © 2018 American Academy of Orthopaedic Surgeons

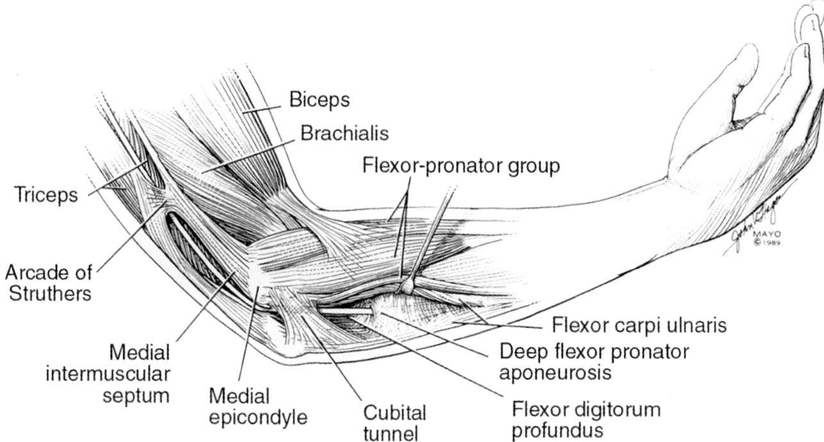

Figure 18.1 Illustration of the course of the ulnar nerve at the elbow, with potential compressive structures. (Reproduced from Elhassan B, Steinmann SP: Entrapment neuropathy of the ulnar nerve. *J Am Acad Orthop Surg*, 2007;15: 674. Reproduced with permission from the Mayo Foundation for Medical Education and Research, Rochester, MN.)

into the anterior compartment. Further, iatrogenic compression or kinking can occur as the nerve reenters the FCU distally (Figure 18.1).

EVALUATION

Evaluation of the patient begins with a thorough history. Patients describe numbness and pain in their hand. Encouraging the patient to localize the numbness to specific digits can be challenging, but immensely helpful. Similarly, isolating activities or arm positions that exacerbate symptoms can help to differentiate the various causes of numbness. Classically, activities in which the elbow is flexed, such as driving, talking on a telephone, texting, reading a newspaper, tasks around the face and head, or sleeping exacerbate symptoms. Similarly, repetitive elbow flexion and extension, or leaning on the elbow, will worsen the patient's pain or numbness. The presence or absence of associated medical conditions such as diabetes, peripheral neuropathy, rheumatoid arthritis, renal disease, or a history of fracture or trauma to the elbow can also help in narrowing the diagnosis.

Physical examination begins with evaluation of the elbow range of motion (ROM), looking for limitations in flexion and extension that may indicate underlying arthritis. The carrying angle of the elbow is observed to identify cubitus valgus, which can increase tension on the ulnar nerve. Any swelling or edema, particularly at the medial elbow, should also be noted. The hand should be evaluated for the presence of atrophy of the ulnar nerve innervated musculature, including the hypothenar mass and the first dorsal interosseous muscle. In severe cases, the ulnar two digits may be in a clawed position—metacarpophalangeal (MCP) hyperextension, proximal interphalangeal (PIP) and distal interphalangeal (DIP) flexion (Figure 18.2, A and B).

Ulnar motor function is assessed with finger abduction and adduction, as well as checking if the patient can cross the index and long fingers. This is a more reliable test, and the examiner is less easily "faked out" by finger extension. Additionally, we have found that finger crossing can be significantly "clumsier" than the unaffected side, even before frank atrophy is noted. The FDP to the ring and small fingers may be affected, resulting in an incomplete fist or weakened grip. Key pinch is often affected in ulnar neuropathy, resulting in the Froment sign. When asked to pinch a piece of paper, the patient with ulnar neuropathy replaces key pinch with tip pinch, flexing the interphalangeal (IP) joint of the thumb. In doing so, the patient utilizes the median nerve innervated flexor pollicis longus (FPL) in lieu of the ulnar innervated adductor pollicis (Figure 18.3, A and B). Strength can be objectively evaluated for grip, using a Jamar dynamometer, and for pinch, including tip, key, and 3-jaw chuck.

Sensation in the ulnar nerve distribution should be evaluated. The pulp of the small finger is predictably innervated by the ulnar nerve, thus should be used for testing. Additionally, the dorsal ulnar hand is innervated by the dorsal cutaneous branch of the ulnar nerve, which branches several centimeters proximal to the wrist. Diminished sensation in the dorsal hand suggests a more proximal lesion, and can help to differentiate ulnar nerve compression at the cubital tunnel from compression at the Guyon canal. Various methods—including light touch, Semmes-Weinstein monofilament, and two-point discrimination—can be utilized. Two-point discrimination is not affected until much later in the disease, while Semmes-Weinstein monofilament testing can be helpful earlier in the course.

In many cases of cubital tunnel syndrome, symptoms are not present unless provoked. Because it is a dynamic process, and can be position and pressure dependent, many patients demonstrate intact motor and sensation on initial testing. To bring about ulnar nerve symptoms, various provocative maneuvers can be performed. A Tinel sign is reproduction of electric shocks or numbness and tingling in the ulnar nerve distribution with percussion over the nerve, either at the cubital tunnel (Figure 18.4) or at the Guyon canal. Note that the Tinel sign can be positive in at least 10% of unaffected individuals. In the elbow compression–flexion test, the examiner places pressure over the ulnar nerve at the cubital tunnel while holding the elbow flexed and the wrist in neutral position to prevent creating secondary pressure at the carpal tunnel or Guyon

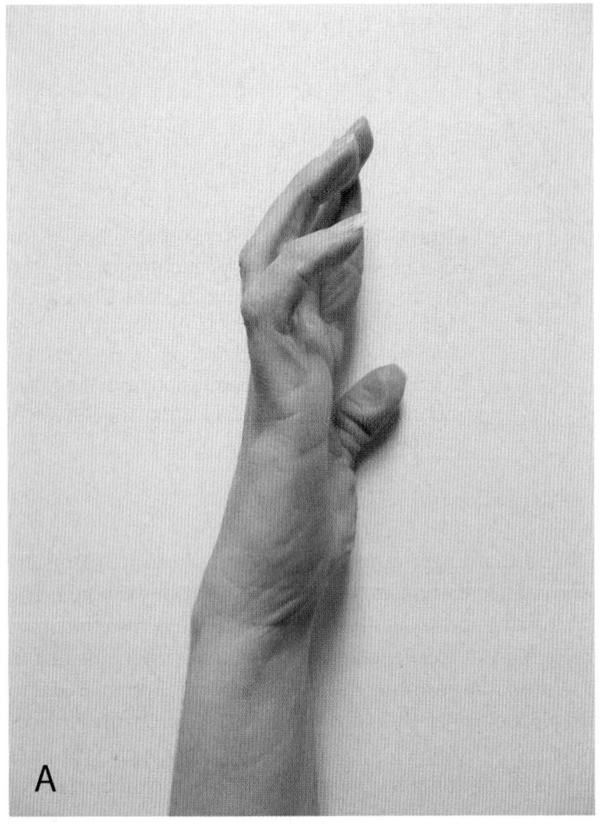

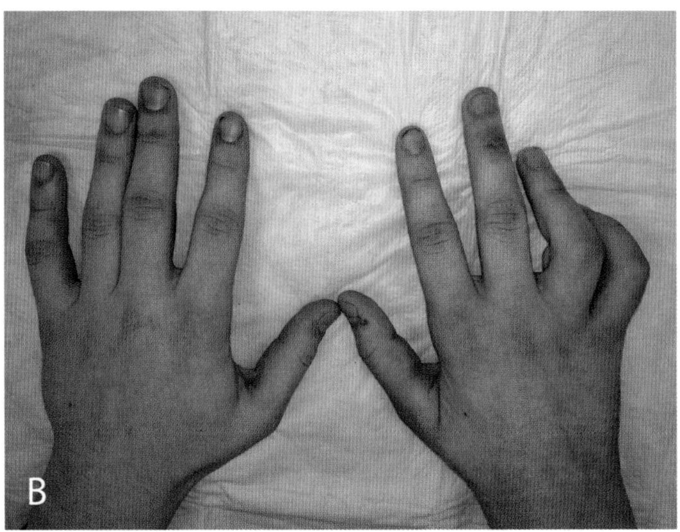

Figure 18.2 **A**, Photograph of the typical ulnar clawing posture of the ring and small fingers, with hyperextension of the metacarpophalangeal joints and flexion of the proximal interphalangeal and distal interphalangeal joints. **B**, Photograph of atrophy of the first dorsal interosseous muscle can be seen along with this clawing (patient's right hand).

canal, which can also cause hand numbness (Figure 18.5). The examiner should also assess for more proximal nerve lesions, including cervical spine and lower brachial plexus lesions that can mimic ulnar neuropathy.

Electrodiagnostic evaluation with electromyography (EMG) and nerve conduction study (NCS) can be used in the evaluation of cubital tunnel syndrome. EMG/NCS testing is often normal because of the dynamic nature of cubital tunnel syndrome, and positive EMG/NCS findings are often only present later in the course of the disease, or in more severe cases. EMG/NCS can be helpful in challenging cases, to help differentiate cervical pathology from peripheral nerve compression, or to help differentiate proximal and distal lesions. We often obtain nerve testing preoperatively to have a baseline study in case

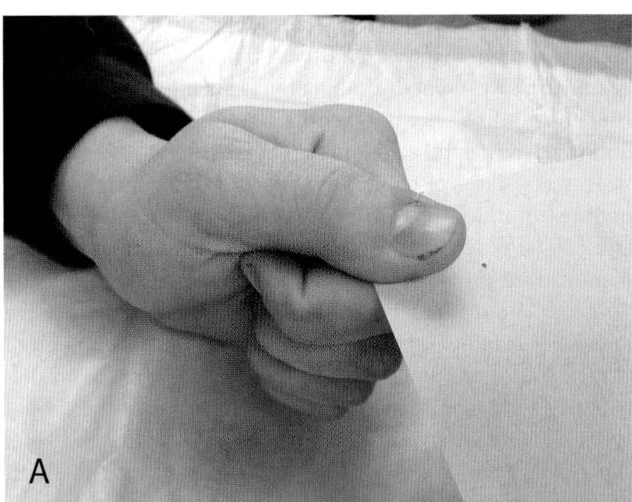

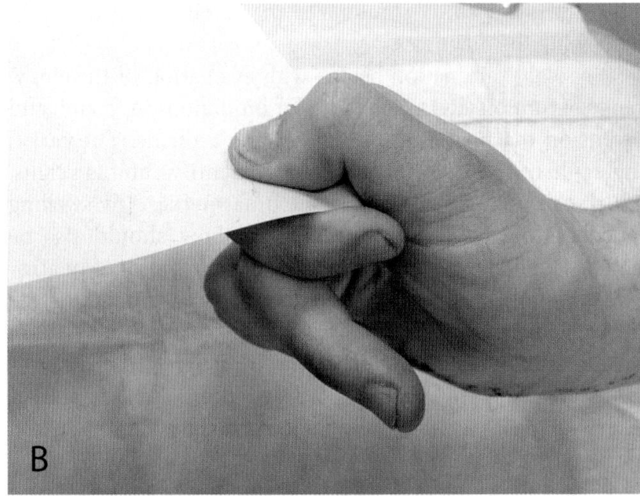

Figure 18.3 Photographs of Froment's sign. The patient is asked to pinch the paper while the examiner tries to pull the paper away. **A**, The patient's left hand shows the normal posture of key pinch. **B**, The patient's right hand shows replacement of key pinch with tip pinch, using the flexor pollicis longus (median innervated) rather than the adductor pollicis and first dorsal interosseous (ulnar innervated).

 © 2018 American Academy of Orthopaedic Surgeons

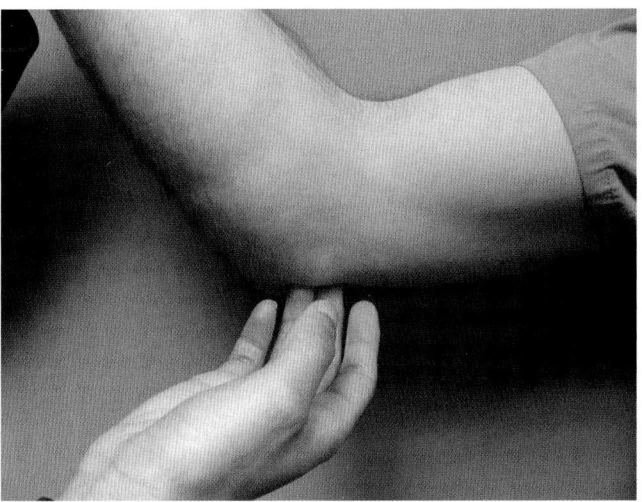

Figure 18.4 Photograph of a Tinel sign, produced by tapping over the ulnar nerve at the cubital tunnel. A positive Tinel sign produces pain or paresthesia into the ring and small fingers.

postoperative symptoms persist, as well as to temper patient expectations in more severe cases. Radiographs or MRI are not a routine part of evaluation of cubital tunnel syndrome; they are reserved only for cases in which there is concern for concomitant arthritis, space occupying lesions, or a history of previous trauma to the elbow that may be contributing to compression of the nerve.

TREATMENT

The primary goals of conservative treatment are to reduce pain, diminish paresthesias or hypersensitivity, improve or compensate for ROM limitations, diminish neural tension, maximize strength, and improve or restore function. In most cases, activity modification can play a major role in resolving the symptoms. Nonoperative treatment is often effective in cases with mild, intermittent symptoms and no weakness or atrophy, with up to 50% of patients with mild cubital tunnel syndrome achieving successful outcomes. However, it is important to note that nonoperative treatment has not been shown to improve strength.

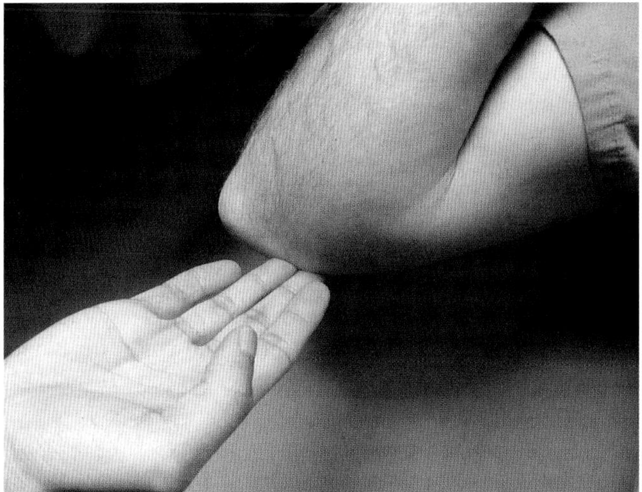

Figure 18.5 Photograph of the elbow compression-flexion test, which is performed by keeping the patient's elbow flexed while keeping the wrist in neutral position. Pressure is placed over the ulnar nerve at the cubital tunnel. A positive test produces numbness, pain, or paresthesia in the ulnar nerve distribution.

Patient education is a large part of treatment. Explaining the relevant anatomy and showing the patient the course of the ulnar nerve allows for an improved understanding of how certain movements or activities may affect the nerve. It reinforces how activity modifications or ergonomic changes may assist in diminishing symptoms and can have a positive impact on outcome. This tends to improve patient compliance with the treatment program.

Modalities may be used in conjunction with treatment techniques. Moist heat can be used for pain relief, as well as soft-tissue preparation prior to exercise or functional activity. Ice can be applied to the symptomatic area to assist in edema and pain reduction. Ultrasound may be utilized to increase blood flow to the area. Specific care should be taken to avoid thermal injury. Close monitoring is advised if applying thermal modalities to an area with altered sensation.

Myofascial mobility may be increased through the use of myofascial release techniques, slow steady stretch, or the use of Kinesio tape, decreasing the tension of the ulnar nerve during functional activities. Neural mobilization techniques can be useful in symptom reduction; care should be taken to not place tension on the nerve. Nerve gliding or flossing techniques are a preferred method to provide neural mobility with limited tension. The use of myofascial release, Kinesio taping, and neural mobilization require an extensive understanding of the evaluation and treatment process beyond the scope of this chapter.

Strengthening proximal muscle groups may be beneficial in those patients who must perform tasks requiring resisted or sustained elbow flexion. Increasing shoulder strength, scapular stabilization, and improving posture allow the stress of lifting to be transferred to more proximal muscle groups, decreasing stresses across more distal affected muscle groups.

Rest from aggravating positions and activities may be quite beneficial. The therapist should evaluate the patient's daily activities—including self-care, work, and leisure pursuits—to identify and target potential areas for modification. Specific areas to focus on include avoidance of compression, avoidance of traction, decreasing overuse of the wrist flexor and pronator muscles, and altering approaches to specific tasks that cause symptoms. On-site assessment of the patient's workplace can be of great benefit. The physical set-up and job requirements are reviewed, and suggestions may be made regarding ergonomic adjustments, environmental alterations, and workflow.

A soft pad worn over the elbow assists in cushioning the cubital tunnel so that increased external pressure or unintentional trauma to the ulnar nerve is avoided during functional use of the involved extremity (Figure 18.6, A and B).

© 2018 American Academy of Orthopaedic Surgeons

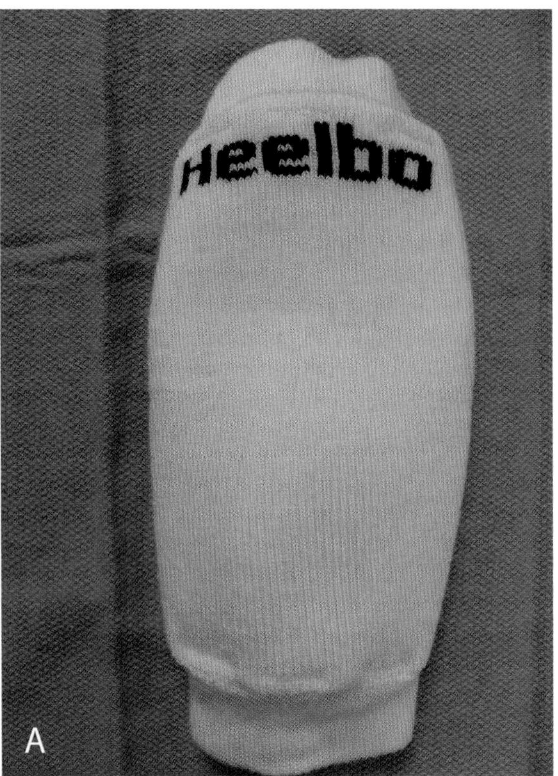

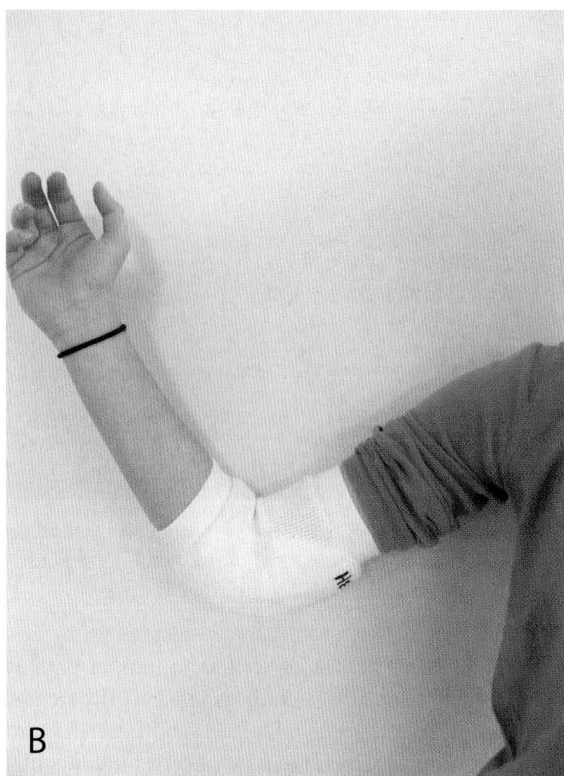

Figure 18.6 **A**, Photograph of a Heelbo, a low-profile elbow pad, which can provide significant relief from external compression of the ulnar nerve (**B**).

- Activity modification suggestions
  - Avoidance of ulnar nerve compression at the cubital tunnel during activities
    - *Driving:* Limit leaning on armrest, window, or door handle. Use elbow pad or pillow to cushion nerve.
    - *Computer station:* Limit leaning on chair armrests, tabletop, or desktop while typing, reading, or writing. Use chair without arms to decrease tendency to rest elbows. Use elbow pad or pillow to cushion nerve. Job rotation with periodic breaks.
    - *Wheelchair users:* Limit leaning on armrests or tray table. Use elbow pad or pillow.
    - *Tool use:* Alter technique or handles to allow for performance in a neutral forearm position.
    - *Lifting:* Position hands so that forearms are neutral.
  - Avoid traction on the ulnar nerve with prolonged elbow flexion
    - *Telephone:* Use shoulder cradle, hands-free headset, or speaker phone.
    - *Computer station:* Place keyboard lower and farther away from body to avoid prolonged elbow flexion beyond 90°. Adjust chair height so that elbows are flexed no farther than 90° when using a keyboard. Use keyboard tray rather than desktop to position keyboard lower, allowing more elbow extension while typing.
    - *Self-care around the face and head:* Take breaks, do in smaller increments. Use blow dryer holder.
    - *Sleeping:* Nocturnal extension orthoses

A particular issue should be discussed regarding sleeping. In our experience, most patients do not tolerate rigid orthoses for the elbow during sleep. A soft elbow brace is better tolerated and accomplishes the same goal of limiting prolonged extreme elbow flexion. A rigid elbow brace for day and night use may be warranted in cases in which symptoms are of greater intensity and duration. Compression of the ulnar nerve is greatest with the elbow at flexed 90° or greater, and minimal with the elbow fully extended. Secondary to poor patient tolerance of elbow immobilization in full extension, the literature suggests positioning at 30° to 45°.

Preoperative Therapy

In patients who are surgical candidates, preoperative therapy can reduce joint contractures, increase ROM, and improve function, enhancing their ultimate postoperative outcomes. If ulnar digit clawing is present, preoperative therapy can greatly improve postoperative hand function. Focus should be on restoration of full passive motion, and placing the hand into a more functional position, particularly improving MCP flexion and PIP and DIP extension, and eliminating small finger abduction.

- Brace or orthosis use to improve digit ROM
  - PIP flexion contractures less than 35°: A dynamic PIP extension brace, such as a prefabricated LMB dynamic extension spring splint may be used.
  - More severe or longstanding PIP flexion contractures: A custom fabricated dynamic or static progressive PIP extension brace may be made.

 © 2018 American Academy of Orthopaedic Surgeons

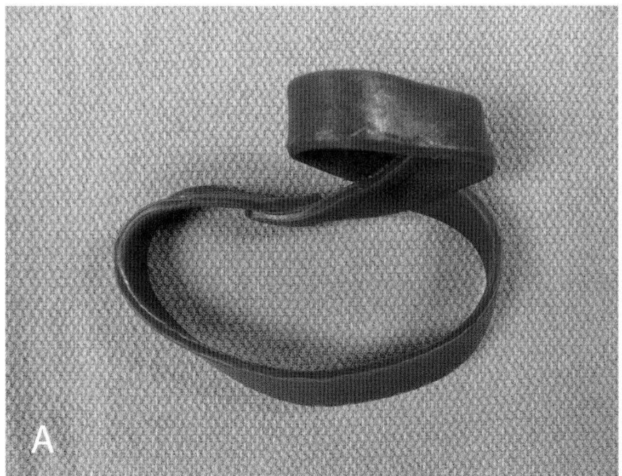

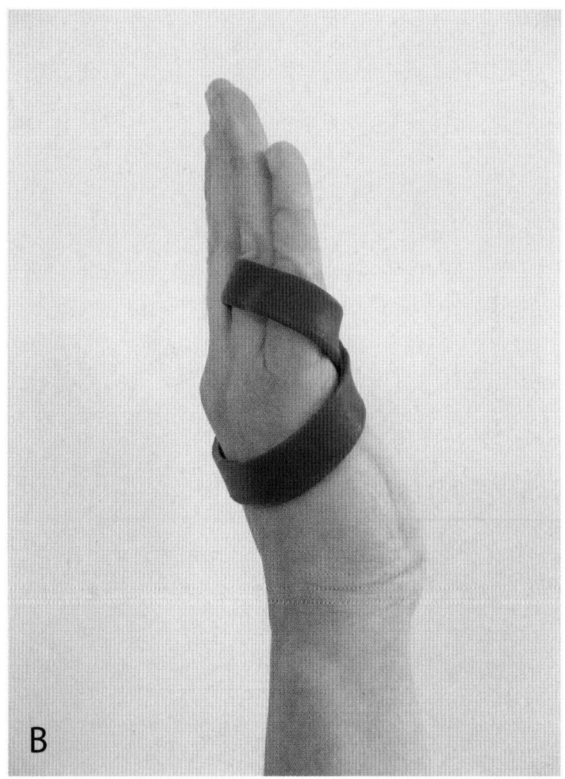

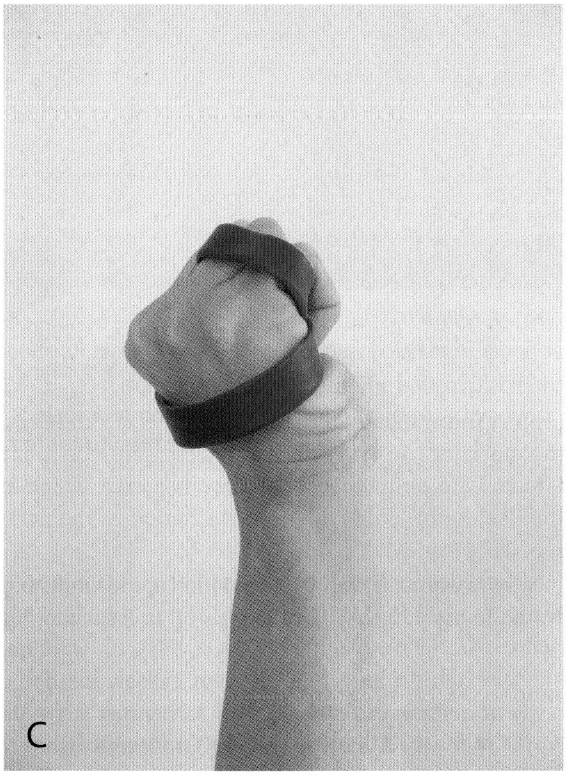

Figure 18.7 **A**, Photograph of a low-profile figure-of-eight brace, which can be effective in patients with clawing. **B**, **C**, The design prevents metacarpophalangeal hyperextension, while allowing full motion.

  - Static night braces can be used to maintain gains achieved during the day through ROM and brace use.
- Functional splinting
  - MCP block or anti-claw brace assists in improving hand function.
  - Blocking MCP hyperextension redirects extrinsic extensor forces, allowing improved PIP and DIP extension.
  - Placing the intrinsic muscles in a more relaxed position improves the initiation of flexion in our experience.
  - Figure-of-eight design is the most efficient and least cumbersome (Figure 18.7).
  - If the small finger rests abducted secondary to the loss of adductor digiti minimi function (Wartenburg sign), buddy straps can keep the small finger adducted, preventing it from being caught during activities (Figure 18.8).

Operative Treatment

Operative intervention is indicated in patients with severe ulnar neuropathy, atrophy of ulnar-innervated musculature, or in milder cases that fail to respond to nonoperative measures. The surgical procedures used to treat ulnar neuropathy at the elbow include simple decompression, anterior subcutaneous transposition, intramuscular or submuscular transposition, and medial epicondylectomy. The selection of which procedure to perform is dependent on the severity of the neuropathy, the presence or absence of ulnar nerve subluxation, and surgeon preference and comfort with the various procedures. There are no absolute contraindications to surgery; however, in the patient with chronic severe neuropathy with wasting, surgery needs to be carefully considered, as there may be little to no chance of meaningful recovery in a severe, long-standing nerve issue.

© 2018 American Academy of Orthopaedic Surgeons

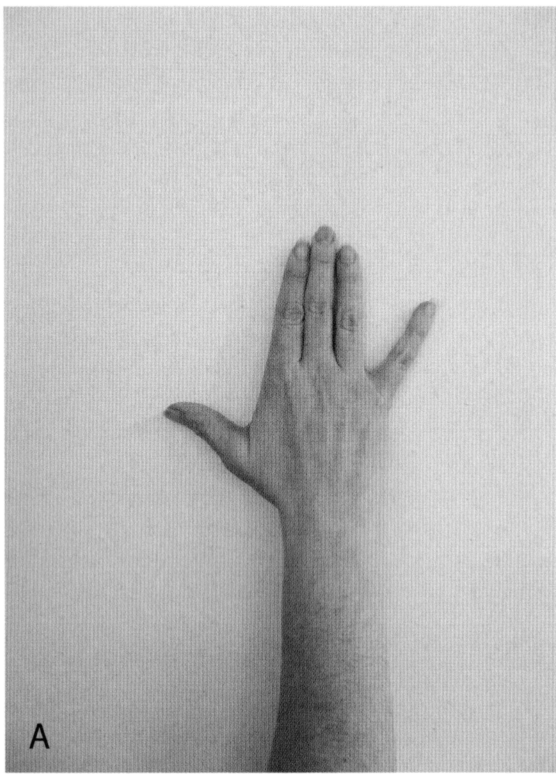

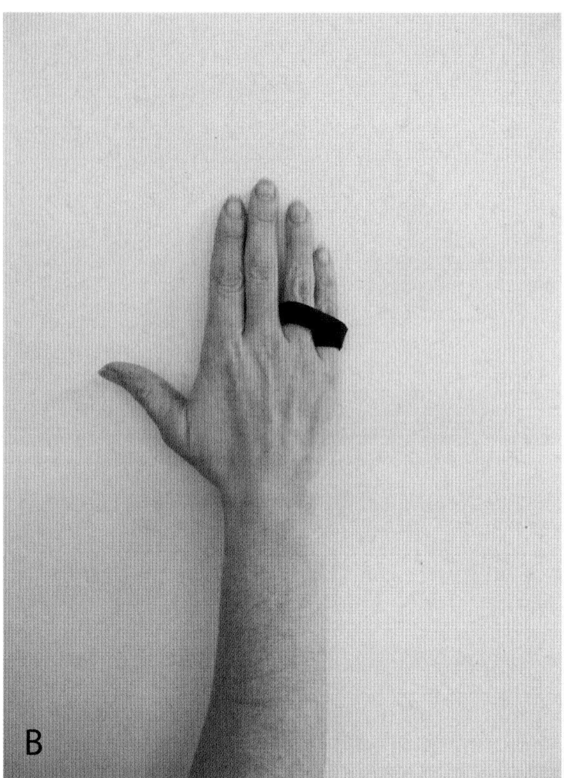

Figure 18.8 **A**, Photograph of hand with loss of adductor digiti minimi function, which can cause abduction of the small finger. **B**, Photograph of use of buddy straps, which can prevent the small finger from being caught on objects, improving function.

In Situ Ulnar Nerve Decompression

In situ decompression can be performed using either open or endoscopic techniques. Endoscopic decompression can be performed either "outside-in" as described by Hoffmann, or "inside-out" as described by Cobb. Open decompression can be performed as described in this section. The principles of decompression remain the same regardless of approach.

A curvilinear incision is made over the course of ulnar nerve, starting about 1 cm proximal to the medial epicondyle and extending 2 to 3 cm distal to the cubital tunnel. The subcutaneous tissue is bluntly dissected, taking care to identify and protect the medial antebrachial cutaneous nerve (MABC). The ulnar nerve is first identified proximal to the cubital tunnel, under the fascia of the triceps. The triceps fascia is released up to and including the Arcade of Struthers (typically found 8 cm proximal to the epicondyle). If an anconeus epitrochlearis muscle (running from the olecranon to the medial epicondyle) is present, it is excised.

Dissection is then continued distally, dividing the Osborne ligament, which overlies the ulnar nerve in the cubital tunnel. The FCU is located at the distal aspect of the Osborne ligament. The superficial fascia of the FCU is incised, remaining superficial to the muscle fibers to protect the nerve. The muscle fibers are then bluntly separated between the two heads of the FCU, exposing the ulnar nerve. Deep to the muscle fibers, the deep fascia overlying the ulnar nerve is identified and divided. Thickenings can be seen 5 to 9 cm distal to the retrocondylar groove, which can compress the nerve. Care must be taken to protect the branches to the FCU. During in situ releases, only the superficial aspect of the ulnar nerve is dissected, as circumferential dissection may destabilize the nerve, which increases the likelihood of perching or subluxation of the nerve at the medial epicondyle.

Once decompression is completed, the elbow is taken through a full ROM. If perching or frank subluxation of the nerve over the medial epicondyle is noted in flexion, a formal anterior transposition is performed.

Anterior Subcutaneous Ulnar Nerve Transposition

The initial portion of the procedure is performed as described earlier for in situ decompression. After completion of decompression, the nerve is then circumferentially dissected along its length to allow mobilization into an anterior position. Some authors have suggested that preservation of longitudinal vessels traveling with the ulnar nerve can improve outcomes.

Once the nerve has been sufficiently mobilized, the intermuscular septum is identified proximal to the medial epicondyle and resected. Failure to do this can cause iatrogenic compression of the nerve, and is a common cause of failed surgery. Several large veins invariably run at the base of the septum. Care should be taken to avoid injury or to appropriately cauterize them. The nerve is then placed anterior to the medial epicondyle. A sling can be created to prevent the nerve from posterior displacement. A proximally based flap of flexor pronator fascia can be secured to the subcutaneous tissues, creating a "backstop" to prevent the nerve from displacing posteriorly. The subcutaneous tissues can

 © 2018 American Academy of Orthopaedic Surgeons

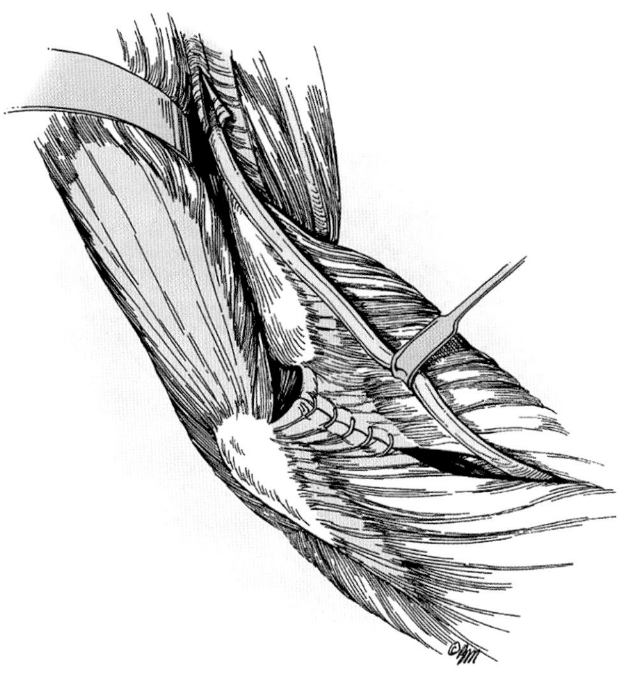

Figure 18.9 Illustration of anterior subcutaneous ulnar nerve transposition. The ulnar nerve is decompressed and transposed anterior to the medial epicondyle. A flap of fascia from the flexor-pronator origin is sutured to the overlying skin to prevent the nerve from returning to its original position within the cubital tunnel. (Illustration by Elizabeth Martin © 2011. Reproduced with permission from Wolfe SQ, Pederson WC, Hotchkiss RN, Kozin SH: *Green's Operative Hand Surgery*, ed 6. Philadelphia, PA, Elsevier, 2011, p. 1000.)

be directly sutured to the flexor-pronator mass. Alternatively, a distally based slip of intermuscular septum can be used as a turn-down flap onto the flexor-pronator fascia. Resection of the proximal portion of the anterior head of the FCU helps to smooth the transition from deep within the FCU to superficial to the flexor pronator fascia, and reduce iatrogenic kinking of the nerve at this critical location.

After transposition and securing the sling, the nerve must be closely inspected. The elbow is then taken through a ROM to ensure that the nerve does not kink throughout the ROM. The nerve should not be compressed by the sling or overlying tissues throughout ROM. It is essential to release the nerve far enough proximally and distally so that it takes a smooth course in the transposed position. Inadequate release during transposition can lead to the nerve appearing as the Greek letter omega (Ω), causing kinking as it exits the triceps fascia or where it reenters the fascia of the FCU, again leading to failed surgery (Figure 18.9).

Intramuscular, Transmuscular, or Submuscular Ulnar Nerve Transposition

Transposition of the ulnar nerve into an intramuscular, transmuscular, or submuscular position has several theoretical advantages. The nerve is placed within a vascular bed, and is better protected in or under the flexor musculature than in a subcutaneous location. Additionally, in this deeper position, the nerve has a more direct path than with subcutaneous transposition, as it remains deep under the triceps, under the flexor-pronator muscles, and deep within the FCU. However, this approach requires significantly more dissection of the flexor pronator musculature, with its resultant morbidity.

For intramuscular or transmuscular transposition, ulnar nerve decompression and mobilization and intermuscular septum resection is performed as described earlier. Next, proximally and distally based flaps of the superficial flexor-pronator fascia are elevated to allow fascial repair in a lengthened position. A trough is made in the muscle fibers along the course of the transposed ulnar nerve, and any vertical fascial bands are resected or incised to prevent iatrogenic nerve compression. The flexor pronator fascial flaps are then repaired to one another in a lengthened fashion; the surgeon's finger should be able to pass under the repaired fascia. Again, after transposition and fascial repair are completed, the elbow is taken through ROM to inspect for iatrogenic compression or kinking (Figure 18.10).

If submuscular transposition is to be performed, the ulnar nerve decompression and intermuscular septum resection are performed as described earlier. The flexor pronator fascia is then incised 1 to 2 cm distal to its origin on the medial epicondyle. However, rather than making a trough within the muscle fibers, the entirety of the flexor mass is elevated off the underlying capsule from proximal to distal using an elevator. The median nerve is visualized deep to the brachialis, and the ulnar nerve is placed under the muscle fibers of the flexor pronator mass, medial and parallel to the course of the median nerve. The flexor-pronator mass is then repaired back to its insertion, either directly (Learmonth technique) or with fascial lengthening to prevent iatrogenic compression by the repaired fascia (Dellon technique). Again, the nerve is inspected for iatrogenic compression or kinking throughout ROM. Special attention should be paid to the intermuscular septal area and the distal edge of the flexor-pronator mass for fascial compression of the nerve (Figure 18.11).

Medial Epicondylectomy

An in situ ulnar nerve decompression is performed as described earlier. The medial epicondyle is exposed subperiosteally and the superficial 5 mm (20%) of the epicondyle is removed using an osteotome. Care must be taken to not remove more than this in order to avoid injuring the origin of the medial collateral ligament (MCL). The bone edges are smoothed with a rongeur or rasp, and the periosteum is closed over the bone. By removing the medial epicondyle, the ulnar nerve is allowed to move freely over the medial elbow, preventing symptomatic snapping as it leaves the cubital tunnel and moves anteriorly over the medial epicondyle (Figure 18.12).

POSTOPERATIVE REHABILITATION

The postoperative rehabilitation after ulnar nerve surgery includes some general principles related to local wound and

© 2018 American Academy of Orthopaedic Surgeons

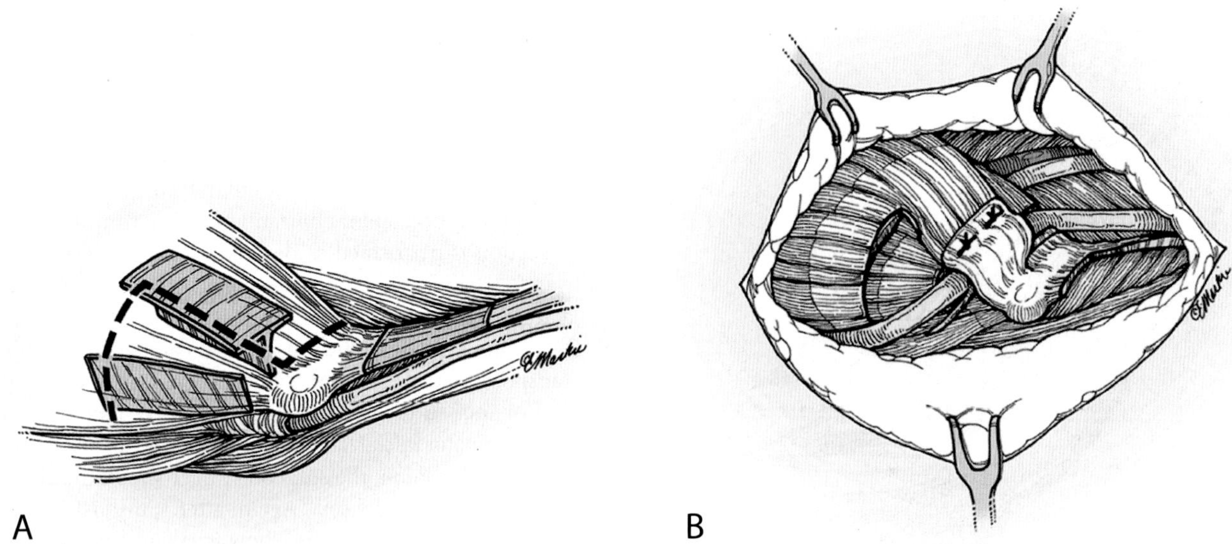

Figure 18.10 Illustrations of intramuscular transposition. **A**, The nerve is decompressed and mobilized. Z-lengthening flaps are elevated from the flexor-pronator fascia. A trough is made in the flexor-pronator muscle fibers, taking care to release all vertical fascial bands to prevent iatrogenic compression. **B**, The fascial flaps are then repaired in a lengthened position over the nerve. (Illustrations by Elizabeth Martin © 2011. Reproduced with permission from Wolfe SQ, Pederson WC, Hotchkiss RN, Kozin SH: *Green's Operative Hand Surgery*, ed 6. Philadelphia, PA, Elsevier, 2011, p. 1002.)

soft-tissue healing, restoration of elbow function and upper extremity function, as well as hand function, especially in cases with more advanced myopathic changes.

A posterior elbow splint is used for the first 7 to 10 days postoperatively, which, in our experience, decreases pain. Short-term immobilization is unlikely to result in significant elbow stiffness, as this is an extra-articular surgery. No splinting is used after the immediate postoperative period. The patient is discharged from surgery with instructions to elevate the extremity and actively use the fingers to minimize

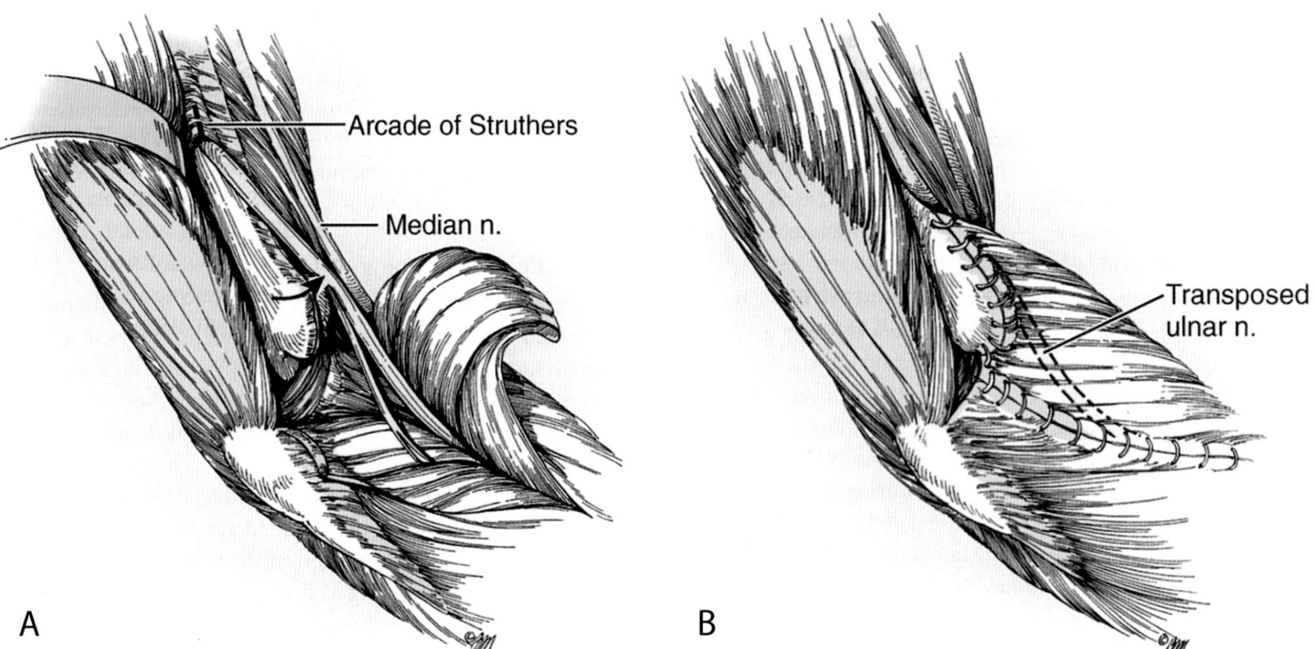

Figure 18.11 Illustrations of submuscular transposition. **A**, The nerve is decompressed and mobilized. The entire flexor-pronator mass is elevated off of the capsule. The nerve is placed deep to the entire flexor-pronator mass, in a path parallel to the median nerve. **B**, The flexor is then repaired to its origin either directly (Learmonth) or in a lengthened position (Dellon). (Illustrations by Elizabeth Martin © 2011. Reproduced with permission from Wolfe SQ, Pederson WC, Hotchkiss RN, Kozin SH: *Green's Operative Hand Surgery*, ed 6. Philadelphia, PA, Elsevier, 2011, p. 1000.)

 © 2018 American Academy of Orthopaedic Surgeons

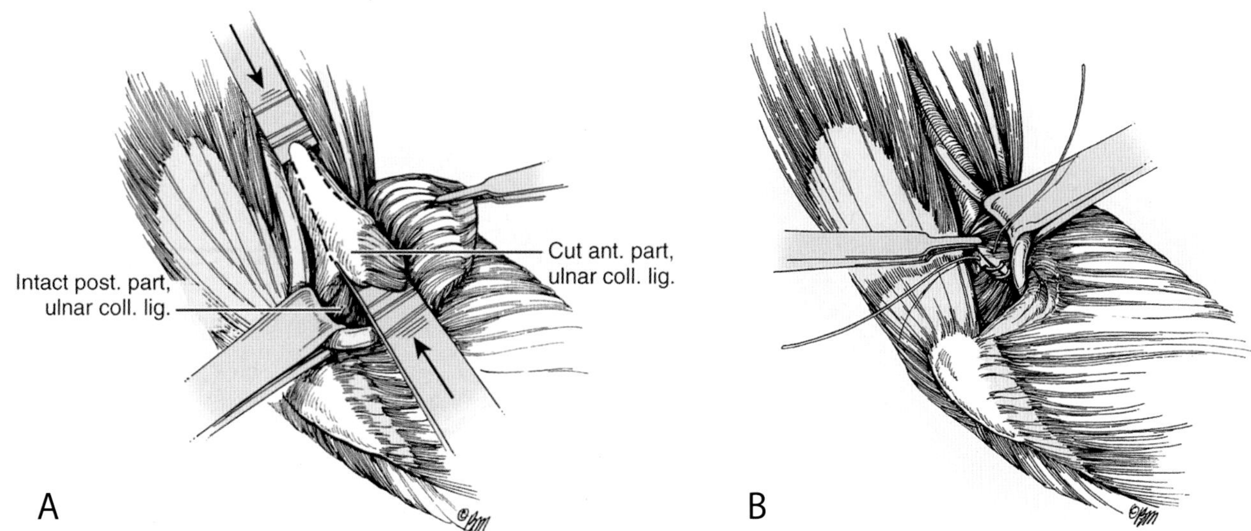

Figure 18.12 Illustrations of medial epicondylectomy. **A**, The superficial portion of the medial epicondyle is removed with an osteotome. **B**, The overlying fascia is repaired over the exposed bone. The ulnar nerve can glide over this repair, and will find its own new resting position. Care must be taken to remove enough medial epicondyle to prevent snapping of the nerve over this prominence, while not removing too much so as to cause instability by excising the insertion of the medial collateral ligament on the humerus. Additionally, the fascia at the entrance of the nerve into the flexor carpi ulnaris must be released to prevent nerve compression (not shown in the figure). (Illustrations by Elizabeth Martin © 2011. Reproduced with permission from Wolfe SQ, Pederson WC, Hotchkiss RN, Kozin SH: *Green's Operative Hand Surgery*, ed 6. Philadelphia, PA, Elsevier, 2011, p. 998.)

swelling and edema. Digit exercises focusing on tendon glides, digit abduction/adduction, and thumb opposition are initiated immediately (Figure 18.13).

At the first postoperative appointment, the splint is removed, sutures are removed, and elbow ROM is initiated. Patients are instructed to work on ROM daily. If there is difficulty achieving full elbow and forearm motion within 7 to 10 days, more specific attention is directed to regaining motion with passive and active-assisted stretching exercises.

If significant hypersensitivity or neuritis is present, either at the MABC or of the ulnar nerve itself, medications may be prescribed, most commonly gabapentin or nonsteroidal anti-inflammatory drugs (NSAIDs). Topical lidocaine gel or patches can also be helpful in decreasing cutaneous sensitivity. In the authors' experience, less than 5% of patients require prescription management of neuritis.

Specific attention to rehabilitation of the hand may be necessary in cases with more advanced preoperative compressive neuropathy and hand-intrinsic dysfunction with clawing and finger contractures.

Authors' Preferred Protocol

- Edema management
  - Immediately postoperatively
    - Elevation
    - Active muscle pumping
  - Beginning after dressing removal
    - Soft-tissue mobilization
    - Retrograde massage
    - Cryotherapy
    - Compression
      - We find that a compressive sleeve, such as Tubigrip, offers more consistent compression and is easier to don than an Ace wrap.
      - If hand edema is present, a compressive glove is issued.
- Scar management is initiated following incisional healing and suture removal to optimize gliding between the surgical scar and surrounding tissues.
  - Soft-tissue mobilization is performed with superficial as well as deep pressure, moving longitudinally, cross-frictionally, and in circles over the incision.
  - Silicone gel sheeting, paper tape, or elastomer with compression can be utilized for very thick or adherent scars.
- Desensitization is initiated after the dressing is removed.
  - Graded stimulation
    - Deep pressure and light touch
    - Tapping
    - Vibration
    - Hot and cold
    - Varying textures (smooth to progressively rougher)
  - A sleeve or pad over the elbow can be used until sensitivity diminishes.
    - It may be used during functional tasks, and occasionally during sleep.
    - Some patients find a thin sleeve, such as Tubigrip (Mölnlycke Health Care, Norcross, GA), helpful in decreasing hypersensitivity from light touch.
    - Some patients prefer thicker padding, such as a HeelBo (Briggs Healthcare, Waukegan, IL) pad.

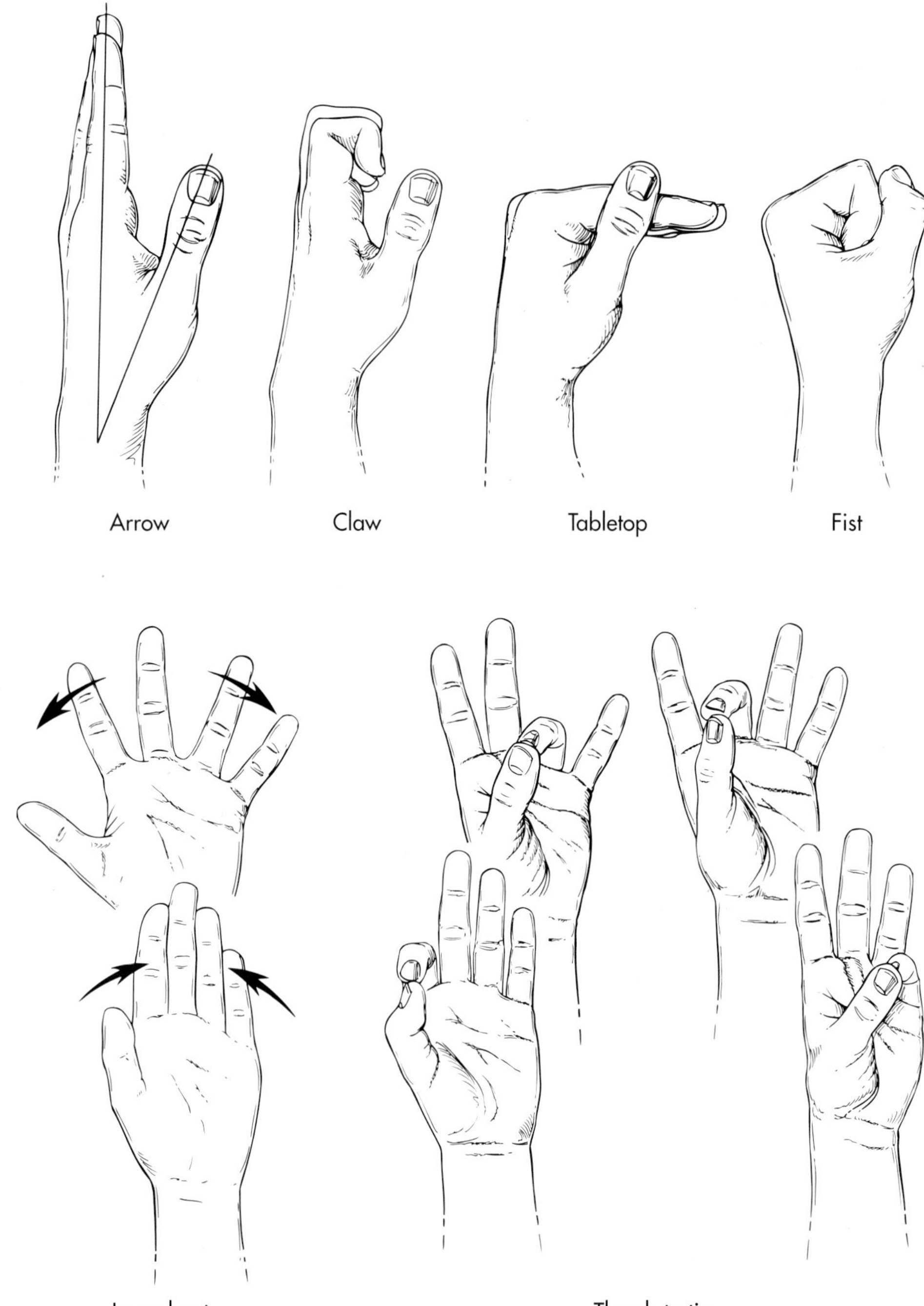

Figure 18.13 Illustration of "Six-pack exercises." All patients are immediately started on digit exercises focusing on tendon gliding, flexion, extension, abduction and adduction, and opposition. (Reproduced with permission from Cooney WP: *The Wrist: Diagnosis and Operative Treatment*, ed 2. Philadelphia, PA, Wolters Kluwer, 2010.)

- Most patients accommodate to MABC numbness, and rarely causes long-term deficiencies.
- Sensory compensation: in cases with long-standing absent or altered sensation, reinnervation may be delayed or unlikely. Education on being cautious when handling sharp or hot items is warranted. Compensating visually by keeping the ulnar side of the hand in direct vision is necessary.
- Modalities are initiated after the dressing is removed.
  - Thermal modalities: Care must be taken to avoid thermal injury; close monitoring is advised when using thermal modalities in areas of altered sensation.
    - Moist heat
      - Increases blood flow
      - Pain relief
      - Increases soft-tissue pliability

 © 2018 American Academy of Orthopaedic Surgeons

- Cryotherapy
  - Pain relief
  - Edema reduction
- Ultrasound
  - Provides deep heat
  - Pain relief
  - Increases blood flow
- Electrical stimulation
  - Neuromuscular reeducation
  - Often difficult to isolate intrinsic muscles with stimulation
  - Transcutaneous electrical nerve stimulation (TENS): Rarely used in our practice
- Range of Motion
  - Active range of motion (AROM) and active-assistive ROM (AAROM) of digits starts immediately postoperatively. Wrist, forearm, elbow, and shoulder ROM is initiated immediately after postoperative dressing removal. If joint contractures are present, passive digit ROM may be initiated immediately.
  - Gentle passive elbow ROM—including forearm rotation, if necessary—is added at 1 to 2 weeks postoperatively.
  - If the wrist flexor/pronator origin has been repaired as part of the operative procedure (such as intra- or submuscular transposition), elbow ROM is initiated with the wrist and forearm in neutral rotation. Forearm rotation and wrist flexion and extension are added at 2 to 3 weeks postoperatively.
  - ROM is progressed as patient tolerance allows.
- Bracing
  - An MCP block brace may be needed to remediate ring and small finger clawing until nerve regeneration occurs (see Figure 18.7).
  - Buddy strapping can be used for small finger adduction until adductor digiti minimi function returns (see Figure 18.8).
- Strengthening
  - Submuscular or intramuscular transposition
    - Strengthening is delayed for 6 weeks to allow healing of the flexor pronator muscles
    - Light strengthening is initiated with grasp, pinch, wrist flexion and extension, forearm supination and pronation, as well as elbow flexion and extension.
    - Resistance is increased as tolerance allows.
  - In situ decompression, anterior subcutaneous transposition, and medial epicondylectomy
    - Strengthening is initiated at 2 to 4 weeks postoperatively.
    - Gentle progressive resistance exercises are initiated once full active ROM is achieved and pain tolerance allows, and resistance is progressed as tolerated.
  - Hand strengthening
    - Grasp: Therapy putty, hand exerciser with rubber band resistance for gross grasp and hook fist
    - Pinch strengthening: Therapy putty to address three-jaw chuck and lateral pinches
    - Hand intrinsics: Therapy putty for digit abduction and adduction, or rubber band can be used for abduction, sponge for adduction
  - Wrist, forearm, elbow, and shoulder strengthening: Free weights, cuff weights, or resistance bands
- Functional tasks
  - General principles
    - Nonresistive functional tasks are initiated first.
    - Resistive activities are added cautiously and advanced as patient tolerance allows.
    - Avoid activities that require prolonged or repetitive elbow motion.
    - Proper postural alignment should be maintained, and position changed frequently to avoid distal strain and overuse.
  - Facilitate active use of affected extremity
    - Encourage return to self-care, light household tasks, and leisure activities
    - Activities to facilitate hand use
      - Coin manipulation
      - Picking up beads with tweezers
      - Picking pegs or beads from buried within putty
      - Games: Mancala, Marbles, Connect Four, Operation
      - Leisure: Needle crafts, puzzles
      - Household tasks: Dishwashing
      - Work tasks: Computer usage, writing
      - Tasks to facilitate elbow flexion
        - Self-care around face and head: Washing hair, applying make-up, shaving, donning/doffing earrings or necklace
      - Tasks to encourage elbow extension
        - Household: Dusting, washing windows
      - Tasks to encourage bilateral upper extremity use
        - Household: Folding laundry, making bed
        - Leisure: Throwing large beach ball, floor loom weaving
      - Activities to promote strength and endurance
        - Household: Carrying laundry baskets, mopping floors, grocery shopping
        - Leisure: Gardening, exercise class, sports pursuits

OUTCOMES

No surgical technique for treating cubital tunnel syndrome has been shown to have superior outcomes over others in primary surgery. Several studies have shown equivalent outcomes for in situ decompression and subcutaneous transposition in patients with normal or mildly positive EMG/NCS. In patients with moderate or severe cubital tunnel syndrome, in situ decompression has poorer outcomes. Dellon reported that submuscular transposition had the best outcomes in cases of severe cubital tunnel syndrome. However, in severe cases, only 50% achieved excellent restoration of sensation, and only 25% achieved excellent results with regard to motor function.

© 2018 American Academy of Orthopaedic Surgeons

Poorer outcomes are expected with older patient age, alcoholism, diabetes, concomitant polyneuropathy, or double-crush phenomenon. Longer duration of symptoms portends poorer results, as does the presence of intrinsic atrophy, clawing, or severe findings on EMG/NCS. Revision surgery has less predictable symptom resolution than primary surgery. Goldfarb reported a 20% revision rate of in situ decompressions, and has reported acceptable results with revision to anterior submuscular transposition. Revision of subcutaneous transposition requires adjunctive procedures, either nerve wrap, vascularized adipose pedicled flap, or placement of the nerve into an intramuscular or submuscular position.

PEARLS

- Nonoperative treatment of ulnar neuropathy includes ergonomic adjustments and activity modifications, and can be enhanced or optimized by therapists.
- Preoperative optimization to minimize clawing, PIP contractures, and small finger abduction, can improve hand function and aid the postoperative recovery.
- The choice of surgical procedure is dependent on the severity of the neuropathy, the presence or absence of ulnar nerve subluxation, and surgeon preference and comfort with the various procedures.
- Complete surgical decompression of all pathologic structures and complete mobilization of the ulnar nerve to avoid iatrogenic compression or kinking is essential.
- Discussion of patient expectations and use of appropriate preoperative and postoperative rehabilitation is critical to achieve optimal outcomes.
- Finger motion should be initiated immediately postoperatively.
- After dressing removal, elbow ROM and desensitization of both the MABC and ulnar nerves should be initiated, supplemented with pharmacologic treatment, if necessary.
- Light activities of daily living can be initiated immediately; however, strengthening should be delayed for 6 weeks if intramuscular, transmuscular, or submuscular ulnar nerve transposition is performed.
- The use of appropriate orthoses or padding can be of great benefit for patients with clawing, small finger abduction, or cutaneous sensitivity.

SUMMARY

A combination of medical intervention and therapeutic techniques can produce positive outcomes of both conservative and surgical treatment of ulnar neuropathy. Patients with recent-onset, mild, or intermittent symptoms may respond favorably to nonsurgical treatment. Surgical intervention is required if nonoperative treatment fails to resolve symptoms, or for those patients presenting with more advanced symptoms (constant altered sensation, motor weakness, and intrinsic atrophy). Individuals with symptoms of less than 12 months and without atrophy generally achieve good outcomes; in cases with preexistent motor loss or muscle wasting, or in patients with chronic disease, recovery may be more limited. Appropriate preoperative and postoperative rehabilitation is critical in achieving optimal results.

BIBLIOGRAPHY

Apfel E, Sigafoos GT: Comparison of range of motion constraints provided by splints used in the treatment of cubital tunnel syndrome—a pilot study. *J Hand Ther* 2006;19(4):384–391; quiz 392.

Cobb TK: Endoscopic cubital tunnel release. *J Hand Surg Am* 2010;35(10):1690–1697.

Coppieters MW, Butler DS: Do 'sliders' slide and 'tensioners' tension? An analysis of neurodynamic techniques and considerations regarding their application. *Man Ther* 2008;13:213–221

Danoff JR, Lombardi JM, Rosenwasser MP: Use of a pedicled adipose flap as a sling for anterior subcutaneous transposition of the ulnar nerve. *J Hand Surg Am* 2014;39(3):552–555.

Day JM, Willoughby J, Pitts DG, McCallum M, Foister R, Uhl TL: Outcomes following the conservative management of patients with non-radicular peripheral neuropathic pain. *J Hand Ther* 2014;27:192–200.

Dellon AL: Review of treatment results for ulnar nerve entrapment at the elbow. *J Hand Surg Am* 1989;14:688–700.

Earle AS, Vlastou C: Crossed fingers and other tests of ulnar nerve motor function. *J Hand Surg Am* 1980;5:560–565.

Goldfarb CA, Sutter MM, Martens EJ, Manske PR: Incidence of re-operation and subjective outcome following in situ decompression of the ulnar nerve at the cubital tunnel. *J Hand Surg Eur* 2009;34(3):379–383.

Hoffmann R, Siemionow M: The endoscopic management of cubital tunnel syndrome.*J Hand Surg Br* 2006;31(1):23–29.

Krogue JD, Aleem AW, Osei DA, Goldfarb CA, Calfee RP: Predictors of surgical revision after in situ decompression of the ulnar nerve. *J Shoulder Elbow Surg* 2015;24(4):634–639.

Lund AT, Amadio PC: Treatment of cubital tunnel syndrome: perspectives for the therapist. *J Hand Ther* 2006;19(2):170–179.

Mackinnon SE, Novak CB: Compression Neuropathies, In Wolfe SW, Hotchkiss RW, Pederson WC, Kozin SH, eds: *Green's Operative Hand Surgery*, ed 6. Philadelphia, PA, Elsevier, 2011.

McAdam SA, Ghandi R, Bezuhly M, Lefaivre KA: Simple decompression versus anterior subcutaneous and submuscular transposition of the ulnar nerve for cubital tunnel syndrome: a metaanalysis. *J Hand Surg Am* 2008;33(8):e1–e12.

Novak CB, Lee GW, Mackinnon SE, Lay L: Provocative testing for cubital tunnel syndrome. *J Hand Surg Am* 1994;19:817–820.

Rayann GM, Jensen C, Duke J: Elbow flexion test in the normal population. *J Hand Surg Am* 1992;17:86–89.

Zlodowski M, Chan S, Bhandari M, Kalliainen L, Schubert W: Anterior transposition compared with simple decompression for treatment of cubital tunnel syndrome. A meta-analysis of randomized, controlled trials. *J Bone Joint Surg Am* 2007;89:2591–2598.

© 2018 American Academy of Orthopaedic Surgeons

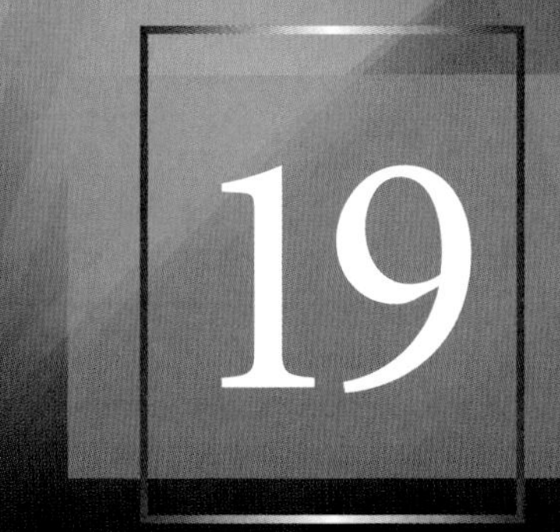

19 Rehabilitation After ORIF of Elbow Dislocations

Cynthia Watkins, PT, DPT, CHT, and Charles L. Getz, MD

INTRODUCTION

Elbow joint stability is dependent on a highly congruent skeletal articulation and collateral ligaments. Dislocations of the elbow are relatively common, being the second most commonly dislocated major joint. Most simple elbow dislocations are managed with closed reduction, a brief period of immobilization, and early protected rehabilitation. Elbow dislocations associated with fractures of the radial head and the coronoid are complex injuries that are much more likely to require surgical intervention.

RELEVANT ANATOMY

The elbow is stabilized by both the bony congruency of the joint and the periarticular soft-tissue structures. The soft-tissue structures on the medial side (Figure 19.1) are the medial collateral ligament (MCL) complex and the flexor pronator mass. The lateral (Figure 19.2) side soft tissues include the lateral collateral ligament complex (LCL) and the extensor and supinator muscular complex. The primary restraint to valgus instability is the radial capitellar joint, while the MCL is a secondary stabilizer that becomes the primary stabilizer if the radial head is removed. The bony congruency of the ulnar trochlear articulation is the primary restraint to varus stress, with the LCL being a secondary stabilizer.

Supination and axial loading of the forearm causes the ulna and radial head to rotate away from the distal humerus, with the radial head translating posterior to the capitellum and the lateral ulna rotating away from the lateral trochlea. The lateral ulnar collateral ligament (LUCL) is the primary stabilizer to prevent this instability pattern, known as posterolateral rotatory instability (PRLI).

Most elbow dislocations occur as a result of a fall onto an outstretched arm. The forearm is forcibly supinated and axially loaded. In addition, the valgus-carrying angle and slight degree of flexion convert the axial load into a valgus thrust. This mechanism results in injury of the stabilizing structures around the elbow. O'Driscoll described the stages of elbow instability as beginning with a failure of the LUCL, with progressive disruption of the anterior and posterior capsule. In severe cases, the medial ulnar collateral ligament (MUCL) is also injured. This unlocks the forearm from the humerus, and allows the radial head to dislocate behind the capitellum.

In cases of complex instability, the radial head is driven into the capitellum and the coronoid into the trochlea before the forearm is fully disengaged, resulting in various degrees of fracture of the radial head and coronoid in addition to the collateral ligament injuries. The terrible triad injury pattern consists of an elbow dislocation, radial head fracture, and coronoid fracture.

PRLI is a relatively rare late sequelae of traumatic elbow dislocation or subluxation. It occurs when the LCL complex fails to heal sufficiently to prevent the forearm from rotating away from the humerus, resulting in either recurrent frank dislocations or subluxations of the elbow. Varus posteromedial rotatory instability (VPRI) is caused by a varus load, which results in failure of the LCL under tension and fracture of the medial ulna joint line due to compression of the coronoid against the medial aspect of the trochlea.

OPERATIVE TREATMENT

Simple Elbow Dislocations

For the majority of patients with simple elbow dislocations, a brief period of immobilization followed by protected early range of motion (ROM) will result in a favorable outcome. In rare cases, the elbow will not be stable even with the elbow in 90° of flexion and the forearm pronated. These patients require operative stabilization of the elbow.

Dr. Getz or an immediate family member is a member of a speakers' bureau or has made paid presentations on behalf of Mitek and Zimmer; serves as a paid consultant to Cayenne Medical; serves as an unpaid consultant to Zimmer; has stock or stock options held in OBERD; and has received research or institutional support from Integra, Rotation Medical, and Zimmer. Neither Dr. Watkins nor any immediate family member has received anything of value from or has stock or stock options held in a commercial company or institution related directly or indirectly to the subject of this article.

© 2018 American Academy of Orthopaedic Surgeons

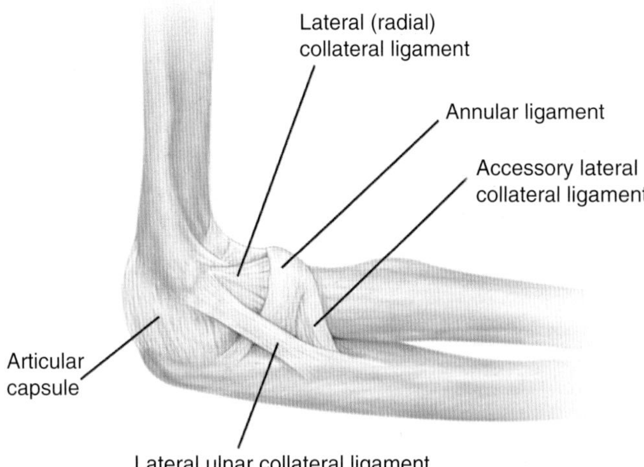

Figure 19.1 Illustration of the medial elbow ligamentous complex. (Reproduced with permission from Gramstad G: Anatomy of the shoulder, arm, and elbow, in Boyer MI, ed: *AAOS Comprehensive Orthopaedic Review 2.* Rosemont, IL, American Academy of Orthopaedic Surgeons, 2014.)

A small number of patients will continue to have radiographic findings of instability at 7 to 14 days or clinical findings of instability at 14 days, thus will be considered for surgical stabilization. In the majority of these cases, the LCL and common extensor origin are found torn away from the lateral epicondyle, and can be anatomically repaired either with sutures through bone tunnels or with suture anchors. If the LCL is torn midsubstance, a ligament reconstruction with a tendon graft may be required (Figure 19.3). Uncommonly, the MCL will also require repair or reconstruction after the lateral repair. If the elbow continues to have instability after both sides of the elbow are addressed, an external fixator is applied to maintain the reduction.

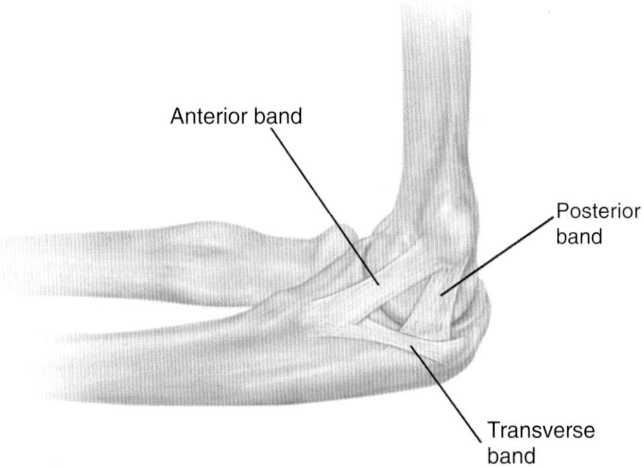

Figure 19.2 Illustration of the lateral elbow ligamentous complex. (Reproduced with permission from Gramstad G: Anatomy of the shoulder, arm, and elbow, in Boyer MI, ed: *AAOS Comprehensive Orthopaedic Review 2.* Rosemont, IL, American Academy of Orthopaedic Surgeons, 2014.)

Ideally, fixation of all of the injuries will be secure enough to start earlier rehabilitation. However, extensive repairs or swelling may require a delay in the initiation of therapy. Wound healing and infection prevention is the highest priority, then joint stability, and finally ROM after complex elbow repairs.

Stabilization surgery can be done through a posterior incision with full-thickness skin and subcutaneous flaps raised to allow access to the lateral and medial sides of the joint. Alternatively, separate direct lateral and medial incisions can be used. The laterally based incision requires less soft-tissue dissection and may lead to less wound healing problems than a posterior incision. The potential need for future additional surgery is also a consideration when planning the surgical approach. A lateral incision may be preferred if future surgical contracture release is planned, while a posterior incision would be preferred for later elbow replacement.

Complex Instability: Fracture Dislocations

Complex instability falls into two main catagories, terrible triad injuries and VPRI. Terrible triad injuries involve fractures in addition to the ligamentous injuries, as described for simple elbow dislocations. Surgery is recommended when the fractures of the coronoid or radial head would require intervention on their own. Surgery is also recommended if the joint is not congruently reduced or the elbow demonstrates clinical instability at greater than 45° of flexion.

Surgery to address terrible triad injuries requires repair of types II and III coronoid fractures, radial head repair or replacement, and repair or reconstruction of the LCL. MCL repair often may be required to stabilize the elbow as well as application of an external fixator. Management of coronoid fractures can be difficult especially if there is comminution. Although the coronoid is most easily accessed from the medial side it can also be reached from the lateral side if a radial head replacement is required. Coronoid fractures can be fixed with a variety of techniques, including screws, small plates and screws, and transosseous sutures. The decision for a single posterior incision or separate lateral and medial incisions is based on surgeon preference. These injuries often include extensive soft-tissue injuries, and swelling can be a problem. Wound healing problems can be a major complication of surgery for these injuries.

VPRI may include subtle injuries and require operative intervention when the trochlea is not congruent and/or the radial capitellar joint is gapped on an anterioposterior elbow radiograph. Computed tomography (CT) is used to assess the joint alignment in suspected cases, as these injuries are often difficult to assess with plain radiographs. The coronoid fracture is addressed through a medial approach to the elbow by elevating the flexor carpi ulnaris muscle (FCU) anteriorly. The ulna nerve is identified and protected during this approach. The LCL requires a separate lateral approach to repair or reconstruct the ligament. If fixation is tenuous, an external fixation will be applied to offload the repaired joint and ligaments, and protect the reduction.

 © 2018 American Academy of Orthopaedic Surgeons

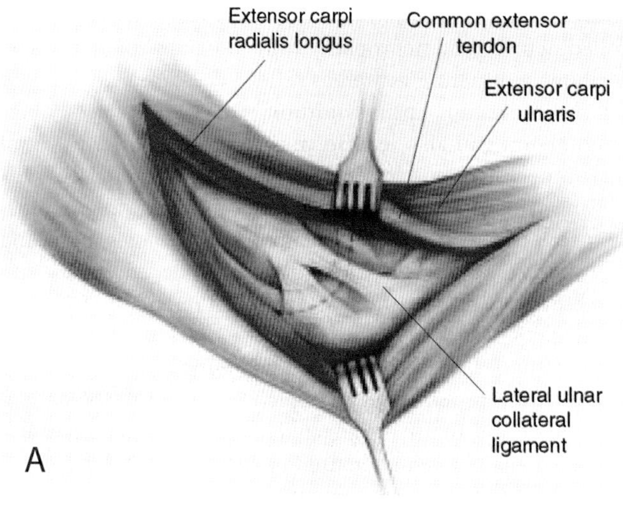

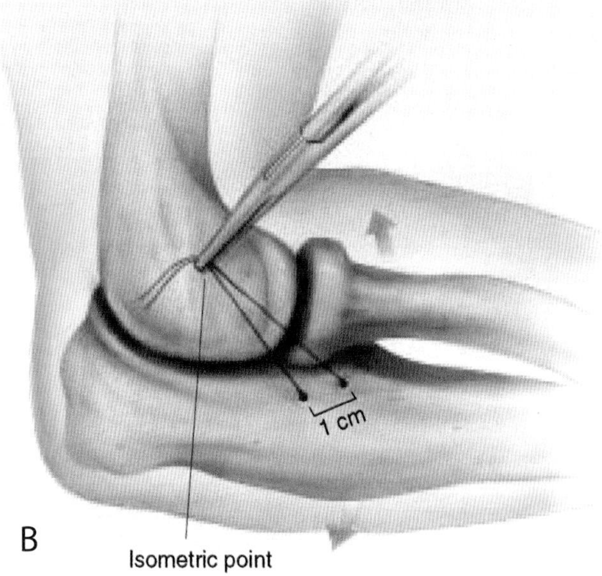

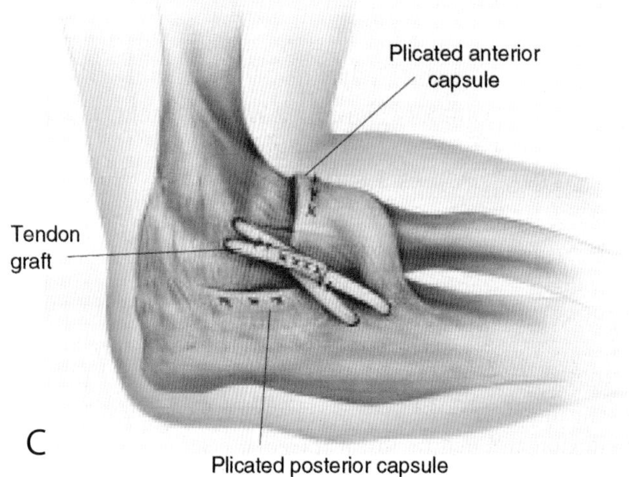

Figure 19.3 **A–C**, Illustrations of reconstruction of the lateral ulnar collateral ligament through an extended Kocher's approach. (Reproduced with permission from Morrey BF. Acute and chronic instability of the elbow. *J Am Acad Orthop Surg* 1996;4(3):117–128, and with permission from the Mayo Foundation for Medical Education and Research, Rochester, MN.)

POSTOPERATIVE REHABILITATION

Although there is no "one-size-fits-all" approach to rehabilitation after operative fixation of elbow instability injuries, there are general principles that can be applied and utilized in individual cases. The initial postoperative management focuses on preventing and decreasing swelling, managing pain, and protecting the repair. The primary rehabilitation goals after surgical treatment of elbow dislocation are restoring joint mobility while protecting the surgical repair, preserving elbow stability, and eventually restoring function. Increases in ROM should not be gained at the expense of joint stability. Restoring a functional arc of motion is essential to enabling the patient to return to normal activities. While normal elbow ROM has been measured as 0° to 140° of flexion and extension, and supination/pronation 80° to 85°, the functional ROM to complete most activities of daily living (ADLs) has been established as 30° to 130° (flexion/extension) and 50°/50° supination/pronation, although some common tasks may require higher degrees of flexion and forearm rotation. It is important to educate the patient early about the expected ROM losses, especially elbow extension. A loss of 15° of elbow extension is not an uncommon sequela of even simple elbow dislocations.

Patients are splinted in the operating room and placed in a sling. The splint rests the soft tissue to help reduce swelling and protect the repair. The splint is typically discontinued 7 to 10 days after surgery. The splint can be replaced with either a custom-molded orthoplast removable splint, or a prefabricated brace, which can be removed for hygiene and permit early ROM exercise while protecting the repair (Figure 19.4).

Gentle active and active assisted exercises are typically initiated within the first 7 to 10 days after surgery. Active range of motion (AROM) rather than passive range of motion (PROM) is advocated to take advantage of the compressive stabilizing forces of the muscles surrounding the elbow. The patient is encouraged to remove the orthosis and perform these exercises at frequent intervals throughout the day. As the bone and soft tissues begin to heal, the ROM can be progressed and light functional activities can be initiated. Strengthening is begun once the joint is declared stable by the physician. In general,

© 2018 American Academy of Orthopaedic Surgeons

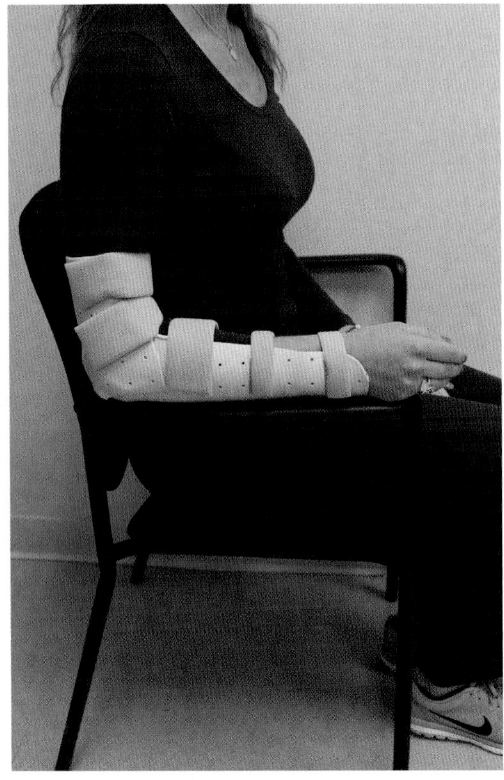

Figure 19.4 Photograph of posterior elbow custom splint.

the elbow has enough healing to tolerate strengthening around 8 weeks after surgery. Comminuted coronoid or radial head fractures may need to be protected for a longer duration.

Dependent on the amount of soft-tissue trauma, there may be substantial swelling and edema in the first 14 days postoperatively. Capsular thickening and co-contracture of the brachialis muscle develops within days of the injury, leading to restricted movement of the elbow, especially with extension. Edema management can include elevation, retrograde massage, and the use of light compressive dressings and sleeves.

Pain also contributes to stiffness and muscle guarding. The therapist needs to distinguish between the normal level of pain associated with the injury and surgery versus pain from nerve irritation. Care must be taken to monitor the ulnar nerve on the medial aspect of the elbow for irritation/instability. Symptoms will include tenderness to palpation of the medial aspect of the elbow and paresthesias in the ring and small fingers. Uncontrolled neuritis and neuropathy with associated pain can lead to elbow contracture as well as reflex sympathetic dystrophy and chronic regional pain syndrome (CRPS). Prolonged ulnar compression can also lead to muscle atrophy or wasting of ulnar innervated muscles, including the hand interossei.

Pain management techniques, including medication, transcutaneous electrical nerve stimulation (TENS), biofeedback, and relaxation techniques may be employed to decrease pain and increase the ability to participate with the therapeutic exercises.

The patient is encouraged to use the affected arm for functional activities, within protected guidelines, throughout the rehabilitation process. For example, if in a splint, the patient may still be able to use the affected hand as a helper for ADLs. When a patient has a weight limit on lifting, it is still beneficial to use the elbow for unweighted ADLs. Since the function of the elbow is to position the hand for functional activities such as dressing, bathing, and eating, patients are usually highly motivated to progress toward these goals.

Authors' Preferred Protocol

Phase 1 (Inflammatory Phase, 0–2 Weeks) (Table 19.1)

Goals

- Protect the repair
- Decrease edema
- Decrease pain
- Influence scar formation/remodeling
- Prevent contracture

Orthosis

- Custom-fabricated long-arm orthosis with elbow in 90° of flexion and neutral forearm (radial head fracture) or pronated forearm (LCL repaired)
- Hinged elbow brace

Exercises

- Supine AA elbow flexion/extension (forearm in pronation if LCL repaired)
- AA supination/pronation (supine or seated)
- AROM/active-assisted range of motion (AAROM) of the wrist
- Tendon gliding exercises

Table 19.1 SUMMARY OF REHABILITATION DURING INFLAMMATORY PHASE

Protection	ROM	Edema Management	Scar Management	Pain Management	HEP	Functional Goal
Long-arm orthosis; hinged brace	AAROM in protected arc	Elevation, retrograde massage, compressive dressings	Scar massage, silicone sheets, desensitization	TENS, IFC, ice, medications as prescribed by physician	Elbow AAROM in protected arc, AROM to unaffected joints	Light use of affected hand while wearing protective orthosis

AAROM = active assisted range of motion, AROM = active range of motion, ROM = range of motion, IFC = interferential current therapy, TENS = transcutaneous electrical nerve stimulation.

© 2018 American Academy of Orthopaedic Surgeons

- AROM of the shoulder (protective orthosis may be worn for comfort)

Edema Management

- Elevate arm above heart level
- Retrograde massage
- Elastic compression sleeve

Scar Management

- Scar massage 2 to 3 times daily with cocoa butter or vitamin E after sutures are removed

Phase 1 (0–2 Weeks Postoperatively)

Protection/Immobilization

Customarily, the patient is placed into a custom-fabricated long-arm orthosis with varying degrees of elbow flexion and forearm rotation, depending on the repaired structures. The elbow is most stable at 90° of flexion. Pronating the forearm will protect lateral ligamentous structures, while supination protects medial structures and stresses the lateral side. Care must be taken to pad the orthosis to protect bony prominences (medial/lateral epicondyles, olecranon, and ulnar styloid), avoid undue pressure, and prevent skin irritation/breakdown. The patient is instructed to remove the orthosis three to four times daily for exercises, hygiene, and light functional activities. The orthosis is worn in this manner for approximately 6 weeks.

Range of Motion

AAROM exercises are begun at the first postoperative visit, generally within 7 to 10 days after surgery. Exercises are started in a supine position. When the primary instability involves the LCL repair, extension is safest with the forearm pronated. If the instability primarily involves MCL repair, extension is safest with the forearm in supination. If both the MCL and LCL are repaired or severely injured or repaired, then extension should be performed with the forearm in neutral rotation. Performing exercises in the supine position allows for scapular stabilization and helps the patient avoid substitution patterns. It also lowers shear forces to the coronoid process (if repaired), decreases the firing of the brachialis muscle, and allows gravity to assist with flexion. When performing supine elbow motion exercises, the patient lies supine, with the shoulder in 90° of forward flexion, and uses the unaffected arm to assist the affected arm through the stable arc of motion (Figure 19.5). If the patient cannot tolerate supine positioning or if the instability is minor, seated extension exercises are also an option. In the same supine position, the patient can use the unaffected hand to gently pronate and supinate the forearm with the elbow in flexion (Figure 19.6).

This position also requires the patient to engage the triceps muscle when extending the elbow against gravity. Activation of the triceps helps to keep the joint stabilized. Usually, the patient will have some amount of an extension deficit, but if the patient has difficulty maintaining extension restrictions set by the physician, then a template orthosis can be fabricated to provide a block, preventing the patient from extending past the limits of stability that were determined at the time of surgery.

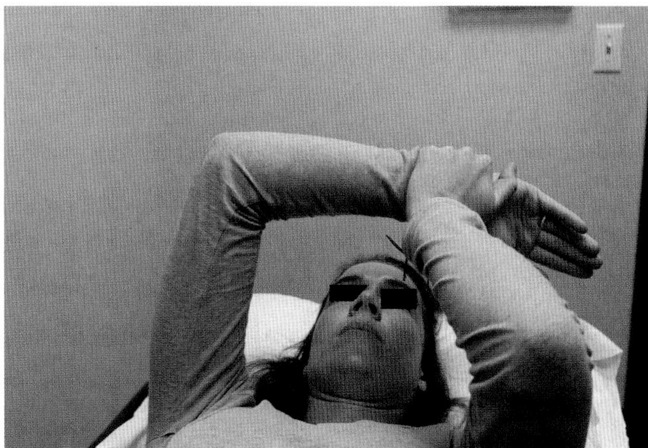

Figure 19.5 Photograph of supine active assisted elbow flexion/extension.

Forearm rotation exercises are performed with the elbow in 90° of flexion and the forearm supported on the table. It is important to initiate rotation early, especially if the radial head has been repaired. These exercises can also be performed in the supine position when increased stability is required due to a LCL repair. Simple functional activities, such as flipping cards or turning pages of a magazine, can be used to reinforce active pronation and supination motion.

Active and active assisted exercises of the shoulder, wrist, and hand are performed to avoid stiffness and muscle atrophy.

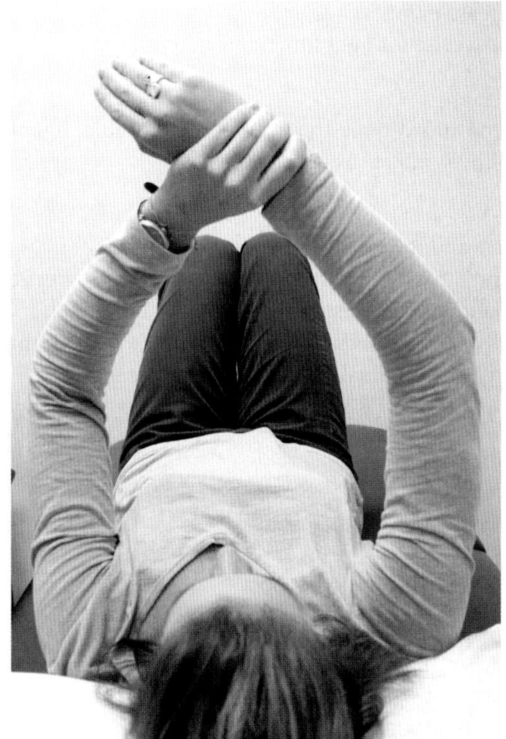

Figure 19.6 Photograph of supine active assisted supination/pronation.

© 2018 American Academy of Orthopaedic Surgeons

Table 19.2 SUMMARY OF REHABILITATION DURING FIBROBLASTIC PHASE

Protection	ROM	Edema Management	Scar Management	Pain Management	HEP	Functional Goals
Orthosis in crowded areas. Avoid activities that cause traction to the joint (carrying a heavy briefcase or bag). Avoid pushing heavy doors.	AROM/AAROM All joints of affected upper extremity, grade I and II joint mobilizations	Ice, retrograde massage, compressive dressings	Scar massage, silicone sheets, desensitization, fluidotherapy	TENS, IFC, ice, medications as prescribed by physician	Moist heat applied at end range prior to exercises. AROM/AAROM with emphasis on end range.	Use of affected arm for light functional activities, typing, donning clothing, tying necktie, eating. Encourage natural position of the arm when walking.

AAROM = active assisted range of motion, AROM = active range of motion, ROM = range of motion, IFC = interferential current therapy, TENS = transcutaneous electrical nerve stimulation.

Phase 2 (Fibroblastic Phase, 2–8 Weeks Postoperatively) (Table 19.2)

Goals

- Increase ROM (add PROM as appropriate if stability of the elbow is no longer a concern)
- Influence soft tissue and joint mobility through controlled stress
- Avoid inflammatory response
- Decrease edema
- Decrease pain
- Improve use for light functional activities

Orthosis

- Discontinued once fracture repair is stable, ligamentous stability is intact (usually 6–10 weeks)

Exercises

- Active and AA elbow flexion and extension
  - Initiate with forearm in pronation and progress to supination. Examples: physioball roll, cane stretch
- Active and AA forearm rotation. Examples: hammer stretch, AA manual stretch, neoprene strap

Edema Management/Pain Management

- Elastic compressive sleeve
- Retrograde massage
- TENS/interferential current

Scar Management

- Silicone sheet, as needed
- Desensitization techniques
- Scar mobilization

Phase 2 (2–8 Weeks Postoperatively)

During this stage of recovery, the patient is weaned out of the orthosis for light activities and has typically discontinued use of the protective orthosis by around 6 weeks. The surgeon assesses ligamentous stability and obtains plain radiographs to confirm that the joint is congruently reduced and that any fractures are healing.

Joint stiffness, especially with extension deficit, is typical at this stage. The use of modalities, such as moist heat, prior to performing ROM increases tissue extensibility, increases blood flow, and relaxes the patient. Positioning the patient in the supine position with the affected elbow at the end range of available extension allows for a prolonged stretch prior to any ROM techniques.

PROM for all joints of the affected upper extremity is now allowed. A low-load, prolonged force is applied to the point of discomfort, not pain, to avoid any inflammatory response. Joint mobilizations (grade I or II) are performed to increase mobility in areas that are lacking end range movement, typically elbow extension and supination. It is important to vary the force and position of the mobilization as the patient exhibits ROM gains. For example, with elbow extension, the force should always be applied perpendicular to the ulna at the ulnohumeral joint. As the patient gains extension, the therapist will need to adjust the patient's hand and body positions during the mobilization to continue to deliver the force in a perpendicular fashion. Likewise, as pain subsides, grades III and IV mobilizations can be used, moving the joint further through the restricted ROM to achieve increases at the end-range points (Figures 19.7 and 19.8). It is also important to avoid overly aggressive PROM techniques. Ballistic, high-force movements can injure soft tissues that are beginning to heal and stimulate heterotopic ossification.

Contract/relax techniques can be utilized during PROM to fatigue the bicep and brachialis muscles, and allow for increased elbow extension. This technique also engages the patient to participate and gives the patient a sense of control when having stretch applied to the arm.

The patient can now start performing AROM and AAROM in sitting or standing positions. Exercises are generally begun

© 2018 American Academy of Orthopaedic Surgeons

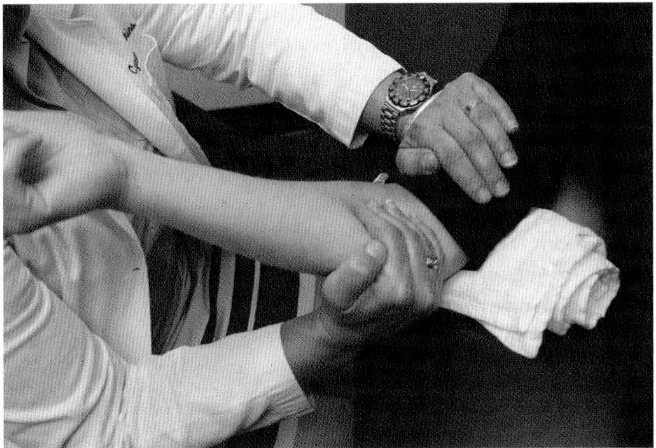

Figure 19.7 Photograph of ulnohumeral joint mobilization.

in protected postures with the forearm in pronation and the elbow moving from flexion/extension, and are progressed to elbow flexion/extension with the forearm in supination. AROM exercises in proprioceptive neuromuscular facilitation (PNF) patterns are also useful at this stage to increase joint proprioception and encourage use of the arm in functional patterns. Manual force can be applied by the therapist and patient to provide graded resistance at varying points throughout the movement. In addition, the patient must perform independent exercises multiple times daily to maintain gains and increase mobility.

Functionally, the patient should be encouraged to use the affected arm for light ADLs, such as self-care and meal preparation. Styling hair, holding a cellphone, and tying neckties encourage elbow flexion. Folding laundry and typing promote forearm rotation. Patients are advised to allow the arm to swing naturally, avoiding the "sling" posture of elbow flexion, shoulder internal rotation, and adduction posture.

Active and Active Assisted Elbow Flexion and Extension

These exercises are begun with the forearm pronated and are progressed to supination as stability allows.

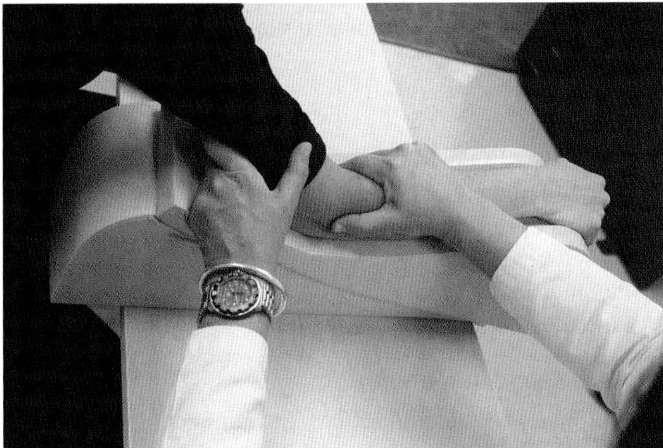

Figure 19.8 Photograph of radiohumeral joint mobilization.

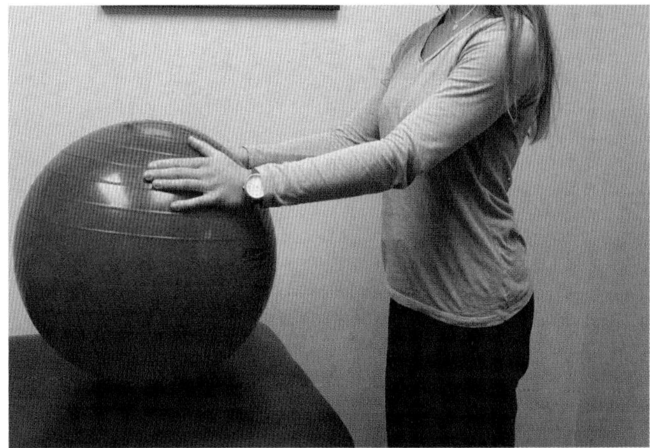

Figure 19.9 Photograph of active assisted elbow extension with a physioball.

1. Physioball roll on plinth with forearm in pronation Patient uses bilateral upper extremities to roll the physioball on the plinth with forearms in pronation. This exercise can also be performed with the affected arm as an active exercise (Figure 19.9).
2. Active Assisted Elbow Extension with Cane Standing with the scapula against the wall, bend and straighten the elbow. A cane can be used to increase extension. Instruct the patient to keep the olecranon in contact with the wall to avoid external rotation from the shoulder. A towel may be placed behind the brachium for feedback to help the patient maintain the correct posture (Figure 19.10).

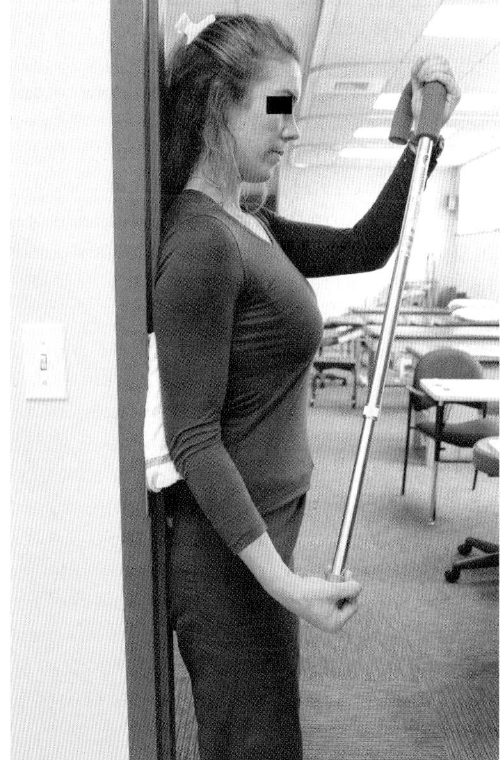

Figure 19.10 Photograph of elbow extension cane stretch.

© 2018 American Academy of Orthopaedic Surgeons

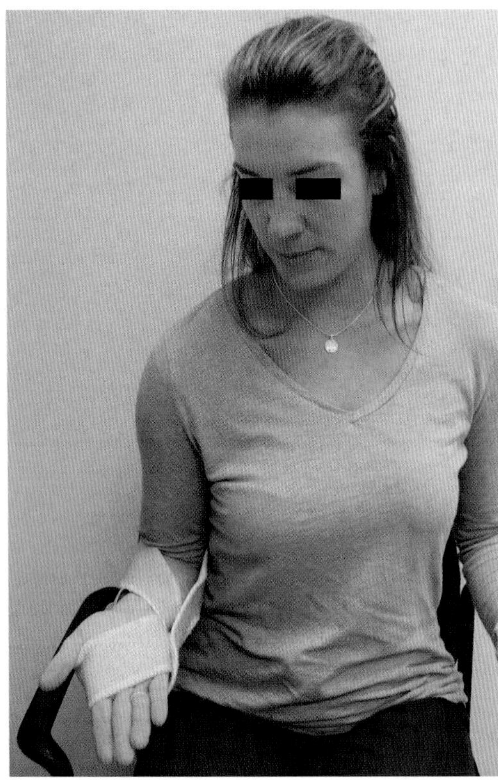

Figure 19.11 Photograph of supination strap stretch, which can be used to improve forearm rotation.

3. AROM/AAROM forearm: keeping the elbow at 90° of flexion Patient performs active pronation/supination seated at a table with the forearm supported. A weighted dowel or hammer can be used to provide stretch at end range. AA manual stretch can be performed with the patient using the uninvolved hand to provide the rotatory force. Also, a neoprene strap can be utilized to maintain the forearm in end-range supination with a low-load prolonged stress to the tissues (Figure 19.11). This is a simple, convenient way for patients to perform this stretch. If tissues do not respond to the strap (hard end feel), static-progressive or dynamic supination orthoses may be used.
4. Joint Mobilizations
   a. Ulnahumeral distraction to increase elbow extension. Patient lies supine with the elbow in a loose packed position, which is the position of maximal joint compression. The distal humerus is stabilized by one of the therapist's hands (or with a Mulligan belt [Mulligan Mobilisation Belt™]) while the opposite hand applies the distracting force 45° to the ulnar diaphysis. As the patient gains increased elbow extension, the therapist must vary the angle of the applied force (see Figure 19.7). Alternating isometrics are performed following the joint mobilizations to increase joint proprioception. The patient then actively uses the arm through the newly available ROM.
   b. Ulnahumeral distraction to increase elbow flexion. The distal humerus is stabilized by the therapist while the therapist's opposite hand distracts the ulna and provides a scooping motion. The patient performs self-mobilizations at home by placing a small rolled-up towel in the elbow crease and applying force to the distal ulna.
   c. Proximal radioulnar mobilizations to increase forearm rotation. The therapist will perform a volar medial glide to increase supination or a dorsolateral glide to increase pronation. Alternating isometrics are performed to increase joint proprioception, followed by AROM exercises, such as card flipping or rotation with a hand-held dowel or light hammer.
5. Grip and Wrist Strengthening: Putty squeezes or light wrist weights
6. Soft-Tissue Mobilization/Scar Management
   Retrograde massage can continue as long as there is edema present in the area. Patients often continue to wear the elastic compression sleeve for 3 to 4 weeks after the orthosis has been discontinued. The patient is instructed to perform scar massage twice daily using vitamin E or cocoa butter. If there is hypertrophic scar, a silicone scar sheet can be used. Scar sensitivity may require desensitization techniques using various textures or immersing the arm in particles (Fluidotherapy®).

Complications

Persistent pain, warmth and edema accompanied by a decrease in ROM may signal heterotopic ossificans. Pain, edema, stiffness in fingers, and skin discoloration may signal CRPS.

Phase 3: Scar Maturation and Fracture Consolidation (Approximately Weeks 8–6 Months) (Table 19.3)

Goals

- Maximize ROM
- Increase strength
- Increase endurance
- Return to functional activities, including recreation and work

Orthosis

- Static-progressive or dynamic splinting, as needed, to achieve end-range motion (especially elbow extension and supination)

Exercises

- AROM/AAROM/PROM, no restrictions
- Strengthening: Graded progressive resistive exercises with weights or resistance band
- Closed-chain activities
- Plyometrics
- Functional/work simulation

Phase 3: Range of Motion

At this phase, AROM and PROM, including composite movements, are allowed. Passive stretching and joint mobilizations may be employed to increase ROM in areas of limitations. If

© 2018 American Academy of Orthopaedic Surgeons

Table 19.3 SUMMARY OF REHABILITATION DURING CONSOLIDATION PHASE

Protection	ROM	Strength and Endurance	Orthosis Management	HEP	Functional Goals
Discontinue use of orthosis	AROM/PROM Goal is full AROM and PROM.	Isometrics progressing to PRES, functional patterns (PNF), proximal muscle strengthening (rotator cuff, scapular muscles), Work-simulated activities, including push/pull, lift/carry. Progress to weight-bearing activities and plyometrics.	Static-progressive orthoses to achieve ROM goals	AROM/PROM, strengthening exercises using weights, resistance bands	Return to ADLs, recreational activities, return to work

AAROM = active assisted range of motion, ADLs = activities of daily living, AROM = active range of motion, IFC = interferential current therapy, PNF = proprioceptive neuromuscular facilitation, PRES = progressive resistive exercises, PROM = passive range of motion, ROM = range of motion, TENS = transcutaneous electrical nerve stimulation.

the patient has significant ROM loss, an orthosis may be used to obtain end-range motion. Custom-fabricated or commercially available splints, such as Dynasplint (Dynasplint System Inc, Severna Park, MD) or JAS (Joint Active Systems Inc, Effingham, IL) may be worn to achieve this goal (Figure 19.12). We prefer custom orthotics that are remolded under the supervision of a therapist.

If the patient has limitation of both elbow flexion and extension, the patient may require two orthoses. In these cases, it is useful to wear the extension orthosis at night and the flexion orthosis at 30-minute intervals throughout the day. It is important to have the patient exercise in the newly available ROM upon orthosis removal to maintain ROM gains.

Strengthening exercises are begun when bony union has occurred and soft tissues are not inflamed. Functional activities and work conditioning are also performed. The work-simulated activities are tailored to the demands of the patient and the patient's specific job.

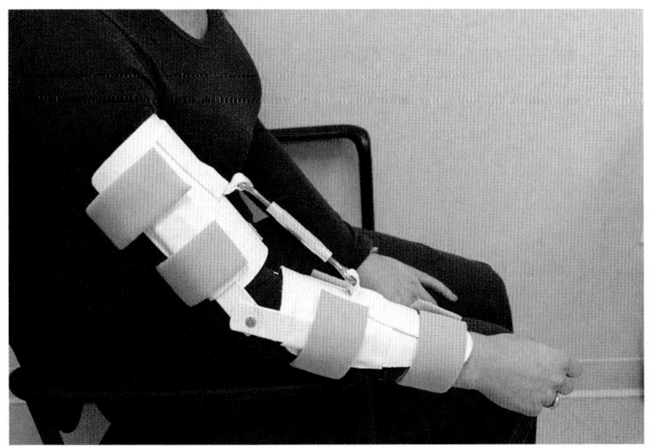

Figure 19.12 Photograph of turnbuckle extension orthosis.

Phase 3: Strengthening

1. Begin with isometrics in midrange
2. Progress to isotonic with light weight
   a. Bicep curls
   b. Tricep kickbacks/overhead tricep extension
   c. Supination/pronation with resistance band/flexbar
   d. Wrist flexion/extension with weight or resistance band
   e. PNF patterns with weight or resistance band (Figure 19.13).
3. Closed-chain activities
   a. Push-ups
      i. Wall
      ii. Counter (Figure 19.14)
      iii. Floor
      iv. BOSU (Bosu Fitness LLC, San Diego, CA) (Figure 19.15)
4. Functional/work simulation
   a. Box lift (Figure 19.16)
   b. Push/pull (Figure 19.17)
   c. Plyometrics-Trampoline toss

OUTCOMES

The approach to surgical treatment of elbow dislocations is determined by the extent of the anatomic injury, and has a bearing on the eventual outcome. For the terrible-triad patient, results were initially reported to be nearly uniformly poor. Improved understanding of the pathology and biomechanics of the elbow has led to about 70% good or excellent results with current treatment. Surgical indications for VPMI are still evolving, and reports of outcomes in these patients involve small case series. Simple elbow dislocations rarely require surgical stabilization, but when the elbow remains unstable

© 2018 American Academy of Orthopaedic Surgeons

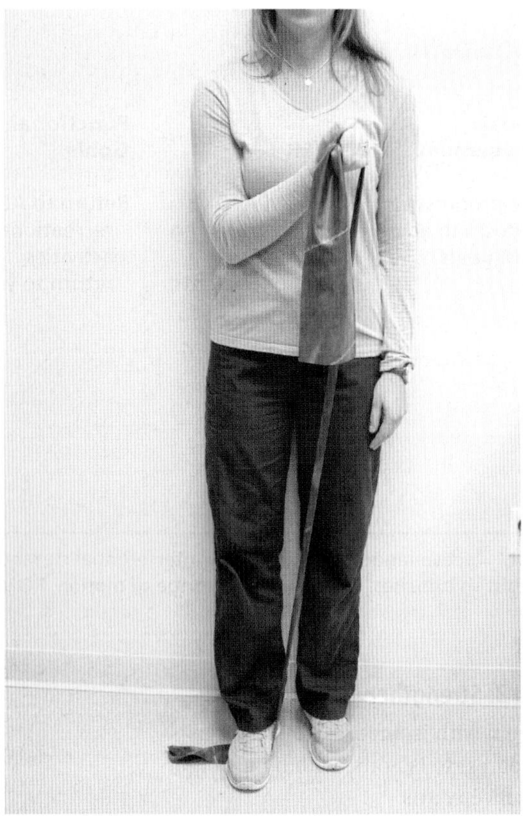

Figure 19.13 Photograph of proprioceptive neuromuscular facilitation with a resistance band.

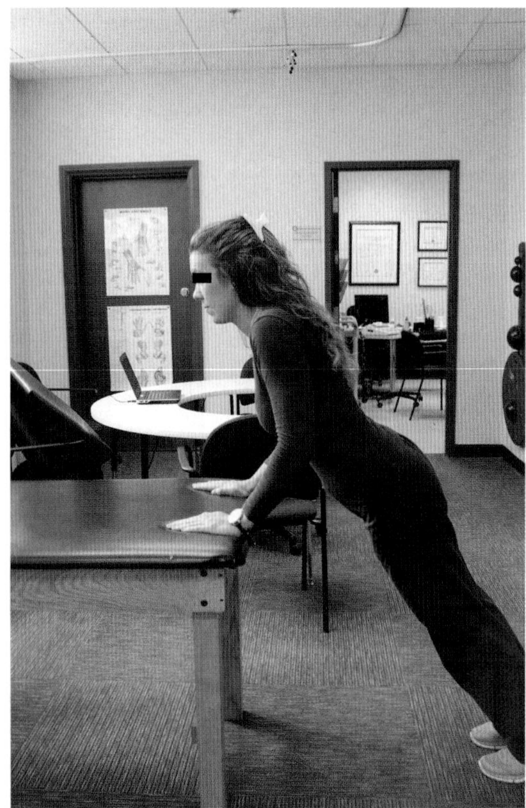

Figure 19.14 Photograph of counter push-ups.

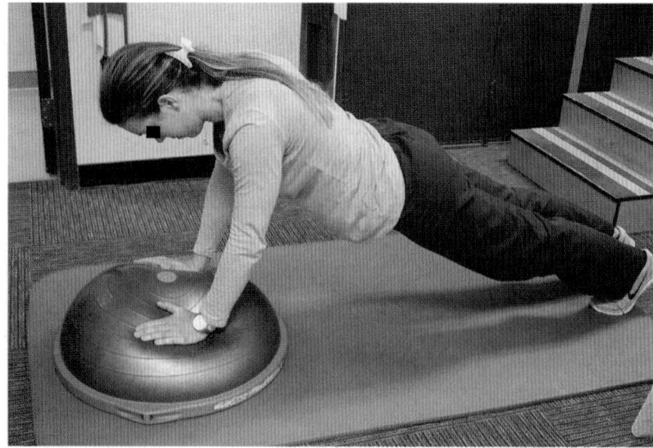

Figure 19.15 Photograph of BOSU push-ups.

after closed reduction, the outcome of operative treatment is reported to be good or excellent results in 90% of cases.

PEARLS

- Healing of the surgical wounds and controlling edema are the first priority after surgical treatment of elbow instability.
- Stability of the joint is more important than ROM; a stiff stable elbow can be surgically improved. The chronically unstable elbow is a difficult treatment dilemma, best treated by prevention.

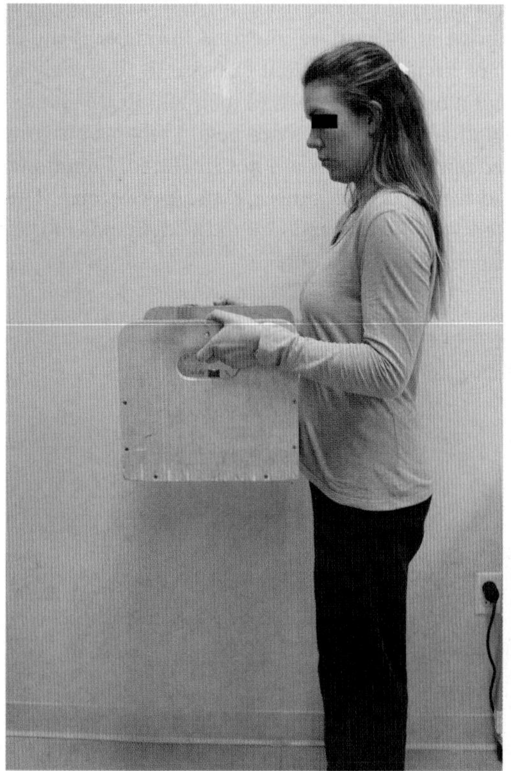

Figure 19.16 Photograph of the box lift exercise.

© 2018 American Academy of Orthopaedic Surgeons

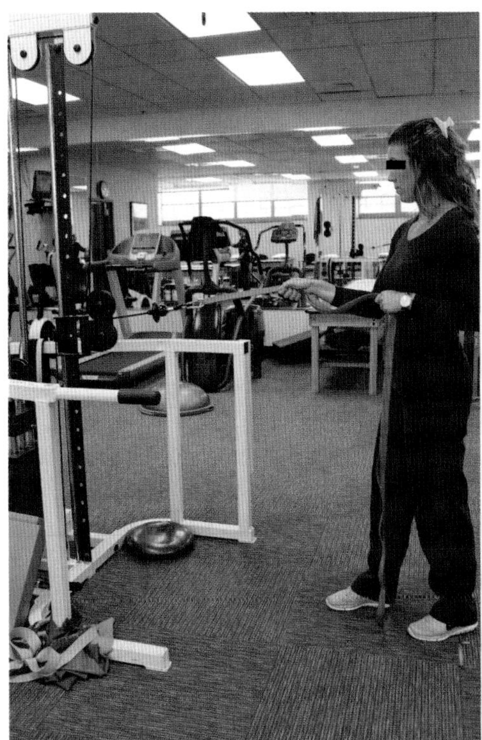

Figure 19.17 Photograph of the push/pull exercise.

- Determining the stable ROM, including the position of the forearm, is essential to determining the early rehabilitation protocol.
- The distracting weight of the forearm on the elbow can be negated by performing AA extension with the patient in the supine position.

SUMMARY

Successful surgical treatment of traumatic elbow instability requires an understanding of the normal anatomy and the underlying instability pattern by both the surgeon and the therapist. The structures repaired must be protected as the elbow is being mobilized. Therefore, it is important to have open communication between the patient, therapist, and surgeon to achieve the desired goals.

BIBLIOGRAPHY

An KN, Zobitz ME, Morrey BF: Biomechanics of the elbow, In Morrey BF, Sanchez-Sotelo J, eds. *The Elbow and its Disorders,* ed 4. Philadelphia, PA, Saunders, 2009, pp 39–63.

Chan K, King GJ, Faber KJ: Treatment of complex elbow fracture-dislocations. *Curr Rev Musculoskelet Med* 2016;9(2):185–189.

Davila S: Therapist's management of fractures and dislocations of the elbow, In Skirven TM, Osterman AL, Fedorczyk JM, Amadio PC, eds. *Rehabilitation of the Hand and Upper Extremity,* ed 6. Philadelphia, PA, Elsevier, 2011.

Doornberg JN, Ring DC: Fractures of the anteromedial facet of the coronoid process. *J Bone Joint Surg Am* 2006;88(10):2216–2224.

Heo YM, Yi JW, Lee JB, Lee DH, Park WK, Kim SJ: Unstable simple elbow dislocation treated with the repair of lateral collateral ligament complex. *Clin Orthop Surg* 2015;7(2):241–247.

Josefsson PO, Johnell O, Gentz CF: Long-term sequelae of simple dislocation of the elbow. *J Bone Joint Surg Am* 1984;66:927–930.

Kaltenborn FM: *Mobilisation of the Extremity Joints.* Oslo, Norway, Olaf Norlis Bokhandel Universitetgaten, 1980.

Lockard M: Clinical Biomechanics of the Elbow. *Journal of Hand Therapy* 2006;19(2):72–81.

Maitland GD: *Maitland's Peripheral Manipulation,* London, England, Butterworths, 1977.

McKee MD, Schemitsch EH, Sala MJ, O'Driscoll SW: The pathoanatomy of lateral ligamentous disruption in complex elbow instability. *J Shoulder Elbow Surg* 2003;12:391–396.

McKee MD, Pugh DM, Wild LM, Schemitsch EH, King GJ: Standard surgical protocol to treat elbow dislocations with radial head and coronoid fractures. Surgical technique. *J Bone Joint Surg Am* 2005;87(1):22–32.

Morrey BF, An KN: Functional anatomy of the ligaments of the elbow. *Clin Orthop Relat Res* 1985;201:84–90.

Morrey BF, Askew LJ, Chao EY: A biomechanical study of normal functional elbow motion. *J Bone Joint Surg Am* 1981;63:872–877.

O'Driscoll SW, Bell DF, Morrey BF: Posterolateral rotatory instability of the elbow. *J Bone Joint Surg Am* 1991;73:440–446.

Richard MJ, Aldridhe JM 3rd, Wiesler ER, Ruch DS: Traumatic valgus instability of the elbow: pathoanatomy and results of direct repair. *J Bone Joint Surg Am* 2008;90(11):2416–2422.

Ring D, Jupiter JB, Zilberfarb J: Posterior dislocation of the elbow with fractures of the radial head and coronoid. *J Bone Joint Surg Am* 2002;84(4):547–551.

Sardelli M, Tashjian RZ, MacWilliams BA: Functional elbow range of motion for contemporary tasks. *J Bone Joint Surg Am* 2011;93(5):471–477.

Wolff AL, Hotchkiss RN: Lateral elbow instability: nonoperative, operative, and postoperative management. *J Hand Ther* 2006;19(2):238–243.

© 2018 American Academy of Orthopaedic Surgeons

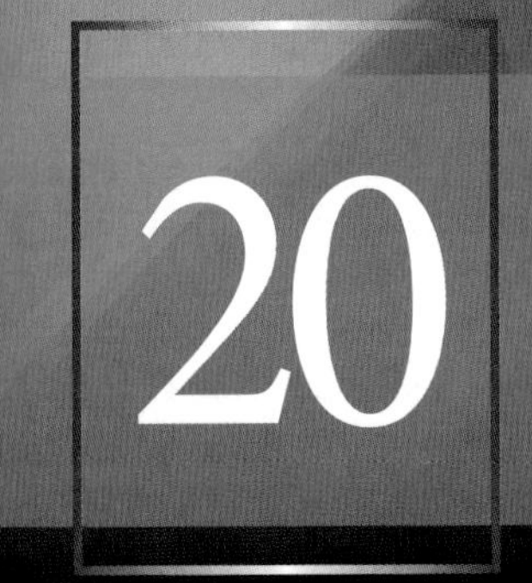

20 Rehabilitation After Distal Humerus Fractures

Gregory N. Nelson, Jr, MD, Laura Walsh, MS, OTR/L, CHT, and Joseph A. Abboud, MD

INTRODUCTION

Fractures of the distal humerus are relatively uncommon injuries. While comprising nearly one-third of all elbow fractures, these injuries make up only 5% to 7% of all fractures. This injury typically has a bimodal distribution occurring from either high-energy trauma in a young population or low-energy injury in the elderly. These two injuries should not be considered as equivalent, however, since each presents with a unique set of challenges. In addition to patient age and injury mechanism, associated traumatic injuries, local soft-tissue condition, medical comorbidities, and fracture pattern are important considerations in the prognosis, timing, and treatment of these injuries. Ultimately, each of these criteria will have an effect on both the treatment and rehabilitation for these patients.

FRACTURE PATTERN

Multiple classification schemes have been used to describe distal humerus fractures. In the end, the primary goal of classification schemes is to provide the health care team with a common vernacular for communication, to guide clinical decision making, and to help predict the prognosis after treatment. Specifics of the most common classification schemes are beyond the scope of this chapter; however, it is important to understand how fracture patterns affect the treatment algorithm.

Distal humerus fractures are generally considered to occur in one of three types: complete extra-articular, partial intra-articular, or complete intra-articular (Figure 20.1). A complete extra-articular fracture involves the distal humeral shaft and variable portions of the columns, but spares the articular surface. Partial and complete articular fractures involve the distal humeral joint surface, but to varying degrees. Each fracture pattern is addressed with different surgical approaches depending on the location of fracture lines and the amount of comminution involved. In all cases, however, the goal of the intervention is to achieve sufficient stability of the fracture in order to allow early range of motion (ROM) and preserve or restore a functional ROM to the elbow joint.

TREATMENT

Nonoperative Management

Unlike midshaft humeral fractures, conservative management is rarely pursued in the setting of a distal fracture, except in rare cases of nondisplaced fracture that are amenable to supervised immobilization. Some authors have reported good results with bracing extra-articular fractures of the distal one-third of the humerus. Unfortunately, bracing often equates to prolonged immobilization, which can result in periarticular contractures and stiffness of the adult elbow. Factors contributing to the development of elbow contracture include the three articulations within one synovial cavity, the intrinsic congruity of the ulnohumeral articulation, and the close relationship of the joint capsule to the surrounding ligaments and musculature. The sequela of prolonged immobilization (stiffness) can be just as debilitating as those of the injury. In some instances, depending on the fracture pattern, custom orthoses will allow protected safe motion, minimizing postinjury

Dr. Abboud or an immediate family member has received royalties from Cayenne, DJ Orthopaedics, Globus Medical, Integra Life Sciences, and Wolters Kluwer Health–Lippincott Williams & Wilkins; serves as a paid consultant to Cayenne, DePuy, A Johnson & Johnson Company, DJ Orthopaedics, Globus Medical, Integra, Mininvasive, and Tornier; has stock or stock options held in Mininvasive; has received research or institutional support from DePuy, A Johnson & Johnson Company, Integra, Tornier, and Zimmer; has received nonincome support (such as equipment or services), commercially derived honoraria, or other non-research–related funding (such as paid travel) from Wolters Kluwer Health–Lippincott Williams & Wilkins; and serves as a board member, owner, officer, or committee member of the American Shoulder and Elbow Surgeons, the Journal of Shoulder and Elbow Surgery, *the Mid Atlantic Shoulder and Elbow Society, and* Orthopaedic Knowledge Online. *Neither of the following authors nor any immediate family member has received anything of value from or has stock or stock options held in a commercial company or institution related directly or indirectly to the subject of this article: Dr. Nelson and Dr. Walsh.*

© 2018 American Academy of Orthopaedic Surgeons

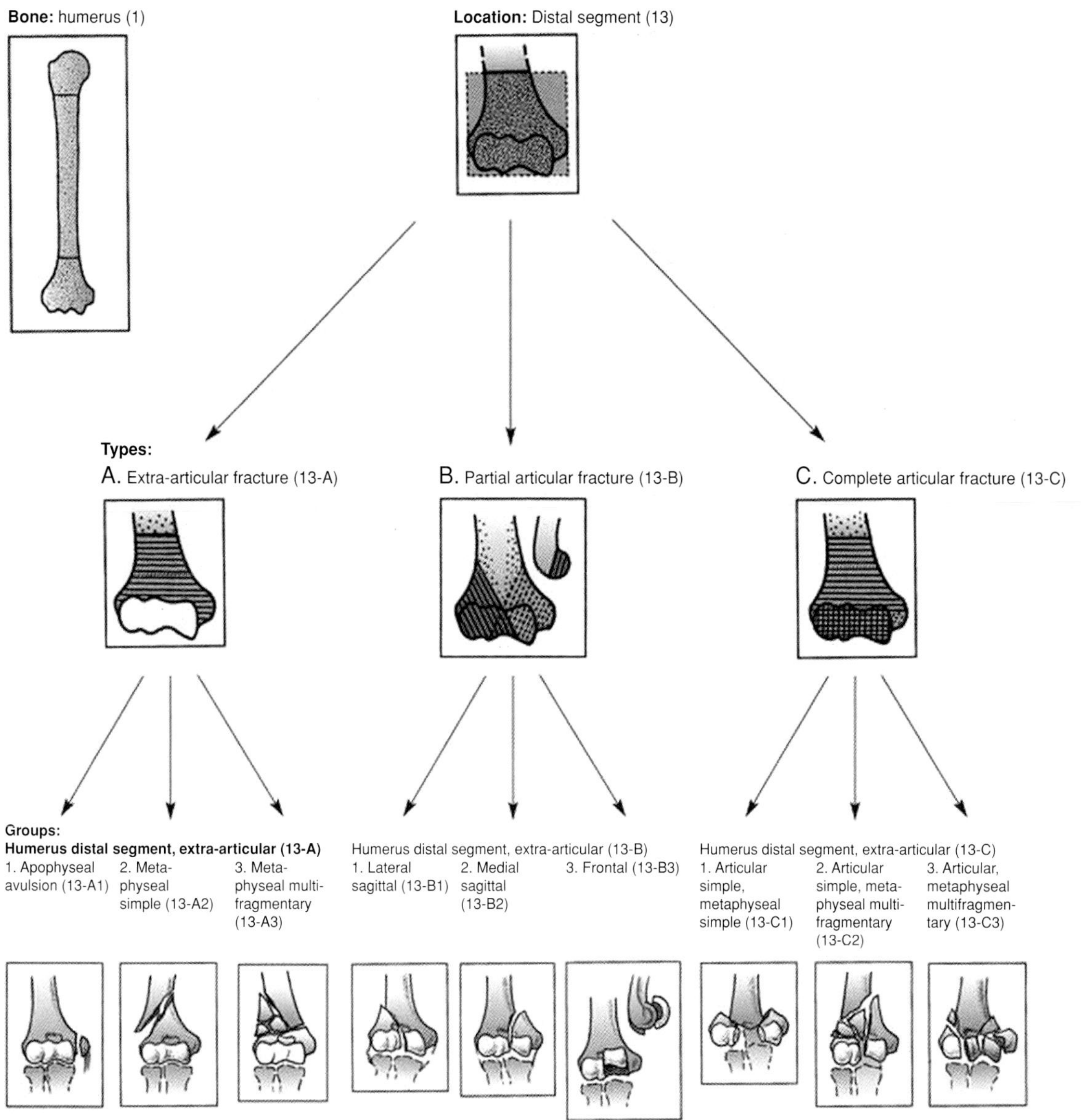

Figure 20.1 Distal humerus fracture patterns and fixation. Fractures that involve the distal humeral shaft and articular surface can present in a variety of patterns. **A**, Illustration of type I, extra-articular. These fractures separate the articular surface as a single unit from the rest of the humeral shaft. **B**, Illustration of type II, partial articular. These fractures leave a portion of the articular surface in continuity with the humeral shaft. Note that fractures can occur in axial, sagittal, coronal, or oblique planes. **C**, Illustration of type III, complete articular. In this pattern, the articular surface is fractured and the entire articulation has been separated from the proximal humeral shaft. (*continued*)

stiffness. Fracture healing through a brace or orthosis requires adequate overlap and proximity of fracture fragments in order to produce bridging callus. Although this can be achieved in a small subset of injuries, most distal humerus fractures are not amenable to nonoperative treatment. In general, surgical intervention is recommended.

Nonoperative treatment may also be appropriate if there are medical comorbidities or associated traumatic injuries (e.g., soft-tissue compromise, wound contamination, anesthetic risk) that render the risks of surgical intervention greater than the benefit. The most common scenario would be an intra-articular fracture in a low-demand, elderly patient with significant comorbidities. In this setting, the elbow is immobilized in an orthosis, then ROM is instituted once initial pain and swelling have improved. This "bag-of-bones" approach often results in a fibrous nonunion of intra-articular fragments or a pseudo-arthrosis at the fracture site. This is sometimes well tolerated in the low-demand population.

Operative Treatment

Indications

In the vast majority of patients, operative treatment is undertaken in order to maximize chances of achieving a stable extremity with a functional arc of elbow motion. The most common operative strategy is open reduction and internal fixation (ORIF), especially in young or high-demand patients.

© 2018 American Academy of Orthopaedic Surgeons

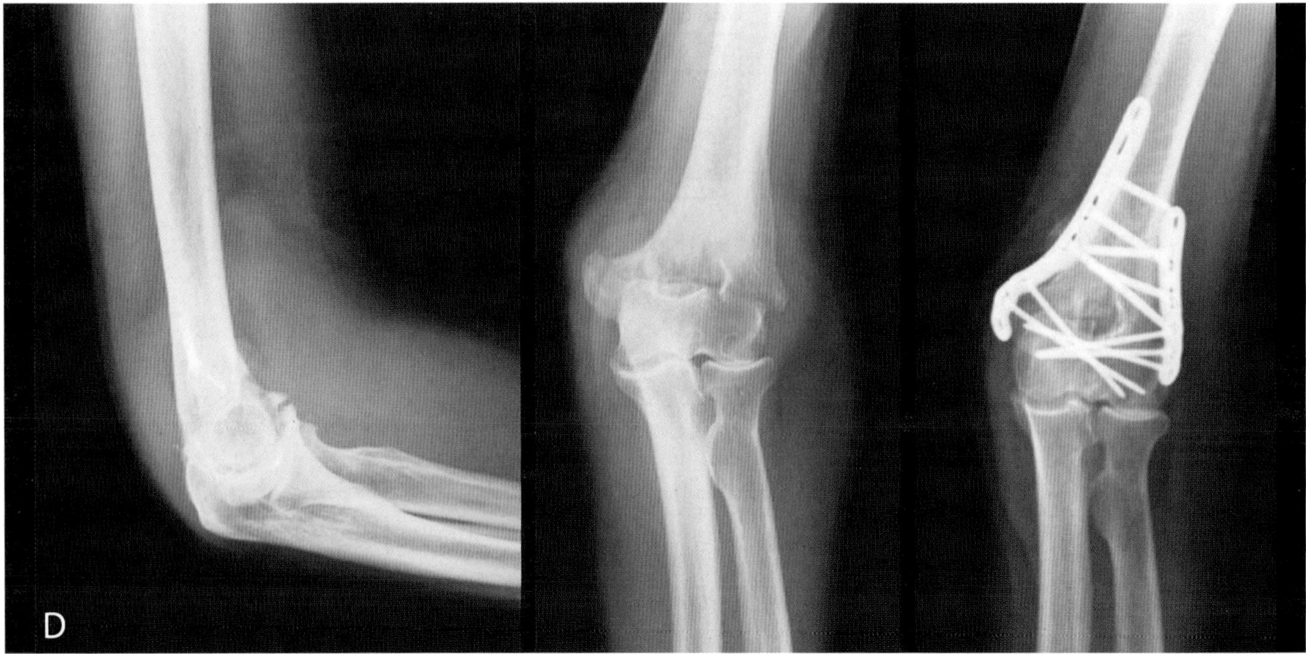

Figure 20.1 (*Continued*) **D**, AP and lateral plain radiographs of a distal humeral transcondylar fracture. The postoperative radiograph demonstrates anatomic reduction of the fracture, bicolumnar plating, multiaxial locking screws, and interdigitating screw paths to maximize fixation rigidity. (Reproduced with permission from Sculco TP, Lim MR, Pearle AD, Ranawat AS. *Hospital for Special Surgery Orthopaedics Manual.* Philadelphia, Lippincott Williams & Wilkins, 2014. Redrawn with permission from Marsh JL, Slongo TF, Agel J, et al. Fracture and dislocation classification compendium–2007: Orthopaedic Trauma Association classification, database, and outcomes committee. *J Orthop Trauma* 2007;21(10 Suppl):S1–133.)

Rigid fixation that can withstand physiologic forces transmitted through the fracture site during rehabilitation is the goal. This permits immediate of ROM exercises in order to minimize postoperative stiffness.

Procedure

The vast majority of ORIF procedures are performed through an extensile posterior approach to the elbow. A longitudinal incision is made along the midline of the posterior arm extending distal to the olecranon. Corresponding full-thickness medial and lateral skin flaps are raised. The ulnar nerve is identified next, and in many cases transposed anteriorly, especially if the fracture involves the medial column. In this case, the nerve is moved in order to place the implants from a medial to lateral direction, or to apply a medially based plate and screws.

The next anatomic structure to address is the extensor mechanism. Assuming that the triceps was not injured in the original trauma, it is preferred to leave the extensor mechanism intact and approach the fracture through a paratricipital approach, triceps splitting, or, in rare cases, a V-Y advancement. However, highly comminuted intra-articular fractures will require the increased surgical exposure that an olecranon osteotomy provides. Proximal reflection of the olecranon and triceps improves visualization of the trochlear spool and, in fractures with severe articular comminution, is the preferred method. In this setting, the olecranon osteotomy will also be repaired with rigid internal fixation.

Once the distal humerus is adequately exposed, the bony injury is addressed. The primary goals of surgery are to achieve perfect alignment of all articular surfaces as well as the extra-articular components of the fracture in order to restore the anatomy of the elbow joint. Secondarily, the surgeon must restore and preserve both the bony and soft-tissue stability of the elbow joint. A comprehensive review of techniques for repair of these fractures is beyond the scope of this chapter. However, there are key fundamental principles for fixation that almost always need to be followed. First, adequate and safe exposure with identification, transposition, and protection of the ulnar nerve is paramount. The next goal is to reconstruct the articular surface by recognizing the injury pattern, associated comminution, and articular relationships. These fragments often need to be provisionally reduced through the use of reduction forceps, Kirschner wires, and headless compression screws. Third, fixation of the fracture progresses from distal to proximal, utilizing bicolumnar locked plating (Figure 20.1, D). Finally, an assessment of the stability of the elbow joint is required. Restoring stability may necessitate formal repair of the collateral ligaments and/or (rarely) the application of an external fixator. At the end of the procedure, the elbow is usually splinted in slight extension to protect the healing posterior soft tissues.

POSTOPERATIVE REHABILITATION

Given that elbow fractures are prone to result in contractures and stiffness, early therapy is advocated. Communication

© 2018 American Academy of Orthopaedic Surgeons

Table 20.1 PHASE I (WEEKS 0–2) THERAPY OVERVIEW

Therapeutic Modalities, Phase I				
Protective Orthoses	Long arm orthosis	Hinge orthosis	External fixator hinge	Over-the-shoulder sling
Edema Control	Cryotherapy	Elevation	Compression	
Early ROM	AROM	AAROM		
Specific Anatomic Considerations	Fracture Stability	Ulnar nerve	Triceps	

AAROM = Active assistive range of motion, AROM = active range of motion, ROM = range of motion.

between the surgeon and therapist regarding stability of the fracture fixation, status of the ulnar nerve, including if the nerve was transposed, and status of the triceps, is imperative. This will enable the therapist to implement a therapy program maximizing early motion while safely protecting the compromised structures and minimizing complications. In the case of ORIF, more often than not, rigid fixation allows the institution of ROM exercises within the first few postoperative days. Lesser rigid fixation may require protected or delayed motion. Due to risk of contracture, elbow motion should be instituted no later than 3 weeks postoperatively, although immediate motion is ideal.

Author's Preferred Protocol

Phase I: Inflammation (Weeks 0–2) (Table 20.1)

- Orthoses: The postoperative splint is exchanged for a removable and lighter thermoplastic molded orthosis fabricated by the therapist at the first postoperative visit. The following are orthosis options:
  - Long-arm orthosis: The injured elbow can be immobilized in a position of protection as determined by the treating surgeon. This type of orthosis prevents all motion when worn (Figure 20.2).
    - Worn for activities of daily living (ADLs) and sleeping
    - May be removed to perform protected ROM exercises as instructed by the therapist and approved by surgeon
  - Hinged orthosis
    - A hinge design allows the therapist to limit motion while still allowing safe motion. The hinge parameters can be set to block flexion or extension at a specific degree without impeding supination and pronation (Figures 20.3 and 20.4). Additionally, the hinge will provide protection from varus and valgus stress, if needed, for ligament protection.
      - Does not require removal for ROM exercises or ADLs given that it allows built-in protected motion.
      - This orthosis is our preference given that the patient does not need to remove it, preventing risk of injury or incorrect reapplication.
  - Hinged external fixator
    - Placed on the elbow in surgery in cases of significant instability pattern.
    - The patient will be able to participate in ROM and functional activities within the parameters of the hinge, which are set by the surgeon during surgery (Figure 20.5).
    - An orthosis can be designed over the hinge for times when the patient feels that the fixator may get bumped (Figure 20.6).
  - Over-the-shoulder sling
    - May be utilized in early stages for extra support in addition to the orthosis, although continuous wear is not recommended due to risk of shoulder stiffness from unnecessary immobilization of the shoulder.
- Edema Control
  - Cryotherapy: 10 to 20 minutes postexercise

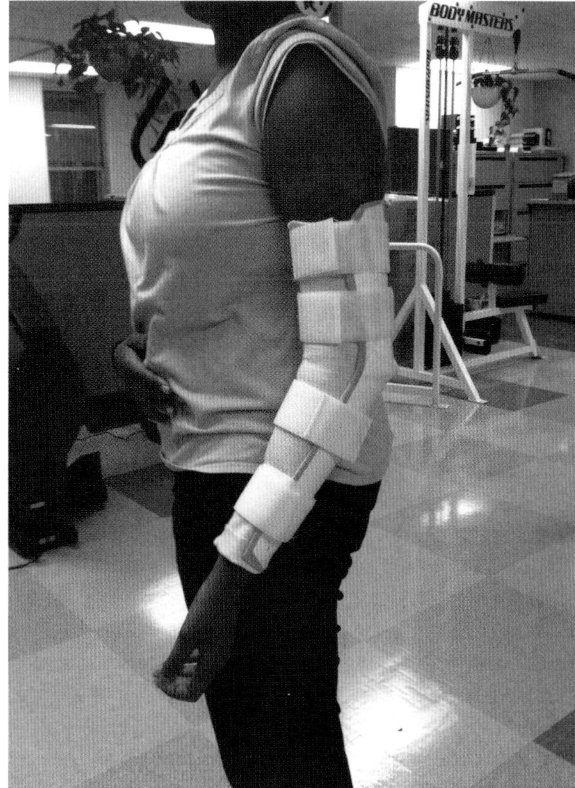

Figure 20.2 Photograph of long-arm orthosis.

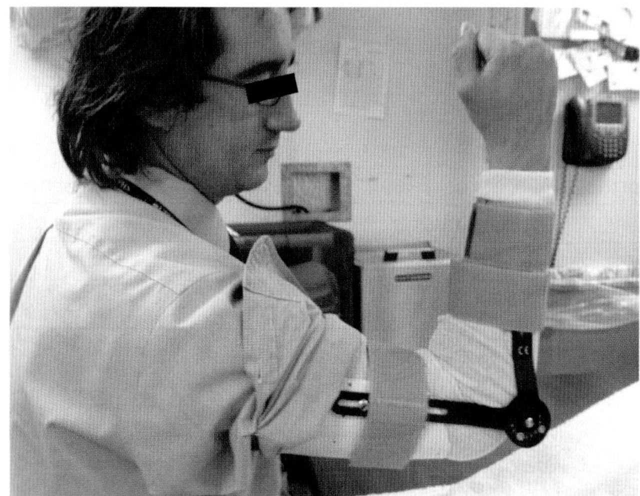

Figure 20.3 Photograph of elbow flexion in hinged splint.

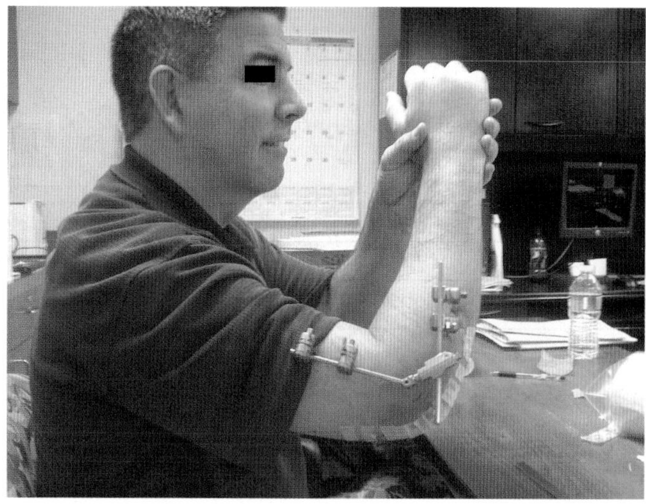

Figure 20.5 Photograph of elbow flexion with external fixator.

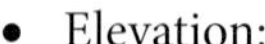

  - Elevation:
    - Educate the patient to elevate injured upper extremity, ideally above heart level for approximately 1 to 2 minutes every hour.
    - Open and close digits to create pumping action.
  - Low-grade elastic compression wraps or sleeves:
    - Applied in a graded fashion
      - Tighter compression distally creates a gradient for fluid
    - Watch for edema pooled in the hand adding to unnecessary stiffness and discomfort.
      - Treat with a compressive glove.
- Early Motion: Limits postoperative stiffness and residual symptoms
  - Begin with moist heat 10 to 20 minutes to increase tissue extensibility.
  - Elbow flexion and extension can be performed in supine or upright (seated or standing) positions. Elbow flexion is the most important movement for ADLs, although elbow extension tends to be more difficult to regain to end range.
    - Initially, patients often feel most comfortable in a supine position, which provides stability to the shoulder girdle and trunk (Figure 20.7).
    - If seated, motion can be performed with the arm resting on a table, providing a gravity-eliminated position for support if needed due to pain and fear (Figure 20.8) with gradual advancement to off-the-table motion.

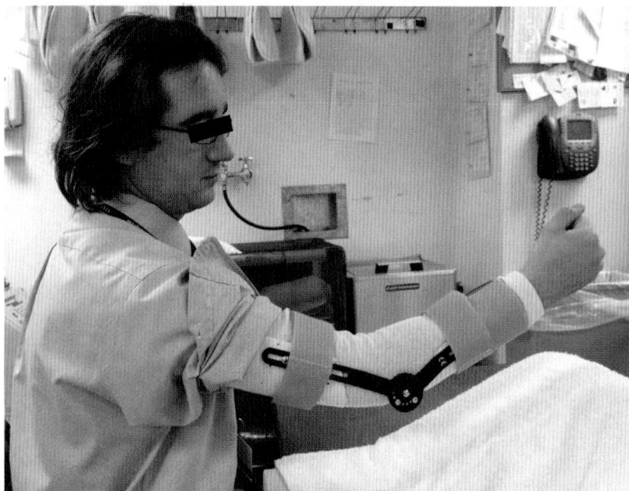

Figure 20.4 Photograph of elbow extension in hinged splint.

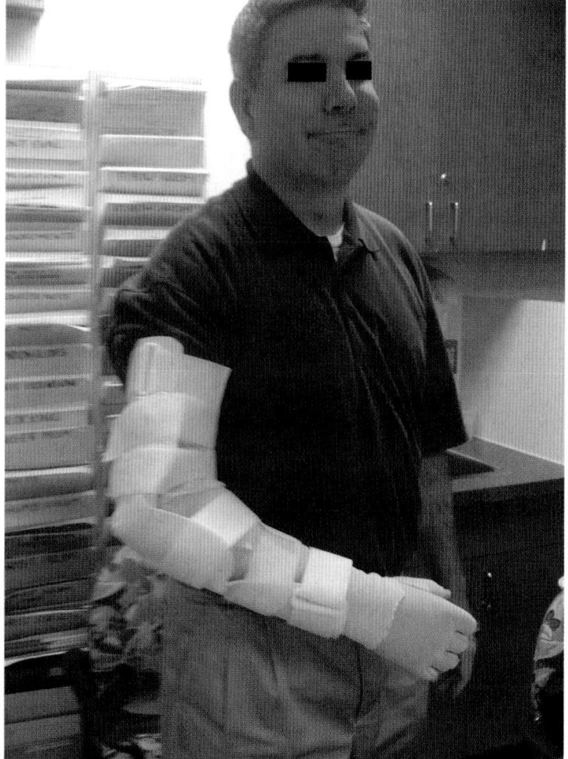

Figure 20.6 Photograph of orthosis to protect external fixator.

© 2018 American Academy of Orthopaedic Surgeons

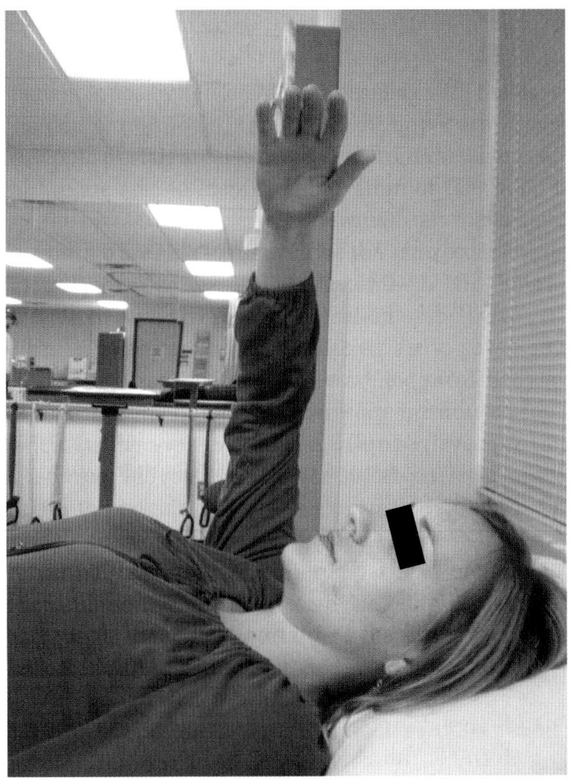

Figure 20.7 Photograph of supine position for elbow ROM.

    - When standing, placing a rolled towel or pillow posterior to the humerus helps to stabilize the shoulder, preventing compensatory shoulder elevation (Figure 20.9).
- Forearm rotational ROM exercises are performed with the shoulder adducted and the elbow flexed to 90°.
- Shoulder, wrist, and hand ROM should also be undertaken in order to prevent stiffness and disability of adjacent joints.
    - ROM should be assessed for gains, loss of motion, or no change. If the results are not positive, the program will need to be adjusted.

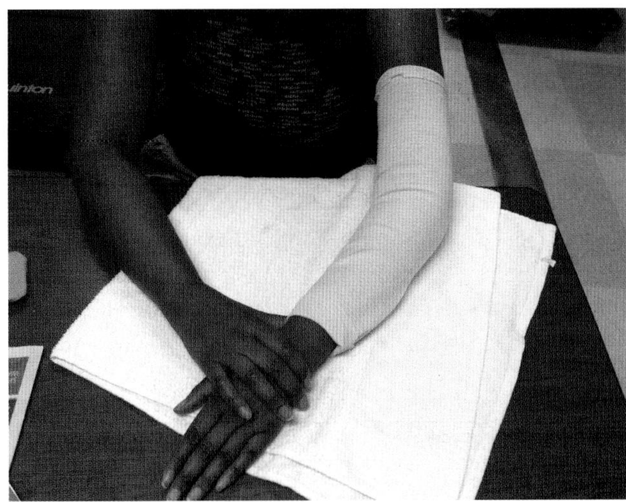

Figure 20.8 Photograph of gravity-eliminated elbow ROM.

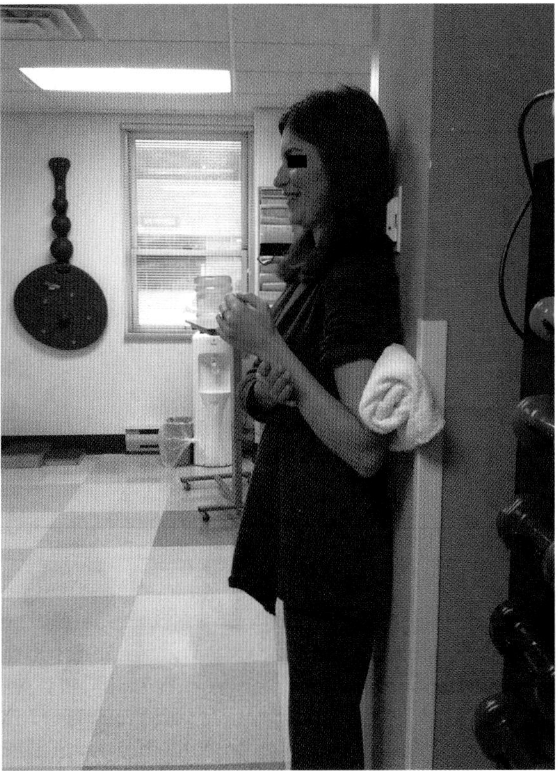

Figure 20.9 Photograph of towel use to support the shoulder with elbow ROM.

    - Although recommended frequency and repetition of exercises has not been documented in literature, we have found that it is important to give the patient a specific program to follow. We recommend a program of 5 to 10 repetitions with a 5- to 10-second hold, five times daily during this initial phase.
- Incorporation of ROM exercises into a home program is crucial for a successful outcome.
    - It is important that the surgeon and the therapist emphasize that home rehabilitation has as much potential to promote or derail functional recovery as the surgical procedure itself.
- Active range of motion (AROM)
    - The patient will gently move the elbow with no assistance or added pressure.
- Active assistive range of motion (AAROM)
    - Using the contralateral limb or a bar (Figure 20.10) to gently assist the effected upper extremity to a tolerable stretch will help increase pain-free motion and limit guarding. The authors prefer bilateral AAROM exercises (Figure 20.10). We find that moving the uninjured limb in the same fashion desired for the injured limb helps to increase motion with less guarding.

- Advanced therapeutic motion, designed to push ROM further and strengthen the elbow
    - Passive range of motion (PROM)
        - Reserved for later stages, after bony healing has progressed.

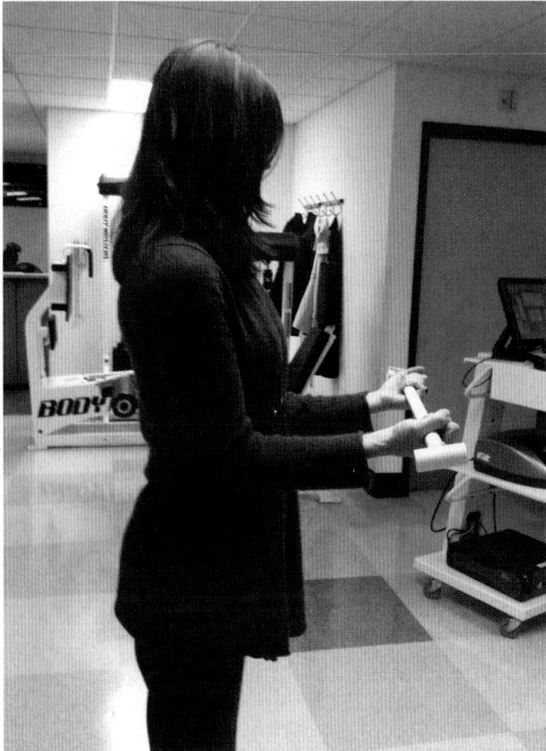

Figure 20.10 Photograph of AAROM with bar.

- Overly aggressive early stretching is not recommended since it can further injure at-risk structures, prolong the inflammation phase, and slow the actual recovery process.
- Strengthening Program
  - Also reserved for later stages, after bony healing has progressed
    - Will focus on resistance exercises (isometric and isotonic) initially closed chain exercises. Generally, closed chain exercise is introduced first, followed by open-chain exercises for strengthening.
    - Patients are always told to progress slowly with strengthening and to spend 60% to 75% of their home rehab time on regaining flexibility, which is the most challenging aspect of elbow trauma recovery.
- Specific Anatomic Considerations
  - Ulnar Nerve
    - If the ulnar nerve is irritable, limit prolonged elbow flexion exercises, which place the ulnar nerve on traction and compress the cubital tunnel. Also, educate the patient to avoid leaning on the injured elbow to avoid additional pressure on the ulnar nerve. Particular attention should be paid to this during seated elbow motion.
    - If the nerve has been decompressed or transposed, early ROM with nerve-gliding exercises may avoid nerve scarring and entrapment, and prevent poor results. If the ulnar nerve has been transposed, the flexor pronator muscle mass may have been elevated surgically. In these patients, the reapproximated flexor pronator attachment may need to be protected. The patient can perform protected motion by avoiding full wrist extension with simultaneous elbow extension for 3 weeks. The patient may perform wrist extension with the elbow maintained in flexion, and elbow extension with the wrist in neutral.
  - Triceps and Extensor Mechanism
    - With a paratricepital approach, the therapist can allow full elbow flexion and extension in order to avoid scarring of the triceps.
    - If an olecranon osteotomy or triceps repair was performed, full elbow flexion may need to be delayed to avoid stress on the olecranon repair. This will be dictated by the surgeon.
      - If the olecranon osteotomy needs protection, a hinge orthosis with the elbow blocked to prevent full flexion will prevent stress on the repaired structures while allowing motion in extension, supination, and pronation. The surgeon will determine the degree of safe motion.

Phase II: Repair (Weeks 1–8) (Table 20.2)

- Scar Management: Commences once incision is satisfactorily healed.
  - Massage scar
    - Remove thin adhesive strips approximately 2 weeks postoperatively.
    - When incision is fully closed, massage with cocoa butter or vitamin E lotion. The authors have seen positive results with scar massage.
      - Recommended routine: Apply firm pressure to the scar and surrounding area, moving in a small

Table 20.2 PHASE II (WEEKS 1–8) THERAPY OVERVIEW

Therapeutic Modalities, Phase II			
Scar Management	Massage	Silicone	Desensitization
Advance Range of Motion	Continue AAROM	Addition of PROM	Functional movement
Orthosis to Increase Motion	Static	Static progressive	Dynamic

AAROM = active assistive range of motion, PROM = passive range of motion.

 © 2018 American Academy of Orthopaedic Surgeons

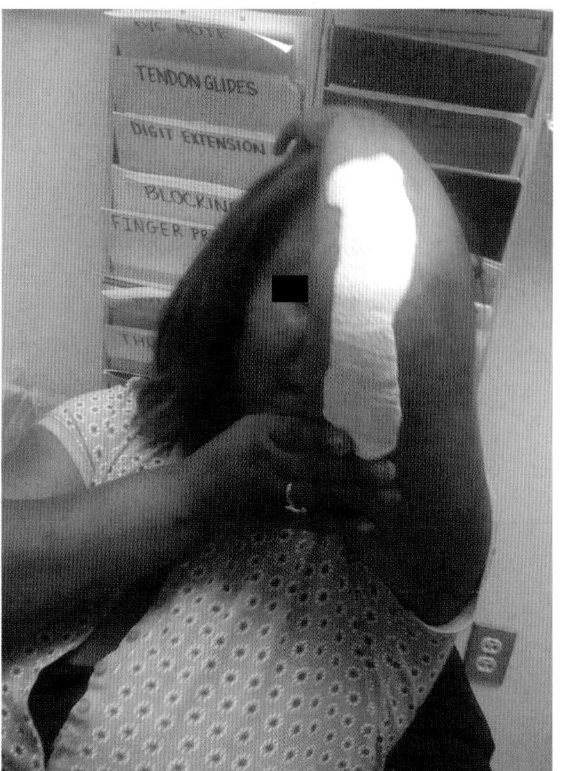

Figure 20.11 Photograph of silicone scar treatment.

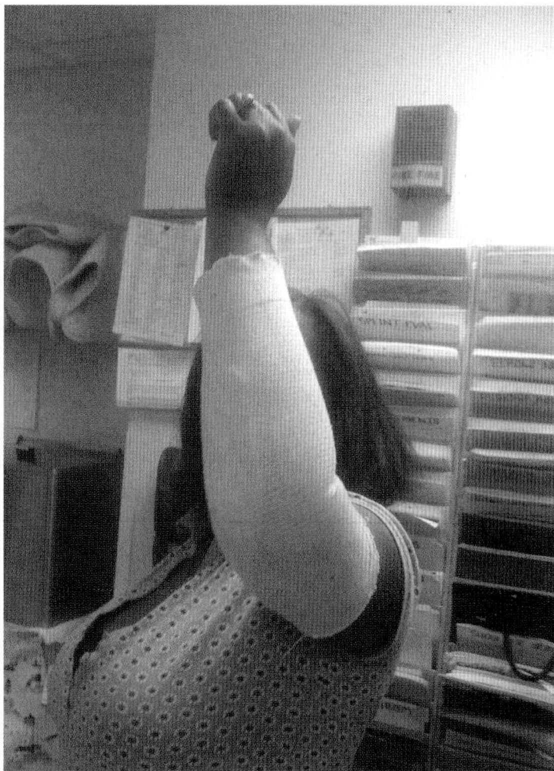

Figure 20.12 Photograph of compression sleeve to hold silicone in place.

circular fashion. This should be performed 5 to 10 minutes five times daily.

- Silicone pad or gel sheet
  - When applied over the scar, typically worn beneath an elastic sleeve, silicone has clinically shown positive results in reducing scar tissue (Figures 20.11 and 20.12). The silicone can be worn during sleep in order to avoid limiting motion during the day. Of note, silicone comes in different forms, such as a clear sheet, or a putty called elastomere or Otoform. The form chosen depends on what works best for the patient. Figure 20.11 shows a representative product.
- Scar desensitization
  - Rubbing varying textures over the sensitive area, beginning with a soft texture and progressing to rougher textures as tolerated, has shown to be effective when performed several times daily for 5 to 10 minutes.
  - In the event that the scar is too sensitive to tolerate pressure during the day, an elbow pad may be issued to further protect the sensitive area (Figure 20.13).

- Range of motion: Regaining motion is paramount during this phase, when the healing response can be most effectively modulated.
  - Week 6 postop or postinjury, orthosis use is weaned and the patient begins to use the limb for light activities. The orthosis is only used at night and in crowded or busy situations to protect the elbow.
    - It may even be discarded completely, depending on the level of healing and stability.
  - Initiate passive ROM if cleared by surgeon (typically when there is clear evidence of bony radiographic healing ~10–12 weeks).
    - Passive motion involves increased stress applied to the repair site; thus, it should be reserved until adequate bony and soft-tissue healing has begun.
    - Passive motion should involve a low-load, steady and prolonged force that may be uncomfortable but

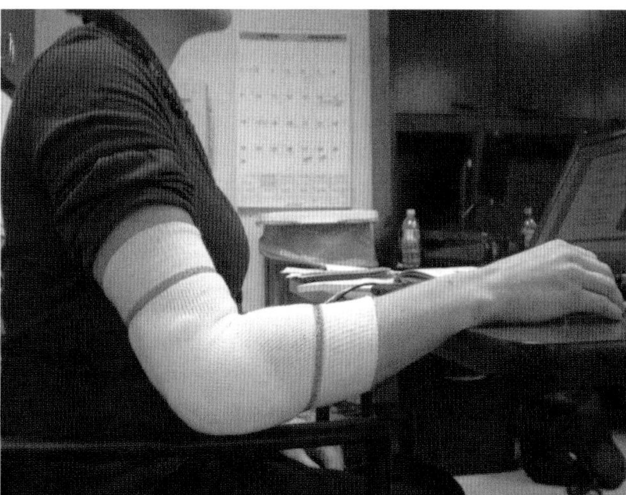

Figure 20.13 Photograph of elbow pad for protection.

© 2018 American Academy of Orthopaedic Surgeons

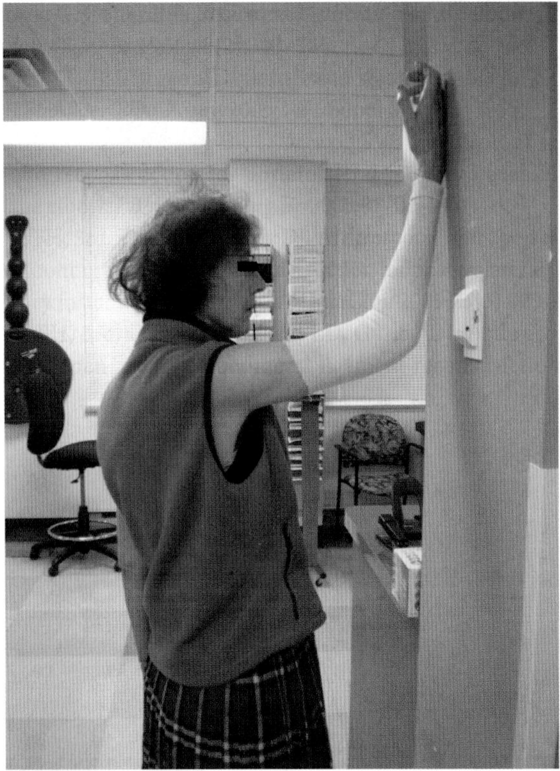

Figure 20.14 Photograph of passive elbow flexion stretch against the wall.

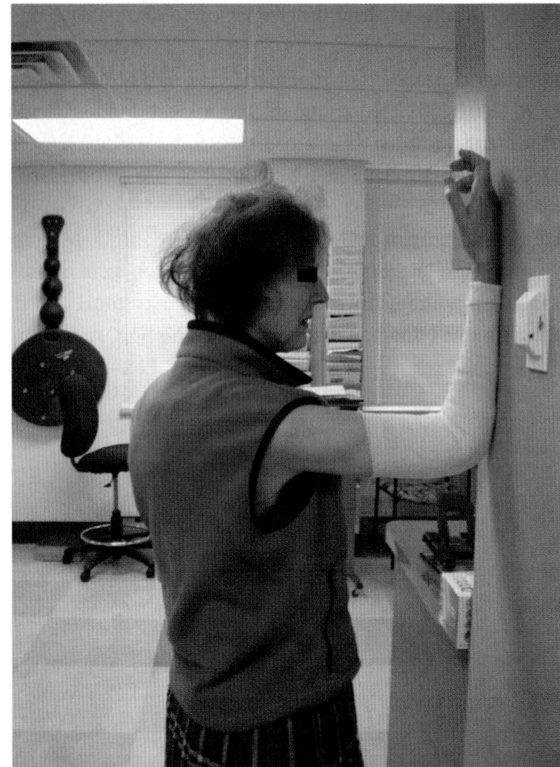

Figure 20.15 Photograph of sliding the elbow downward to increase passive flexion.

should not be painful. Pain may cause co-contraction, which is counterproductive to the stretching process.

- Add passive ROM as needed, depending on the level of stiffness. There are many different ways to perform passive stretch.
    - Figures 20.14 and 20.15 show the "wall stretch" for elbow flexion. The patient places the flexed elbow and forearm against a wall, and gradually slides the elbow into flexion, maintaining contact with the wall.
    - We have found this particular passive stretch to be very effective and easy for patients to perform correctly. The therapist will work with the patient to determine the optimal stretching program for the particular patient considering comfort level, avoiding guarding postures, and advancing motion.
    - Passive motion involves increased stress applied to the repair site; thus, it should be reserved until adequate bony and soft-tissue healing has begun.

- Orthoses to increase motion
    - If early postoperative stiffness persists, splinting with tension applied to the tissue at maximal length for a longer period of time is helpful to increase motion.
    - Available orthoses include serial static orthoses, static progressive orthoses, or dynamic orthoses.
        - Serial static orthoses have no movable parts and are adjusted by the therapist as motion is gained. We prefer this type of orthosis for elbow extension deficits. The orthosis should be the entire length of the arm to provide optimal distribution of pressure.
        - Straps are applied at the wrist and upper arm to hold the orthosis in place. Straps at the elbow can be tightened or loosened depending on the desired amount of stretch. This orthosis can be fabricated with a slight "bump-out" at the anterior elbow, allowing increased ease with stretch. This is called a belly gutter orthosis (Figure 20.16).
        - Static progressive orthoses generate a mobilizing force on the tissue, utilizing nonelastic traction.

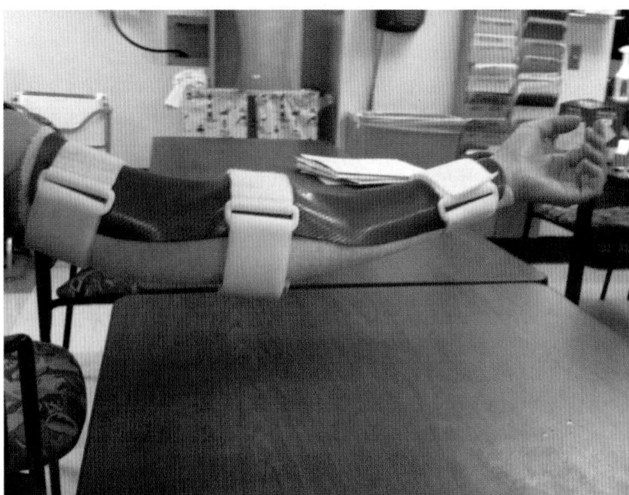

Figure 20.16 Photograph of thermoplastic elbow extension splint.

© 2018 American Academy of Orthopaedic Surgeons

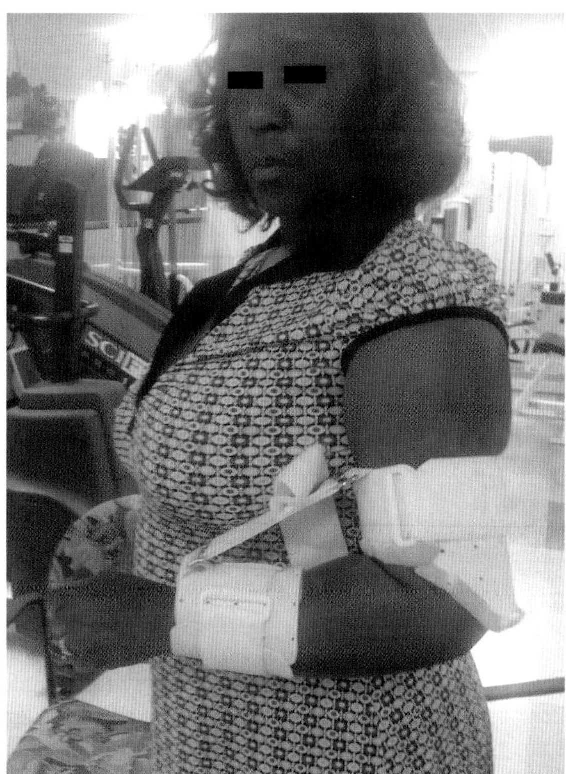

Figure 20.17 Photograph of static progressive elbow flexion splint, cuff design.

- The tension can be adjusted by the patient as tolerated. This type of orthosis is very helpful for gaining elbow flexion. The authors prefer the cuff design. It is simple to fabricate and easy for the patient to use. One cuff is placed at the wrist and the other cuff is placed on the upper arm. A strap between the two cuffs is attached using D rings. The patient can simply pull the strap tighter, flexing the elbow to toleration (Figure 20.17).
- Dynamic orthoses generate force on the tissue through elastic traction.
- A dynamic orthosis will allow the patient to adjust the tension; however, the authors have found that, at times, when wearing dynamic orthoses, patients guard against the constant dynamic tension.
- Despite the chosen preferred method of utilizing static progressive versus dynamic orthoses to increase motion, the literature supports that both dynamic and static progressive orthoses help to improve motion and that there is no significant difference in outcome between the two designs.
- Our recommendation is that motion orthoses be worn for prolonged periods of end-range stretch since the goal is to affect a change in the tissue structure through stretch. The literature supports that the splint should be worn at least 6 hours a day.

Phase III: Remodeling (Week 6–Month 6) (Table 20.3)

- Maintain and increase motion: Precautions that may have limited the aggressiveness of therapy are lifted.
  - Scar management
    - Continue as needed until scar and surrounding area remains soft.
  - Range of motion
    - Continue present ROM program as needed.
    - Progressive static or dynamic splints are continued for maximizing end ROM.
    - Add closed-chain activities to promote ROM while providing proximal and distal stabilization with light resistive use. Rolling a ball on the table is a great closed-chain activity that the patient can easily perform as part of the home program (Figure 20.18).
- Strengthening program (~10–12 weeks postop)
  - A graduated strengthening program can be instituted once fracture and muscle origin healing is deemed adequate.
    - Elbow flexion and extension, forearm pronation and supination, shoulder, wrist, and hand should all be addressed. The therapist will focus on areas of weakness.
    - Particular attention should be paid to the triceps if compromised in surgery. We find that the triceps can be very weak after an elbow surgery (Figure 20.19). Performing triceps exercises in a supine position helps to isolate the triceps and decrease compensatory movements.
- Functional use
  - Patients are encouraged to begin ADLs and resistive use of the injured arm with all ADLs.

Table 20.3 PHASE III (WEEK 6–MONTH 6) OVERVIEW

Therapeutic Modalities, Phase III			
Maintain and Increase Motion Gains	Continue with scar management	Continue with ROM	Continue with orthosis to increase motion
Promote Strength and Endurance	Precautions for strengthening lifted	Add formal strengthening program	Focus on areas of weakness
Regain Full Functional Use of Upper Extremtiy	Encourage use of upper extremity for all ADLs		

ADLs = activities of daily living, ROM = range of motion.

© 2018 American Academy of Orthopaedic Surgeons

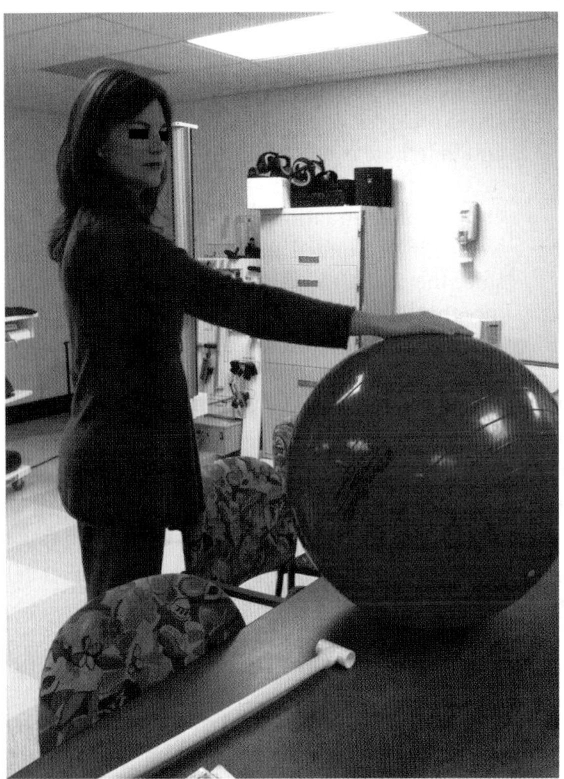

Figure 20.18 Photograph of closed-chain elbow ROM.

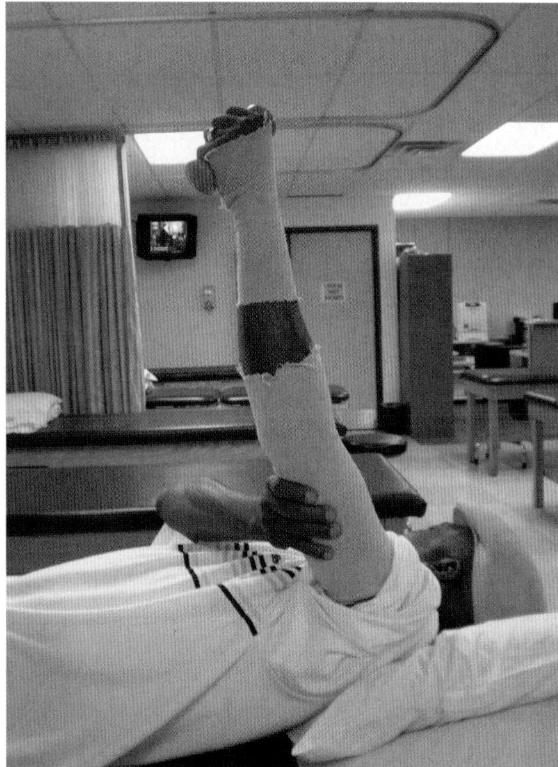

Figure 20.19 Photograph of isolated triceps strengthening.

- Work conditioning therapy is an option as needed for those patients who seek to return to careers in manual labor.

COMPLICATIONS

Historically, treatment of intra-articular distal humerus fractures has resulted in mixed results due to the high rate of complications (11%–48%). These include stiffness, infection, hematoma formation, wound complications, hardware failure, and nerve injury. When associated injuries and posttraumatic arthrosis are added to this list, it is clear why the postoperative course in these patients can be so difficult. It is not uncommon for a patient who suffers a severe elbow injury, whether soft-tissue or bony in nature, to develop significant stiffness, especially in terminal extension. All patients should be counseled to this reality at the time of injury to help temper expectations with treatment and rehabilitation.

One hundred degrees The minimum functional flexion–extension arc needed for ADLs has been reported to be 100°, although many patients will not be satisfied with even this level of function. Causes of postoperative motion loss vary from intra-articular incongruity, adhesions, and loose bodies to capsular contracture, heterotopic ossification, bony impingement, and prominent hardware. Each of these should be kept in mind as potential causes for an early plateau in rehabilitative gains, especially because repeat surgical intervention can be of use in addressing these impediments. The treating therapist should be alert to these possible anatomic causes of limited gains, particularly if a patient has a hard end-feel with motion, loses motion, or becomes increasingly painful as time progresses rather than making steady progress.

The patient who appears to make early gains but quickly plateaus or begins to lose motion should also raise concern for the therapist. If the patient is trustworthy and has been consistent with a home program in between therapy visits, the early rehabilitation failure may be due to heterotopic ossification (HO). A reevaluation by the surgeon can help to clarify this. In early stages, HO may not appear radiographically; however, once the diagnosis is confirmed, stiffness due to HO will not improve appreciably unless the HO is addressed surgically. This is undertaken after the HO matures (usually 3–6 months) to prevent a recurrence. It is important, however, to keep in mind that many instances of HO are asymptomatic and its presence does not always equate with stiffness and a poor functional prognosis. An experienced surgeon should be able to determine whether heterotopic ossification is of any real significant consequence. Patients who feel dissatisfied with their outcome secondary to stiffness after a full course of therapy should be referred back to their surgeon for discussion of surgical treatment for postoperative or postinjury contracture. Late capsular release or excision of heterotopic ossification for postoperative stiffness has been used successfully to improve motion after ORIF of distal humerus fractures. However, it is important to remember that repeat surgery is not without risks as well; thus, it is reserved for persistent stiffness after failure of a prolonged course of therapy. Further details can be found in Chapter 13: Contracture Release.

© 2018 American Academy of Orthopaedic Surgeons

Unfortunately, there are patients who never progress well and have persistent stiffness and pain. Although they may lack clear signs of infection, such as constitutional symptoms, erythema and swelling, drainage, and wound dehiscence, there should be concern for infection. These patients may have radiographic findings that suggest this as well, including delayed bony union and/or early diffuse arthritic changes. As with any joint infection, this can be very challenging and requires a team approach with the infectious disease specialist and the surgeon for decision making about antibiotics, revision surgery, and possible need for staged surgical treatment.

PEARLS

- Rigid fixation that allows for early motion is desired, whenever possible.
- Reconstruct the intra-articular segments first, since these can tolerate the least amount of incongruity.
- Protect the ulnar nerve at all times. The surgeon should have a low threshold to transpose the nerve.
- An olecranon osteotomy greatly increases visualization for intra-articular fractures.
- Early postoperative ROM is the goal of both surgery and rehabilitation.
- Overly aggressive stretching can prolong the inflammatory stage and slow recovery.

SUMMARY

Distal humeral fractures can be difficult injuries to treat. Surgical intervention is the mainstay of treatment for most patients, although a few exceptions exist. Stiffness is the most common rehabilitation challenge. However, with an appropriate therapy protocol emphasizing early protected motion, functional outcomes can be maximized, thus preserving patient independence.

BIBLIOGRAPHY

Blackmore, S: Splinting for elbow injuries and contractures. *Atlas of Hand Clinics* 2001;6:21–50.

Brouwer KM, Guitton TG, Doornberg JN, Kloen P, Jupiter JB, Ring D: Fractures of the medial column of the distal humerus in adults. *J Hand Surg Am* 2009;34(3):439–445.

Charalambous CP, Morrey BF: Posttraumatic elbow stiffness. *J Bone Joint Surg Am* 2012;94(15):1428–1437.

Cheung EV, Steinmann SP: Surgical approaches to the elbow. *J Am Acad Orthop Surg* 2009;17(5):325–333.

Dávila SA, Johnston-Jones K: Managing the stiff elbow: operative, nonoperative, and postoperative techniques. *J Hand Ther* 2006; 19(2):268–281.

Doornberg JN, van Duijn PJ, Linzel D, Ring DC, Zurakowski D, Marti RK, Kloen P: Surgical treatment of intra-articular fractures of the distal part of the humerus. Functional outcome after twelve to thirty years. *J Bone Joint Surg Am* 2007;89(7):1524–1532.

Flowers KR, LaStayo PC: Effect of total end range time on improving passive range of motion. 1994. *J Hand Ther* 2012;25(1): 48–54; quiz 55.

Galano GJ, Ahmad CS, Levine WN: Current treatment strategies for bicolumnar distal humerus fractures. *J Am Acad Orthop Surg* 2010;18(1):20–30.

Glasgow C, Wilton J, Tooth L: Optimal daily total end range time for contracture: resolution in hand splinting. *J Hand Ther* 2003;16(3):207–218.

Lindenhovius AL, Doornberg JN, Brouwer KM, Jupiter JB, Mudgal CS, Ring D: A prospective randomized controlled trial of dynamic versus static progressive elbow splinting for posttraumatic elbow stiffness. *J Bone Joint Surg Am* 2012;94(8):694–700.

Lund AT, Amadio PC: Treatment of cubital tunnel syndrome: perspectives for the therapist. *J Hand Ther* 2006;19(2):170–178.

Mustoe TA: Evolution of silicone therapy and mechanism of action in scar management. *Aesthetic Plast Surg* 2008;32(1):82–92.

Wolf JM, Athwal GS, Shin AY, Dennison DG: Acute trauma to the upper extremity: what to do and when to do it. *Instr Course Lect* 2010;59:525–538.

© 2018 American Academy of Orthopaedic Surgeons

21 ORIF for Olecranon Fractures: Simple Olecranon Fractures, Transolecranon Fracture-Dislocations and Posterior Monteggia Variant

Robert Z. Tashjian, MD

INTRODUCTION

Olecranon fractures account for about 10% of all adult upper extremity fractures and a majority of fractures, approximately 85%, are simple displaced transverse fractures. Dislocation associated with olecranon fractures is much less commonly reported in the literature. In general, olecranon fracture-dislocations can be categorized into two different groups: transolecranon fracture-dislocations and Monteggia fracture-dislocations. Each pattern has a unique injury mechanism, at-risk patient population, structural injury pattern, repair technique, postoperative rehabilitation, and functional outcomes.

The complexity of bony and soft-tissue injury has a substantial impact on the details of surgical management. With regard to the simple olecranon and transolecranon fracture-dislocation, only the ulna is injured and requires fixation if displaced. In the Monteggia fracture-dislocation, the olecranon similarly needs repair if displaced, and the associated radial head fractures should be treated with open reduction and internal fixation (ORIF) in the setting of Mason type 2 injuries and either repaired or replaced in the setting of Mason type 3 injuries. Excision of a comminuted radial head fracture should be considered only if the lateral collateral ligament (LCL) complex is intact. If the lateral ligament complex is injured, then surgical repair should also be performed. Similarly, the details of postoperative rehabilitation are dictated by the overall complexity of the injury as well as the specifics of the surgical treatment. Understanding the differences and nuances will allow for optimization of treatment and final clinical outcomes.

OLECRANON AND PROXIMAL ULNA FRACTURES

Simple Olecranon Fractures

Simple olecranon fractures (without instability) are very common injuries in all age groups. Fractures either result from a trauma forcing the proximal ulna into the distal humerus or a forceful contraction of the triceps. Olecranon fractures can be classified into stable (transverse, oblique, or comminuted) or unstable (fracture-dislocation) patterns (Figure 21.1). Most olecranon fractures require surgical fixation; however, nondisplaced, stable, noncomminuted fractures can be considered for nonoperative treatment. Displaced transverse fractures can be treated using a variety of surgical constructs, including tension-band, intramedullary screw, or plate and screw fixation with the goals of restoring appropriate ulnar length and anatomic articular congruity (Figure 21.2, A and B). Comminuted or oblique fractures require dorsal plate fixation often with possible addition of interfragmentary screws outside the plate. The primary goal of surgery is to provide stable, rigid fixation, allowing immediate protected motion in order to optimize final range of motion (ROM) and strength.

Transolecranon Fracture-Dislocations

Transolecranon fracture-dislocations typically occur as a result of a blow to the dorsum of the forearm. These injuries occur in the young with good bone quality as a result of a high-energy injury. Typically, a highly comminuted fracture of the olecranon process occurs with subluxation or dislocation of the radial head anteriorly on the distal humerus (Figure 21.3, A and B). The proximal radioulnar joint is not injured in this pattern, which is an important difference between transolecranon fracture-dislocations and posterior Monteggia fracture-dislocations. Both the radial shaft and the ulnar shaft translate anteriorly and in the same direction; in a Monteggia injury, the radius and ulna translate in opposite directions. Radial head and neck fractures are uncommon with transolecranon fracture-dislocations, and if coronoid fractures occur, they are typically basal injuries. The medial collateral ligaments (MCLs) and LCLs are typically spared in this injury compared to a typical elbow dislocation or a

Dr. Tashjian or an immediate family member has received royalties from Cayenne Medical, IMASCAP, and Shoulder Innovations; serves as a paid consultant to Cayenne Medical and Mitek; has stock or stock options held in Conextions, INTRAFUSE, and KATOR; has received nonincome support (such as equipment or services), commercially derived honoraria, or other non-research–related funding (such as paid travel) from the Journal of Bone and Joint Surgery–American*; and serves as a board member, owner, officer, or committee member of the* Journal of Orthopaedic Trauma.

© 2018 American Academy of Orthopaedic Surgeons

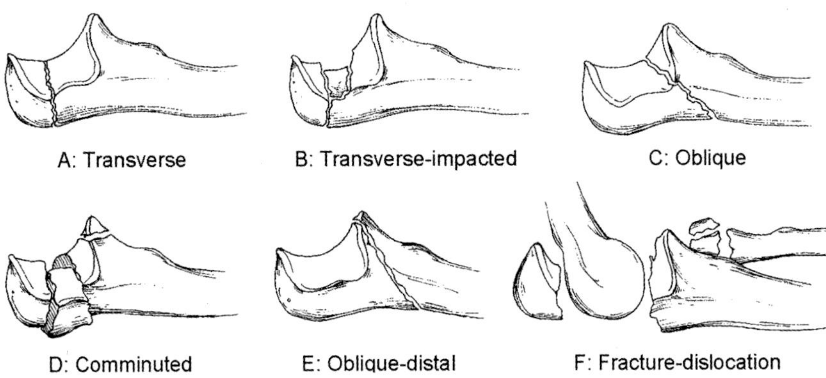

Figure 21.1 Shatzker classification of olecranon fractures. (Reproduced with permission from Hak DJ, Golladay GJ. Olecranon fractures: treatment options. *J Am Acad Orthop Surg* 2000;8(4):266–275.)

Monteggia fracture-dislocation. The primary lesion in a transolecranon fracture-dislocation is disruption of the ulnohumeral joint. The key to treatment of these injuries is restoration of the trochlea notch with stable fixation (Figure 21.4, A and B). A dorsally applied 3.5-mm reconstruction, precontoured, or compression plate is the implant of choice for these injuries with a higher failure rate if a tension-band device or one-third tubular plate is utilized. In general, outcomes of these injuries are very good, with a low level of posttraumatic arthritis as long as the contour and dimensions of the trochlea notch are restored independent of comminution. As long as stable fixation is achieved, very aggressive postoperative therapy can be performed with limited protection since there is no reliance on soft-tissue ligamentous healing. Early stretching will optimize clinical outcomes.

Monteggia Fractures

Fractures of the ulna with a dislocation of the proximal radioulnar joint are known as Monteggia fractures. The traditional classification of Monteggia fractures is according to the direction of the radial head dislocation (anterior, lateral, or posterior). In the adult, posterior Monteggia fracture-dislocations are the most common injury classified as a Bado type 2. In this injury pattern, the proximal radioulnar joint is disrupted, with the radial head dislocating posteriorly and the apex of the proximal ulna fracture directed anteriorly. Jupiter has further classified the Bado type 2 injuries by location of the ulna fracture: A—the distal olecranon and coranoid process, B—at the metaphyseal–diaphyseal junction, C—diaphyseal, D—extending along the proximal third to half of the ulna. These injuries typically occur in the elderly and osteoporosis is often present, which can compromise stable internal fixation. A low-energy fall onto an outstretched arm is the most common injury mechanism. A comminuted fracture of the olecranon typically occurs and is commonly associated with fractures of the coronoid process (frequent) and the radial head (almost always) (Figure 21.5, A and B). Associated LCL complex injuries occur in up to

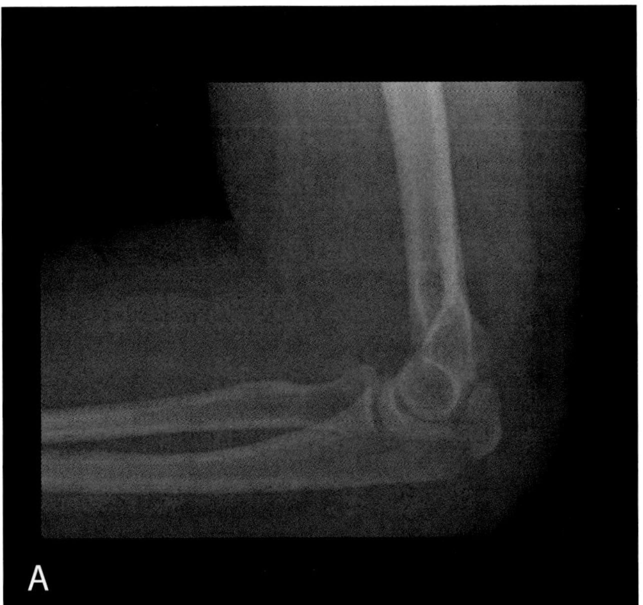

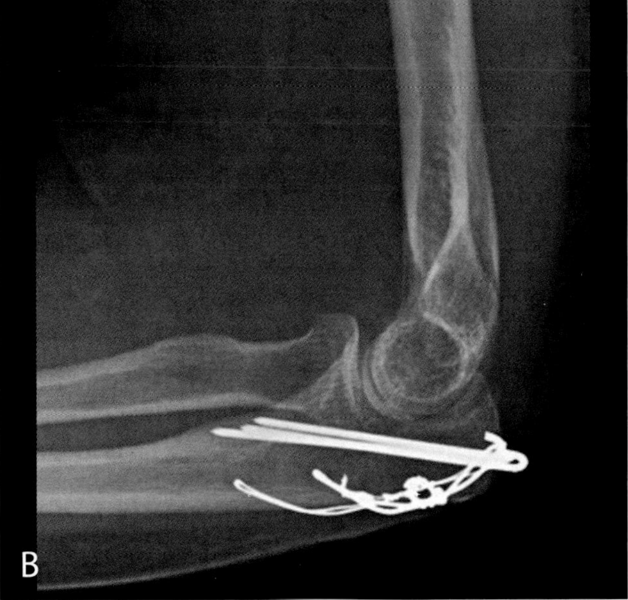

Figure 21.2 Lateral radiographs of a simple displaced transverse olecranon fracture: **A,** preoperative and **B,** posteroperative after tension-band fixation.

© 2018 American Academy of Orthopaedic Surgeons

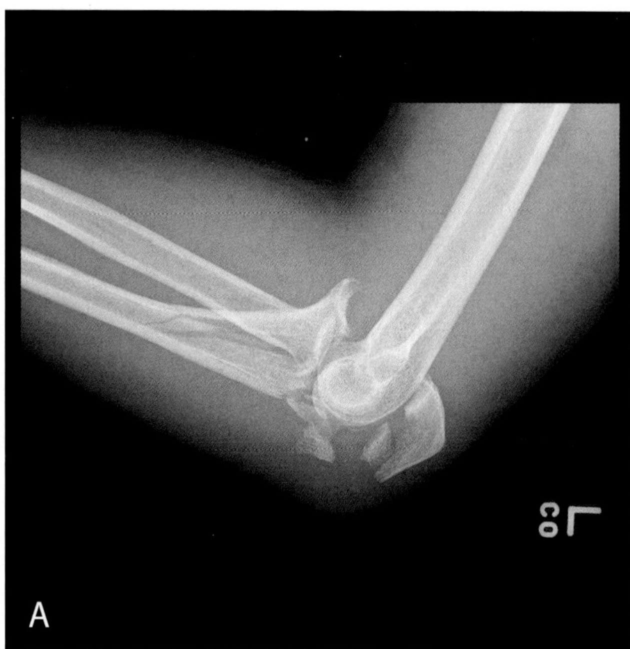

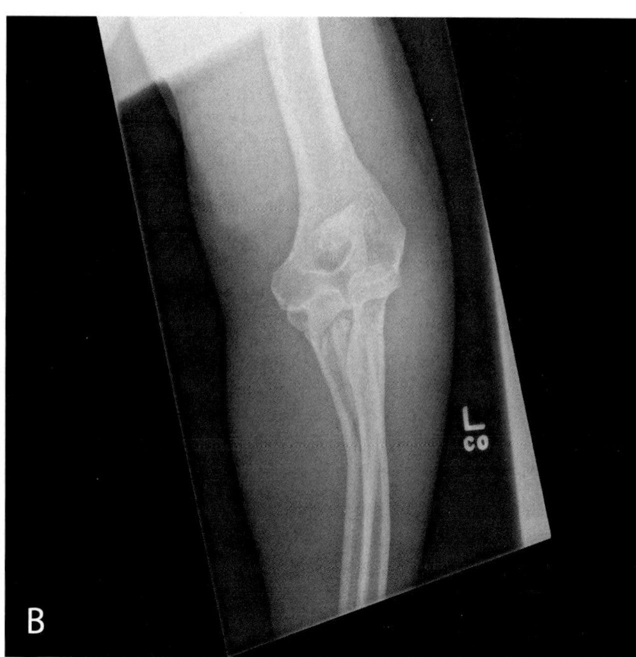

Figure 21.3 **A**, AP and **B**, lateral radiographs of a transolecranon fracture-dislocation.

two-thirds of patients and associated ulnohumeral instability can occur as well. Surgical treatment typically involves treating all of the pathologic structures, including the anatomic axial alignment of the ulna fracture (primary goal), repair or replacement of radial head and coronoid fractures, and repair of the injured LCL complex (Figure 21.6, A and B). Ulna fractures should be treated with a dorsally applied 3.5 reconstruction, precontoured, or compression plate. Overall results are slightly worse than the results of transolecranon fracture-dislocations due to increased risk for complications, including proximal radioulnar synostosis, ulnar malunion, posterolateral rotatory instability, and fixation failure due to

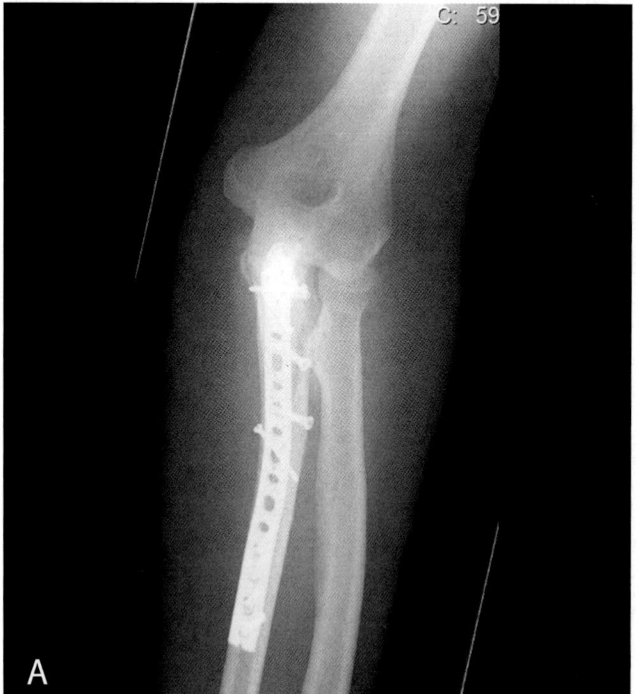

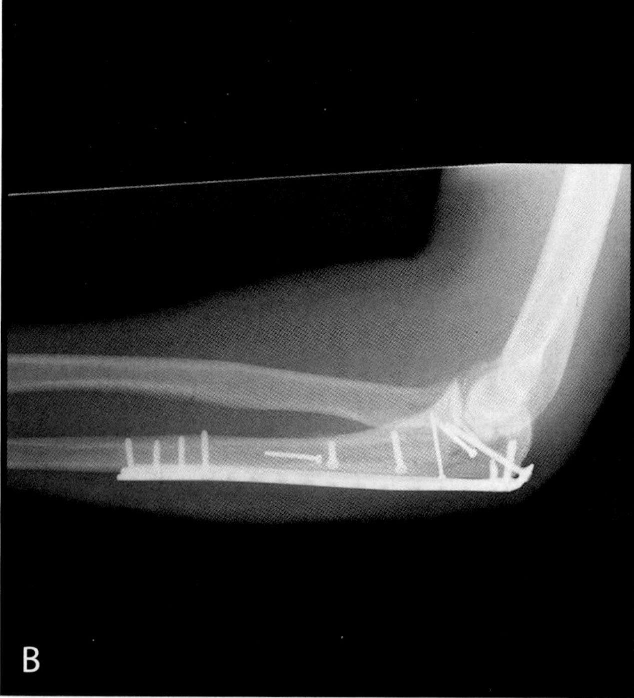

Figure 21.4 **A**, AP and **B**, lateral radiographs of a transolecranon fracture-dislocation surgically repaired with multiple small interfragmentary screws and a long dorsal 3.5-mm contoured olecranon plate.

© 2018 American Academy of Orthopaedic Surgeons

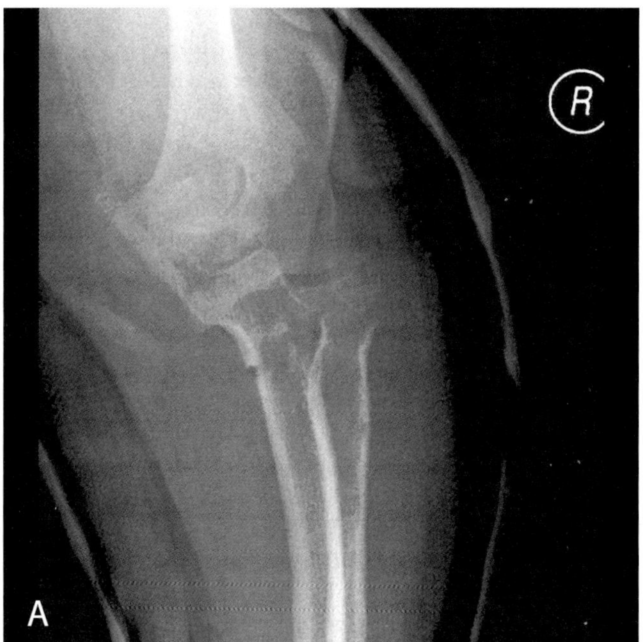

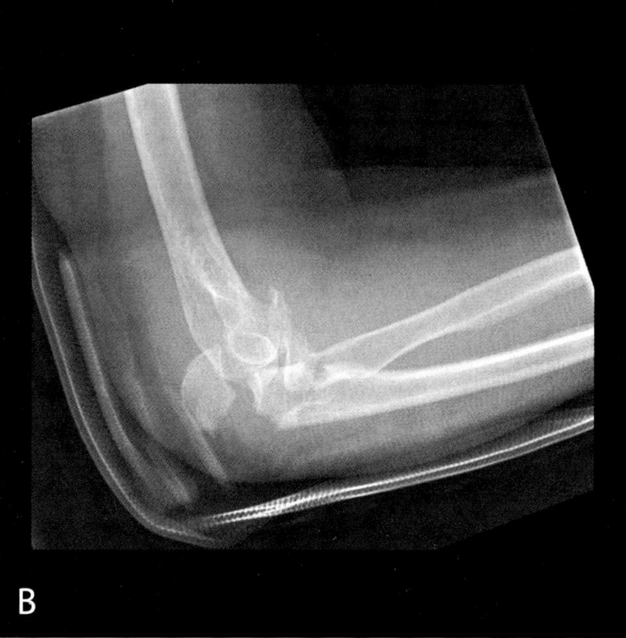

Figure 21.5 **A**, AP and **B**, lateral radiographs of a posterior Monteggia fracture-dislocation.

osteoporotic bone. Associated radial head and coronoid fractures negatively affect the surgical outcomes of these injuries. Postoperative rehabilitation therapists need to practice more cautious with these injuries compared to transolecranon fracture-dislocations due to less stable fixation associated with osteoporosis and the protection required for a repaired LCL complex. Despite these limitations, reasonable outcomes can still be achieved with a structured rehabilitation program.

SURGICAL PROCEDURE: ORIF FOR OLECRANON FRACTURES—SIMPLE OLECRANON FRACTURES, TRANSOLECRANON FRACTURE-DISLOCATIONS AND POSTERIOR MONTEGGIA VARIANT

Indications

The indications for operative fixation of an olecranon fracture—simple stable patterns with or without comminution,

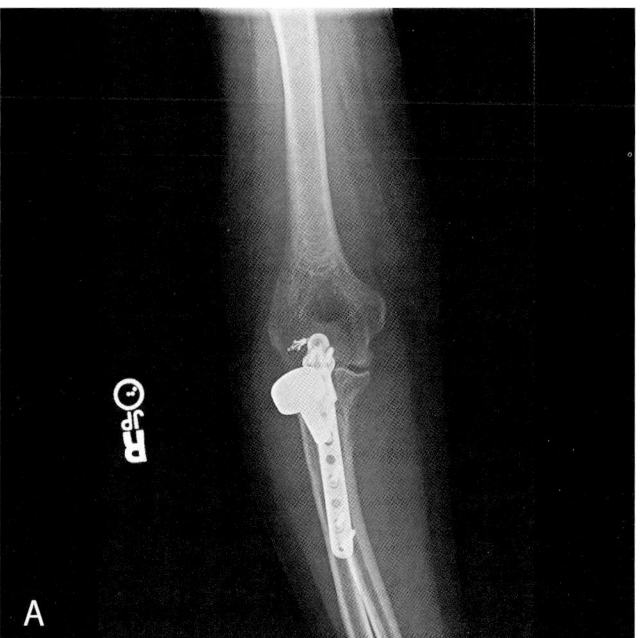

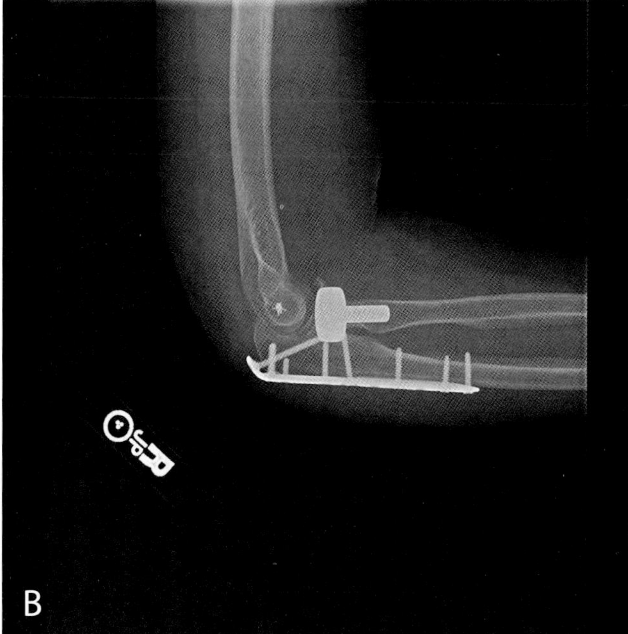

Figure 21.6 **A**, AP and **B**, lateral radiographs of a posterior Monteggia fracture-dislocation surgically repaired with a contoured 3.5-mm dorsally applied olecranon plate, suture fixation of a small type I coronoid fracture, radial head arthroplasty, and LCL repair.

© 2018 American Academy of Orthopaedic Surgeons

transolecranon fracture-dislocation, and a posterior Monteggia fracture-dislocation—are fairly straightforward. In general, displaced fractures of the olecranon generally require surgical fixation and nonoperative management has a minimal role except for nondisplaced stable injuries or in patients who are not surgical candidates due to other comorbid conditions.

Contraindications

In general, there are few contraindications to surgical repair for these injuries. If a patient is medically unfit and cannot tolerate an anesthetic, that may be considered a contraindication. Open fractures will require definitive fixation, but initial fixation may be deferred until adequate debridement and wound management has been performed.

Procedure

The setup, patient positioning, and superficial approach are identical for surgical procedures to treat all variants of olecranon and proximal ulna fractures. The deep approach and aspects of the fixation differ depending on the specific injury pattern. The patient can be positioned "lazy lateral" with soft padding behind the ipsilateral chest and thorax and the arm draped across the chest, or full lateral decubitus. Either setting provides access to the posterior and lateral aspects of the elbow and forearm while still allowing medial access if required. A mini C-arm or full-sized image intensifier is used throughout the case and brought in from the same side as the operative arm. A sterile tourniquet is used for bleeding control throughout the case.

It is important to have a full complement of plates and screws available. For simple stable fractures, tension band and intramedullary screw fixation are options and having appropriately sized Kirschner wires (K-wires; 1.6 or 2 mm), wire (18- or 20-gauge), and intramedullary screws (7.3-mm partially threaded cancellous) available is recommended (Figure 21.2, A and B). For more comminuted stable fractures as well as the dislocation patterns, plate-and-screw fixation is recommended. Current precontoured locking olecranon plates provide advantages over traditional reconstruction and compression plates. Additionally, smaller screws of various lengths may be needed to fix small fracture fragments. Long K-wires and reduction clamps are required to gain provisional fixation. If a displaced radial head fracture is part of the injury pattern, radial head and neck plates, headless screws, and radial head arthroplasty implants should be available. Finally, small screws and plates are used to fix coronoid fractures.

A medial approach is often required for reduction and fixation of significant coronoid fractures. The commonly utilized medial approaches include the flexor carpi ulnaris (FCU) split between the humeral and ulnar heads of the FCU and the Taylor-Scham approach between the ulnar shaft and the ulnar head of the FCU.

Simple Olecranon Fracture ORIF

Isolated simple olecranon fractures can be managed with a tension band, intramedullary screw, or plate fixation. Tension-band or intramedullary screw fixation is reasonable for noncomminuted, nonoblique fractures. Plate fixation may be used for these injuries as well as for oblique and comminuted fractures.

A direct posterior approach to the dorsal aspect of the olecranon is preferred. The proximal and distal fracture fragments need to be cleared of soft tissue at the fracture line to allow for anatomic reduction. Visualization of the joint reduction can be most easily achieved laterally through elevation of the anconeus from the olecranon. The ulnar nerve does not usually need transposition, but it should be identified and protected during fixation. The reduction is usually maintained using a bone reduction clamp. If a tension band is utilized, two or three smooth 1.6 or 2.0-mm K-wires are inserted from the proximal olecranon tip to engage the anterior ulna cortex after passing across the fracture line. After engagement of the anterior cortex, the wires are backed out slightly and bent. One or two 18-gauge wires are passed deep to the triceps tendon and crossed in a figure-of-8 pattern over the dorsal cortex of the ulna. One limb of the wire is then passed through a 2-mm transverse hole located 2 cm distal to the fracture site, dorsal to the mix-axis of the ulna (Figure 21.7). The 18-gauge wires are tensioned and the pins are impacted over the tension band, burying the ends in the triceps.

A locking precontoured or nonlocking 3.5-mm reconstruction or LCDC plate can also be utilized (Figure 21.8, A and B). Tension-band fixation does not provide enough stability in comminuted fractures and does not create dynamic compressive forces across oblique fractures; therefore, plate fixation should be used in these cases.

Transolecranon Fracture-Dislocations

For the treatment of transolecranon fracture-dislocations, medial and lateral surgical windows are not typically required.

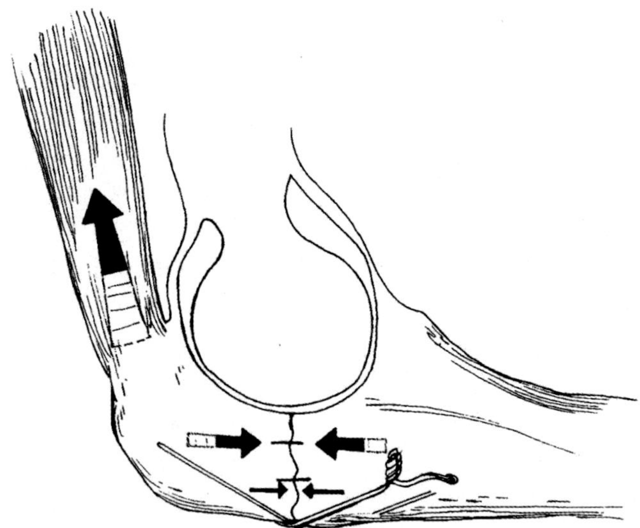

Figure 21.7 Tension band wire fixation of an olecranon fracture. Static compression is achieved dorsally (*paired thin arrows*). The extensor force of the triceps (*single thick arrow*) is converted into dynamic compression just below the articular surface (*paired thick arrows*). (Reproduced with permission from Hak DJ, Golladay GJ. Olecranon fractures: treatment options. *J Am Acad Orthop Surg* 2000;8(4):266–275.)

© 2018 American Academy of Orthopaedic Surgeons

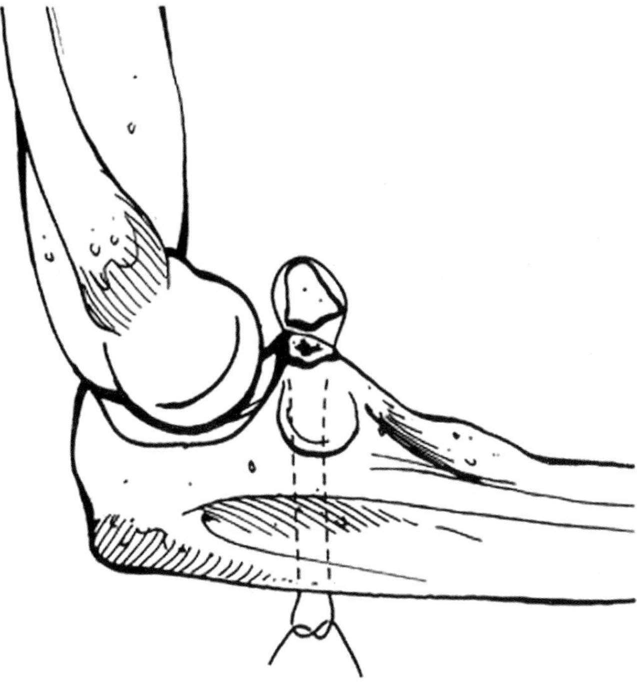

Figure 21.13 Illustration of coronoid fracture fixation using a Lasso repair, in which the suture is placed around a small coronoid piece, then passed through drill holes posteriorly in the ulna. (Reproduced with permission from Tashjian RZ, Katarincic JA. Complex elbow instability. *J Am Acad Orthop Surg* 2006;14(5):278–286.)

of the posterior Monteggia variant, then slight pronation of the forearm can aid in stability. There is no need for this maneuver after fixation of a transolecranon fracture-dislocation.

Author's Preferred Protocol

Simple Olecranon and Transolecranon Fracture Dislocations

- If excellent bone quality and intact ligaments, splint in neutral rotation and 90° of elbow flexion for 1 week to allow the wound to stabilize.
- Initiate active assisted and passive stretching of the elbow with full extension and flexion (Figure 21.14, A and B) as well as supination and pronation at 90° of elbow flexion (Figure 21.15, A and B) at 1 week postoperative but still protect the elbow with a sling between exercise sessions.
- Several sets of stretches should be performed four to five times per day.
- Discard the sling at 3 weeks postoperative and allow activities of daily living (ADLs) with no lifting over 2 to 3 pounds and continued active, active assisted, and passive stretching in all directions without restrictions.
- At 6 weeks, allow lifting between 5 and 10 pounds, continuing to work on stretching.
- If significant stiffness is present at 6 weeks, static progressive stretching can be introduced with a Joint Active Systems (JAS) brace to aid in motion (typically, if flexion is less than 110° and extension limit is greater than 40°).
- Isometric strengthening of the upper extremity is initiated after 6 weeks.

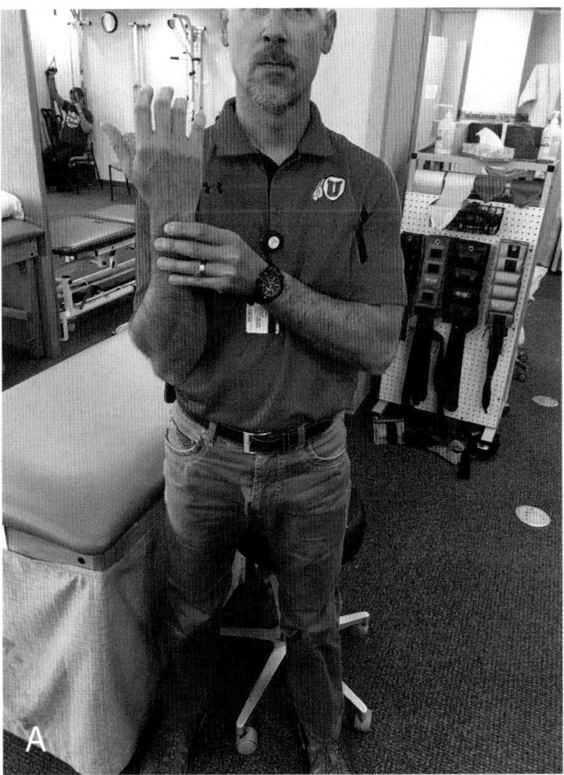

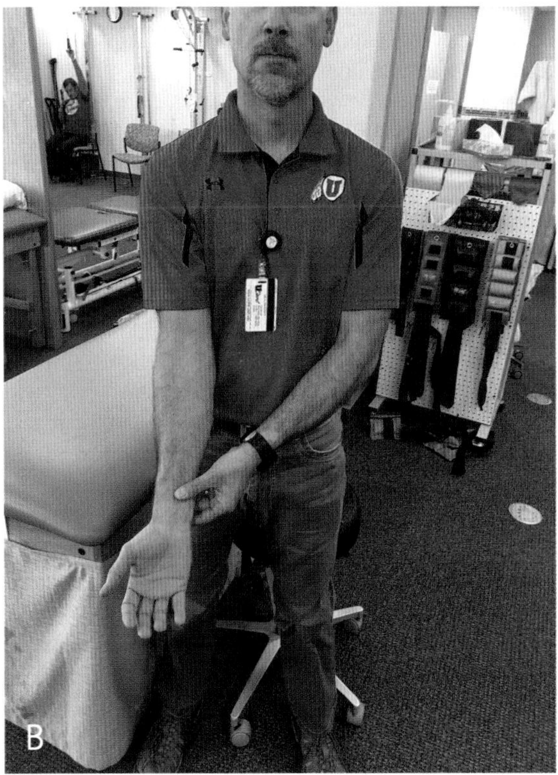

Figure 21.14 Photographs demonstrating active assisted and passive stretching exercises: **A**, flexion and **B**, extension.

© 2018 American Academy of Orthopaedic Surgeons

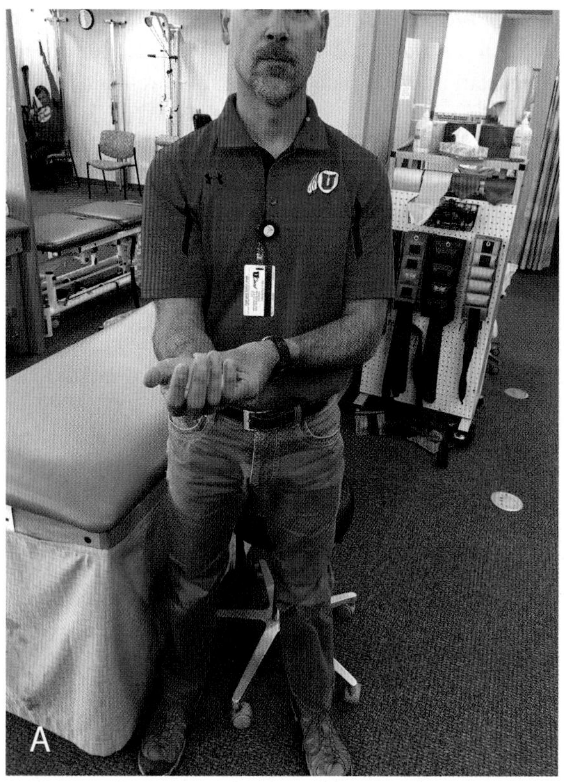

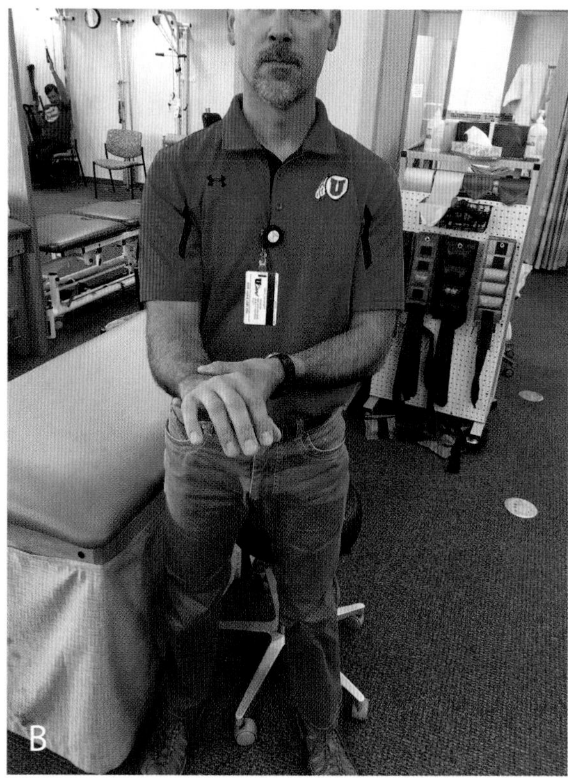

Figure 21.15 Photographs demonstrating active assisted and passive stretching exercises: include **A**, supination and **B**, pronation at 90° of elbow flexion.

- Resistive strengthening of the upper extremity is initiated after 3 months, when the fracture is typically healed.
- After 5 months, the patient is allowed to return to all activities, including contact sports, without restrictions.
- Full recovery may take up to 1 year.

Posterior Monteggia Variant Fracture Dislocations

- If no LCL repair and excellent bone quality, then protocol is identical to that for a transolecranon fracture-dislocation.
- Rehabilitation is slowed if there is repair of the LCL complex.
- Splint in neutral rotation and 90° of elbow flexion for 1 week in slight pronation.
- Hinged elbow braced applied when the splint is removed. The brace is locked with a 30° extension limit.
- A sling is worn for the first 3 weeks in addition to the brace.
- The sling and brace are removed daily to perform stretching exercises, including active assisted and passive supine elbow flexion and extension to limit varus stress on the elbow with a 30° extension block (Figure 21.16)
- The forearm is also held in pronation during extension to protect the lateral ligament repair.
- Active assisted and passive pronation and supination are allowed without restriction, but only at 90° of elbow flexion.
- The sling is discarded after 3 weeks, but the brace is still worn full time.
- The extension limit of the brace after 3 weeks is 15°; then, at 5 weeks postoperative, go to full extension.

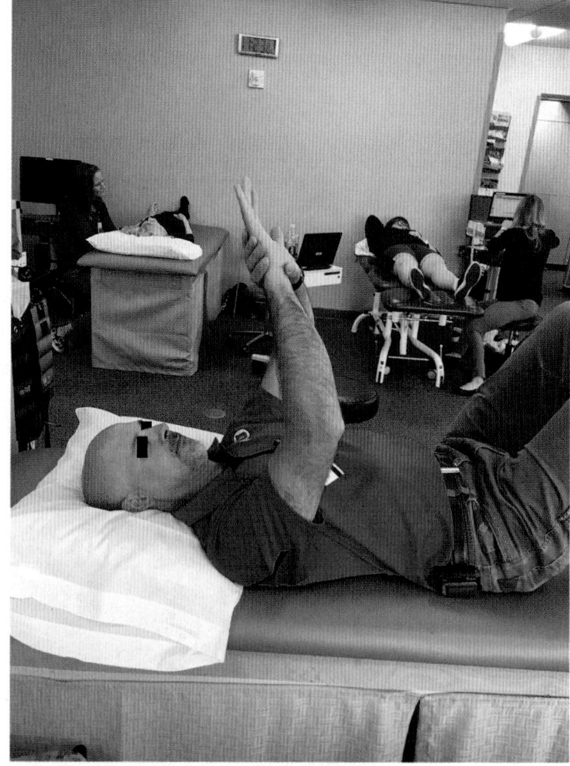

Figure 21.16 Photograph demonstrating supine passive elbow flexion and extension with the elbow in pronation, which allows unloading and protection of the LCL after repair.

© 2018 American Academy of Orthopaedic Surgeons

- If significant stiffness is present at 6 weeks, static progressive stretching can be introduced with a JAS brace to aid in motion (typically, if flexion is less than 110° and extension limit is greater than 40°).
- Lifting up to 2 to 3 pounds and daily activities are allowed at 3 weeks.
- At 6 weeks postoperative, lifting up to 5 to 10 pounds is allowed as well as light isometric strengthening of the upper extremity.
- At 3 months, the brace is discarded and resistive strengthening of the arm is initiated, with no lifting over 20 to 30 pounds.
- At 4.5 months, 40- to 50-pound lifting is allowed.
- At 6 months, return to all activities and contact sports, and heavy lifting is allowed.

COMPLICATIONS

Various complications—including loss of fixation, nonunion, elbow joint incongruity and instability, stiffness, heterotopic ossification, ulnar neuropathy, and painful hardware—can occur after surgical treatment of olecranon fractures or fracture-dislocations. Elbow stiffness is very common after surgical fixation of even simple fractures. The key to avoidance of stiffness is early mobilization within a week of the surgery. If stiffness occurs, early management includes static progressive splinting. If a patient has not achieved extension within 30° of full extension and flexion to 120° by 6 weeks postoperative, static progressive splinting using the JAS brace is initiated as long as the radiographs confirm progressive healing. Bracing is continued until 3 to 6 months postoperative. If at 4 to 6 months postoperative a functional ROM (30°–130° of a flexion-extension arc) has not been achieved, then open or arthroscopic capsular release can be considered to improve motion. If elbow flexion is restricted to less than 100° or preoperative ulnar nerve symptoms exist, a concomitant ulnar nerve in situ release or transposition should be performed to prevent postoperative ulnar neuropathy.

Some degree of heterotopic ossification is not uncommon after olecranon fracture-dislocations. In general, if there is not a significant restriction in ROM, then heterotopic ossification can be ignored. If significant restriction of motion remains in the setting of heterotopic ossification, the ossification can be excised at the same time as open capsular release is performed. The earliest that heterotopic ossification should be removed is about 4 months postoperative, when the ossification typically matures on plain radiographs. Extreme care and planning needs to be performed before excision, as the neurovascular structures are at high risk during the procedure.

Postoperative ulnar neuropathy in isolation is relatively uncommon, but if it occurs can be initially treated with night extension splinting for isolated sensory changes or paresthesias only. If there is motor involvement or a patient fails splinting for sensory changes, in situ ulnar nerve decompression or transposition can be performed depending on surgeon preference. If instability of the nerve is present with flexion after decompression, a transposition should be performed.

Finally, painful hardware is very common after olecranon fracture fixation due to the subcutaneous nature of the proximal ulna. Hardware removal should not be considered prior to 12 months postoperative. Radiographs should reveal complete remodeling of the fracture site and the patient should not have localized tenderness at the fracture site. Pain with pressure over the hardware should be the indication for removal. If there is any concern regarding fracture healing, a preoperative CT scan should be performed to confirm union. After hardware removal, the arm should be protected for about 4 weeks using a sling, but therapy should be initiated immediately to regain motion. Heavy lifting or contact sports should be restricted for about 12 weeks to eliminate the possibility of refracture.

OUTCOMES

Overall, there is relatively limited information on outcomes of treatment after transolecranon fracture-dislocations, with slightly more data after posterior Monteggia fracture dislocations. Ring et al. originally reported on the outcome for 17 patients with a transolecranon fracture-dislocation who underwent ORIF. Thirteen patients were treated with ORIF with a dynamic compression plate or reconstruction plate, one patient was treated with a one-third tubular plate and three patients were treated with a tension band construct. The patient treated with a one-third tubular plate needed early revision for fixation failure. At an average of 25 months postoperative, 15 patients had good or excellent results and two patients had fair results, with those two having significant arthritis. Large coronoid fragments and extensive comminution of the trochlear notch did not preclude a good result provided that stable anatomic fixation was achieved. The authors concluded that the goal of treatment should be restoration of the appropriate contours and dimensions of the trochlear notch of the ulna, as this will typically lead to good results in most cases.

Moushine et al. also reported on 14 patients with transolecranon fracture-dislocations treated with a variety of techniques, including ORIF with dynamic compression plates or reconstruction plates (four patients) or a tension band construct or one-third tubular plate (10 patients). Three patients required early revision for fixation failure, all of which had fixation with a tension band construct. At an average of 3.6 years postoperative, 10 patients had good or excellent results, two had fair results, and two had poor results based on the Broberg and Morrey score. Four patients showed signs of degenerative arthritis on follow-up radiographs. The authors recommended avoiding tension band reconstruction in these injuries due to their high failure rate and requirement for revision.

Outcomes assessment has been performed after surgical treatment of posterior Monteggia fracture-dislocations by several authors. Overall, the results of surgical treatment are slightly worse than those reported for transolecranon

© 2018 American Academy of Orthopaedic Surgeons

fracture-dislocations. Ring et al. reported on a series of 38 Bado type II injuries treated with ORIF of the ulna fracture treated with a plate (35 cases) or a tension-band construct (three cases). Radial head fractures were associated with the injury in 28 of 38 cases treated with complete or partial excision (12 cases), ORIF (10 cases), no intervention (four cases), or silicone arthroplasty (two cases). Coronoid fractures were present in 10 of 38 cases. Revision surgery was required in nine of 38 cases within 3 months due to revision of loose ulna fixation (five cases), radial head nonunion or failure leading to excision (three cases), or painful hardware requiring removal (one case). Fair or poor results were seen in six' of 38 cases, and all cases had an associated radial head fracture. These fair/poor results were secondary to malunited coronoid fractures, proximal radioulnar synostosis, or malunited ulna fractures. In general, problems relating to the fractures of the coronoid or radial head were the most challenging elements of treatment of these injuries.

Konrad et al. also reported on 27 Bado type II injuries treated with ORIF of the ulna fracture. Radial head fractures were present in 11 of 27 cases and coronoid fractures were present in 11 of 27 cases. Overall, 4 ulna fractures went on to nonunion. Four patients had a complication as a result of the radial head fractures. Five patients developed significant heterotopic ossification. Final functional outcomes included an average Mayo Elbow Performance Score of 81, an average flexion-extension arc of 103° and an average Disability of the Arm, Shoulder, and Hand (DASH) questionnaire of 22. Poor clinical outcomes were associated with Jupiter IIa fractures as well as injuries with concomitant radial head and coronoid fractures.

PEARLS

- Stable anatomic reduction and fixation of the ulna is key.
- Oblique, comminuted, or unstable fractures require plate fixation. Do not use a tension-band construct to treat these fractures.
- If there is any concern regarding LCL injury in a posterior Monteggia variant, perform either a radial head fracture repair or arthroplasty, and do *not* excise the radial head.
- Coronoid fractures in posterior Monteggia variants and transolecranon fracture-dislocations must be addressed. Have a low threshold to transpose the ulna nerve and make a medial approach to gain a reduction.
- Be aware of osteoporosis, especially in the posterior Monteggia variants, and utilize fixation techniques, including locking plates, to maximize stability.
- Perform rehabilitation of the elbow (flexion and extension exercises) when there is a concomitant LCL repair in the supine position overhead and with the forearm pronated to protect the lateral ligaments from gravitational varus stress during rehabilitation.
- Utilize a hinged elbow brace during the first 3 months postoperative to further protect the lateral ligament repair in posterior Monteggia variant fracture-dislocations.

SUMMARY

Proximal ulna fractures range from relatively simple transverse olecranon fractures to complex proximal ulna fractures that can be associated with comminution that can involve and extend distal to the coronoid process, as well as involve the lateral ligament complex and radial head. The most important goal of surgical treatment is to achieve a stable and anatomic reduction that minimizes the risk of fixation failure and permits early ROM exercises. With accurate reduction and stable internal fixation, as well as appropriate and coordinated rehabilitation, successful outcomes can be achieved.

BIBLIOGRAPHY

Bado JL: The Monteggia lesion. *Clin Orthop* 1967;50:71–76.

Baecher N, Edwards S. Olecranon fractures. *J Hand Surg Am* 2013; 38:593–604.

Jupiter JB, Leibovic SJ, Ribbans W, Wilk RM: The posterior monteggia lesion. *J Orthop Trauma* 1991;5(4):395–402.

Konrad GG, Kundel K, Kreuz PC, Oberst M, Sudkamp NP: Monteggia fractures in adults. Long-term results and prognostic factors. *J Bone Joint Surg Br* 2007;89:354–360.

Mortazavi SM, Asadollahi S, Tahririan MA: Functional outcome following treatment of transolecranon fracture-dislocation of the elbow. *Injury Int J Care Injured* 2006;37:284–288.

Moushine E, Akiki A, Castagna A, Cikes A, Wettstein M, Borens O, Garofalo R: Transolecranon anterior fracture dislocation. *J Shoulder Elbow Surg* 2007;16:352–357.

Ring D, Jupiter JB, Sanders RW, Mast J, Simpson NS: Transolecranon fracture-dislocation of the elbow. *J Orthop Trauma* 1997;11(8):545–550.

Ring D, Jupiter JB, Simpson NS: Monteggia fracrures in adults. *J Bone Joint Surg Am* 1998;80(12):1733–1744.

Ring D: Monteggia fractures. *Orthop Clin N Am* 2013;44:59–66.

Strauss EJ, Tejwani NC, Preston CF, Egol KA: The posterior Monteggia lesion with associated ulnohumeral instability. *J Bone Joint Surg Br* 2006;88:84–89.

© 2018 American Academy of Orthopaedic Surgeons

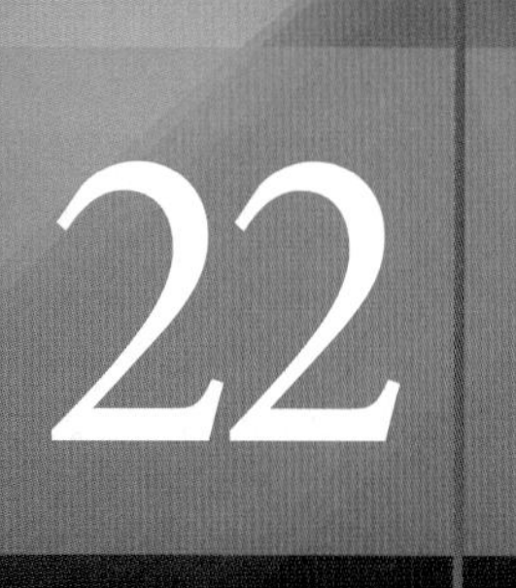

ORIF and Radial Head Replacement for Radial Head Fractures

Kevin Chan, MD, MSc, FRCSC, Joey G. Pipicelli, PhD Student, MScOT, CH, Shrikant J. Chinchalkar, MThO, BScOT, OTR, CHT, and George S. Athwal, MD, FRCSC

INTRODUCTION

Fractures of the radial head are the most common adult fracture around the elbow. The radial head acts as a stabilizer against valgus, axial, and posterolateral forces. Surgery aims to restore joint congruity and stability with either open reduction and internal fixation (ORIF) or radial head arthroplasty. This permits early, stable postoperative elbow range of motion (ROM) and forearm rotation to prevent stiffness and long-term disability. The specific rehabilitation regime after surgery depends heavily on the associated osseous and/or ligamentous injuries.

OPEN REDUCTION INTERNAL FIXATION

Indications

Surgical indications for radial head fractures is an area of controversy. In general, ORIF is offered to patients with radial head fractures that are displaced ≥2 to 3 mm and involve >30% of the articular surface, even if they do not impede forearm rotation. Radial head fractures that cause a mechanical block to motion should be fixed, regardless of their size. Fixation is also indicated during the surgical treatment of complex elbow fracture-dislocations to provide additional stability. The radial head is described as a secondary elbow stabilizer; however, when injuries occur to the primary stabilizers (medial collateral ligament [MCL] and lateral collateral ligament [LCL] and ulnohumeral articulation), its importance is elevated. Isolated nondisplaced and minimally displaced radial head fractures generally do not cause any mechanical blocks to rotation, thus can be treated nonoperatively.

Contraindications

A relative contraindication to ORIF is a comminuted radial head fracture with more than three displaced articular fragments. Although ORIF can be attempted, radial head arthroplasty is often preferred in these cases.

Procedure

The patient is typically positioned supine, with the affected arm placed over the chest or extended on an arm table. A "universal posterior" or lateral skin incision can be used, depending on surgeon preference and associated injuries. Deep dissection can be performed laterally through different intervals, depending on the status of the LCL. In cases of an isolated radial head fracture, we recommend a common extensor tendon-splitting approach, since it protects the LCL and provides a more direct exposure for fixation of partial articular radial head fractures, which are typically located in the anterolateral quadrant with the forearm in neutral rotation (Figure 22.1). If the LCL is ruptured, a classic Kocher approach (extensor carpi ulnaris-anconeus interval) may be preferable. The posterior interosseous nerve (PIN) is at risk with lateral exposures of the elbow; it can be protected by avoiding excessive distal dissection and placing the forearm in a pronated position.

Displaced fracture fragments should be carefully reduced and secured using small headless or countersunk headed interfragmentary screws. An obliquely oriented screw inserted from the radial head into the radial neck is a described technique to avoid placement of plates for fractures involving the entire articular surface or extending into the radial neck. Plate-and-screw constructs are avoided if possible because they are associated with postoperative stiffness, need for subsequent hardware removal, and disruption of periosteal vascularization of the radial head. However, if a plate is considered necessary for additional stability, it should be contoured to the patient's anatomy and placed on the nonarticular portion of the radial head.

Repair of associated injuries is carried out as indicated, including collateral ligaments or other bony structures, such

Dr. Athwal or an immediate family member has received royalties from IMASCAP and Wright Medical Technology; serves as a paid consultant to DePuy, A Johnson & Johnson Company, Smith & Nephew, and Wright Medical Technology; has received research or institutional support from DePuy, A Johnson & Johnson Company, Exactech, Smith & Nephew, Tornier, and Zimmer; and serves as a board member, owner, officer, or committee member of the Journal of Shoulder and Elbow Surgery. *None of the following authors or any immediate family member has received anything of value from or has stock or stock options held in a commercial company or institution related directly or indirectly to the subject of this article: Dr. Chan, Dr. Chinchalkar, and Dr. Pipicelli.*

© 2018 American Academy of Orthopaedic Surgeons

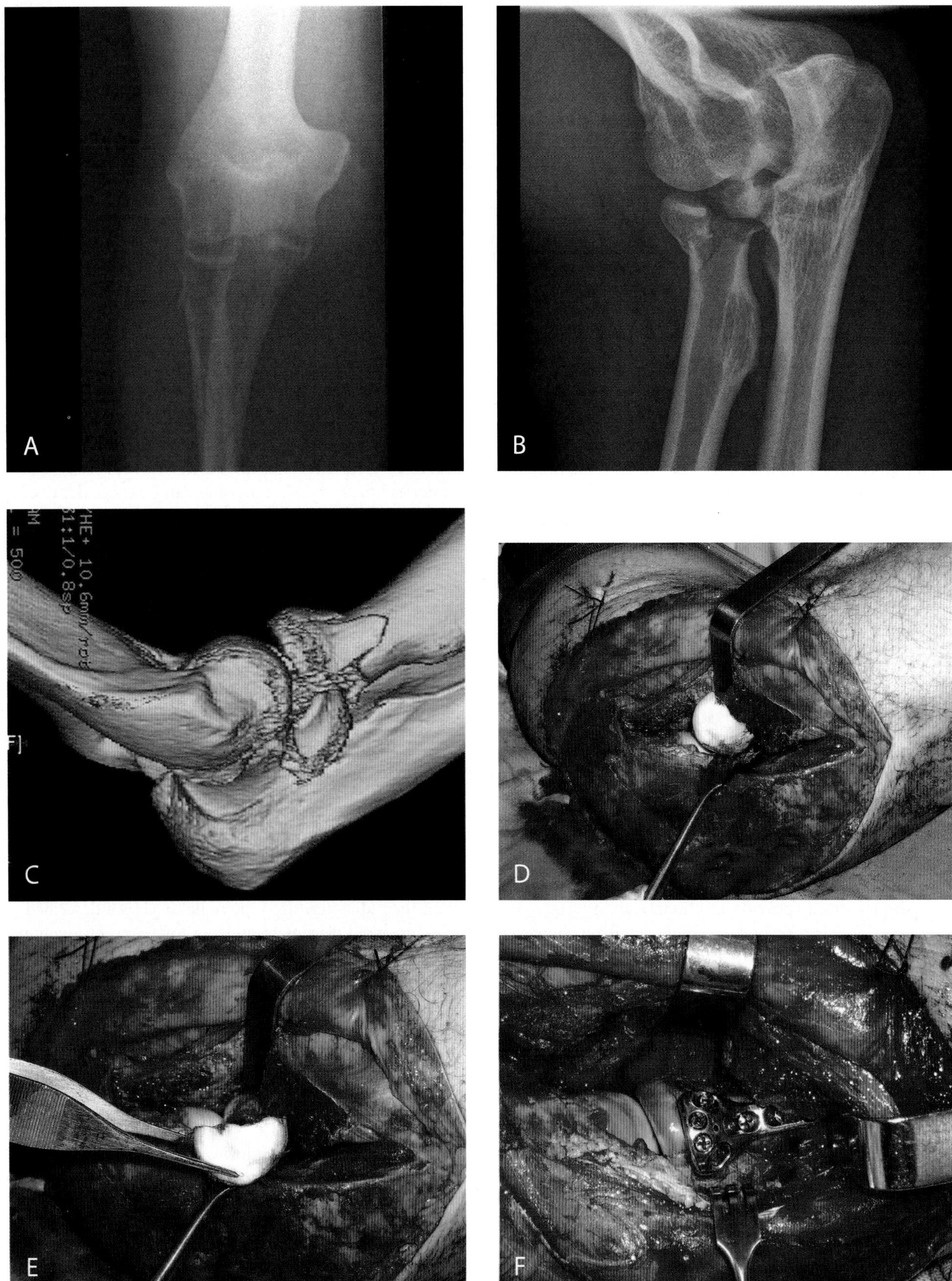

Figure 22.1 **A**, Anteroposterior and **B**, oblique radiographs of a comminuted radial head and neck fracture in a 27-year-old male. **C**, The 3-dimensional CT scan demonstrates the comminution. **D**, **E**, **F**, Clinical photographs of a Kocher approach, open reduction and internal fixation, done with an anatomic radial head/neck plate.

 © 2018 American Academy of Orthopaedic Surgeons

as the coronoid. All injuries, repaired or not, should be documented and communicated to collaborating therapists, since this will influence postoperative rehabilitation. Specifically, the status of the MCL (repaired or not) and the status of the LCL (solid repair or poor-quality repair) should be documented. The wound is then closed in layers. The elbow is typically immobilized and elevated after surgery for a brief period to decrease swelling and pain prior to therapy.

Complications

Elbow stiffness is a common complication after ORIF of the radial head. Possible etiologies include prominent hardware, capsular scarring and adhesions, heterotopic ossification (HO), prolonged immobilization, or noncompliance with postoperative rehabilitation. Physical examination should assess whether the end ROM is firm or soft. The latter finding may be managed successfully with therapy using stretching and static-progressive splinting. However, firm endpoints should be investigated to determine the cause. Mature capsular scarring and adhesions may require open or arthroscopic capsular releases.

Other less common complications may include infection, ulnar nerve or PIN injury, malunions, nonunions, and persistent elbow instability.

RADIAL HEAD ARTHROPLASTY

Indications

Radial head arthroplasty is indicated for comminuted, displaced fractures for which stable internal fixation cannot be achieved. For complete articular radial head fractures, there is some evidence that arthroplasty is superior to ORIF.

Procedure

Patient positioning and surgical approach are similar to ORIF. Arthroplasty is typically performed using metallic implants. Although the specific technique will vary depending on the prosthesis used, optimal sizing of all implants is critical to avoiding complications, such as pain, postoperative stiffness, and arthrosis. Articular fragments should be retained and reassembled to help determine the appropriate implant diameter and length. The diameter can be chosen based on the minimum outer diameter of the native radial head. The use of the lesser sigmoid notch for implant diameter sizing may be unreliable. An alternative method is to use the ipsilateral capitellar dimensions on preoperative radiographs to estimate radial head diameter. Similarly, implant length can be approximated using the excised radial head. When the prosthesis is inserted, its articular surface should be even with the proximal edge of the lesser sigmoid notch. Contralateral elbow radiographs can further aid in identifying over- or under-lengthening of the radial head prosthesis. Inappropriate length can be difficult to diagnose using radiographs of the injured elbow only. Local landmarks have been shown to be inaccurate, including the lateral ulnohumeral joint space, which can be nonparallel on anteroposterior radiographs in normal patients due to anatomic variability. The medial ulnohumeral joint space is also unreliable because it may not demonstrate widening on anteroposterior radiographs until significant over-lengthening has occurred.

Once a trial implant is inserted, the elbow is placed through ROM, with stability testing and fluoroscopic assessment. The tracking of the radial head implant on the capitellum is observed to ensure that it is congruent. As in the case of ORIF, the associated injuries are repaired, if required, and documented.

Complications

Possible complications after radial head replacement include infection, loosening, radial head "over-lengthening" or "overstuffing," radiocapitellar arthritis, instability, HO and fractured components. In a retrospective review of 47 failed metallic radial head arthroplasties, 31 (66%) were caused by aseptic loosening. Other causes included stiffness, instability, and deep infection. Prophylaxis against HO remains controversial. In the authors' opinion, prophylaxis may be unnecessary in isolated radial head fractures with minimal soft-tissue trauma.

POSTOPERATIVE REHABILITATION

Rehabilitation following elbow trauma can be a challenging proposition for the surgeon and therapist, as well as the patient. The elbow is a notoriously unforgiving joint. The literature on postoperative therapy following radial head fractures managed by ORIF or radial head arthroplasty is limited. A comprehensive understanding of the specific anatomy and supporting structures is essential to facilitate communication between the surgeon and therapist. This will allow for the implementation of a systematic rehabilitation program that encourages early mobilization within a safe arc of motion while maintaining joint stability.

AUTHORS' PREFERRED PROTOCOL

Key Information Required for Therapists from Surgeons

Prior to initiating postoperative rehabilitation, the therapist must be aware of the following:

- Type of procedure performed
- Rigidity of the bony fixation
- Status of the soft-tissue structures surrounding the elbow, including ligaments, nerves, muscles, and joint capsule
- Presence of any radiographic abnormalities, such as a drop sign (≥4 mm in ulnohumeral joint space seen on unstressed lateral radiographs of the elbow)

These important details allow the therapist to create a custom-tailored rehabilitation program (Figure 22.2). Ideally,

© 2018 American Academy of Orthopaedic Surgeons

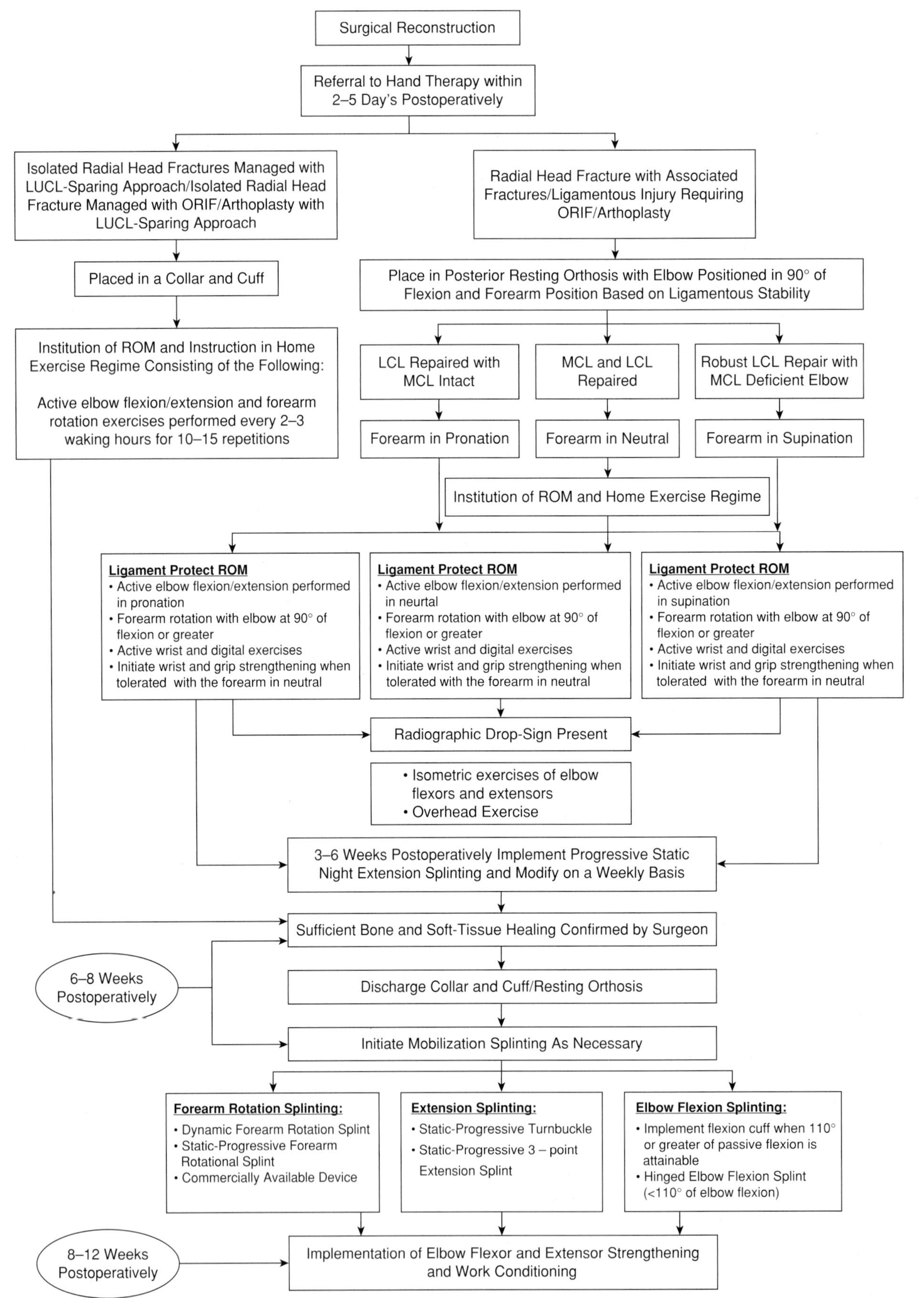

Figure 22.2 Radial head fracture rehabilitation algorithm.

 © 2018 American Academy of Orthopaedic Surgeons

patients should be seen in specialized outpatient therapy 48 to 72 hours following surgery.

Postoperative Positioning and Immobilization

Isolated radial head fractures managed with a lateral ulnar collateral ligament (LUCL)–sparing approach can be placed in a sling or a collar and cuff (Figure 22.3) with the elbow maintained at 80° to 90° of flexion. These are used for comfort during the day and in between exercise sessions.

Patients with associated ligamentous injuries or fractures should be placed in a posterior elbow resting orthotic, with the elbow positioned in approximately 80° to 90° of flexion. The forearm rotation should be specific to the injury pattern to provide optimal ligament protection:

- If the LCL was repaired and the MCL was intact, the elbow is positioned with the forearm in pronation.
- With associated MCL injuries, but a robust LCL repair, the elbow may be positioned in supination.
- If both the MCL and LCL are disrupted, the elbow should be positioned in an orthosis, with the forearm in neutral rotation.

Early Mobilization

Although the optimal time for initiation of ROM after radial head fracture is unknown, the stability of fixation is critically important. We usually advocate that patients begin controlled active and passive mobilization 2 to 5 days postoperatively. Modifications to the exercise regime are made in cases with associated injuries:

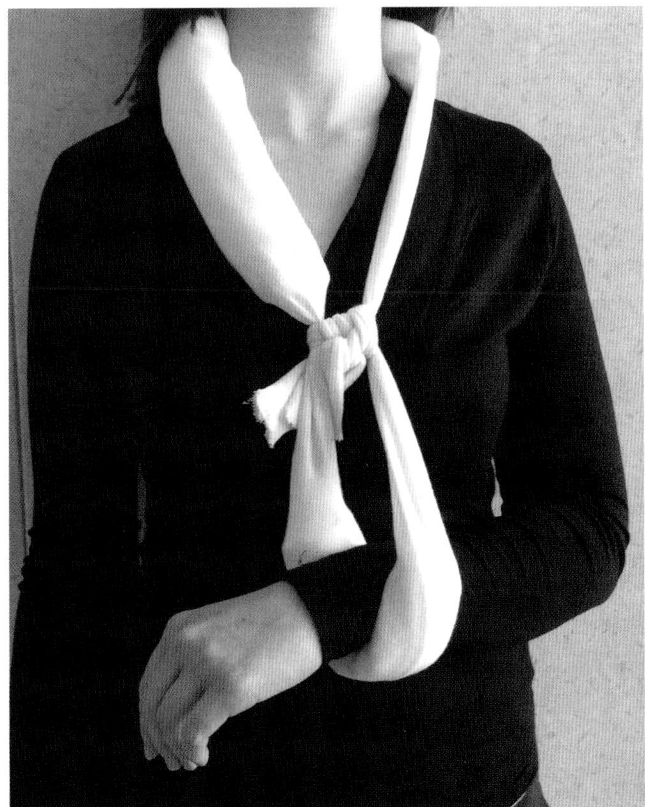

Figure 22.3 Photograph of a collar and cuff for positioning the elbow between 80° and 90° of flexion following elbow trauma.

- If the LCL was repaired and the MCL was intact, active elbow extension and flexion are to be performed with the forearm in full pronation exclusively until 6 weeks post-repair to ensure that adequate ligamentous healing has occurred. Active forearm rotation exercises are to be performed with the elbow in >90° of flexion to protect the LCL complex.
- If the LCL repair is stable and robust, but the integrity of the MCL is in question, positioning the patient in full supination may be considered. In such cases, active elbow extension/flexion exercises are performed with the forearm in supination. Active forearm rotation exercises are to be performed with the elbow in >90° of flexion to protect both the LCL and MCL.
- If the LCL repair is not robust and the MCL is deficient, the patient should be positioned in neutral rotation to protect both the MCL and LCL. Elbow flexion and extension exercises are to be performed with the forearm in the neutral position exclusively. Initially, terminal extension is limited to 30° to 45° and advanced by 10° increments on a weekly basis. Forearm rotation exercises are performed with the elbow in >90° of flexion.

ROM Exercise Progression and Strengthening

The optimal frequency of ROM exercises is unknown. We advocate that patients perform 10 to 15 repetitions of active elbow and forearm ROM exercises every 2 to 3 waking hours initially during the early phases of healing. The frequency and repetition of exercise can be increased to 15 to 25 repetitions hourly. However, therapists must ensure that exercise frequency and duration do not cause pain, inflammation, or muscle fatigue. Patients are not given instructions on home passive ROM exercises until proficiency is demonstrated in supervised therapy.

Forearm rotation exercises are performed with the elbow in >90° of flexion to minimize stress on the medial and/or lateral ligamentous structures. Passive forearm rotational exercises should not be instituted until sufficient ligamentous healing has occurred, which is typically between 6 to 8 weeks post-repair. A simple way to self-stretch the forearm is to use the towel stretch for pronation/supination (Figure 22.4). In cases of isolated radial head fractures without ligamentous injuries, ROM and physiotherapy may be advanced more rapidly (Figure 22.2).

At about 6 to 8 weeks postsurgery, after radiographs demonstrate signs of healing, active and passive ROM in all directions can be instituted. At 8 weeks postoperatively, gentle strengthening exercises for the elbow flexors, extensors, forearm rotators, and shoulder are instituted. Light weights are incorporated into the rehabilitation program. However, emphasis should be placed on strengthening the triceps, as this will help minimize elbow flexion contracture formation.

© 2018 American Academy of Orthopaedic Surgeons

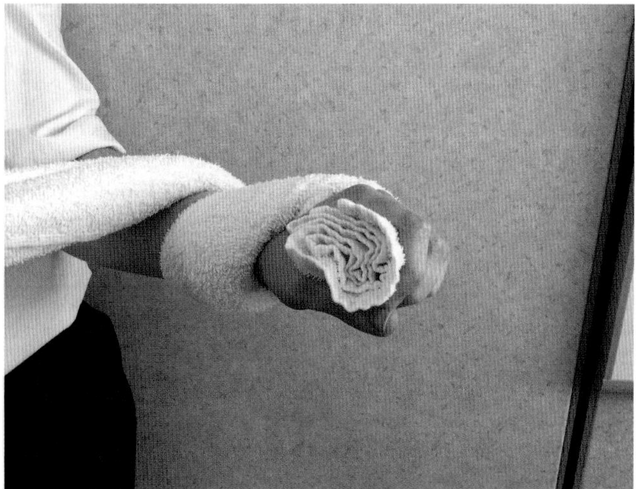

Figure 22.4 Photograph of towel stretch for pronation. This is an easy way to self-stretch the forearm. Reverse the direction of pull to enhance supination.

Radiographic Drop Sign

A radiographic drop sign is an objective, measurable increase in ulnohumeral joint distance that is evident on a static lateral radiograph (Figure 22.5). he normal ulnohumeral joint distance is 2 to 3 mm; an ulnohumeral joint distance of greater than >4 mm would be considered a positive drop sign. A drop sign can be present after simple or complex elbow dislocations treated with or without surgery, and indicates a persistent instability of the elbow joint. If a drop sign is present, modifications are made to the controlled mobilization program, which include the following:

- Isometric exercise of the triceps, biceps, and brachialis. Isometric exercise should be performed at regular intervals throughout the day while the affected arm is resting within the sling, collar and cuff, or orthosis. Isometric exercise enhances compressive joint forces across the ulnohumeral joint, reducing ulnohumeral joint sagging. Exercises are performed four to six times per day for 5 to 10 repetitions, holding each repetition for 5 to 10 seconds.
- Overhead elbow and forearm active ROM exercises (Figure 22.6). Overhead ROM is performed while supine with the shoulder flexed to 90°. Overhead exercise reduces the gravitational forces distracting the ulnohumeral joint and enhances ulnohumeral joint tracking during flexion and extension exercises. This will minimize ulnohumeral joint sagging, joint hinging, and impingement during early ROM exercises.
- Instruction in active wrist and digital motion. This will provide a compressive force to the ulnohumeral joint as the wrist and digital flexors and extensors cross the elbow joint. As no ulnohumeral joint motion occurs with such exercises, they do not need to be performed in the overhead manner.

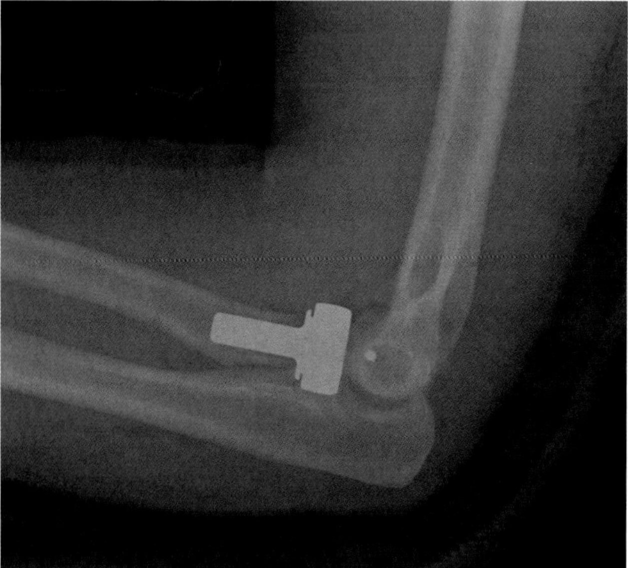

Figure 22.5 A radiographic drop sign is apparent on this lateral radiograph and is an objective, radiographically measurable increase in ulnohumeral joint distance.

It is our experience that the radiographic drop sign spontaneously reduces within the first 2 to 4 weeks after initiation of the aforementioned modifications to rehabilitation. Once the correction of the drop sign is observed radiographically, the patient can discontinue performing overhead exercise and can be progressed to active ROM in all planes based on the stages of healing of the involved structures.

ORTHOTIC CONSIDERATIONS

Extension Orthoses

Progressive static extension orthoses can be applied during the first 3 to 6 weeks postoperatively (Figure 22.7). Typically, such orthoses are prescribed for nighttime usage. Progressive static extension orthoses do not apply overpressure, allowing the patient to maintain any extension gains made during the day with frequent ROM exercise. The orthosis is serially adjusted on a weekly basis until satisfactory extension is achieved. If a firm flexion contracture is developing, the progressive-static extension orthosis can be worn intermittently throughout the day to provide a low-load, long-duration stretch.

Typically, application of progressive static extension orthoses produces adequate extension results. However, if minimal improvements are made, then a static-progressive turnbuckle extension orthosis should be fabricated. Such devices have been shown to be effective at regaining elbow ROM. The patient is instructed to serially self-adjust extension by adjusting the turnbuckle. These devices can be custom fabricated by elbow therapists or are available commercially in a prefabricated form (Figure 22.8).

Static-progressive extension orthotics should not be applied until the surgeon feels that sufficient osseous and soft-tissue healing has occurred. As extension improves, it may be necessary to modify custom-made versions to create a 3-point extension orthosis (Figure 22.9), which has been shown

© 2018 American Academy of Orthopaedic Surgeons

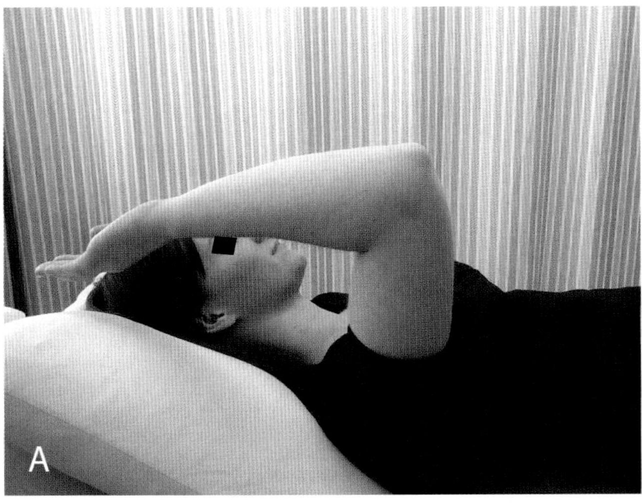

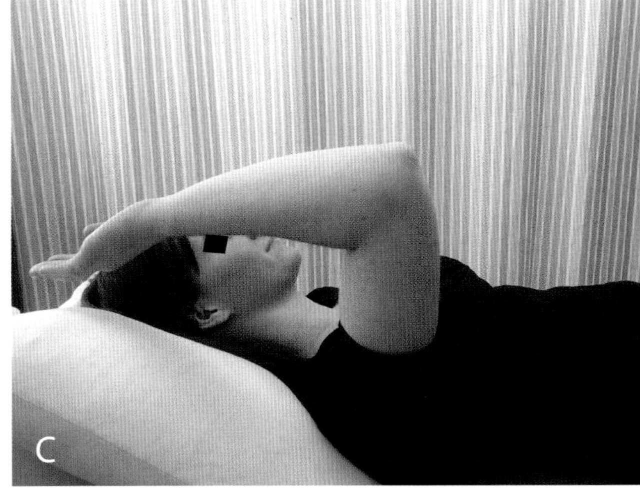

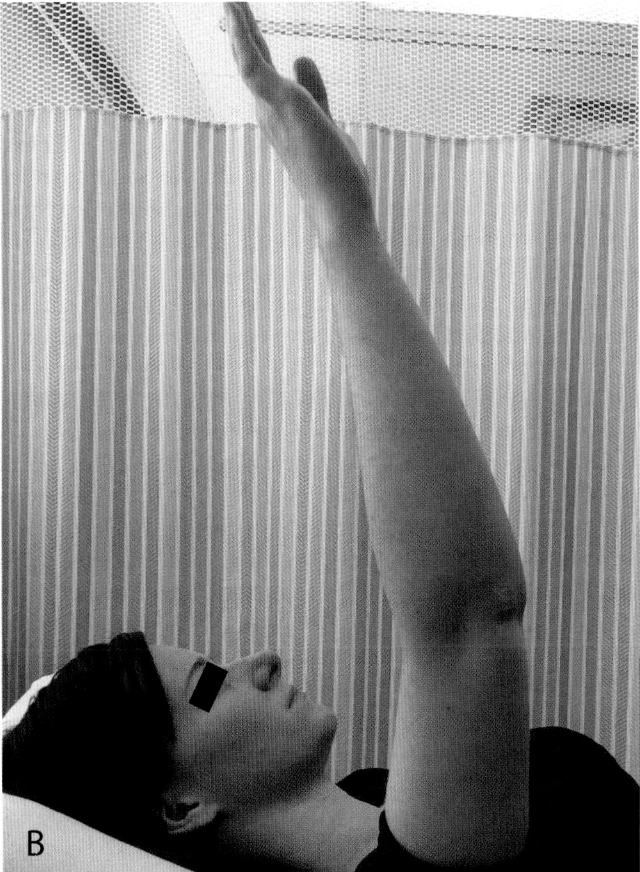

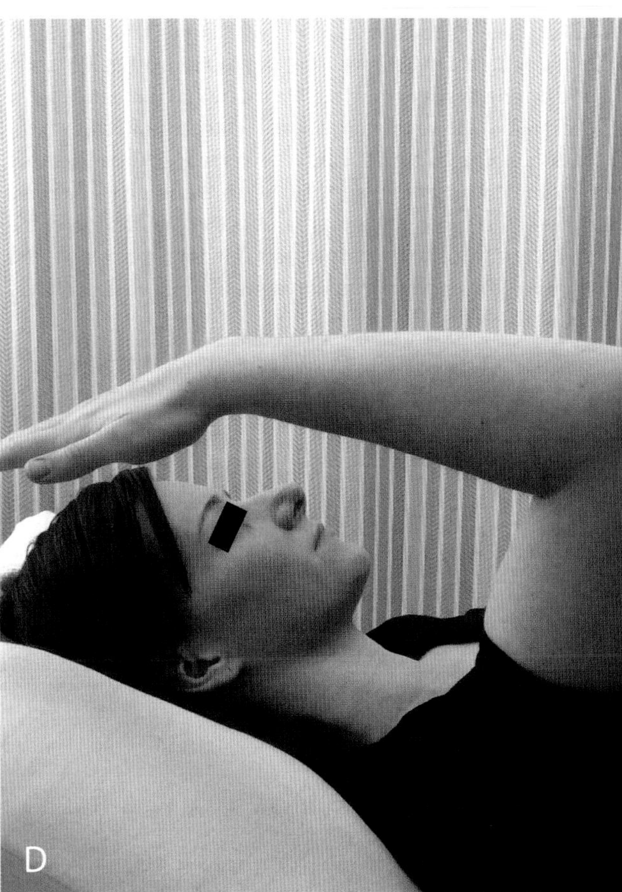

Figure 22.6 **A**, **B**, Photographs demonstrating overhead active flexion and extension exercises performed supine with the forearm positioned in pronation. The position of the forearm during this exercise is dependent on ligamentous stability. **C**, **D**, Photographs demonstrating forearm rotation exercises performed in the overhead position with the elbow positioned in 90° of elbow flexion to protect ligamentous structures.

mathematically to be more effective at producing greater rotational force to improve extension.

Flexion Orthoses

Elbow flexion is typically regained in a predictable fashion following radial head fractures. However, if limitations in elbow flexion occur, a static-progressive elbow flexion orthosis can be utilized. Use of such devices early during the rehabilitation program can lead to injury, ligamentous insufficiency, and possibly heterotopic bone formation, and should only be applied after sufficient osseous and ligamentous healing, in around 6 to 8 weeks.

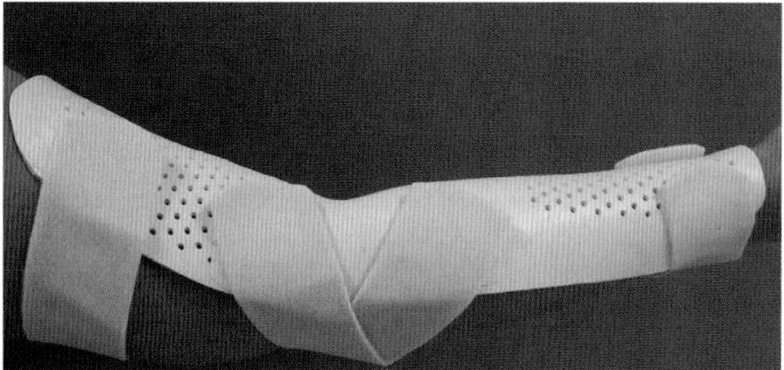

Figure 22.7 Photograph of progressive static elbow extension orthosis. The forearm is positioned in neutral to protect both the MCL and LCL complexes.

Several orthotic designs exist; however, we typically fabricate custom static-progressive elbow flexion cuffs or hinged elbow flexion turnbuckle orthoses (Figure 22.10). Decision making is critical when choosing the type of flexion device to apply. When a patient can achieve ≥110° of flexion, a flexion cuff is a good option to apply an effective rotational force to enhance elbow flexion. However, for patients who cannot achieve 110° of flexion, a hinged turnbuckle is preferred, as the hinges will minimize compressive loads placed on the joint while maximizing rotation force. Static-progressive elbow flexion orthoses are worn three to four times per day for a period of 15 to 40 minutes while monitoring for signs of ulnar neuropathy.

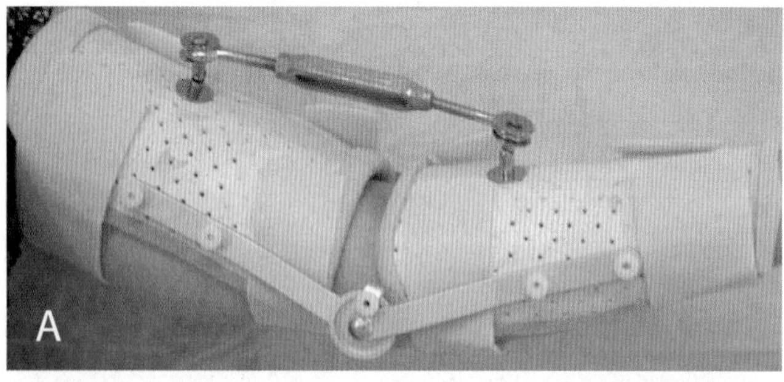

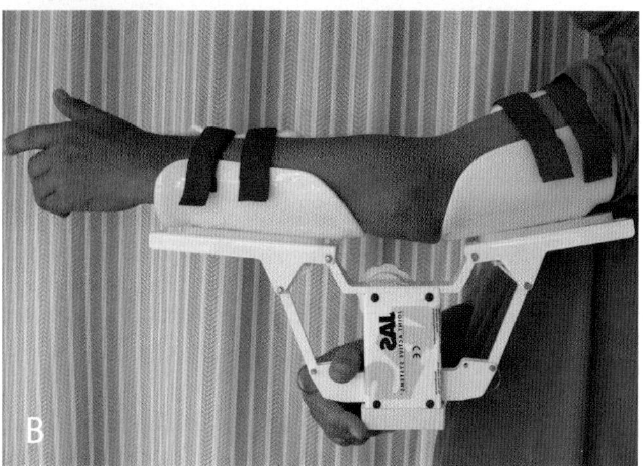

Figure 22.8 **A**, Photograph of custom-fabricated static progressive turnbuckle elbow extension orthosis. **B**, Photograph of commercially available static-progressive elbow extension-flexion orthosis from Joint Active Systems.

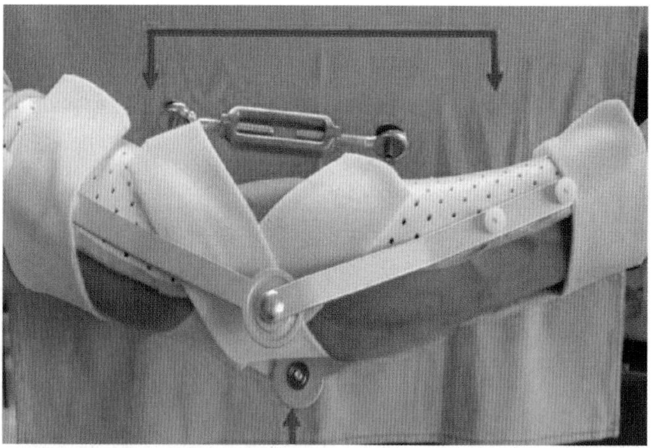

Figure 22.9 The 3-point static progressive elbow extension orthosis produces greater rotational force by simply cross crossing the straps posterior to the elbow joint.

Forearm Rotation Orthoses

Forearm rotation can be limited following radial head fractures. When the patient is having difficulty attaining sufficient rotation, various forms of dynamic and static-progressive orthoses have been found to be successful. However, these devices should not be instituted until at least 8 weeks postoperatively to ensure that sufficient osseous and ligamentous healing has occurred. At our facility, we typically employ dynamic forearm orthoses first (Figure 22.11). However, if limited improvement is achieved, we often progress to a commercially available static-progressive orthosis. We find the stress-relaxation principle of static–progressive orthotic application to be successful at improving forearm rotation when the creep principle of dynamic loads has produced minimal improvement. Patients are typically instructed to wear such devices two to four times per day for 15 to 45 minutes while monitoring for increases in pain and inflammation.

Orthotic Considerations in the Presence of a Radiographic Drop Sign

Despite our best efforts when managing a radiographic drop sign, it may not spontaneously reduce within the first 2 to 4 weeks following surgery. In such instances, mobilization orthotic application must be implemented with caution to prevent hinging of the articular structures, which leads to joint damage, pain, inflammation, and greater stiffness. Static-progressive extension orthoses should be applied with caution with flexion contractures of ≤30°, as hinging may be profound with this orthotic application (Figure 22.12). Also, static-progressive flexion splinting may be contraindicated in patients who can achieve 130° of flexion, as joint hinging may occur between the coronoid and coronoid fossa (Figure 22.13). However, this form of flexion splinting may be used cautiously when the patient is unable to achieve 130° of flexion. In contrast, forearm rotation splinting can be used to regain terminal rotation, as this motion occurs at the proximal and distal radioulnar joints, which should be in proper alignment.

 © 2018 American Academy of Orthopaedic Surgeons

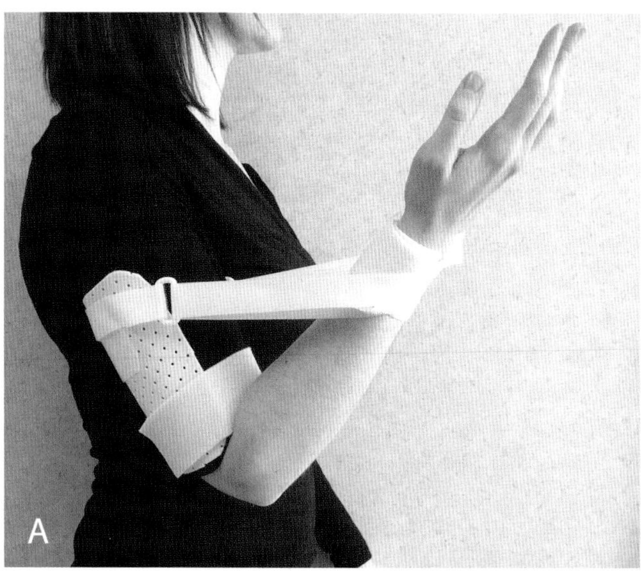

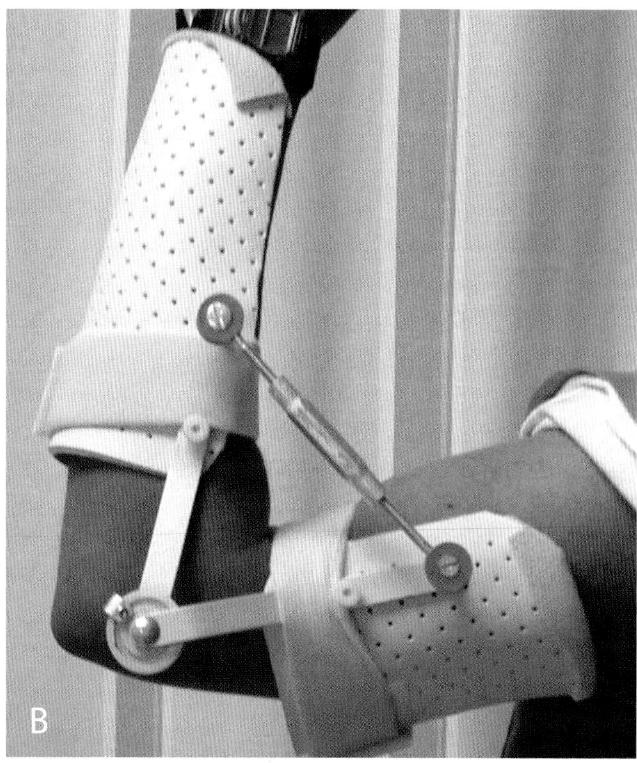

Figure 22.10 **A**, Photograph of custom-made static-progressive elbow flexion cuff. Appropriate for use in patients who can achieve >110° of flexion. **B**, Photograph of custom-fabricated turnbuckle static-progressive elbow flexion orthosis. Appropriate for use in individuals with <100° of flexion. (Reproduced with permission from Pipicelli JG, Chinchalkar SJ, Grewal R, Athwal GS: Rehabilitation considerations in the management of terrible triad injury to the elbow. *Tech Hand Up Extrem Surg.* 2011;15:198–208.)

THERAPEUTIC TECHNIQUES

Progressive manual joint mobilization therapy has a role in the rehabilitation of radial head fractures, as it assists with pain reduction, decreases muscle spasm, and is beneficial to regain motion. However, these treatment maneuvers are performed with caution to minimize stress to the healing bony structures, ligaments, and surrounding soft tissues.

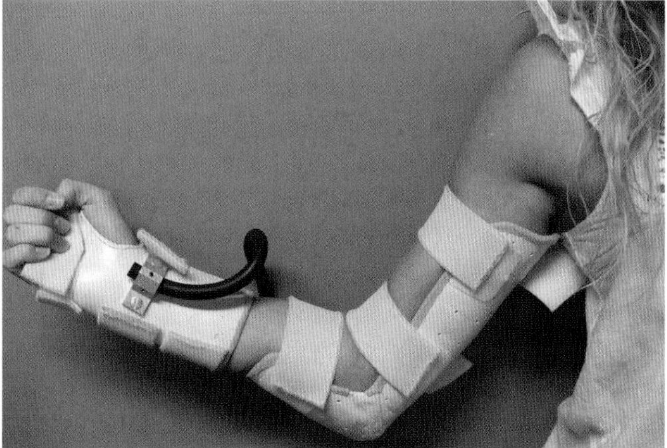

Figure 22.11 Photograph of custom-fabricated dynamic pronation and supination orthosis. (Reproduced with permission from Pipicelli JG, Chinchalkar SJ, Grewal R, Athwal GS: Rehabilitation considerations in the management of terrible triad injury to the elbow. *Tech Hand Up Extrem Surg.* 2011;15:198–208.)

Heat is typically applied during therapy sessions in order to precondition the soft tissues to allow for adequate muscle relaxation and increase tissue extensibility. Heating agents that are effective for soft tissues include hot packs, whirlpools, or fluidotherapy. If stretching is also desired, an effective method of increasing elbow extension is to position the elbow at a tolerable end range for the duration of the heating application. Once bone and soft-tissue healing are deemed adequate, the same technique can be utilized while applying a light load for the duration of the heating application, which is typically 15 to 20 minutes.

Muscular guarding caused by co-contraction of the antagonist muscles or muscle spasms during ROM exercise can occur, especially at end range in certain patients. This co-contraction limits ROM and is a challenging task to manage. Although not completely understood, it is postulated that the neural receptors around the elbow joint—which detect change in tension, joint position, and muscle length—are often injured following elbow trauma. Simply, this leads to abnormal programming of the joint receptor system. EMG biofeedback can be added to the rehabilitation program to help manage abnormal muscular guarding. A dual channel EMG biofeedback instrument should be used. During application, patients are encouraged to inhibit co-contraction of the antagonist by using verbal cues

© 2018 American Academy of Orthopaedic Surgeons

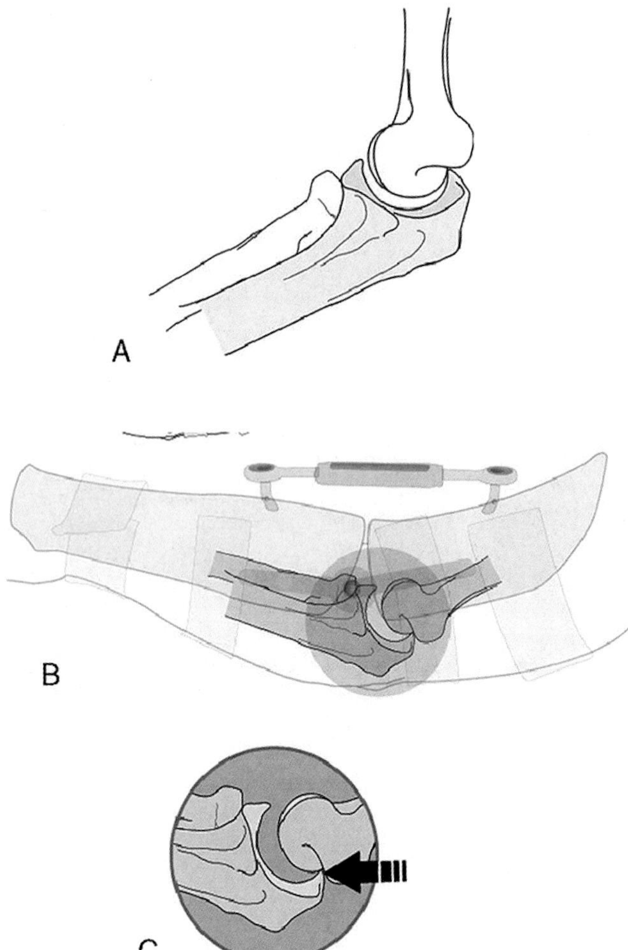

Figure 22.12 **A**, Illustration of an elbow in approximately 30° of flexion with a drop sign. **B**, Illustration of a static-progressive turnbuckle elbow extension orthosis applied to improve a 30° flexion contracture in the presence of an unresolved drop sign. **C**, Illustration demonstrating that this form of orthotic application will likely cause posterior joint impingement, hinging, inflammation, and pain. (Reproduced with permission from Pipicelli JG, Chinchalkar SJ, Grewal R, Athwal GS: Rehabilitation considerations in the management of terrible triad injury to the elbow. *Tech Hand Up Extrem Surg.* 2011;15:198–208.)

and proprioceptive facilitation stimulation while elbow motion is performed. Once desired gains in ROM have been achieved, triggered electrical stimulation EMG biofeedback can be utilized to enhance strength of the muscles surrounding the elbow. Combined active muscular contraction with electrical stimulation produces forceful contractions, which can be utilized for the purpose of strengthening and enhanced active ROM.

OUTCOMES

Nonoperative treatment of isolated undisplaced or minimally displaced fractures of the radial head are generally acceptable. Duckworth et al. reviewed 100 patients with a Mason type 1 and 2 radial head fracture and reported excellent outcomes with

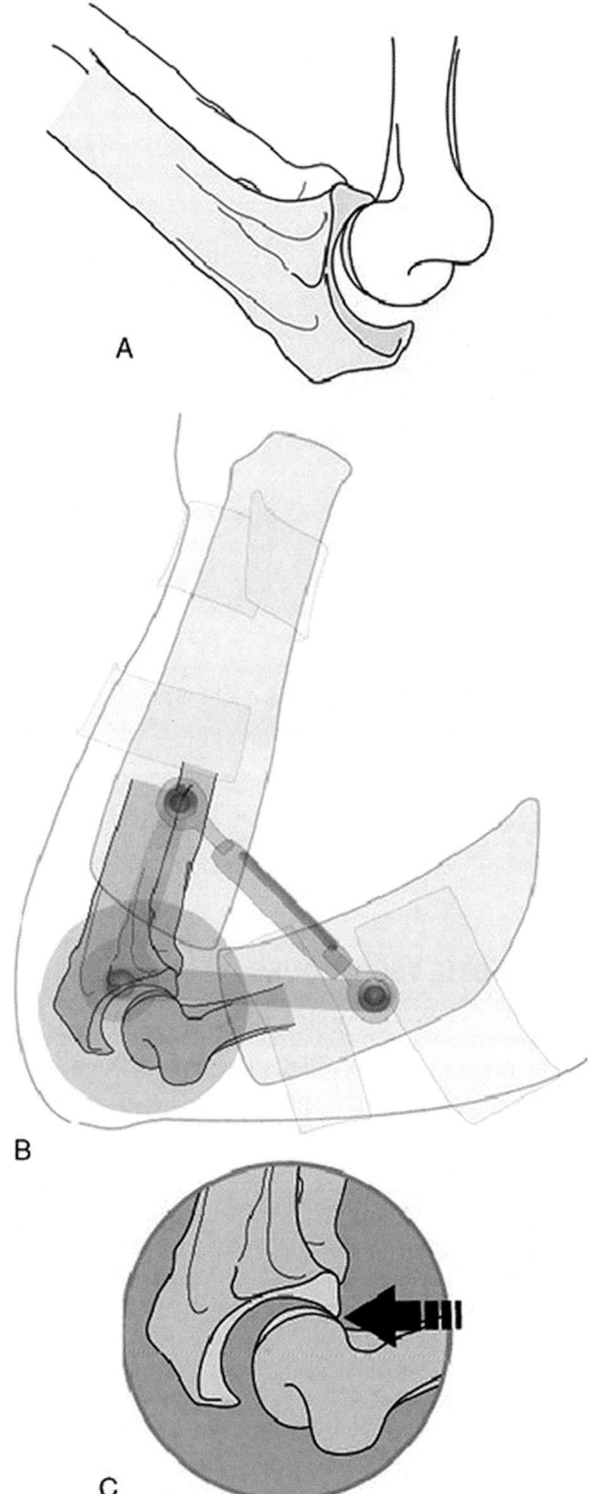

Figure 22.13 **A**, Illustration of an elbow in approximately 115° of elbow flexion with an unresolved drop sign. **B**, Illustration of the application of a static-progressive elbow flexion orthosis with an unresolved drop sign. **C**, Illustration demonstrating that this form of orthotic application will likely cause anterior joint impingement, hinging, inflammation, and pain. (Reproduced with permission from Pipicelli JG, Chinchalkar SJ, Grewal R, Athwal GS: Rehabilitation considerations in the management of terrible triad injury to the elbow. *Tech Hand Up Extrem Surg.* 2011;15:198–208.)

© 2018 American Academy of Orthopaedic Surgeons

a mean Disabilities of the Arm, Shoulder and Hand (DASH) score of 5.8. A total of 92% of patients were satisfied with their results of conservative treatment. Only two patients required subsequent surgical intervention; one of these patients with a Mason type 2 radial head fracture had ORIF for a block to forearm rotation 10 days after injury, while the other patient received a radial head excision for persistent pain and clicking 8 years after injury.

While it is generally accepted that complete articular radial head fractures with more than three displaced fragments have more favorable outcomes with radial head arthroplasty compared to ORIF, less is known about the optimal treatment of partial articular fractures. Yoon et al. retrospectively compared ORIF with nonoperative treatment for patients with partial articular radial head fractures displaced between 2 mm and 5 mm. They found no difference in results, but noted age ≥60 years as an independent predictor of better outcome. Further well-designed studies are needed to clarify the optimal treatment for these fractures.

PEARLS

- ORIF can be attempted for comminuted radial head fractures with more than three fragments, but radial head arthroplasty is generally preferred.
- The choice of a deep surgical exposure should depend on the status of the LCL.
- Optimal sizing of implants during radial head arthroplasty is critical to avoid overstuffing and complications such as pain, stiffness, and arthrosis.
- Close communication between the surgeon and therapist is essential in order to custom-tailor rehabilitation programs and optimize outcomes.
- Early referral to therapy within the first 2 to 5 days postoperatively to initiate controlled mobilization of the elbow and forearm will prevent profound stiffness and the need for lengthy rehabilitation.
- Postoperative positioning of the elbow and forearm is dictated based on the injury pattern to provide optimal ligamentous protection.
- Therapists must be aware if a radiographic drop sign is present, as this has direct implications for rehabilitation.
- The application of progressive static nighttime orthoses as early as 3 to 6 weeks can prevent the development of a flexion contracture.
- In the presence of postoperative stiffness, static-progressive or dynamic splinting is effective to regain motion.
- Superficial heating modalities such as hot packs, whirlpools, or fluidotherapy is helpful to precondition the soft tissues prior to performing ROM exercises at home and in therapy.

SUMMARY

Radial head fractures are common. Evaluation of patients with these injuries begins with a thorough assessment for potential associated osseous and ligamentous disruptions. Acceptable outcomes can be obtained by adhering to basic principles of achieving a stable elbow joint and early ROM. Collaboration with knowledgeable therapists can greatly facilitate a patient's return to premorbid function after radial head fractures.

BIBLIOGRAPHY

Alolabi B, Studer A, Gray A, Ferreira LM, King GJ, Johnson JA, Athwal GS: Selecting the diameter of a radial head implant: an assessment of local landmarks. *J Shoulder Elbow Surg* 2013;22(10):1395–1399.

Armstrong AD, Dunning CE, Faber KJ, Duck TR, Johnson JA, King GJ: Rehabilitation of the medial collateral ligament-deficient elbow: an in vitro biomechanical study. *J Hand Surg Am* 2000;25(6):1051–1057.

Athwal GS, Rouleau DM, MacDermid JC, King GJ: Contralateral elbow radiographs can reliably diagnose radial head implant overlengthening. *J Bone Joint Surg Am* 2011;93(14):1339–1346.

Bonutti PM, Windau JE, Ables BA, Miller BG: Static progressive stretch to reestablish elbow range of motion. *Clin Orthop Relat Res* 1994;(303):128–134.

Chinchalkar SJ, Pearce J, Athwal GS: Static progressive versus three-point elbow extension splinting: a mathematical analysis. *J Hand Ther* 2009;22(1):37–42; quiz 3.

Coonrad RW, Roush TF, Major NM, Basamania CJ: The drop sign, a radiographic warning sign of elbow instability. *J Shoulder Elbow Surg* 2005;14(3):312–317.

Duckworth AD, Clement ND, Jenkins PJ, Aitken SA, Court-Brown CM, McQueen MM: The epidemiology of radial head and neck fractures. *J Hand Surg Am* 2012;37(1):112–119.

Duckworth AD, Wickramasinghe NR, Clement ND, Court-Brown CM, McQueen MM: Long-term outcomes of isolated stable radial head fractures. *J Bone Joint Surg Am* 2014;96(20):1716–1723.

Dunning CE, Zarzour ZD, Patterson SD, Johnson JA, King GJ: Muscle forces and pronation stabilize the lateral ligament deficient elbow. *Clin Orthop Relat Res* 2001;(388):118–124.

Gelinas JJ, Faber KJ, Patterson SD, King GJ: The effectiveness of turnbuckle splinting for elbow contractures. *J Bone Joint Surg Br* 2000;82(1):74–78.

Green DP, McCoy H: Turnbuckle orthotic correction of elbow-flexion contractures after acute injuries. *J Bone Joint Surg Am* 1979;61(7):1092–1095.

Lapner M, King GJ: Radial head fractures. *J Bone Joint Surg Am* 2013;95(12):1136–143.

Li N, Chen S: Open reduction and internal-fixation versus radial head replacement in treatment of Mason type III radial head fractures. *Eur J Orthop Surg Traumatol* 2014;24(6):851–855.

Pipicelli JG, Chinchalkar SJ, Grewal R, Athwal GS: Rehabilitation considerations in the management of terrible triad injury to the elbow. *Tech Hand Up Extrem Surg* 2011;15(4):198–208.

Pipicelli JG, Chinchalkar SJ, Grewal R, King GJ: Therapeutic implications of the radiographic "drop sign" following elbow dislocation. *J Hand Ther* 2012;25(3):346–353; quiz 354.

© 2018 American Academy of Orthopaedic Surgeons

Ring D, Quintero J, Jupiter JB: Open reduction and internal fixation of fractures of the radial head. *J Bone Joint Surg Am* 2002;84-A(10):1811–1815.

Shulman BS, Lee JH, Liporace FA, Egol KA: Minimally displaced radial head/neck fractures (Mason type-I, OTA types 21A2.2 and 21B2.1): are we "over treating" our patients? *J Orthop Trauma* 2015;29(2):e31–e35.

Smith AM, Morrey BF, Steinmann SP: Low profile fixation of radial head and neck fractures: surgical technique and clinical experience. *J Orthop Trauma* 2007;21(10):718–724.

Szekeres M: A biomechanical analysis of static progressive elbow flexion splinting. *J Hand Ther* 2006;19(1):34–38.

van Riet RP, Sanchez-Sotelo J, Morrey BF: Failure of metal radial head replacement. *J Bone Joint Surg Br* 2010;92(5):661–667.

Yoon A, Athwal GS, Faber KJ, King GJ: Radial head fractures. *J Hand Surg Am* 2012;37(12):2626–2634.

Yoon A, King GJ, Grewal R: Is ORIF superior to nonoperative treatment in isolated displaced partial articular fractures of the radial head? *Clin Orthop Relat Res* 2014;472(7): 2105–2112.

 © 2018 American Academy of Orthopaedic Surgeons

23 Total Elbow Arthroplasty

Michael Szekeres, OT Reg (Ont.), CHT, and Graham J.W. King, MD, MSc, FRCSC

INTRODUCTION

Total elbow arthroplasty was first described in the literature over 40 years ago. Advances in implant design and surgical technique, combined with increased knowledge of elbow biomechanics and rehabilitation, have made elbow arthroplasty a viable option for treatment of elbow arthritis and distal humerus fractures. Rehabilitation is dependent on several aspects of the surgical procedure, making communication between the surgeon and treating therapist essential for success. Therapy programs vary considerably in relation to the type of implant and surgical approach. Thus, two separate rehabilitation programs are suggested here based on intraoperative implant selection.

SURGICAL PROCEDURE (TOTAL ELBOW ARTHROPLASTY)

Indications

The most common indications for total elbow arthroplasty are rheumatoid arthritis or other types of inflammatory arthritis, primary or posttraumatic osteoarthritis, and acute fractures. Recent advances in the medical management of inflammatory joint diseases has resulted in a relative decrease in the numbers of total elbow arthroplasties performed for inflammatory arthritides while there has been a simultaneous increase in the use of elbow arthroplasty to treat primary and posttraumatic conditions, as well as acute fractures. Less common conditions treated with total elbow arthroplasty include osteonecrosis, hemophilic arthropathy, comminuted distal humeral fractures, distal humeral nonunions, and periarticular tumors.

Contraindications

Active infection is an absolute contraindication, as with any other joint arthroplasty. A history of remote infection, an inadequate soft-tissue envelope, a nonfunctional hand, and the unwillingness of a patient to be compliant with long-term postoperative activity restrictions and limitations are considered relative contraindications.

Procedure

Identification and protection of the ulnar nerve is critical when performing an elbow replacement, as it is at risk throughout the operation. The procedure can be simplified by detaching the triceps from the olecranon to improve exposure for placement of the implant components. However, triceps insufficiency is not uncommon, prompting many surgeons to leave some or all of the triceps attached to the olecranon when possible. The medial collateral ligament (MCL) and lateral collateral ligament (LCL) are typically released to allow access to the joint for proper implant placement. Ligament repair is not required if a linked arthroplasty is performed since the mechanical connection between the humeral and ulnar components prevents instability (Figure 23.1). However, a secure anatomic ligament repair is required when using an unlinked prosthesis due to the risk of postoperative elbow instability. Unlinked arthroplasties are prone to instability because there is no connection between the humeral and ulnar components (Figure 23.2). These implants are typically used in younger patients with good bone and ligamentous integrity with a lack of significant bony deformity. The advantage of an unlinked implant is that there is no dependence on a mechanical hinge that may be prone to wear and mechanical failure. This may allow slightly greater loads to be safely applied through the elbow, provided that the collateral ligaments, radial head, and other soft tissues around the elbow are structurally sound. The potential of unlinked arthroplasty to withstand higher loads is the primary reason that it tends to be used in younger patients with higher functional demands. All implants replace the articulation of the ulnohumeral joint. Some implants include the option to retain or replace the radial head, which

Dr. King or an immediate family member has received royalties from Wright Medical Technology; serves as a paid consultant to Wright Medical Technology; and serves as a board member, owner, officer, or committee member of the American Shoulder and Elbow Surgeons, the Journal of Hand Surgery–American, *and the* Journal of Shoulder and Elbow Surgery. *Dr. Szekeres or an immediate family member serves as a board member, owner, officer, or committee member of the* Journal of Hand Therapy.

© 2018 American Academy of Orthopaedic Surgeons

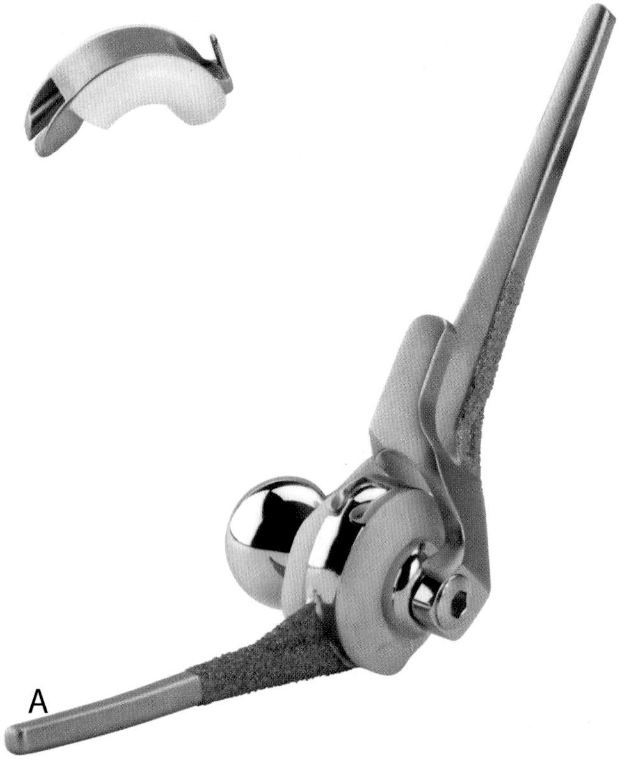

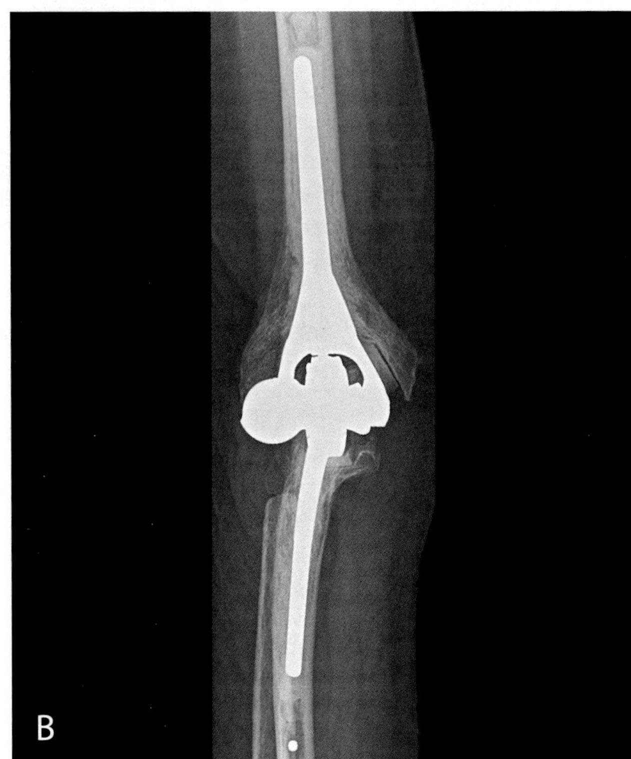

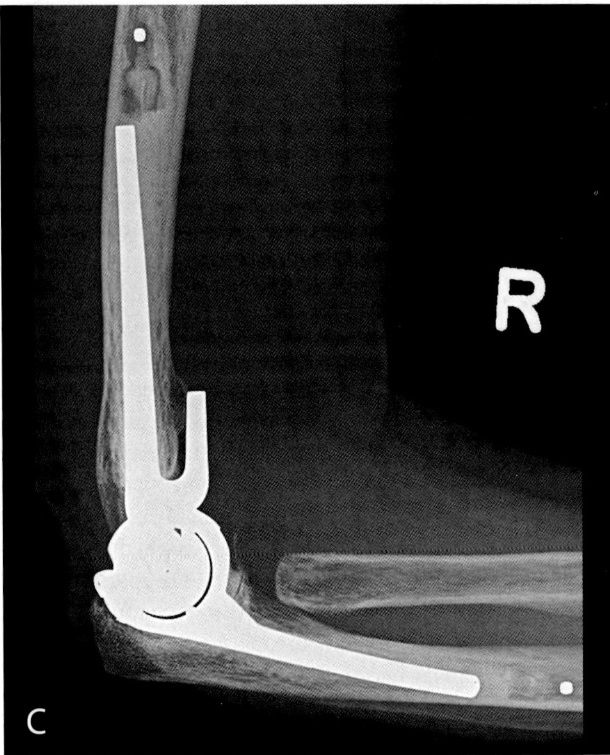

Figure 23.1 **A**, **B**, **C**, Linked total elbow arthroplasty. Note cap on ulnar component links the ulna to the humeral component. (Courtesy Wright Medical, Bloomington MN)

contributes to joint stability if an unlinked arthroplasty is selected. Retaining the native radial head or using a radial head implant theoretically reduces wear of the ulnohumeral bearing, and may improve implant longevity. The use of a radial head implant increases cost and complexity of the procedure, and adds another potential source of implant failure. The role of radial head replacement in total elbow arthroplasty remains controversial.

Unlinked implants have become less popular in recent years with the advent of improved reliability of linked devices.

© 2018 American Academy of Orthopaedic Surgeons

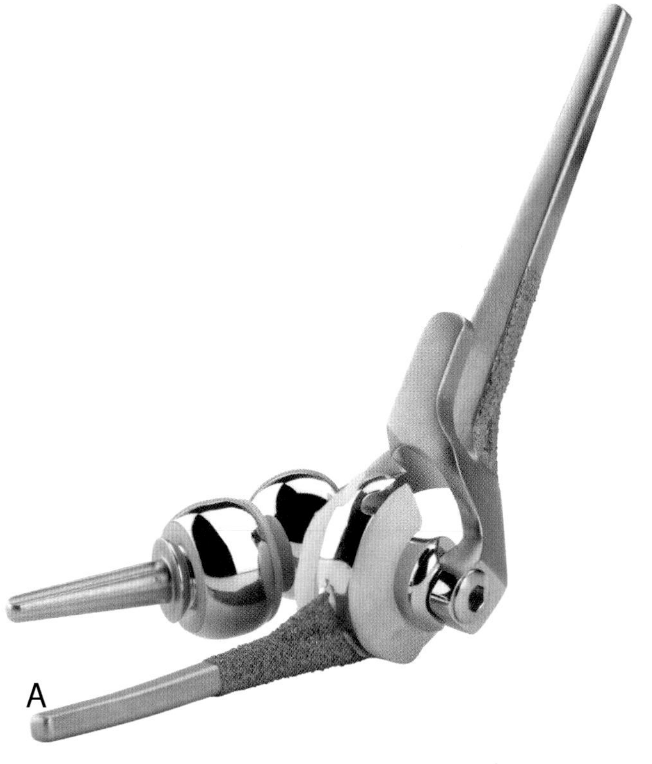

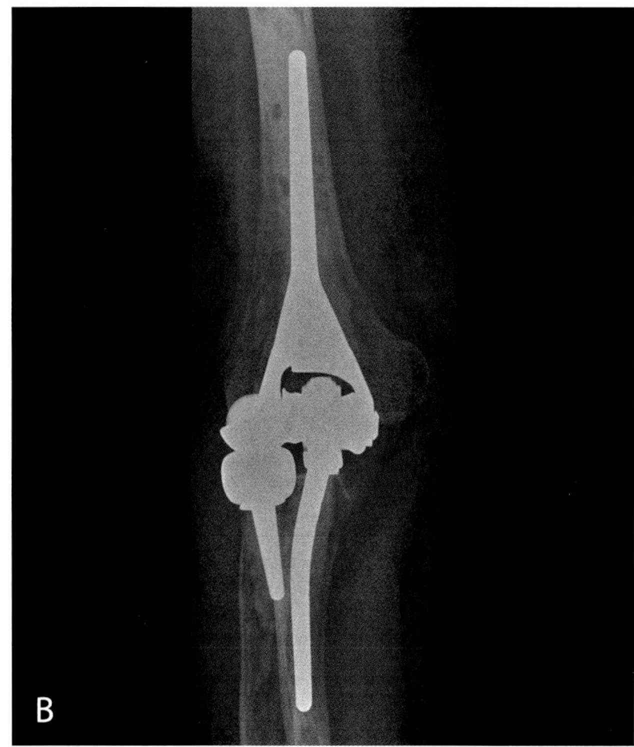

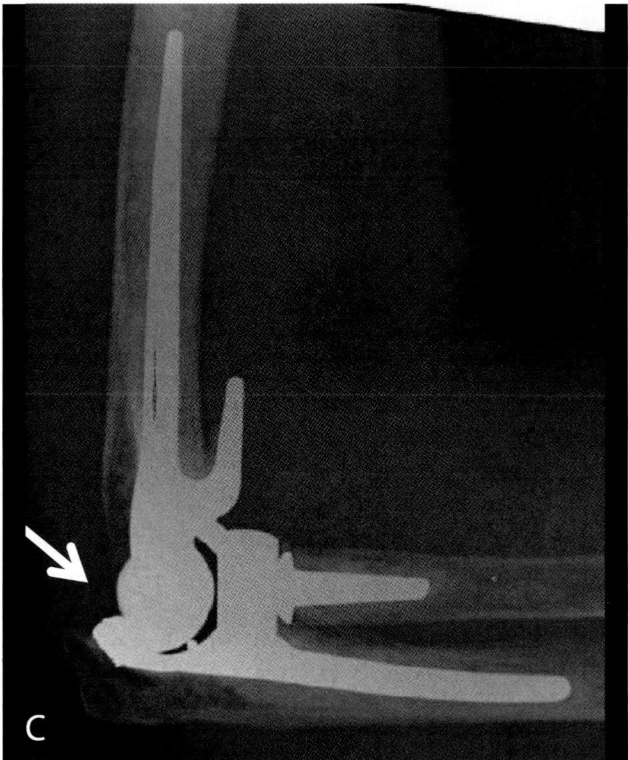

Figure 23.2 **A**, **B**, **C**, Unlinked total elbow arthroplasty. Note there is no connection between the humeral and ulnar components (white arrow). This implant system offers the option of using a bipolar radial head arthroplasty to improve elbow stability and load transfer. (Courtesy Wright Medical, Bloomington MN)

Many have been withdrawn from the market, and only one is currently available in North America. More recently, convertible implants have been developed that provide the option to link an unstable unlinked device without the need to remove the components. This may increase the use of unlinked devices in younger and more active patients in the future since the salvage of an unstable convertible implant can be quick and reliable. Most total elbow implants currently employed are linked, reducing the risk of postoperative instability and allowing expanded indications for the replacement of the elbow in the setting of periarticular bone loss and ligament insufficiency.

Surgical Technique

The surgical technique will depend on the elbow arthroplasty system employed. Elbow arthroplasty is typically performed in the supine position; however, some surgeons prefer using a lateral decubitus option. Patients should receive standard prophylactic intravenous antibiotics. A general or regional anesthetic is employed. A sterile tourniquet is recommended to expand the sterile field and allow proximal extension of the incision if required. A posterior midline incision is placed medial to the tip of the olecranon to prevent injury to longitudinally running cutaneous nerves. To reduce the incidence of flap necrosis, full-thickness flaps are elevated on the deep fascia to optimize skin perfusion. The ulnar nerve should be identified and transposed.

The deep surgical approach to the elbow is at the surgeon's discretion. In the setting of distal humeral bone loss, a paratricipital approach should be considered as it avoids detachment of the triceps from the olecranon, preserving extension strength and allowing for a more rapid functional recovery. This is particularly useful in patients with comminuted distal humeral fractures, in which adequate access to the proximal ulna can be achieved once the distal humeral bone fragments are removed. The paratricipital approach follows the medial–lateral margins of the triceps. In the setting of elbow stiffness and where distal humeral bone stock is preserved, detachment of the triceps from the olecranon facilitates exposure for preparation and insertion of a total elbow arthroplasty. The triceps can be elevated from the olecranon in a medial–lateral direction (Bryan-Morrey) or from the lateral to medial direction (extended Kocher). Alternatively, a triceps-splitting approach can be employed, in which the triceps is split centrally and elevated both medially and laterally off the proximal ulna. Some surgeons prefer the use of a triceps tongue approach, in which a portion of the triceps is left attached to the olecranon to facilitate later repair. All surgical approaches that detach the triceps from the olecranon allow for improved visualization, thus easier and more accurate ulnar component placement. Detachment of the triceps tendon delays return to function, as resisted extension must be avoided until tendon healing is secure; otherwise, disabling extension weakness can compromise outcome. This is particularly problematic for patients who require lower extremity walking aids such as crutches, a walker, or wheelchair.

More recently, a lateral paraolecranon approach has been described. This is a compromise between a triceps-reflecting and paratricipital approach. Exposure of the proximal ulna is improved without the need to restrict postoperative activities or compromising extension strength. The LCL and MCL are sectioned from the humeral epicondyles and the elbow is dislocated by hyperflexion, allowing the olecranon to move away from the humerus. The anterior capsule is elevated off the humerus to allow for placement of a bone graft behind the anterior flange of the humeral component.

An appropriately sized implant is selected. Bony cuts on the distal humerus, proximal ulna, and proximal radius (if applicable) are made using the supplied instruments, and trial prostheses are inserted (Figure 23.3). The radial head is retained in acute fractures or when there is mild arthritic involvement. A trial reduction is performed to ensure that the implants track correctly. If articular tracking is suboptimal, repositioning of an unlinked implant is needed. An unlinked implant should only be considered in younger patients in the setting of good flexor and extensor mechanisms, adequate collateral ligaments, absence of significant preexisting deformity, and retention or replacement of the radial head. A linked implant should be performed when these prerequisites are not met or the trial unlinked implants are maltracking. A radial head component should not be employed if the radial head cannot be made to articulate congruously with the capitellum throughout motion. Linked implants are recommended in elderly low-demand patients because wear and loosening are less of a concern.

In most cases, the implants are cemented. When possible, a cancellous bone graft is placed between the anterior flange of the humeral component and the humerus. Secure the linkage mechanism if a linked arthroplasty is to be performed. The collateral ligaments are repaired back to the epicondyles and the implant if an unlinked arthroplasty is employed. If the triceps was detached, it is repaired to the olecranon through drill holes using locking nonabsorbable Krackow sutures. The ulnar nerve can be transposed into the subcutaneous tissues anterior to the medial epicondyle. The wound is closed in layers over a closed suction drain.

The elbow is initially immobilized with an anterior splint in near full extension if a linked component is used and at 70° of flexion if an unlinked component is used to avoid posterior wound pressure. The drain is removed 1 day postoperatively. Elbow motion exercises are initiated when soft-tissue healing is secure, typically in 10 to 14 days. Rehabilitation can be initiated within 1 to 2 days of surgery to review edema control and to initiate shoulder, wrist, and digital exercises as outlined later.

Complications

Unfortunately, complications remain common following total elbow arthroplasty. Intraoperative complications include cortical perforations, fractures, and nerve injuries. Postoperative complications include delayed wound healing, flap necrosis, infection, and triceps insufficiency. Sensory ulnar neuropathy is a relatively common postoperative finding. Instability can occur with unlinked arthroplasties. Infection, aseptic loosening, polyethylene wear, stem fractures, linkage failure, and periprosthetic fractures occur with longer follow-up.

POSTOPERATIVE REHABILITATION

General Therapy Considerations

Although the efficacy of rehabilitation after total elbow arthroplasty has been questioned in the literature, the authors have found therapy beneficial for their patients. The therapist assists

© 2018 American Academy of Orthopaedic Surgeons

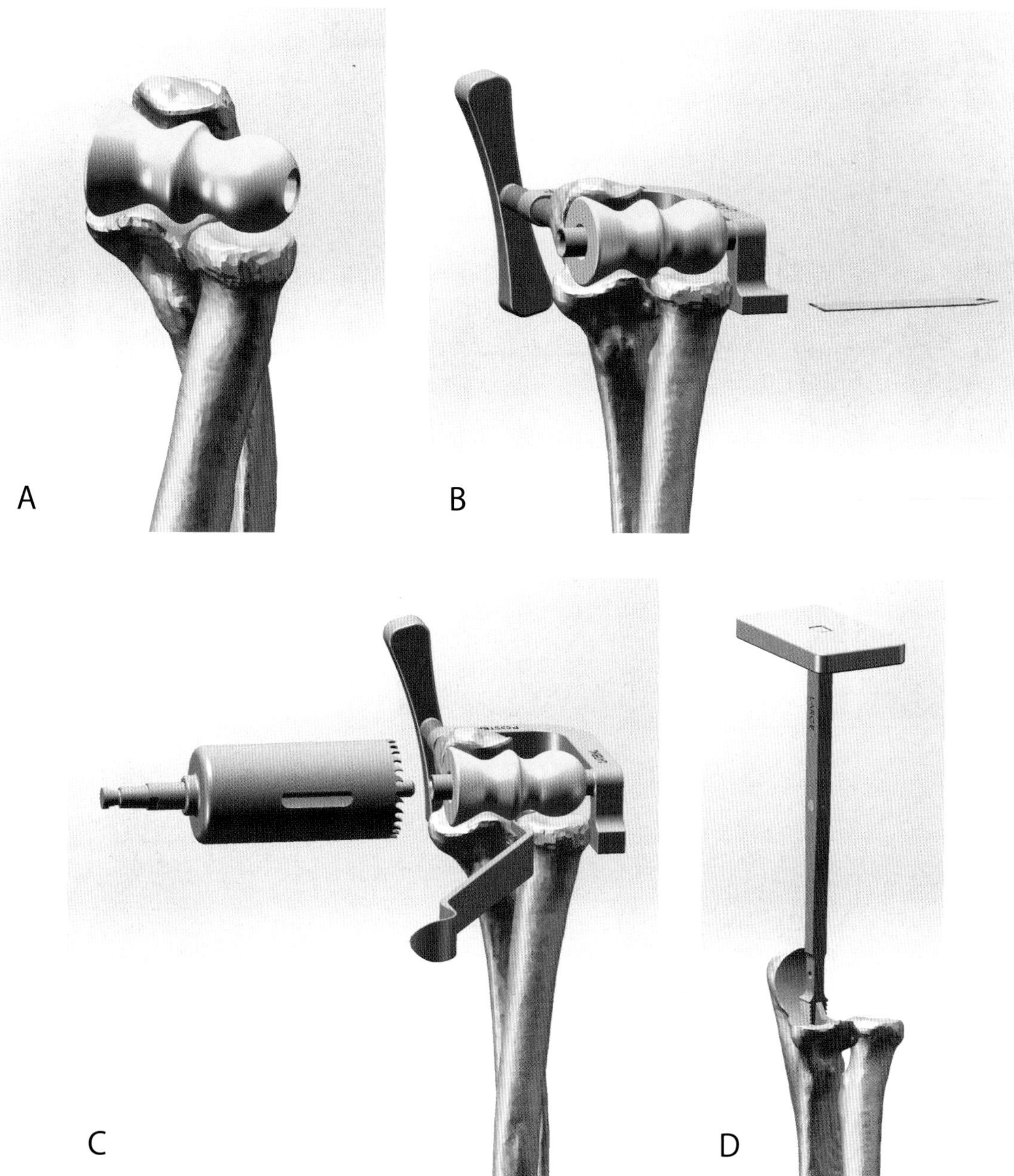

Figure 23.3 Illustrations of total elbow arthroplasty procedure. **A**, Measurement of articular width using spool to size elbow arthroplasty. **B**, Radial head excision, if indicated. **C**, Resection of proximal ulna using bell saw. **D**, Preparation of ulnar medullary canal using rasp. *(continued)*

with edema control, fabricates appropriate orthoses, educates patients regarding restrictions, reviews range of motion (ROM) exercises, and implements gentle passive stretching if stiffness occurs.

Regardless of the type of implant used, there are a few consistent and important factors to consider during rehabilitation after elbow arthroplasty. The first general consideration is the status of the triceps muscle. Triceps insufficiency is a potential complication after arthroplasty, and has been shown to occur in 2% to 5% of cases in which triceps has been reflected off of the olecranon during surgery in spite of reattachment prior to closure. Triceps weakness is much more common than complete failure and is correlated with lower patient satisfaction. The triceps is an important dynamic elbow stabilizer; contraction of this muscle helps maintain the joint reaction forces necessary to prevent gapping of the ulnohumeral articulation. If the triceps was reflected or detached during surgery, modifications to therapy programs are necessary to protect the triceps reattachment and prevent triceps insufficiency. These modifications include limiting elbow flexion during the early postoperative period and minimizing contraction of the triceps by performing extension exercises in a gravity-assisted position. Furthermore, lower extremity walking aids should not be used until triceps healing is secure.

© 2018 American Academy of Orthopaedic Surgeons

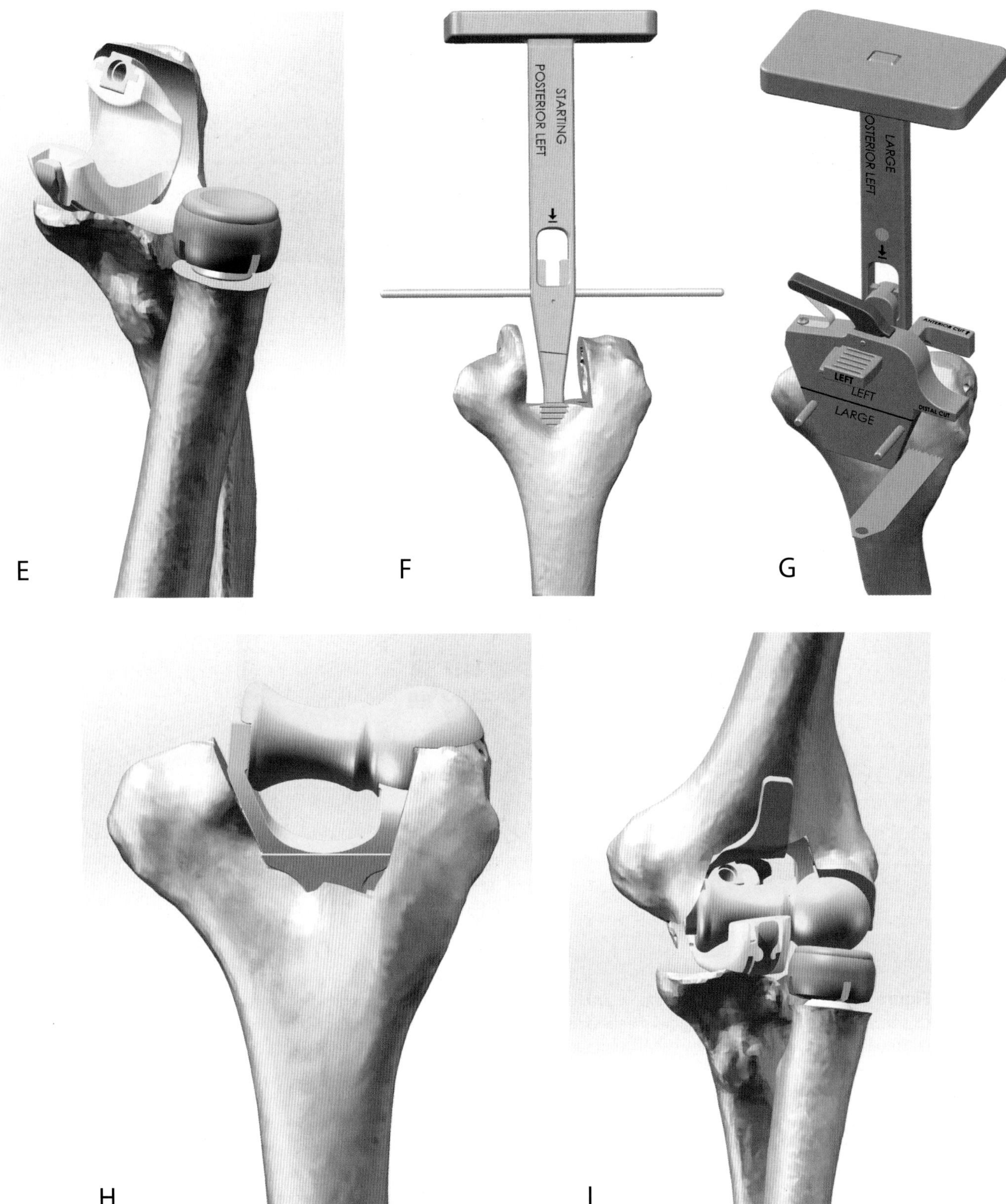

Figure 23.3 (*Continued*) **E**, Trial ulnar and radial component insertion. **F**, The intercondylar portion of the distal humerus is resected and the humeral rasp is inserted into the medullary canal in the correct rotational orientation and to the correct depth to replicate the axis of motion. **G**, Humeral preparation completed using cutting block and sagittal saw. **H**, Trial humeral component insertion. **I**, Trial reduction of prosthesis. (Courtesy Wright Medical, Bloomington MN)

© 2018 American Academy of Orthopaedic Surgeons

The implant type is also an important consideration during postoperative rehabilitation. Total elbow arthroplasty implants are either linked or unlinked. Linked systems connect at the ulnohumeral articulation and elbow stability depends primarily on the bearings and hinge components. Patients are unlikely to have instability postoperatively unless the linkage mechanism fails. In contrast, unlinked implants depend on the collateral ligaments and soft-tissue envelope for stability and require protection during the early postoperative period to prevent subluxation. More recently, convertible implants have been developed that allow the surgeon to choose between an unlinked or linked implant intraoperatively or to easily salvage an unlinked implant that develops postoperative instability.

Patients who have linked arthroplasty are less prone to developing stiffness since they can usually begin full ROM as soon as the postoperative dressing is removed as long as the triceps was not detached during surgery. If the triceps was detached, ROM in flexion should be controlled and progressive to facilitate triceps healing. In addition, unrestricted active use should be avoided for the first 6 weeks. These patients are fit with a collar and cuff for comfort during the day and an extension orthosis for night (Figure 23.4A, B). There is a lack of high-level evidence to support the use of extension orthoses following linked arthroplasty, but we use them regularly in an effort to minimize tension on the posterior wound during healing and to optimize elbow extension. Flexion stiffness is uncommon, and can usually be overcome with exercise. It is important that therapy focus on functional restrictions early on since the period of immobilization is short and patients are often using their upper extremities within 2 weeks following surgery.

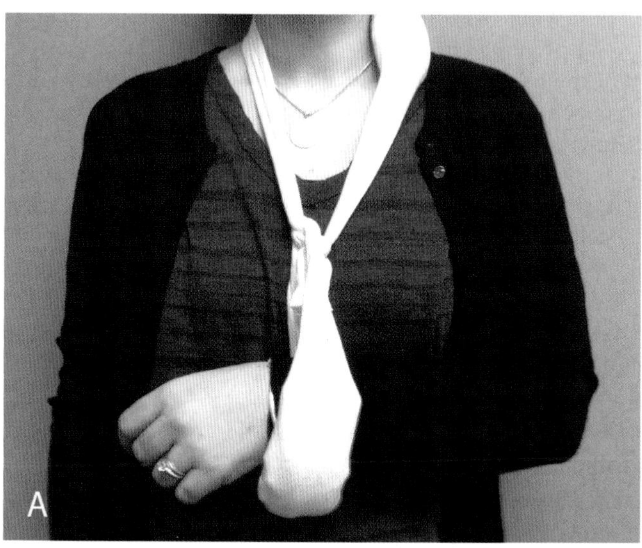

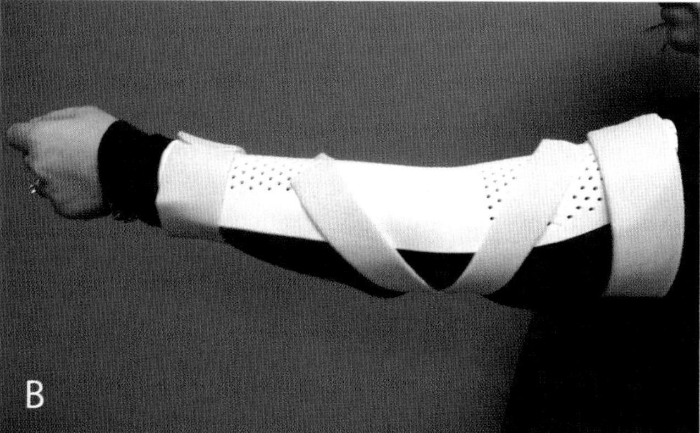

Figure 23.4 Photographs of postoperative orthoses. **A**, Collar and cuff. **B**, Static-progressive extension orthosis.

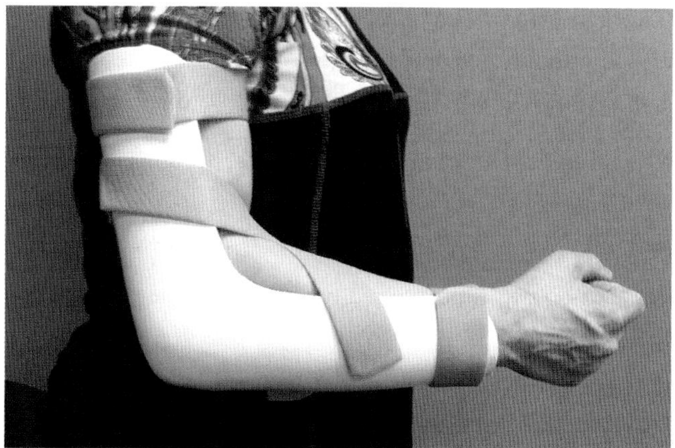

Figure 23.5 Photograph of resting 90° orthosis. (Reproduced with permission from Szekeres M: A biomechanical analysis of static progressive elbow flexion splinting. *J Hand Ther.* 2006;19:34–38.)

Patients with unlinked implants and a triceps on approach are allowed to perform early full active flexion, and forearm rotation (with the elbow in a flexed position) motion exercises because triceps healing is not an issue. Extension is initially limited to 40° to protect the healing collateral ligaments and prevent elbow subluxation. Extension is progressed by 10° per week until full extension is achieved. Patients are immobilized in a posterior resting elbow orthosis at 90° of flexion that is worn for 6 weeks at all times except for exercises and skin care (Figure 23.5). Since motion is restricted and protection is required with full-time orthotic use, patients tend to be stiffer during the initial postoperative period than those with a linked arthroplasty. Instability after unlinked arthroplasty is primarily a problem during the first 6 to 8 weeks following surgery. If properly managed with careful patient selection, meticulous surgical technique, and appropriate therapy, this complication can be minimized.

General therapy techniques used for most postoperative care are relevant after elbow arthroplasty, including early swelling and edema control and scar management. Swelling and edema control include arm elevation as well as frequent finger motion to encourage contraction of the long flexor and extensor origins. A light compressive sleeve can also be used. Patients are encouraged to use ice during the first 2 weeks following surgery. Ice can be applied after exercise sessions to prevent inflammation. Once wound healing is secure, patients are instructed to perform scar massage to help soften and mobilize the scar, improve cosmesis, and minimize hypersensitivity.

© 2018 American Academy of Orthopaedic Surgeons

General Considerations

- Edema control is implemented immediately after surgery; it includes frequent finger ROM and arm elevation when the patient is sedentary.
- Apply ice for 15 minutes after exercise sessions during the first 2 weeks.
- Wounds are kept dry and clean until sutures are removed 10 to 14 days post-op.
- Scar massage is performed two to three times per day for 5 minutes once wound healing is secure.

Linked Total Elbow Arthroplasty

Protection/Immobilization

- Patients are fit with a collar and cuff (Figures 23.3A to 23.4A) for rest and comfort during the day for 4 weeks.
- Patients can easily remove this for exercises and very light functional use as long as the triceps tendon was not detached during surgery.
- An extension orthosis (Figures 23.3B to 23.4B) is used at night for 8 to 12 weeks depending on ROM.
- The extension orthosis is adjusted every 7 to 10 days to accommodate increases in extension if unable to achieve full extension immediately postop due to pain, swelling, or muscle tension.

Range of Motion Exercises (Table 23.1)

- Exercises are performed five to six times per day. Perform 10 repetitions of each position, holding for 10 seconds each—but this depends on swelling, pain, and amount of motion patient is able to achieve.
- All exercises should be performed slowly, using the other hand to support if needed.
- Small amounts of discomfort are acceptable while performing elbow ROM, as long as this resolves upon completion of exercises. If any pain persists, patients should reduce the number of repetitions or decrease intensity.
- See Table 23.1 for specifics related to performing exercises. Exercises include active shoulder flexion and external rotation, active wrist flexion/extension, active forearm pronation/supination, and elbow motion as outlined here:
  - *If triceps tendon insertion was preserved (triceps on):* Full active range of motion (AROM) once the postoperative bulky dressing is removed (Table 23.1, 1.5).
  - *If triceps was detached (Bryan-Morrey; triceps splitting):* active flexion to 90° during week 1, and progress flexion by 10° per week. Extension is performed using the contralateral hand to assist, in a gravity-assisted position (Table 23.1, 1.6).
- Other exercises (not shown) should include active composite finger flexion, hook fist, and thumb opposition.
- Gentle passive range of motion (PROM) for elbow flexion/extension is initiated at week 4 if the patient is not making expected gains in ROM.
- Superficial heat using hot packs or therapeutic whirlpool can be used prior to exercise once edema has reduced sufficiently (usually after 4 weeks) to improve tissue elasticity and minimize pain/co-contracture while stretching.
- For cases in which the elbow remains stiff 8 weeks postop, static-progressive orthoses can be used as a supplement to stretching. Our preferred orthoses are the static-progressive flexion cuff and a turnbuckle for flexion or extension (Figures 23.3 to 23.6). These orthoses are worn three to four times for per day for 1 hour after stretching.

Strengthening

- Strengthening exercises are not always prescribed. Since patients who receive a linked arthroplasty usually have lower functional demands, functional use of the upper extremity is often an adequate strengthening program in itself.
- Strengthening can begin at week 6 if triceps was preserved and at week 10 if detached depending on the quality of the repair.
- A weight limit of 5 pounds is implemented during exercise sessions.
- Strengthening should be pain-free and is performed once per day. Exercises include resisted gripping, wrist and elbow flexion/extension.

Functional Restoration

- Since postoperative stability is less dependent on soft-tissue healing, patients may begin earlier functional use with a linked arthroplasty than with unlinked if the triceps was preserved in surgery.
- If the triceps was preserved and wound healing is secure, patients can begin light functional use within 2 weeks of surgery and use a collar and cuff for comfort only.
- If the triceps was detached, patients are advised to wear the collar and cuff at all times during the day for 6 weeks, except while exercising. An extension orthosis is used at night.
- A lifetime weight-lifting restriction of 5 pounds is reviewed with the patient before surgery and during rehabilitation. Heavier loading of the elbow may lead to mechanical wear and loosening.

Unlinked Total Elbow Arthroplasty

Protection/Immobilization

- Posterior elbow orthosis (Figure 23.4) at 90° of elbow flexion to be worn at all times for approximately 6 weeks, except exercises and skin care.
- The daytime splint is discontinued after 6 weeks provided that radiographs and clinical assessment confirm elbow stability.
- A nighttime extension orthosis is added after 6 weeks if elbow extension is not progressing as expected.
- Maintaining muscle tone is important in order to preserve elbow stability. Early isometric contractions are encouraged within the postoperative splint. Patients are encouraged to flex and extend the wrist and elbow (provided that the triceps was preserved) against the splint several times per day.

Range of Motion Exercises (Table 23.2)

- Exercises are performed six times per day. Usually perform 10 repetitions of each position, holding for 10 seconds each—but this depends on swelling, pain, and amount of motion the patient is able to achieve.

© 2018 American Academy of Orthopaedic Surgeons

Table 23.1 LINKED TOTAL ELBOW ARTHROPLASTY EXERCISE PROGRAM

1.1 Active Shoulder Flexion • Position the patient seated on a hard surface, arms resting at the side. • While maintaining the forearm in neutral or slight supination, ask the patient to lift the arm overhead. • Ensure slow, pain-free ROM with good posture and anterior pelvic tilt while seated. • Discourage any shoulder "hiking" or substitution patterns.	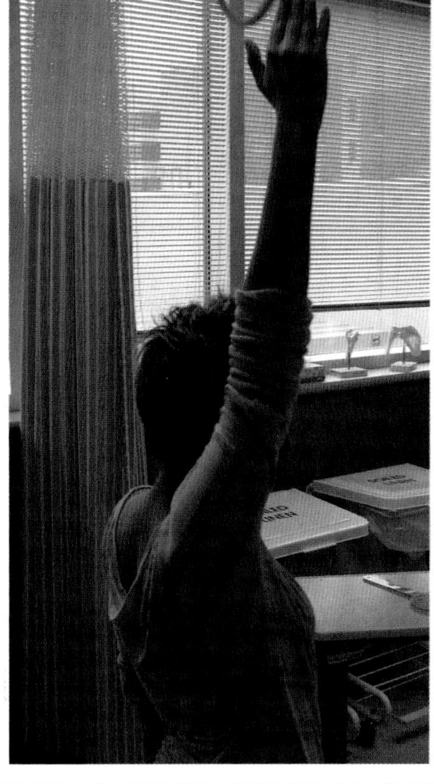
1.2 Active Shoulder External Rotation • Position the patient in either sitting or standing, elbow at 90°, shoulder in neutral rotation. • Ask the patient to externally rotate at the shoulder. • If the patient is unsure, sit or stand in front of the patient and mirror the desired motion. • Discourage trunk rotation, as this will decrease stretch to the anterior shoulder capsule.	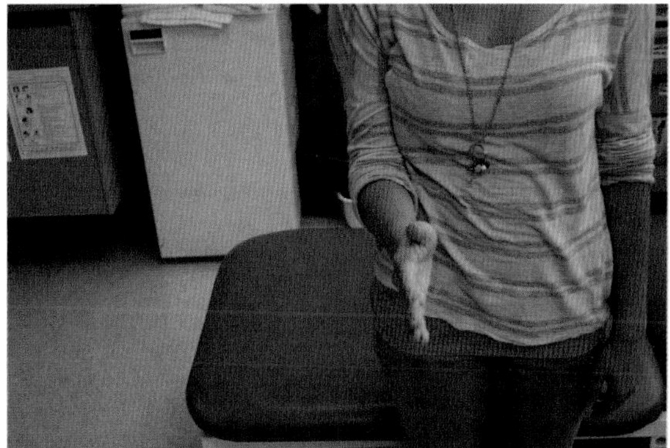 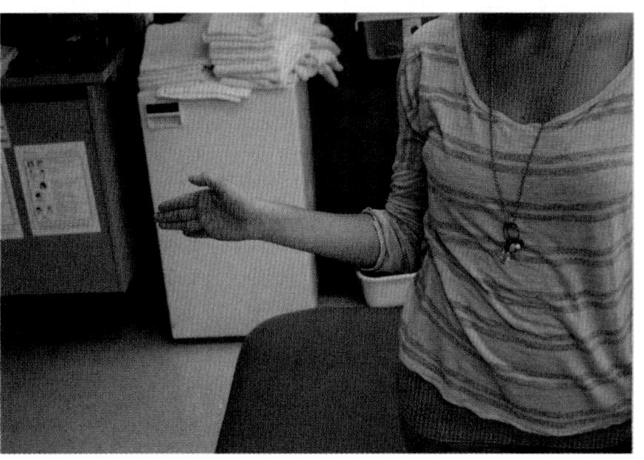

Continued on following page

© 2018 American Academy of Orthopaedic Surgeons

Table 23.1 LINKED TOTAL ELBOW ARTHROPLASTY EXERCISE PROGRAM *(Continued)*

1.3 Active Wrist Flexion and Extension • Position the patient seated beside a table with the forearm resting on the surface and the hand over the edge. • Ask the patient to flex the wrist with the fingers relaxed. • Once 10 repetitions are complete, move to wrist extension. • Ask the patient to make a gentle fist while extending to isolate the wrist extensors.	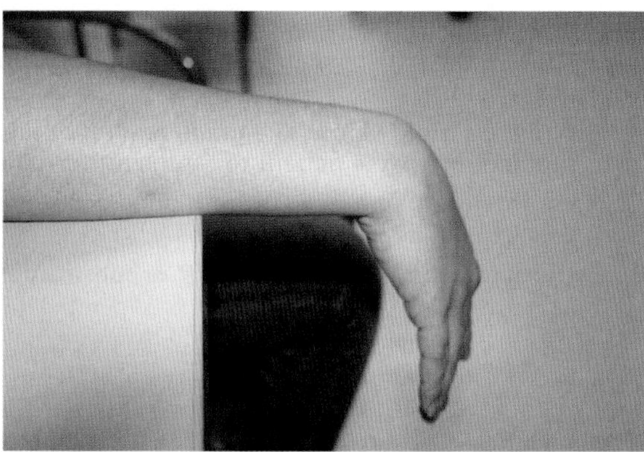 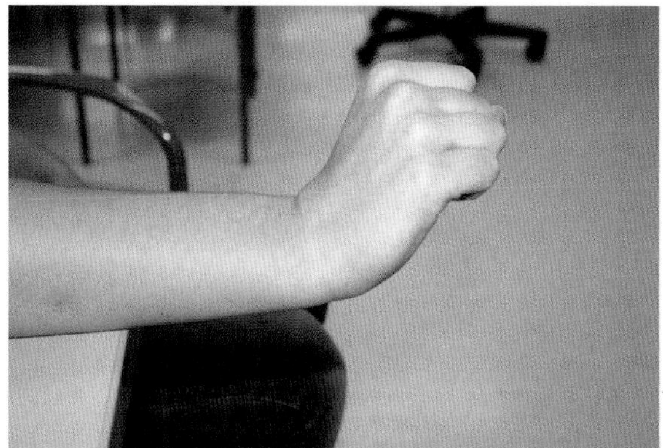
1.4 Active Forearm Supination and Pronation • Preferred position of the patient is supine. • This discourages trunk motion and helps isolate forearm rotation. • If the wound is sensitive, this exercise may be done in a seated position. • Starting in neutral forearm rotation with the elbow flexed to 90° degrees, ask the patient to rotate and "look" at the palm. • Once 10 repetitions are complete, move to pronation by asking the patient to "look" at the back of the hand.	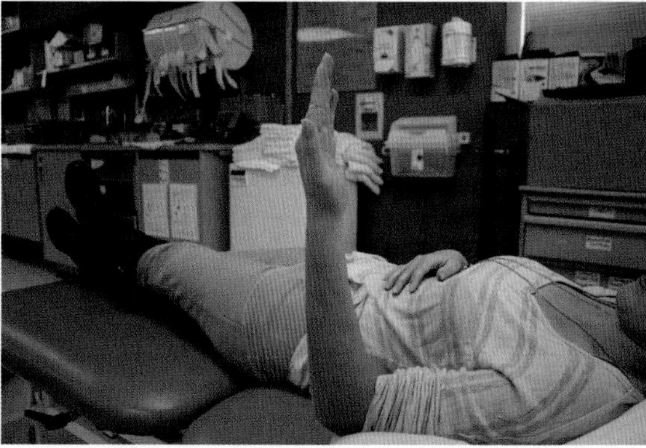 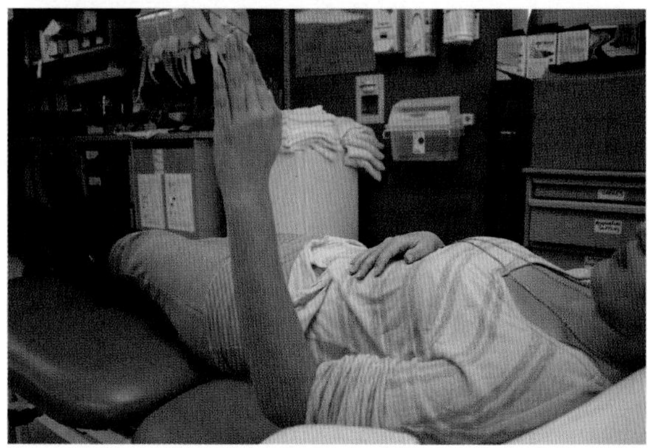

© 2018 American Academy of Orthopaedic Surgeons

Table 23.1 **LINKED TOTAL ELBOW ARTHROPLASTY EXERCISE PROGRAM** *(Continued)*

1.5 Active Elbow Flexion and Extension (Triceps Intact)

- Position the patient supine, with the posterior arm resting on a small pillow or rolled towel.
- Supine is preferred, as this position discourages substitution motion of the shoulder.
- With the forearm in neutral, ask the patient to flex the elbow to touch the shoulder.
- Encourage the patient to remain in full flexion for 10 seconds.
- Once 10 repetitions are complete, ask the patient to straighten the elbow. Encourage contraction of the triceps muscle by palpating if necessary. Ask the patient to contract and hold maximum extension for 10 seconds.

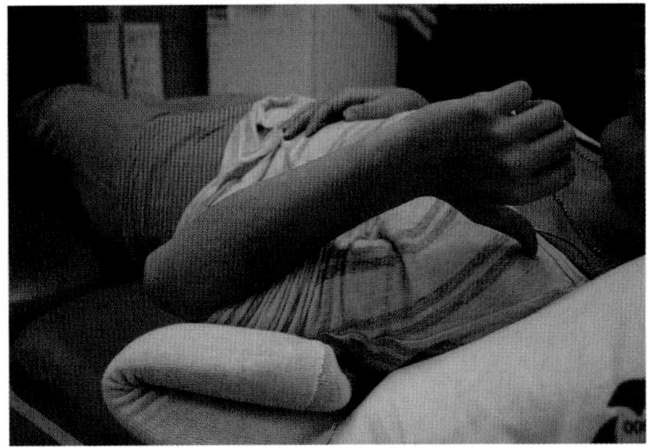

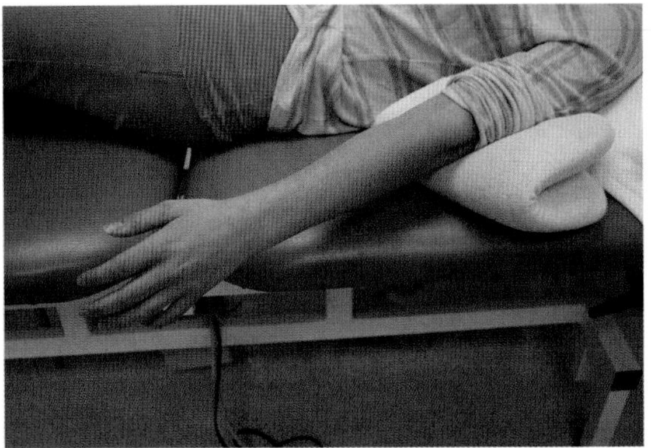

1.6 Active Elbow Flexion and Extension (Triceps Detached)

- Position the patient supine, with the posterior arm resting on a small pillow or rolled towel.
- Supine is preferred to allow gravity to assist extension.
- Using the contralateral arm for assistance, ask the patient to flex the elbow to 90° and hold for 10 seconds. The amount of flexion can be increased by 10° per week.
- Once 10 repetitions of flexion are complete, work on assisted extension.
- Using the contralateral arm for assistance, ask the patient to use the other hand to extend the arm to full elbow extension.
- Discourage any contraction of triceps. Use palpation to ensure that the patient is not activating triceps and that the contralateral arm is doing the work.

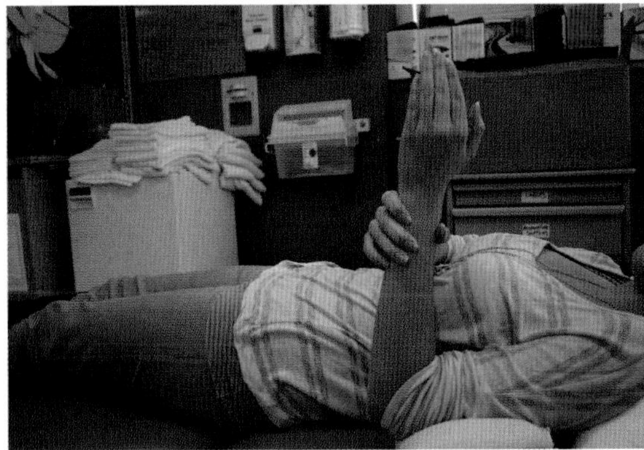

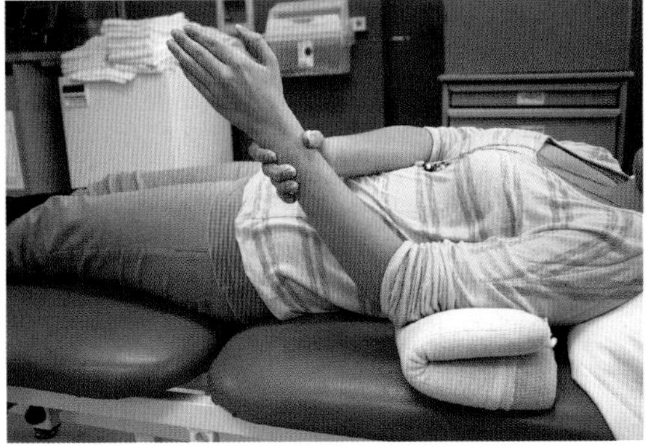

© 2018 American Academy of Orthopaedic Surgeons

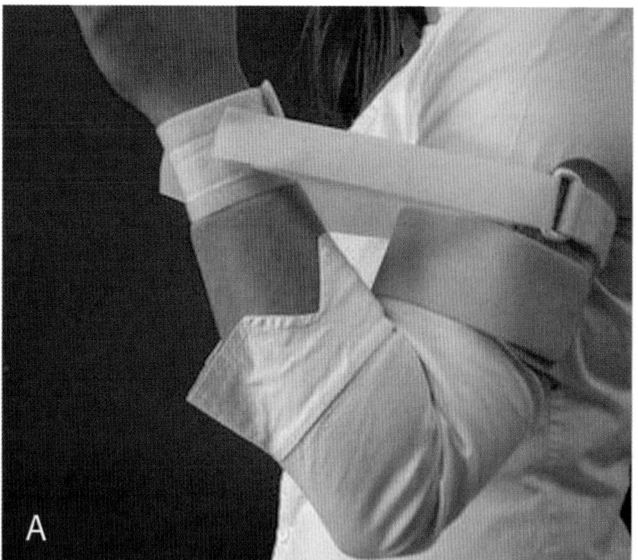

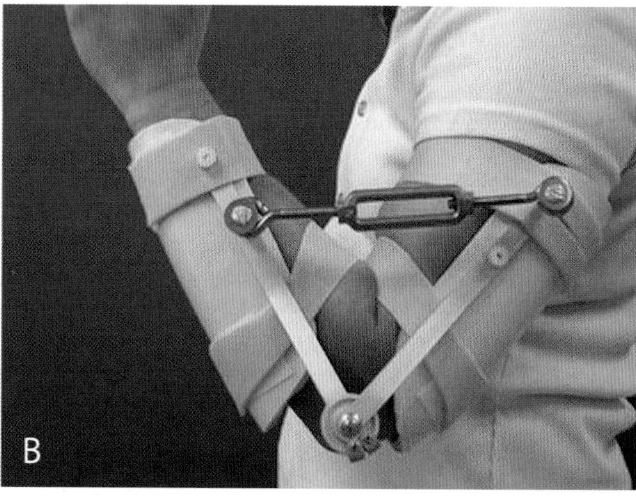

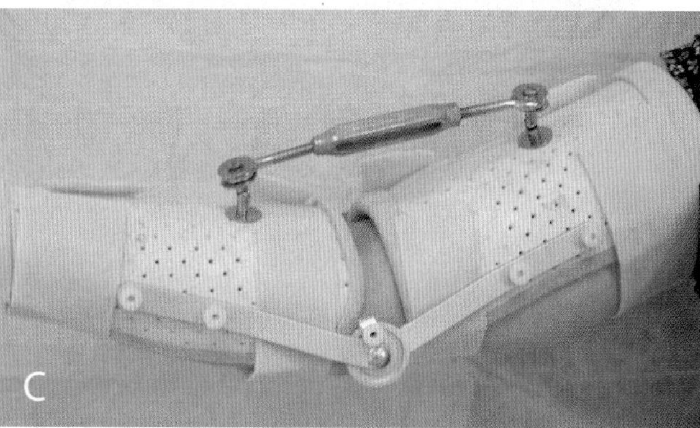

Figure 23.6 Photographs of static-progressive elbow flexion and extension orthoses. **A**, Flexion cuff. **B**, Static-progressive flexion turnbuckle. **C**, Static-progressive extension turnbuckle.

- Shoulder, wrist, and finger ROM exercises are performed with the protective orthosis on. Shoulder ROM should be performed in a position that avoids varus or valgus loads through the elbow.
- Exercises include active shoulder flexion and external rotation, active wrist flexion/extension, active forearm pronation/supination, composite finger flexion/extension, hook fist, and thumb opposition.
- Once these exercises are complete, the orthosis is removed for elbow ROM.
- Elbow exercises are usually performed in the supine position and include the following:
    - *If triceps was preserved (triceps on):* Full active elbow flexion allowed. Extension to 40° in the first week and increased by 10° each week (Table 23.2, 2.5).
    - *If the triceps was detached (Bryan-Morrey; triceps splitting):* active flexion to 90° during week 1, and progress by 10° per week. Extension is performed in a gravity-assisted position. Extension to 40° in the first week and increased 10° per week (Table 23.2, 2.6).
- Gentle passive elbow flexion/extension is initiated at week 6 if the patient is not making expected gains in ROM.
- Nighttime extension splinting is initiated at week 6 if the patient is not making expected gains in ROM and remain more than 20° to 30° short of full extension.
- For cases in which the elbow remains stiff 8 weeks postop, static-progressive orthoses can be used as a supplement to stretching. Our preferred orthoses are the static-progressive flexion cuff and a turnbuckle for flexion or extension (Figures 23.5 to 23.6). These orthoses are worn four times for per day for 1 hour after stretching.

Strengthening

- Early isometric strengthening of the wrist flexors and extensors is initiated in the postop splint and continues throughout rehabilitation. Gentle active isometric contraction of the elbow flexors and triceps (if intact) are encouraged 3 to 5 days postoperatively to increase joint reaction forces and enhance elbow stability.
- Isotonic elbow strengthening can begin at week 8 if the triceps is intact, week 12 if detached depending on quality of repair.
- If patients have functional limitations due to weakness and strengthening is prescribed, a weight limit of 5 pounds is implemented.

© 2018 American Academy of Orthopaedic Surgeons

Table 23.2 UNLINKED TOTAL ELBOW ARTHROPLASTY EXERCISE PROGRAM

2.1 Active Shoulder Flexion

- Performed with the posterior resting orthosis on.
- Position the patient seated on a hard surface, arms resting at the side.
- Ensuring that the shoulder is not internally rotated, ask patient to lift the arm overhead.
- Ensure slow, pain-free ROM with good posture and anterior pelvic tilt while seated.
- Discourage any shoulder "hiking" or substitution patterns.

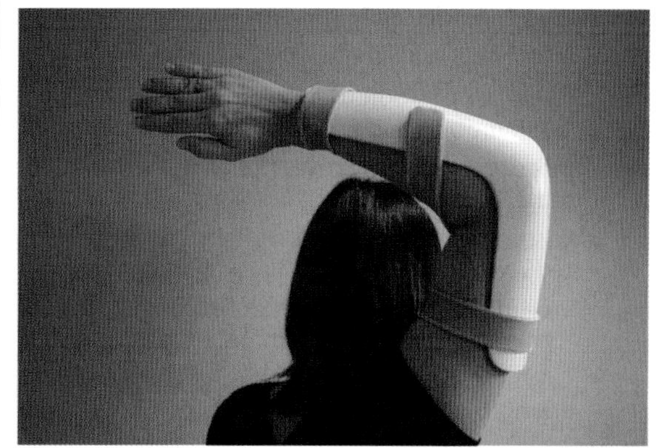

2.2 Active Shoulder External Rotation

- Performed with the posterior resting orthosis on.
- Position the patient either sitting or standing, elbow at 90°, shoulder in neutral rotation.
- Ask the patient to externally rotate at the shoulder.
- If the patient is unsure, sit or stand in front of the patient and mirror the desired motion.
- Discourage trunk rotation, as this will decrease stretch to the anterior shoulder capsule.

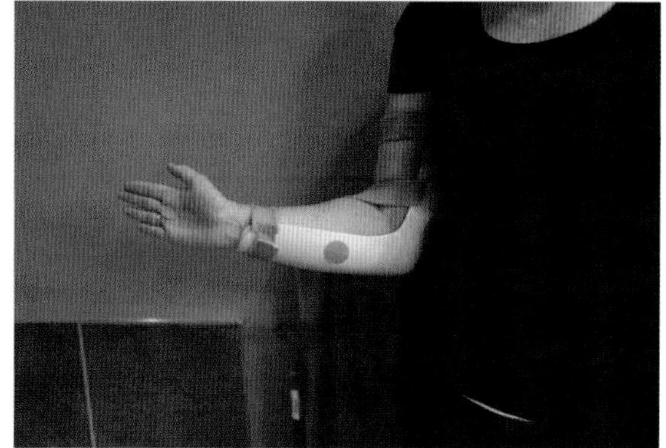

2.3 Active Wrist Flexion and Extension

- Performed with the posterior resting orthosis on.
- Position the patient seated with forearm resting on the lap.
- Ask the patient to flex the wrist with the fingers relaxed.
- Once 10 repetitions are complete, move to wrist extension.
- Ask the patient to make a fist while extending to isolate the wrist extensors.

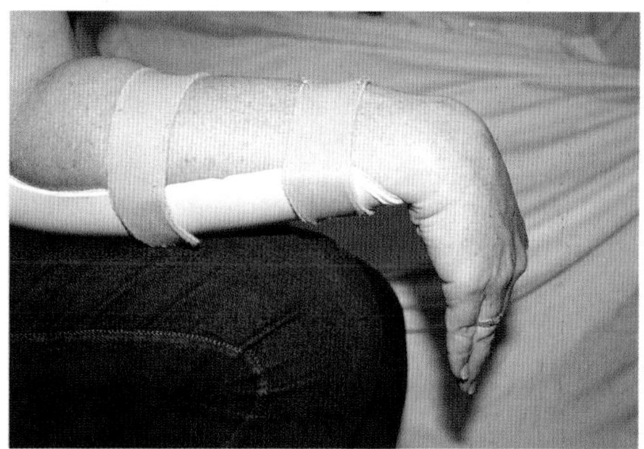

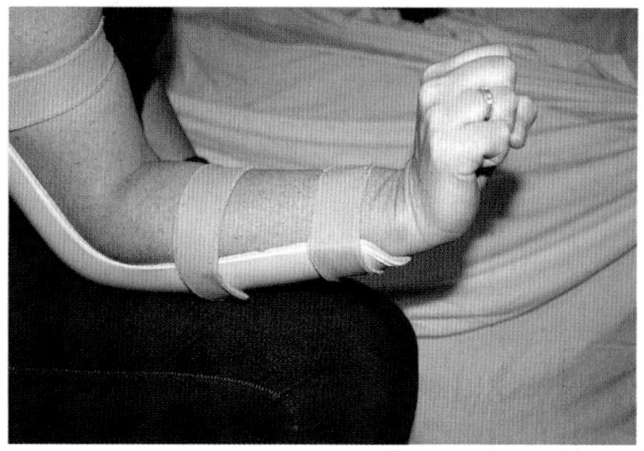

Continued on following page

© 2018 American Academy of Orthopaedic Surgeons

Table 23.2 UNLINKED TOTAL ELBOW ARTHROPLASTY EXERCISE PROGRAM *(Continued)*

2.4 Active Forearm Supination and Pronation

- Performed with the posterior resting removed.
- Preferred position of the patient is supine. This discourages trunk motion and helps isolate forearm rotation.
- If the wound is sensitive, this exercise may be done in a seated position.
- Ensure that the elbow is as flexed as possible (past 90°) to reduce tension on the collateral ligaments.
- Starting in neutral forearm rotation, ask the patient to rotate to "look" at the palm.
- Once 10 repetitions are complete, move to pronation by asking the patient to "look" at the back of the hand.

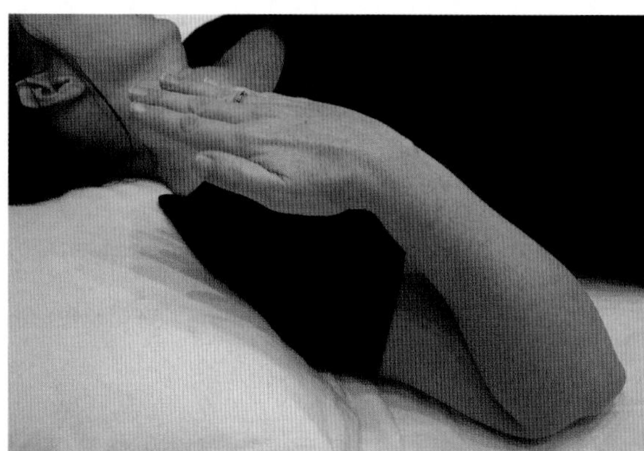

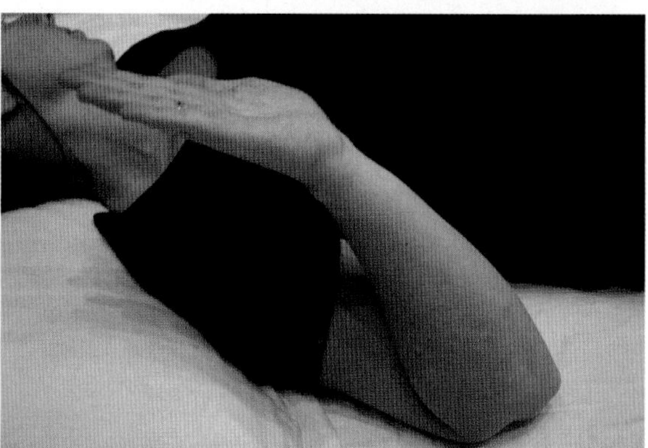

2.5 Active Elbow Flexion and Extension (Triceps Intact)

- Position the patient supine, with the posterior arm resting on a small pillow or rolled towel.
- Supine is preferred, as this position discourages substitution motion of the shoulder.
- For individuals with increased instability, an overhead program may be used to enhance stability. If this is the case, keep the patient in the supine position and simply flex the shoulder to 90° prior to initiating elbow motion.
- With the forearm in neutral, ask the patient to flex the elbow to touch the shoulder.
- Encourage the patient to remain in full flexion for 10 seconds.
- Once 10 repetitions are complete, ask the patient to straighten the elbow.
- Extension is usually to 40° and is progressed 10° per week, but the amount of extension depends on the stability of the elbow. Encourage contraction of the triceps muscle by palpating if necessary. Ask the patient to contract and hold maximum extension for 10 seconds.

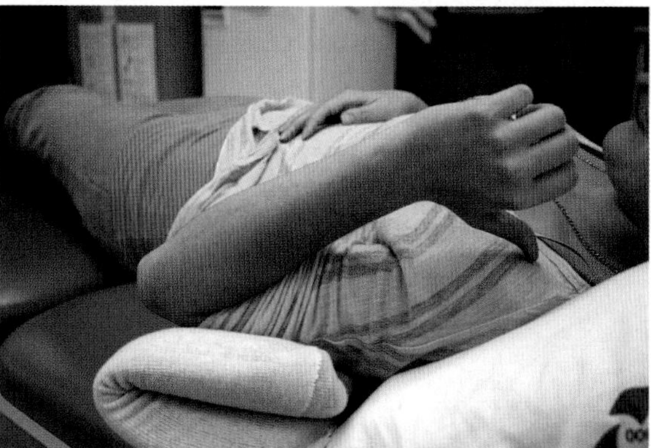

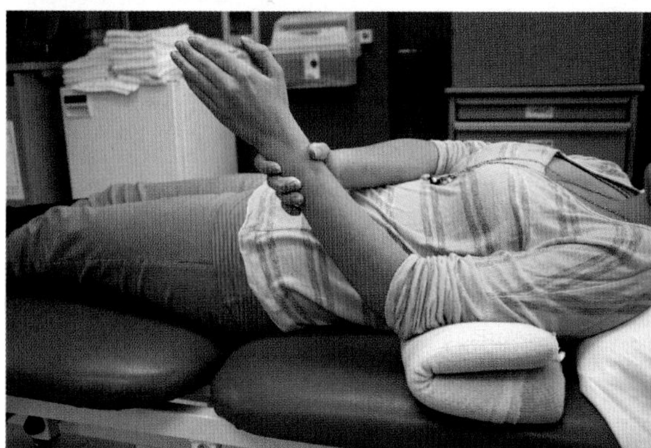

© 2018 American Academy of Orthopaedic Surgeons

Table 23.2 UNLINKED TOTAL ELBOW ARTHROPLASTY EXERCISE PROGRAM *(Continued)*

2.6 Active Elbow Flexion and Extension (Triceps Detached) • Position the patient supine, with the posterior arm resting on a small pillow or rolled towel. • Supine is preferred to allow gravity to assist extension. • Using the contralateral arm for assistance, ask the patient to flex the elbow just past 90° and hold for 10 seconds. The amount of flexion can be increased by 10° per week. • Once 10 repetitions of flexion are complete, work on assisted extension. Extension is usually limited to 40° and is progressed 10° degrees per week.	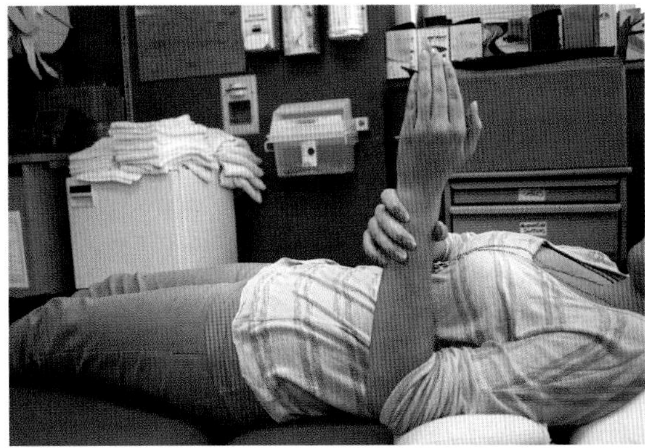 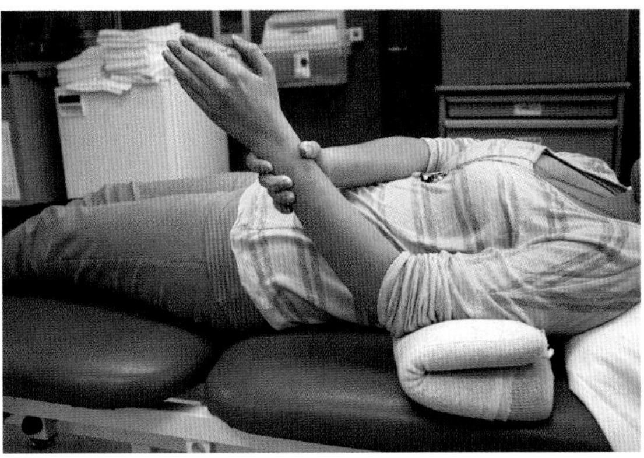

- Strengthening is performed once per day and includes resisted gripping, wrist and elbow flexion/extension.

Functional Restoration

- Since postoperative stability is dependent on healing of the collateral ligaments, patients require protection and immobilization for 6 weeks after surgery.
- With unlinked arthroplasty, rehabilitation is similar to an elbow dislocation, in which preservation of stability is an important goal in the early postoperative period.
- Once stability is achieved, patients may use their arm for functional use as tolerated, provided they adhere to weight restrictions.
- A lifetime weight-lifting restriction of 10 pounds is reviewed with the patient before surgery and during rehabilitation. Patients with unlinked implants tend to be younger and more active than those with linked designs. For this reason, education is important regarding joint protection and limiting loads through the elbow as much as possible during functional use.

OUTCOMES

The early outcome of total elbow arthroplasty is rewarding in most patients, with restoration of functional motion, stability, and little if any pain. The medium to long-term outcomes in patients with generalized rheumatoid arthritis have been favorable. Implant loosening and bearing wear have been more problematic in younger, more active, patients and those with posttraumatic conditions of the elbow with otherwise well-functioning upper extremity joints. Perioperative complication rates remain higher than hip and knee replacement, particularly the risk of infection, ulnar neuropathy, and wound healing problems.

PEARLS

Top Five Surgical Pearls

1. Preserve the triceps insertion to the olecranon when possible.
2. Unlinked arthroplasty is reserved for younger, more active, patients with good bone stock and ligament integrity.
3. Ensure correct component positioning and avoid impingement of the coronoid or olecranon process on the humeral component, as this may lead to ulnar component loosening.
4. Secure ligament repair and preservation or replacement of the radial head is needed when performing an unlinked total elbow arthroplasty.
5. Immobilize elbow until skin healing is secure.

© 2018 American Academy of Orthopaedic Surgeons

Top Five Therapy Pearls

1. Communicate with surgeon as to
   a. whether an unlinked or linked elbow arthroplasty was performed
   b. motion achieved at surgery
   c. integrity of the triceps tendon
   d. intraoperative stability of the elbow and the quality of collateral ligaments
2. Early isometric contractions are important to recover muscle tone, especially with unlinked arthroplasty.
3. If the triceps was detached, avoid early aggressive elbow flexion exercises.
4. Avoid splint pressure over the tip of the olecranon, as delayed wound healing impairs progression of therapy and increases the risk of deep infection.
5. Educate patients regarding functional restrictions on the first therapy visit to prevent potential complications associated with instability, triceps insufficiency, and implant failure.

BIBLIOGRAPHY

Brownhill JR, Pollock JW, Ferreira LM, Johnson JA, King GJ: The effect of implant malalignment on joint loading in total elbow arthroplasty: an in vitro study. *J Shoulder Elbow Surg* 2012;21(8):1032–1038.

Bryan RS, Morrey BF: Extensive posterior exposure of the elbow. A triceps-sparing approach. *Clin Orthop Relat Res* 1982;(166):188–192.

Celli A, Arash A, Adams RA, Morrey BF: Triceps insufficiency following total elbow arthroplasty. *J Bone Joint Surg Am* 2005;87(9):1957–1964

Davis RF, Weiland AJ, Hungerford DS, Moore JR, Volenec-Dowling S: Nonconstrained total elbow arthroplasty. *Clin Orthop Relat Res* 1982;(171):156–160.

Dowdy PA, Bain GI, King GJ, Patterson SD: The midline posterior elbow incision. An anatomical appraisal. *J Bone Joint Surg Br* 1995;77(5):696–699.

Ewald FC, Simmons ED Jr, Sullivan JA, Thomas WH, Scott RD, Poss R, Thornhill TS, Sledge CB: Capitellocondylar total elbow replacement in rheumatoid arthritis. Long-term results. *J Bone Joint Surg Am* 1993;75(4):498–507.

Gay DM, Lyman S, Do H, Hotchkiss RN, Marx RG, Daluiski A: Indications and reoperation rates for total elbow arthroplasty: an analysis of trends in New York State. *J Bone Joint Surg Am* 2012;94(2):110–117.

Gill DR, Morrey BF: The Coonrad-Morrey total elbow arthroplasty in patients who have rheumatoid arthritis. A ten to fifteen-year follow-up study. *J Bone Joint Surg Am* 1998;80(9):1327–1335.

Kocher T: Textbook of Operative Surgery, ed 3. London, Adam and Charles Black, 1911.

Mehta JA, Bain GI: Surgical approaches to the elbow. *Hand Clin* 2004;20(4):375–387.

Schneeberger AG, Adams R, Morrey BF: Semiconstrained total elbow replacement for the treatment of post-traumatic osteoarthrosis. *J Bone Joint Surg Am* 1997;79(8):1211–1222.

Studer A, Athwal GS, Macdermid JC, Faber KJ, King GJ: The lateral para-olecranon approach for total elbow arthroplasty. *J Hand Surg Am* 2013;38:2219–2226.

© 2018 American Academy of Orthopaedic Surgeons

SECTION 3

Hand and Wrist

24 Introduction to Hand and Wrist Anatomy

Jun Matsui, MD, and Ryan P. Calfee, MD, MSc

INTRODUCTION

A detailed understanding of anatomy is the basis of safely and efficiently performing surgery in the hand and wrist. Here, we review surgical anatomy relevant to the procedures discussed in this region.

WRIST

Bones and Joints

The distal radius has three articular facets: the scaphoid facet, the lunate facet, and the sigmoid notch, which articulates with the distal ulna. The normal distal radius is characterized by several measurements: radius inclination (22°), lateral tilt (11° volar), radius height (12 mm of styloid height relative to the ulnar corner of the lunate facet), and length relative to the ulna (normal is neutral ulnar variance; Figure 24.1). Change from these normal values is assessed following fracture; this, along with articular displacement, often dictates treatment. There is a prominent transverse ridge 2 mm proximal to the volar rim of the lunate facet and 12 mm proximal to the scaphoid facet (Figure 24.2). Volar plate placement on the fractured distal radius is preferably done proximal to this ridge so that this bony prominence is the most volar surface contacting the flexor tendons.

The carpal bones are arranged in two rows: the proximal (scaphoid, lunate, triquetrum, pisiform) and distal (trapezium, trapezoid, capitate, hamate) rows. These bones interact in a complex but coordinated fashion to produce wrist motion as described subsequently in the Kinematics section. Notable from a surgical standpoint, the scaphoid derives a retrograde vascular supply from a dorsal branch of the radial artery entering the dorsal ridge of the scaphoid. Thus, the most extensive dissection for scaphoid fracture is accomplished from the volar wrist to avoid disrupting the vascular supply. Second, the lunate is wider volarly than dorsally, making it more susceptible to palmar dislocation. This contributes in part to the preponderance of volar lunate dislocations compared to dorsal dislocations as the final step in perilunate instability.

Ligaments

The primary volar ligamentous stabilizers of the carpus include the radioscaphocapitate and long and short radiolunate ligaments (Figure 24.3). These ligaments originate from the volar articular margin of the distal radius and must be preserved during volar approach to the distal radius for fracture fixation. Violation of these volar ligaments can result in iatrogenic ulnar carpal translation. Preservation of the radioscaphocapitate ligament origin is the limiting factor for volar bony excision (4 mm) during radial styloidectomy.

The dorsal intercarpal and dorsal radiocarpal ligaments are the key spanning dorsal ligaments (Figure 24.3). The dorsal radiocarpal ligament originates from the distal radius to insert on the triquetrum, and the dorsal intercarpal ligament originates on the triquetrum to insert on the scaphoid, trapezium, and trapezoid. These ligaments can be identified and incised in line with their fibers to allow a ligament-sparing approach to the dorsal aspect of the distal radius and carpus. The primary intrinsic carpal ligaments of the proximal carpal row are the scapholunate and lunotriquetral. The scapholunate interosseous ligament is strongest dorsally, while the lunotriquetral interosseous ligament is most substantial volarly. Care should

Dr. Calfee or an immediate family member has received research or institutional support from Medartis; and serves as a board member, owner, officer, or committee member of the American Society for Surgery of the Hand and the Journal of Hand Surgery–American. *Dr. Matsui or an immediate family member has received research or institutional support from Arthrex.*

© 2018 American Academy of Orthopaedic Surgeons

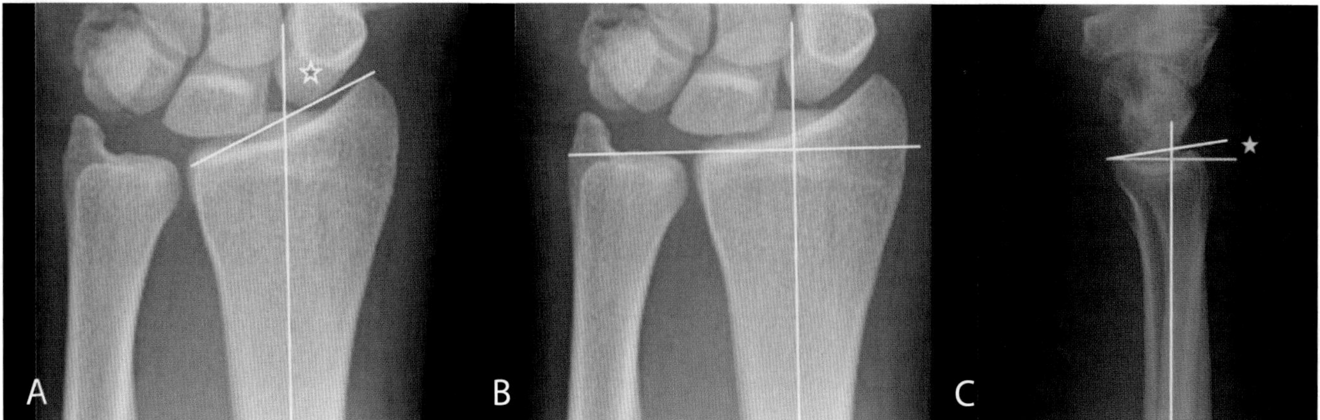

Figure 24.1 Plain radiographs illustrating characteristic distal radius measurements. **A**, radius inclination. **B**, ulnar variance (neutral in this case). **C**, Lateral tilt (volar in this case).

be taken during a dorsal exposure of the wrist to prevent iatrogenic injury to the scapholunate ligament, which is routinely located slightly ulnar to the longitudinal axis of the radius passing through Lister's tubercle.

On the ulnar aspect of the wrist, the triangular fibrocartilage complex (TFCC) is the confluence of an articular disc, ulnocarpal meniscus homolog, dorsal and volar radioulnar ligaments, the floor of the extensor carpi ulnaris (ECU) tendon sheath, and the volar ulnocarpal ligaments (Figure 24.4). The TFCC runs from the ulnar fovea to the radius and triquetrum. It is biconcave in shape. The dorsal and volar radioulnar ligaments are the primary stabilizers of the distal radioulnar joint (DRUJ). The dorsal radioulnar ligament is preserved when exposing the dorsal wrist by carefully elevating the fourth extensor compartment without dissecting deep to the fifth extensor compartment overlying the DRUJ. The fact that only the peripheral 10% to 40% of the TFCC is vascularized dictates routine repair of peripheral TFCC tears versus débridement of central tears of the articular disc.

Tendons

The extensor tendons run in six separate fibro-osseous sheaths under the extensor retinaculum at the level of the wrist. From radial to ulnar, the six compartments are: (1) abductor pollicis longus/extensor pollicis brevis (APL/EPB), (2) extensor carpi radialis longus and brevis (ECRL/ECRB), (3) extensor pollicis longus (EPL), (4) extensor digitorum communis/extensor indicis proprius (EDC/EIP), (5) extensor digiti minimi (EDM), and (6) extensor carpi ulnaris (ECU). The muscle bellies of the first compartment cross dorsal to the second compartment tendons 6 cm to 7 cm proximal to the wrist crease. Within the first dorsal compartment, the APL commonly consists of multiple tendinous slips, and the EPB may be contained within a separate subsheath prior to its insertion

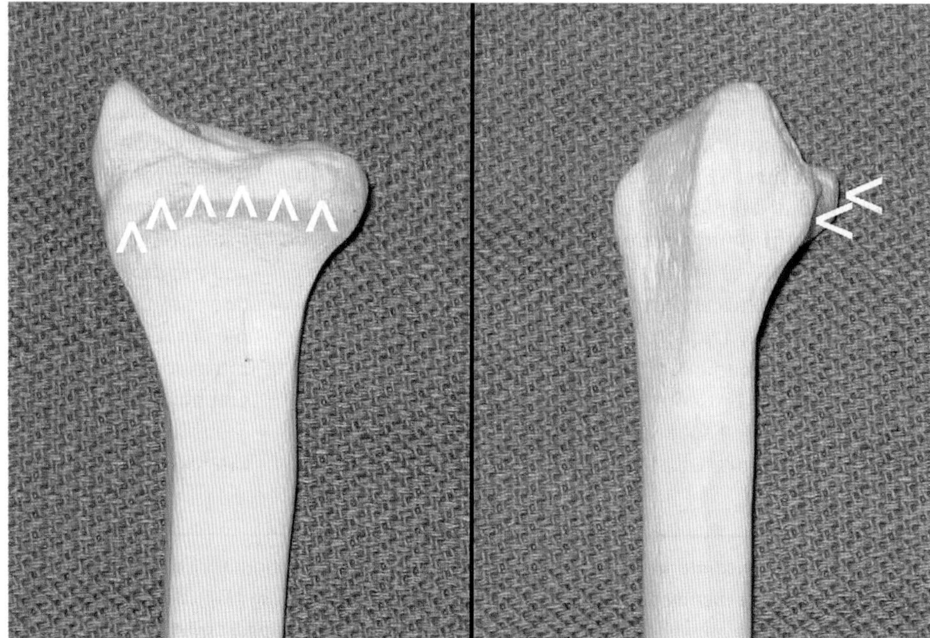

Figure 24.2 Photographs showing the watershed line of the distal radius, marked by arrows. (Reproduced with permission from Soong M, Earp BE, Bishop G, Leung A, Blazar P: Volar locking plate implant prominence and flexor tendon rupture. *J Bone Joint Surg* 2011;93:328–335.)

© 2018 American Academy of Orthopaedic Surgeons

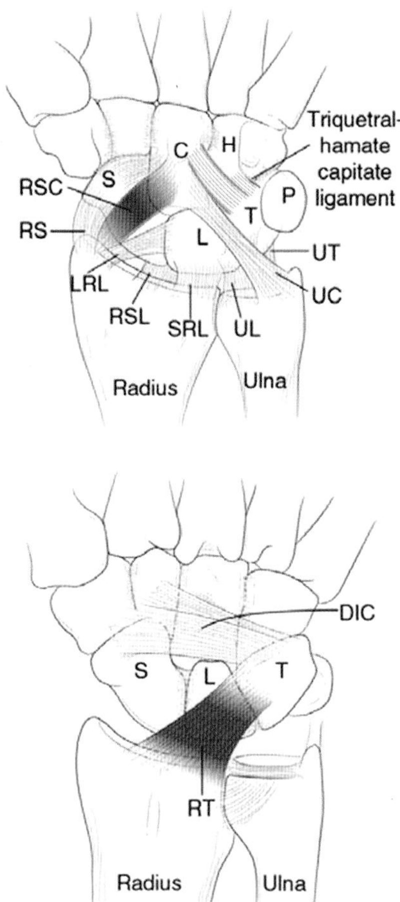

Figure 24.3 Illustrations of the volar (*top*) and dorsal (*bottom*) wrist ligaments. (Reproduced with permission from Wolfe SW, Garcia-Elias M, Kitay A: Carpal instability nondissociative. *JAAOS* 2012;20:575–585.)

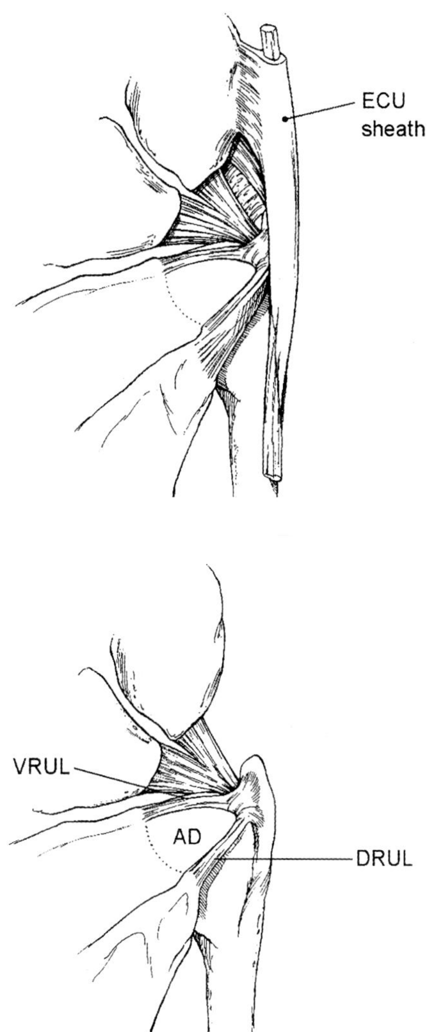

Figure 24.4 Illustrations of triangular fibrocartilage complex anatomy. (Reproduced with permission Chidgey LK: The distal radiounlar joint: problems and solutions. *JAAOS* 1995;3:95–109.)

on the proximal phalanx of the thumb. The EPL angles 45° radially from its origin on the ulna as it passes around the ulnar aspect of Lister's tubercle to insert on the distal phalanx of the thumb, where it extends and retropulses the thumb. During the utilitarian dorsal approach to the wrist between the third and fourth extensor compartments, care must be taken to identify and protect the EPL, as it is the only extensor tendon deviating substantially from a longitudinal course. Thus, most dorsal exposures of the wrist—whether for arthrodesis, arthroplasty, or traumatic reconstruction—are performed by opening the extensor retinaculum into the third extensor compartment to first identify and then protect the EPL tendon before elevating surrounding extensor compartments off the radius (Figure 24.5). The fourth extensor compartment contains the posterior interosseous nerve in its radial-sided floor. The posterior interosseous nerve is commonly excised during dorsal wrist exposures to provide pain relief as a partial wrist denervation—although some argue for preservation, as the nerve provides proprioceptive information for the carpus. Also, within the fourth extensor compartment and commonly used for tendon transfers, the EIP can be differentiated from the EDC to the index finger by its more distal muscle belly, a lack of tendon juncturae, and its location typically ulnar and deep to the EDC tendon. Clinically, presence of the EIP is confirmed by independent active extension of the index metacarpal-phalangeal joint while all other fingers remain in a fist. Within the fifth compartment, the EDM tendon typically has two slips that course directly over the distal radial-ulnar joint. The EDM is the landmark for operative exposure of the DRUJ and TFCC. The sixth compartment containing the single ECU tendon is typically exposed to débride tendonitis or to stabilize the ECU tendon. Importantly, the extensor retinaculum is expansive and anchored to the more volar-ulnar surface of the ulna, with ECU stability dependent on a competent ECU subsheath.

Neurovascular Structures

The median nerve enters the hand through the carpal tunnel, running under the transverse carpal ligament, which spans from the scaphoid tubercle and trapezial ridge to the pisiform and hook of the hamate. The carpal tunnel is, on

© 2018 American Academy of Orthopaedic Surgeons

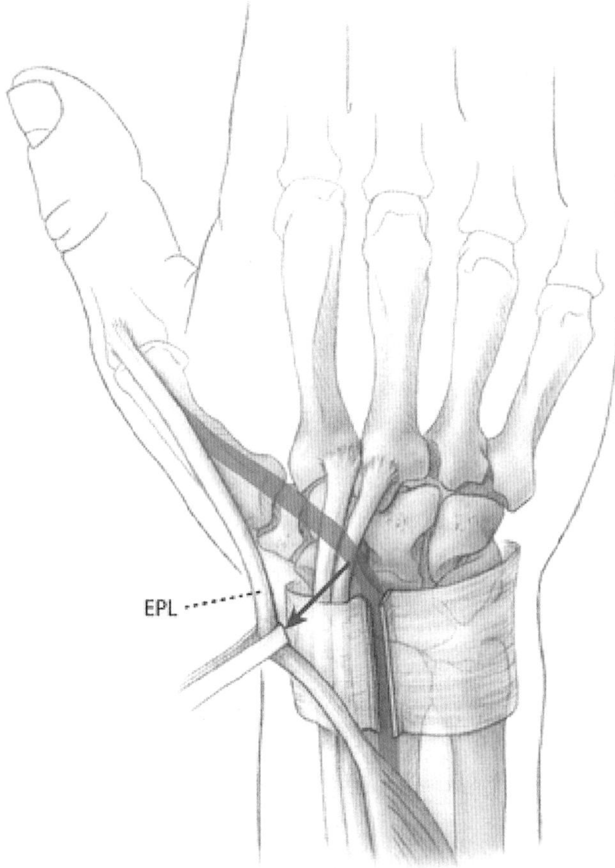

Figure 24.5 Illustration of exposure of the dorsal wrist transposing the EPL tendon for protection. (Reproduced with permission Stern PJ1, Agabegi SS, Kiefhaber TR, Didonna ML: Proximal row carpectomy. *J Bone Joint Surg Am* 2005 Sep;87 Suppl 1(Pt 2):166–174.)

average, 22 mm wide and 26 mm long. The carpal canal contains the median nerve, which is the most superficial structure, four tendons of the flexor digitorum superficialis (FDS), four tendons of the flexor digitorum profundus (FDP), and the flexor pollicis longus (FPL) tendon (Figure 24.6). At the carpal tunnel, the median nerve is 94% sensory and 6% motor. The palmar cutaneous branch of the median nerve arises 5 cm to 7 cm proximal to the wrist crease and travels within the median nerve epineurium for 16 mm to 25 mm before passing superficial to the transverse carpal ligament to supply sensation to the thenar eminence. Injury to the palmar cutaneous branch of the median nerve produces a small area of paresthesia, but, more important, often produces substantial pain and hypersensitivity over the course of the nerve.

The ulnar nerve gives off a dorsal cutaneous branch approximately 6 cm proximal to the ulnar head, then enters the hand through the distal ulnar tunnel, or Guyon's canal, radial to the FCU tendon. It courses ulnar and volar to the ulnar artery. The ulnar nerve divides into superficial sensory and deep motor branches 11 mm distal to the proximal aspect of the pisiform. The distal ulnar tunnel may be divided into three zones (Figure 24.7). In Zone I, between the proximal edge of the volar carpal ligament and the bifurcation of the ulnar nerve,

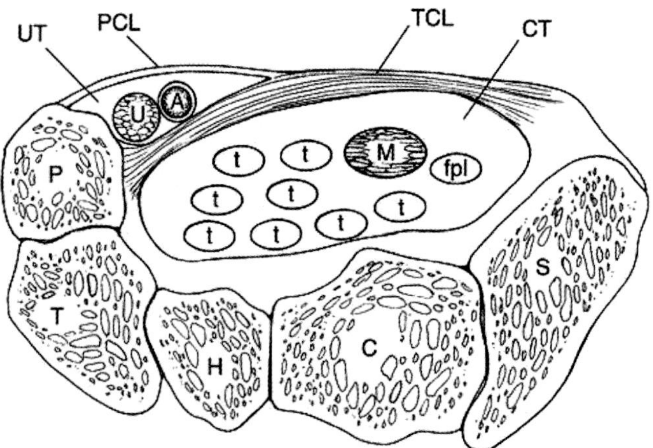

Figure 24.6 Cross-sectional illustration of the carpal tunnel. (Reproduced with permission Szabo RM, Steinberg DR. Nerve entrapment syndromes in the wrist. *JAAOS* 1994;2:115–123.)

the ulnar nerve has both motor and sensory function. Zone II is the area encompassing the deep motor branch as it passes around the hook of the hamate. Nerve injury in Zone II produces a motor deficit of the interossei, third and fourth lumbricals, adductor pollicis, and flexor pollicis brevis muscles. Ganglion cysts and fractures (e.g., hook of the hamate) can cause injury to the ulnar nerve in Zones I and II. In Zone III, the area encompassing the sensory branch of the ulnar nerve, the most common causes of neurologic symptoms are arterial thrombosis or compression from anomalous muscles, which may cause sensory deficits to the small and ring fingers.

The superficial branch of the radial nerve becomes subcutaneous as it exits dorsally from underneath the brachioradialis tendon in the distal forearm and courses in the subcutaneous

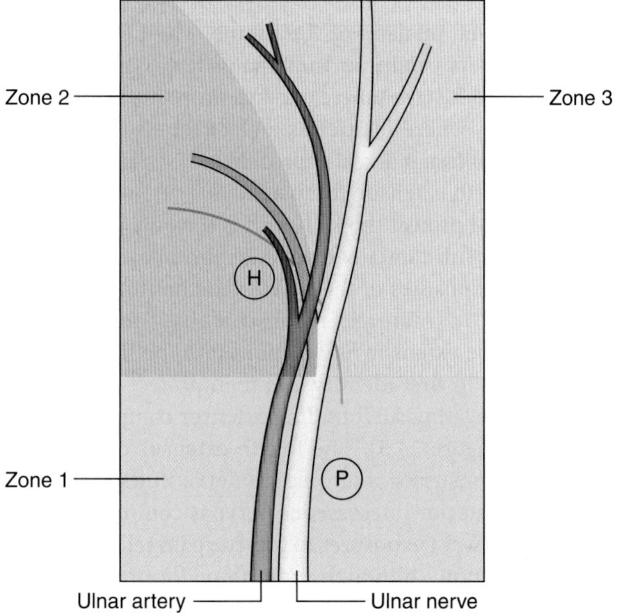

Figure 24.7 Illustration of the zone of Guyon's canal. (Reproduced with permission from Szabo RM, Steinberg DR: Nerve entrapment syndromes in the wrist. *JAAOS* 1994;2:115–123.)

© 2018 American Academy of Orthopaedic Surgeons

tissues over the radial side of the wrist. This nerve has multiple branches that are both susceptible to sharp and blunt (traction or compression during retraction) iatrogenic injury.

The radial artery divides at the wrist into the superficial branch that contributes to the superficial palmar arch, and the more dominant deep dorsal branch, which passes through the floor of the anatomic snuff box overlying the scaphotrapezotrapezoidal (STT) joint. During thumb carpometacarpal (CMC) joint surgery, the dorsal branch of the radial artery can be readily identified by dissection just dorsal to the first extensor compartment tendons deep in the fatty tissue over the dorsal STT joint. There, several small articular branches can be cauterized to allow safe retraction of the artery.

The ulnar artery courses across the wrist without major branching. The artery is located radial and deep to the FCU tendon. The artery is superficial and radial to the ulnar nerve. The ulnar artery will provide the dominant contribution to the superficial palmar arch in most people.

Kinematics

The stability of the wrist is primarily determined by the complex relationships between the bony articulations, ligaments, and tendons of the wrist. Wrist range of motion (ROM), from 70° of extension to 80° of flexion, is produced by tendons that pass over the carpus and attach to the metacarpal bases, with the exception of the pisiform, which acts as a sesamoid bone within the FCU. With ulnar deviation of the wrist, the proximal row extends relative to the distal row, and with radial deviation, the proximal row flexed. With axial loading, in neutral position, approximately 80% of the force is transmitted through the distal radius, and 20% through the distal ulna. However, this relationship changes with every 2 mm of increased ulnar variance, increasing the force through the distal ulna and TFCC by 20%.

HAND AND FINGERS

Bones and Joints

The unique anatomy of the metacarpophalangeal (MCP) and proximal interphalangeal (PIP) joints specifies the function of the joints, but also makes the joints vulnerable to deformity from injury. The MCP joint is a condyloid joint capable of triaxial motion in flexion–extension, abduction–adduction, and circumduction. The collateral ligaments are taut in flexion, due to the eccentric origin of the collateral ligament dorsal to the axis of rotation as well as the volarly wider metacarpal head, producing a CAM effect. The volar plate of the MCP joint connects to the deep transverse metacarpal ligament, and tends to rupture proximally. The deep transverse metacarpal ligament, also known as the interpalmar plate ligament, passes between the MCP joints, with the interossei running dorsal to the ligament, and the lumbricals and neurovascular bundles pass volar to the ligament. Provided minimal mechanical stability imparted by bony articulations, capsuloligamentous support is critical for the MCP joint. This support is often compromised in inflammatory arthritic conditions, which dictates the use of hinged silicone spacer arthroplasty as opposed to resurfacing implants.

The PIP joint is a bicondylar, single-axis hinge moving only in flexion and extension, with its collateral ligaments taut throughout all positions. The many ligament and tendon insertions include the central slip onto the dorsal base of the middle phalanx, the collateral ligaments, the FDS, and the A4 pulley (Figure 24.8). Dorsal exposure of the PIP joint is most limited by the central slip of the extensor mechanism due to its small bony footprint that closely approximates the articular surface and the thin nature of the tendon at that level. The volar plate of the PIP joint, which prevents joint hyperextension, is stabilized by the check ligaments proximally, and tends to rupture distally.

The CMC, or basal, joint of the thumb is unique in its ROM, shape, and the stresses that it bears. Formed by the reciprocally opposed saddles of the trapezium and base of the thumb metacarpal, it can move in three planes: flexion–extension, adduction–abduction, and pronation–supination. The bony structure of the joint does not provide substantial stability. The five primary ligamentous stabilizers of the thumb CMC joint include three intracapsular ligaments (anterior oblique or volar beak ligament, posterior oblique ligament, dorsoradial ligament) and two extracapsular ligaments (ulnar collateral ligament and the intermetacarpal ligament). It is stabilized

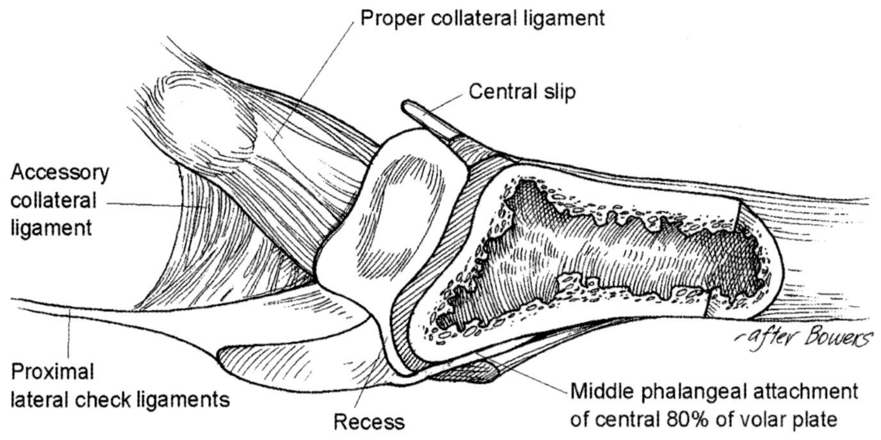

Figure 24.8 Illustration of the anatomy of the proximal interphalangeal joint. (Reproduced with permission from Blazar PE, Steinberg DR: Fractures of the proximal interphalangeal joint. *JAAOS* 2008;8:383–390.)

on either side by the radial and ulnar collateral ligaments (and their accessory collateral ligaments). As pinch forces at the thumb tip are magnified 13× at the thumb CMC joint, operative salvage or reconstruction of this joint must remain durable over time.

Tendons and Fascia

The extensor mechanism is a delicately balanced system of ligaments and tendon that converge to extend the fingers. The EDC tendons are connected by the junctura tendinae at the level of the metacarpals, which can result in preservation of active MCP joint extension (usually weaker and somewhat incomplete) despite tendon laceration at this level. At the level of the MCP joints, the sagittal bands, thickenings of the dorsal intertendinous fascia keep the digital extensor tendons centered over the midline of the metacarpal heads and contribute to MCP extension through their attachments to the palmar plate. Just distal to the sagittal bands, the continuation of the interossei, the transverse fibers, cause flexion of the MCP joint. The continuation of the lumbricals, the oblique fibers, add further stability to the tendon, flex the MCP joints, and extend the PIP joint.

Just proximal to the PIP joint, the EDC trifurcates into the central slip, inserting onto the base of the middle phalanx, and the two lateral slips. These lateral slips then converge with the oblique fibers of the lumbricals to form the conjoined lateral bands, which then reunite at the distal end of the middle phalanx to insert onto the base of the distal phalanx as the terminal tendon, which extends the distal interphalangeal (DIP) joint. The transverse retinacular ligament is a fibrous sheath at the PIP joint that prevents dorsal subluxation of the conjoined lateral bands, which may be deficient in swan-neck deformities. The triangular ligament stabilizes the lateral bands and maintains their dorsal position. In boutonniere deformities, attenuation of the triangular ligament causes volar subluxation of the lateral bands, which may contribute to the formation of a PIP joint flexion deformity.

In the hand, the FDS tendons course volar to the FDP tendons. The FDS tendons function independently to flex the PIP joints, while the FDP tendons work from a common muscle belly to flex the DIP joints. Over the midshaft of the proximal phalanx, the FDS flattens and bifurcates and the FDP emerges volarly to course distally. At this level, a laceration to the volar aspect of a finger can commonly lacerate the FDP, causing a loss of active DIP flexion while preserving active PIP flexion. At Camper's chiasm, the FDS medial and lateral slips rejoin dorsal (deep) to the FDP tendon over the distal aspect of the proximal phalanx and PIP joint to insert at the base of the middle phalanx.

The flexor tendons are enclosed by synovial sheaths in the digits, which consist of two distinct layers with specific functions. The retinacular portion, which overlies the membranous portion, forms the five annular and three cruciate pulleys that prevent tendon bowstringing and maximize the biomechanical pull of the flexor tendon force (Figure 24.9). In the fingers, the most critical pulleys for these functions are the A2 and A4, which overlie the proximal and middle phalanges and are the

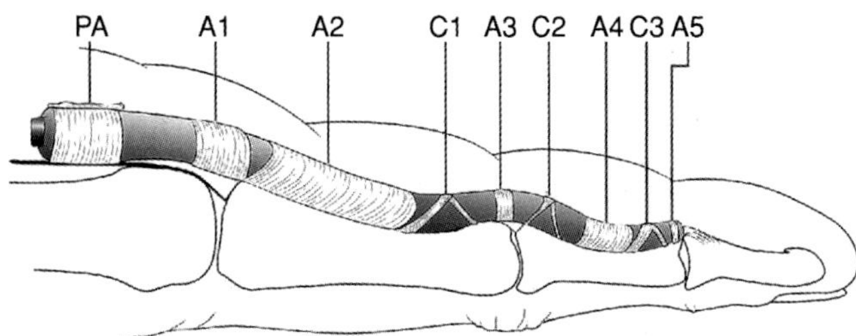

Figure 24.9 Illustration of the anatomy of the flexor tendon sheath. (Reproduced with permission from Draeger RW, Bynum DK: Flexor tendon sheath infections of the hand. *JAAOS* 2012;20:373–382.)

strongest and longest pulleys, at 17 mm and 7mm, respectively. Biomechanically, while the A2 and A4 pulleys remain intact, the tendon excursion required for full ROM is minimally increased. In the thumb, the A1 and oblique pulleys are the most important biomechanically. The A1 pulley is at the level of the MCP joint, in proximity with the radial digital nerve, which runs an oblique course at this level. The membranous or synovial layer provides vascularity, nutrition, and lubrication to the tendons. The limited space within the tendon sheathes necessitates precise repair of lacerated flexor tendons without increasing the bulk of the tendon at the repair site.

The vascular supply to the flexor tendons derives from two sources: the vinculae and synovial diffusion. Transverse digital arteries, or "ladder branches," from the digital arteries supply the vinculae, which are vascular networks on the dorsal surfaces of the FDS and FDP tendons. The relatively hypovascular zones of the FDS and FDP within the flexor tendon sheath rely on intratendinous canaliculi to provide nutrition via synovial diffusion.

On the volar aspect of the hand, the palmar fascia is composed of the palmar aponeurosis, pretendinous bands, superficial and transverse metacarpal ligaments, natatory ligaments, and the vertical septa of Legeau and Juvara. The palmar aponeurosis is the terminal extension of the palmaris longus tendon, superficial to the transverse carpal ligament. When using the palmaris longus for an opposition transfer, the central palmar fascia should be harvested for several centimeters in continuity with the palmaris longus. The ulnar border of the palmar fascia generally overlies the ulnar side of the transverse carpal ligament, marking an appropriate location for carpal tunnel release.

Pretendinous bands are the longitudinal fascial bands of the palm, run volar to the palmar aponeurosis, and insert into the skin at the level of the MCP joint. The vertical septa of Legeau and Juvara divide the palm into seven longitudinal compartments, four containing flexor tendons and three containing neurovascular bundles and lumbricals. The palmar fascia and its associated bands become thickened and contracted in Dupuytren's disease.

Neurovascular Structures

The hand is mostly innervated by the median and ulnar nerves, while the superficial and deep arches are supplied by the radial and ulnar arteries.

 © 2018 American Academy of Orthopaedic Surgeons

In the hand, the median nerve gives rise to a recurrent motor branch to the thenar muscles, in addition to a proper radial digital nerve to the index finger and three common digital nerves (thumb, and second and third webspaces), innervating the radial and ulnar aspects of the thumb, index, and long finger, as well as the radial border of the ring finger. The first and second lumbrical muscles are innervated by branches of the common digital nerves. There is variability in the course of the recurrent motor branch of the median nerve, which may run volar to, dorsal to, or within the transverse carpal ligament. It is most commonly extraligamentous, coursing volar to the transverse carpal ligament, and innervates the abductor pollicis brevis, flexor pollicis brevis, and opponens pollicis.

On the ulnar side of the hand, the superficial sensory ulnar nerve branches to form the proper ulnar nerve to the ulnar border of the small finger and a common digital nerve to the radial border of the small finger and ulnar border of the ring finger. The digital nerves are small, purely sensory nerves containing three to six fasciculi, and trifurcate at the DIP joint. At the level of the finger, the nerves are volar to the arteries. As discussed is the Wrist section, the deep motor branch of the ulnar nerve innervates the interossei, third and fourth lumbricals, adductor pollicis, and flexor pollicis brevis muscles after coursing around the hook of the hamate.

Sensibility on the dorsum of the hand and proximal fingers is produced by the superficial branch of the radial nerve and the dorsal cutaneous branch of the ulnar nerve. These nerves have multiple branches on the dorsal hand and are most notably causalgic nerves imparting substantial morbidity when injured.

The ulnar artery, which passes ulnar to the hook of the hamate, is most commonly the dominant contribution to the superficial palmar arch, which then provides a proper digital artery to the small finger as well as three common digital arteries and a branch to the deep palmar arch (Figure 24.10). The superficial palmar arch lies volar to the median nerve and branches. The proper digital nerves first become volar to the digital arteries at the level of the metacarpal necks and continue to be volar/superficial throughout the length of the fingers. The superficial palmar arch is complete, indicating anastomoses between the vessels that constitute the arch, in 84%. The deep palmar arch, proximal to the superficial palmar arch, is primarily derived from the radial artery and gives branches to the radial index digital artery and the arterial supply to the thumb (princeps pollicis artery). The proximal-distal location can be estimated using Kaplan's cardinal line, drawn from the apex of the interdigital fold between the thumb and index finger to the hook of the hamate. The superficial palmar arch is located proximal to the distal palmar crease.

The radial artery divides into three main branches at the wrist: the volar carpal branch; the superficial branch, which contributes to the superficial palmar arch; and the deep dorsal branch, which passes through the floor of the anatomic snuff box, passes superficial to the STT joint, and dives between the heads of the first dorsal interosseous muscle to form the deep palmar arch.

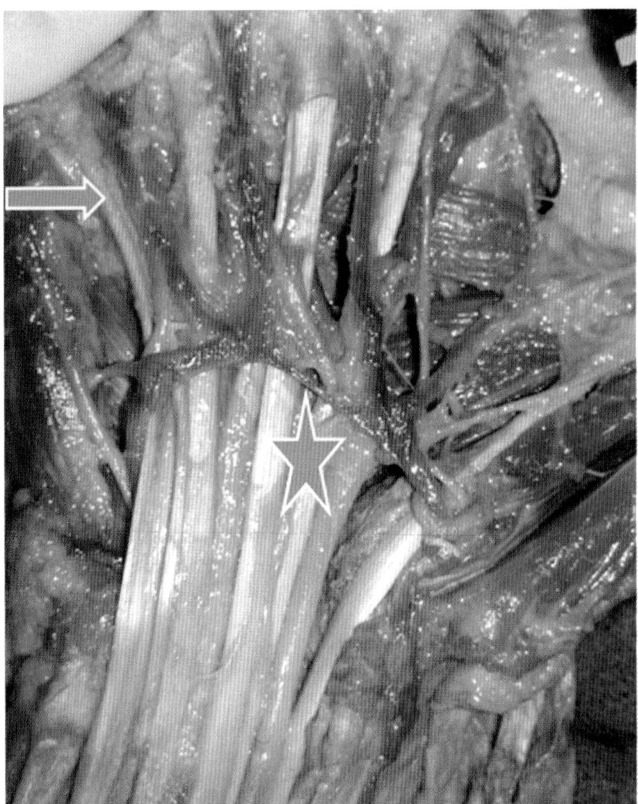

Figure 24.10 Photograph of the superficial palmar arch (*star*) with exiting common digital arteries (*one marked with arrow*).

Grayson's and Cleland's ligaments hold the neurovascular bundles in place in the finger from their positions volar and dorsal to the bundles, respectively. They insert into the skin dorsally and volarly. Both Grayson's and Cleland's ligaments contribute to the lateral digital sheet, along with the spiral band and natatory ligament. The spiral band originates at the pretendinous band and passes dorsal to the neurovascular bundle to insert onto the lateral digital sheet, and the natatory ligaments are transverse fibers at the palmodigital crease.

SUMMARY

The anatomy of the wrist, hand, and fingers is complex. Likewise, function of the hand is dependent on the integrity of the anatomy. The postoperative rehabilitation of the wrist, hand and fingers is critically important to the outcome. Having a thorough and clear understanding of the anatomy and the specifics and details of the surgical procedure is an integral part of determining the appropriate rehabilitation to ensure a successful outcome.

BIBLIOGRAPHY

Berger RA: The anatomy of the ligaments of the wrist and radioulnar joints. *Clin Orthop Relat Res* 2001;(383):32–40.

© 2018 American Academy of Orthopaedic Surgeons

Bettinger PC, Linscheid RL, Berger RA, Cooney WP 3rd, An KN: An anatomic study of the stabilizing ligaments of the trapezium and trapeziometacarpal joint. *J Hand Surg Am* 1999;24:786–798.

Boyer MI, Gelberman RH: Operative correction of swan-neck and boutonniere deformities in the rheumatoid hand. *J Am Acad Orthop Surg* 1999;7(2):92–100.

Doyle JR: Anatomy of the finger flexor tendon sheath and pulley system. *J Hand Surg Am* 1988;13(4):473–484.

el-Badawi MG, Butt MM, al-Zuhair AG, Fadel RA: Extensor tendons of the fingers: arrangement and variations–II. *Clin Anat* 1995;8:391–398.

Gross MS, Gelberman RH: Anatomy of distal ulnar tunnel. *Clin Orthop Relat Res* 1985;238–247.

Harris C Jr, Rutledge GL Jr: The functional anatomy of the extensor mechanism of the finger. *J Bone Joint Surg Am* 1972;54: 713–726.

Kauer J: Functional anatomy of the carpometacarpal joint of the thumb. *Clin Orthop Relat Res* 1987;7–13.

Leversedge FJ, Ditsios K, Goldfarb CA, Silva MJ, Gelberman RH, Boyer MI: Vascular anatomy of the human flexor digitorum profundus tendon insertion. *J Hand Surg Am* 2002; 27(5):806–812.

Leversedge FJ, Goldfarb CA, Boyer MI: *A Pocketbook Manual of Hand and Upper Extremity Anatomy Primus Manus.* Philadelphia, PA, Lippincott Williams and Williams, 2010.

Palmer AK, Werner FW: The triangular fibrocartilage complex of the wrist – anatomy and function. *J Hand Surg* 1981;6: 153–162.

Schmidt H and Lanz U: Anatomy of the Median Nerve in the CT- Ch. 61. In: Richard H. Gelberman. *Operative Nerve Repair and Reconstruction.* Philadelphia, PH: Lippincott; 1991:889–898.

Smith RJ: Intrinsic muscles of the fingers: function, dysfunction, and surgical reconstruction. In: *AAOS Instructional Course Lecture,* St. Louis, MO, C. V. Mosby, vol. 24, 1975, 200–220.

 © 2018 American Academy of Orthopaedic Surgeons

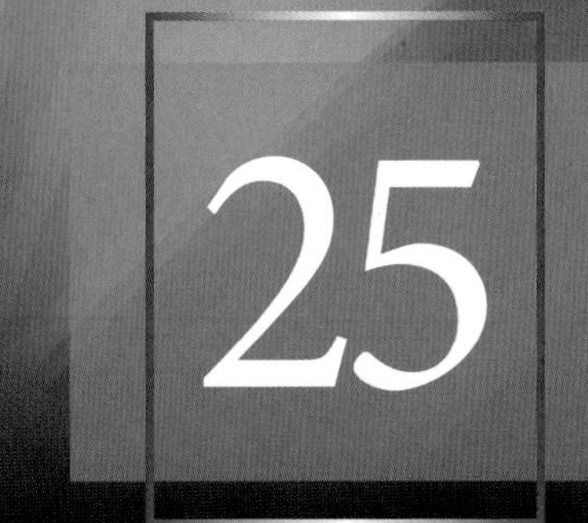

25 Dupuytren Disease

Charles Eaton, MD

INTRODUCTION

Dupuytren disease is the most common hereditary disorder affecting connective tissue. It is most common in senior Caucasian men and affects at least 10 million Americans. There is no biologic cure, all current treatments are palliative, and recurrence is common. The single biggest risk factor for developing Dupuytren disease is having a close relative with the condition—parent, grandparent, or sibling. The hallmarks of Dupuytren disease are nodules in the palm or on the extensor surfaces of the finger joints, and cords in the palm, which may cause finger deformity and limit finger extension.

Until a laboratory biomarker of Dupuytren disease is developed, the diagnosis can only be made clinically, after the development of secondary changes. The increasingly recognized association of Dupuytren disease with other medical issues (hypothyroidism, depression, cardiovascular disease, early mortality, cancer) underscores the need to study Dupuytren disease as a systemic disorder, not simply a local hand problem.

The basic biology is an abnormal response of the fascia to mechanical stress (Figure 25.1). The key cell is the myofibroblast, which is not usually present in a normal fascia, but appears in response to new mechanical strain in injury. Myofibroblasts have characteristics of both fibroblasts and smooth muscle cells. They manufacture and remodel collagen strands along lines of mechanical tension. This increases strength and stiffness of the fascia, which is the normal adaptive response to activity-related strain on supporting tissues. Myofibroblast tissue shortening involves cell contraction, rearrangement of individual collagen strands attached to myofibroblasts, and the action of extracellular enzymes (Figure 25.2). The end result of fibrotic tissue changes resembles scar tissue.

There is controversy as to whether, on a cellular level, Dupuytren tissue remodeling more resembles wound scar contracture or immobilization fibrosis (Figure 25.3). Most patterns of Dupuytren contracture bring the fingers into flexion resembling the resting posture of the hand. In contrast, the same biology affecting the extensor aspect of the fingers (dorsal Dupuytren nodules or “knuckle pads”) does not usually produce extension contracture, because that is not their resting posture—these joints rest in flexion.

The clinical presentation varies greatly. At one end of the spectrum, most patients with Dupuytren disease have mild involvement and never develop contractures. On the other end, some patients have aggressive biology with severe, recurrent contractures and all of the associated conditions. Patients with more severe biology are more likely to develop contractures and to require treatment. Patients referred for hand therapy after a procedure for Dupuytren contracture represent a subgroup of Dupuytren patients with more severe biology than average Dupuytren disease patients.

Patients diagnosed before the age of 50 years have a greater risk of progression to contracture and recurrence after treatment. Recurrent contractures are not uncommon, but not all recontractures are recurrent Dupuytren contracture. The achievable goal of Dupuytren contracture procedures is not to cure the patient of Dupuytren disease, but to improve deformity and trigger a period of prolonged disease stability before the contracture recurs. This goal is not always achieved. Postoperative rehabilitation plays an important role in the final outcome of surgical management of Dupuytren disease.

Anatomy

Most patterns of Dupuytren cords follow the course of normal anatomic structures (Figure 25.4). Common cord patterns are shown in Figure 25.5. Cords may be confined to the palm, the digit, or span both. Common central palm cords are the central palmar, spiral, and proximal first web. Common border palm cords are the natatory, distal first web, hypothenar, and thenar cords. Thenar and hypothenar cords are uncommon, and usually associated with diffuse disease or aggressive biology. The majority of metacarpophalangeal (MCP) joint contractures are due to the effect of an isolated central cord. In contrast, the majority of proximal interphalangeal (PIP) contractures have involvement of multiple cords in the digit. In the digit, the relationship of the neurovascular bundle to the cord is determined

Neither Dr. Eaton nor any immediate family member has received anything of value from or has stock or stock options held in a commercial company or institution related directly or indirectly to the subject of this article.

© 2018 American Academy of Orthopaedic Surgeons

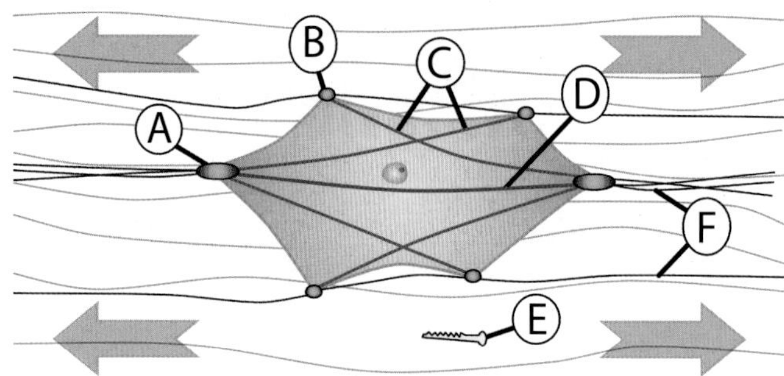

Figure 25.1 Illustration of the components involved in myofibroblast contraction shown in Figure 25.2. The central structure is a myofibroblast. The *pink arrows* show how tension placed on tissues is transmitted to individual myofibroblasts through attachments (adhesions) of extracellular collagen strands to the myofibroblast cell membrane and internal cell structures. **A**, Large adhesion complex in the cell membrane, attached to both extracellular and intracellular stress fibrils. **B**, Focal adhesion in the cell membrane, attached to both extracellular matrix fibrils and subcellular stress fibrils. **C**, Subcellular stress fibrils responsible for periodic (weak, brief) contraction. **D**, Global stress fibrils responsible for isometric (strong, sustained) contraction. **E**, Extracellular matrix proteolytic enzyme and cross-linker that joins adjacent collagen strands. **F**, Collagen fibrils in the extracellular matrix.

A

B

C

D

E

F

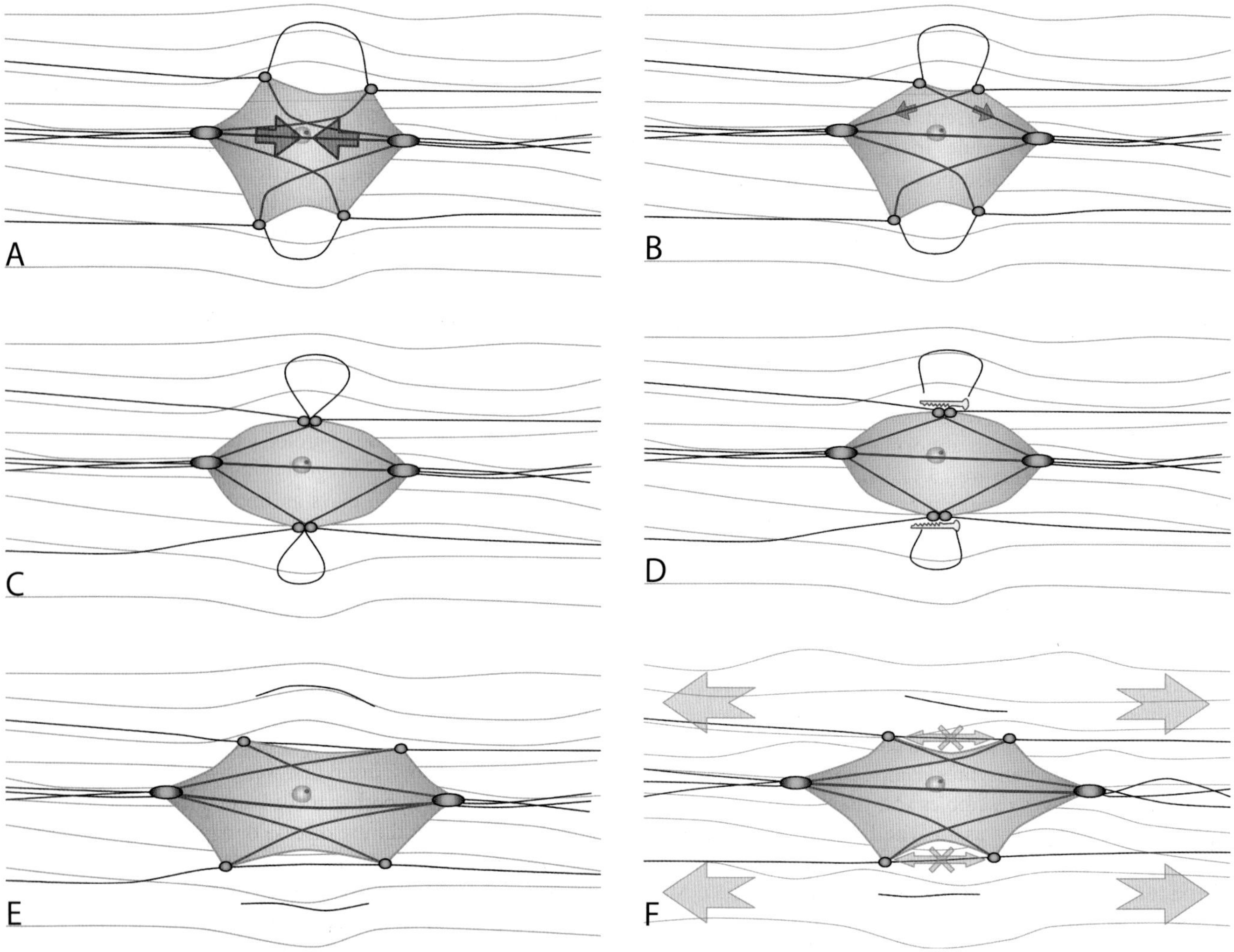

Figure 25.2 Illustration of contracting mechanism that shortens collagen. **A**, Isometric contraction of the global stress fibrils deforms the matrix, pulling collagen strands at each end of the myofibroblast and creating slack in strands in each side of the cell. **B**, **C**, Periodic contractions of the subcellular stress fibrils remove collagen strand slack beyond the cell, creating collagen strand loops on the side of the cell. **D**, While in this position, extracellular proteolytic and cross-linking enzymes divide overlapping collagen loops and join segment ends. **E**, Isometric contractions end, and the cell shape re-equilibrates. **F**, Newly shortened collagen strands sustain the matrix deformity created by active cell contraction.

© 2018 American Academy of Orthopaedic Surgeons

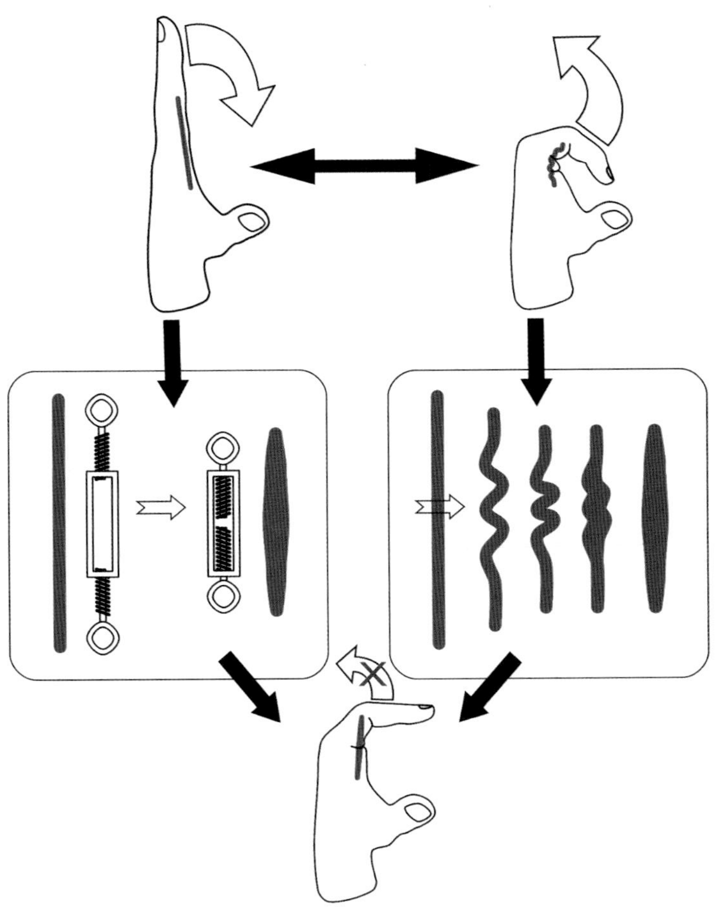

Figure 25.3 Illustration comparing Dupuytren contracture biology concepts. The *blue lines* in the diagram represent connective tissues affected by Dupuytren disease. *Top:* Fascia accommodates full finger flexion and extension by conformational changes similar to folding and unfolding. Fingers rest in flexion. *Left:* Active contracture concept of tissue shortening, similar to that of the healing and scarring that draws closed an open wound. The turnbuckle represents tissue contraction independent of the posture of the finger. *Right:* Passive contracture concept of tissue remodeling, similar to that of immobilization fibrosis. At rest, depending on the posture of the finger, shortening conformational changes from tissue slack are made permanent by tissue remodeling, which removes posture-related slack in individual collagen strands. *Bottom:* The end result of each mechanism has the same tethering effect, limiting finger extension.

by whether the cord is central, lateral, spiral, or retrovascular (Figure 25.5). Neurovascular bundles may be abnormally displaced by a spiral cord, which occurs in about a quarter of digital contractures.

Patient Evaluation

The extent of Dupuytren involvement varies considerably from minimal contracture and deformity to severe involvement. Measurements of contractures are affected in two ways specific to Dupuytren disease. First, although the cords themselves are not elastic, they are often anchored to elastic tissues. This may lead to significant differences between active and passive measurements and to examiner bias in passive range of motion (PROM) measurements. Second, cords that span multiple joints may produce dynamic contractures, in which measurements of one joint are

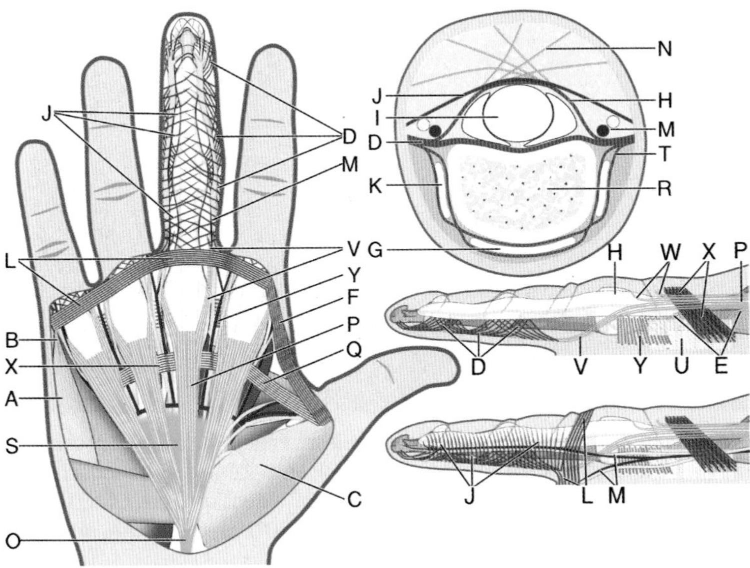

Figure 25.4 Illustration of normal fascial anatomy. **A**, Abductor digiti minimi fascia. **B**, Abductor digiti minimi tendon. **C**, Abductor pollicis brevis fascia. **D**, Cleland ligament. **E**, Deep pretendinous fibers. **F**, Distal first web space ligament. **G**, Extensor tendon. **H**, Flexor tendon sheath. **I**, Flexor tendons. **J**, Grayson ligament. **K**, Lateral band. **L**, Natatory ligament. **M**, Neurovascular bundle. **N**, Palmar anchoring fibers. **O**, Palmaris longus tendon. **P**, Pretendinous band. **Q**, Proximal first web space ligament. **R**, Proximal phalanx. **S**, Proximal pretendinous band coalescence. **T**, Retinacular ligaments. **U**, Septum of Legueu and Juvara. **V**, Spiral band. **W**, Superficial pretendinous fibers. **X**, Superficial transverse palmar ligament. **Y**, Transverse metacarpal ligament.

© 2018 American Academy of Orthopaedic Surgeons

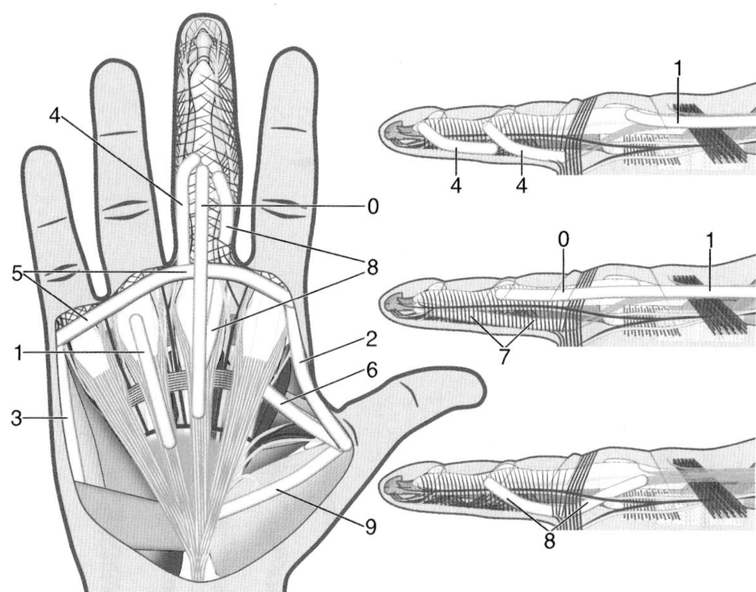

Figure 25.5 Illustration of common cord patterns. 0, central digital; 1, central palmar; 2, distal first web space; 3, hypothenar; 4, lateral digital; 5, natatory; 6, proximal first web space; 7, retrovascular; 8, spiral; 9, thenar.

influenced by the position of the adjacent joint. Dynamic contractures spanning the palm and the carpometacarpal (CMC) joints can result in large variations in measurements (Figure 25.6). A Dupuytren-specific diagram designed to allow documentation of findings and measurements is shown in Figure 25.7.

SURGICAL MANAGEMENT

Despite pilot studies suggesting use of splinting as the sole treatment for Dupuytren contracture in compliant patients, there is no agreement on the effectiveness of preventive or non-operative therapy for Dupuytren disease. Studies of the effect

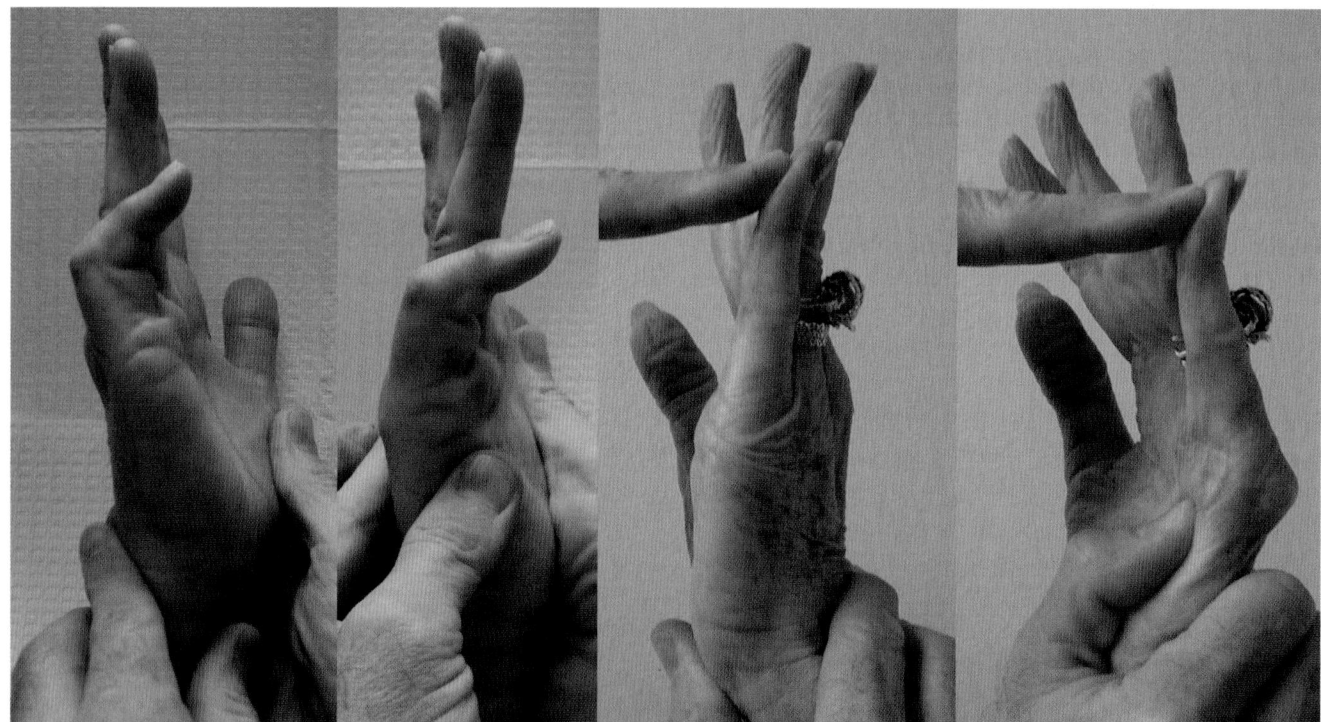

Figure 25.6 Photpgraphs demonstrating dynamic contractures with carpometacarpal (CMC) fasciodesis. Patients use a trick motion to compensate for a tight fascia. When cords span the MCP and PIP, patients flex their MCP to extend their PIP and vice versa. The same is true with cords extending into the proximal palm, in which flexing the ring and small CMC joints increases MCP extension. *Left:* CMC flexion allows 10° of active MCP hyperextension. When CMC flexion is blocked, active MCP extension is limited to 20°, which, in turn, improves active PIP extension by 10°. *Right:* Blocking CMC flexion changes passive MCP extension from 0° to 65°.

© 2018 American Academy of Orthopaedic Surgeons

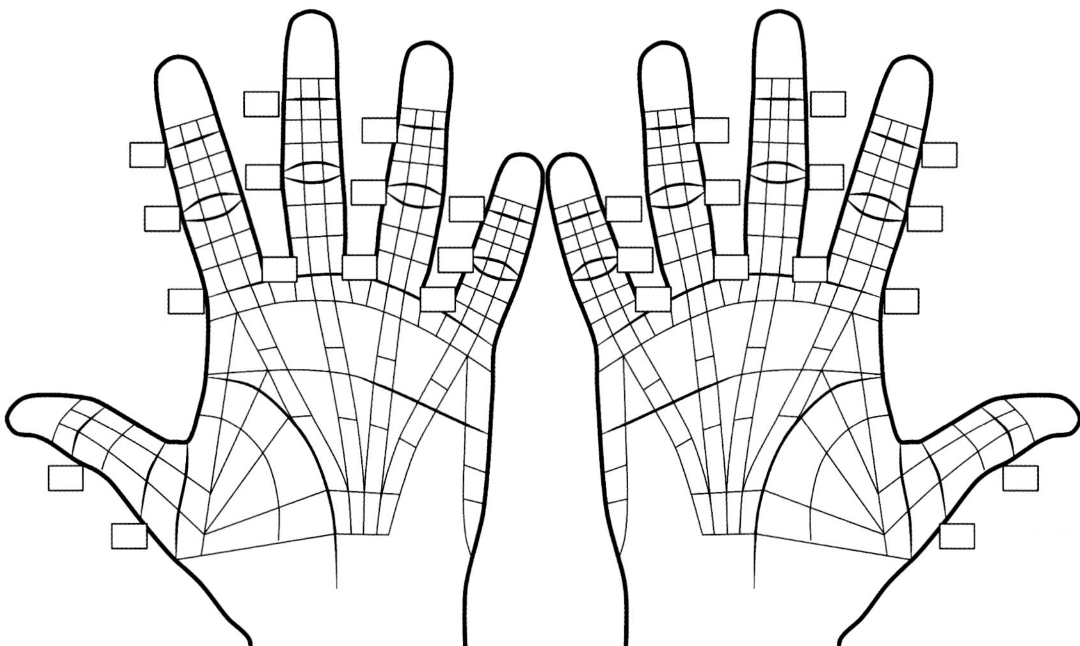

Figure 25.7 This diagram is based on common zones of involvement and allows standard documentation of the location of physical findings, procedures, and joint measurements. PDF versions of this as evaluation and procedure forms are available at http://Dupuytrens.org/forms.

of occupation and rock climbing on the incidence of Dupuytren contracture are consistent with cell biology research in that high-stress/shear manual activities may provoke the core biology. This is difficult to translate into lifestyle or activity recommendations for all patients, but should be discussed.

There are three types of procedures used to treat primary Dupuytren contracture (Figure 25.8). Minimally invasive procedures disrupt cords without removing tissue. Examples of this are percutaneous needle fasciotomy (PNF) and enzymatic fasciotomy with collagenase *Clostridium histolyticum* (Xiaflex®, Auxilium Pharmaceuticals, Inc., Chesterbrook PA). Fasciectomy, the most common procedure, is removal of some or all of the affected cord tissue. Dermofasciectomy is removal of affected cord tissue and the overlying skin and resurfacing the area with skin graft. Salvage procedures for failed surgery include flap reconstruction, PIP arthrodesis, and amputation. The three procedures for primary disease have similar outcomes in terms of initial correction of deformity. Recovery time, complication rate, and average time before recurrence are least for minimally invasive procedures and greatest for dermofasciectomy.

One goal of all procedures is to remove tension on cord tissue, either by removing the cord or completely dividing all cord tissues at one or more levels. Dupuytren contracture is provoked by mechanical tension; releasing tissue tension turns the local biology off, at least temporarily. It may not be possible to remove or release all involved tissues in patients with severe contractures or very aggressive disease biology. If Dupuytren tissues are not adequately released, even if stretched out by passive manipulation at the time of the procedure, they will remain active as progressive Dupuytren contracture.

Percutaneous Needle Fasciotomy (PNF)

Indications

PNF is indicated for treatment of a contracture from a palpable Dupuytren cord in a cooperative patient with mild to moderate biologic severity with no skin shortage, and for whom rapid recovery is more important than earlier recurrence risk. With experience, PNF may be used for complex involvement of multiple cords involving multiple rays, both palm and digit, all in a single setting.

Contraindications

PNF is contraindicated for patients who cannot tolerate an awake procedure, who have tight skin or scars preventing extension, diffuse skin involvement, lack of a palpable cord, or who have biologically aggressive or rapidly recurrent disease. PNF is an extra-articular approach, and does not address fixed joint contractures due to joint capsule or ligament changes.

Procedure

PNF can be performed as a single office visit. The surgeon injects the skin over a cord with small amounts (0.1 ml) of intradermal local anesthesia, avoiding a digital nerve block. Although the cords are insensate, the neurovascular bundle and flexor tendon sheath remain sensitive. Thus, the patient can feel and report if the surgeon veers too close to these structures. The surgeon then passes a small (e.g., 25-gauge) needle through the anesthetized skin, feels the surface of the cord with the needle tip, then, with a series of sweeping and perforating moves, divides the cord. Once weakened enough, passive extension ruptures the remaining cord fibers, allowing extension of the previously tethered joint.

© 2018 American Academy of Orthopaedic Surgeons

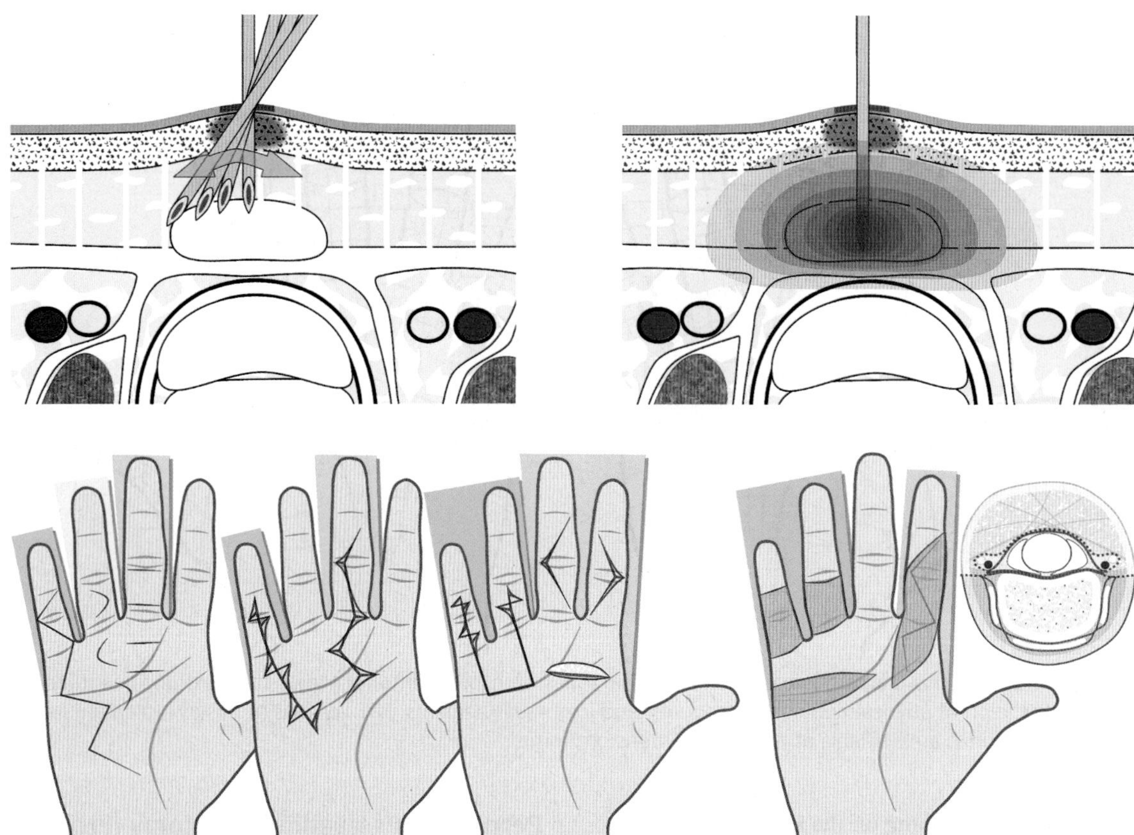

Figure 25.8 Illustration of treatment options for primary Dupuytren disease. *Top left:* Percutaneous needle fasciotomy of a cord in the palm. *Top right:* Xiaflex® injection of a cord in the palm. *Bottom left (from left: incisions are red lines, closures are blue lines):* Incisions for segmental or regional fasciectomy; Z plasty and Y-V plasty; combinations for multiple fingers with either primary closure or McCash open-palm technique. *Bottom right (tissue excision covered with skin graft is orange):* Dermofasciectomy and skin graft for primary or recurrent disease; cross-section of tissue excised in the finger.

Complications

Skin tears that occur in about one out of ten treated hands are treated with dressing changes and usually heal within 1 to 2 weeks, even if fairly large. Nerve and tendon injury each have a less than 1% incidence. Infection is rare, as are postoperative flare reaction (see Fasciectomy section) or complex regional pain syndrome reactions. Pain is uncommon, and patients should be cautioned to avoid strenuous use or gripping for the first week after release to avoid provoking local inflammation.

Collagenase Injection

Indications

The indications for collagenase injection are the same as for PNF.

Contraindications

Xiaflex® is contraindicated in patients with a history of severe allergic reaction to it or to collagenase used in any other therapeutic application or application method. As of this writing, severe allergic reaction to Xiaflex® has not been reported. The safety of Xiaflex® is unknown in patients who are pregnant, plan to become pregnant, are breastfeeding, plan to begin breastfeeding, have a bleeding problem, have other medical conditions, are on any anticoagulant medications, have had prior mild allergic reaction to Xiaflex®, or are less than 18 years old. Otherwise, the contraindications are the same as for PNF.

Procedure

Xiaflex® injection is performed over the course of two closely spaced office visits, typically two consecutive days per hand, with additional injections spaced a minimum of 30 days apart.

Technique

The central substance of the chosen cord segment is injected at three closely spaced points with the recommended dose of the reconstituted drug. After injection, the hand is wrapped in a soft immobilizing bandage. The patient is instructed to keep the hand elevated and avoid moving the fingers until the next office visit. On return the next day, manipulation is performed by the physician, optionally using local anesthetic.

Complications

Bruising and swelling are common reactions. Pain in the hand, lymph node tenderness, and hemorrhagic skin blebs are also common self-limited reactions to the medication and resolve within the first week. These events are expected temporary

 © 2018 American Academy of Orthopaedic Surgeons

responses to the medication rather than complications. As with PNF, skin tears may occur during manipulation and are managed with local wound care. Although sometimes described as nonoperative treatment, Xiaflex® is a minimally invasive enzymatic fasciotomy, which can result in surgical complications.

Fasciectomy

Indications

Fasciectomy is indicated for failed minimally invasive treatment, for diffuse disease, for concurrent treatment of secondary pathology, or based on surgeon and patient preference.

Contraindications

Fasciectomy is contraindicated in patients who cannot tolerate a long procedure, a long recovery, or have biologically aggressive or rapidly recurrent disease.

Procedure

Technique

Fasciectomy is performed as an outpatient procedure in a surgical setting. There are three versions of fasciectomy. Regional (or local) fasciectomy involves removing all diseased fasciae, and is the most common practice in the United States. Regional fasciectomy may be performed through extensile incisions or a series of transverse incisions. *Segmental fasciectomy,* more popular in Europe, involves removing enough of the diseased fasciae to restore finger extension. Segmental fasciectomy is performed through a series of short incisions along the length of the cord. Radical fasciectomy, removing all normal and diseased fasciae, has a higher complication rate but the same recurrence rate and is no longer recommended.

Zigzag or longitudinal incisions are closed, but transverse incisions or the transverse limbs of zigzag incisions may be left open and allowed to heal by secondary intent, referred to as the McCash or open palm technique (Figure 25.8).

Immobilization varies with surgeon preference and with tissue laxity at procedure completion. Transarticular pins may be inserted (and ends buried under the skin) to immobilize PIP joints with or without skin grafting. Plaster, fiberglass, or thermoplastic materials may be incorporated into bandages. There is a trend away from pins and rigid bandaging in cases without skin grafting to reduce stress and improve vascularity of skin flaps.

Complications

Fasciectomy has a high complication rate compared to other elective hand procedures for benign conditions. Complications fall into three categories. The most troublesome operative technical complications are nerve or vascular injury, common because anatomic landmarks and the anatomy of the digital neurovascular bundle are changed by the disease. The most common postoperative technical complications of regional fasciectomy are delayed healing (Figure 25.9), wound marginal necrosis, or flap necrosis. These arise because subdermal disease forces the surgeon to raise thin skin flaps, and because the skin itself can become fibrotic from the disease. In addition, splinting the fingers in extension at the end of the procedure may provoke ischemia by placing stress on the flaps.

The most troublesome postoperative biological complication is the postfasciectomy flare reaction. Because the Dupuytren core biology resembles that of wound contracture, it can be provoked by the skin wounds and flap elevation of fasciectomy.

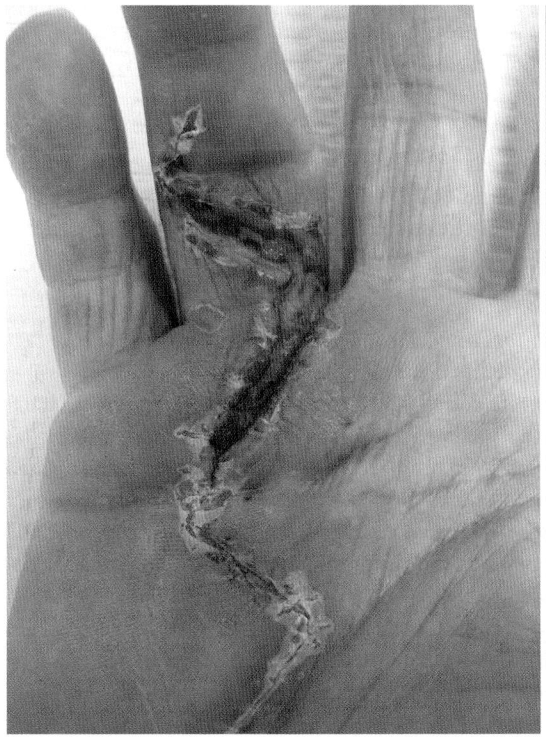

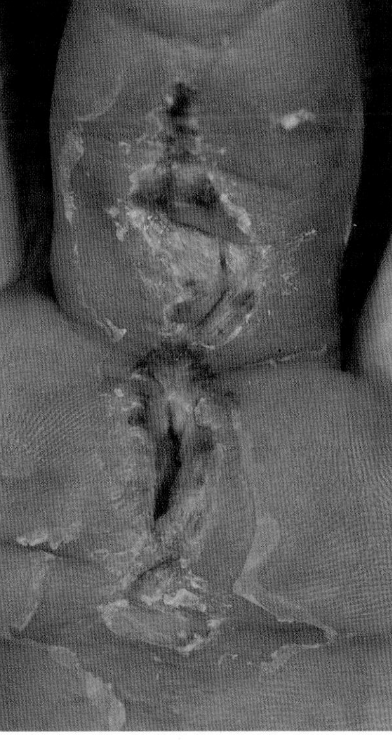

Figure 25.9 Photographs of delayed wound healing after fasciectomy. *Left:* Fasciectomy with zigzag incision. Sutures were removed at 3 weeks, and wound edges were not adherent. *Right:* Five weeks after fasciectomy with Z plasties. Epithelialization of the central wound opening in the distal palm required repeated débridement to prevent sinus formation. Despite these appearances, final scars and range of motion were excellent.

© 2018 American Academy of Orthopaedic Surgeons

The flare reaction is disproportionate and prolonged swelling, stiffness, and pain occur, worsening several weeks after an initially uneventful postoperative course and continuing for months thereafter. Postfasciectomy flare reaction occurs in up to one in ten patients, leading to permanent flexion loss in about 1 out of 20 hands. Minimally invasive procedures are not commonly associated with flare reaction.

Dermofasciectomy

Indications

Dermofasciectomy is indicated for recurrent contracture with diffuse skin involvement or extensive scarring, or as the first procedure in selected young patients with aggressive disease.

Contraindications

Dermofasciectomy is contraindicated in patients who cannot tolerate a long procedure, a long recovery, or for whom skin grafting is contraindicated.

Procedure

Technique

Dermofasciectomy is performed as an outpatient surgical procedure. Technically, dermofasciectomy is replacement of a block of fascia and overlying skin with a large full-thickness skin graft. It is *not* simply fasciectomy plus skin graft. If performed for primary disease, tissue blocks in the distal palm and the proximal phalanx pulp are excised and grafted. For recurrent disease, areas of scarred skin are also replaced (Figure 25.8).

Intraoperative immobilization varies with surgeon preference. The surgeon may insert transarticular pins to immobilize PIP joints, and may bury the pin ends under the skin. Plaster, fiberglass, or thermoplastic materials are usually incorporated into bandages.

Complications

Complications are similar to those described for fasciectomy, and similar to other procedures involving skin grafting the palm. In addition, because dermofasciectomy is often performed for recurrent disease diffuse postoperative scarring, the risk of nerve or vascular injury is greater. Overall recovery time for dermofasciectomy is about 50% longer than for fasciectomy, and the long-term recurrence rate is less than half of that for fasciectomy.

POSTOPERATIVE REHABILITATION

Therapy requirements vary dramatically according to the procedure used to treat the Dupuytren contracture. Minimally invasive treatments do not routinely require intervention to increase dexterity, strength, range of motion (ROM), endurance, or programs to reduce sensitivity. In contrast, these needs are common in the postoperative fasciectomy or dermofasciectomy patient. The role of splinting is controversial. Routine posttreatment extension splinting is widely used despite evidence of lack of effectiveness. All studies comparing postfasciectomy splinting versus no splinting have demonstrated no added benefit when evaluated 3 months or longer after surgery. This seems counterintuitive, but reflects the complex biology of Dupuytren disease. Studies that only compare splinting outcomes in compliant versus noncompliant patients do not demonstrate the effectiveness of splinting. Rather, they demonstrate splinting intolerance in patients experiencing early or progressive recontracture, as described earlier. Gains in extension from splinting may be matched by loss of flexion. Extension deficit often improves without therapy in the months that follow minimally invasive procedures. There is considerable experience that aggressive splinting, prolonged passive composite extension splinting, or splinting that produces pain increases the incidence of postfasciectomy flare reaction, stiffness, and flexion loss.

Communication and coordination of care between the surgeon and therapist is important. Specific details about the pathology, preoperative motion and contracture, surgical findings, and the procedure should form the basis of postoperative care and rehabilitation.

Percutaneous Needle Fasciotomy

Formal therapy is recommended only for a minority of patients with specific indications that include desensitization for procedure-related nerve irritation and wound management after skin tear in patients who are unable to care for themselves.

Collagenase Injection

The manufacturer of Xiaflex® recommends use of a static extension night splint for up to 4 months after the final joint manipulation. Patients perform active range of motion (AROM) exercises during the day, and are instructed to avoid strenuous activities with the treated hand for several weeks. Therapy is otherwise recommended only as for PNF.

Fasciectomy

Based on the available evidence, routine postoperative splinting is not recommended for routine fasciectomy. Splinting may be indicated for the concurrent treatment of other conditions, or according to the surgeon's preference.

A common therapy protocol after fasciectomy is as follows:

- *First postoperative visit* (1 day to 1 week postop).
  - Remove the postoperative dressing.
  - Measure active joint motion and reassess weekly. Unexpectedly rigid joints may mean that the surgeon has pinned joints, buried the pins, and not communicated this situation.
  - Assess any areas of anesthesia and, if present, instruct the patient regarding protection of insensate areas.
  - Provide the patient with wound care instructions, a light dressing, and supplies as needed. If the open-palm technique has been used, instruct the patient to change dressings daily, if soiled, or as often as needed to prevent maceration.

© 2018 American Academy of Orthopaedic Surgeons

- Instruct the patient on blocked and composite flexion and extension exercises (distal interphalangeal [DIP] flexion/extension, PIP flexion/extension, MCP flexion/extension, as shown in Table 25.1), have the patient demonstrate them, and provide written instructions for these to be performed as a set four to six times daily. Encourage elevation and light active painless use of the hand.
- *First two weeks*
  - Schedule therapy 2 to 3 times per week for supervision, wound care, and reinforcement of the ROM program.
  - Begin wound desensitization and instruct the patient on a home program of percussive desensitization to add to the four to six times daily exercises. Percussive desensitization is performed as follows. The patient identifies areas of tenderness to light touch. Each tender area is treated separately, starting with the most tender spot. The patient uses a fingertip of the opposite hand or the corner of a folded gauze or washcloth to tap on the skin of the most tender area: lightly (just enough to feel the touch), rapidly (two to three times a second), and steadily (for 1–2 minutes). This is then repeated for the next most tender area, until all tender areas are treated.

Table 25.1 HOME EXERCISE PROGRAM AFTER SURGERY FOR DUPUYTREN CONTRACTURE: ACTIVE EXERCISES

Before exercise: Heat may help make these exercises more comfortable. To warm up, submerge the hand in a sink filled with comfortably hot (no hotter than 102°F/39°C) water for 3 to 5 minutes.

After exercise: Apply a cold pack to the hand for 5 to 10 minutes to prevent inflammation.

These exercises should not be painful to do or make the hand ache or throb afterward.

Exercise Type	Number of Reps/Sets	Days per Week	Number of Weeks
DIP Flexion/Extension	4 repetitions/4–6 sets per day	Daily	6 or until motion plateau
PIP Flexion/Extension	4 repetitions/4–6 sets per day	Daily	6 or until motion plateau
MCP Flexion/Extension	4 repetitions/4–6 sets per day	Daily	6 or until motion plateau
Composite Flexion/Extension	4 repetitions/4–6 sets per day	Daily	6 or until motion plateau
Abduction–Adduction	4 repetitions/4–6 sets per day	Daily	6 or until motion plateau

The diagrams for the following exercises show what the helping hand is doing with *white arrows,* and what the recovering hand should try to do with *black arrows.*

DIP Flexion/Extension

With the helping hand, hold the MCP and PIP joints comfortably straight and keep them from bending. The patient should actively flex the tip of the finger and hold for 5 seconds, then straighten and hold for 5 seconds.

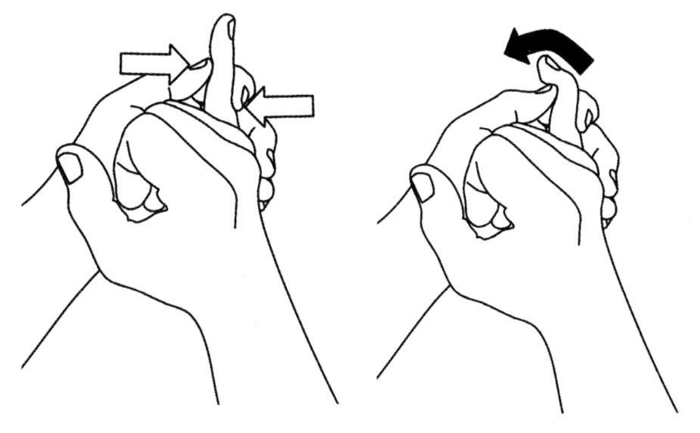

PIP Flexion/Extension

With the helping hand, hold the MCP joint comfortably straight and keep it from bending. Have the patient actively flex the PIP joint and hold for 5 seconds, then straighten and hold for 5 seconds.

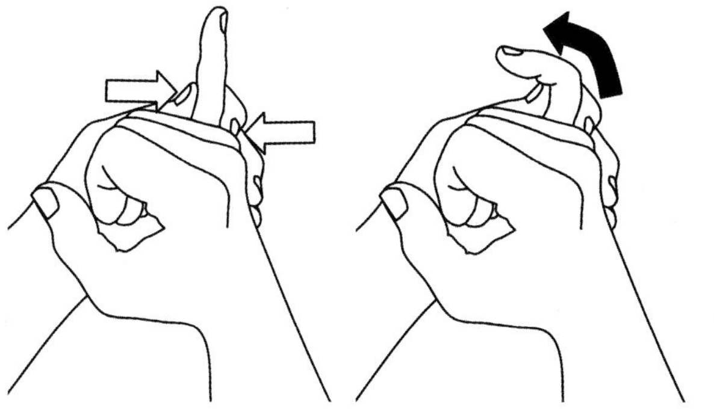

Continued on following page

© 2018 American Academy of Orthopaedic Surgeons

Table 25.1 HOME EXERCISE PROGRAM AFTER SURGERY FOR DUPUYTREN CONTRACTURE: ACTIVE EXERCISES *(Continued)*

MCP Flexion/Extension Use the helping hand to put comfortable pressure across the middle of the palm. While doing this, have the patient flex the MCP and try to keep the interphalangeal joints straight. Hold for 5 seconds, then straighten back and hold for 5 seconds.	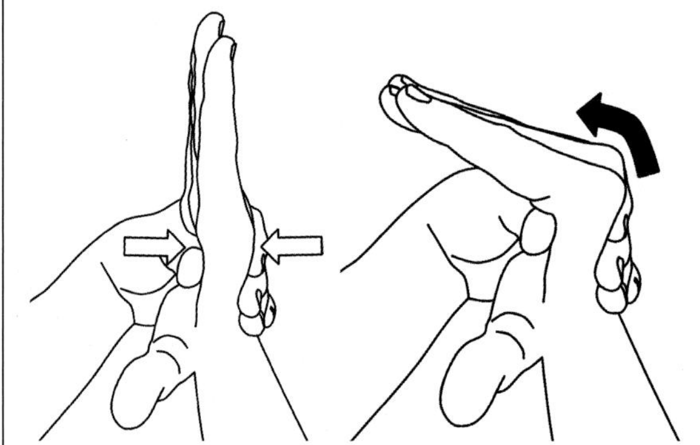
Composite Flexion/Extension Start with all fingers as straight as is comfortably possible. Have the patient flex just the interphalangeal joints into a hook position, hold this for 5 seconds, then curl the fingers into a full fist and hold for 5 seconds.	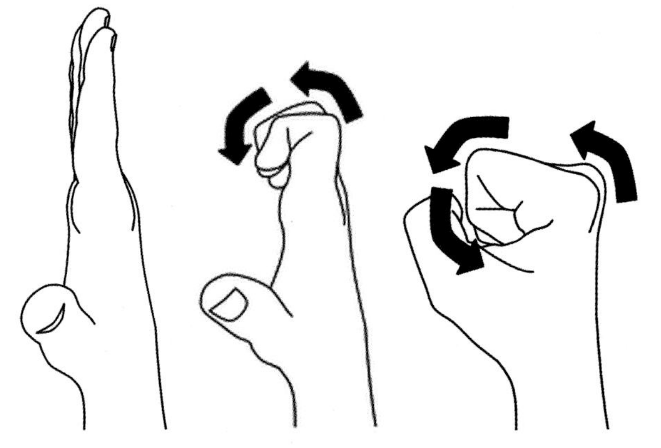
Abduction–Adduction Start with all fingers as straight as is comfortably possible and adducted together. Hold for 2 seconds. Abduct the fingers and thumb apart and hold for 2 seconds.	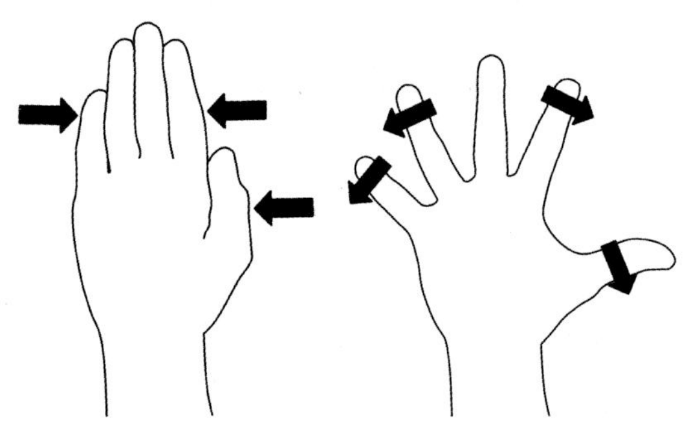

DIP = distal interphalangeal, MCP = metacarpophalangeal, PIP = proximal interphalangeal.

- *Two to 8 weeks*
  - Sutures are removed at 2 to 3 weeks after surgery because of the tendency for delayed healing.
  - Taper to weekly sessions if the patient's performance allows.
  - If passive stiffness remains a problem, add thermal modalities (hot packs to initiate therapy, cold packs at the conclusion of the session).
  - Intrinsic stretch, oblique retinacular ligament stretch and composite flexion stretch (as shown in Table 25.2) if active flexion is poor after edema has subsided. Passive extension is not recommended.
  - Once wounds are healed and swelling and pain permit, add strengthening within comfort level using foam or putty.
  - Treat scar hypertrophy with continuous paper taping or adhesive silicone gel sheeting.
- *Beyond 8 weeks*
  - Continue only if the patient requires longer supervision or reinforcement of the home program (as shown in the Home Exercise Program instruction sheet).

Complications and Problems

Delayed healing (failure of primary edge to edge wound healing) occurs in a minority of patients. Wound edges may remain separated long enough to develop epithelialized sinuses (Figure 25.9). This may require freshening the skin edges by peeling off the new epithelial edge at dressing change to prevent

© 2018 American Academy of Orthopaedic Surgeons

Table 25.2 HOME EXERCISE PROGRAM AFTER SURGERY FOR DUPUYTREN CONTRACTURE: PASSIVE STRETCH EXERCISES

Exercise Type	Number of Reps/Sets	Days per Week	Number of Weeks
Intrinsic Stretch	3 repetitions/4 times daily	Daily	4–6 or motion plateau
ORL Stretch	3 repetitions/4 times daily	Daily	4–6 or motion plateau
Flexion Stretch	3 repetitions/4 times daily	Daily	4–6 or motion plateau

These are optional exercises to help improve motion when stiffness limits the ability to do active exercises. These should be done *before* doing the active exercises shown on the other sheet. These should be done slowly and gently with enough force to feel the stretch, but *not enough to cause pain.* Hold the positions steadily and don't "bounce" the joints during these stretches. The diagrams for these exercises show what the helping hand is doing with *white arrows.*

Intrinsic Stretch

Intrinsic muscle tightness makes it difficult to flex the interphalangeal joints and to extend the MCP joints. This exercise stretches the intrinsic muscles. Hold the recovering finger to bend both of the interphalangeal joints. Once they are bent, stretch the entire finger backwards at the MCP joint. Hold this position for 30–60 seconds.

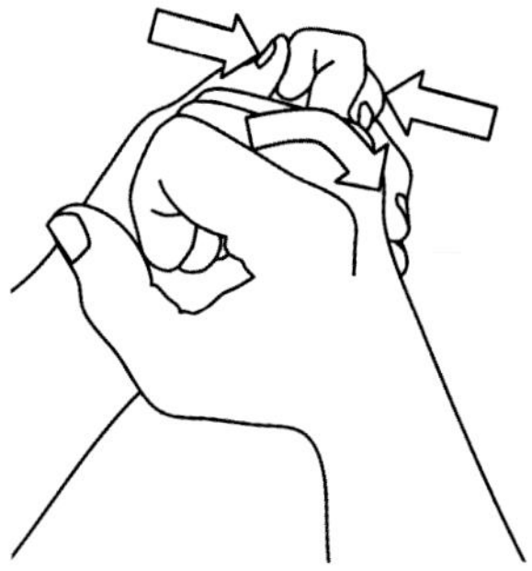

ORL Stretch

ORL tightness makes it difficult to extend the PIP joint and to flex the DIP joint. This exercise stretches the ORL. Hold the PIP joint comfortably straight and at the same time passively flex the DIP joint. The MCP joint can be in any comfortable position. Hold this position for 30–60 seconds.

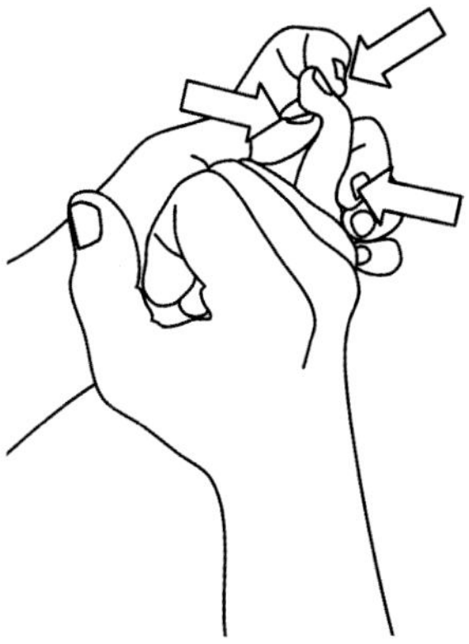

Composite Flexion Stretch

Hold the finger to passively flex both interphalangeal joints. The MCP joint knuckle can be in any comfortable position, but is usually most comfortable flexed as well. Once in this position, hold for 30–60 seconds.

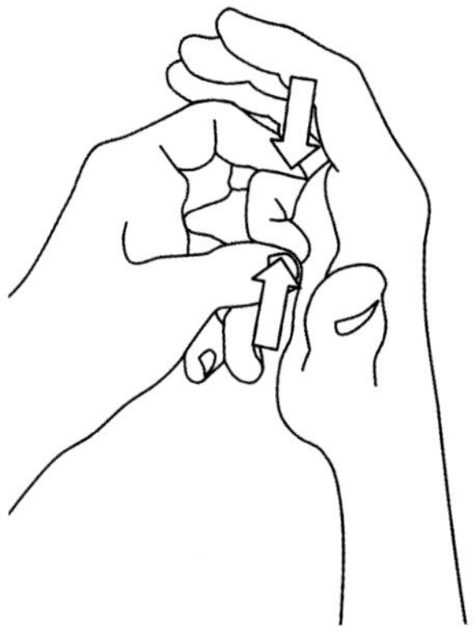

MCP = metacarpophalangeal, ORL = oblique retinacular ligament, PIP = proximal interphalangeal.

sinus formation. Marginal necrosis (wound edge necrosis) and flap loss are managed with wound care, débridement, and, if extensive, may require skin grafting.

Flare reaction with disproportionate swelling and stiffness may become obvious in the first days after surgery, or not be obvious until several weeks postoperatively. Flare may be indistinguishable from complex regional pain syndrome. Some, but not all, patients benefit from a course of oral steroids. The biggest risk posed by flare reaction is long-term stiffness. The highest-priority goal is restoration of active flexion.

© 2018 American Academy of Orthopaedic Surgeons

Edema control measures include retrograde massage, contrast baths, active use, avoiding dependent positioning, and avoiding circumferential dressings (including compression gloves). The safest step at any time is to initiate a stress loading program and notify the physician if the patient develops signs of vasomotor instability, excessive sweating, temperature change, worsening pain, or progressive stiffness and swelling.

Early recontracture is loss of initial correction beginning days to weeks after a procedure, and plateauing after 6 to 12 weeks. This is *not* recurrent Dupuytren contracture, but instead persistence of secondary effects of contracture. PIP joint contractures greater than 45° result in tightness of the accessory collateral ligaments; contractures of 60° or greater result in incompetence of the extensor mechanism. The effects of these problems may appear to be corrected by manipulation at the time of the procedure, but their underlying mechanics remain. Such fingers have their best correction at the time of the initial procedure, only to undergo recontracture in the weeks that follow. Because these are static persistent mechanical abnormalities, their effects quickly plateau after treatment, and they are resistant to temporary splinting.

Progressive recontracture is loss of initial correction beginning shortly after the procedure, then continuing to progress over the following year. This is *not* recurrent Dupuytren contracture, but rather persistent ongoing contraction without interruption of residual active disease remaining after treatment.

Late recontracture is loss of correction following an initial period of stability lasting a year or more. This is true recurrence, new disease in an area that was previously inactive. Dupuytren disease extension, described earlier, is similar to this: new Dupuytren disease in the treated hand arising in an area that did not previously have active disease.

Dermofasciectomy

The approach to postoperative therapy differs from fasciectomy only by the surgeon's preference regarding skin graft immobilization, which ranges from light active motion at 1 week to temporary joint pinning to cast immobilization for 6 weeks. Because of the more extensive nature of the procedure, recovery after dermofasciectomy often takes 3 to 4 months, as for fasciectomy, final plateau is not expected until 1 year after surgery.

OUTCOME

The patient and the healthcare provider often have very different perspectives of the outcome of treatment of Dupuytren contracture. For most patients, the starting reference point is painless awkwardness of an otherwise normal hand. Patients judge outcome by comparing their improvement from this reference point to the perceived ordeal of their treatment and permanent complications from their treatment. Partial improvement may be seen as a complete success in the context of a relatively painless minimally invasive procedure with a short uncomplicated recovery while complete correction of contracture may be seen as a failure in the context of fasciectomy with a prolonged painful recovery and areas of permanent abnormal palm sensibility. Patient Reported Outcome Measures (PROMs) have not yet settled this complex issue. Disability of Arm, Shoulder and Hand (DASH) scores do not correlate with the severity of Dupuytren flexion contractures. Dupuytren-specific PROMs, such as the Unité Rhumatologique de Affections de la Main scale (URAM), are in progress in an area that still needs work.

The most common objective Dupuytren outcome metrics used by therapists and surgeons are ROM and time until recurrence. These are easy to measure, but difficult to interpret. In Dupuytren patients, functional adaptation to a slowly changing deformity results in poor correlation between severity of flexion contracture and functional loss. Many factors influence recurrence rate. On average, recurrences occur earlier in PIP than in MCP joints, in younger than in older patients, after minimally invasive treatment compared to fasciectomy, and with partial correction compared to complete correction of contracture. Definitions of recurrence vary widely and are procedure-specific. The definition of recurrence used in Xiaflex® studies excludes patients having partial correction of contracture, resulting in lower reported rates of "recurrence" compared to definitions used for other procedures. Pooling data from many studies, fasciectomy lasts about twice as long before recurrence when compared to minimally invasive procedures, and less than half as long before recurrence when compared to dermofasciectomy.

PEARLS

- Recovery after a procedure for Dupuytren disease depends on
  - patient's individual biologic severity.
  - type of procedure performed.
  - secondary anatomic changes from long-standing pretreatment immobility.
  - stress placed on the hand during therapy.
- Splinting is commonly used, but has no proven benefit for routine use. Splinting may be helpful for specific secondary changes.
- Recontracture is not always recurrence of Dupuytren disease. Patterns of recontracture are
  - *Early:* First 6 to 12 weeks, then plateau (residual secondary changes).
  - *Progressive:* First 6 to 12 weeks, then progressive worsening (residual active disease).
  - *Late:* One year or longer posttreatment after an initial plateau (true recurrence).
- Aggressive hand therapy, passive extension stretching, and splinting provoking the biology that aggravates pain or swelling may be worse than no therapy.

SUMMARY

Dupuytren disease is a chronic systemic disorder of inflammation and scar regulation that results in Dupuytren contracture. The patient recovering from treatment of Dupuytren

© 2018 American Academy of Orthopaedic Surgeons

contracture still has Dupuytren disease. Expectations and care requirements after Dupuytren contracture release are very different than after scar contracture release. Delayed wound healing and prolonged inflammation are common after fasciectomy and dermofasciectomy. There is an abnormally low threshold for mechanical stress to trigger disproportionate and prolonged inflammation. Postoperative inflammation, pain, and loss of flexion may be indistinguishable from the spectrum of sympathetic mediated pain. Recurrence is common, occurring in the majority of patients within a decade of fasciectomy or minimally invasive treatment.

These aspects of Dupuytren disease need to guide rehabilitation efforts both by the therapist and by the patient. The effects of Dupuytren biology are unintuitive for patients, who may downplay the details of the preoperative discussion of recovery. Such patients often provoke inflammation in their own efforts to speed up their recovery away from therapy, or feel that slow recovery is an unexpected complication. Therapy-guided patient education of these issues and close adaptive supervision through the period of recovery are critical to achieving the best results and patient satisfaction after treatment of Dupuytren contracture.

BIBLIOGRAPHY

Ball C: The use of splinting as a non-surgical treatment for Dupuytren's disease: a pilot study. *British Journal of Hand Therapy* 2002;7(3):6–8.

Ball C, Pratt AL, Nanchahal J: Optimal functional outcome measures for assessing treatment for Dupuytren's disease: a systematic review and recommendations for future practice. *BMC Musculoskelet Disord* 2013;14:131.

Collis J, Collocott S, Hing W, Kelly E: The effect of night extension orthoses following surgical release of Dupuytren contracture: a single-center, randomized, controlled trial. *J Hand Surg Am* 2013;38(7):1285–1294.e2.

Ebskov LB, Boeckstyns ME, Sorensen AI, Soe-Nielsen N, Sørensen AI: Results after surgery for severe Dupuytren's contracture: does a dynamic extension splint influence outcome? *Scand J Plast Reconstr Surg Hand Surg* 2000;34(2):155–160.

Evans RB, Dell PC, Fiolkowski P: A clinical report of the effect of mechanical stress on functional results after fasciectomy for Dupuytren's contracture. *J Hand Ther* 2002;15(4): 331–339.

Jerosch-Herold C, Shepstone L, Chojnowski A, Larson D: Severity of contracture and self-reported disability in patients with Dupuytren's contracture referred for surgery. *J Hand Ther* 2011;24(1):6–10.

Jerosch-Herold C, Shepstone L, Chojnowski AJ, Larson D, Barrett E, Vaughan SP: Night-time splinting after fasciectomy or dermo-fasciectomy for Dupuytren's contracture: a pragmatic, multi-centre, randomised controlled trial. *BMC Musculoskelet Disord* 2011;12:136.

Kemler MA, Houpt P, van der Horst CM: A pilot study assessing the effectiveness of postoperative splinting after limited fasciectomy for Dupuytren's disease. *J Hand Surg Eur* 2012; 37(8):733–737.

Larson D, Jerosch-Herold C: Clinical effectiveness of postoperative splinting after surgical release of Dupuytren's contracture: a systematic review. *BMC Musculoskelet Disord* 2008;9:104.

© 2018 American Academy of Orthopaedic Surgeons

26 Thumb CMC Osteoarthritis: LRTI Procedure, Simple Trapeziectomy, CMC Arthrodesis

Jennifer Moriatis Wolf, MD, and Katherine Barnum Baynes, MS, OTR, CHT

INTRODUCTION

Trapeziometacarpal (TM) osteoarthritis is common, appearing most frequently in middle-aged women and increasing in prevalence with age. This degenerative condition is thought to be due to attenuation of the stabilizing ligaments of the thumb base, as well as to chronically stressing this saddle-shaped joint during use of the thumb. After failing nonoperative treatments, including opponens splinting and corticosteroid injections, there are several surgical treatment options.

Ligament reconstruction and tendon interposition (LRTI), as described by Eaton and Littler and modified by Burton and Pellegrini, remains the most commonly performed surgical procedure. The trapezium is removed and half or all of the flexor carpi radialis (FCR) tendon is used to reconstruct the stabilizing ligaments and form an "anchovy" to cushion the base of the first metacarpal. Simple trapeziectomy is similar, but does not require tendon transfer or specifically reconstruct the ligaments. Finally, TM arthrodesis, with fusion of the trapezium to the first metacarpal, is typically chosen in young laborers and is performed using fixation with wires or plate/screw constructs.

All of these procedures typically require an initial period of immobilization which contributes to stiffness in the tissues around the TM joint. Postoperative rehabilitation is a key adjunct for these procedures, necessary for recovery from the surgical dissection and the subsequent immobilization. The goals of hand therapy after TM surgery reflect a graded return to activities, including increased range of motion (ROM), restoration of functional pinch and grasp, and strengthening.

SURGICAL PROCEDURES

Ligament Reconstruction and Tendon Interposition and Simple Trapeziectomy

The indications for both LRTI and simple trapeziectomy are similar. These procedures are typically performed in patients with moderate to advanced-stage TM osteoarthritis who have failed nonoperative treatment such as activity modification, opponens splinting, and corticosteroid injections.

Collagen vascular diseases, with excessive joint laxity, are a contraindication for simple trapeziectomy, as these patients may require ligament reconstruction to avoid instability.

Procedure

The two most common surgical approaches are the volarly based Wagner approach (Figure 26.1), which exposes and peels up the thenar musculature to expose the joint capsule, and the longitudinal dorsal approach between the abductor pollicis longus and extensor pollicis longus (Figure 26.2), exposing the anatomic snuffbox. Recognition and protection of the deep branch of the radial artery at the proximal portion of the snuffbox and the branches of the superficial radial nerve are important. In LRTI, a separate forearm incision or incisions are placed to harvest either half or all of the FCR tendon.

In both approaches, the trapezium is removed either piecemeal or whole. If the FCR tendon is used, a drill hole is placed from the dorsal radial side of the first metacarpal obliquely into its base, and the tendon is passed through the base and sutured to itself to suspend the metacarpal, with the remaining tendon fashioned into an "anchovy" spacer and placed into the joint. The capsule is then closed with resorbable suture. The subcutaneous tissues are approximated with resorbable sutures and the skin closed with a running subcuticular suture.

The thumb is immobilized in a bulky dressing and thumb spica splint holding the thumb in a functional opposition position immediately postoperatively, then is changed into a short-arm thumb spica cast, which is maintained for 4 additional weeks for a total of 6 weeks of immobilization.

Potential surgical complications that may impact rehabilitation include damage to the superficial radial nerve branches with neuroma formation and incisional pain, or FCR tendinitis when half the tendon is harvested.

Ms. Barnum or an immediate family member is an employee of Falcon Rehab Products. Dr. Wolf or an immediate family member has received nonincome support (such as equipment or services), commercially derived honoraria, or other non-research–related funding (such as paid travel) from Elsevier, the Journal of Hand Surgery; *and serves as a board member, owner, officer, or committee member of the American Society for Surgery of the Hand, the* Journal of Bone and Joint Surgery–American, *the* Journal of Hand Surgery–American, *and* Orthopedics.

© 2018 American Academy of Orthopaedic Surgeons

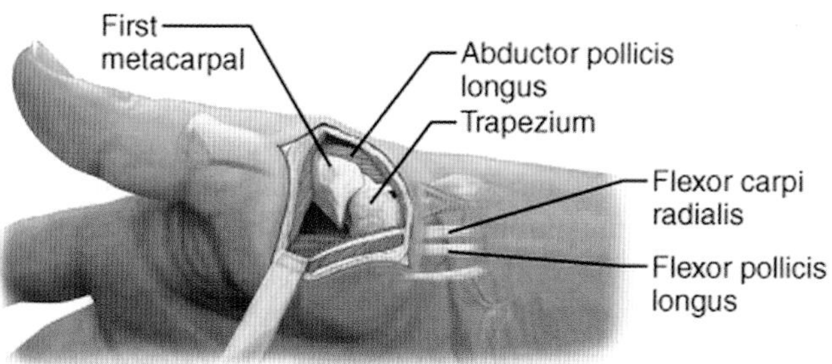

Figure 26.1 Illustration of volar Wagner approach to the thumb carpometacarpal joint, with the thenar musculature retracted ulnarly to expose the volar capsule, which is opened longitudinally over the trapezium. (Reproduced with permission from Wiesel S, ed: *Operative Techniques in Orthopaedic Surgery*. Philadelphia, PA, Lippincott Williams & Wilkins, 2010.)

Trapeziometacarpal Arthrodesis

TM arthrodesis in indicated in the young laborer or other worker who needs a stable joint to tolerate heavy loads. Previous arthrodesis of the thumb metacarpophalangeal (MCP) joint is a contraindication to TM fusion, as more proximal arthrodesis would severely limit any thumb mobility. Relative contraindications include patients with occupations requiring a high degree of thumb mobility, such as musicians, dentists, and graphic designers.

Fusion of the TM joint is typically performed using the dorsal approach described earlier. The TM joint is exposed and decorticated. The joint is positioned to allow the distal phalanx of the thumb to contact the middle phalanx of the index finger, with the thumb rotated into sufficient opposition to allow

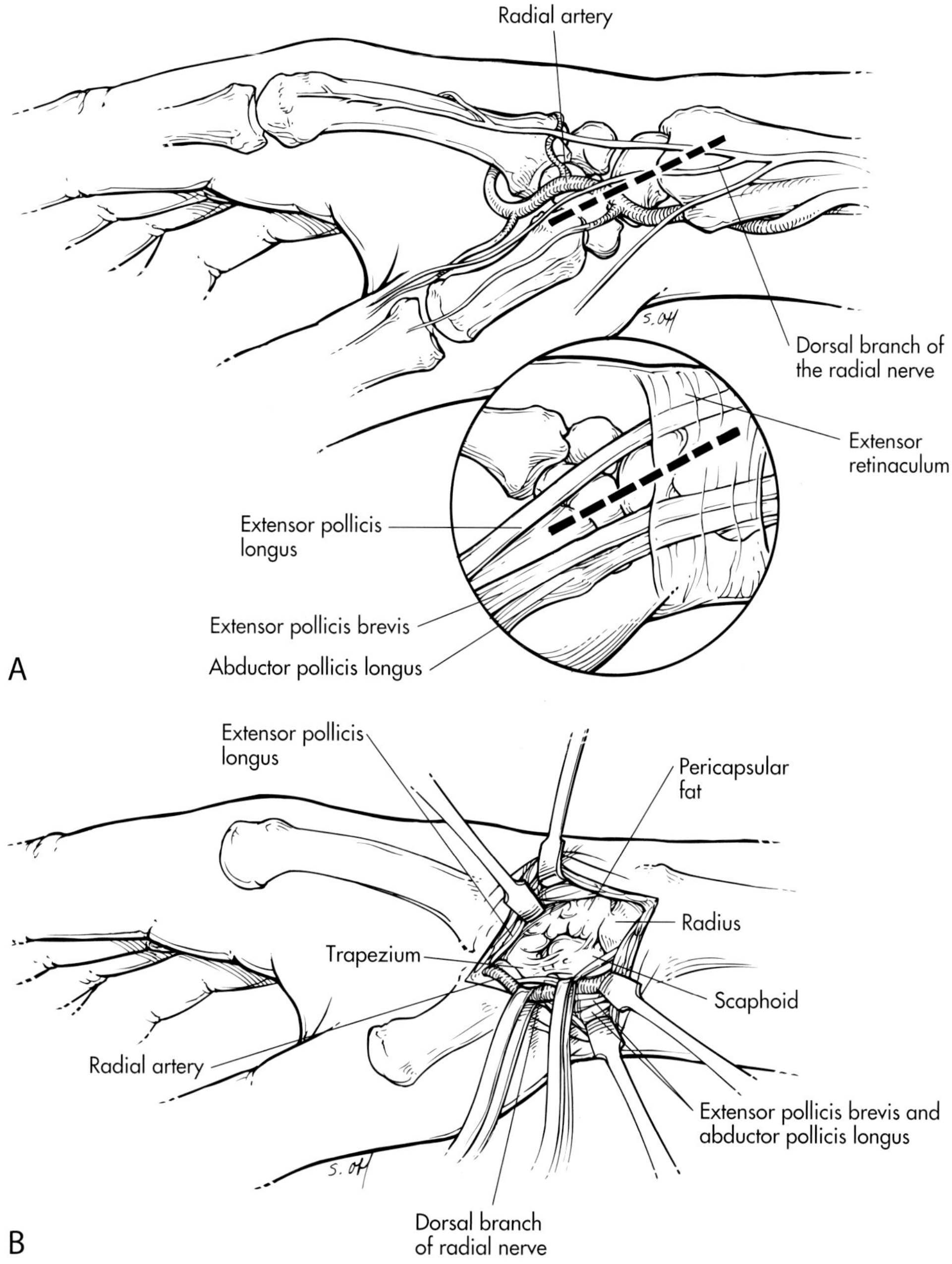

Figure 26.2 Illustration of dorsal approach to the thumb carpometacarpal joint. **A** and **B**, The interval between the abductor pollicis longus and extensor pollicis longus is opened, exposing the dorsal capsule. This is opened, with careful protection of the radial artery at the base of the anatomic snuffbox. (Reproduced with permission from Cooney WP: *The Wrist: Diagnosis and Operative Treatment*, ed 2. Philadelphia, PA: Lippincott Williams & Wilkins, 2010.)

© 2018 American Academy of Orthopaedic Surgeons

circumduction across the palm. The joint is then stabilized with Kirschner wires (K-wires), staples, screws, or plates placed on the dorsal surface of the thumb metacarpal and trapezium. The periosteum is then closed over the construct chosen, followed by closure of the tendon interval and skin. As described earlier, the patient is placed into a bulky dressing and thumb spica splint, which is then converted to a thumb spica cast at 10 to 14 days.

Trapeziometacarpal Implant Arthroplasty

Multiple implant options have been described for use in the TM joint, including silicone, metal-polyethylene, and pyrocarbon constructs, with either stemmed (placed into the first metacarpal base) or spacer options. The surgical approach is either through a dorsal or volar Wagner interval, per the surgeon's preference. After removal of the joint surfaces and implant placement, it is critical to repair the capsular interval securely, as dislocation of TM implants is a well-described complication. The patient is typically immobilized in a thumb spica splint for 2 to 3 weeks at a minimum before mobilization is allowed, and a removable thumb spica splint is used to support the joint while the soft tissues heal to provide implant stability.

POSTOPERATIVE REHABILITATION FOLLOWING TRAPEZIOMETACARPAL JOINT PROCEDURES

Postoperative rehabilitative care of the patient should begin early after surgery in ensure the best possible outcome, recognizing the balance between immobilization for stability and healing and motion to maintain function. Early interventions include adequate postoperative immobilization with functional positioning of the thumb, edema management, and ROM beginning at the initial postoperative visit. Patients who undergo TM joint procedures often have adjacent joints affected by osteoarthritis, or pain and symptoms in the contralateral hand and thumb that may be exacerbated by increased use and stress as the patient becomes predominantly dependent on the nonoperative hand during the postoperative immobilization period. The ultimate goal of the rehabilitation process is to assist the patient in a customized program that allows the patient to return to the activities that were previously limited by a painful, unstable thumb. An older patient who performs basic homemaking tasks will require a different postoperative program than a person whose hands have greater physical demands. Recovery time from surgery typically is between 3 and 6 months depending on the patient's level of hand function.

Unless surgically corrected, altered preoperative prehension patterns will likely reappear postoperatively. Encourage the patient to adopt balanced thumb postures to reduce the stress on the postoperative site, which allows the appropriate musculature to perform the task. Patients who had been primarily using the adductor pollicis muscle to perform prehension tasks due to joint collapse need to be retrained through instruction in prehension patterns and in strengthening of the opponens pollicis, abductor pollicis brevis, and first dorsal interosseous muscles. Encouraging balanced prehension patterns of thumb MCP flexion and interphalangeal (IP) flexion with dynamic stabilization of the thumb during light tasks, with progression to activities with loading, is part of a postoperative neuromuscular re-education program.

A staged and graded program is designed to provide the following:

- Functional ROM for tasks
- Functional strength for grip-and-pinch activities and patient-specific tasks
- Neuromuscular re-education to encourage balanced pinch postures for tasks with loaded pinch for long-term protection of the procedure
- Joint protection education

POSTOPERATIVE REHABILITATION FOR LRTI AND SIMPLE TRAPEZIECTOMY PROCEDURES—AUTHORS' PREFERRED PROTOCOL

Postoperative Immobilization

- *Casting* (weeks 0–4)
  - Initial postoperative dressing is replaced with a thumb spica cast.
  - Optimal thumb position is midway between radial and palmar abduction, while preserving the web space.
  - MCP joint is placed in 30° of flexion and the IP joint is left free.
- *Splinting* (weeks 4–8)
  - Volar-based or circumferential forearm-based thumb spica splint (Figure 26.3) allows wrist and thumb active ROM and passive ROM exercises to begin.
  - Wean out of the splint for light tasks between weeks 6 and 8.
  - Transition may include progressing to a hand-based protective splint, as desired.
- *Hand-based splints* (week 8 and beyond)
  - Thermoplastic (Figure 26.4) or soft supports (Figure 26.5) that provide continued protection at the surgical site and splinting for positioning of the MCP and IP to encourage optimal positioning may be used as long as needed for comfort after surgery.

Postoperative Assessment and Intervention

- *Edema management, beginning immediately after surgery*
  - Coban wraps and compressive finger socks
  - Retrograde massage (Figure 26.6)
  - Icing and elevation
  - Additional compression techniques including the use of Isotoner™ gloves and compression sleeves can be used once the patient is out of the cast.

© 2018 American Academy of Orthopaedic Surgeons

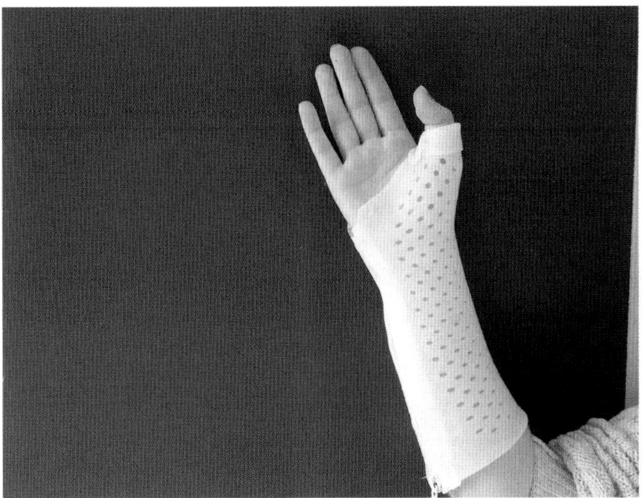

Figure 26.3 Photograph of perforated thermoplastic forearm-based, radially-based thumb spica splint with thumb in opposition.

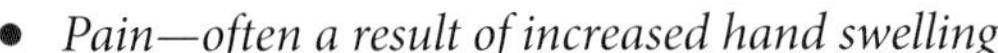

- *Pain—often a result of increased hand swelling*
  - Cast or splint should also be assessed to ensure that poor fit or undue pressure is not a cause of pain, and modified as needed.
- *Scar adherence*
  - An adherent scar will limit ROM.
  - Scar massage is performed along the entire area of the scar by gently mobilizing the scar
    - Using a circular pattern
    - Perpendicular to the scar
    - Parallel to the scar
  - It is preferable that scar massage is performed without lotion to improve traction on the skin.
  - To reduce the stress on the contralateral hand, nonslip material such as Dycem™ (Figure 26.7) or a pencil eraser can be used if the skin is fully healed. These devices increase the traction on the skin and reduce the amount of force applied by the patient's other hand.

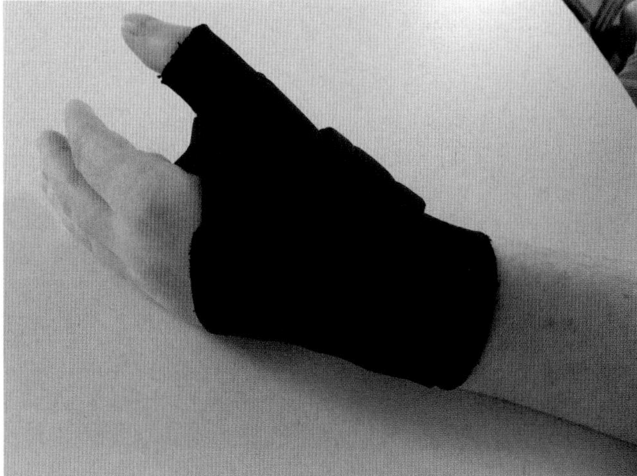

Figure 26.4 Photograph of thermoplastic thumb-based splint to position thumb in slight abduction and extension.

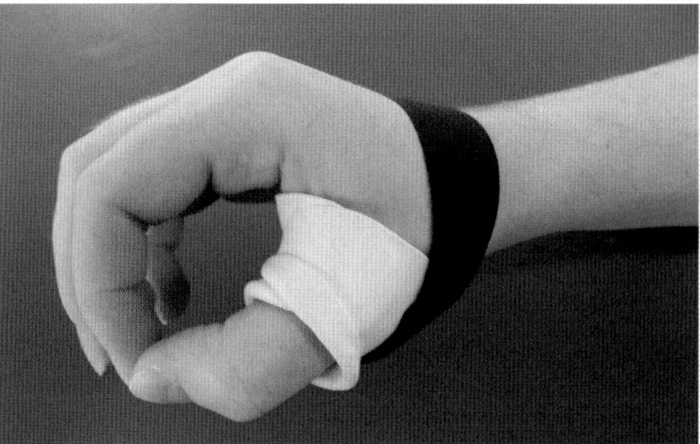

Figure 26.5 Photograph of soft supportive hand-based thumb spica splint, to be used later in the rehabilitation course.

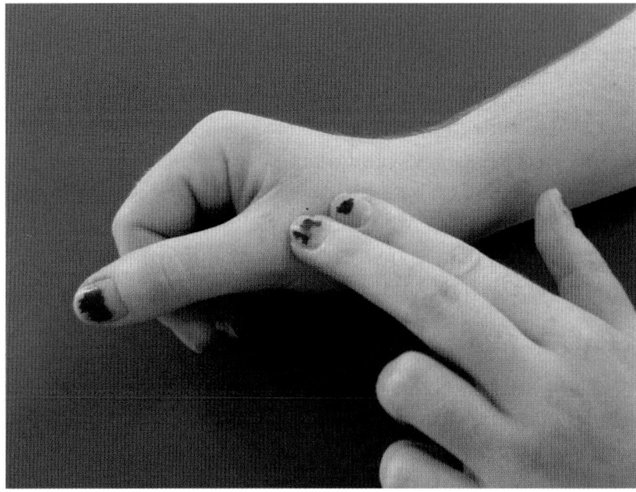

Figure 26.6 Photograph of retrograde massage to manage edema.

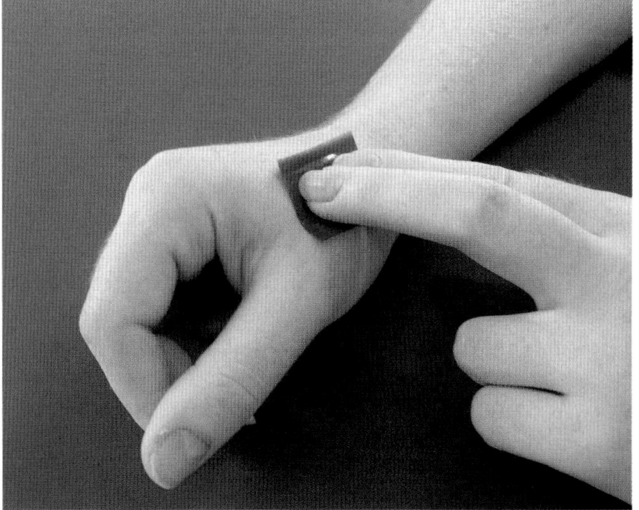

Figure 26.7 Photograph of example of scar massage with Dycem™ nonslip material.

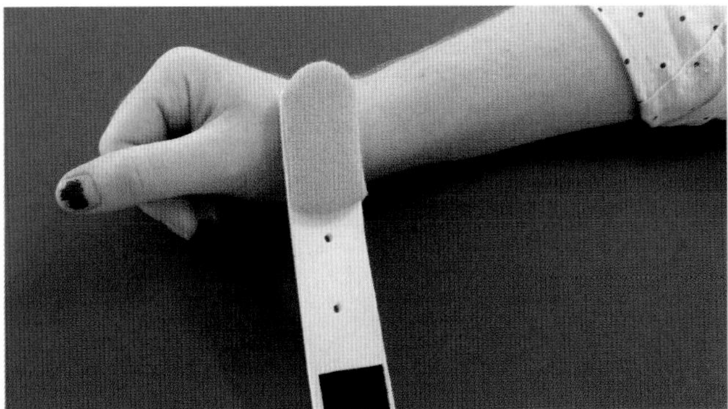

Figure 26.8 Photograph of scar desensitization using different materials, including soft cotton and Velcro.

- *Scar and skin sensitivity—a relatively common issue*
  - Scar massage techniques may be too uncomfortable for the patient to perform due to a hypersensitive postoperative scar.
  - Irritation of the superficial branch of the radial nerve can cause skin sensitivity.
  - Desensitization program
    - Scar massage with lotion
    - Tapping the scar
    - Gently touching the scar with textured materials, including progression from cotton and cloth to carpet and Velcro (Figure 26.8).

Range of Motion

- *Active range of motion (AROM) in cast (weeks 0–4)*
  - The patient is instructed to move uninvolved joints of the upper extremity, including the shoulder and elbow, as well as the index finger through small fingers.
  - Digit blocking exercises
  - Tendon glides
  - Thumb IP joint flexion
- *ROM postcasting (after week 4)*
  - Initial AROM continued
  - Wrist ROM exercises are added and continued until full AROM is achieved.
- *Thumb ROM*
  - Increasing isolated MCP and IP motion of the thumb
  - Passive thumb abduction exercises for radial palmar abduction with the goal of stretching the adductor prior to beginning active thumb abduction (Figure 26.9)
  - Adductor release technique (Figure 26.10)
  - Early active thumb motions to emphasize composite thumb motions of abduction and extension of the thumb and limited composite motions of the thumb in adduction and flexion are begun.
  - At 6 to 8 weeks postoperatively, AROM in thumb circumduction, as well as active radial and palmar thumb abduction, are begun. Thumb opposition to the index and long finger to emphasize the motion of the opponens pollicis in preparation for prehension tasks are initiated.

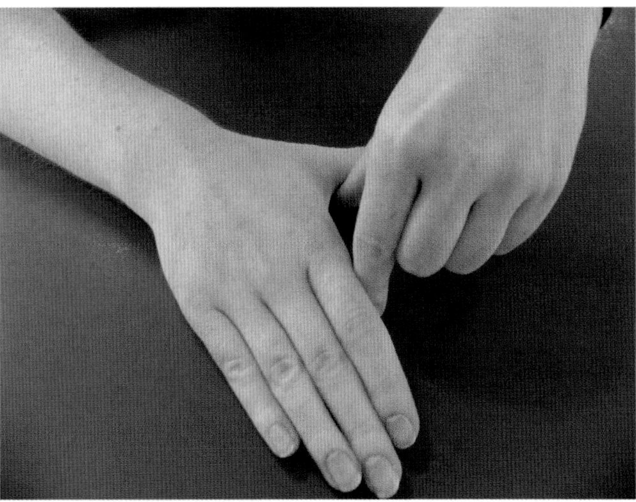

Figure 26.9 Photograph of passive abduction stretching exercises, which increase flexibility of the first dorsal interosseous and thenar musculature.

Functional Goals/Restrictions

- Incorporate activities of daily living into therapy program.
- Instruct the patient in the refinement of prehension or grasping/gripping patterns.
- At 6 weeks, the patient should be encouraged to begin dressing and bathing activities with the hand out of the splint as well as folding clothes and using utensils.
- Retraining in prehension with grasp of larger objects (Figure 26.11)
- Retraining in prehensile grasp using smaller objects (Figure 26.12)
- The patients gradually increase activities as long as they are pain-free.
- Orthotics may be needed during the period of retraining and return to function.

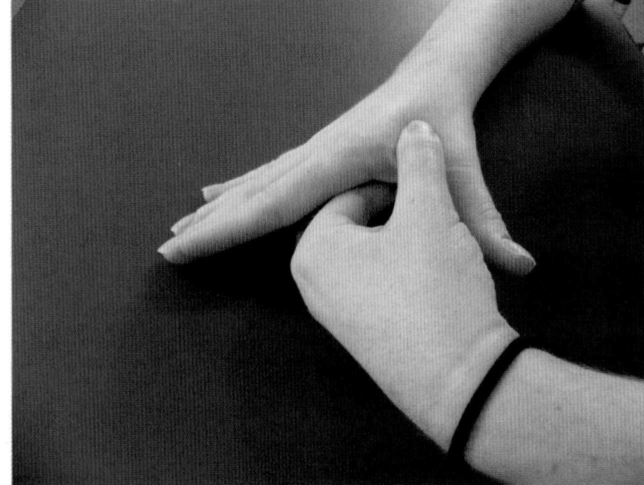

Figure 26.10 Photograph of adductor release technique: application of dorsal and volar compressive force to soften and stretch the adductor muscle.

 © 2018 American Academy of Orthopaedic Surgeons

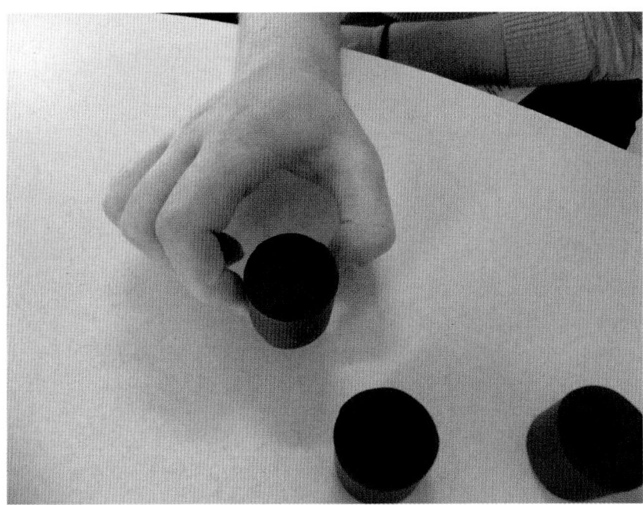

Figure 26.11 Photograph of retraining in prehension with grasp of larger objects.

Joint Protection

Joint protection techniques should be reviewed with the patient as part of a lifelong habit.

- Techniques and devices that reduce stress on the thumb and hand joints are key components (Figures 26.13–26.17): using scissors for opening packaging, modified can openers, jar openers, hemostats to assist with power pinching tasks, and tools for reducing joint stress when gardening and cooking.
- The program is personalized based on the patient's individual needs or hobbies.

Strengthening

- *Isometrics*
    - Wrist isometrics begin once the patient is in the removable splint.

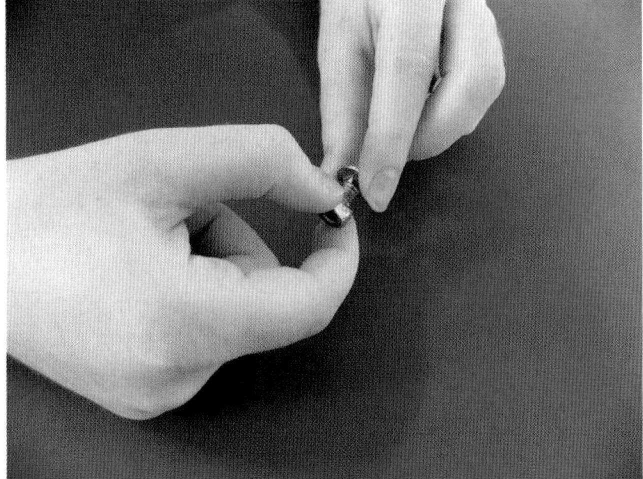

Figure 26.12 Photograph of progressive retraining in prehensile grasp using smaller objects.

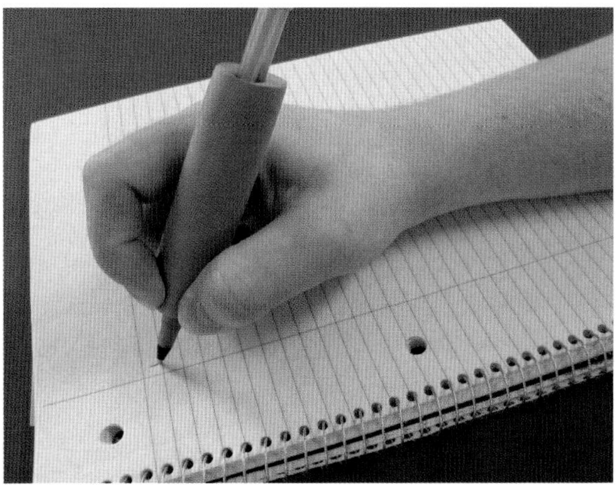

Figure 26.13 Photograph of pen holder to decrease stress on thumb basilar joint.

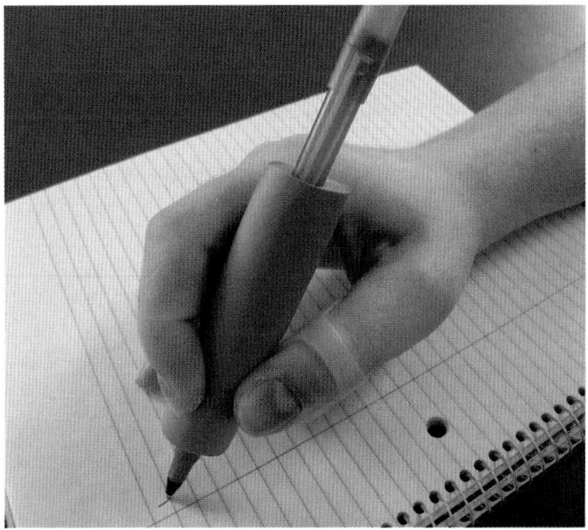

Figure 26.14 Photograph of use of a pen holder combined with an interphalangeal support splint to provide joint protection.

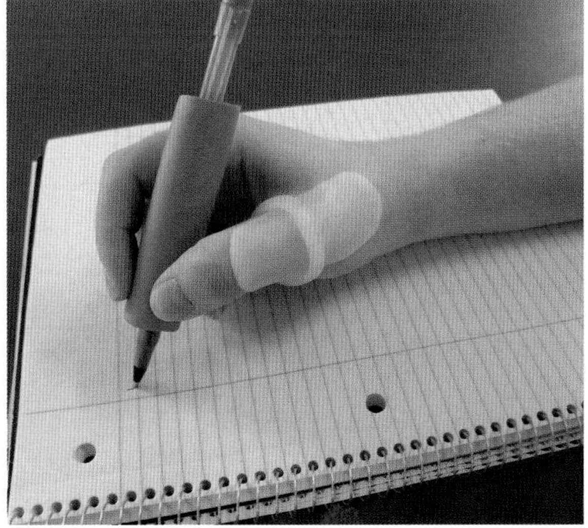

Figure 26.15 Photograph of use of a custom thermoplastic splint to prevent thumb MCP hyperextension.

© 2018 American Academy of Orthopaedic Surgeons

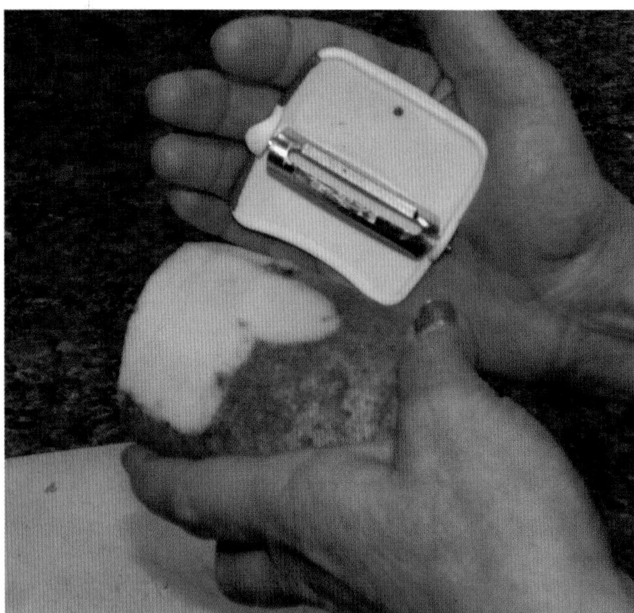

Figure 26.16 Photograph of a handheld peeler that is used in the palm to prevent stress and grasp at the thumb CMC joint.

- Thumb isometrics, initiated in the postoperative splint after initial ROM is gained
  - Thumb abduction (Figure 26.18)
  - Thumb opposition to the index (Figure 26.19)
- First dorsal interosseous motions (Figure 26.20)
- *Finger strengthening*
  - Can be performed in the splint
  - Using a foam roll (Figure 26.21)
  - Using light rubber band (Figure 26.22)
  - Theraputty™ (Figure 26.23)

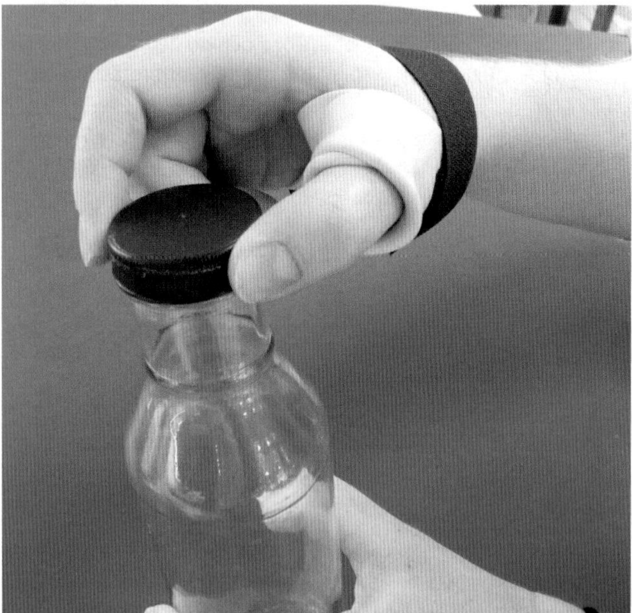

Figure 26.17 Photograph of wearing a small thumb-based splint while removing a bottle cap to stabilize the thumb CMC joint and decrease painful loading.

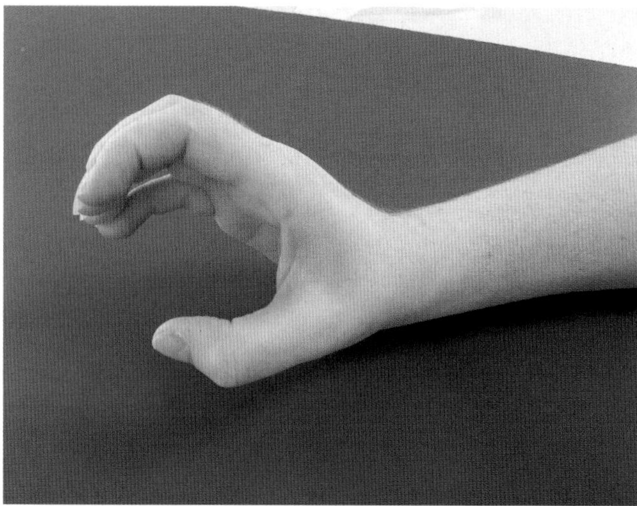

Figure 26.18 Photograph of thumb abduction rehabilitation exercise. The thumb is placed into abduction, then trained for functional grasp.

- Pinch strengthening—gentle pain-free pinch strengthening exercises can be done between 10 and 12 weeks using Theraputty™ (Figure 26.24)
- A patient unable to perform these exercises without pain should be deferred and the isometric exercises continued.
- Strengthening will increase with functional use of the hand and thumb.

POSTOPERATIVE REHABILITATION AFTER TRAPEZIOMETACARPAL ARTHRODESIS—AUTHORS' PREFERRED PROTOCOL

Although the ultimate outcome goals of this procedure are in general similar to those of the CMC arthroplasty procedures described earlier, arthrodesis is typically performed in patients who intend to use their hand for more physical activities.

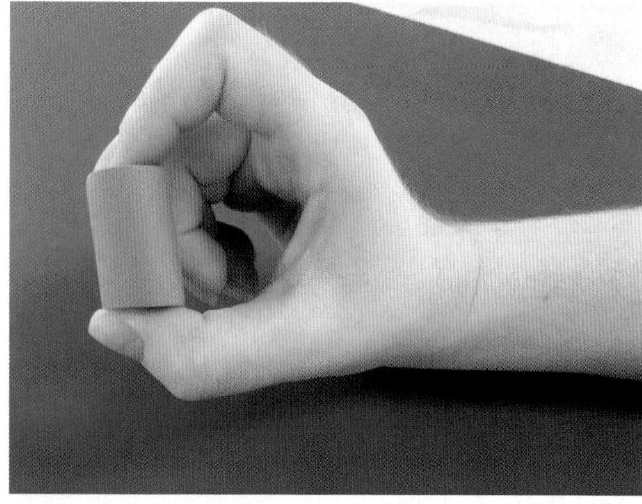

Figure 26.19 Photograph of isometric thumb opposition.

© 2018 American Academy of Orthopaedic Surgeons

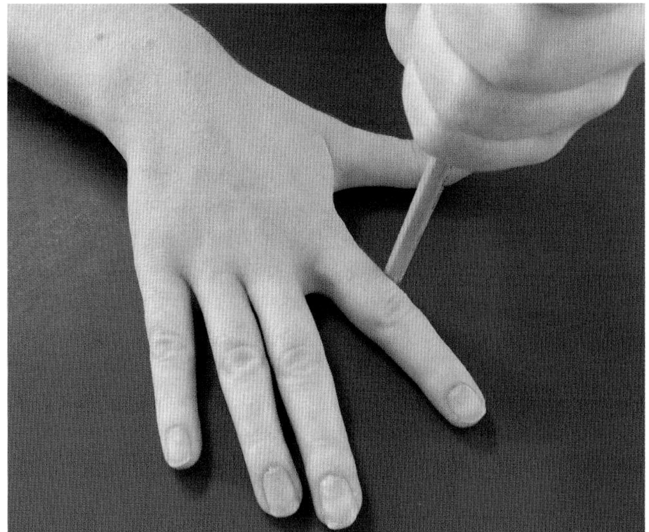

Figure 26.20 Photograph of rehabilitation by strengthening the first dorsal interosseous.

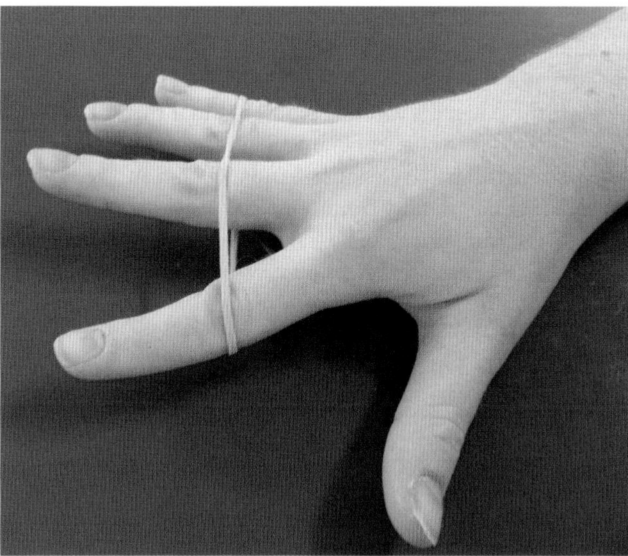

Figure 26.22 Photograph of abduction strengthening using rubber bands for resistance.

- *Immobilization*
  - Thumb spica cast for up to 2 months with the IP joint free
  - Circumferential or volar-based splint until radiographic healing is evident
- Edema is evaluated and treated as noted earlier.
- AROM begins in the cast with finger ROM and thumb IP joint motion as noted earlier.
- Thumb MCP motion and thumb to fingertip opposition are initiated in a splint.
- The patient will generally achieve some radial and palmar abduction over time.

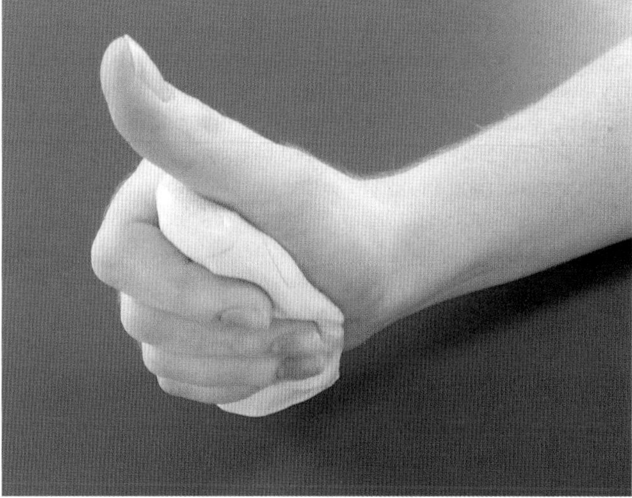

Figure 26.23 Photograph of use of putty to improve hand grasp and grip.

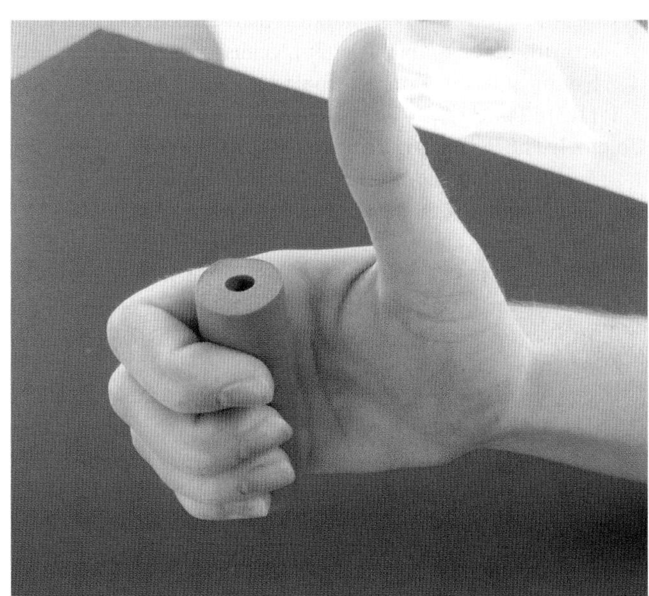

Figure 26.21 Photograph of finger strengthening using a foam roll.

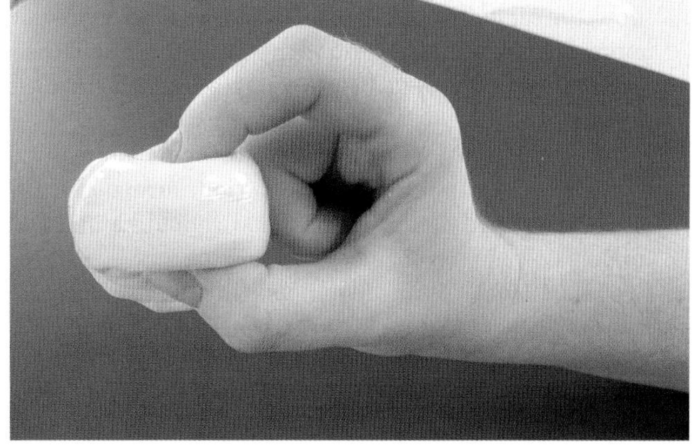

Figure 26.24 Photograph of use of putty to work on thumb pinch exercises with proper positioning.

- Using the techniques noted earlier to release the thumb adductor may be beneficial.
- *Strengthening*
  - If the patient is a young laborer, initial therapy sessions that assist the patient in maintaining shoulder and elbow strength using resistance bands will aid in keeping the affected extremity conditioned.
  - Wrist isometrics can be started once the patient is out of the cast with a progression to wrist strengthening, with a modified grip if needed to reduce the amount of pressure over the surgical site.
  - Once cleared by the hand surgeon for full strengthening, a more aggressive grip and pinch strengthening program as well as upper extremity strengthening and conditioning program should be devised that will prepare the patient to meet the physical demands of his or her job.

OUTCOMES

The outcomes of surgery for TM joint osteoarthritis are generally good, with high patient satisfaction and pain relief as measured by standardized outcome measures. A systematic review of outcomes after a variety of surgical procedures has shown no differences in outcomes among patients undergoing trapeziectomy alone compared to trapeziectomy with ligament reconstruction or TM arthrodesis. Trapeziectomy alone is associated with a significantly lower complication rate, while arthrodesis is associated with a higher rate of complications, including hardware failure and nonunion. Studies of long-term outcomes after the most common procedure—trapeziectomy with LRTI—have shown excellent pain relief and function.

PEARLS

- Smaller incisions and sharp dissection are associated with less postoperative pain and decreased narcotic requirements.
- In the volar Wagner approach, the thenar musculature should be carefully reapproximated and repaired to provide optimal recovery of strength and motion at the thumb base.
- Strict elevation should be encouraged for 3 to 5 days postoperatively.
- If the patient is not spontaneously moving the uninvolved digits in the early postoperative period, formal therapy is key to prevent digital stiffness and should be initiated immediately upon recognition of this issue.
- Keep the IP joint free in all immobilizing splints or casts to allow the patient to move it.
- A longer period of immobilization is used in patients with ligamentous laxity, as these patients tend to take longer to stabilize the arthroplasty site with scar tissue.
- The extended period of immobilization after this surgery can make tissue edema and stiffness difficult to control. It is critical to recognize the patient who is not moving the rest of the hand to mobilize edema and increase blood flow, and as stated earlier, early therapy is suggested in these cases.
- The clinician should be vigilant for early signs of chronic regional pain syndrome (CRPS). In particular, the patient with pain out of proportion to examination, persistent swelling, or color changes or abnormal sweating should be identified early and prompt referral to pain management for medication, stellate ganglion blocks, and other modalities should be considered.

SUMMARY

The role of therapy in the treatment of patients with thumb CMC osteoarthritis is critical, both before and after surgical treatment. Specialized splinting and exercises are used to treat pain and dysfunction of the base of the thumb, and to allow strengthening and functional recovery after surgery.

BIBLIOGRAPHY

Avisar E, Elvey M, Wasrbrout Z, Aghasi M: Long-term follow-up of trapeziectomy with abductor pollicis longus tendon interposition arthroplasty for osteoarthritis of the thumb carpometacarpal joint. *J Orthop* 2013;10(2):59–64.

Bamburger JB, Stern PJ, Kiefhaber TR, McDounough JJ, Cantor, RM: Trapeziometacarpal joint arthrodesis: a functional evaluation. *J Hand Surg Am* 1992;17:605–611.

Beatus J, Beatus RA: Management of the basal joint of the thumb following interposition arthoplasty for pain and instability. *Physiother Theory Pract* 2008;24(4)299–309.

Burton RI, Pellegrini VD Jr: Surgical management of basal joint arthritis of the thumb. Part II. Ligament reconstruction with tendon interposition arthroplasty. *J Hand Surg Am* 1986; 11(3):324–332.

Colditz J: The Perplexing Thumb and CMC Joint Osteoarthritis. Available at: http://myemail.constantcontact.com/HandLab-Clinical-Pearl—23.html?soid=1102126638168&aid=tW6VIZU83hc. Accessed June, 2013.

De Smet LD, Meir V, Verhoeven N, Degreef I: Is there still a place for arthrodesis in the surgical treatment of basal joint osteoarthritis of the thumb? *Acta Orthop Belg* 2010;76: 719–724.

O'Brien VH, Giveans MR: Effects of a dynamic stability approach in conservative intervention of the carpometacarpal joint of the thumb; a retrospective study. *J Hand Ther* 2013;26:44–52; quiz 52.

Patel TJ, Beredjiklian PK, Matzon JL: Trapeziometacarpal joint arthritis. *Curr Rev Musculoskelet Med* 2013;6(1):1–8.

Roberts RA, Jabaley ME, Todd NG: Results following trapeziometacarpal arthroplasty of the thumb. *J Hand Ther* 2001; 14:202–207.

© 2018 American Academy of Orthopaedic Surgeons

Valdes K, von der Heyde R: An exercise program for carpometacarpal osteoarthritis based on biomechanical principles. *J Hand Ther* 2012;25:251–263.

Vermeulen GM, Slijper H, Feitz R, Hovius SE, Moojen TM, Selles RW: Surgical management of primary thumb carpometacarpal osteoarthritis: a systematic review. *J Hand Surg Am* 2011;36(1):157–169.

Wajon A, Carr E, Edmunds I, Ada L: Surgery for thumb (trapeziometacarpal joint) osteoarthritis. *Cochrane Database Syst Rev* 2009;(4):137–142.

Weiss S, LaStayo P, Mills A, Bramlet D: Prospective analysis of splint the first carpometarpal joint; an objective, subjective and radiographic assessment. *J Hand Ther* 2000;13: 218–226.

© 2018 American Academy of Orthopaedic Surgeons

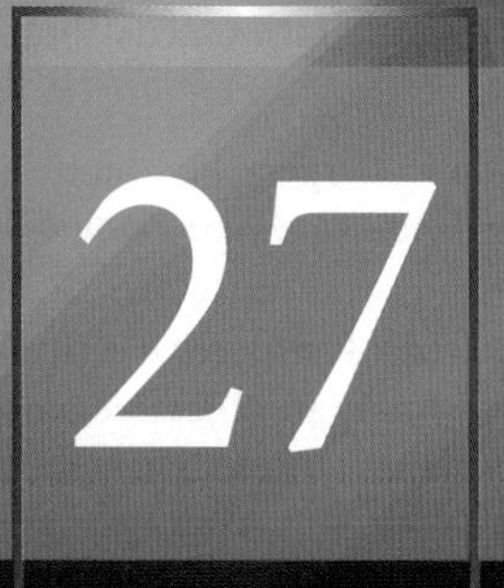

27 MP and PIP Joint Arthroplasty

Lindley B. Wall, MD, and Rhonda K. Powell, OTD, OTR/L, CHT

INTRODUCTION

Function of the metacarpophalangeal (MCP) and proximal interphalangeal (PIP) joints of the hand are important for activities of daily living (ADLs) and are susceptible to degenerative changes. Arthroplasty of the small joints of the hand, specifically the MCP and PIP joints, is an established and accepted treatment for symptomatic arthritis. Small joint arthroplasty can reliably treat pain, restore joint motion, and improve overall hand function. Silicone and resurfacing (pyrocarbon or metallic) implants are available for both the MCP and PIP joints.

METACARPOPHALANGEAL JOINT ARTHROPLASTY

Relevant Anatomy

The MCP joint has a CAM-like structure that is stabilized by the proper and accessory collateral ligaments. The joint is more stable to varus and valgus stress in a flexed position compared to extension. The volar plate also stabilizes the MCP joint by limiting joint hyperextension. The extensor tendon is located dorsal to the joint, and is maintained in a central position by the radial and ulnar sagittal bands.

Patient Evaluation

The preoperative evaluation assesses digit range of motion (ROM), grip-and-pinch strength, as well as consideration of functional needs and overall goals. The alignment, active range of motion (AROM) and passive range of motion (PROM), stability, and degree of laxity of the involved joints are evaluated. Radiographs of the hand, including a posterior-anterior (PA) and lateral image, are also obtained to assess for degenerative changes, including joint space narrowing, osteophyte formation, and subchondral sclerosis.

Indications and Contraindications

Silicone MCP arthroplasty has been utilized for over 50 years with acceptable levels of pain relief and restoration of joint motion. Silicone is a synthetic polymer that can be fashioned into different structures and provides a flexible rubber-like form. The silicone arthroplasty is a constrained implant that bridges from the metacarpal to the proximal phalanx and acts as a hinge joint while providing inherent stability. This arthroplasty is most commonly utilized in the setting of rheumatoid arthritis and other conditions with ligament or capsular laxity and deficiency. Patients must have adequate bone stock to support the implant and functioning flexor and extensor tendons to allow for active joint ROM.

Resurfacing arthroplasties are a newer-generation arthroplasty for the painful arthritic MCP joint, fabricated from pyrocarbon, cobalt chrome with polyethylene, or other composite materials. Pyrocarbon is a synthetic material consisting of a graphite core coated by a pyrolytic carbon layer. These implants are unconstrained and require stability from the surrounding collateral ligaments and capsule. Therefore, these implants are ideal for osteoarthritic joints or posttraumatic joints with competent ligamentous support. Joints affected by inflammatory arthritis and compromised soft-tissue structures are a relative contraindication to pyrocarbon implants because of the risk of instability.

Arthroplasty is generally contraindicated in a previously infected joint because of increased risk of joint loosening and failure.

Surgical Procedure

The surgical techniques used for silicone and resurfacing arthroplasty are similar. A dorsal approach to the MCP joint is utilized. A longitudinal incision is made centrally over a single involved joint. If all or multiple MCP joints are being addressed at one time, then a transverse incision centered over the joints is preferred. Care is taken to preserve small sensory nerves.

Neither of the following authors nor any immediate family member has received anything of value from or has stock or stock options held in a commercial company or institution related directly or indirectly to the subject of this article: Dr. Powell and Dr. Wall.

© 2018 American Academy of Orthopaedic Surgeons

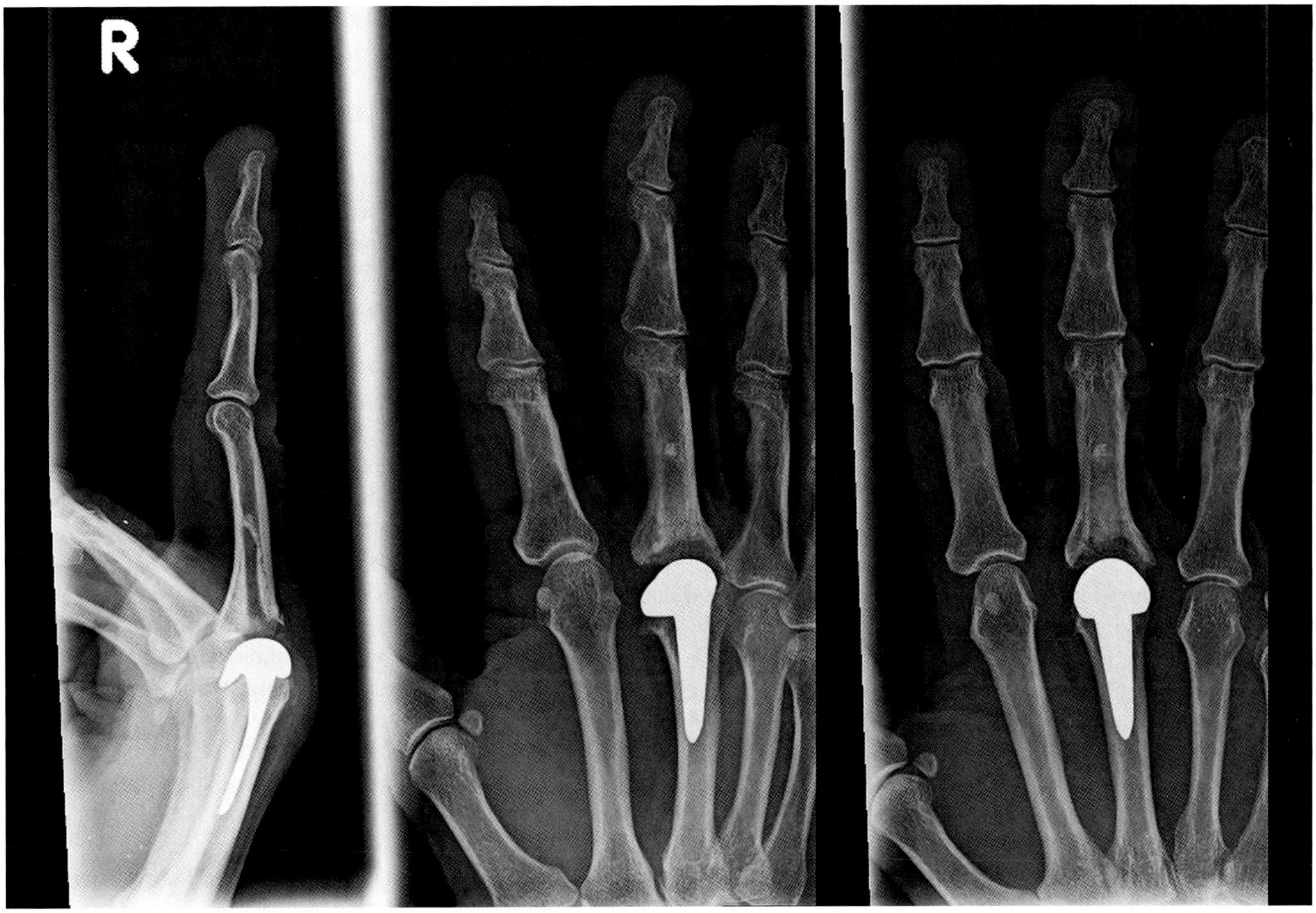

Figure 27.1 Lateral, oblique, and posteroanterior radiographs of a metacarpophalangeal joint pyrocabon arthroplasty of the middle finger.

In the rheumatoid patient, the extensor tendon is usually subluxated ulnarly, thus the extensor hood is incised on the ulnar side of the extensor tendon. If the tendon is not subluxated, it can be incised longitudinally and repaired at closure. The joint capsule is then incised and synovectomy is performed to remove any extensive synovitis.

The metacarpal bone resection is performed just distal to the origin of the collateral ligaments. With silicone implants, the distal portion may simply be placed in the proximal phalanx canal without resection of the subchondral bone. For resurfacing implants, an alignment awl is used with fluoroscopic assistance to make both the metacarpal and phalanx osteotomies. An awl and sequentially increasing-sized broaches are used to open the intramedullary canals. Trial implants are used to assess the appropriate implant size. The joint is assessed for stability and ROM. Implant placement is confirmed with fluoroscopy; both the PA and lateral images are used to assess the implant position. The dorsal capsule and extensor tendon are repaired. The hand is placed into a bulky padded postoperative volar slab splint with the MCP joints flexed and PIP joints extended. If a joint is felt to be looser than intended, then the implant size should be reconsidered or postoperative rehabilitation should be more conservative. Radiographic images of the two MCP arthroplasties can be seen in Figures 27.1 and 27.2.

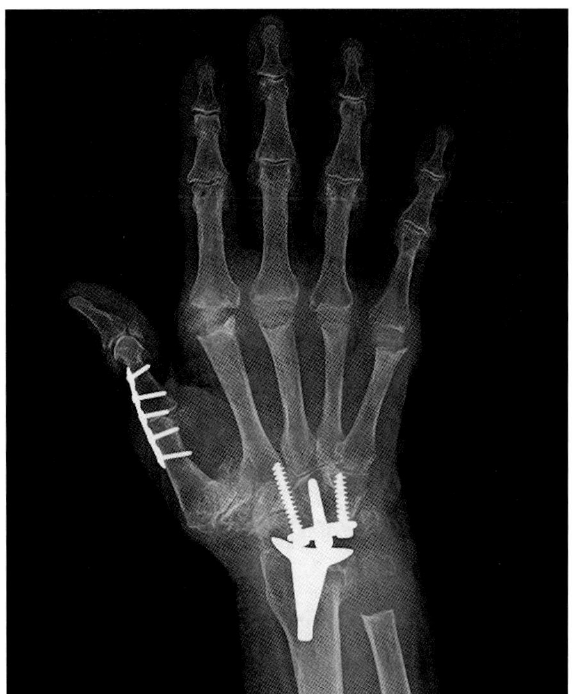

Figure 27.2 Posteroanterior radiograph of 4 silicone metacarpophalangeal joint arthroplasties involving the index, middle, ring, and small finger metacarpophalangeal joints.

© 2018 American Academy of Orthopaedic Surgeons

Complications

Potential complications in small joint arthroplasty include dislocation, instability, neuroma formation, infection, and stiffness. Specifically, silicone arthroplasties can fracture over time and can result in a silicone synovitis that can necessitate revision arthroplasty or joint arthrodesis. Resurfacing implants can also fracture, but are more likely to fail secondary to loosening of the implant, thus requiring revision or arthrodesis.

Postoperative Rehabilitation

Introduction

The goal of surgery and therapy is to reduce pain in the MCP joints and improve hand function. Patient goals also may include improving the appearance of their hands. Patient education should include potential difficulty with ADLs immediately postoperatively and an overall description of the rehabilitation program, including interventions provided, orthoses that will be worn by the patient, and approximate frequency and duration of therapy visits. Patients may need to consider arranging for transportation to therapy appointments, or planning for expected copayments of therapy visits.

Collaboration and communication between the therapist, surgeon, and patient are important to coordinate the postoperative care and rehabilitation. Details of the surgical procedure help to identify points of concern that will help to safely guide the recovery. Consideration of other related comorbidities and functional limitations—especially in patients with polyarticular involvement, such as with inflammatory arthritis—is also important.

Therapy is usually initiated 1 to 2 weeks postoperatively, depending on surgeon preference. As the initial goal is to allow the implant to become encapsulated, the main reason to start therapy sooner than the date of suture removal is to provide wound care. Initial postoperative evaluation includes assessment of wound healing (including swelling and edema), alignment of digits, ROM (including active flexion and passive extension of digits), and ADL status.

Interventions

- *Wound care:* After the bulky dressing is removed, a light compressive dressing is applied. Dressings are changed in the therapy or physician clinics, and are maintained until the wound is sealed. Scar massage is initiated after suture removal, which usually occurs at 2 weeks, when the wounds are fully closed.
- *Edema management:* Light compressive wraps such as a self-adherent wrap can be applied to the digits and hand. Active ROM of the shoulder, elbow, wrist, and digits will assist in minimizing edema of the upper extremity. The patient should continue to keep the hand elevated while sedentary for the first few weeks after surgery.
- *Orthoses:* Two orthoses are fabricated; one for daytime use and one for sleeping.
  - Day orthosis for ROM (Figure 27.3)
    - A dorsal forearm-based dynamic digit extension orthosis is fabricated.
    - Dynamic MCP extension is achieved through an outrigger attachment with finger slings that encompass the proximal phalanges, and rubber band tension that passively extends the MCP joints.
    - Orthosis supports the wrist in neutral, MCP joints at 0° to slight flexion, and allows active MCP joint flexion to 70° with dynamic return to the resting position, while maintaining neutral coronal plane alignment of the digits.
    - It is imperative that the dynamic extension tension is adjusted to avoid any hyperextension of the MCP joints, with careful attention to the small finger, which is most vulnerable to hyperextension.
    - Imaging with plain radiographs or fluoroscopy can be used to confirm that the MCP joint is not resting in hyperextension within the orthosis.
    - Patients should be able to demonstrate and report ease of flexion against the rubber band tension as forceful flexion can create deforming forces through the joints. Forty percent more force is required to actively flex the fingers with the low-profile outrigger (see Figure 27.3). However, most patients prefer the appearance of the lower-profile outrigger. Force application needs to be carefully monitored.
    - A supinator attachment may be added to protect radial collateral ligament repair to the index finger (Figure 27.4). This attachment should be worn between exercise sessions.

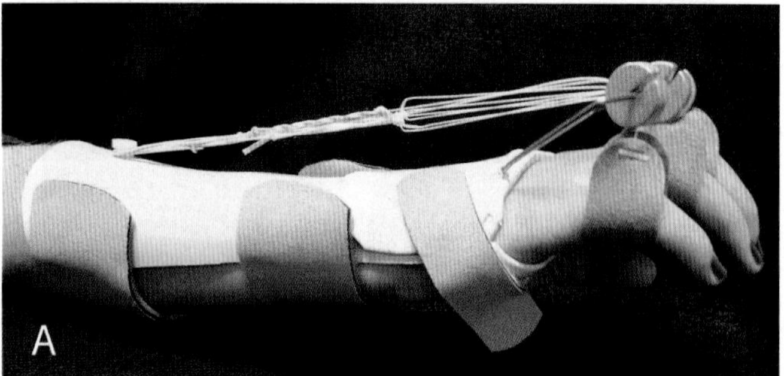

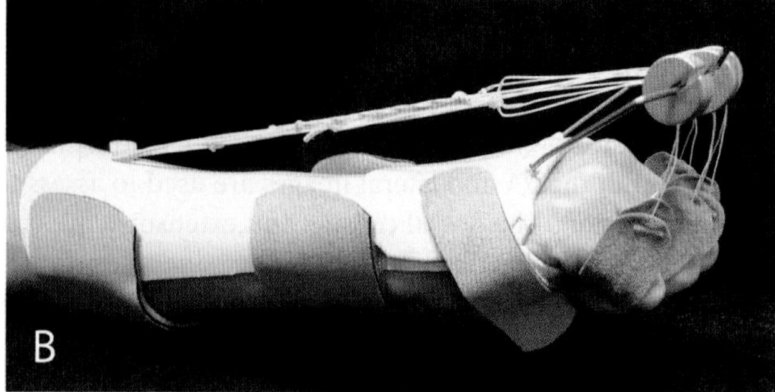

Figure 27.3 **A,** Photograph of a dynamic metacarpophalangeal joint extension orthosis with low-profile outrigger for day wear until 6 to 8 weeks following arthroplasty. **B,** The orthosis allows full metacarpophalangeal joint flexion.

© 2018 American Academy of Orthopaedic Surgeons

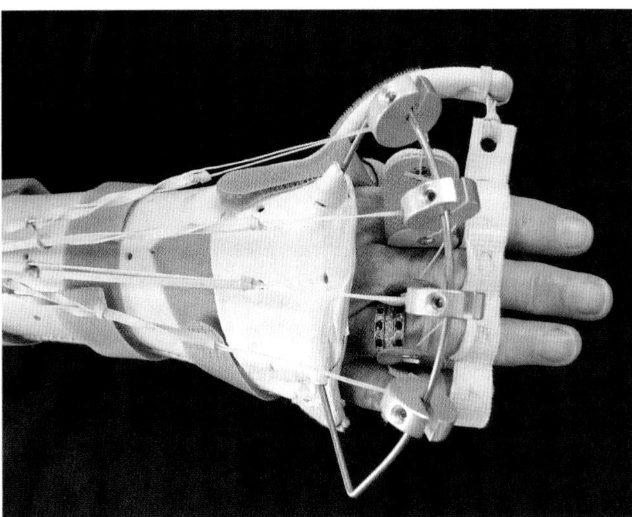

Figure 27.4 Photograph of a supinator attachment used to protect the radial collateral ligament.

- Night orthosis for positioning (Figure 27.5): Because the outrigger orthosis can be cumbersome to sleep in, a volar resting orthosis is fabricated to hold the wrist and digits in neutral alignment.
  - A high ulnar return on the orthotic pan will assist in preventing ulnar drift. Strapping and individual digital guides attached to the finger pan will facilitate neutral alignment.
  - A night orthosis is often worn for several months after surgery to allow the collateral ligaments to rest in neutral and maximize the potential for long-term joint alignment through ligamentous balance.
- Exercise—MP joint motion is the focus
  - *Initial visit to week 4*
    - Active and gentle passive ROM exercises begin at the first therapy visit.
    - All ROM will influence scar modeling around the joint. Active ROM will assist in edema management. Exercises are performed hourly.
    - ROM measurements are obtained at each therapy visit to monitor for extension lag. If an unacceptable extension lag (>30°) develops, passive flexion should be discontinued.
    - 2 to 3 weeks: MCP flexion should be at least 50°. If this has not been achieved, an additional orthotic intervention may be required.
      - PIP cuff to block PIP motion (Figure 27.6) and emphasize MCP joint motion
      - Static progressive or dynamic MCP flexion assist.
    - 3 weeks: the encapsulation process should provide enough joint stability to allow AROM out of the dynamic orthosis.
  - *Weeks 4 to 6:* Light ADLs within safe parameters are initiated out of the orthosis.
    - Safe parameters include no tight or sustained gripping or pinching activities, and avoidance of ADLs requiring ulnar forces to digits.

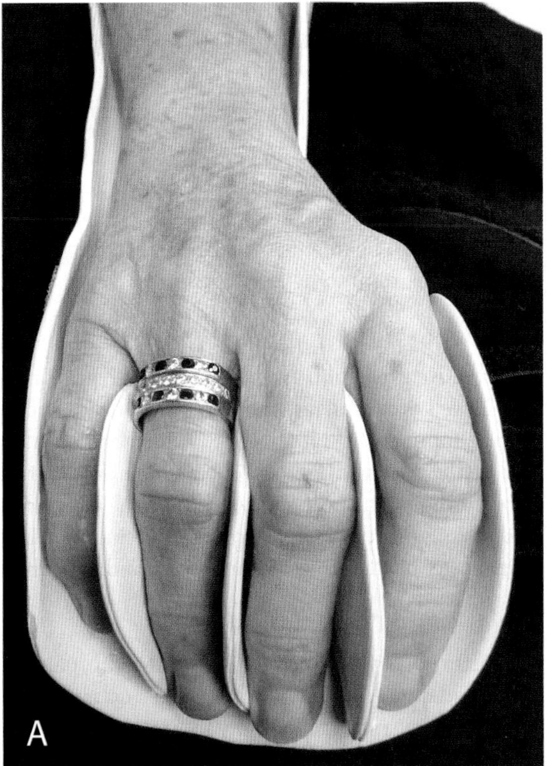

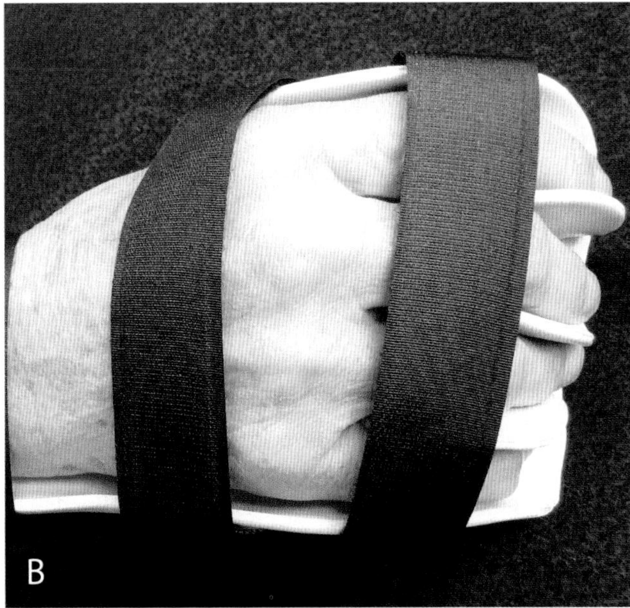

Figure 27.5 **A**, Photograph of a night orthosis with digit guides to maintain neutral alignment. **B**, Straps assist with maintaining alignment.

© 2018 American Academy of Orthopaedic Surgeons

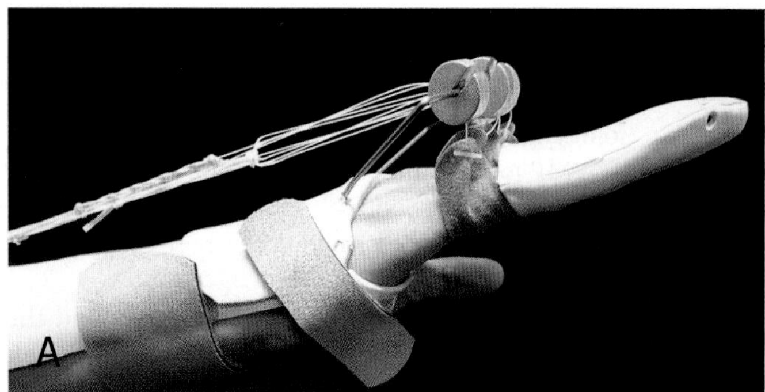

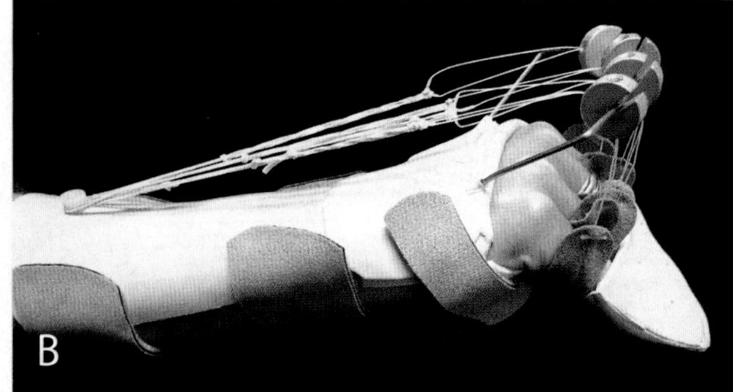

Figure 27.6 **A**, Photograph of proximal interphalangeal cuff blocking PIP and DIP motion, directing motion forces to the metacarpophalangeal joints. **B**, The cuff allows full metacarpophalangeal joint motion.

    - Joint protection principles are reviewed with the patient and practiced in therapy. These can include activity modification, enlarged grips, pain management techniques, and built-up grips.
    - If ulnar drift is noted with activities, a hand-based orthosis that allows active ROM and maintains neutral alignment is worn.
    - If an extensor lag greater than 30° is present, the dynamic extension orthosis is continued between exercise and light ADL sessions.
- *Weeks 6 to 8*
    - Continue exercises from weeks 0 to 6.
    - ROM and edema management continues, as described earlier.
    - The dynamic daytime orthosis is discontinued.
    - The night positioning orthosis is maintained.
- *Weeks 8 to 12*
    - If needed, light functional strengthening can be implemented. The priority is to maintain good alignment of the digits while performing activities and exercises that demonstrate avoidance of deforming forces.
    - Dynamic flexion orthosis is continued if flexion is inadequate for function and active extension is adequate.
- *Final home program*
    - Night positioning orthosis is continued until at least 6 months postarthroplasty. There are no activity limitations or precautions long term.

This therapy program is intended to serve as a general guide. Notably, at this time there is no consensus on when to start therapy, whether a dynamic orthosis is required, or if alternating between a static flexion and static neutral extension is sufficient. Likewise, specifics about discontinuation of a dynamic day and night positioning orthosis are not clearly defined. Rehabilitation following MCP joint arthroplasty requires a skilled hand therapist who can integrate each patient's tissue response to surgery and therapy interventions with clinical reasoning to determine parameters for an individualized therapy program.

Pearls

- Joint stability and pain-free function, not ROM or strength, are the ultimate goals.
- Fit the choice of orthosis to the patient, not the patient to the orthosis.
- Patient education on joint protection principles is as important postarthroplasty as prearthroplasty.
- Progressive stiffness despite therapy could represent fibrosis.
- Clicking and catching can represent extensor tendon subluxation or dislocation.
- Watch for deviation of the joint, which can lead to progressive instability.
- Progressive hyperextension can lead to joint instability.

PROXIMAL INTERPHALANGEAL JOINT ARTHROPLASTY

Relevant Anatomy

The PIP joint is a concentric hinge joint with an equal degree of lateral stability throughout the full ROM. The proper and accessory collateral ligaments provide this stability. The volar plate provides restraint to hyperextension.

Patient Evaluation

The preoperative evaluation assesses digit ROM, grip and pinch strength, as well as consideration of functional needs and overall goals. The alignment, AROM and PROM, stability, and degree of laxity of the involved joints are evaluated. Radiographs of the involved digits, including a PA and lateral image, are also obtained to assess for degenerative changes, including joint space narrowing, osteophyte formation, and subchondral sclerosis.

Indications and Contraindications

PIP joint arthroplasty is indicated in the arthritic, painful joint that has failed conservative nonoperative treatment. Arthroplasty treats pain and allows joint motion. Indications and contraindications are similar to those listed earlier for MP arthroplasty. Additionally, the central slip must be competent for arthroplasty placement. A relative contraindication to

© 2018 American Academy of Orthopaedic Surgeons

silicone arthroplasty is use in the index finger because of the lateral stress that occurs with pinch.

Procedure

Similar to MCP arthroplasty, the surgical technique for PIP arthroplasty is the same for silicone or resurfacing implants. A dorsal approach is most commonly utilized, with a longitudinal incision centered over the PIP joint. The extensor mechanism is exposed and an interval is created between the central slip and the lateral band, taking care to preserve the central slip. Some advocate a Chamay approach, with elevation of the central slip and repair at closure. A saw is used to remove the end of the phalanges, preserving the collateral ligaments. The canal of the phalanx is found by use of a starting awl; then, a reamer is used to open the canal. A broach is used to create a fit for the prosthesis, after which a trial prosthesis is tested. The joint is taken through ROM and stability is assessed. Fluoroscopic imaging is used to confirm position. Before the final implant is impacted into place, drill holes are made for suture repair of the collateral ligaments. Then the implant is placed, collaterals are repaired, the capsule is repaired, and the skin is closed with nonabsorbable suture. We do not advocate the use of cement with pyrocarbon arthroplasty. The hand is placed into a bulky padded postoperative volar slab splint with the MCP joints flexed and PIP joints extended. Figure 27.7 depicts a radiograph of a well seated PIP arthroplasty.

Complications

Complications are similar to those seen with MCP joint arthroplasty.

Postoperative Rehabilitation

The goal of PIP joint arthroplasty is a pain-free joint that moves in a functional range. Patient goals also may include improving the appearance of the hands. Patient education should include potential difficulty with ADLs immediately postoperatively and an overall description of the rehabilitation program, including interventions provided, orthoses that will be worn by the patient, and approximate frequency and duration of therapy visits. Patients may need to consider arranging for transportation to therapy appointments or planning for expected copayments of therapy visits.

Therapy is usually initiated 1 to 2 weeks postoperatively. As the initial goal is to allow the implant to become encapsulated, the main reason to start therapy sooner than the date of suture removal is to provide wound care and maintain the motion of the adjacent digits and joints. Initial postoperative evaluation includes assessment of wound healing (including swelling and edema), alignment of digits, ROM (including active flexion and passive extension of digits), and ADL status.

Interventions

- *Wound care:* After the bulky dressing is removed, a light, compressive dressing is applied. Dressings are changed in the therapy or physician clinics, and are maintained until the wound is sealed. Scar massage is initiated after suture removal, which usually occurs at 2 weeks, when the wounds are fully closed.
- *Edema management:* Light compressive wraps, such as self-adherent wrap, can be applied to the digits and hand. AROM of the shoulder, elbow, wrist, and digits will assist

A

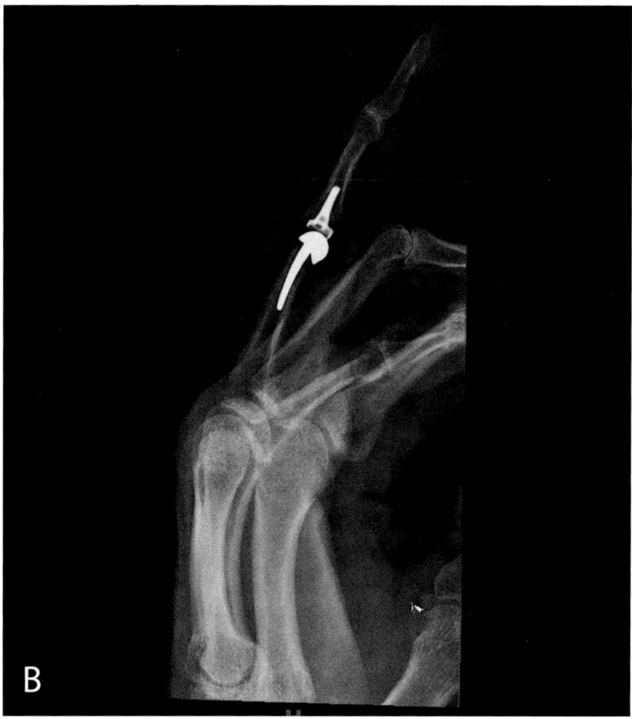

Figure 27.7 **A**, Posteroanterior radiograph of a proximal interphalangeal joint arthroplasty. **B**, Lateral radiograph of a proximal interphalangeal joint arthroplasty.

© 2018 American Academy of Orthopaedic Surgeons

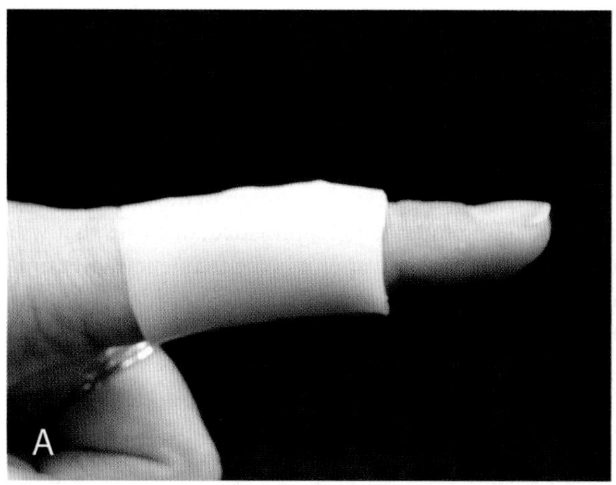
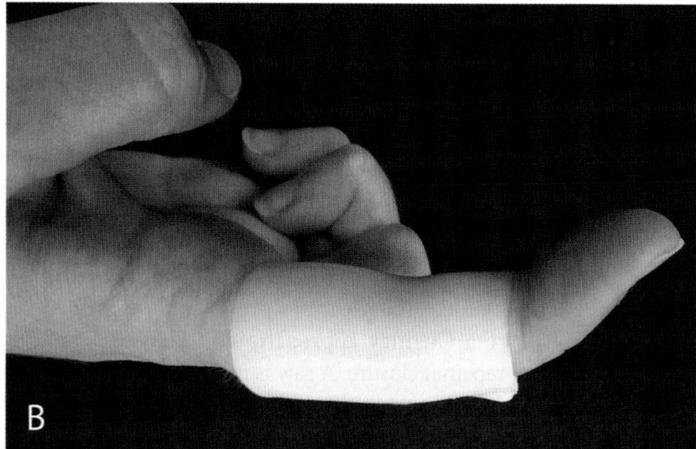

Figure 27.8 A, Photograph of a circumferential static orthosis, which blocks proximal interphalangeal motion while allowing full metacarpophalangeal and distal interphalangeal motion (**B**).

in minimizing edema of the upper extremity. The patient should continue to keep the hand elevated while sedentary for the first couple of weeks.

- Orthoses
  - *Weeks 1 to 5*
    - Static hand-based splint
    - MCP joint in 15° flexion
    - PIP joint in 15° to 30° flexion to increase opportunity for the joint to stabilize in position, which prevents hyperextension.
    - A recent study shows that the results of static orthoses are equivalent to dynamic orthoses, at lower cost to the patient and more easily managed by therapists not experienced in dynamic extension orthosis fabrication and management.
    - The patient should be evaluated in a splint under fluoroscopy to ascertain that the PIP joint is not hyperextended.
  - *Weeks 6 to 11*
    - Continue resting orthosis at night and as needed for rest for 2 more weeks. This will allow the joint to rest after onset of hand use for ADLs.
    - Discontinue day orthosis. The patient is using the hand for light activity and can exercise without extension block, as scar tissue should have encapsulated joint in slight flexion by 6 weeks postoperatively.
- Exercise
  - MCP and DIP joint AROM (Figure 27.8). Zones 3 to 4 extensor tendon repair requires PIP immobilization only due to minimal glide of the extensor in that zone with motion at the MCP or DIP joint.
  - Short arc motion (SAM) for PIP: –15°/35° AROM in exercise orthosis; MCP held in extension and wrist in slight flexion (Figure 27.9). Early AROM decreases edema and tendon adhesions. Limits on extension should prevent implant hyperextension. Active

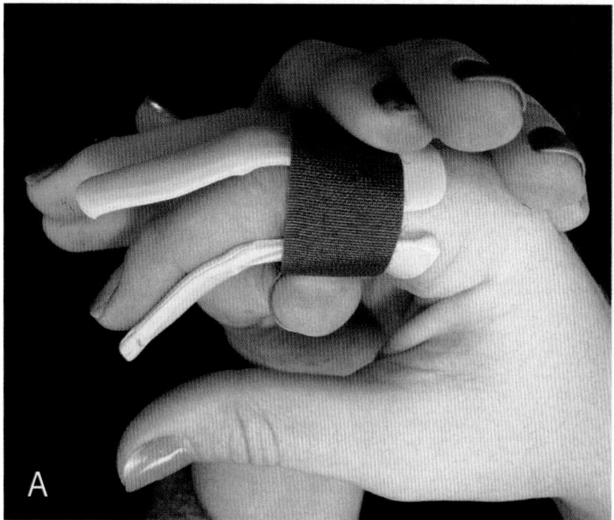
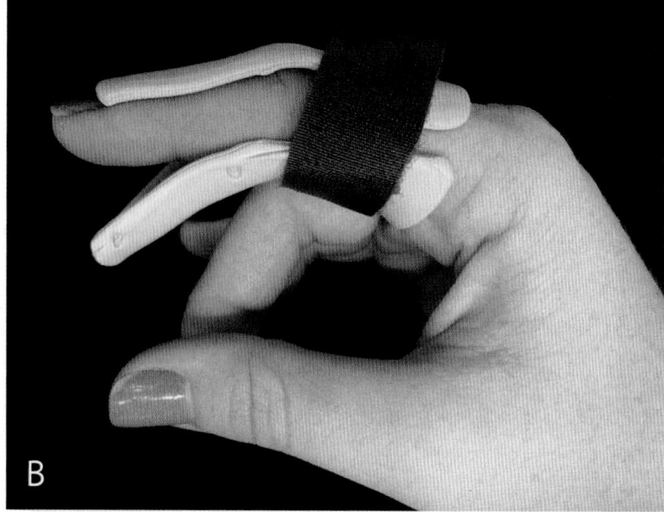

Figure 27.9 A, Photograph of a short arc motion (SAM) orthosis, which allows the proximal interphalangeal joint to actively flex to 35° and extend to –15° (**B**).

© 2018 American Academy of Orthopaedic Surgeons

flexion can be progressed 10° weekly if no extensor lag develops.

- *Weeks 6 to 11*
  - Orthoses
  - Exercise
    - Light ADL use will assist in regaining functional strength without undue stress that could lead to an increase in edema and pain.
    - Avoid resistive activities if collateral ligaments have been compromised through surgery because resistance at 6 weeks may encourage instability. Resistance may also result in pain.
- *Week 12:* Until patient is satisfied with functional strength
  - Exercise: Initiate light resistance (soft putty or hand helper) if needed to assist with return to functional strength.

Pearls

- Compression wraps may create undesired torque at the joint, unlike at the MCP joint, where the wrap is applied volar and dorsal only, as the MP joints are linked.
- Lack of full extension is preferable to avoid any chance of hyperextension.
- Patients often report satisfaction with the procedure due to decreased pain and increased functional status, even with minimal change in ROM following arthroplasty.
- Progressive stiffness despite therapy could represent fibrosis.
- Watch for deviation of the joint, which can lead to progressive instability.
- Progressive hyperextension can lead to joint instability.

SUMMARY

Arthroplasty of the MCP and PIP joints can provide excellent clinical outcomes in the appropriately chosen patient. Surgical indications should be followed and patient expectations set preoperatively by the surgeon. Care must be taken to follow the postoperative protocol, working closely with the hand therapist with regard to the appropriate progression of motion and splinting. This combination of care, surgical and rehabilitative, will effectively maximize clinical outcomes, improving function and pain of the involved joint.

BIBLIOGRAPHY

Bielefeld T, Neumann DA: The unstable metacarpophalangeal joint in rheumatoid arthritis: anatomy, pathomechanics, and physical rehabilitation considerations. *J Orthop Sports Phys Ther* 2005;35(8):502–520.

Boozer JA, Sanson MS, Soutas-Little RW, Coale EH Jr, Pierce TD, Swanson AB: Comparison of the biomechanical motions and forces involved in high-profile versus low-profile dynamic splinting. *J Hand Ther* 1994;7:171–182.

Burr N, Pratt AL, Smith PJ: An alternative splinting and rehabilitation protocol for metacarpophalangeal joint arthroplasty in patients with rheumatoid arthritis. *J Hand Ther* 2002;15:41–47.

Estes JP, Bochenek C, Fasler P: Osteoarthritis of the fingers. *J Hand Ther* 2000;13:108–123.

Evans RB, Thompson D: An analysis of factors that support early active short arc motion of the repaired central slip. *J Hand Ther* 1992;5(4):187–201.

Evans RB: Managing the injured tendon: current concepts. *J Hand Ther* 2012;25:173–189; quiz 190.

Luther C, Germann G, Sauerbier M: Proximal interphalangeal joint replacement with surface replacement arthroplasty (SR-PIP): functional results and complications. *Hand (NY)* 2010;5(3):233–240.

Massy-Westropp N, Krishnan, J: Postoperative therapy after metacarpophalangeal arthroplasty. *J Hand Ther* 2003;16:311–314.

Michlovitz S: Arthroplasty of the hand and wrist: therapist's commentary. *J Hand Ther* 1999;2:133–134.

Riggs JM, Lyden AK, Chung KC, Murphy SL: Static versus dynamic splinting for PIP joint pyrocarbon implant arthroplasty: a comparison of current and historical cohorts. *J Hand Ther* 2011;24(3):231–239.

© 2018 American Academy of Orthopaedic Surgeons

28 Acute Flexor Tendon Injuries

Christopher H. Judson, MD, Mark E. Warren, OTR/L, CHT, and Craig M. Rodner, MD

INTRODUCTION

Flexor tendon injuries of the hand have historically been a difficult problem to treat, with unpredictable outcomes. Flexor tendon injuries are typically caused by open trauma, resulting in laceration of the tendons. Less commonly, closed injuries can occur, such as with a "Jersey finger" (flexor digitorum profundus tendon avulsion). These injuries are seen in all age groups and pose several challenges in returning normal strength and range of motion (ROM) to the involved digits. After repair is performed, immobilization promotes adhesions within the tendon sheath, limiting long-term function. On the other hand, excessive early motion can subject the tendon to forces that result in disruption of the repair. Therefore, the central dilemma involves determining the optimal surgical repair and rehabilitation regimen that will avoid these complications. Consequently, these injuries require a coordinated effort between the surgeon and hand therapist.

SURGICAL PROCEDURE: ACUTE DIGITAL FLEXOR TENDON REPAIR

Indications/Contraindications

Complete tendon lacerations in all five flexor tendon zones require operative repair to restore active digital flexion (Figure 28.1). Although primary repair is recommended within the first week after injury to limit tendon retraction and scarring, primary repair can be reasonably attempted even for injuries that are up to 4 weeks old. Beyond this time point, a staged flexor tendon reconstruction should be considered. For partial tendon lacerations, repair is indicated if greater than 60% of the tendon is involved.

Contraindications to primary repair include severe wound contamination, multiple points of injury in the tendon, or substantial skin loss over the flexor tendon sheath. Concomitant fractures do not represent a contraindication to tendon repair if they can be stabilized at the same time of the repair. Likewise, neurovascular injuries are repaired at the same time as the tendon.

Relevant Anatomy

Flexor tendon injuries can occur in any of the five zones in the hand and forearm (Figure 28.1). In the forearm, or Zone V, the flexor digitorum superficialis (FDS) is volar to the flexor digitorum profundus (FDP) and the flexor pollicis longus (FPL). After passing through the carpal tunnel (Zone IV) and through the palm (Zone III), the FDS and FDP to all the digits except the thumb become encased within fibro-osseous synovial sheaths beginning at the level of the metacarpophalangeal joint (Zone II). Zone II injuries are the most difficult to treat, as the two tendons occupy nearly all of the relatively small space beneath multiple fibrous pulleys. Within Zone II, the FDS starts as a superficial structure, then divides into two slips that proceed deep to and on either side of the FDP as the slips insert onto the volar aspect of the middle phalanx. After the insertion of the FDS, the FDP proceeds to insert at the volar distal phalanx (Zone I). There are numerous annular and cruciate pulleys in Zones I and II, the most important being the A2 and A4 pulleys that prevent tendon bowstringing with flexion (Figure 28.2).

Repair Technique

Surgical Approach

In Zones I, II, and III, a zigzag, or Bruner, incision can be made to expose the injured area (Figure 28.3). Alternatively, a midlateral incision can be used. In either case, the incisions can be modified slightly to incorporate the traumatic laceration. These approaches allow visualization of the neurovascular bundles and assessment of any other injury that might require concomitant repair. It may be necessary to release one or more of the flexor pulleys to expose the injury site, as long as the integrity of the A2 and A4 pulleys is maintained. After tendon repair, if passive flexion or extension of the digit causes impingement of the repair site on the A2 or A4 pulleys, these can be vented to facilitate postoperative ROM. If these pulleys

Neither of the following authors nor any immediate family member has received anything of value from or has stock or stock options held in a commercial company or institution related directly or indirectly to the subject of this article: Dr. Rodner, Dr. Judson, and Mr. Warren.

 © 2018 American Academy of Orthopaedic Surgeons

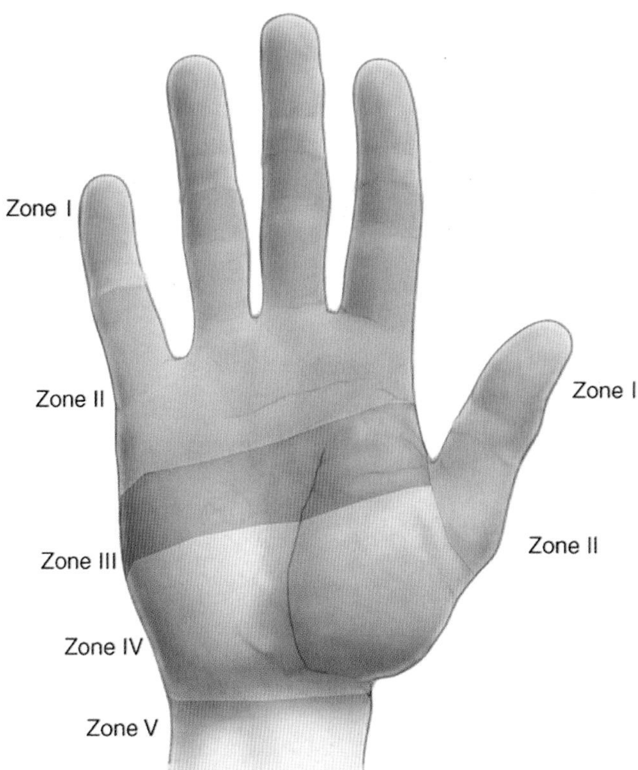

Figure 28.1 Illustration of the five flexor tendon zones. (Reproduced with permission from Hunt TR, Wiesel SW: *Operative Techniques in Hand, Wrist, and Forearm Surgery.* Philadelphia, Lippincott Williams & Wilkins 2011.)

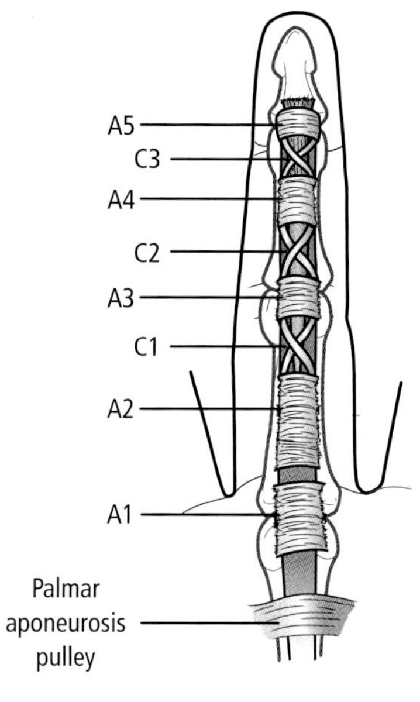

Figure 28.2 Illustration of the anatomy of the flexor tendon sheath. There are five annular pulleys (A1–A5) and three cruciform pulleys (C1–C3). (Reproduced with permission from Bindra R, Sinclair M: Trigger Finger Release, in Flatow E, Colvin AC, eds: *Atlas of Essential Orthopaedic Procedures.* Rosemont, IL, American Academy of Orthopaedic Surgeons, 2013, pp. 253–257.)

are completely disrupted by the injury or are iatrogenically released, they should be repaired prior to closure. However, the A1 and A3 pulleys should be left unrepaired to improve tendon gliding at the repair site. For Zones IV and V, a volar Henry approach to the forearm with extension to the carpal tunnel can be used.

Procedure

Prior to any flexor tendon repair, identification and retrieval of the severed tendon ends must be performed with as little trauma as possible to the surrounding tissue to minimize subsequent adhesions within the tendon sheath. All injuries can result in retraction of the proximal tendon end, especially with increasing time from injury. This becomes less likely in distal injuries, in which the vincula to the tendons may prevent retraction to the palm. For Zone I injuries, the Leddy classification is used to describe the level to which the FDP tendon has retracted and whether any bony avulsion is present (Figure 28.4).

In both Zone I and II injuries, retrieval of the proximal tendon end can sometimes be accomplished by milking the forearm and palm, and a small, narrow instrument can be passed beneath the pulleys to attempt to grasp the tendon. If this is unsuccessful, it may be necessary to extend or make a separate proximal incision to identify and retrieve the tendon. Once the lacerated tendon is identified proximally, we prefer to

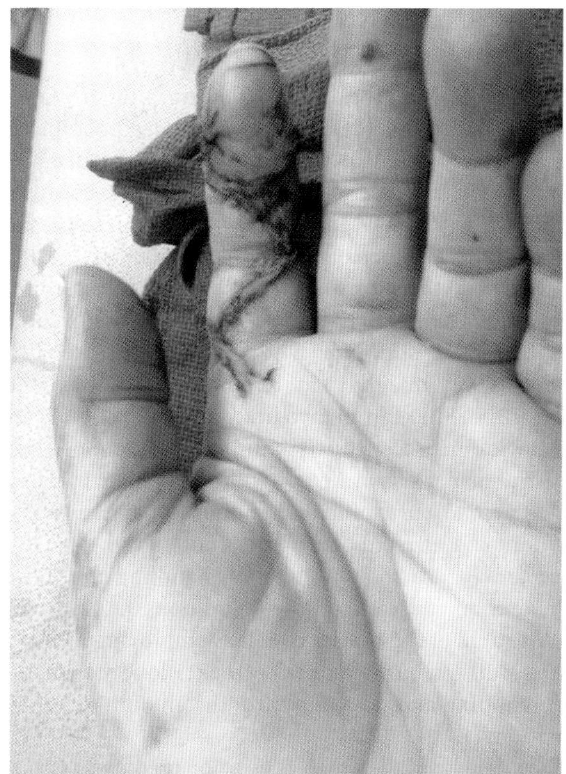

Figure 28.3 Photograph of a zigzag, or Bruner, incision that has been closed following flexor tendon repair.

© 2018 American Academy of Orthopaedic Surgeons

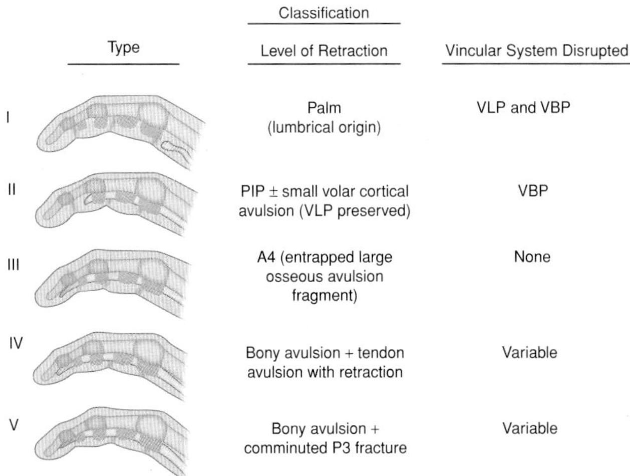

Figure 28.4 Illustration of the Leddy classification of flexor digitorum profundus tendon avulsion injuries. (Redrawn from Ruchelsman DE, Christoforou D, Wasserman B, et al: Avulsion injuries of the flexor digitorum profundus tendon. *JAAOS* 201;19(3): 152–162.)

pass a pediatric feeding tube from distal to proximal though the pulleys (Figure 28.5). The feeding tube is then sutured to the tendon and helps guide passage back to the site of injury. The tendon ends can then be held in place for repair using a small-gauge needle. In Zones II, III, and IV injuries, the distal tendon stump will often be more distal than the skin laceration if the fingers were flexed at the time of injury; therefore, the approach must be extended distally accordingly.

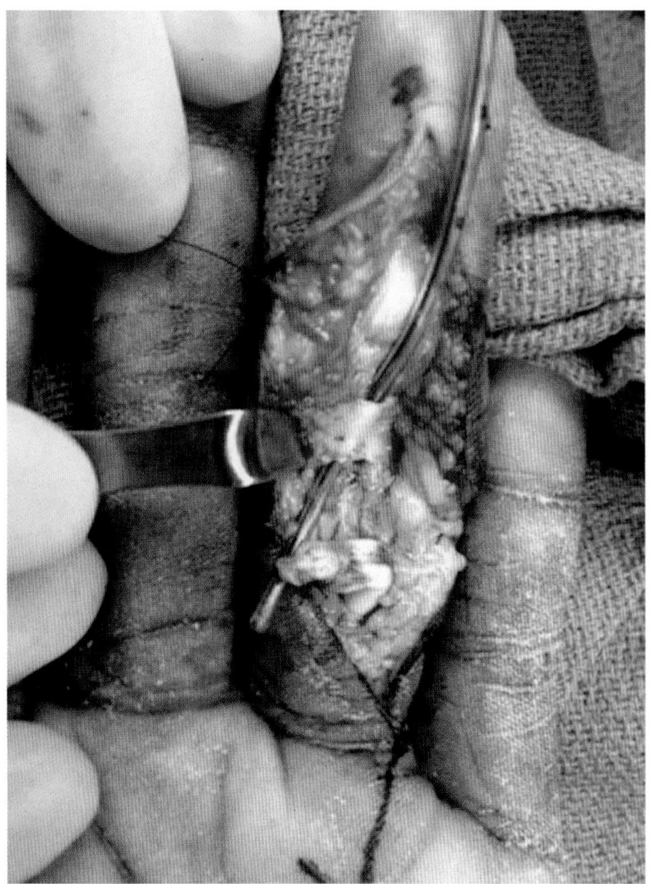

Figure 28.5 Photograph showing a pediatric feeding tube that has been passed from distal to proximal under the pulley system and will be sutured to the tendon end to assist passage under the pulleys.

Authors' Preferred Protocol

An ideal repair of the injured tendon will provide the maximal strength to resist failure during postoperative rehabilitation, while still allowing adequate vascularity and contact of the tendon ends to facilitate healing. For injuries in Zones II through V, there have been numerous studies regarding the number of core sutures to cross the repair site, the size of the suture, and the type of suture technique. The author's preferred method uses 3-0 monofilament, non-absorbable suture in a four-strand core repair. To create this we prefer the suture configuration depicted in Figure 28.6, although many suture configurations can be used, including a Kessler-style suture with a looped suture (two strands per pass). An epitendinous repair is also performed with 6-0 monofilament, nonabsorbable suture with attention paid to avoid placing the knot on the volar side of the repair (Figure 28.7). Meticulous handling and suturing of the tendon ends, using an epitendinous suture to minimize the bulk of the repair, as well as employing techniques such as pulley venting or FDS slip excision, may facilitate tendon gliding and help minimize the amount of adhesion formation.

The strength of the repair is a major predictor of rupture risk. The number of suture strands that cross the repair site is directly proportional to the repair strength. For instance, a

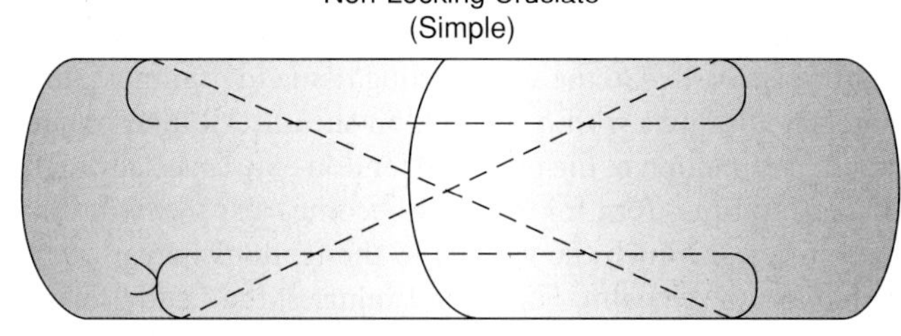

Figure 28.6 Illustration of a four-strand repair for end-to-end tendon repair. (From Chauhan A, Palmer BA, Merrell GA: Flexor tendon repairs: techniques, eponyms, and evidence. *J Hand Surg Am* 2014;39(9):1846–1853. doi: 10.1016/j.jhsa.2014.06.025)

© 2018 American Academy of Orthopaedic Surgeons

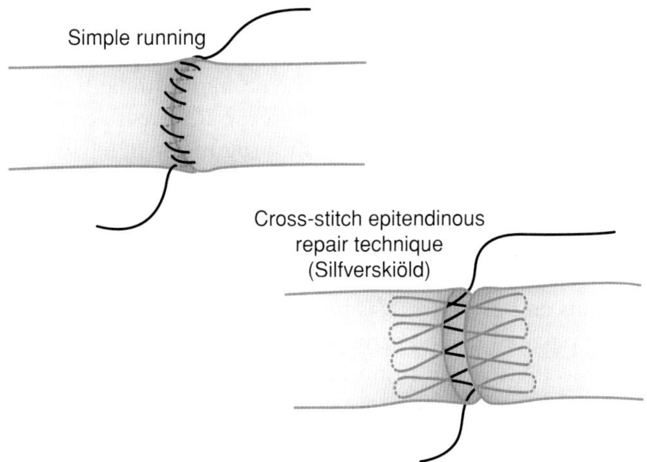

Figure 28.7 Illustration of an epitendinous repair, which increases strength of the repair and decreases gapping. (Reproduced with permission from Hammer WC, Boyer MI, Bozentka DJ, Calfee RP: *ASSH Manual of Hand Surgery.* Philadelphia, Lippincott Williams & Wilkins, 2010.)

four-strand repair has been shown to be twice as strong as a two-strand repair. Strickland estimates from prior studies that repairs have 50% of their strength at 1 week, 67% at 3 weeks, and, finally, 120% strength at 6 weeks. The addition of an epitendinous repair has been shown to decrease gapping at the repair site and increase the strength of the repair by 10% to 50%. Therefore, the combination of a four-strand repair and an epitendinous suture should provide enough strength to withstand light active grip even at the weakest time point of 1 week. Studies have shown no definitive consensus for the recommended suture, material, or size that is most optimal for repair strength and healing.

For Zone II injuries in which the FDS and FDP are both injured, there is some debate regarding whether the FDS should be repaired. Repair of both slips of FDS may inhibit tendon gliding beneath the A2 pulley and promote adhesions. However, even though the loss of FDS does not cause a major functional deficit, it may serve as an important source of blood flow to the FDP. The authors therefore prefer to repair at least one slip of the FDS as long as it does not cause significant gliding resistance; otherwise, it is excised. The repair should then be observed as it glides beneath the pulley system. The A1, A3, and A5 pulleys can potentially be sacrificed to improve gliding. For the A2 and A4 pulleys, if the pulley impedes full passive flexion or extension of the digit, partial venting of the pulley may be appropriate to allow full motion to be achieved.

Zone I injuries are unique and the repair method varies depending on the presence or absence of a bony avulsion fracture. The most common repair methods include suture anchors, sutures tied over a dorsal button, or sutures tied directly over the bone. If the avulsed bony fragment is large enough for open reduction and internal fixation, this can be accomplished with either small screws or Kirschner wires.

Wound Closure

After repairing the tendon, thorough irrigation of the wound is performed. For Zone V, the subcutaneous layer can be loosely closed with absorbable suture, followed by skin closure. For all other zones, we suture the skin only with 4-0 monofilament, absorbable or nonabsorbable interrupted sutures.

Complications

The most common complication following flexor tendon repair is adhesion formation and resulting limitation of finger motion and function. If adhesions develop, early recognition by the hand surgeon or hand therapist is important so that therapy can focus on separating the differential gliding of the FDS and FDP tendons. Ultimately, flexor tenolysis may occasionally be indicated if months of exercises do not lead to an acceptable ROM.

Joint stiffness, or contractures, of the proximal interphalangeal (PIP) and/or distal interphalangeal (DIP) joints are relatively common after flexor tendon repairs. This occurs in approximately 15% of cases, and is even more common for Zone I injuries. Addressing a patient's postoperative joint stiffness with early motion regimens—and splinting when the repair can tolerate it—are the best methods to combat this complication. Just as is the case in treating postoperative tendon adhesions, the development of joint stiffness after a flexor tendon repair may necessitate a modification of the rehabilitation protocol to best suit an individual patient's clinical course. In some patients with persistent contractures, a joint release may be required if conservative treatments are unhelpful.

Tendon repair rupture remains one of the most feared complications after flexor tendon repair for patients, surgeons, and therapists alike. The postoperative rupture rate has been estimated at approximately 4% in a large series. It is important to note that the repair will be weakest from 6 to 18 days following repair. Poor surgical technique, aggressive rehabilitation, or patient noncompliance (such as attempting a strong grasp or removing the splint before recommended) can predispose to repair failure. If rupture is identified, surgical exploration is indicated within 1 to 2 weeks. If complete rupture is recognized and the original repair was performed within 4 weeks, primary repair can be attempted. If longer than 4 weeks have passed since initial repair, a staged reconstruction or tendon grafting should be performed. If no rupture is identified but the repair is attenuated, scar can be resected and a primary repair performed if the scar is less than 1 cm in length. If the scar is greater than 1 cm, tendon grafting is recommended to avoid shortening of the tendon.

Postoperative triggering may occur secondary to the repair site impinging underneath a pulley during tendon gliding. If this is observed, therapeutic ultrasound or massage can be performed by the therapist. On the other end of the spectrum, tendon bowstringing may result from complete release of either the A2 or A4 pulleys.

Last, since the FDP tendons share a common muscle belly, the overall excursion of each tendon is limited by the shortest tendon. Therefore, the phenomenon of quadriga can occur if the injured FDP tendon has a defect that requires excessive

© 2018 American Academy of Orthopaedic Surgeons

tensioning, resulting in overall shortening after repair. In this scenario, the patient cannot make a full fist with the nonoperative fingers and has a weak grip secondary to a relatively shorter FDP of the operative finger. Surgical tenolysis or release of the repaired tendon may be indicated for this issue if it is persistently symptomatic.

POSTOPERATIVE REHABILITATION

Introduction

The postoperative rehabilitation of flexor tendon injuries presents a myriad of challenges that can ultimately affect functional outcome. Current approaches to rehabilitation have evolved steadily over the years concurrent with improved surgical techniques. When designing a rehabilitation regimen for a patient, there are three broad categories of factors that must be considered: patient-related, injury-related, and surgery-related.

- *Patient-related:* Underlying medical comorbidities, cognitive capacity, age, and lifestyle choices (such as cigarette smoking, drug use, or alcohol use) may affect the patient's ability to follow certain rehabilitation protocols and may also influence the rate of postoperative tendon and skin healing. In addition, patient expectations, goals, and functional requirements should be considered.
- *Injury-related:* A laceration caused by a lawnmower is a very different entity from one caused by a kitchen knife, with vastly different rehabilitative expectations. Higher-energy injuries often have associated injuries that may affect rehabilitation, including loss of skin, concomitant fractures, and neurovascular injuries.
- *Surgery-related:* The design of the postoperative rehabilitation program is dependent on the surgical technique and strength of the repair, as a four-strand repair with epitendinous suture can withstand a more aggressive rehabilitation regimen than an isolated two-strand repair.

The primary goal in the rehabilitation of a flexor tendon repair is to protect the repair during its vulnerable healing stages, while preventing tendon adhesions and joint stiffness. Information about the extent of the injury and the details about the flexor tendon repair and any associated procedures must be communicated to the therapist.

The information contained in this chapter describes how we rehabilitate flexor tendon repairs in our practice based on a four-strand repair with an epitendinous suture. It is important to note that this is not intended to be a dogmatic "one-size-fits-all" approach. We do gravitate primarily to an early-motion, place-and-hold approach, as evidence has shown better results with this than passive motion protocols. A prospective randomized trial demonstrated greater finger ROM after an early active motion protocol compared to a passive ROM protocol without an increase in rupture rate. However, a recent systematic review on flexor tendon rehabilitation protocols did show a slightly higher rupture rate with early active protocols, although this was highly dependent on number of core sutures.

Each patient's rehabilitation is constantly reevaluated and adjusted based on an individual patient's progress, tissue response, the mechanism and zone of injury, strength of the repair, and amount of time since surgery. If there is persistent edema or wound healing issues, the progression in rehabilitation needs to be altered, and may ultimately affect outcome.

In our practice, the patient is seen approximately 3 days postoperatively for removal of the dressing, wound assessment, application of an immobilizing orthosis, and education in precautions and exercises. It is important to begin mobilization of the repaired tendon early, whether passively or actively, in order to increase nutrition to the repaired tendon through synovial diffusion, improve tendon excursion, and minimize the development of adhesions. The therapeutic regimen followed in the course of the recovery is dependent on the location of the flexor tendon injury.

Zones I to III

3 Days to 4 Weeks

- A dorsal blocking orthosis (DBO) is fit to the patient, with the wrist in 0° to 20° of flexion, the metacarpophalangeal (MCP) joints in 40° to 50° of flexion, and the interphalangeal (IP) joints in full extension. This will keep the healing tendon slack, while allowing full IP joint extension up to the limit of the orthosis, thereby limiting potential for flexion contractures at the IP joints (Figure 28.8)
- Passive flexion of digit(s) within the orthosis; active extension of (IP) joints to limit of DBO (Figures 28.9–28.11).
  - We believe that education of the patient at this point is crucial for a good outcome, utilizing exercise handouts and photo and/or video technology as needed.
- Once edema is decreased and there is good passive range of motion (PROM), synergistic place-and-hold exercises are initiated (Figure 28.12). The patient is instructed to passively flex the digits while simultaneously extending the wrist. Once this position is obtained, the patient is instructed to let go of the involved hand and hold the

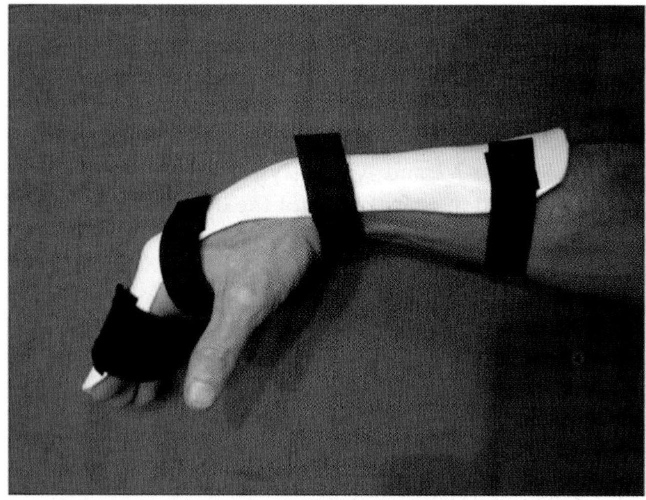

Figure 28.8 Photograph of a dorsal blocking orthosis (DBO).

© 2018 American Academy of Orthopaedic Surgeons

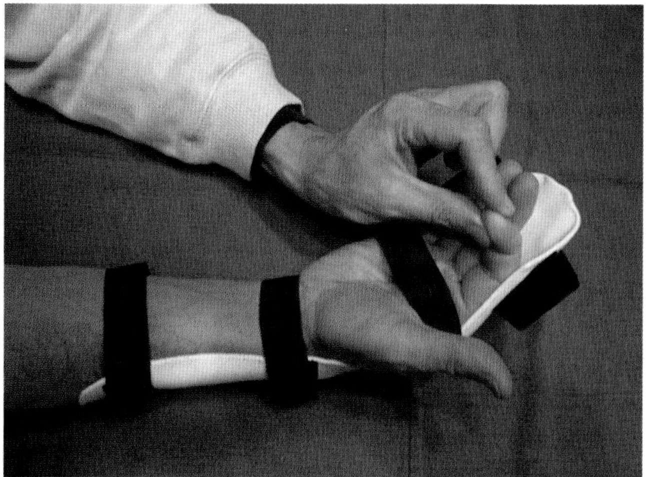

Figure 28.9 Photograph of passive flexion of the distal interphalangeal joint.

placed position for 5 seconds. The patient then releases the position, allowing the wrist to fall into flexion, which physiologically allows the digits to open into extension. The differential excursion between the two digital flexors is increased with the use of this synergistic motion, while minimizing the force required to achieve full active flexion.

4 Weeks to 7 or 8 Weeks

- The DBO is worn between exercise sessions and at night. If the original position of the DBO was flexed at the wrist, it should be brought to a neutral position.
- Active range of motion (AROM) of the digit in flexion and extension outside the orthosis with wrist in neutral. No composite (simultaneous) wrist and finger extension is performed.
- FDS gliding exercises, which involve active flexion of the PIP joints while maintaining DIP joints in extension. This can be done by flexing the PIP joint of the finger while maintaining the other fingers in extension.

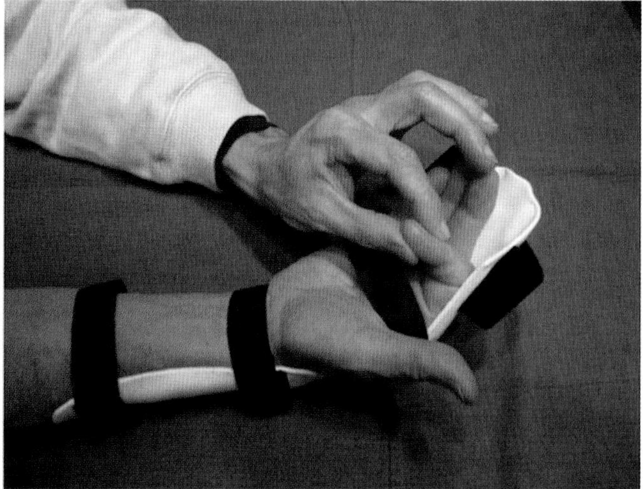

Figure 28.10 Photograph of passive flexion of the proximal interphalangeal joint.

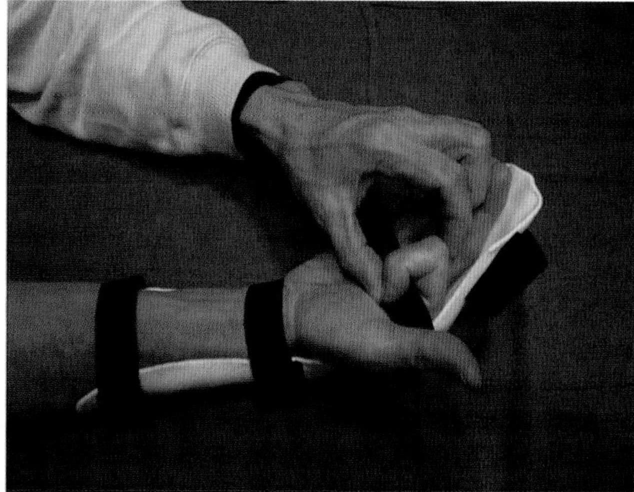

Figure 28.11 Photograph of composite, or simultaneous, passive flexion of the distal interphalangeal and proximal interphalangeal joints.

- Hook fisting, which involves maintaining the MCP joints in extension, while actively flexing the IP joints. This allows maximum glide between the FDS and the FDP.
- Composite flexion, which is simultaneous active flexion of all joints in the fingers.
- Blocking exercises at 5 to 6 weeks if tendon gliding is not sufficient; otherwise, these are held until 7 weeks postoperatively. Blocking exercises involve manually holding the MCP joint in extension while active flexing the PIP joint to isolate FDS glide, or holding both the MCP and PIP joints in extension while flexing the DIP joint to isolate FDP glide. Determination of appropriate gliding can be performed using either of the two methods to follow.
    - Total active motion (TAM) measurements are advocated by the American Society for Surgery of the Hand to better assess functional outcomes, but can also be used in the decision to advance exercises. TAM is determined by the sum of the degrees of active flexion at the MCP, PIP, and DIP joints, minus the degrees from full extension. Comparison of TAM and total passive motion (TPM) measurements can be used in the decision making process for the start of blocking exercises. If there is a 50° difference between TAM and TPM, then there are dense adhesions present, and blocking exercises can be initiated.
    - Another method for determining the start of flexion blocking exercises is to determine whether there is an active tendon lag (the difference between active and passive motion) and how responsive the lag is to the current exercise regime of tendon glides. If there is less than a 10% resolution of active lag between therapy sessions, then progression to blocking exercises is indicated.
- If flexion contractures are present, nighttime static-progressive extension splinting can be initiated at approximately 7 to 8 weeks postoperatively (Figure 28.13).

© 2018 American Academy of Orthopaedic Surgeons

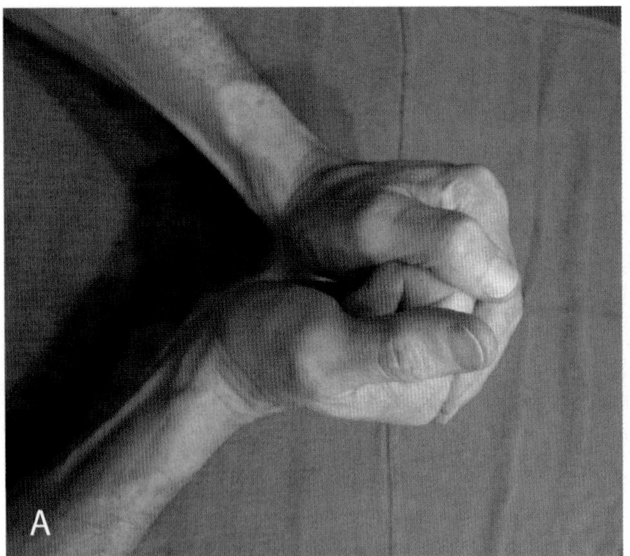

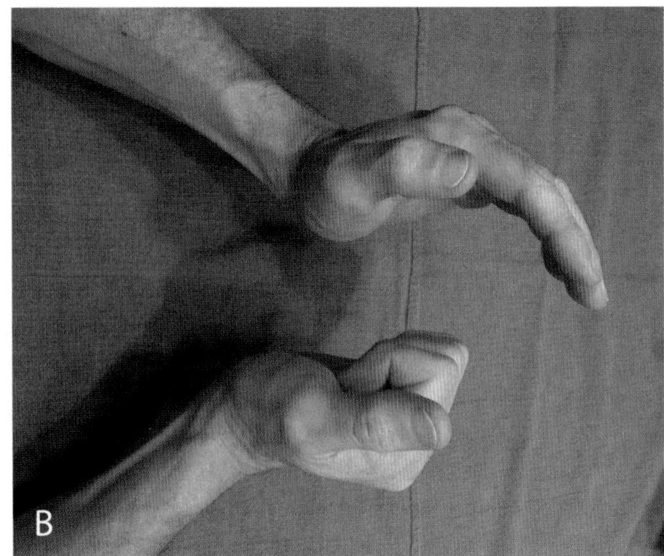

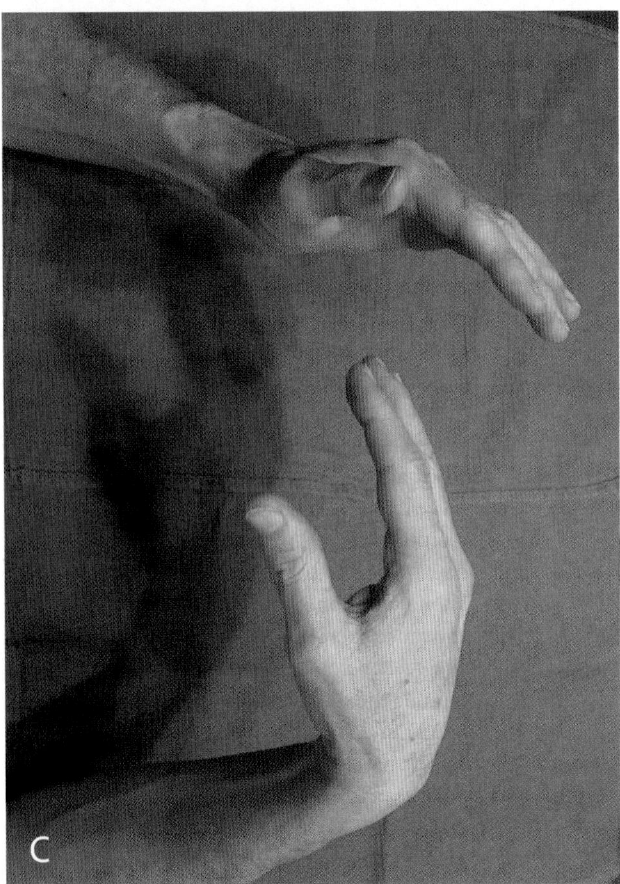

Figure 28.12 Photographs of synergistic place-and-hold exercises of the digits for the right hand. **A**, The patient passively flexes the digits and extends the wrist. **B**, The patient is instructed to hold this position for five seconds. **C**, The patient releases this position, allowing the wrist to fall into flexion, which passively extends the digits.

7 Weeks to 12 to 14 Weeks

- Discontinue the DBO. Continue nighttime extension splinting if needed.
- Hand use in light activities of daily living (ADLs) is encouraged, but no heavy sustained grasping.
- Progressive resistive exercises with gradually increased use of the hand each week. Exercises should begin with light grasping of handfuls of beans, crumpling paper, towel gathering, or sustained grasping of variously sized cylinders. The patient can be progressed to resistance exercises utilizing graded therapy putty or grippers.
- No restrictions at 12 to 14 weeks, allowing heavy hand use.

Complications

Even with the best surgical repair and postoperative rehabilitation, there are complications that may develop that can affect

© 2018 American Academy of Orthopaedic Surgeons

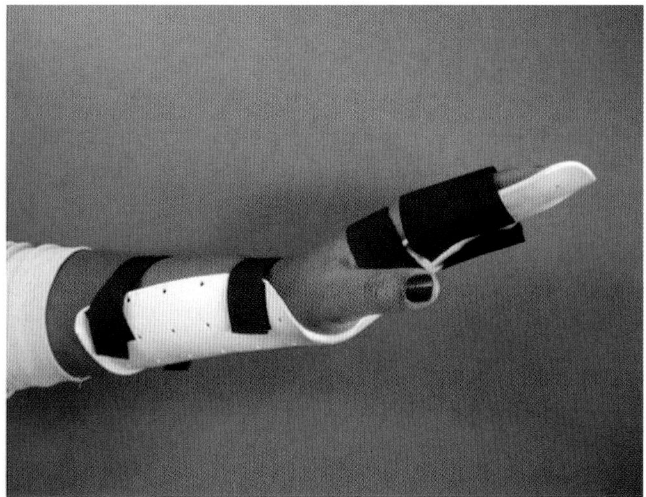

Figure 28.13 Photograph of a static-progressive extension splint, which can be used if flexion contractures have developed.

the ultimate functional outcome of the digit, including swelling/edema, tendon adhesions, joint contractures, infections, tendon gaps, and tendon ruptures. All of these situations must be closely monitored and treated appropriately for the best functional outcome.

Edema should be brought under control as quickly as possible after surgery, especially before active motion is begun. Edema increases friction and the work of flexion, which can disrupt the repair. Use of early compressive dressings, finger socks, self-adherent wrap, and elevation are all reasonable methods to decrease edema.

Tendon adhesions are the most common complication that is faced during postoperative rehabilitation. Postoperatively, methods to decrease adhesion formation include early motion, which can be either active or passive depending on the regimen. Although early motion programs have minimized the development of adhesions after flexor tendon surgery, it unfortunately remains a relatively common complication despite the therapist's and patient's best efforts. If adhesions are evident early in a patient's postoperative rehabilitation, advancement of the program could be considered. Groth describes a grading system for adhesions based on whether the adhesions are responsive or unresponsive to the current therapy modalities. The program is advanced or held back based on the therapist's determination of tissue response. This system is helpful in preventing and treating adhesions, but is also just as important in preventing gapping or ruptures of repairs, when there is insufficient development of scar. Therapeutic techniques for scar adhesions include, but are not restricted to, deep friction massage, ultrasound, use of electrical stimulation for stronger contractions, scar mobilizations with tendon pulls, therapy putty utilizing scraping motions, towel gathering, isolated tendon glides, and blocking exercises. Caution needs to be taken in repairs involving both the FDS and FDP, as blocking a PIP joint too vigorously to increase FDP function can rupture the FDS. It should be emphasized that these techniques must be utilized at the appropriate point in time based on the individual patient's postoperative course, as well as the strength of the repair.

Zones IV and V

3 Days to 4 Weeks

- The DBO is fit to the patient, with the wrist in 0° to 20° of flexion, the MCP joints in 40° to 50° of flexion, and the IP joints fully extended.
- Passive flexion of digits within the orthosis.
- Synergistic place and hold exercises as described above.
- Do not extend the wrist past neutral if a wrist flexor tendon was repaired in addition to a finger flexor tendon.

4 Weeks to 7 to 8 Weeks

- Continue DBO between exercise sessions and at night.
- At 6 to 7 weeks, wrist/hand/finger extension orthosis if extrinsic flexor tightness is evident.
- AROM of the wrist and fingers outside the orthosis, including composite extension.
- Gentle blocking exercises.
- Differential tendon gliding to avoid development of adhesions between the tendons. This is performed so that the tendons develop maximum excursion and move individually from one another. These exercises involve a series of motions, including a hook, full and straight fist (Figure 28.14).

7 to 12 Weeks

- Start light progressive strengthening, with unrestricted hand and wrist use by 12 weeks.

Complications

In Zone IV injuries, the development of intertendinous adhesions is a relatively common postoperative complication. In Zone V repairs, tendon adhesions to the overlying distal forearm soft tissues may cause skin dimpling with digital movement. In addition, owing to the relatively higher prevalence of concomitant median and/or ulnar nerve repairs in Zone V injuries, prolonged postoperative wrist immobilization may be necessary, which can lead to joint stiffness or contracture. In such cases, corrective splinting may be indicated once the nerve repair can tolerate stretch.

Flexor Pollicis Longus

With regard to rehabilitation, lacerations to the flexor pollicis longus (FPL) tendon are treated in a similar fashion to Zones I to III injuries of the digits.

3 Days to 4 Weeks

- A wrist/hand/thumb DBO is fit to the patient, with the wrist at 0° to 20° of flexion, the thumb in carpometacarpal (CMC) flexion, palmar abduction, MCP flexion, and IP extension (Figure 28.15).
  - Passive flexion of the thumb within the orthosis.
  - Active thumb IP extension to the limit of the orthosis.
  - Synergistic place-and-hold exercises, using the tenodesis concept. The wrist is passively extended while the thumb is simultaneously passively flexed. The patient is asked to hold that position for 5 seconds, then allow the wrist

© 2018 American Academy of Orthopaedic Surgeons

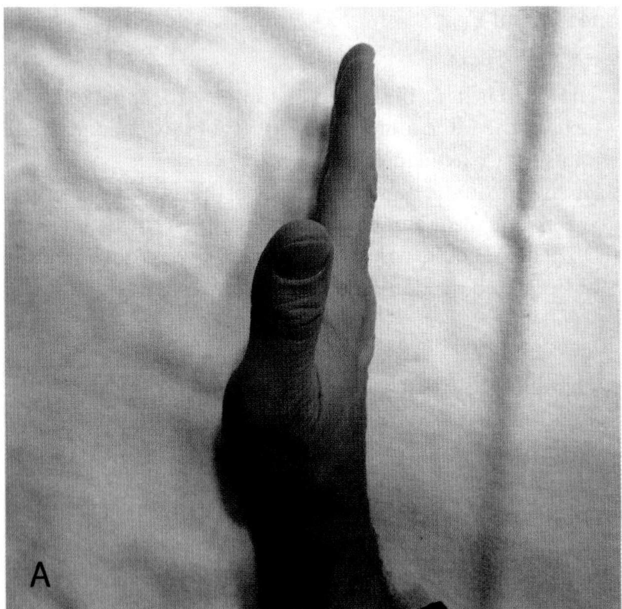

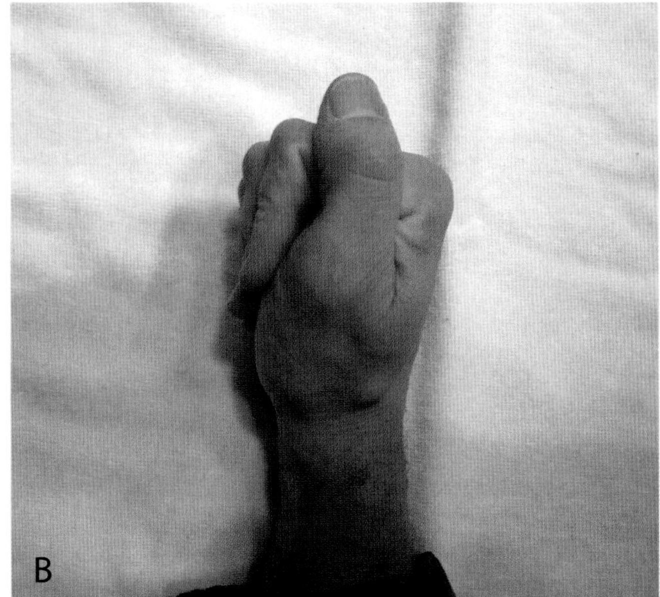

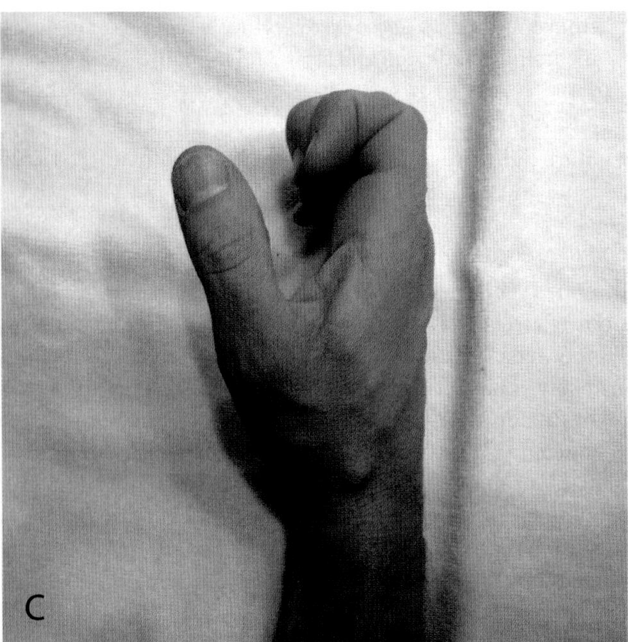

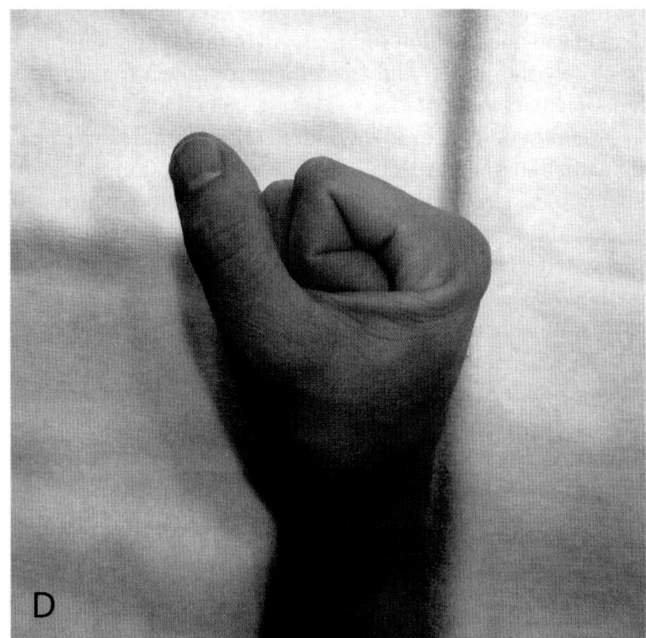

Figure 28.14 Photographs of differential tendon gliding exercises. Progression is performed from straight hand (**A**), to straight fist (**B**), to claw fist (**C**), to composite fist with simultaneous distal interphalangeal, proximal interphalangeal, and metacarpophalangeal flexion (**D**).

to relax into flexion, which physiologically causes the thumb to extend (Figure 28.16).

4 Weeks to 7 to 8 Weeks

- Continue the DBO at night and in between exercise sessions.
- AROM of the wrist and thumb outside the orthosis.
- Blocking exercises at 5 weeks if excursion is not good; otherwise, hold blocking if excursion is optimal.
- PROM of the thumb if extrinsic flexor tightness is noted.
- Nighttime static thumb and wrist extension orthosis if extrinsic tightness.

7 to 12 Weeks

- Discontinue the DBO.
- Continue static-extension orthosis if needed.
- Gradual strengthening exercises, with avoidance of heavy hand use and sustained strong pinch activities.
- Unrestricted hand use by 12 weeks.

Complications

Just as with all the flexor tendon zones that we have discussed, postoperative tendon adhesions are the most common complication after FPL repairs. It is important to note that, with FPL injuries, there may also be additional adhesions at the wrist if

© 2018 American Academy of Orthopaedic Surgeons

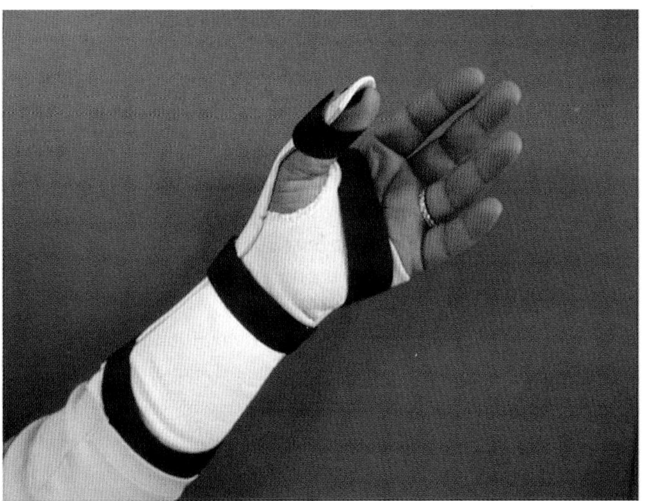

Figure 28.15 Photograph of a dorsal blocking orthosis used after a flexor pollicis longus repair.

the tendon had retracted far proximally and was retrieved intraoperatively from the level of the wrist, which is quite common.

TAKE-HOME PEARLS

Surgical Repair

- Minimizing the amount of time between injury and surgery (less than 1 week) can decrease the difficulty of the repair and optimize outcomes.
- Gentle and atraumatic surgical technique is helpful in preventing postoperative adhesions within the tendon sheath.
- Repair with a four-strand core suture and an epitendinous suture allows for light active grip during the weakest time for the repair, which occurs between 6 and 18 days postoperatively.
- In concomitant FDS/FDP injuries, an attempt is made to repair at least one slip of the FDS. After repair, it should be verified that this does not cause resistance to FDP tendon gliding.
- The A1, A3, and A5 pulleys can be sacrificed intraoperatively to decrease resistance to tendon gliding, while the A2 and A4 pulleys should be preserved to prevent bowstringing, but can be partially vented to improve gliding.

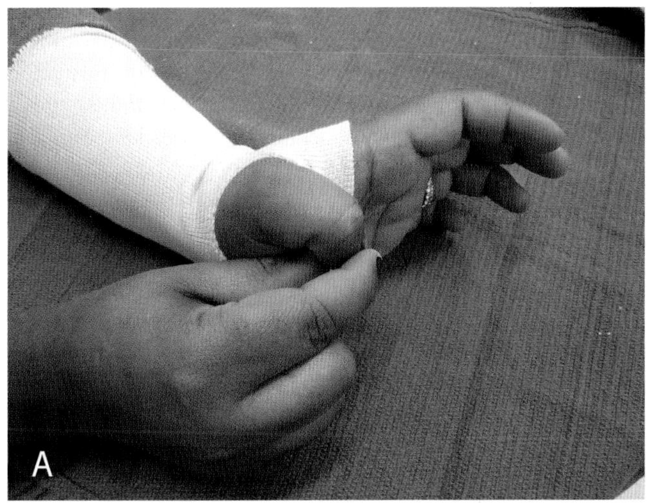

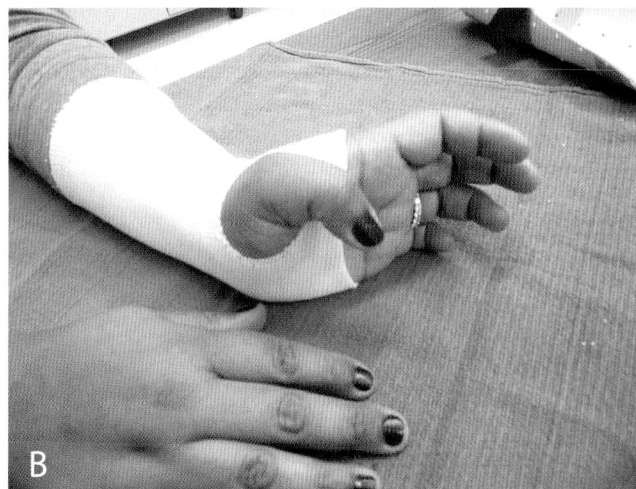

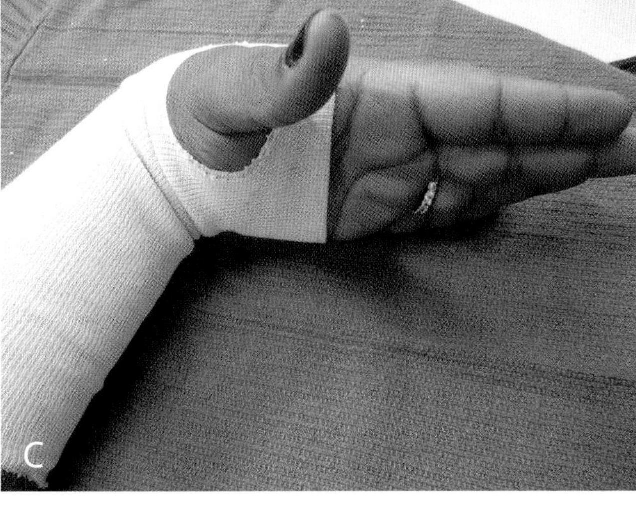

Figure 28.16 Photographs of synergistic place-and-hold exercises for the flexor pollicis longus. **A**, The wrist is passively extended while the thumb is passively flexed at the interphalangeal joint. **B**, The patient holds this position for five seconds. **C**, This position is then released, allowing the wrist to flex, which causes passive extension of the thumb.

© 2018 American Academy of Orthopaedic Surgeons

Rehabilitation

- Use edema control methods to decrease edema and inflammation prior to initiating early motion, which will reduce the work of flexion.
- To enhance understanding of the postoperative exercise regime and precautions, include photo/video instruction that the patient can take home.
- Prevent flexion contractures before they develop. Be sure to position the IP joints in full extension in the DBO.
- Utilize TAM measurements to assist in the decision-making process for the start of blocking exercises.
- Flexor tendon rehabilitation is not a "one-size-fits-all" approach. An individual's response to rehabilitation must be closely monitored.
- Active communication efforts between the hand surgeon and the hand therapist are vital to obtaining a good outcome, especially if complications develop during the rehabilitation process.

BIBLIOGRAPHY

Bishop AT, Cooney WP 3rd, Wood MB: Treatment of partial flexor tendon lacerations: the effect of tenorrhaphy and early protected mobilization. *J Trauma* 1986;26(4):301–312.

Groth GN: Pyramid of progressive force exercises to the injured flexor tendon. *J Hand Ther* 2004;17(1):31–42.

Harris SB, Harris D, Foster AJ, Elliot D: The aetiology of acute rupture of flexor tendon repairs in zones 1 and 2 of the fingers during early mobilization. *J Hand Surg Br* 1999;24(3): 275–280.

Lilly SI, Messer TM: Complications after treatment of flexor tendon injuries. *J Am Acad Orthop Surg* 2006;14(7):387–396.

Ruchelsman DE, Christoforou D, Wasserman B, Lee SK, Rettig ME: Avulsion injuries of the flexor digitorum profundus tendon. *J Am Acad Orthop Surg* 2011;19(3):152–162.

Savage R: In vitro studies of a new method of flexor tendon repair. *J Hand Surg Br* 1985;10(2):135–141.

Starr HM, et al: Flexor Tendon Repair Rehabilitation Protocols: a Systematic Review. *J Hand Surg Am* 2013;38-A(9):1712–1717. e1–e14.

Strickland JW: Flexor tendon repair: Indiana method. *Indiana Hand Center Newsletter* 1993;1:1–12.

Strickland JW: Flexor Tendon Injuries: I. Foundations of Treatment. *J Am Acad Orthop Surg* 1995;3(1):44–54.

Taras JS, Gray RM, Culp RW: Complications of flexor tendon injuries. *Hand Clin* 1994;10(1):93–109.

Trumble TE, Vedder NB, Seiler JG 3rd, Hanel DP, Diao E, Pettrone S: Zone-II flexor tendon repair: a randomized prospective trial of active place-and-hold therapy compared with passive motion therapy. *J Bone Joint Surg Am* 2010;92(6): 1381–1389.

Zhao C, Amado PC, Momose T, Couvreur P, Zobitz ME, An KN: Effect of synergistic wrist motion on adhesion formation after repair of partial flexor digitorum profundus tendon lacerations in a canine model in vivo. *J Bone Joint Surg Am* 2002;84-A(1):78–84.

© 2018 American Academy of Orthopaedic Surgeons

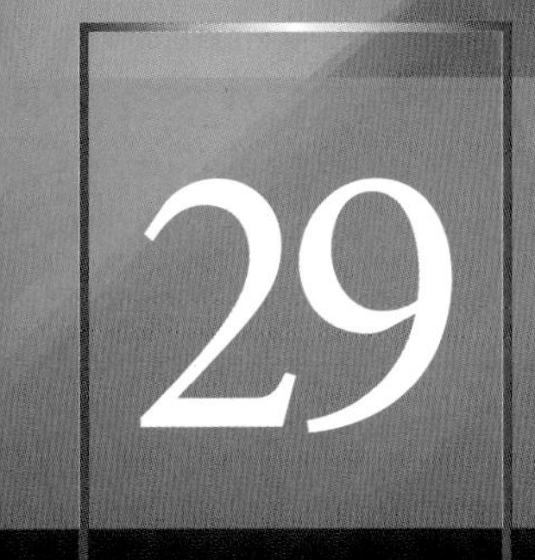

Extensor Tendon Repairs

Carol Recor, OTR/L, CHT, and Jerry I. Huang, MD

INTRODUCTION

Extensor tendon injuries of the fingers are quite common. However, since many extensor tendon lacerations are repaired in the emergency department, it is easy to disregard the impact and potential disability from an extensor tendon injury. While there is extensive published research regarding rehabilitation protocols following flexor tendon repairs, rehabilitation outcomes for extensor tendon repairs has received less attention.

The anatomy of the extensor tendons, with a flat profile and short distal excursion, combined with close approximation to bony structures and adjacent structures, requires thoughtful rehabilitation programs. In addition, the reduced size and tensile strength of finger extensor repairs, compared to that of flexor tendon repairs, require further consideration when advancing extensor tendon repair protocols. Failure of the extensor tendon repair leads of loss of digit extension, which can be quite disabling in activities of daily living (ADLs). Moreover, extensor tendon injuries can also lead to loss of finger flexion from scarring.

Due to the complex extensor tendon anatomy, there are a variety of injuries that present different scenarios for both surgical treatment and postoperative rehabilitation. Early intervention, with appropriate attention to the details and timing of therapy, is critical to achieving excellent functional outcomes. Communication between the surgeon and therapist is also critical, and the therapist's role in patient education and monitoring for any early extensor lag cannot be understated.

RELEVANT ANATOMY

The extensor mechanism of the hand is divided into eight anatomic zones. The odd-number zones are over the joints, starting with the distal interphalangeal (DIP) joint, and progress proximally; the even-numbered zones are over the bones. Zone VIII is over the distal forearm and contains the musculotendinous junction. In Zone VI, the junctura tendinae connect the extensor tendons of the middle, ring, and small fingers. Injuries proximal to the junctura are often missed, as patients can retain some extensor function. The location of an extensor tendon injury is important to consider in surgical decision-making, and directs the postoperative rehabilitation protocol.

SURGICAL TREATMENT

Indications

Extensor tendon injuries can occur from direct lacerations, complex open wounds, or from closed means with forced hyperflexion of the proximal interphalangeal (PIP) and DIP joints. Depending on the amount of tendon involvement and overlying soft-tissue injury, as well as associated bony injuries, operative intervention may be indicated. In general, surgical repair should be performed for tendon lacerations involving more than 50% of the tendon, or partial tendon lacerations with loss of finger extension strength. Injuries in Zones I through VI can often be irrigated and repaired primarily in the emergency department. If there is significant wound contamination or joint involvement, as in a Zone 5 "fight bite" injury over the metacarpophalangeal (MCP) joint, or soft-tissue loss, surgical débridement and repair should be performed in an operating room. More proximal injuries in Zones VII and VIII should also be treated in the operating room, as they often involve more extensive dissection for adequate surgical exposure. Surgical repair should be performed with 3-0 or 4-0 nonabsorbable sutures. Horizontal mattress or figure-of-eight sutures are used for more distal injuries, as the tendon is quite thin and flat. More proximally, if there is enough tendon substance, a core suture technique, such as a modified Bunnell or modified Kessler repair, is recommended.

Dr. Huang or an immediate family member is a member of a speakers' bureau or has made paid presentations on behalf of Arthrex and Trimed; serves as a paid consultant to Acumed and Arthrex; and serves as a board member, owner, officer, or committee member of the American Association for Hand Surgery, *the American Society for Surgery of the Hand, and the* Journal of Hand Surgery–American. *Neither Ms. Recor nor any immediate family member has received anything of value from or has stock or stock options held in a commercial company or institution related directly or indirectly to the subject of this article.*

© 2018 American Academy of Orthopaedic Surgeons

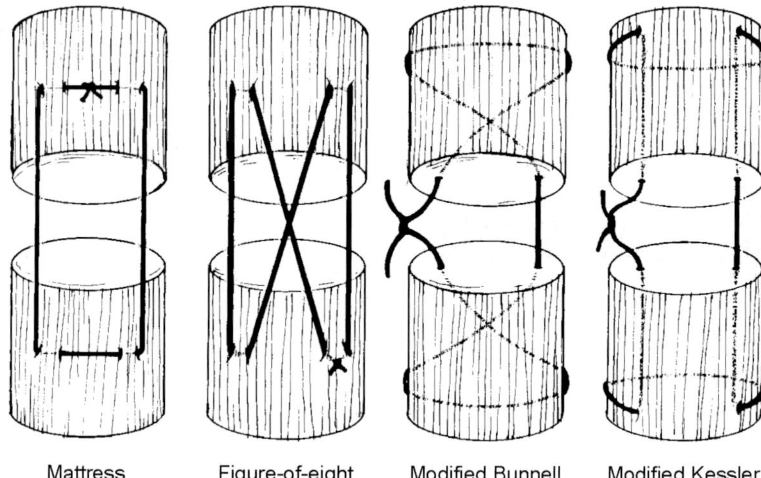

Figure 29.1 Illustration of four commonly used repair techniques for extensor tendon lacerations. (Reproduced with permission from Newport ML: Extensor tendon injuries in the hand. *J Am Acad Orthop Surg* 1997;5: 59–66.)

LACERATIONS AND OPEN INJURIES

Zones I and II

Procedure

We prefer performing extensor tendon lacerations in Zone I under local anesthesia with a digital nerve block. Our preferred skin incision is Y-shaped with a transverse limb over the DIP joint with midaxial incisions distally and proximal extensions dorsally over the midline. The terminal extensor injury in Zone I and Zone II lacerations is usually repaired with a figure-of-eight or horizontal mattress suture with nonabsorbable suture (4-0 nylon) (Figure 29.1). In more distal lacerations, the tendon is very thin and flat, and tenodermodesis is recommended, suturing the tendon and skin as one single layer. As it is very difficult to maintain the DIP joint in extension and protect the repair, it is best to pin the joint in extension with a 0.045-inch Kirschner wire (K-wire) and leave the PIP joint free. We bury the pin below skin and remove it at 8 weeks postoperatively under local anesthesia in the office.

Postoperative Rehabilitation

- A static thermoplast DIP splint is fitted at 5 to 7 days postoperatively to protect the distal tip of the digit and the K-wire until the K-wire is removed (Figure 29.2). The splint may be removed for showering.
- Use of the hand for heavy lifting or gripping is discouraged during this time until the K-wire is removed.
- PIP joint active range of motion (ROM) exercises are initiated at 2 weeks.
- Gentle active range of motion (AROM) is encouraged after pin removal.
- Specific instructions provided to the patient, to monitor for development of extensor lag.
- Orthosis should be resumed if extensor lag recurs, with progressive weaning of orthosis over the next 4 weeks.
- Active functional hand use will allow the patient to regain grip strength without applying additional stress to the extensor tendon.
- Home strengthening programs, such as Theraputty or similar strengthening modalities, should be avoided. Full unrestricted activities may be resumed at 8 weeks postoperatively in the absence of any extensor lag at the DIP joint.

Clinical Pearls

- Full thickness skin flaps should be elevated to minimize flap necrosis and wound problems. Careful elevation of the distal skin flap is performed to avoid injury to the germinal matrix.
- If mild extensor lag develops, we recommend use of an Oval-8 splint (3-Point Products, Stevensville, MD), which is adjusted to keep the PIP joint in slight flexion. This splint can be used for reverse blocking exercises to improve DIP joint extension (Figure 29.3).

Zone III

Procedure

Extensor lacerations of the central slip in this zone are often associated with open fractures and contaminated wounds;

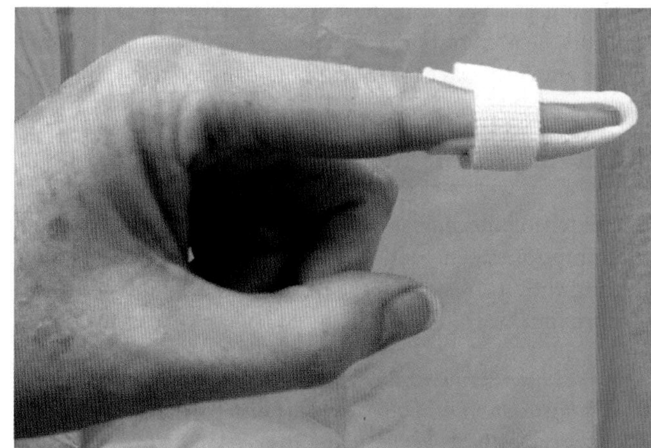

Figure 29.2 Photograph of a thermoplast clam-shell orthosis, which helps protect the K-wire tip over the fingertip as well as providing support to the distal interphalangeal joint.

 © 2018 American Academy of Orthopaedic Surgeons

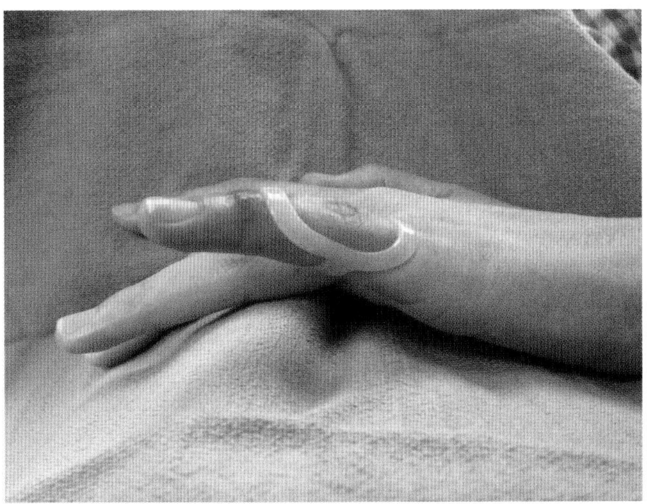

Figure 29.3 Photograph of an oval 8 splint to keep the proximal interphalangeal joint in slight flexion, allowing for reverse blocking extension exercises for the distal interphalangeal joint.

care should be taken to address the concomitant injuries. Thorough irrigation of the joint should be performed as well as repair of collateral ligament injuries. The surgical exposure is performed through a dorsal longitudinal incision over the PIP joint, incorporating the laceration. Alternatively, some surgeons prefer a curvilinear skin incision to avoid an incision directly over the lacerated tendon and repair sutures. Extensor tendon repair is performed with horizontal mattress or figure-of-eight sutures using nonabsorbable 3-0 or 4-0 sutures (Figure 29.1). Avulsion fractures off the dorsal base of the middle phalanx are common. With large fragments, fixation can be performed with 1.2-mm or 1.5-mm lag screws. With smaller fragments, surgical repair can be performed with 1 to 2 small suture anchors (1.8-mm or 2.2-mm anchors; Figure 29.4). If lacerated, the lateral bands are repaired separately using 5-0 or 6-0 sutures in a figure-of-eight fashion.

Postoperative Rehabilitation

- Thermoplastic orthosis is used with the PIP joint in full extension to avoid extensor lag and the DIP joint left free for active motion (Figure 29.5). The authors prefer a three-quarter circumferential thermoplastic orthosis, which provides adequate support on both the dorsal and volar surfaces of the digit, with easy accommodation for fluctuations in edema.
- Orthosis is used continuously for 6 weeks.
- Active DIP joint ROM is initiated immediately, with the orthosis in place. This provides a mechanism for blocking exercises to isolate the DIP joint only. Active DIP joint flexion will pull the lateral bands dorsally and allow reapproximation of the central slip.
- Protected isolated active PIP flexion is initiated at 2 weeks, beginning with 15° of active flexion and increasing flexion an additional 15° each week. This is accomplished with a

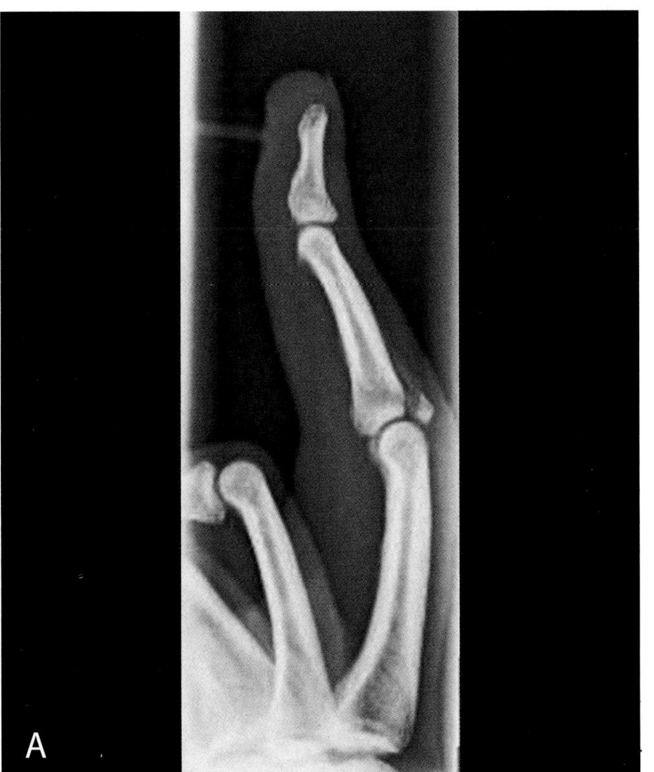

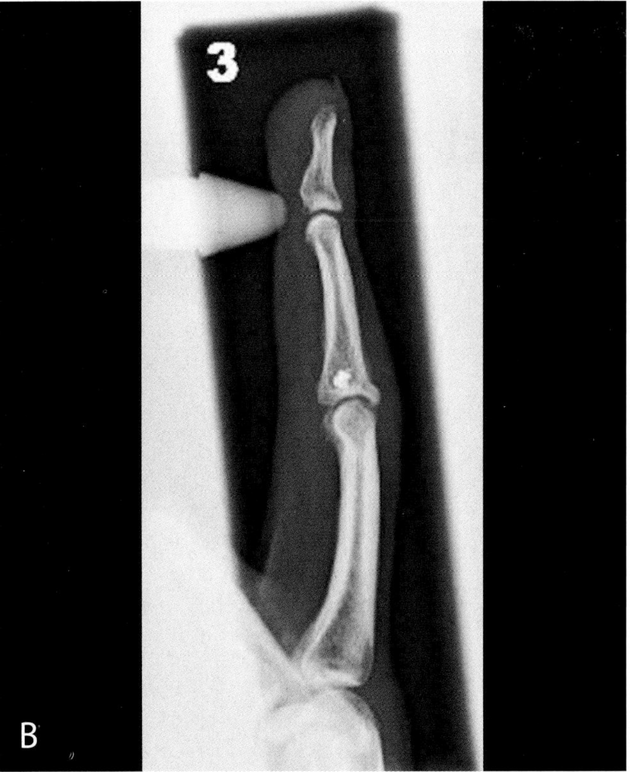

Figure 29.4 **A**, Plain radiograph of the base of a middle phalanx avulsion fracture of the central slip. **B**, Plain radiograph of fracture in **A** showing treatment with suture anchors with intraosseous sutures passed through the avulsion fragment.

© 2018 American Academy of Orthopaedic Surgeons

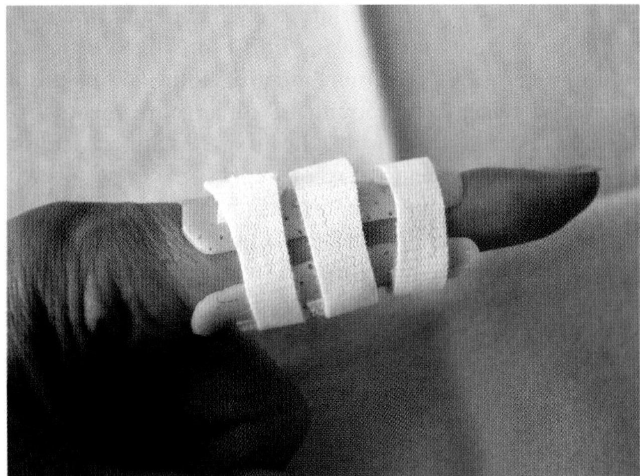

Figure 29.5 Photograph of thermoplast orthosis with proximal interphalangeal joint in full extension.

progressive exercise orthosis, which the patient is using as a guide to block excessive flexion (Figure 29.6). Not only will this prevent a tendon rupture, it will also minimize the development of an extensor lag from early dorsal scar adhesions from immobilization.

- If an extensor lag is noted, early protected active motion is discontinued for at least 1 week while the PIP joint is immobilized in full extension.
- Combined IP joint flexion is initiated at 6 weeks postoperatively.
- Orthosis is discontinued during the day at 6 weeks, with continued use of static PIP extension splinting at night for an additional 2 to 4 weeks.
- Gentle passive composite flexion may be initiated at 8 weeks postoperatively, with careful monitoring for development of extensor lag.
- A static-progressive flexion orthosis may be required if composite flexion is limited and there is no evidence of extensor lag. Use of orthosis should be limited to short duration (no longer than 20 minutes per session) and low tension to avoid recurrent extensor lag.
- Gentle strengthening program, using light-resistance Theraputty, is initiated at 8 weeks postoperatively.
- Return to full, unlimited activity at 12 weeks postoperatively.

Clinical Pearls

- Reverse blocking exercises may be performed at 6 weeks, if an extensor lag has developed.
- Use of a relative motion flexion orthosis as a method for reverse blocking exercises allows AROM of all digits, with the affected digit positioned in relative flexion to the unaffected digits (Figure 29.7).

Zones IV through VII

Procedure

Extensor tendon lacerations in Zones IV through VII are repaired with nonabsorbable 3-0 or 4-0 core sutures. The authors' preferred technique is a 4-strand repair with 3-0 nonabsorbable sutures using a modified Kessler technique, augmented with a figure-of-eight suture. In Zones IV and V or in smaller tendons, 4-0 nylon sutures are used. In Zones VI and VII, where the tendon is wider more proximally, 3-0 Ethibond is used. Zone VI tendon lacerations are often missed and not recognized, as extension (albeit weak and sometimes incomplete) of the injured digit is still possible through the junctura

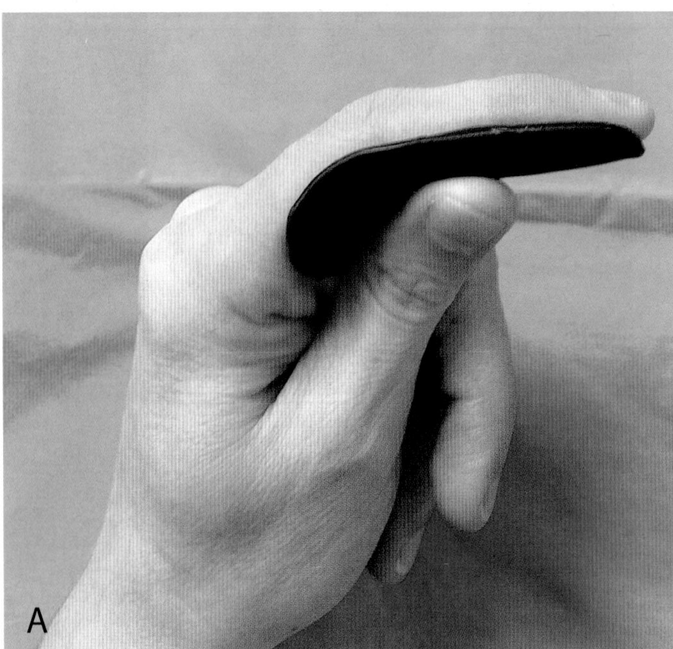

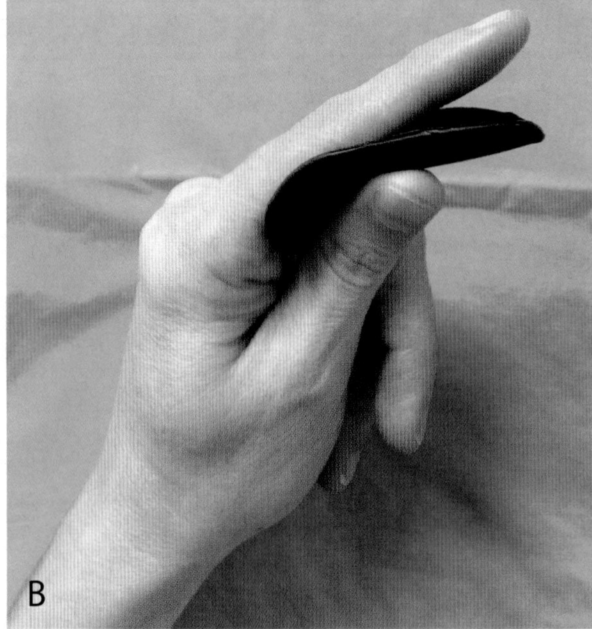

Figure 29.6 **A**, **B**, Photographs of progressive exercise templates, which allow for block against excessive flexion and reverse blocking exercises for proximal interphalangeal joint extension.

 © 2018 American Academy of Orthopaedic Surgeons

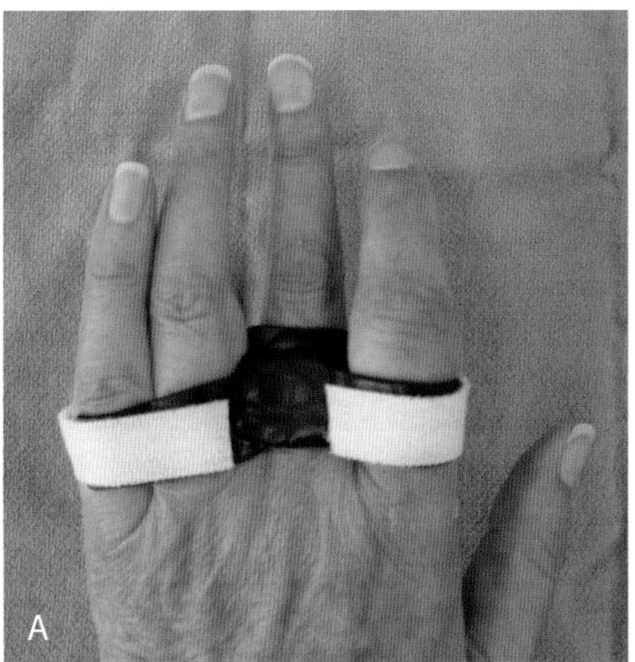

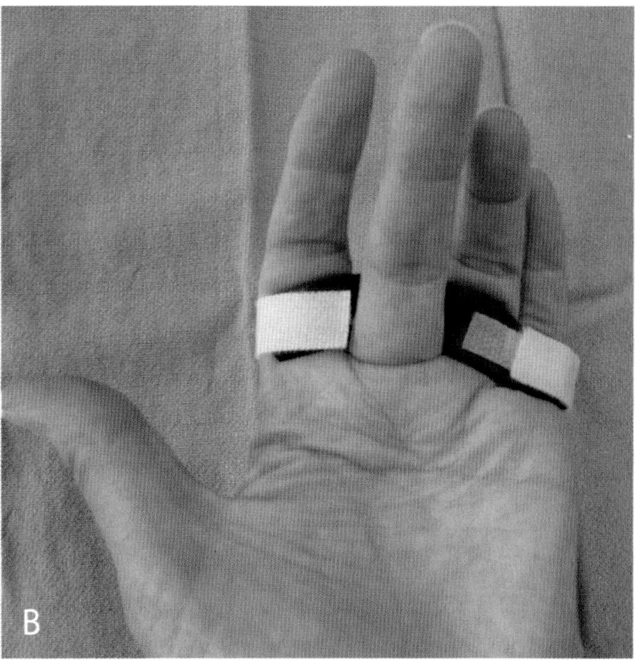

Figure 29.7 **A**, **B**, Photographs of relative motion flexion orthoses, which allow for reverse blocking exercises to improve proximal interphalangeal and distal interphalangeal joint extension.

tendinae from the adjacent digits. It is important to examine extension of the digit with the other uninjured digits in full MCP flexion in order to isolate the tendon in question.

Postoperative Rehabilitation

Historically, extensor tendon repairs in Zones IV to VII were treated postoperatively with either a dynamic or static-extension orthosis. Dynamic orthoses are cumbersome and more difficult to fabricate. A static forearm–based orthosis that immobilizes the wrist and MCP joints in extension but allows for early interphalangeal (IP) joint motion is more popular for the simplicity in orthosis fabrication and the rehabilitation protocol (Figure 29.8). However, early protected active motion, with the use of the relative motion orthosis, as described by Howell et al., provides an alternative approach for the compliant patient. This protocol requires use of a finger yoke and a wrist orthosis (Figure 29.9). The finger yoke orthosis positions the affected digit(s) in 25° of MP joint hyperextension relative to the adjoining digits. Active digit flexion and extension is allowed within the limits of the orthosis.

Relative Motion Orthosis Protocol

- Begin early active motion protocol with use of a relative motion orthosis at 5 to 7 days postoperatively, allowing

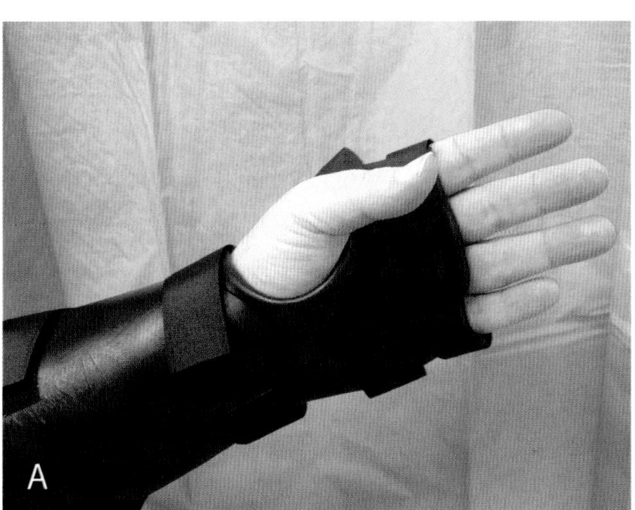

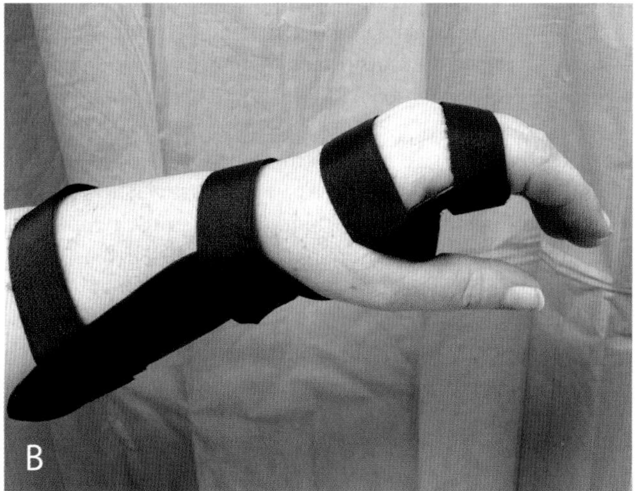

Figure 29.8 **A**, **B**, Photographs of static forearm-based orthoses with metacarpophalangeal joints immobilized and interphalangeal joints left free for active ROM.

© 2018 American Academy of Orthopaedic Surgeons

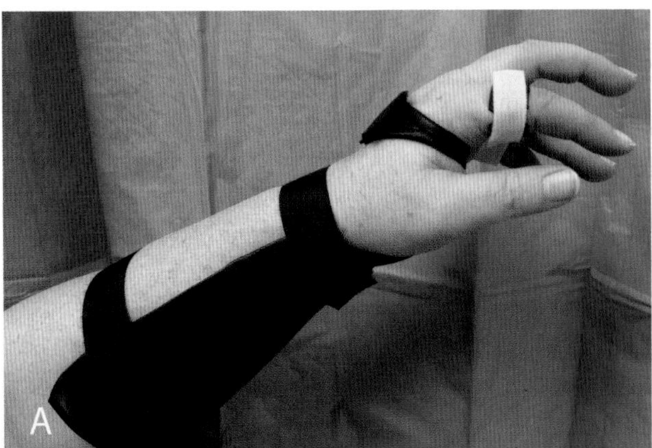

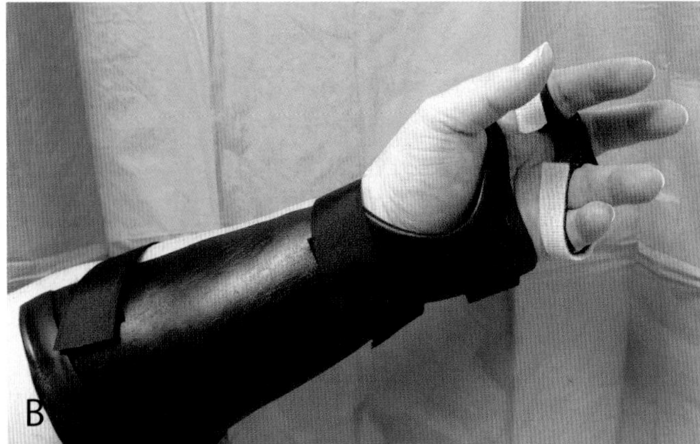

Figure 29.9 **A**, **B**, Photographs of relative motion extension orthosis protocol, allowing early protected motion for extensor tendon repairs in Zones IV to VII.

early digit flexion and extension within the limits of the finger orthosis.

- The wrist orthosis is discontinued at 3 weeks postoperatively, with continued use of the finger yoke orthosis for 2 more weeks. The patient uses the wrist orthosis for risky, heavy activities only.
- At 5 weeks postoperatively, the wrist orthosis is completely discontinued for all activities, with continued use of the finger orthosis. The finger yoke orthosis is continued for the next 1 to 2 weeks.
- Composite wrist and digit flexion is gradually increased at 6 weeks postoperatively.
- Return to full activity at 8 weeks post-op.

Static Extension Orthosis Protocol

- The relative motion orthosis and protocol cannot be used when all four digits are involved. In this situation, the forearm-based static orthosis is fabricated, with the wrist in 30° of extension and MP joints in 30° of flexion. IP joints are left free for immediate active flexion and extension.
- Orthosis is worn continuously, with removal under supervision of the therapist for the first weeks. Gentle tenodesis exercises are allowed under guidance of the therapist during this time, to increase tendon excursion and minimize dorsal adhesions.
- Gentle progression of AROM of digits is allowed for the next 2 weeks.
- AROM and passive range of motion (PROM) of the wrist and digits is allowed at 6 weeks postoperatively.
- Early intervention may be required if there is evidence of extensor lag, including immobilization in full extension for an additional 2 weeks.
- Zone VII repairs require the wrist to be positioned at neutral in the orthosis, to allow tendon excursion in relation to the retinaculum.

Clinical Pearls

- Paper tape or stretch athletic tape can be applied to dorsal scar adhesions, creating a gentle shear force and decreasing extensor lag in Zones V to VII (Figure 29.10).

CLOSED EXTENSOR TENDON INJURIES

Zone I Mallet Finger

The majority of closed mallet injuries with avulsion fracture of the dorsal base of the distal phalanx are treated conservatively with splint immobilization, which can be effective even in subacute injuries that are up to 3 months old. Excellent outcomes with minimal extensor lag can be expected from nonoperative management even with large bony fragments involving more than 40% to 50% of the articular surface. A wide variety of splints or orthoses are available to manage acute mallet deformities. All splints should position the DIP joint in full extension, avoiding excessive hyperextension and blanching of the skin to protect vascular integrity of the distal tip. Nevertheless, there are occasional instances when operative treatment is pursued.

Indications

Reduction and pinning of mallet fingers is recommended for patients whose occupation makes continuous splint wear challenging, such as dentists and surgeons, and those

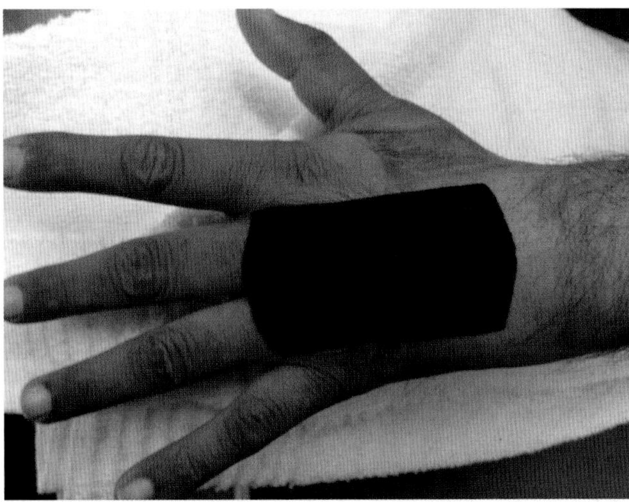

Figure 29.10 Photograph of tape applied over scar, which can create gentle shear forces to decrease adhesions.

© 2018 American Academy of Orthopaedic Surgeons

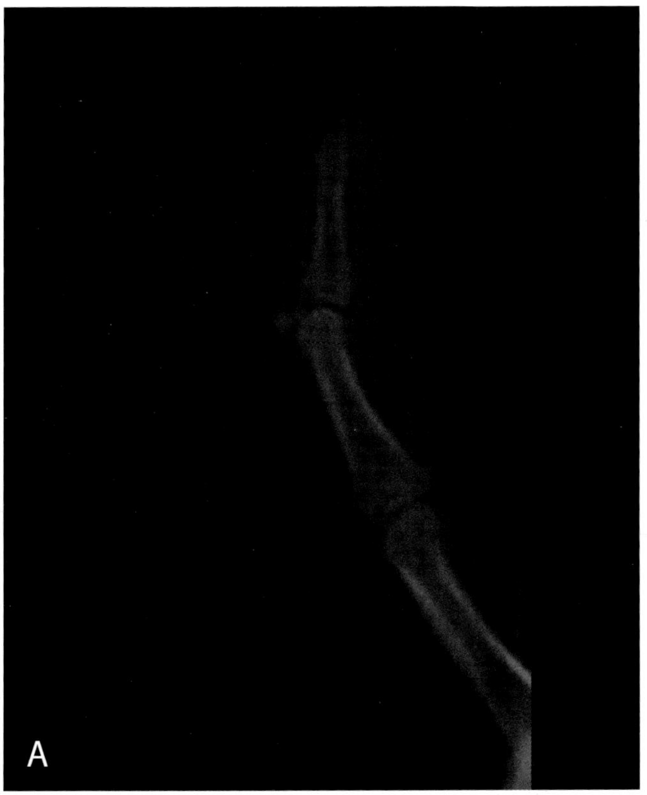

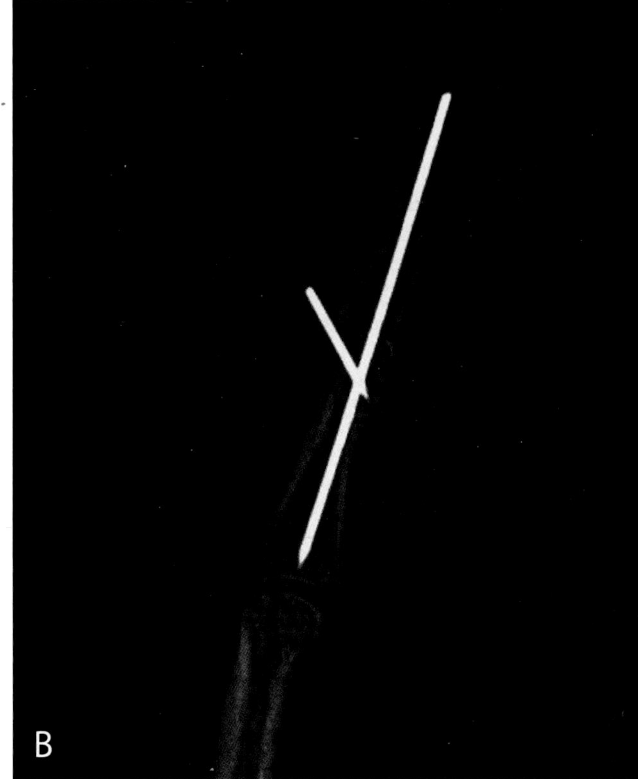

Figure 29.11 **A**, Plain radiograph of a patient with a bony mallet involving 40% of the articular surface. **B**, Plain radiograph of the same patient" extension block pinning was performed with a 0.045-inch K-wire through the head of the middle phalanx, followed by extension of the distal interphalangeal joint, and pinning of the distal interphalangeal joint with a second 0.045-inch K-wire.

who have failed a trial of conservative management for over 12 weeks. Open surgical treatment of bony mallet injuries is recommended if there is subluxation of the DIP joint.

Nonoperative Treatment

- Multiple orthoses options
- Over-the-counter Stax™ splints (Brown Medical Industries, Hartley, IA) may apply excessive pressure along the edge of the nailbed, especially if there is significant postinjury edema.
- Dorsal mallet splints or orthoses allow more functional use of the affected digit, with the volar pad of the digit partially exposed. However pressure ulcers can be a problem as well as skin maceration.
- Volar aluminum splints not as effective in maintaining full extension.
- Volar thermoplast orthoses (authors' preferred protocol) can achieve slight hyperextension positioning of the DIP joint without excess pressure on the dorsal skin.
- Volar orthosis can be used at night while sleeping, alternating with a dorsal orthosis during the day.
- Orthosis should be used for a full 8 weeks.
- Maintain the DIP joint in hyperextension while changing splints.
- Gradually weaning from the orthosis will provide the best outcome, with removal of the splint by one additional hour every 2 to 3 days and continued use of the splint at night for 4 more weeks.
- Strengthening exercises should be avoided, as the strength of the flexors can easily create an imbalance and a recurrent extensor lag.

Procedure

With closed soft-tissue mallet injuries, the joint should be positioned in neutral extension or slight hyperextension and fixed with a 0.045-inch K-wire. It is important to avoid excessive dorsal position of the K-wire to avoid injury to the nail matrix. In a bony mallet injury, extension block pinning is recommended rather than open reduction and internal fixation (ORIF) of the mallet fragment (Figure 29.11). First, a 0.045-inch K-wire is placed through the head of the middle phalanx, just dorsal to the bony fragment while the DIP joint is being held in flexion. The DIP joint is slightly hyperextended to reduce the joint, and fixed with a 0.045-inch K-wire. The K-wires can be buried just below the skin and removed in the office at 8 weeks with local anesthesia. Complications of pinning of mallet fingers include nail deformity, pin traction infection, osteomyelitis, and post-traumatic arthritis of the DIP joint (Figure 29.12).

Postoperative Rehabilitation

- Five to 7 days postoperatively, dressings are removed and patient is fitted with a custom thermoplastic clam-shell orthosis for protection.
- The orthosis may be removed for hygiene and light ADLs, but should be worn for heavy activities.

© 2018 American Academy of Orthopaedic Surgeons

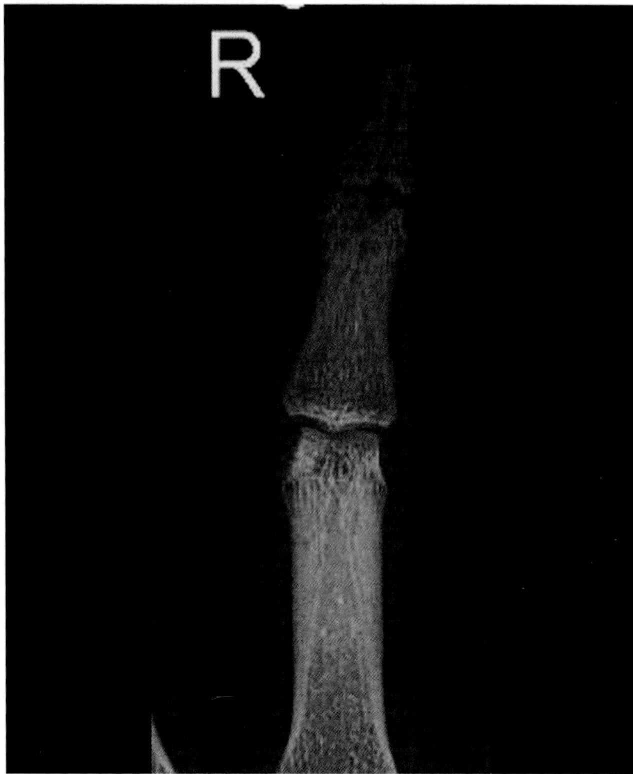

Figure 29.12 Plain radiograph of a patient who developed post-traumatic arthritis of the distal interphalangeal joint following pinning of a mallet injury.

- Following K-wire removal at 8 weeks, the patient may discontinue use of the orthosis during the day, but may benefit from its continued use for an additional 2 weeks at night.
- Begin gentle active isolated DIP joint motion, as well as composite digit flexion following K-wire removal.

Strengthening exercises should be avoided, as the strength of the flexors can easily create an imbalance and a recurrent extensor lag.

Clinical Pearl

- If preexisting hypermobility is present, use of a full-finger orthosis in a boutonnière position can prevent early swan-neck deformity (Figure 29.13).

Zone V Sagittal Band Rupture

Procedure

Acute sagittal band ruptures rarely require surgery and do well with referral to hand therapy and orthotic management. Most commonly, the radial sagittal band ruptures with ulnar subluxation of the central extensor tendon. Patients present to clinic with inability to extend the MCP joint of the affected digit. Specifically, patients are unable to attain full MCP extension from a flexed posture, but when placed in MCP extension, patients are able to maintain extension as the tendon is located in extension. Surgery is recommended for patients who fail a trial of conservative management with use of an orthosis. In subacute injuries, primary repair of the radial sagittal band can be performed using 4-0 nonabsorbable sutures in a figure-of-eight fashion. In chronic sagittal band injuries, reconstruction of the sagittal band can be performed using the lateral one-third of the central tendon. A longitudinal incision is made over the dorsum of the hand, centered over the MCP joint and full thickness skin flaps are elevated with identification of the extensor mechanism. A distally based slip of the lateral one-third of the central tendon is routed from proximal to distal, deep to the intermetacarpal ligament, then sutured back to the central tendon.

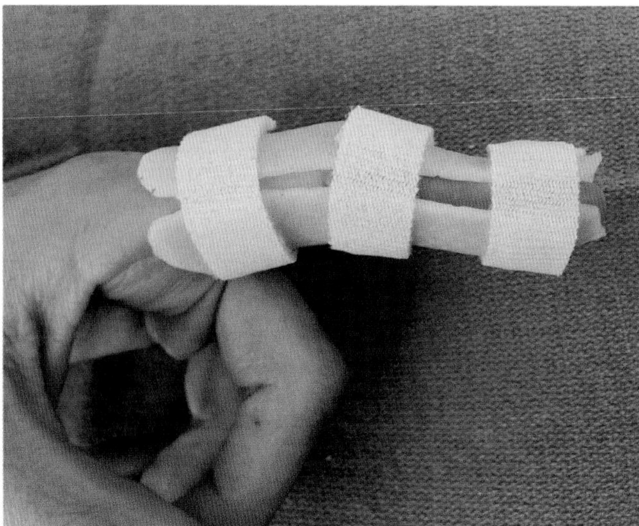

Figure 29.13 Photograph of the use of a boutonnière position in a patient with Zone I injury with preexisting hypermobility, which can avoid early swan-neck deformity.

Postoperative Rehabilitation

For those patients who failed conservative management and required surgical intervention of acute sagittal band ruptures, use of the relative motion finger extension orthosis is advocated post-operatively.

- The affected digit is positioned in 25° of hyperextension relative to the unaffected digits. The orthosis must be worn for 6 weeks continuously.
- Strengthening exercises are not advised.
- For those patients who may not be considered a good candidate for the relative motion orthosis protocol, a hand-based thermoplastic orthosis is used, positioning the MP joint in slight hyperextension and leaving the IP joints free for active motion (Figure 29.14).

Patients with a static extension orthosis would be expected to demonstrate significant MP joint stiffness following removal of the orthosis, from prolonged immobilization. These patients may require more extensive rehabilitation to correct an extension contracture of the MP joint.

Authors' Preferred Protocol

- Relative motion finger extension orthosis for 6 weeks, with careful monitoring of extensor tendon alignment with digit

© 2018 American Academy of Orthopaedic Surgeons

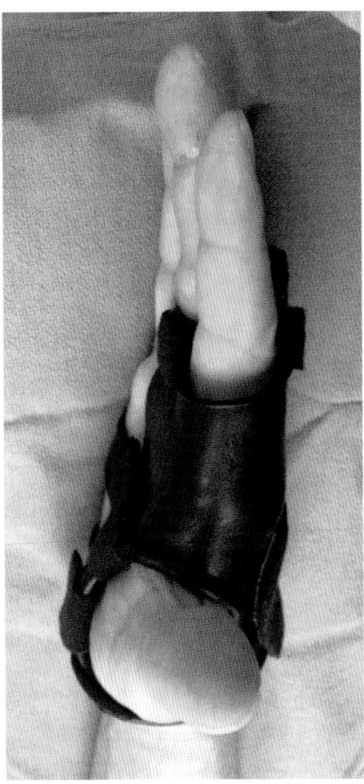

Figure 29.14 Photograph of immobilization of the metacarpophalangeal joint in full extension following sagittal band rupture and surgical repair.

flexion. With the orthosis on, there should not be any tension applied to surgical repair with active flexion. If tension is noted, the MP joint of the affected digit should be placed in greater hyperextension relative to adjacent digits.

Clinical Pearl

- For patients with MP joint extension contracture, use of an IP joint extension orthosis while performing active MP joint flexion will allow more efficient exercises (Figure 28.15).

Thumb Extensor Pollicis Longus Repair (EPL)

Procedure

Lacerations of the EPL tendon are repaired with modified Kessler core sutures using 3-0 or 4-0 nonabsorbable sutures. With Zone I injuries, the repair is protected by pinning the IP joint in slight hyperextension with a 0.045-inch K-wire. With EPL tendon ruptures, which often occur in the setting of conservative management of nondisplaced distal radius fractures, primary repair is not possible. Treatment options include tendon reconstruction with an intercalary palmaris tendon autograft or an extensor indicis propius to extensor pollicis longus tendon transfer.

Postoperative Rehabilitation

Postoperative treatment of surgical repairs of the thumb extensor tendon requires an initial period of splinting with early protected motion, forearm-based static extension orthosis,

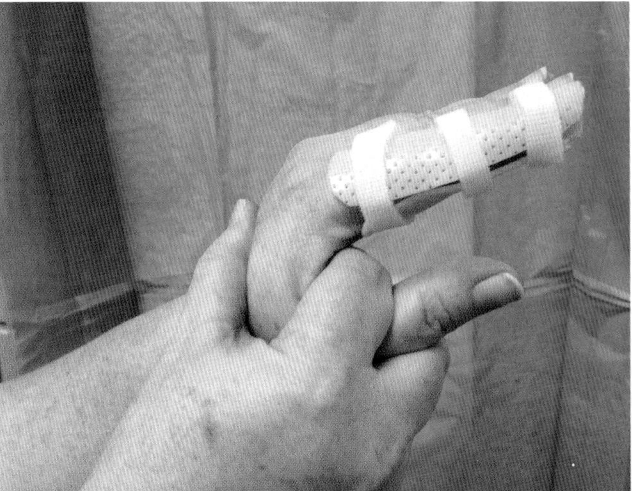

Figure 29.15 Photograph of immobilization of the interphalangeal joints with active metacarpophalangeal joint flexion, which can decrease metacarpophalangeal joint extension contracture.

with the wrist positioned in 30° of extension, and thumb MP and IP joint in full extension.

- Forearm-based static extension orthosis; wrist 30° of extension and thumb MP and IP joints in full extension (Figure 29.16).
- A hand-based thermoplastic thumb spica orthosis can also be used, with the orthosis extended distally on the thumb to allow for no more than 30° to 40° of IP joint flexion.

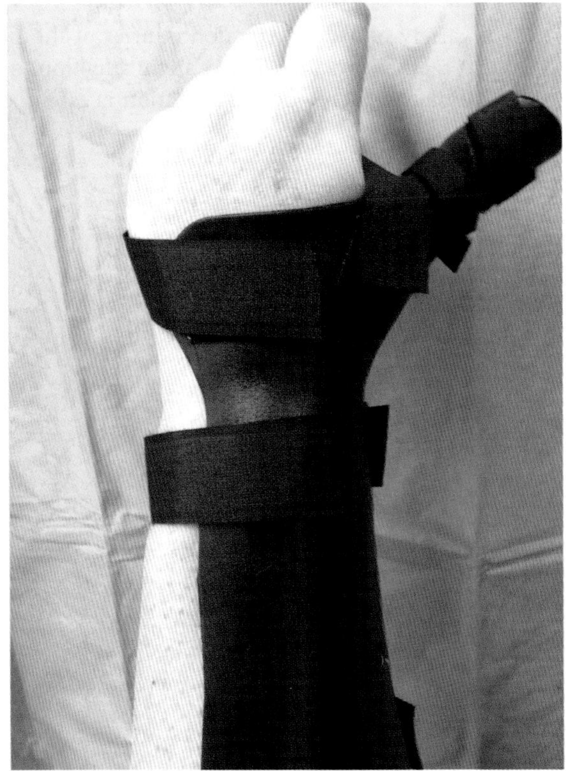

Figure 29.16 Photograph of a protective dorsal forearm-based orthosis following extensor pollicis longus laceration and repair.

© 2018 American Academy of Orthopaedic Surgeons

- Early protected motion can be initiated at 2 weeks postoperatively, allowing 10° of isolated flexion of the thumb MP and IP joints, followed by passive extension. Exercises are performed in the therapy clinic only for the first week, until the patient is able to demonstrate the home program.
- As with Zone I and Zone III extensor tendon repairs of the digits, an exercise splint can be provided to the patient to prevent flexion of the joints beyond the desired amount. Flexion is increased 10° each week.
- At 4 weeks postoperatively, gentle tenodesis exercises are initiated.
- At 6 weeks postoperatively, the orthosis is discontinued during the day. If there is evidence of extensor lag, night time orthosis is continued for an additional 2 to 4 weeks.
- At 8 weeks postoperatively, a home strengthening program may be initiated.
- At 10 weeks postoperatively, return to full activity, without limitations.

Clinical Pearls

- Patients require approximately 30° of thumb IP joint flexion to be able to perform pinch activities.
- Prolonged immobilization without early protected motion may create dorsal adhesions that would limit IP joint flexion and, therefore, making it functionally difficult to perform fine motor tasks.

SUMMARY

There are a variety of extensor tendon injuries of the hand and wrist that require surgical repair. Careful attention to the postoperative management and rehabilitation is essential to the successful outcome. Specific therapy protocols and time frames can provide a foundation for therapists, but strict adherence to protocols is not always in the best interest of the patient. Decisions regarding early active motion should be based on each patient's physiologic healing response, with early stiffness and scar formation used as a guide to advance protected motion more quickly. In addition, a patient's ability to comply with a home exercise program and orthotic use must be factored in to the rehabilitation program.

BIBLIOGRAPHY

Chester DL, Beale S, Beveridge L, Nancarrow JD, Titley OG: A prospective, controlled, randomized trial comparing early active extension with passive extension using a dynamic splint in the rehabilitation of repaired extensor tendons. *J Hand Surg Br* 2002;27:283–288.

Evans, RB: Immediate active short arc motion following extensor tendon repair. *Hand Clin* 1995;11(3):483–512.

Howell JW, Merritt WH, Robinson, SJ: Immediate controlled active motion following zone 4–7 extensor tendon repair. *J Hand Ther* 2005;18:182–190.

Howell JW, Peck F: Rehabilitation of flexor and extensor tendon injuries in the hand: current updates. *Injury, Int J Care Injured* 2013;44:397–402.

O'Brien LJ, Bailey MJ: Single blind, prospective, randomized controlled trial comparing dorsal aluminum and custom thermoplastic splints to stack splint for acute mallet finger. *Arch Phys Med Rehabil* 2011;92:191–198.

Pike J, Mulpuri K, Metzger M, Ng G, Wells N, Goetz T: Blinded, prospective, randomized clinical trial comparing volar, dorsal, and custom thermoplastic splinting in treatment of acute mallet finger. *J Hand Surg Am* 2010;35:580–588.

© 2018 American Academy of Orthopaedic Surgeons

30 Tenolysis: Flexor and Extensor

Gleb Medvedev, MD, and Elisa J. Knutsen, MD

INTRODUCTION

Trauma to flexor and extensor tendons can cause adhesion formation that inhibits motion. Early motion therapy protocols following tendon injury are aimed at disrupting these adhesions. However, when the results of therapy have been exhausted, tenolysis is a salvage procedure to remove those adhesions and improve motion. Tenolysis should not be undertaken lightly since it is another insult to an already traumatized finger, and carries the risk of tendon rupture as well as decreased innervation and blood supply to the previously injured digit. Following tenolysis, the patient must be active in the postoperative treatment at home and with the therapist. To that end, the patient must demonstrate a history of compliance with therapy prior to tenolysis, and have confirmed access to a hand therapist. Before proceeding to tenolysis, the patient must have anatomically aligned and healed fractures, coverage of any open wounds with soft and supple skin, intact tendons, good muscle strength, and near full passive range of motion (ROM).

FLEXOR TENOLYSIS

Indications

Flexor tendons need to be able to glide within the flexor tendon sheath to function properly. Adhesions, which form as part of the healing process following trauma—such as a crush injury, infection, or laceration of the tendon—interfere with tendon gliding and can cause loss of motion. The indication for tenolysis is decreased active flexion ROM compared to passive flexion in patients who have reached a plateau in their rehabilitation. The timing of tenolysis is generally 3 months after the injury or tendon repair, with a 4- to 8-week plateau of progress in hand therapy. This allows adequate time for healing of tendon repairs and softening of the covering tissues. Other prerequisties to tenolysis include healing of all finger fractures, mobilization of joint contractures, and the patient must be compliant and motivated to actively participate in the postoperative rehabilitation. The decision to proceed with tenolysis should be made in conjunction with the patient based on the patient's expectations and other factors, such as his or her functional demands and other concominant injuries or arthritis of the hand or digit.

Procedure

Local anesthesia, either a regional block or subcutaneous infiltration, is recommended with use of intravenous sedation and analgesics. This allows for patient interaction with active flexion examination at the conclusion of tenolysis.

The procedure is performed through wide exposure of the flexor tendon using a Bruner incision or a midlateral incision. The approach is often dictated by prior wounds and incisions. During dissection, care is taken to preserve the annular pulleys, especially the A2 and A4, to prevent bowstringing. Next, the flexor tendons are identified and the superficialis and profundus are separated. This can be achieved through multiple transverse windows in the retinaculum and by using special tenolysis knives, elevators, or braided suture to release adhesions (Figure 30.1). If a flexor tendon repair was performed, the site should be examined and débrided as needed to allow for smooth tendon gliding. If more than 30% of the width of the tendon is lost or if the tendon is not in continuity, then staged reconstruction must be pursued.

Once tenolysis is achieved along the entirety of the tendon in the digit and palm, the patient under local anesthesia can be asked to actively flex the digits. Under general anesthesia, it is necessary to create a separate proximal incision and manually pull the tendons for a "traction flexor check."

Complications

Complications from tenolysis include wound healing problems and failure to maintain motion due to recurrent adhesions. Tendon rupture is infrequent but obviously a disastrous complication that requires either staged reconstruction or repair, depending on the tendon quality.

Neither of the following authors nor any immediate family member has received anything of value from or has stock or stock options held in a commercial company or institution related directly or indirectly to the subject of this article: Dr. Knutsen and Dr. Medvedev.

© 2018 American Academy of Orthopaedic Surgeons

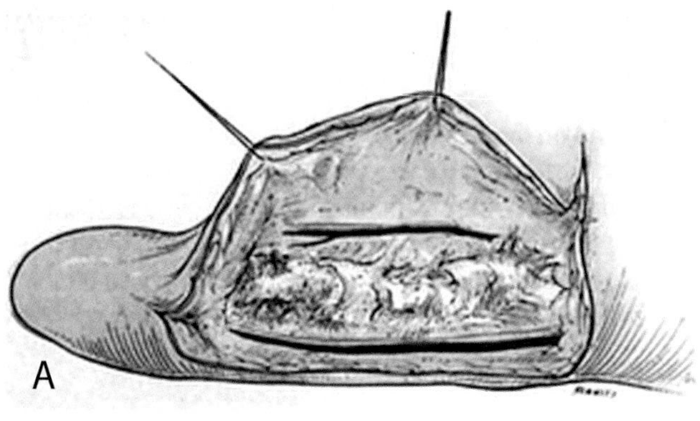

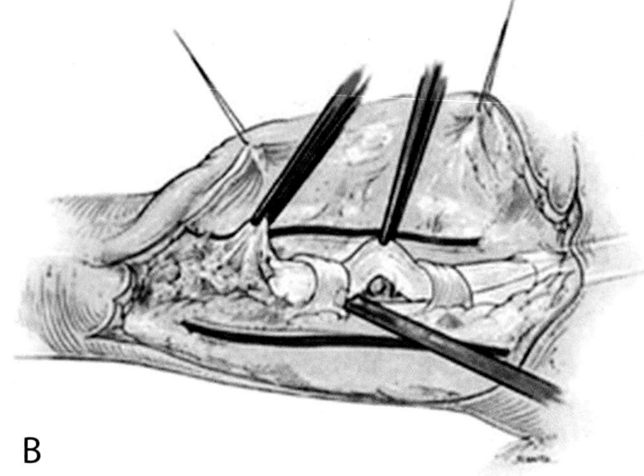

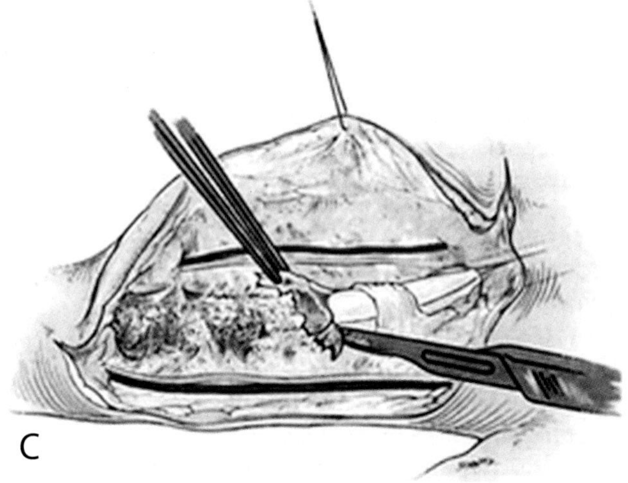

Figure 30.1 Illustration of flexor tenolysis performed by identifying the scarred tendon and sheath (**A**), followed by release of adhesions and careful preservation of the pulley system (**B**). **C**, Release may be facilitated by passing a small elevator or dental probe through windows in less critical portions of the sheath (e.g., proximal to A2, or between A2 and A4 pulleys). (Reproduced with permission from Strickland JW: Flexor tenolysis, in Strickland JW, ed: *Master Techniques in Orthopaedic Surgery: The Hand.* Philadelphia, PA, Lippincott Raven, 1998, pp 525–538. Illustrations copyright © Gary Schnitz and the Indiana Hand Center.)

Postoperative Rehabilitation

Dedication to vigorous and early therapy is necessary to keep gains made intraoperatively, and is dictated by the quality of the tendon after tenolysis. For frayed tendons, we recommend focusing on active place-and-hold exercises (explained later) initially with full active extension, but avoiding active flexion exercises for 4 weeks postoperatively. This should minimize the risk of rupture while maintaining as much tendon excursion as possible.

Postoperative pain control is crucial for patient participation in therapy. Occasionally, a regional block catheter can be left in place postoperatively for up to 5 to 7 days to facilitate immediate therapy participation. A number of variables can make pain control difficult, including edema and the pain from the extensive dissection.

For patients with normal or near-normal tendons after tenolysis, an immediate motion protocol is started within 12 to 24 hours after surgery. The therapy regimen should include edema control, wound management, active range of motion (AROM) and passive range of motion (PROM), and a home exercise program. As the patient progresses, these elements should be advanced or modified to maintain and increase motion and strength.

Active Range of Motion

- AROM is begun immediately with the goal of replicating intraoperative motion at the first therapy visit.
- "Place-and-hold" tendon gliding exercises is the method of placing the digits passively into a position and having the patient actively hold that position. Three positions are maintained: slight, moderate, and maximal finger flexion. This exercise is performed by using the nonoperative hand to place the operative hand in the desired position, which is then held with the muscle power of the operated hand. It requires activation and excursion of the flexor tendons to maintain position without high tension on the tendons. In the initial weeks, this exercise is more tolerable than tendon gliding exercises.
- Tendon gliding exercises are AROM that prevent adhesion formation between the flexor digitorum superficialis and profundus tendons by providing maximal differential gliding. They are performed by flexion of the fingers through a set of positions: (1) straight hand, (2) hook fist, (3) table top, (4) straight tip fist, and (5) full fist (Figure 30.2). As the patient advances, the patient may begin performing these exercises with the wrist in flexion and in extension to increase excursion of the tendons.
- Blocking exercises are started within the first week to isolate motion at individual joints and tendons. First, the metacarpophalangeal (MCP) should be held in extension and perform active proximal interphalangeal (PIP) motion. Then, hold (or block) the distal interphalangeal (DIP) joint in extension while actively flexing the DIP joint

 © 2018 American Academy of Orthopaedic Surgeons

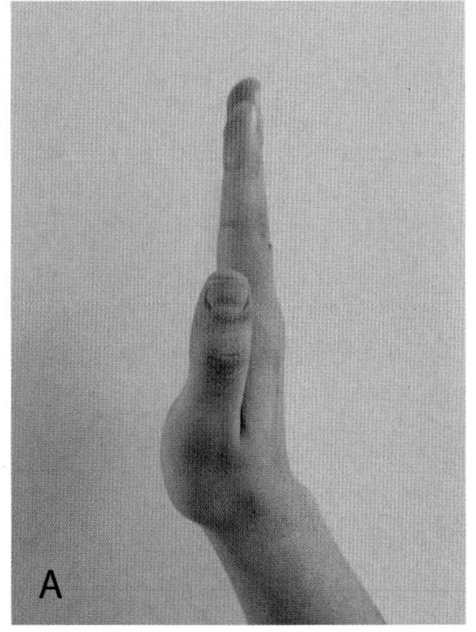

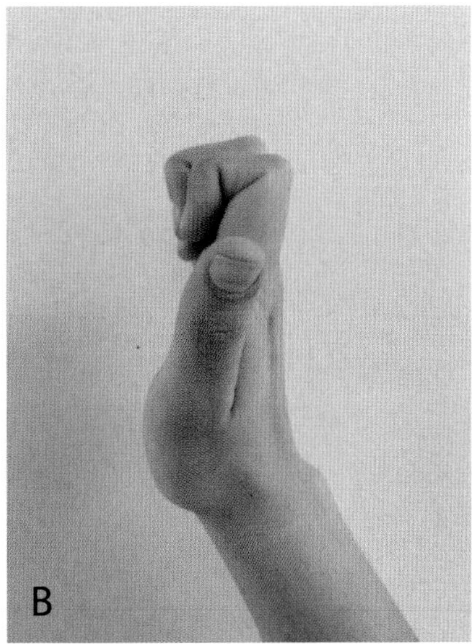

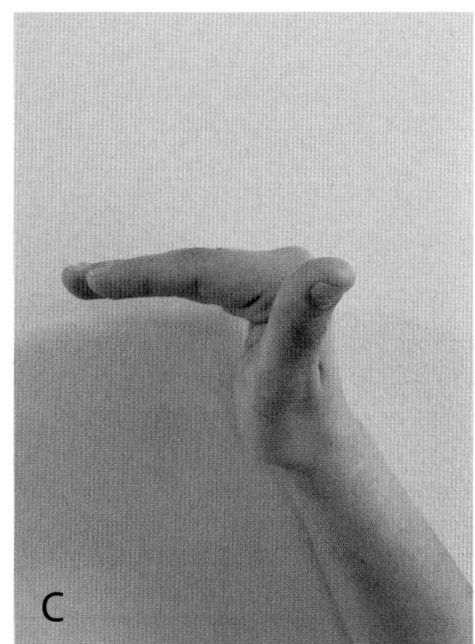

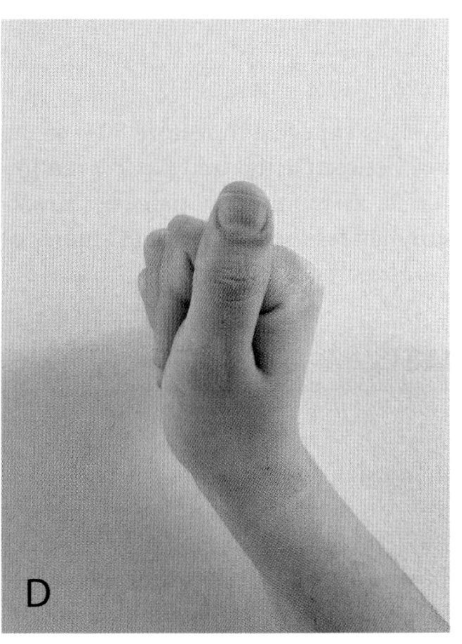

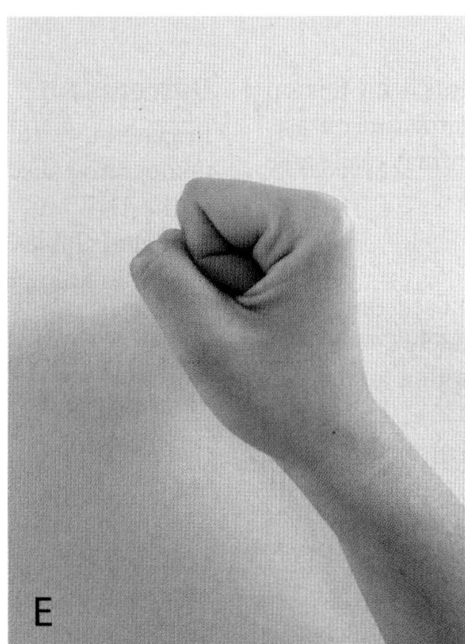

Figure 30.2 Illustrations of tendon gliding exercises: Straight hand (**A**), hook fist (**B**), table top (**C**), straight tip fist (**D**), and full fist (**E**).

(Figure 30.3). This will direct excursion of the tendon to the unblocked joint.

Passive Range of Motion

- PROM is a useful adjunct for patients who have concurrent joint contractures.
- PROM exercises that isolate each joint (MCP, PIP, and DIP) should be performed in addition to composite motion.
- Care must be taken not to be overly vigorous, as this can cause pain and incite inflammation.

Edema Control

- Edema and swelling can decrease ROM and increase pain, making cooperation with therapy difficult.
- Elevation of the operative hand above the level of the heart is an effective means to decrease edema.
- Overhead exercises, such as fist pumps, can achieve both ROM and edema control.
- Coban, lightly wrapped in a figure-of-eight pattern from distal to proximal, can also be used to control edema.
- Bulky dressings should be removed prior to performing exercises.

Home Program

- Exercises should be performed hourly during waking hours with 5 to 10 repetitions each.
- After sutures have been removed, patients should also start deep friction scar massage in line with the incision several times a day to soften the scar and improve tissue mobility.

Splinting

- Splinting is a useful adjunct to therapy. It can protect repairs, allow soft-tissue rest, and increase or maintain ROM.
- If there is concern for tendon quality, the fingers can be splinted in flexion for the first 3 weeks when not performing controlled exercises.

© 2018 American Academy of Orthopaedic Surgeons

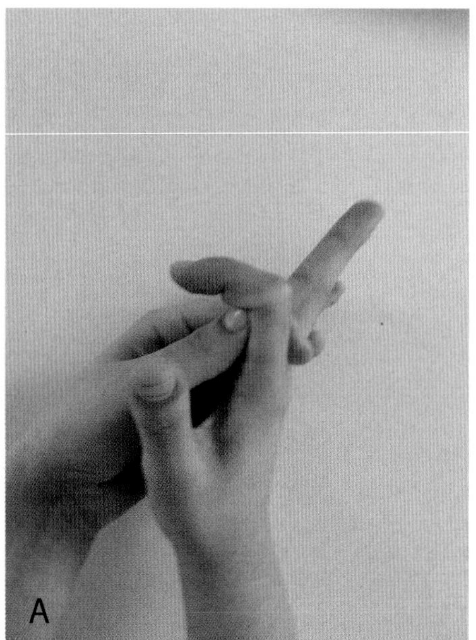

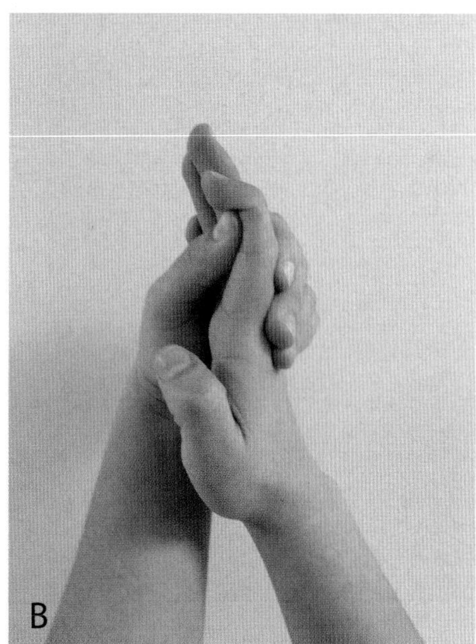

Figure 30.3 Illustrations of blocking exercises: **A**, The patient blocks the middle phalanx while actively flexing the distal interphalangeal joint. **B**, The patient block the proximal phalanx while actively flexing the proximal interphalangeal joint.

- Extension splinting can be used in patients with flexion contractures to maintain extension after contracture release.
- Splints should be removable so that patients may easily take them on and off for hourly exercises.

Continuous Passive Motion

- Continuous passive motion (CPM) can be used after tenolysis to increase tendon excursion immediately.
- No significant difference in total active motion after CPM compared to standard therapy.
- CPM can acutely increase pain if used inappropriately and possibly cause tendon rupture. We do not recommend its standard use.

Strengthening

- Resistive exercises and grip strengthening should begin around 6 weeks after surgery to allow for adequate tendon healing. This is important for eventual return to work.

Outcomes

In general, flexor tenolysis is expected to restore 50% of the preoperative discrepancy between active and passive motion at the DIP and PIP joints, as reported initially by Strickland et al. Table 30.1 summarizes the four relevant studies of outcomes following flexor tenolysis.

EXTENSOR TENOLYSIS

Indications

Similar to flexor tendon injuries, adhesions are one of the primary complications after extensor tendon injury. However, early AROM protocols following extensor tendon repair have improved motion following extensor tendon repair. More often, it is the extensor tendon adhesions that develop following crush injuries or finger fractures that need to be addressed surgically. Adhesions on the extensor side can be concomitant

Table 30.1 OUTCOMES FOLLOWING FLEXOR TENOLYSIS

Authors	Year	Study Group	Results	Complications
Schneider and Hunter	1975	60 patients	72% improved AROM, 48% good to excellent results	4 flexor tendon ruptures
Whitaker and Strickland	1977	77 digits	50% of restoration of TAM in 65% of digits	8% flexor tendon ruptures
Goloborod'ko	1999	20 digits	18 excellent results, 1 fair, 1 poor*	3 tendon ruptures
Jupiter et al.	1989	41 replanted digits	Mean TAM improved from 72° to 130° 13 excellent, 11 good, 6 fair, and 11 poor results*	Only in zone II injuries: 1 infection, 2 tendon ruptures

AROM = active range of motion, TAM = Total Active Motion.
*Results are reported as excellent, good, fair, and poor according to Strickland et al.

 © 2018 American Academy of Orthopaedic Surgeons

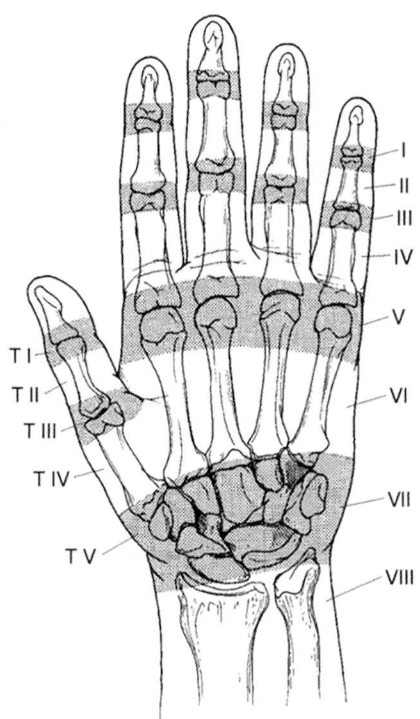

Figure 30.4 Illustration of the eight extensor tendon zones. T = Thumb. (Reproduced with permission from Newport, M: Extensor tendon injuries in the hand. *J Am Acad Orthop Surg* 1997;5(2):59–66.)

with joint contractures, and cause limitation of passive flexion as well as occasional active extension. Extensor tenolysis requires the same patient involvement in postoperative rehabilitation as flexor tenolysis, and is indicated when progress with therapy has plateaued 3 months following injury or surgery. As with flexor tenolysis, all finger fractures must be well aligned and healed, and all scars must be stable and soft prior to embarking on extensor tenolysis.

Procedure

Wide exposure of the tendon is necessary, starting at an unaffected area to determine normal anatomy and proceeding with care to preserve the tendon during tenolysis. Dorsal full-thickness skin flaps are created and dissected off the extensor tendon. The extensor tendon is then sharply freed from the underlying bone with care to not injure the insertion of the terminal tendon or the central slip into the middle phalanx. The lateral bands should be mobilized from the MCP to the PIP joint. The relevant anatomy is demonstrated in Figures 30.4 and 30.5. If full passive flexion is not restored, it may be necessary to perform dorsal capsulotomies. If motion is observed to consist more of open hinging of the affected joint as opposed to congruent gliding into flexion following the capsulotomy, the volar plate may need to be released as well. In more proximal procedures, care should be taken to preserve the extensor retinaculum at the wrist.

Postoperative Rehabilitation

Postoperative care of extensor tenolysis is different from flexor tenolysis because the extensors are weaker and thinner tendons. They are also prone to overstretching from overly aggressive rehabilitation, which can cause an extensor lag. A balance must be achieved when striving to regain digital flexion to avoid injury or overstretching of the extensors. The rehabilitation protocol for extensor tenolysis focuses on the same aspects as flexor tenolysis, including AROM, PROM, edema control, and splinting, and should begin within 1 to 3 days after tenolysis to avoid formation of adhesion and provide maximal extensor tendon excursion. As in the descriptions to follow, often the progression of AROM and PROM exercises are dictated by the lack or presence of an extensor lag. Extensor lag is a complication of overstretching. Recognition of this complication is important, so that appropriate intervention can be taken. Strengthening of the extensors can decrease lag but should not begin until 6 weeks after surgery to allow for tendon healing. As motion and strength improve, patients can progress to more intense activities.

Active Range of Motion

- Begin AROM immediately postoperatively.
- Use place-and-hold techniques (see description in Flexor Tenolysis section).
- "Reverse blocking" is an exercise specific to PIP extension. It is performed with the patient using the nonoperative hand to hold the MCP in hyperflexion while extending the interphalangeal joints. This allows easier extension at the PIP as tension from the flexor tendon is relieved (Figure 30.6).

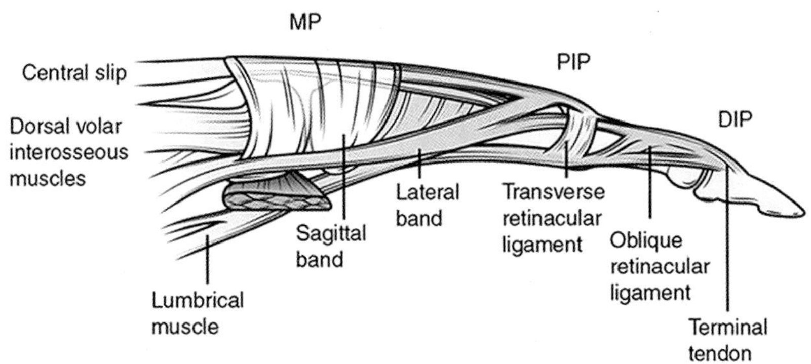

Figure 30.5 Illustration of the lateral view of the anatomy of the extensor mechanism at the metacarpophalangeal joint. The sagittal band arises from the volar plate and intermetacarpal ligament, and stabilizes the extensor tendon. DIP = distal interphalangeal, MCP = metacarpophalangeal, PIP = proximal interphalangeal. (Reproduced with permission from Kleinhenz, BP: Adams, BD: Closed sagittal band injury of the metacarpophalangeal joint. *J Am Acad Orthop Surg* 2015;23(7):415–423.)

© 2018 American Academy of Orthopaedic Surgeons

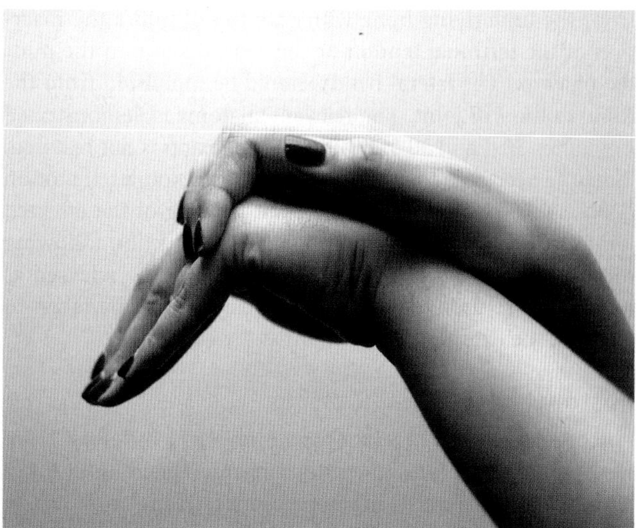

Figure 30.6 Photograph of the "reverse blocking" exercise. The patient hypreflexes the metacarpophalangeal joint and extends the interphalangeal joints.

- Active MCP extension is performed by having the patient hang the fingers over the edge of a table, then actively extending them at the MCP joint (Figure 30.7).
- Extensor tendon gliding exercises are essentially the reverse of flexor exercises. The patient begins in a full fist position, moves to a hook fist, and then straight hand (see Figure 30.2). This facilitates maximal extensor digitorum communis excursion. It can also be advanced to include wrist flexion when the patient can tolerate it.

Passive Range of Motion

- PROM is useful to prevent joint contractures. Care must be maintained not to injure the weakened extensor tendons. This is especially a concern with more distal injury, such as Zones I and II.
- Aggressive PROM can also impede progress by causing inflammation.

Splinting

- Splinting is used when there was a preoperative flexion contracture or postoperative extension lag.
- Splints are initially worn at all times, except for when doing therapy exercises.
- Splints should be weaned as gains in motion are made.
- Splinting varies depending on the zone of initial injury.
  - Zones I and II: DIP extension splints (Figure 30.8).
  - Zones III and IV: PIP dynamic extension splints (Figure 30.9).
  - Zone V and proximal: MCP extension splints (Figure 30.10).
  - Flexion splinting is occasionally used to achieve full flexion when extensor contractures are present. However, overstretching of the extensor tendons and extensor lag can occur with flexion splinting (Figure 30.11).

Strengthening

- Strengthening should be delayed for 6 weeks. This allows for appropriate wound healing and avoids the proliferative healing stage.

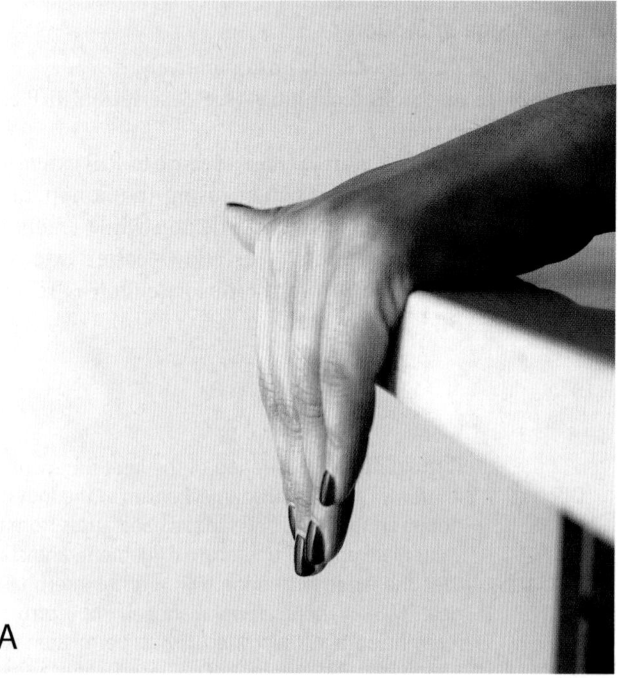

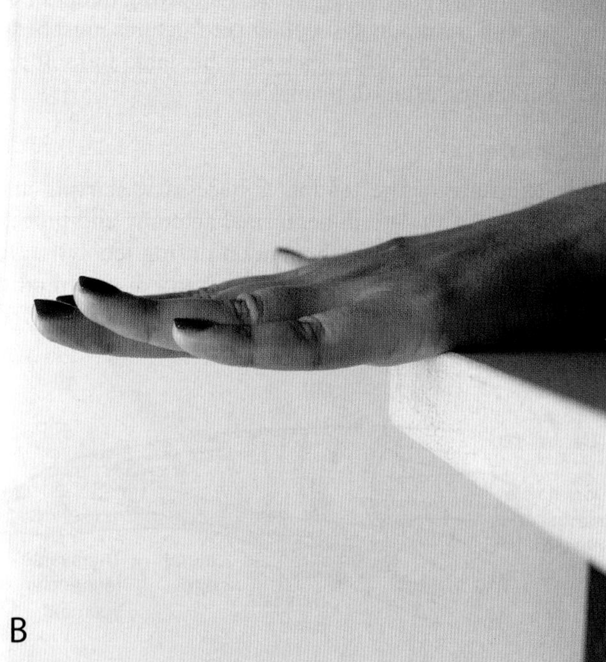

Figure 30.7 Photograph of active metacarpophalangeal extension. The patient places the hand at the edge of the table (**A**) and actively extends at the metacarpophalangeal joint (**B**).

 © 2018 American Academy of Orthopaedic Surgeons

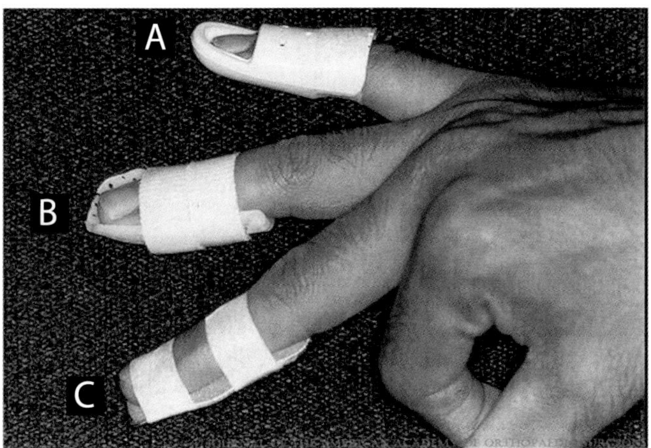

Figure 30.8 Three different finger extension splints. **A**, Stack splint (Stax Finger Splint, Sammons Preston Rolyan, Bolingbrook, IL). **B**, Perforated thermoplastic splint (Aquaplast Splinting Material, Sammons Preston Rolyan). **C**, Aluminum foam splint. (Reproduced with permission from Bendre AA, Hartigan BJ, Kalainov DM: Mallet Finger. *J Am Acad Orthop Surg* 2005;13(5):336–344.)

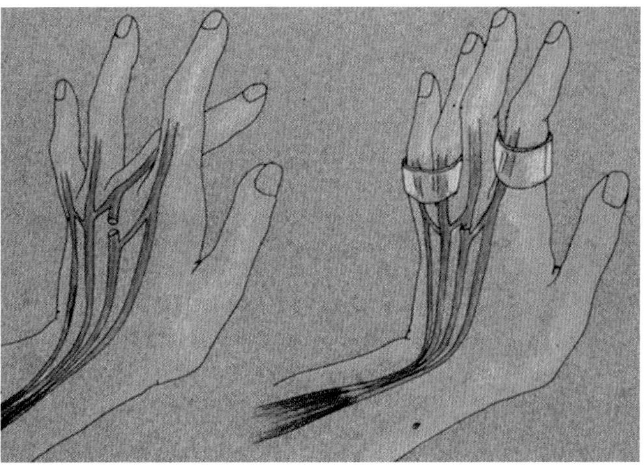

Figure 30.10 Illustration of relative motion extension splint, which allows for range of motion at the metacarpophalangeal and decreases tension on repairs. (Reproduced with permission from Merritt WH: Relative motion splint: active motion after extensor tendon injury and repair. *J Hand Surg* 2014;39(6):1187–1194.)

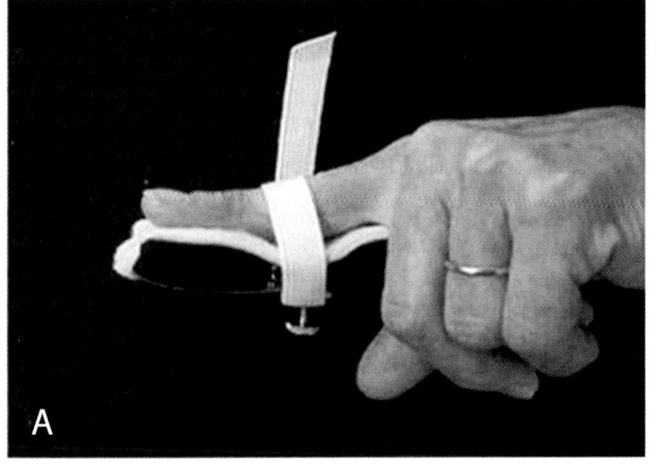

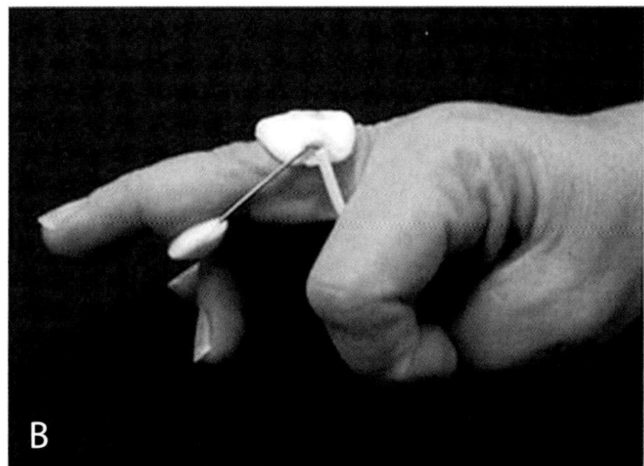

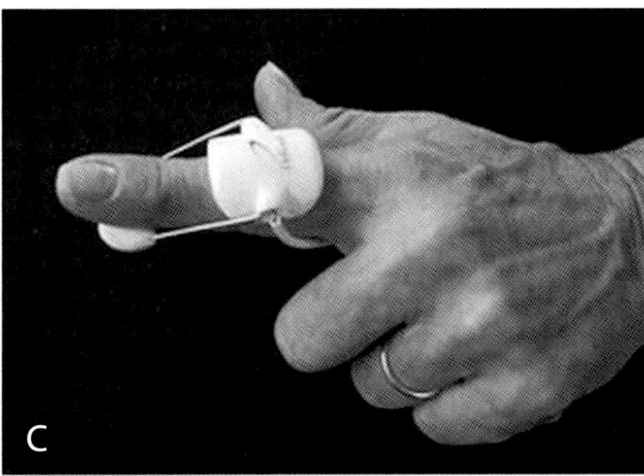

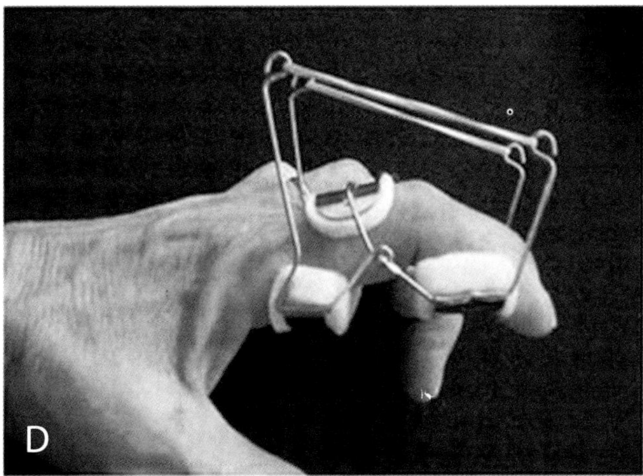

Figure 30.9 Photographs of finger splints. **A**, Joint-Jack. Lateral (**B**) and dorsal (**C**) views, DeRoyal splint. **D**, Reverse finger knuckle bender. (Reproduced with permission from Hogan CJ, Nunley JA. Posttraumatic proximal interphalangeal joint flexion contractures. *J Am Acad Orthop Surg* 2006;14(9):524–533.)

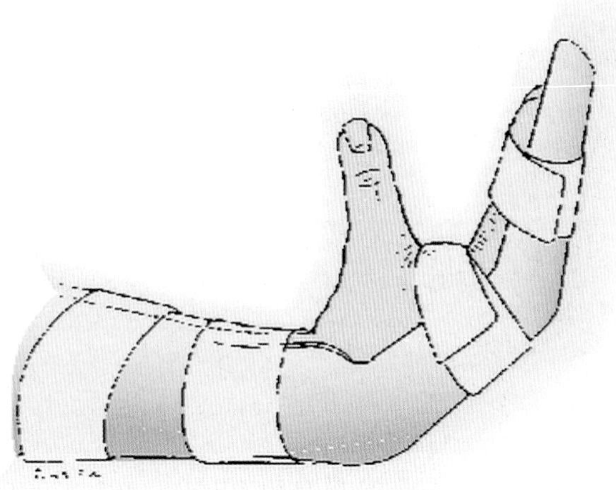

Figure 30.11 Dorsal hand flexion splint. (Reproduced with permission from Seiler JG, Taras JS, Kaufmann RA: Flexor Tendon Injury,in Wolfe SW, ed: *Green's Operative Hand Surgery*, ed 6. Philadelphia, PA, Elsevier, 2011, pp 189–238.)

- Exercises are graded with time, beginning with light ADLs, then progressing to resistive exercises and grip strengthening.
- After 8 weeks, the focus turns to return to work. This includes work simulation and work hardening.
- Throughout this time, improving overall fitness is important for return to work. This can include aerobic/cardiovascular conditioning.

Outcome

The reported evidence on outcomes following extensor tenolysis is limited. Creighton and Steichen reported an average improvement in total active motion of 54° and improvement in extension lag in 50% of patients. They also found that the best results in active motion after tenolysis occurred when no joint contracture releases were necessary. Overall, one must expect to lose some of the ROM gained in surgery, particularly when performing concurrent capsulotomy or both flexor and extensor tenolysis. However, functionally, most patients are satisfied and able to return to work.

SUMMARY

Flexor and extensor tenolysis are salvage procedures that require close collaboration between the surgeon, the hand therapist, and the patient. For a motivated patient who has exhausted hand therapy following a trauma and tendon injury, these procedures can be quite successful.

BIBLIOGRAPHY

Azari KK, Meals RA: Flexor tenolysis. *Hand Clin* 2005;21:211–217.

Cannon NM, Strickland JW: Therapy following flexor tendon surgery. *Hand Clin* 1985;1:147–165.

Creighton JJ Jr, Steichen JB: Complications in phalangeal and metacarpal fracture management. Results of extensor tenolysis. *Hand Clin* 1994;10:111–116.

Derby BM, Wilhelmi BJ, Zook EG, Neumeister MW: Flexor tendon reconstruction. *Clin Plastic Surg* 2011;38:607–619.

Feldscher SB, Schneider LH: Flexor tenolysis. *Hand Surg* 2002; 7:61–74.

Goldfarb CA, Gelberman RH, Boyer MI: Flexor tendon reconstruction: current concepts and techniques. *J Am Soc Surg Hand* 2005;5:123–130.

Goloborod'ko SA: Postoperative management of flexor tenolysis. *J Hand Ther* 1999;12:330–332.

Jupiter JB, Pess GM, Bour CJ: Results of flexor tendon tenolysis after replantation in the hand. *J Hand Surg* 1989;14:35–44.

McCarthy JA, Lesker PA, Peterson WW, Manske PR: Continuous passive motion as an adjunct therapy for tenolysis. *J Hand Surg* 1986;11:88–90.

Schneider LH: Tenolysis and capsulectomy after hand fractures. *Clin Orthop Relat Res* 1996:72–78.

Schneider LH, Hunter JM: Flexor tenolysis, in *AAOS Symposium on Tendon Surgery in the Hand. St.* Louis, MO, Mosby, 1975.

Schwartz DA, Chafetz R: Continuous passive motion after tenolysis in hand therapy patients: a retrospective study. *J Hand Ther* 2008;21:261–266.

Strickland JW: Delayed treatment of flexor tendon injuries including grafting. *Hand Clin* 2005;21:219–243.

Strickland JW: Flexor tendon surgery. Part 2: Free tendon grafts and tenolysis. *J Hand Surg* 1989;14:368–382

Whitaker JH, Strickland JW, Ellis RK: The role of flexor tenolysis in the palm and digits. *J Hand Surg* 1977;2:462–470.

© 2018 American Academy of Orthopaedic Surgeons

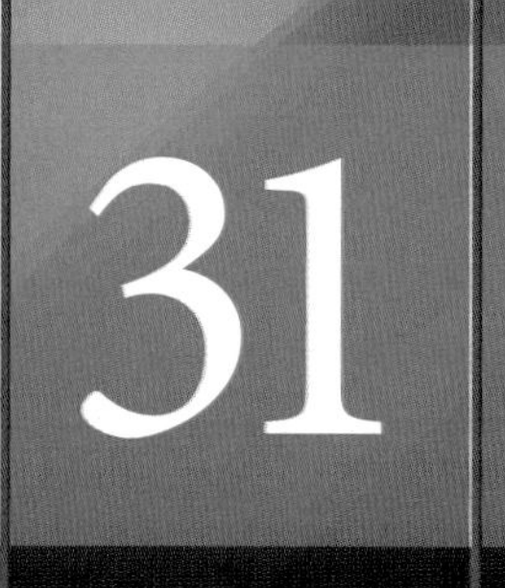

Principles of Tendon Transfers

David M. Brogan, MD, MSc, Stephanie Kannas, OTD, OTR/L, CHT, CLT-LANA, and Sanjeev Kakar, MD, MRCS

INTRODUCTION

Tendon transfers are a reconstructive tool to restore function in the setting of impaired intrinsic and/or extrinsic muscles affecting the hand and wrist. In patients with radial nerve dysfunction, the goal of tendon transfer surgery is the restoration of active wrist, thumb, and finger extension. Although the flexor musculature for the fingers is unaffected, these patients lose grip strength, as they are unable to effectively stabilize their wrist in extension during finger flexion. Therefore, they have poor transmission of flexor power to their fingers. Sensory disturbance is not routinely of functional consequence to these patients, unless they develop a symptomatic neuroma. This chapter presents the general principles of tendon transfers and details transfers for radial nerve palsies as a representative example.

RELEVANT ANATOMY

The radial nerve originates from the posterior cord of the brachial plexus and constitutes the largest terminal branch of the plexus. It travels along the posterior wall of the axilla and through the triangular space, continuing deep to the long and lateral head of the triceps as it spirals around the posterior-lateral humerus. The radial nerve pierces the lateral intermuscular septum at a relatively constant distance proximal to the lateral epicondyle (known as the lateral nerve height), thereby entering the anterior compartment of the arm between the brachioradialis and brachialis. This height can be determined as a function of the trans-epicondylar distance (TED). The TED is the distance between the lateral and medial epicondyle; the ratio of lateral nerve height to TED averages 1.7. The nerve then crosses the elbow and continues deep to the brachioradialis, splitting into the superficial branch of the radial nerve (SBRN) and the posterior interosseous nerve (PIN). The SBRN provides sensory innervation to the radial aspect of the forearm and hand, while the PIN travels deep to the supinator (the radial tunnel) to innervate the extensors of the wrist and fingers (Table 31.1).

HIGH VERSUS LOW PALSY

Radial nerve palsies may occur from a variety of causes: a penetrating wound, a closed or open fracture of the humerus, or iatrogenic injuries during surgical procedures around the distal humerus and elbow. Regardless of the cause, it is important to distinguish the level of the radial nerve injury (high vs. low), as this will dictate remaining function and availability of possible donor muscles and tendons. A low injury is typically classified as a lesion distal to the elbow, namely the PIN, whereas a high injury involves the proper radial nerve proximal to its bifurcation. A low injury or isolated PIN lesion will result in lack of finger metacarpophalangeal (MCP) extension and radial deviation with wrist extension, due to loss of extensor carpi ulnaris (ECU) with persistent activity of extensor carpi radialis longus (ECRL) ± extensor carpi radialis brevis (ECRB). Thumb retropulsion and interphalangeal hyperextension are lost secondary to losing the extensor pollicis longus (EPL) function. A high lesion will also lose all wrist extension (ECRB and ECRL) and brachioradialis. Extension at the proximal and distal interphalangeal (PIP and DIP) joints will remain intact following any radial nerve paralysis, as these joints are extended by the lumbrical and interosseous muscles, which are innervated by the median and ulnar nerves.

PRINCIPLES OF TENDON TRANSFER SURGERY

There are several basic requirements that must be met when planning tendon transfer surgery. These include (1) supple joints; (2) soft-tissue equilibrium; (3) similar excursion

---

Dr. Brogan or an immediate family member has received nonincome support (such as equipment or services), commercially derived honoraria, or other non-research–related funding (such as paid travel) from Arthrex and Axogen. Dr. Kakar or an immediate family member serves as a paid consultant to AM Surgical, Arthrex, and Skeletal Dynamics. Dr. Toomey or an immediate family member serves as a paid consultant to Celleration.

© 2018 American Academy of Orthopaedic Surgeons

Table 31.1 MUSCLES INNERVATED BY THE RADIAL NERVE AND ITS BRANCHES

Nerve	Muscle	Function
Radial N.	Long, Lateral and Medial Head of Triceps	Elbow Extension
Radial N.	Brachioradialis	Elbow Flexion
Distal to the Elbow (in order of innervation)		
Radial N.	Brachioradialis	Elbow Flexion
Radial N. vs. PIN	**ECRL**	Wrist Extension
Radial N. vs. PIN	**ECRB**	Wrist Extension
PIN	Supinator	Supination
PIN	**EDC**	MCP Extension*
PIN	ECU	Wrist Extension*
PIN	EDM	MCP Extension*
PIN	APL	Thumb CMC extension*
PIN	EPB	Thumb MCP extension*
PIN	EPL	Thumb IP extension*
PIN	EIP	MCP Extension*

APL = abductor pollicis longus, EDC = extensor digitorum communis, EDM = extensor digiti minimi, ECRB = extensor carpi radialis brevis, ECRL = extensor carpi radialis longus, ECU = extensor carpi ulnaris, EIP = extensor indicus proprius, EPB = extensor pollicis brevis, EPL = extensor pollicis longus, PIN = posterior interosseous nerve.
* = Affected with low nerve palsy.
(Adapted from Mazurek MT, Shin AY: Upper extremity peripheral nerve anatomy: current concepts and applications. *Clin Orthop Relat Res* 2001;383:7–20.)

between donor and target muscles; (4) adequate strength; (5) expendable donor muscles and tendons; (6) similar straight line of pull between transferred tendons; (7) synergy; (8) one tendon for one function; and (9) the fact that all fractures must be healed. Each of these will be examined in more detail, as it is imperative that the surgeon address these conditions prior to proceeding in order to maximize postoperative function.

Supple Joints

Supple joints may be obtained by passive range of motion (PROM) exercises, capsular release and splinting (to be covered later). Postoperative ROM will not exceed passive preoperative ROM; therefore, maintaining a supple joint with full PROM after nerve palsy is crucial to restoration of maximal motion.

Soft Tissue Equilibrium

The condition of the soft tissues through which the tendon will glide is critically important to the success of any procedure. All wounds must be mature and appropriately soft to maximize tendon movement—a scarred or infected tissue bed must be allowed to heal or consideration should be given to the use of a flap to resurface the bed and its gliding surface.

Excursion

The surgeon must consider the strength and excursion of the donor tendon/muscle to ensure that it will meet the demands of its recipient. The work capacity of a muscle is related to the force exerted by the muscle multiplied by the distance over which it moves (excursion). To restore full function, the excursion of a donor should be similar to the recipient, or the ROM of the affected joint will be altered. The excursion of a muscle is related to the average length of the resting muscle fibers, and can be thought of as the amplitude over which the tendon can affect motion. Wrist flexors and extensors have an average excursion ranging from 15 to 33 mm, finger extensors and the EPL average 50 mm of excursion, and finger flexors are generally thought to have an average excursion of 70 mm. A useful aid to remember this is the 3–5–7 rule (the excursion in cm for tendons of the wrist, finger extensors, and finger flexors, respectively). On the basis of excursion alone, wrist flexors may be a poor substitute for finger extensors, but excursion can be relatively increased by releasing any fascial attachments and by taking a tendon that crosses one joint and transferring it so that it crosses two joints. In that manner, wrist flexion will, in effect, amplify the excursion of a wrist flexor transferred to provide digit extension.

Strength

Assuming that excursion is appropriately matched between donor and recipient, consideration must also be given to a donor muscle's strength. The work capacity of a muscle is proportional to its mass, and while the absolute values of muscle strengths vary considerably from one person to the next, the

© 2018 American Academy of Orthopaedic Surgeons

Table 31.2 COMPARISON OF POTENTIAL DONOR AND RECIPIENT MUSCLE STRENGTHS FOR TENDON TRANSFER

Muscles/Groups	Relative Strength
Brachioradialis, FCU	2
FCR, wrist extensors, digital flexors, PT	1
Digital extensors	0.5
Palmaris, abductor pollicis longus	0.1

FCR = flexor carpi radialis, FCU = flexor carpi ulnaris muscle, PT = pronator teres.
(Data from Youm Y, Thambyrajah K, Flatt AE: Tendon excursion of wrist movers. *J Hand Surg* 1984;9A:202–209.)

ratio of strength between muscles in the same limb is relatively constant. The strengths of various tendons in the forearm have been measured and are listed in Table 31.2.

Expendable Donor Tendons

When a possible donor is well matched in terms of its strength and excursion, it must have redundant functionality to be an ideal candidate for transfer. Tendon transfers seek to restore balance to the extremity; therefore, redundant functionality of donor muscles is essential to allow sacrifice of a tendon without developing a new functional deficit. Examples of this include the use of the flexor carpi radialis (FCR) or flexor carpi ulnaris (FCU) assuming the other to function, or pronator teres (PT) if a functioning pronator quadratus exists.

Line of Pull

A straight line of pull is crucial to maximize the length tension relationship of the muscle. The maximum work capacity of the muscle will be realized when the direction of contraction and muscle shortening is in line with the vector required to pull the recipient tendon. Still, this is not always possible; fixed, smooth structures can be utilized as pulleys when needed to alter the line of pull of the tendon. An example of this is the extensor indicis proprius (EIP) transfer to restore thumb opposition in either a high or low median nerve palsy. By being transferred around the ulnar side of the wrist, the line of pull is directed to restore thumb opposition as the tendon is transferred into the abductor pollicis brevis insertion.

Synergy

Synergy is the inherent nature for certain muscles and tendon units to work concurrently; an example of this is finger extension with wrist flexion, which naturally allows the hand to release its grip when the wrist is flexed. Transferring a wrist flexor to a finger extensor takes advantage of this natural synergy. Another example of synergy is the enhancement of finger flexion (grip strength) with wrist extension–wrist extension places the finger flexors at their optimal length–tension relationship, which yields maximum grip.

One Tendon for One Function

Function can be maximized by utilizing one tendon for one function. Attempting to restore multiple functions of a joint by a single transfer will likely yield disappointing results. An example that violates this rule would be attempting the use of the FCU for restoration of both wrist and finger extension.

Healed Fractures

All fractures should be healed prior to surgery to permit early mobilization of tendon transfers if desired.

NONSURGICAL TREATMENT

Nonoperative treatments (physical therapy and splinting) may be offered to patients who have evidence of radial nerve neurapraxia (for which recovery of the nerve is expected) or for those who are unsuitable candidates for surgery. The goals of splinting are to maintain a stable wrist, and preserve passive finger extension as well as thumb abduction and extension. Multiple splint designs have been described, one of the most popular being a dynamic outrigger splint (Figure 31.1). The dynamic external outrigger functions to keep the wrist at neutral or above, augmenting the normal tenodesis effect of the hand (as described earlier). Active flexion of the fingers allows extension of the wrist by placing a stretch on the tension bands. Relaxation of the wrist out of extension, accompanied by gravity, allows extension of the MCPs via the brace and subsequent extension of the PIP and DIP joints through the use of the intrinsics.

OPERATIVE INDICATIONS

Timing of Surgery

Much controversy exists in the timing of surgery for radial nerve palsy. The rationale behind performing an early tendon

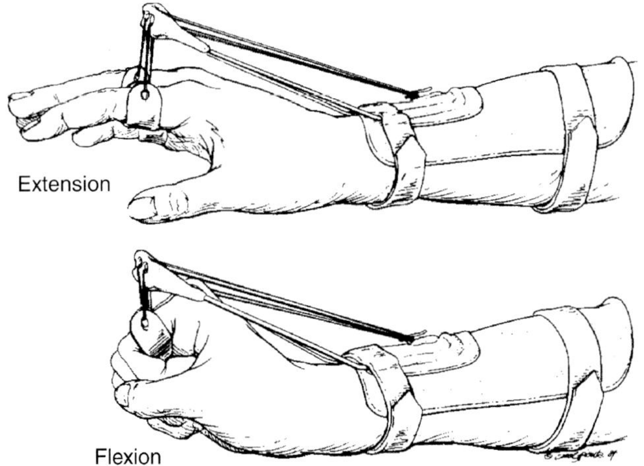

Figure 31.1 Illustration of a dynamic external outrigger splint, which augments the tenodesis effect, promoting wrist extension with flexion of the fingers. (Reproduced with permission from Colditz JC: Splinting for Radial Nerve Palsy. *J Hand Ther* 1987;1(1):18–23.)

© 2018 American Academy of Orthopaedic Surgeons

Table 31.3 COMPARISON OF EARLY VERSUS LATE TENDON TRANSFERS

	Early Transfer	Late Transfer
Timing	Perform 1–4 weeks after injury.	6–18 months
Number of Tendons	Transfer single tendon to maintain wrist extension. Transfer multiple tendons if nerve recovery has a poor prognosis (nerve gap >4 cm, extensive scarring).	Transfer multiple tendons to address major deficits: wrist extension, finger extension, and thumb extension.
Advantages	Restore power grip early on.	Wait for several months after nerve repair to allow demonstration of nerve recovery, which may obviate need for tendon transfers.

(Adapted from Ingari JV, Green DP: Radial nerve palsy. In: Worlfe SW, Hitchkiss RN, Pederson WC, Kozin SH, eds. *Green's Operative Hand Surgery*, ed. 6. Philadelphia, Elsevier, 2011.)

transfer is for the transfer to act as an internal splint, placing the fingers and thumb in a position of biomechanical advantage to maintain wrist extension and power grip while the radial nerve recovers. Historically, this has involved transfer of the PT to the ECRB. Proponents claim that this allows power grip prior to nerve regeneration, maintains a supple wrist joint, and supplements wrist extension in cases of poor nerve recovery. Dabas et al. reported on a series of 10 patients who underwent PT to ECRB transfer for radial nerve palsy within 10 weeks of injury. They found an increase of 48% in grip strength from preop to postop, as well as a 162% increase in tip pinch and 90% increase in key pinch.

Recovery of brachioradialis function is an important predictor of continued radial nerve reinnervation, as it is the first muscle to be innervated within the extensor compartment of the arm. Once restored, it is likely that reinnervation of wrist and finger extensors will ensue. Failure to do so indicates a poor chance of recovery of wrist and finger extension; thus, "late" radial nerve tendon transfers may be considered. Table 31.3 shows a comparison of early and late tendon transfers.

TYPES OF TENDON TRANSFERS

Several tendon transfer options exist for the management of radial nerve palsy. Specific transfers are chosen based on the level of nerve injury, the dysfunction caused, and suitable donor tendons available. A proximal or high radial nerve injury requires transfers to restore elbow extension, wrist extension, MCP extension, and thumb extension and abduction. In low radial nerve injuries (PIN palsy), the patient retains elbow extension, and possibly wrist extension depending on whether the lesion is above or below the motor branches to ECRL and ECRB, but lacks finger extension and thumb extension and abduction.

Various combinations of tendon transfers to restore wrist extension, finger extension, and thumb extension have been described. Currently, one of the most popular sets of transfers uses the palmaris longus to the EPL to restore thumb extension, and the PT into the ECRB to restore wrist extension. Transfers of the PT and palmaris longus closely follow the principles outlined at the beginning of this chapter—there is little functional morbidity associated with their use, excursion and strength suitably match the donor tendons, and they can be made to have an appropriate vector of pull. All of these benefits make their use widely accepted in tendon transfers for radial nerve palsies. More controversial, however, is the choice of transfer to the extensor digitorum communis (EDC) to restore finger extension (FCU, FCR or flexor digitorum superficialis [FDS]).

The FCU is a prime stabilizer of the ulnar side of the wrist and needed for the "dart throwing" wrist motion from radial-extension toward ulnar-flexion and power grip. Given this, some have cautioned against use of the FCU, and instead recommended use of FCR transfer to the EDC. Further, transfer of the FCU into the ECRL, in the setting of ECU and ECRB paralysis, may result in significant radial deviation. A potential solution to this is to transfer the PT into the ECRB for a more central line of pull along the longitudinal axis of the forearm. Alternatively, the PT can be transferred into the ECRL and ECRB, with transfer of the insertion of the ECRL into the fourth metacarpal.

In an effort to negate the morbidity associated with FCU transfer, Brand, Starr, and Tsuge have advocated transfer of the FCR either through a subcutaneous tunnel or via the interosseous membrane to the EDC. The PT is transferred to the ECRB, and the palmaris longus is utilized for transfer to the EPL.

Boyes advocated the use of the FDS of the long and ring fingers for restoration of finger extension. Given that the native excursion of the FCR and FCU is 30 mm and that of the EDC is 50 mm, Boyes suggested that the greater excursion amplitude of the FDS tendons (70 mm) would provide a more suitable transfer for the EDC. The FDS to the fourth finger is transferred to the EDC by dividing the FDS proximal to the chiasm to decrease PIP joint hyperextension, then passed through the interosseous membrane between the FDP and FPL. The FDS to the third finger may be transferred to the EIP and EPL through the interosseous membrane on the ulnar side of the FDP. The advantages of the FDS transfer are that the patient can extend the wrist and fingers at the same time and the excursion match between finger extensors and finger flexors is much closer than

 © 2018 American Academy of Orthopaedic Surgeons

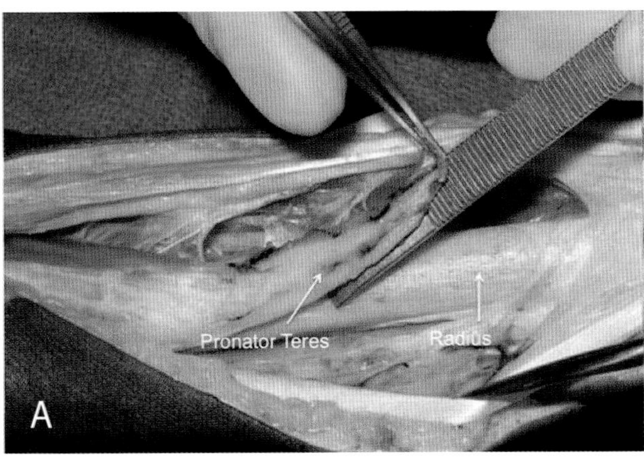

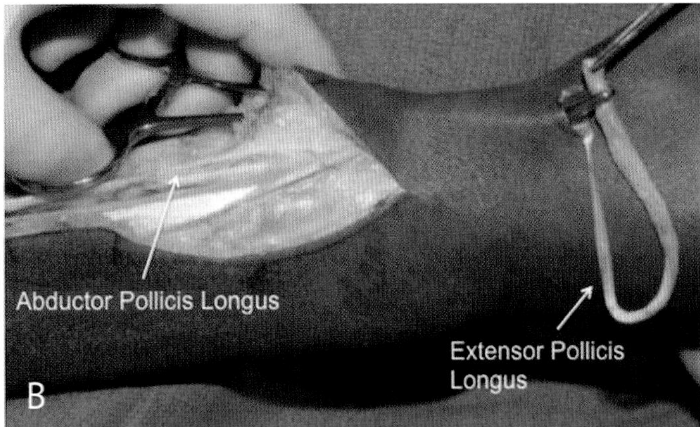

Figure 31.2 **A**, Photograph of the pronator teres being harvested with a periosteal sleeve; **B**, Clinical photograph: the extensor pollicis longus is found, isolated, and transposed from the third compartment radially to decrease its adduction vector and promote extension. (Photos courtesy of A. Shin, MD.)

when utilizing wrist flexors. However, this transfer has two downsides: the first is that the FDS is an out of phase donor; the second is that passage of the tendon through the interosseous membrane carries the risk of possible adhesions. A solution to mitigate this last problem is to create a large opening in the membrane.

SURGICAL TECHNIQUE

Given the potential dysfunction with use of the FCU as a donor tendon, our preferred transfers for radial nerve palsy are FCR to EDC, PL to EPL and PT to ECRB. Adhering to the principles as detailed earlier, the procedure starts by isolating the donor tendons through a volar radial incision including the PL (with care to ensure that this is found superficial to the antebrachial fascia to prevent inadvertent median nerve injury), FCR, and PT. To ensure maximal length of the PL and FCR tendons, these are cut at the distal wrist crease and any proximal fascial adhesions released to increase their relative excursions. To increase the relative length of the PT, it is harvested with a strip of periosteum off the distal radius. Attention is then directed dorsally where the EPL, EDC, and ECRB tendons are identified. To ensure adequate thumb extension and decrease the natural adduction moment of the EPL, the EPL tendon is transected proximally and rerouted from the third to first dorsal compartment, radial to the APL tendon (Figure 31.2).

Transfer of the volar compartment donor tendons to the dorsal compartment can either be through the interosseous membrane or via a radial subcutaneous tunnel that connects the volar and dorsal compartments. The subcutaneous tunnel lies deep to the cutaneous sensory nerves (SBRN, lateral antebrachial) but dorsal to the ECRL and brachioradialis.

After transfer of the donor tendons dorsally, the sequence of transfer is FCR to EDC, PL to EPL, and PT to ECRB. The purpose of doing the PT to ECRB transfer last is to enable one to use the tenodesis effect of the wrist to check for the correct tension of transfer of FCR to EDC and PL to EPL (Figure 31.3).

The EDC is often placed superficial to the extensor retinaculum to allow a straight line of pull. An assistant helps to position the hand such that the wrist is in neutral to 20° of extension, the MCP joints are fully extended and the FCR is at its resting tension. A tendon weaver is utilized to perform a Pulvertaft weave and supplemental stitches are placed after each pass with the tendon weaver utilizing 2-0 nonabsorbable suture. The FCR is woven into the EDC first, then the palmaris longus to the EPL. The tension of the tendon transfers is then tested by using wrist tenodesis principles. If the tension appears satisfactory, with passive extension of the MCP joints occurring with wrist flexion, the PT is then woven into the ECRB with the wrist maintained at 45° of extension. The ECRB can be transected at the musculotendinous junction, or imbricated in a side-to-side fashion if there is a chance of motor recovery of the radial nerve. Testing for appropriate intraoperative tensioning of the tendon transfers is critical to a successful outcome (Figure 31.4, A and B). Freehafer et al. determined that the muscle length after transfer should be equivalent to the muscle length before transfer in order to maximize contractile function. Wounds are closed per standard protocol with a combination of absorbable and nonabsorbable sutures. A well padded, above elbow plaster splint is applied with the elbow flexed at 90°, wrist extended to 45° and the MCP joints at 45° of flexion and the PIP and DIP joint in full extension. The thumb is placed in extension and palmar abduction. This is continued for up to 3 to 6 weeks, after which a supervised rehabilitation program is started.

POSTOPERATIVE REHABILITATION

Communication between the surgeon, therapist, and patient during rehabilitation is critically important. It is vital for the therapist to know the date of surgery, the transferred tendons, and the quality of repair of the tendon transfer. Rehabilitation after a tendon transfer is typically divided into different phases in order to protect the transfer, reduce scarring to allow

© 2018 American Academy of Orthopaedic Surgeons

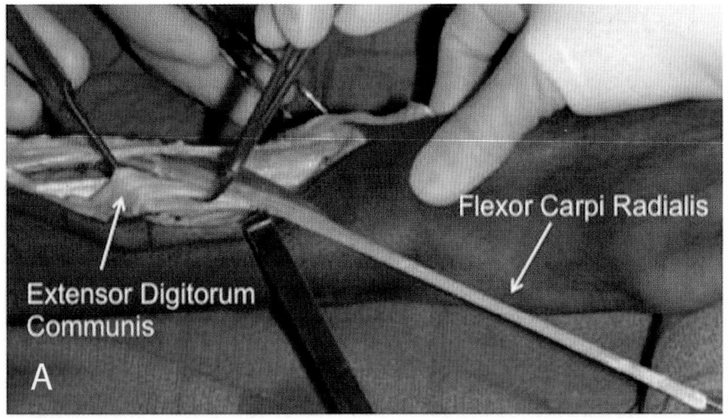

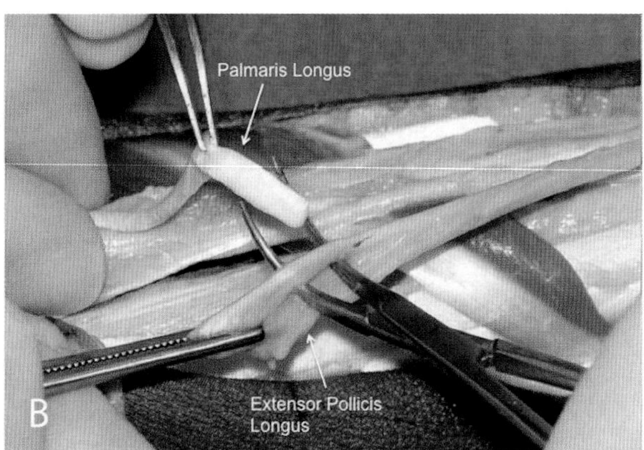

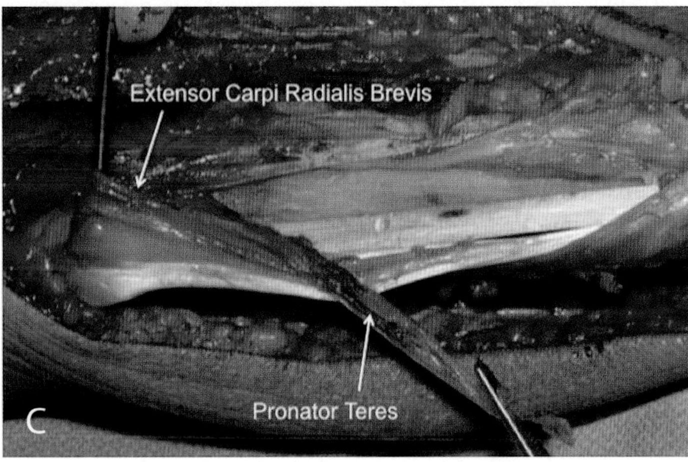

Figure 31.3 **A**, Photograph of the flexor carpi radialis being transferred dorsally towards the extensor digitorum communis; **B**, Photograph of the palmaris longus being woven into the extensor pollicis longus utilizing a Pulvertaft weave; **C**, Photograph of the PT then being transferred into the extensor carpi radialis brevis after ensuring appropriate tensioning of the previous transfers. (Photos courtesy of A. Shin, MD.)

the transfer appropriate gliding, and, finally, restore function through re-education techniques and strengthening. The three phases are immobilization, mobilization, and light functional use in conjunction with strengthening.

Immobilization Phase

This phase typically lasts up to 6 weeks. The length of immobilization is dependent on the type of transfer, quality of tissue, and compliance of the patient. A strong repair with at least three intertendinous weaves may permit early mobilization. In this phase, the tendon needs to be protected from overstretching or rupturing. Initially, the extremity should be immobilized in a position that places the least amount of stress/tension on the transfer. During this immobilization phase, edema control, pain management, and ROM of unaffected joints should be addressed. If the patient is in a removable orthosis, scar

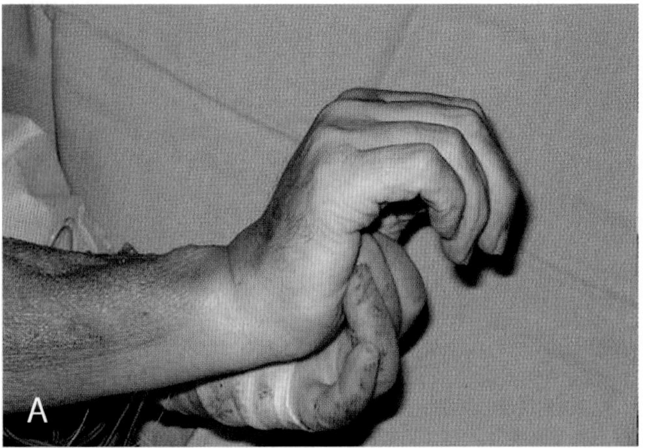

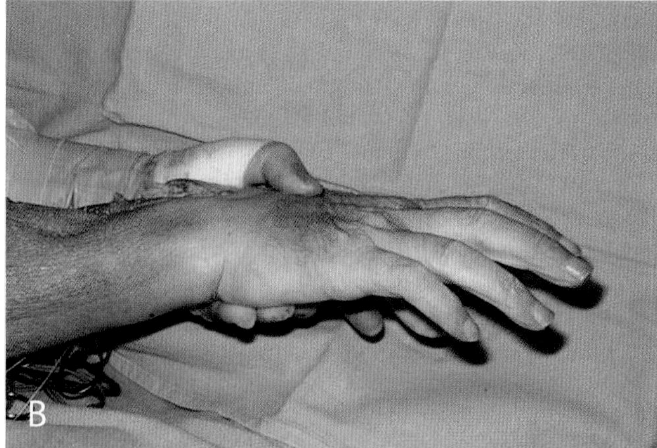

Figure 31.4 Photographs of tensioning of the transfers being checked with the wrist in extension (**A**) and flexion (**B**). (Photos courtesy of A. Shin, MD.)

 © 2018 American Academy of Orthopaedic Surgeons

management strategies should be initiated to assist with tendon excursion. Attention is directed at both the incision and deeper scar to promote motion. Superficial scar massage (incision) includes using circular motion directly over the incision for 3 to 5 minutes at a time. At the end of the scar massage, lotion may be applied. In addition, silicone or elastomer sheets may be used to guard against hypertrophic or keloid scar formation. Deep scar management aims to prevent adhesion formation that may limit tendon excursion. This can comprise of early tendon gliding techniques (providing that the repair is strong, as dictated by the surgeon) and ultrasound after 6 weeks once early tendon healing has occurred. During this phase, the surgical extremity should not be used for functional activities.

Mobilization Phase

In a typical rehabilitation program, mobilization and consistent activation of the tendon transfer typically lasts for 3 to 4 weeks. The patient will require a protective orthosis that is worn between therapy sessions for 4 to 6 weeks after surgery or longer if still demonstrating limited activation of the transfers. The orthosis needs to have the tendon transfer in a tension-free position. Following surgery for FCR to EDC, PL to EPL, and PT to ECRB, the orthosis will be forearm based, positioning the wrist in 30° to 45° of extension, the MCP joints in full extension, the IPs are left free. and the thumb positioned midway between radial and palmer abduction with the IP in 0° to 10° of hyperextension (Figure 31.5).

The exercise sessions will focus on neuro-re-education techniques to activate the transfer. To activate the transfer, one must learn to activate the donor muscle at the same time as moving the recipient muscle in its previous pattern. For example, if the PT is transferred to the ECRB, the patient will pronate the forearm and extend the wrist at the same time or the patient will pretend to tell time on a wristwatch. Some patients benefit from trying the activation technique on the unaffected extremity first or performing the activation technique simultaneously with both extremities. Biofeedback, mirror visual feedback, vibration, and neuromuscular electrical stimulation (NMES) may also be used to assist with activation of the transfer. Exercise sessions should begin in a gravity-eliminated plane. Exercise sessions during the day should be frequent. To avoid fatigue and substitution patterns, a 10- to 20-second rest period in between each activation attempt is highly encouraged. Once the tendon transfer is consistently activated, light functional activities may be initiated. Light functional activities include washing the face, brushing teeth, and eating. No heavy use of the surgical extremity should be done during this phase. PROM to stretch the transfers is generally avoided throughout rehabilitation.

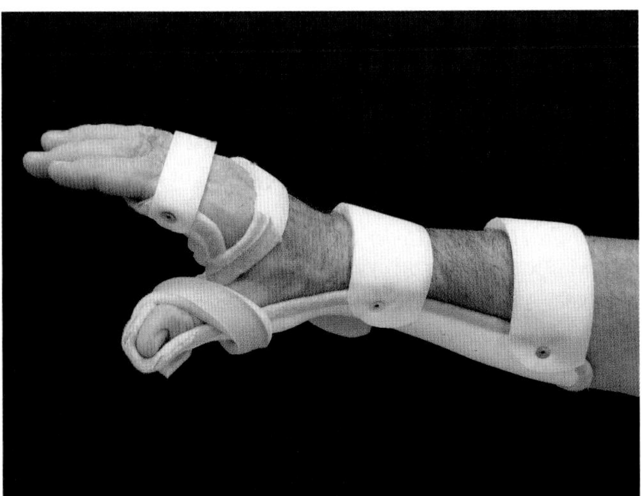

Figure 31.5 Photograph of typical orthosis fashioned for radial nerve palsy. Note that the wrist is in 30° to 45° of extension, metacarpophalangeal joints are placed in full extension, and interphalangeal joints are left free.

Complications that may be suspected or seen during this phase include scar adhesions and weakness of the tendon transfer. Scar management techniques need to be utilized (as noted earlier). Place-and-hold and active assisted ROM are helpful. At approximately 6 weeks, electrical stimulation and ultrasound may also be used to assist with tendon excursion.

Strengthening Phase

The third and final phase of therapy is strengthening and functional use of the involved extremity. This phase starts when the transferred tendon's insertion is strong enough to withstand resistance, which is typically between 6 and 12 weeks after surgery. Progressive strengthening of the extremity should be initiated specifically for the donor muscle as well as the extremity overall. Functional use of the hand should be encouraged during this stage of rehabilitation. Compensatory motions need to be avoided. During this phase, the patient may discontinue the orthosis as long as weakness and flexion/extension lags are not present. Gradual return to all activity should be encouraged during this final stage.

During each phase of rehabilitation of the tendon transfer, patient education is critical for success. The patient must understand the focus of each phase of therapy as well as restrictions at each phase of therapy. The rehabilitation phases outlined here are meant as a guide for surgeons and hand therapists.

EXPECTATIONS AND OUTCOMES

Historically, tendon transfers have proven very effective in restoring function after radial nerve palsies, although the choice of procedures and the length of postoperative immobilization have been controversial. In one series of 35 patients undergoing transfer of FCR to EDC, PL to EPL, and PT to ECRB, average postop wrist extension was 54°, wrist flexion averaged 42°, and thumb radial abduction was 36°. Patients were followed for an average of 11.3 years, and radial wrist deviation was noted in three patients, bowstringing of the PL to EPL transfer was found in 12 patients, and grip strength was noted to be 63% of the contralateral hand. Another series of tendon transfers in 14 patients with isolated radial nerve

© 2018 American Academy of Orthopaedic Surgeons

palsies resulted in grip strength of 20 kg, 38° of wrist extension and 40° opening of the first web space. The transfers in these patients were PT to ECRB, FCU to ED + EPL and PL to APL + EPB. The authors did note that radial deviation of the wrist secondary to FCU transfer resulted in diminished grip strength. This was further demonstrated in a mixed series of tendon transfers for 15 patients with either high or low radial nerve palsies. The authors used either the FCR or FCU for finger extension and PT or ECRL augmentation for wrist extension (for high or low palsies, respectively). Four of the five patients with FCU transfer had ulnar deviation with gripping, compared to 4 out of 10 patients with FCR transfers. Greater average wrist flexion was preserved in the patients with FCR transfer when compared to FCU transfer (41° vs. 21°). Average wrist extension was 38° with the MCP joints flexed, and 13 of the 15 patients were able to actively extend the thumb. The authors graded their results according to a scale developed by Bincaz (2002), and reported 11 patients with excellent results, 2 with good results, one with fair results, and one with bad results.

As discussed earlier, appropriate postoperative rehabilitation can be as critical to success as choice of tendon transfer. Early mobilization studies for tendon transfers have demonstrated decreased length of therapy services, and reduced costs. When possible, these protocols are typically initiated during the first week after surgery. Rath studied an immediate active motion protocol (IAMP) in five hands with a low median nerve paralysis. These five patients underwent opposition transfers with IAMP and were compared to a retrospective control of seven patients following a traditional tendon transfer protocol. This study found that there were no ruptures of the tendon transfers with the IAMP. The study found no differences between ROM and pinch strength outcomes between the early active motion protocol versus the traditional tendon transfer protocol. Sultana et al. performed a systematic review on the efficacy of early mobilization. A total of six studies were included in the results. Three studies focused on patients with Hansen disease who underwent tendon transfers for ulnar, median, or a combined nerve paralysis. One study found significant improvement in total active motion, deformity correction, improved intrinsic plus position, and improved closed fist for early mobilization at late follow-up. Two studies found no difference in outcomes between early mobilization and immobilization groups. Another study assessed claw deformity correction. This study found that the early mobilization group had less pain and quicker return to function. The other two studies focused on thumb extension using the EIP or the ECRL. Both of these studies found that the early controlled motion groups had quicker recovery, increased cost-effectiveness, and shorter time off from work. Further research is required to fully understand and support early mobilization after a tendon transfer.

Ultimately, the timing of each phase of rehabilitation is dependent on many variables, but not limited to the following: type of tendon transfer, quality of tendon transfer, patient's ability to actively participate in therapy, and patient's or caregiver's learning ability to perform a home exercise program. Regardless of the technique chosen or the rehabilitation protocol, close communication between the surgeon, therapist, and patient is critical to ensure optimal results.

CONCLUSION

With careful adherence to preoperative planning, selection of donor tendons, surgical technique, and postoperative rehabilitation, tendon transfers may enhance function for patients with peripheral nerve or spinal cord injuries. While debate exists regarding exact tendon selection in each case, the basic principles of tendon transfers and rehabilitation following transfers may be applied to any number of tendon transfers. Similarly, close collaboration between the hand therapist and surgeon is crucial to maximize postoperative motion while protecting the integrity of the transfer.

BIBLIOGRAPHY

Bincaz LE, Cherifi H, Alnot JY: Les transferts palliatifs de réanimation de l'extension du poignet et des doigts. A propos de 14 transferts pour paralysie radiale et dix transferts pour lésion plexique. *Chirurgie de la Main* 2002;21(1):13–22.

Brand PW, Beach RB, Thompson DE: Relative tension and potential excursion of muscles in the forearm and hand. *J Hand Surg Am* 1981;6(3):209–219.

Burkhalter WE: Early tendon transfer in upper extremity peripheral nerve injury. *Clin Orthop Relat Res* 1974;(104):68–79.

Cannon NM: *Diagnosis and treatment manual for physicians and therapists,* ed 8. Indianapolis, Ind, Hand Rehabilitation Center of Indiana, 2001, p vi, 296.

Colditz JC: Splinting for radial nerve palsy. *J Hand Ther* 1987; 1(1):18–23.

Dabas V, Suri T, Surapuraju PK, Sural S, Dhal A: Functional restoration after early tendon transfer in high radial nerve paralysis. *J Hand Surg Eur vol* 2011;36(2):135–140.

Dorf ER, Chhabra AB: Chapter 19—Tendon transfers, in T. Trumble T, et al, eds: *Principles of Hand Surgery and Therapy.* Philadelphia, PA, Saunders, 2010, pp 302–313.

Duff SV, Humpl, D: Therapist's management of tendon transfers, in Skirven TO, A; Fedorczyk, J; Amadio, P, eds: *Rehabilitation of the Hand and Upper Extremity,* Philedelphia, PA, Elsevier Mosby, 2011, pp 781–791.

Freehafer AA, Peckham PH, Keith MW: Determination of muscle-tendon unit properties during tendon transfer. *J Hand Surg Am* 1979;4(4):331–339.

Ingari JV, Green DP: *Radial Nerve Palsy, in Green's Operative Hand Surgery,* Wolfe SW, Pederson WC, Kozin SH, eds, Philadelphia, PA, Elsevier, 2011.

Ishida O, Ikuta Y: Analysis of Tsuge's Procedure for the Treatment of Radial Nerve Paralysis. *Hand Surg* 2003;8(1):17–20.

Jones NF, Machado GR: Tendon Transfers for Radial, Median, and Ulnar Nerve Injuries: Current Surgical Techniques. *Clin Plast Surg* 2011;38(4):621–642.

© 2018 American Academy of Orthopaedic Surgeons

Kamineni S, Ankem H, Patten DK: Anatomic relationship of the radial nerve to the elbow joint: Clinical implications of safe pin placement. *Clin Anat* 2009;22(6):684–688.

Kozin SH: Tendon transfers for radial and median nerve palsies. *J Hand Ther* 2005;18(2):208–215.

Mazurek MT, Shin AY: Upper extremity peripheral nerve anatomy: current concepts and applications. *Clin Orthop Relat Res* 2001;(383):7–20.

Naeem R, Lahiri A: modified camitz opponensplasty for severe thenar wasting secondary to carpal tunnel syndrome: Case Series. *J Hand Surg Am* 2013;38(4):795–798.

Raskin KB, Wilgis EF: Flexor carpi ulnaris transfer for radial nerve palsy: functional testing of long-term results. *J Hand Surg* 1995;20(5):737–742.

Rath S: immediate active mobilization versus immobilization for opposition tendon transfer in the hand. *J Hand Surg Am* 2006;31(5):754–759.

Ratner JA, PeljovichA. Kozin SH: Update on tendon transfers for peripheral nerve injuries. *J Hand Surg Am* 2010;35(8): 1371–1381.

Richards RR: Tendon transfers for failed nerve reconstruction. *Clinics in Plastic Surgery* 2003;30(2):223–45, vi.

Ropars M, Dreano T, Siret P, Belot N, Langlais F: Long-term results of tendon transfers in radial and posterior interosseous nerve paralysis. *J Hand SurgBr* 2006;31(5):502–506.

Sammer DM, Chung KC: Tendon transfers: part I. Principles of transfer and transfers for radial nerve palsy. *Plastic Reconstr Surg* 2009;123(5):169e–177e.

Smith RJ: Tendon transfers to restore wrist and digit extension, in Smith RJ, ed: *Tendon Transfers of the Hand and Forearm,* Boston, MA, Little, Brown and Company, 1987, p. 35–56.

Starr CL: Army experiences with tendon transference. *J Bone Joint Surg* 1922;4(1):3–21.

Sultana SS, MacDermid JC, Grewal R, Rath S: The effectiveness of early mobilization after tendon transfer in the hand: a systematic review. *J Hand Ther* 2013;26:1–20.

Toth S: Therapist's management of tendon transfers. *Hand Clin* 1986;2:239–246.

Youm Y, Thambyrajah K, Flatt AE: Tendon excursion of wrist movers. *J Hand Surg Am* 1984;9(2):202–209.

© 2018 American Academy of Orthopaedic Surgeons

32 Distal Radius Fractures

Corey McGee, PhD, MS, OTR/L, CHT, Agnes Z. Dardas, MD, Msc, and Ryan P. Calfee, MD, MSc

INTRODUCTION

Distal radius fractures present to orthopaedic surgeons with a bimodal patient distribution of younger, predominantly male, patients with high-energy trauma, such as motor vehicle accidents, and older, predominantly female, patients with high- or low-energy trauma, such as same-level falls. The incidence is reported to be 195.2/100,000 persons per year. Patients present with pain, tenderness, swelling, deformity over the wrist, and potentially symptoms attributable to either median neurapraxia (paresthesia since injury either stable or improving) or acute carpal tunnel syndrome (worsening paresthesia and acute pain after injury). The goal of treatment is return the patient to baseline functional status.

Careful consideration of individual patient goals and expectations, and the various treatment options (nonoperative and operative) in combination with appropriate postinjury and postoperative management, are essential to optimize the functional outcome after these relatively common injuries.

SURGICAL TREATMENT

The AO/OTA Classification System identifies three main types of fracture pattern: A, extra-articular; B, partial articular; and C, complete articular. Fractures with any of the following postreduction characteristics are indicated for operative fixation as opposed to nonoperative treatment: radial shortening >3 mm, dorsal tilt >10°, intra-articular displacement or step-off >2 mm, or associated neurovascular injury. The majority of distal radius fractures are treated nonoperatively, with cast immobilization. Operative treatments include closed reduction and percutaneous pinning, closed reduction and external fixation, and open reduction and internal fixation (ORIF) using volar or dorsal plates. ORIF is the preferred technique in the United States. In older adult patients with unstable fracture characteristics, operative management offers the advantages of earlier return to function, better radiographic fracture alignment, and stronger grip strength. However, there is no clearly documented difference between ultimate functional outcomes at 1 year or later and return to activities of daily living (ADLs) between nonoperatively and operatively treated older adult patients. ORIF is contraindicated when a patient's medical conditions are not amenable to safe surgical intervention, and is relatively contraindicated in grossly contaminated open fractures.

Surgical Procedure

ORIF of distal radius fractures can be accomplished through volar or dorsal approaches, the most common procedure being volar plate fixation. Volar plates are applied for the majority of operatively treated distal radius fractures, but are believed to produce similar outcomes to dorsal plating except when volar plates are mechanically superior for buttressing volar partial articular fractures of the distal radius associated with palmar translation of the carpus. Dorsal plating is most advantageous when addressing intra-articular incongruity that requires direct visualization.

Volar Plate Fixation

After prepping and draping the arm, the limb is exsanguinated and a tourniquet is inflated. A volar longitudinal incision is made over the distal aspect of the flexor carpi radialis (FCR) tendon and carried through the skin (Figure 32.1, A), cauterizing small veins in the subcutaneous tissue. The FCR tendon sheath is opened, and the palmar cutaneous branch of the median nerve is identified within the sheath and avoided. The floor of the sheath is incised, and the interval just radial to the flexor pollicis longus (FPL) muscle is entered. The pronator quadratus is then identified and released distally and radially. The brachioradialis tendon fibers are elevated off of the radial styloid if needed to help with gaining length and radial inclination during the reduction. The fracture is manually reduced (Figure 32.1, B) and the volar plate is positioned on the distal radius, keeping it proximal to the watershed line distally. We tend to fix the plate with an initial screw through the oblong hole proximal to the fracture in the shaft, allowing adjustment of the plate (Figure 32.1, C), and a provisional Kirschner wire

Dr. Calfee or an immediate family member has received research or institutional support from Medartis; and serves as a board member, owner, officer, or committee member of the American Society for Surgery of the Hand and the Journal of Hand Surgery–American.

 © 2018 American Academy of Orthopaedic Surgeons

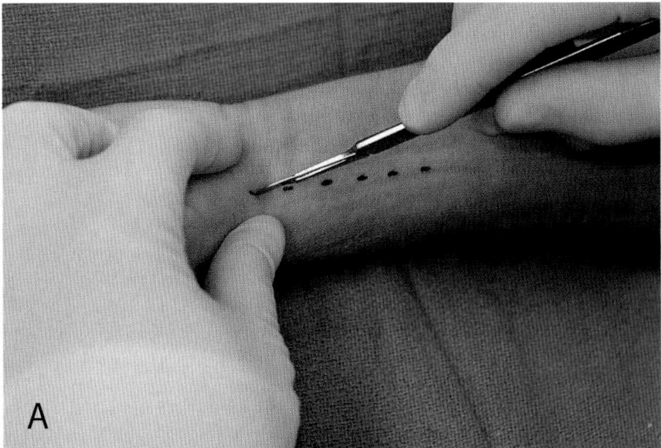

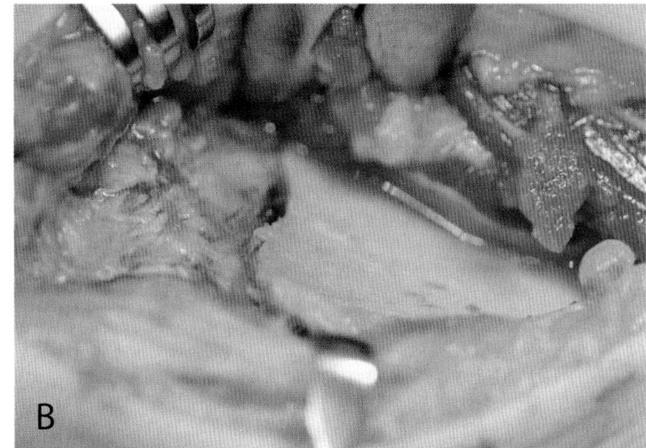

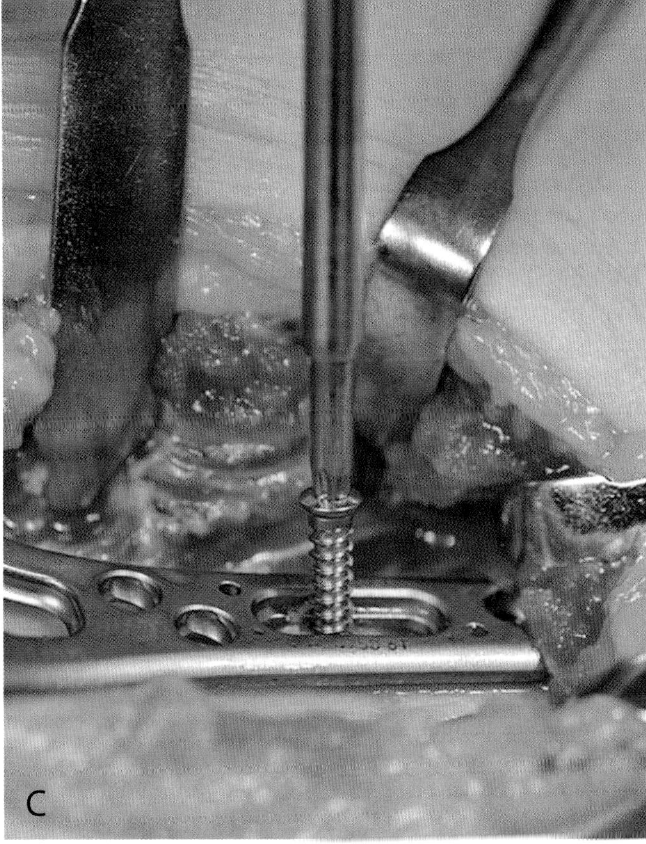

Figure 32.1 Photographs of the volar approach to distal radius incision (**A**), exposure of the fracture (**B**), and plate application (**C**).

(K-wire) through a wire hole typically located in the distal aspect of the plate. The fracture reduction and placement of the plate is confirmed with fluoroscopy. The fracture is re-reduced if necessary, and a second and third screw are placed into the radial diaphysis. For all metaphyseal fractures, we place distal screws unicortically to minimize the chance of rupturing extensor tendons. Unless the carpus is subluxating dorsally with intra-articular dorsal fracture fragments, all other dorsal comminution is ignored. After fixation, we again review the distal radius alignment, distal radioulnar joint (DRUJ) stability, and evaluate motion in forearm supination and pronation, as well as wrist flexion and extension. Any crepitus raises concern for intra-articular hardware. The final alignment and appropriate hardware placement are verified with fluoroscopy. We let down the tourniquet before closing the skin to confirm hemostasis. Patients are routinely placed into a short-arm volar splint before leaving the operating room.

Dorsal Plate Fixation

After prepping and draping the arm, the limb is exsanguinated and a tourniquet is inflated. A dorsal longitudinal incision is made centered at the distal radius over the dorsal aspect of the wrist. The dissection is carried sharply down from the skin to the extensor retinaculum. The extensor retinaculum is opened

© 2018 American Academy of Orthopaedic Surgeons

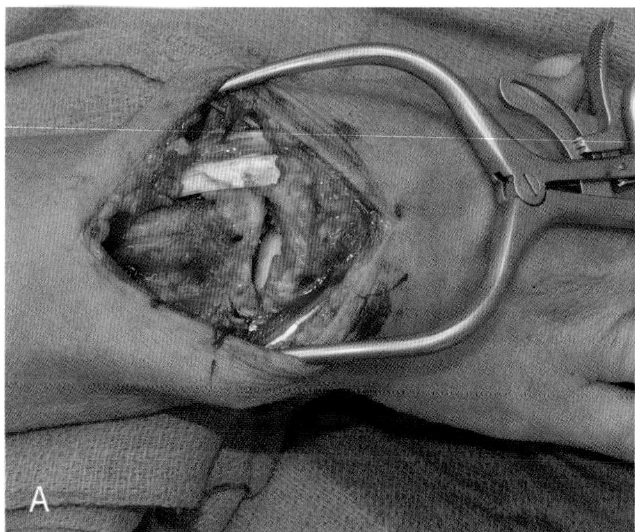

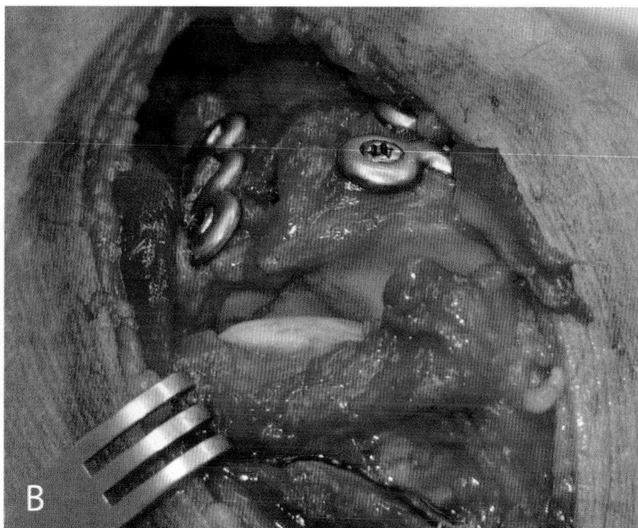

Figure 32.2 Photographs of the dorsal exposure of the distal radius (**A**), and plates applied with good reduction of the articular fracture (**B**).

with a step cut in order to allow closure over the dorsal plates. The extensor pollicis longus (EPL) tendon is identified and transposed radially. The second and fourth compartments are raised off the dorsal distal radius subperiosteally and off the wrist capsule distally (Figure 32.2, A). A transverse radiocarpal arthrotomy is made off the distal radius, providing visualization of the cartilage surfaces of the scaphoid and lunate, keeping the remaining capsule distally attached. A longitudinal capsular incision can be made to elevate the capsule off the carpal bones to give more exposure as needed. The scaphoid and lunate are examined to identify associated chondral injury. In addition, the scapholunate ligament is evaluated for associated injury. This exposure provides direct visualization of intra-articular fractures and allows for reduction. Displaced fragments are aligned with minimal step-off and gap, placing provisional K-wires as needed. The reduction is verified with direct visualization and confirmed with fluoroscopy. When reduction is achieved, the dorsal plate is positioned on the distal radius to span the fragments (Figure 32.2, B). We typically first place one screw through an oblique hole proximal to the fracture and into the radial shaft. The position of the plate can be fine-tuned to capture the fragment pieces without entering the DRUJ. Distal screws are placed within the fracture fragments, then additional bicortical proximal screws are placed into the shaft. We then do final visual and fluoroscopic checks of alignment, wrist and forearm motion, DRUJ stability, and for proper hardware placement (nothing excessively prominent). The extensor retinaculum is repaired, leaving the EPL transposed in the subcutaneous tissues. We let down the tourniquet before closing the skin to confirm hemostasis. A short-arm volar splint is the applied before leaving the operating room.

Other Surgical Options

Other surgical options rely on ligamentotaxis to reduce distal radius fractures followed by maintenance of reduction with either K-wires or spanning fixation (external fixation or spanning plate fixation). When performing isolated K-wire fixation, incisions are recommended as there are no true safe zones free of nerves or tendons. Postoperatively, patients are immobilized until healing (4–6 weeks). Spanning fixation also obligates absolute wrist immobility until hardware is removed. External fixators are typically removed at 6 weeks while spanning plates that have less risk of infection can be maintained for up to 3 months. During healing, it is imperative to rehabilitate the fingers to prevent digit stiffness.

Complications

Complications associated with distal radius fractures include late tendon ruptures, carpal tunnel syndrome, and chronic regional pain syndrome (CRPS). The two most common flexor tendon ruptures are the FPL and flexor digitorum profundus (FDP) to the index finger, with FPL ruptures reported as late as several years after volar plating. This is thought to be due to plates distal to the volar rim and transverse ridge of the volar radius, plates palmar to the bone distally, or residual dorsal tilt causing increased pressure on the flexor tendons as they course over a volar plate. Extensor tendon rupture can occur with either volar or dorsal plates, most commonly involving the EPL, extensor digitorum communis (EDC), or radial wrist extensors (extensor carpi radialis brevis [ECRB] and longus [ECRL]). This is thought to occur due to vascular insult to the tendons imparted by the fracture or drill or screw penetration during volar plate fixation, or direct tendon irritation from the plate after dorsal plate fixation. If signs of tendonitis present postoperatively, patients should undergo surgery to remove the offending hardware in order to prevent further irritation and tendon rupture. Ulnar wrist pain may also occur after distal radius fracture; patients should be specifically examined for lunotriquetral ligament injury, signs of ulnar impaction (pain with ulnar deviation of the wrist), and extensor carpi ulnaris (ECU) tendonitis or instability. In our experience, ulnar wrist pain without clear cause or mechanical instability will often

© 2018 American Academy of Orthopaedic Surgeons

resolve within 6 months. If persistent, we typically proceed with corticosteroid injection into the ulnar carpal joint.

The most common postoperative neurologic complications are carpal tunnel syndrome and CRPS. CRPS is suggested by a constellation of symptoms, including persistent disproportionate pain, excessive swelling, dysesthesias, and limited finger motion. In the distal radius fracture population, CRPS most commonly presents as type II, in a median-nerve-like distribution. In either case (type I or II), patients should be managed operatively with a carpal tunnel release. Women with high-energy trauma or severe fracture type are at higher risk of developing CRPS type I. Early diagnosis and multidisciplinary treatment are key to a successful recovery. It is currently debatable whether Vitamin C supplementation can assist in preventing CRPS, but there is little risk in recommending 500 mg per day for 5 weeks when initially evaluating the patient with a distal radius fracture.

REHABILITATION AFTER DISTAL RADIUS FRACTURE

Recent advances in the surgical fixation of distal radius fractures have allowed for improved outcomes and, in some instances, earlier postoperative mobilization of the wrist and forearm. For example, after volar plating, early therapist-supervised mobilization of the wrist and forearm has resulted in improved outcomes, including reduced disability and improved wrist range of motion (ROM) and forearm supination at 8 weeks. In addition to traditional exercises used to regain ROM, Movement Representation Techniques (i.e., mirror therapy or Graded Motor Imagery) may assist in pain management (perhaps even preventing the development of CRPS) as well as retaining distal upper extremity representation in the brain (Figure 32.3, A, B). Mirror therapy involves taking the uninjured wrist and hand through the therapeutic exercises with the injured hand resting behind a mirror that is reflecting the uninjured hand's function. To the patient, it appears visually as if the injured hand is moving symmetrically with the uninjured hand in a pain-free fashion.

Successful postsurgical hand therapy is contingent on early communication between the surgeon and therapist with discussion of the surgical approach, success of reduction and restoration of alignment, any associated complications, and postoperative restrictions. This helps the therapist to plan intervention, assist with goal setting, and to be proactive in addressing or anticipating associated problems or complications.

Rehabilitation following distal radius fracture can be considered in three functional phases: protective (0–5 weeks), mobilization (6–8 weeks), and weight-bearing (9–12 weeks).

Closed Reduction and Casting: Nonoperative Treatment

Protection Phase

- Cast-immobilization for 4 to 8 weeks depending on fracture comminution and bone quality
- Cast fit check and any related symptomatology (i.e., superficial branch of the radial nerve or median nerve irritation)
- Evaluate disability and instruct on task modification to ensure that patient is able to engage in ADLs while adjusting to upper limb immobilization and weight-bearing restrictions.
- Pain management, edema management
- Active motion/tendon gliding to digits, and active range of motion (AROM) to all upper limb joints proximal to the forearm

Mobilization Phase

- Supervised hand therapy may be necessary for older patients, patients with pain, or those with impaired upper limb strength and mobility, which impede daily function. This is generally initiated in the mobilization phase and entails weekly visits for up to 6 to 8 weeks, with emphasis placed on home program competency.
- Initiate active assisted and active wrist ROM.

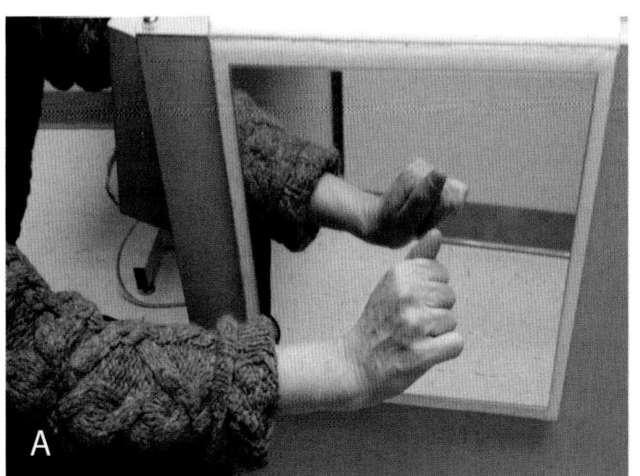

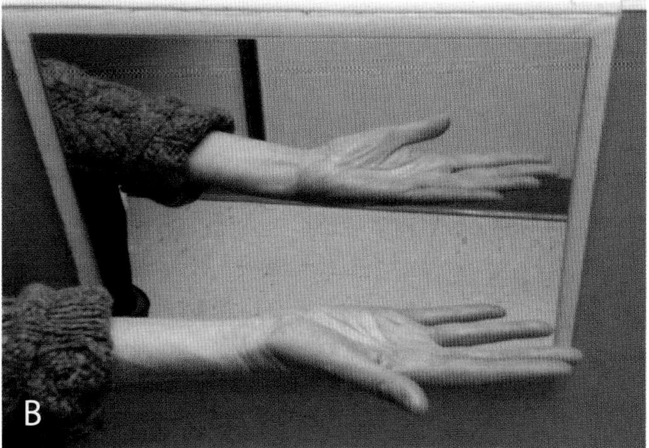

Figure 32.3 Photographs of Movement Representation Techniques (i.e., mirror therapy). Affected hand is occluded from vision. **A**, synergistic fist; **B**, finger extension and supination.

© 2018 American Academy of Orthopaedic Surgeons

- Depending on alignment, the therapist's interventions may involve compensatory training when adequate ROM cannot be restored.

Closed Reduction With External Fixation and Percutaneous Pin Fixation

Protection Phase

- Follow protocol for nonoperative treatment outlined earlier.
- Training on pin site care
- Assess for signs/symptoms of pin site infection
- Splint or orthoses to protect wrist and external fixator until removal
- Active-assisted forearm rotation with overpressure applied proximal to fracture site
- Early emphasis on active and passive finger ROM
- Composite fist/thumb opposition, intrinsic minus, and thumb palmar/radial abduction stretches should be incorporated immediately to prevent intrinsic, long finger/thumb extensor, and first webspace tightness (Figure 32.4, A–D).

Mobilization and Weight-Bearing Phases

- Initiate AROM and gentle passive range of motion (PROM) wrist motion around week 6 when pins/fixators are removed.
- Pin site scar massage should precede AROM/PROM in each rehabilitation session and should be incorporated into home programming.
- Adjust fit of and gradually wean wrist orthosis, generally by week 8.
- Static-progressive wrist orthoses may be necessary to regain wrist PROM should capsular tightness be present.
- When bony healing has completed or neared completion (~8 weeks), initiate more aggressive passive wrist ROM. Progressive resistive exercises (PREs) can generally be initiated at this time. Home programming should be adjusted to include passive stretching and PRE.
- Activity restrictions are generally lifted by 10 to 12 weeks.

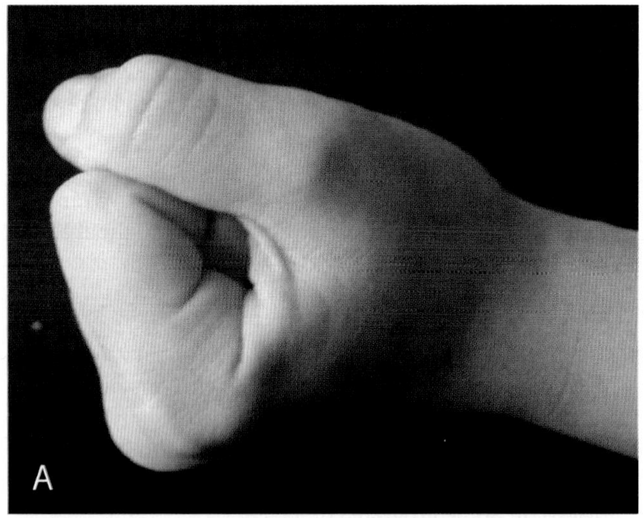

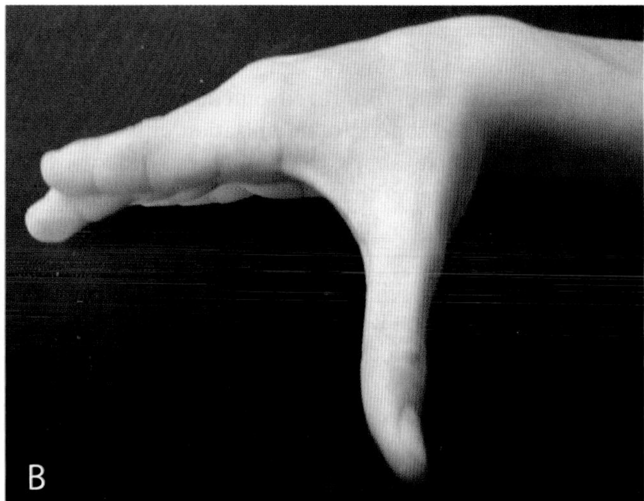

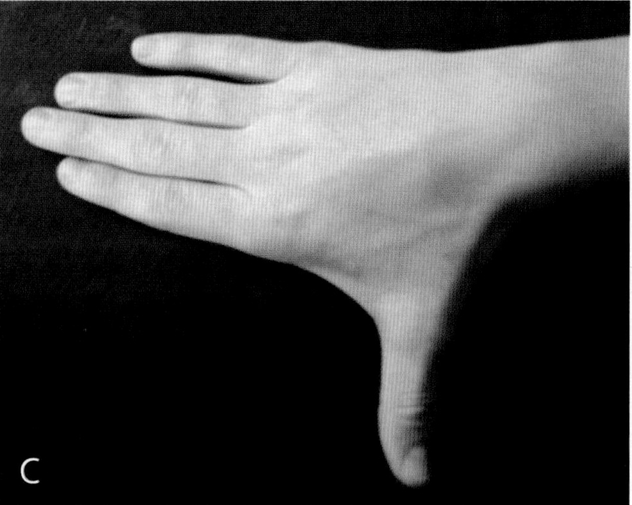

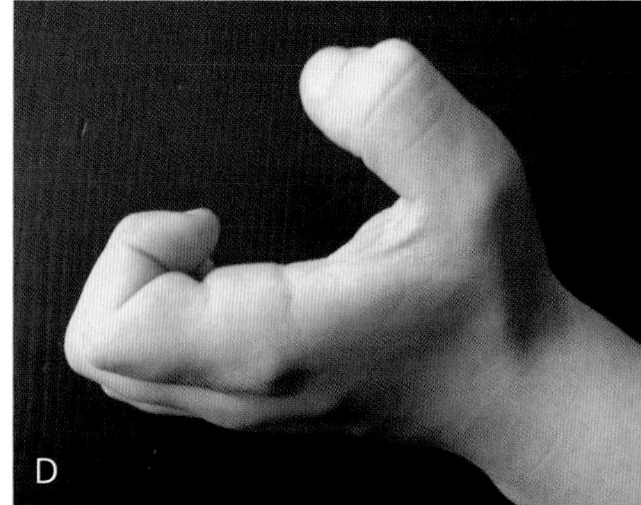

Figure 32.4 Photographs of composite fist (**A**), thumb palmar abduction (**B**), thumb radial abduction (**C**), and intrinsic minus active stretches (**D**).

© 2018 American Academy of Orthopaedic Surgeons

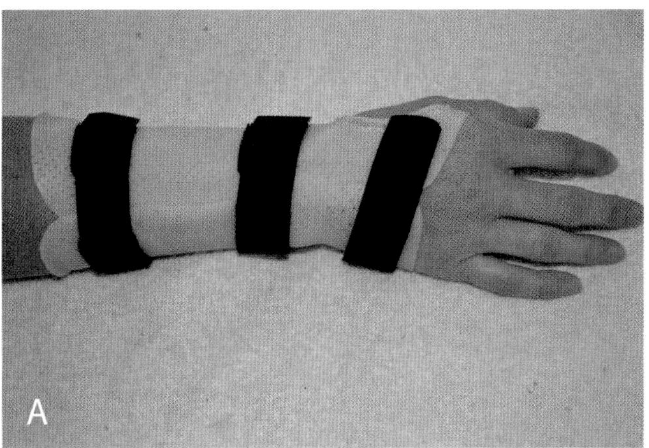

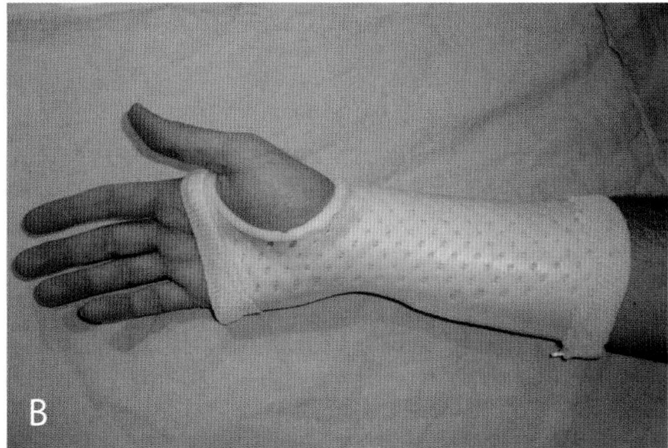

Figure 32.5 Photographs of circumferential forearm-based static wrist protection orthoses. **A**, dorsal view; **B**, volar view.

Open Reduction and Internal Fixation

When volar or dorsal plating techniques are used for noncomminuted fractures with good bone quality, an early motion program can usually be instituted. The decision to initiate an early motion program is dependent on the surgeon's satisfaction with the fracture fixation and the absence of concomitant injuries or comorbid medical conditions that might complicate bone healing and responsiveness to hand therapy. In an early motion program, the progression to functional outcome is often faster, and formal rehabilitation may be discontinued earlier compared to traditional approaches. In addition to the therapy interventions used following closed reduction and nonoperative treatment, the early motion protocol after ORIF includes the following:

Protective Phase (0–4 Weeks)

- A custom circumferential orthosis is fabricated (Figure 32.5, A, B) and worn when not performing exercises. This orthosis is typically weaned between weeks 4 and 6.
- Active wrist and forearm motion exercises as soon as 3 to 5 days postoperatively.

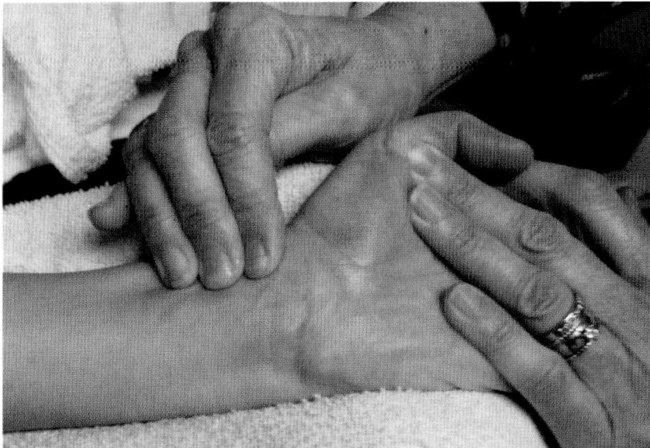

Figure 32.6 Photograph of scar massage with flexor pollicus longus glide.

- Initiate early tendon gliding for the FPL and long finger flexors at 3 to 5 days to prevent tendon adherence.
- After suture removal, scar management consists of scar massage to assist in softening scar tissue, decreasing tenderness, and reducing adherence of skin to underlying tendons (Figure 32.6).
- Silicon sheeting may be applied to the surface of the incisional scar to enhance cosmesis and increase scar pliability.
- Gentle passive motion (Figure 32.7, A, B).
  - Gentle traction to the radiocarpal joint during PROM may reduce discomfort and enhance patient responsiveness.
  - Active assisted forearm rotation should be facilitated by adding overpressure to the midproximal radius as opposed to distally in order to avoid stressing the fixation construct.
- Early phase strengthening (2–4 weeks). This should be limited to grip forces less than 3 to 5 lbs to avoid excessive stress on the healing radius. A lightly resistant sponge and therapy band can be used.

Mobilization Phase (4–8 Weeks)

- Moist heat/fluidotherapy to prepare for stretch when edema is resolving
- Barring any DRUJ involvement, more aggressive "towel" and "hammer" forearm stretches (Figure 32.8) are initiated in the mobilization phase.
- Continue active and gentle passive stretching of the wrist in flexion/extension and radial/ulnar deviation motion.
- Emphasis on initiating wrist movements with wrist flexors and extensors rather than long finger extensors or flexors. This can be accomplished by encouraging the patient to hold fingers in a fist when extending the wrist and fully extend the digits when flexing the wrist (Figure 32.9, A, B). This promotes effective synergistic movement patterns that are used during most daily tasks.
- With evidence of healing, implement medium resistance and isotonic exercise. This can be initiated as early as 4 weeks with progressive isotonic strengthening on hold until 6 to 8 weeks.

© 2018 American Academy of Orthopaedic Surgeons

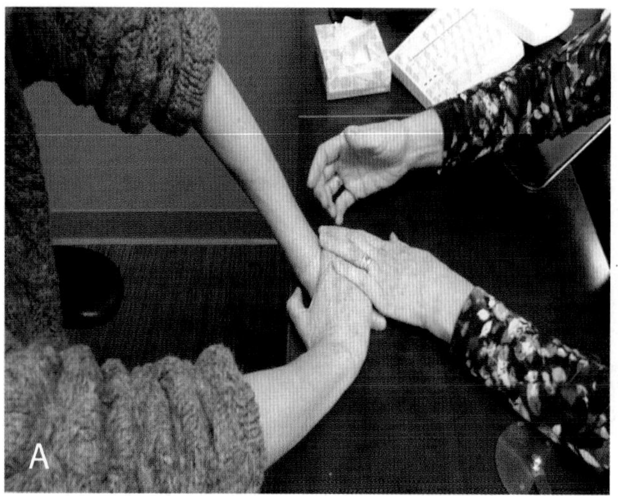

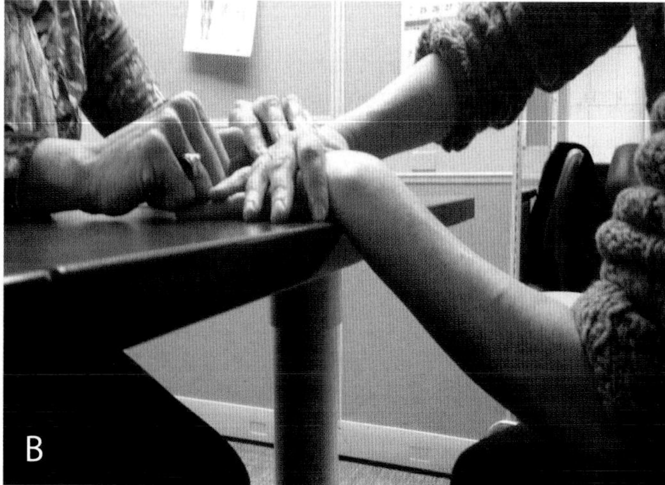

Figure 32.7 Photographs of tabletop-assisted gentle passive wrist extension (**A**) and flexion (**B**) stretches.

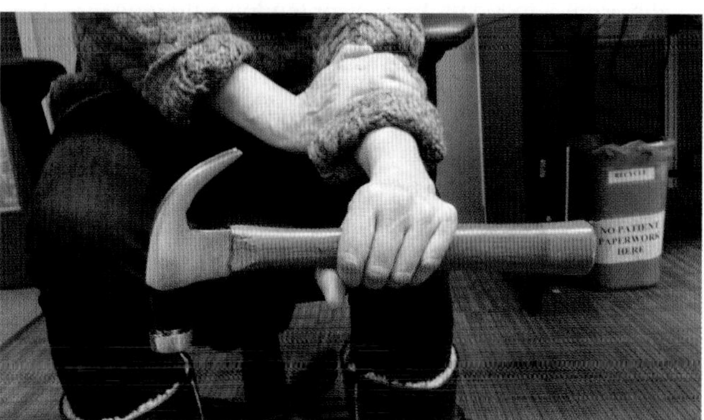

Figure 32.8 Photographs of hammer stretch to promote forearm rotation.

Weight Bearing Phase (6–12 Weeks)

- Return to weight-bearing ADLs at 6 to 8 weeks.
- Increase lifting according to tolerance without specific limits. Strengthening and functional use are typically recovered before impact activities.
- Activity restrictions are generally lifted by 10 to 12 weeks.
- Preparation for discontinuation of formal therapy (i.e., focus on home program and symptom management independence).

PEARLS

All Distal Radius Fractures

- Early focus should be on addressing disability rather than presuming that resolution of pain and physical impairments

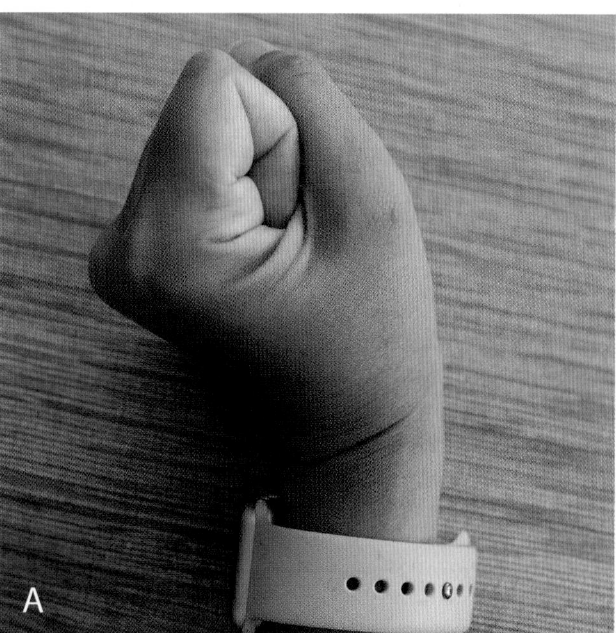

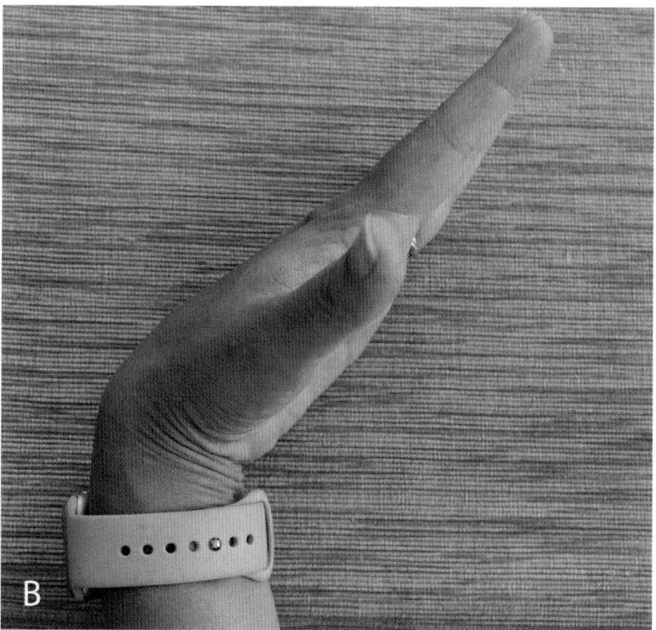

Figure 32.9 Photographs of use of prime movers during wrist flexion and extension AROM to avoid atypical movement patterns. **A**, wrist extension with finger flexion; **B**, wrist flexion with finger extension.

© 2018 American Academy of Orthopaedic Surgeons

will ultimately resolve disability; it should be recognized that patients need to engage in ADLs sooner than 6 to 8 weeks postoperatively.
- Early finger motion is crucially important.
- Be alert to sensory changes that might indicate posttraumatic carpal tunnel syndrome
- Be aware of early signs of CRPS.
- Following radiographic and clinical bony union, low-load-long-duration static progressive splinting to the wrist may also be necessitated when not responsive to stretching.

Closed Reduction With External Fixation/Percutaneous Pins

- Early finger motion incorporated immediately to prevent intrinsic, long finger/thumb extensor, and first webspace tightness.
- Superficial branch of the radial nerve irritation/injury can occur with external fixation; assessment with monofilaments, desensitization, and re-education may be necessary.

Open Reduction and Internal Fixation

- Early ROM protocol if there is no comminution and fracture fixation is secure.
- Initiate early tendon gliding for the FPL and long finger flexors to prevent tendon adherence.

OUTCOMES

Despite regaining most function in the first 3 months after ORIF of distal radius fracture, wrist motion, strength, and patient-reported function continues to improve for 1 year after distal radius fracture. The ultimate function is unaffected by the duration of immobilization during healing as outcomes are not significantly different when wrist motion is started before 2 weeks versus waiting 6 weeks. However, the inability to make a composite fist can impart more impairment than any wrist stiffness. Final wrist motion is frequently mildly restricted versus the uninjured wrist (0°–15° in each direction) but function is expected to be well preserved after most distal radius fractures. Barring complication, patients infrequently report inability to complete vocational or hobby activities after distal radius fractures.

Long-term follow-up reveals that most patients have radiographic evidence of posttraumatic arthrosis by 7 to 15 years after intra-articular distal radius fractures. However, in this nonweight–bearing joint, arthrosis has not correlated with either objective or patient-reported outcomes. The incidence of radiocarpal joint arthrosis is correlated with residual articular displacement. Similarly, long-term evaluations of distal radius fractures associated with untreated scapholunate ligament injuries (Geissler I–IIIB) or triangular fibrocartilage complex (TFCC) tears occasionally necessitates subsequent surgical treatment for these associated injuries. Therefore, despite a high incidence of associated injuries within the carpus, the majority of these are partial injuries that will not impair final function.

SUMMARY

Distal radius fractures are a common injury in patients of all ages. The decision to treat nonoperatively with immobilization or surgical reduction and fixation is dependent on individual fracture characteristics, patient preferences, and patient medical health. In all fractures, early full-finger motion is critical to the ultimate outcome and is emphasized starting at the initial encounter. Both objective and patient-reported outcomes after distal radius fracture plateau at 1 year after injury.

ACKNOWLEDGMENTS

We thank Virginia O'Brien, OTD, OTR/L, CHT for her assistance with photography, and Logan and Avery McGee for serving as hand models.

BIBLIOGRAPHY

Arora R, Lutz M, Deml C, Krappinger D, Haug L, Gabl M: A prospective randomized trial comparing nonoperative treatment with volar locking plate fixation for displaced and unstable distal radial fractures in patients sixty-five years of age and older. *J Bone Joint Surg Am* 2011;93(23):2146–2153.

Bell JS, Wollstein R, Citron ND: Rupture of flexor pollicis longus tendon: a complication of volar plating of the distal radius. *J Bone Joint Surg Br* 1998;80:225–226.

Brehmer JL, Husband JB: Accelerated rehabilitation compared with a standard protocol after distal radial fractures treated with volar open reduction and internal fixation: A prospective, randomized, controlled study. *J Bone Joint Surg Am* 2014; 96(19):1621–1630.

Chen NC, Jupiter JB: Management of distal radial fractures. *J Bone Joint Surg Am* 2007;89(9):2051–2062.

Court-Brown CM, Caesar B: Epidemiology of adult fractures: A review. *Injury* 2006;37(8):691–697.

Ipaktchi K, Livermore M, Lyons C, Banegas R: Current concepts in the treatment of distal radial fractures. *Orthopedics* 2013; 36(10):778–784.

Koval KJ, Harrast JJ, Anglen JO, Weinstein JN: Fractures of the distal part of the radius. The evolution of practice over time. Where's the evidence? *J Bone Joint Surg Am* 2008;90(9):1855–1861.

Lee DS, Weikert DR: Complications of distal radius fixation. *Orthop Clin North Am* 2016;47(2):415–424.

Putnam MD, Meyer NJ, Nelson EW, Gesensway D, Lewis JL: Distal radial metaphyseal forces in an extrinsic grip model: implications for postfracture rehabilitation. *J Hand Surg Am* 2000;25(3):469–475.

Roh YH, Lee BK, Noh JH, Baek JR, Oh JH, Gong HS, Baek GH: Factors associated with complex regional pain syndrome type I in patients with surgically treated distal radius fracture. *Arch Orthop Trauma Surg* 2014;134(12):1775–1781.

Rostami H, Arefi A, Tabatabaei S: Effect of mirror therapy on hand function in patients with hand orthopaedic injuries: A randomized controlled trial. *Disabil Rehabil* 2013;35(19):1647–1651.

© 2018 American Academy of Orthopaedic Surgeons

Soong M, Earp BE, Bishop G, Leung A, Blazar P: Volar locking plate implant prominence and flexor tendon rupture. *J Bone Joint Surg Am* 2011;93(4):328–335.

The Treatment of Distal Radius Fractures: Guideline and Evidence Report. AAOS 2009.

Thieme H, Morkisch N, Rietz C, Dohle C, Borgetto B: The Efficacy of Movement Representation Techniques for Treatment of Limb Pain—A Systematic Review and Meta-Analysis. *J Pain* 2016;17(2):167–180.

Valdes K, Naughton N, Burke, CJ: Therapist-supervised hand therapy versus home therapy with therapist instruction following distal radius fracture. *J Hand Surg Am* 2015;40(6): 1110–1116.e1.

 © 2018 American Academy of Orthopaedic Surgeons

Total Wrist Arthroplasty

Rowena McBeath, MD, PhD, Annie Ashok, MD, and Terri Skirven, OTR/L, CHT

INTRODUCTION

Total joint arthroplasty has defined the modern era of orthopaedic surgery. In the wrist, total wrist arthroplasty (TWA), though innovative, has yet to match the successful patient outcomes provided by hip and knee arthroplasty. However, notwithstanding differences in joint anatomy, mechanics, and, thus, kinematics, novel TWA designs have proven promising for the appropriate patient.

INDICATIONS AND CONTRAINDICATIONS

As with many surgical interventions, the success of TWA depends on patient selection. The ideal candidate for TWA has painful, destructive arthritis of one or both wrists, and/or coexistent multilevel upper extremity arthritis. Patients must be willing to accept a low-demand lifestyle in return for a stable, pain-free joint with functional range of motion (ROM) and the ability to perform activities of daily living (ADLs) that require wrist motion such as writing, fastening buttons, and perineal care.

The primary indication for TWA is painful, debilitating pancarpal arthritis. TWA has traditionally been employed in patients with advanced rheumatoid arthritis, a disease that commonly affects bilateral wrists and multiple joints of the upper extremity. In addition, studies have shown that TWA is beneficial to patients with severe nonrheumatoid inflammatory arthritis, osteoarthritis, and posttraumatic arthritis. TWA is also indicated in patients with advanced avascular necrosis of the carpal bones.

TWA is contraindicated in those unable to adhere to strict activity limitations, such as physical laborers or patients who require the use of walking aids and must bear weight on their wrists. Other contraindications include active infection, a history of sepsis or osteomyelitis, a hand lacking neurologic function, rupture of the radial wrist extensors, and ligamentous laxity. Relative contraindications to TWA include immunosuppression, systemic lupus erythematosus, proximal row carpectomy, and other conditions resulting in poor carpal bone stock.

PROCEDURE

Relevant Anatomy

The wrist moves in three planes of motion: flexion-extension, radial-ulnar deviation, and prono-supination. Normal ROM of the wrist includes volar flexion of 85° to 90°, extension (or dorsiflexion) of 80° to 85°, radial deviation of 20° to 25° and ulnar deviation of 30° to 35°. The movements of the wrist take place along an axis through the capitate, and pronation and supination occur about the distal radioulnar joint.

The mechanical axes of the wrist are oriented obliquely to the anatomic axes, with the primary mechanical direction of the wrist being radial extension and ulnar flexion. The ROM of the wrist that is required for most functional ADLs is flexion and extension of 30°, and ulnar and radial deviation of 10°, thus facilitating a hand position that contributes to fine motor control of the fingers and grip strength.

Technique

The surgical approach to TWA is similar across implants, with some variation based on the specific prosthesis used. Postoperative rehabilitation is similar across implants without any specific alterations according to the implant used (Figure 33.1).

Prior to surgery, radiographs of the wrist are used to template and estimate the size of the implant, as well as the amount of distal radius to be resected. The operation is performed on a hand table with the use of an upper arm tourniquet and either general or regional anesthesia. The arm and hand are prepped and draped in the standard fashion, and an Esmarch bandage is used to exsanguinate the limb. Loupe magnification is used for all dissection.

A longitudinal dorsal incision is made from the middle of the third metacarpal extending to 2 cm proximal to the Lister tubercle on the distal radius. Skin flaps are created and bleeding is controlled with a clamp and microcautery. Care must

None of the following authors nor any immediate family member has received anything of value from or has stock or stock options held in a commercial company or institution related directly or indirectly to the subject of this article: Dr. McBeath, Dr. Ashok, and Dr. Skirven.

© 2018 American Academy of Orthopaedic Surgeons

be taken to protect the sensory branches of the radial nerve, which course over the anatomic snuffbox, and dorsal ulnar cutaneous nerve branches, which become dorsal distal to the ulnar styloid. The dissection is carried down to the extensor retinaculum, the third dorsal compartment is opened, and the extensor pollicis longus (EPL) tendon is released and radialized. Extensor tenosynovectomy is performed in all compartments.

Next, capsular flaps are elevated from the radius through a longitudinal incision based on the third metacarpal. Carpal resection is performed using rongeurs. The carpal guide is placed parallel to the longitudinal axis of the long finger metacarpal and stabilized with two 0.062-inch Kirschner wires (K-wires). The proximal carpal row, edge of the hamate, and proximal capitate head are resected according to each implant's requirement. The carpal component is then trialed.

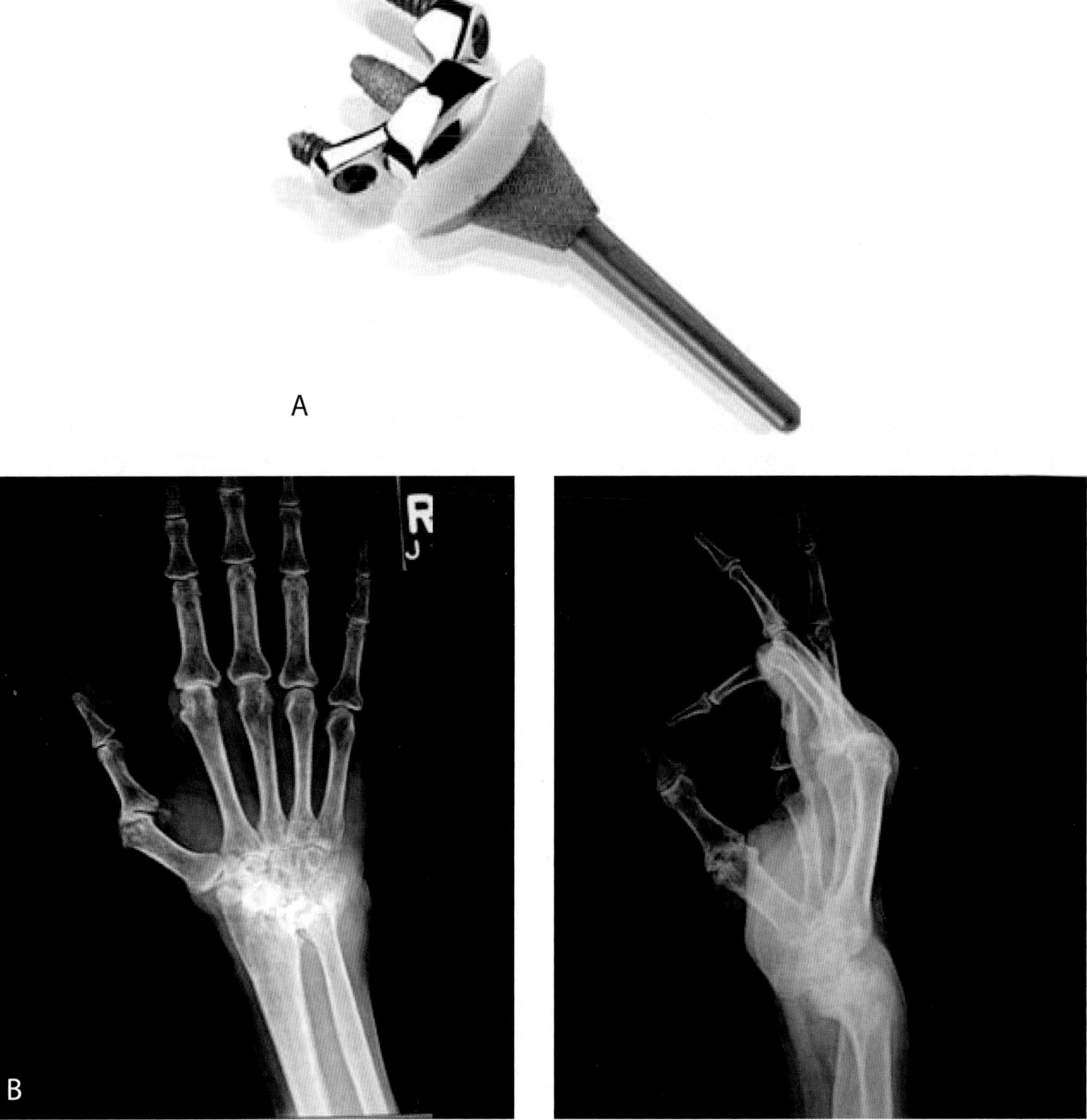

Figure 33.1 **A**, Photograph of an example of total wrist arthroplasty implants. **B**, Preoperative wrist radiographs of a patient with rheumatoid arthritis.

 © 2018 American Academy of Orthopaedic Surgeons

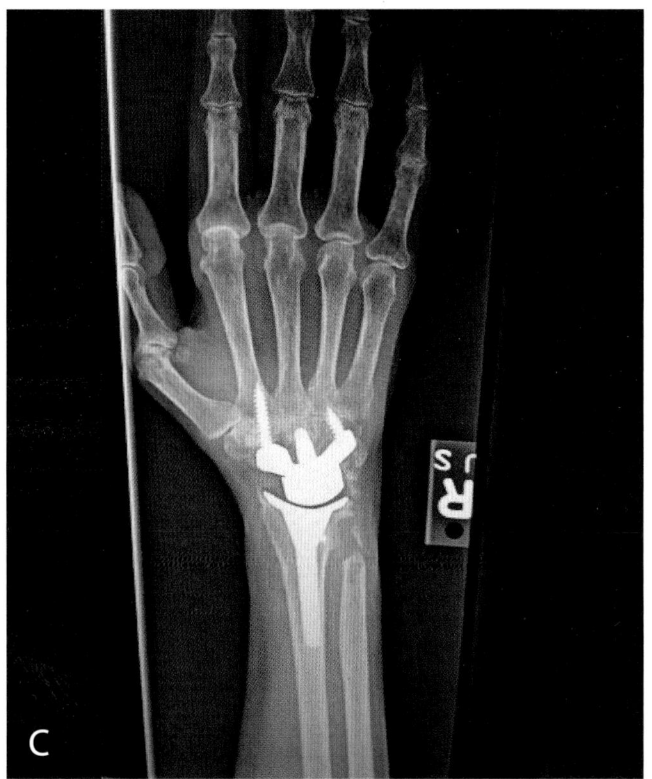

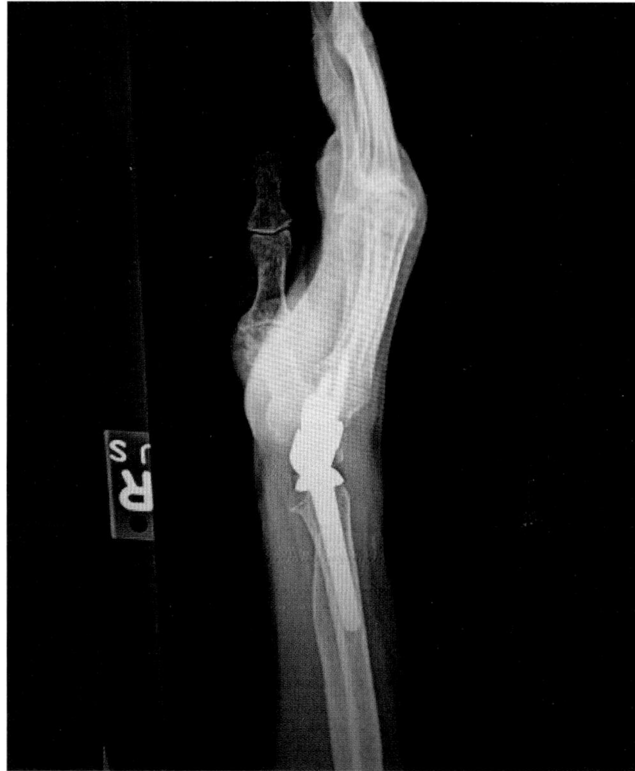

Figure 33.1 (*Continued*) **C**, Postoperative radiographs of a total wrist arthoplasty in a patient with rheumatoid arthritis.

Turning attention to the radial component, the wrist is then palmar flexed and a K-wire is driven into the center of the distal radius intramedullary canal and the position is confirmed by fluoroscopy. The distal articular surface of the radius is resected, broached, and trialed, paying close attention to protect the surrounding soft-tissue structures, including the volar radiocarpal ligaments. The wrist with trial carpal and radial components is then reduced to examine stability and ROM, both clinically and fluoroscopically.

The trials are then exchanged for implants, and screw fixation to the long finger metacarpal shaft and hamate is performed. After ensuring adequate ROM and stability, the wound is irrigated, the EPL is radialized, and the extensor retinaculum is repaired. The wounds are closed in a layered fashion and postoperative radiographs are obtained to confirm alignment of the prosthesis. The wrist is typically immobilized with a volar wrist neutral splint, and the hand is elevated to prevent and minimize swelling.

Complications

In addition to general complications of operative procedures, including bleeding and damage to nearby structures, many of the complications of TWA are related to the nature of the disease process. Infection is an especially severe problem, with the potential for substantial morbidity. Patients with rheumatoid arthritis may be particularly susceptible to infection because of the immunosuppressive effects of medical therapy for this condition.

The most common cause of failure of TWA is metacarpal loosening, with dorsal perforation of the stem. Additional complications include hardware failure, pin migration, and persistent pain. These outcomes may result from inadequate alignment and fixation of the prosthesis and/or improper soft-tissue balancing. Factors contributing to TWA failure also include patient-specific factors such as poor bone stock and progressive bony disease, ligamentous laxity or contracture, and failure to adhere to low-demand activities. Salvage operations for a failed TWA include revision arthroplasty or arthrodesis.

POSTOPERATIVE REHABILITATION

Introduction

The overall goal of rehabilitation after TWA is to maximize ROM to enable performance of ADLs within the constraints of maintaining prosthesis stability. The rehabilitation protocol should be tailored to reflect individual patient goals regarding self-care, household responsibilities, work, and leisure activities. Reasonable rehabilitation expectations, the timetable of recovery, and ultimate functional limitations should be discussed with the patient preoperatively. The initiation and timing of new exercises may be adjusted according to patient comfort and ability, and according to the integrity of soft tissues and the surgical approach, which should be determined by the surgeon. The final outcome is generally achieved between 6 and 12 months after surgery.

© 2018 American Academy of Orthopaedic Surgeons

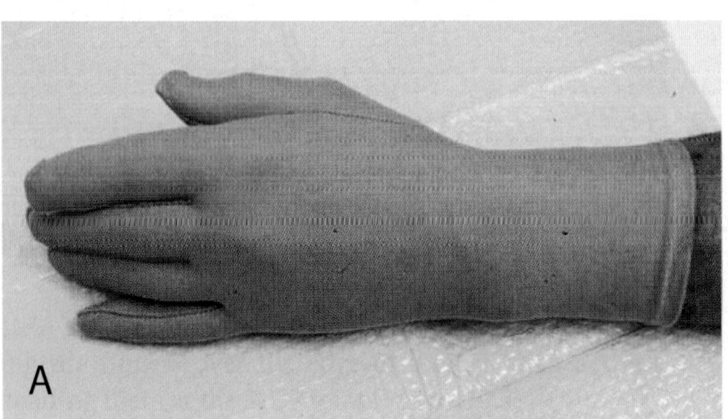

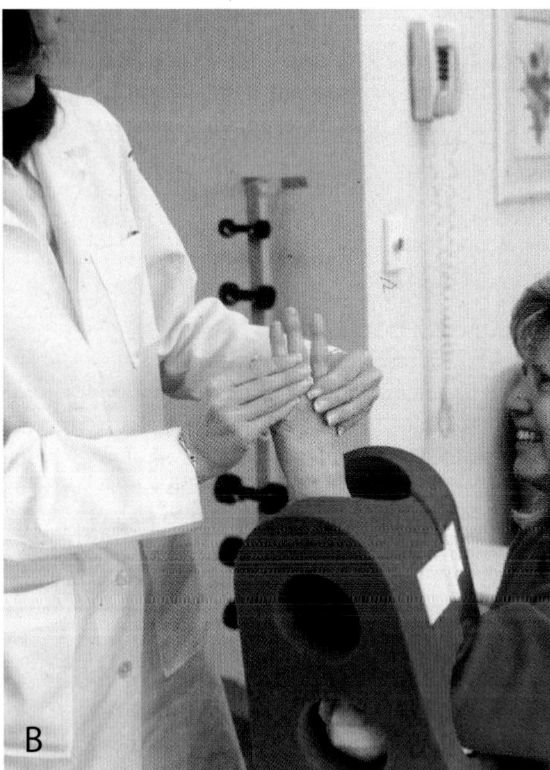

Figure 33.2 Photographs of edema control techniques: **A**, Compression gloves. **B**, Retrograde massage.

Authors' Preferred Protocol

Initial Healing and Protective Phase (Weeks 1 to 2)

- Edema control techniques including elevation, compression sleeves or gloves, and gentle retrograde massage may be employed throughout the rehabilitation process (Figure 33.2.)
- Pain management techniques, including the use of cold compresses or transcutaneous electrical nerve stimulation (TENS) may be used as needed.
- Custom fabricated thermoplastic volar wrist orthosis (Figure 33.3) in 15° of dorsiflexion worn full-time except for hygiene and exercises
- Thumb and finger active range of motion (AROM) and passive range of motion (PROM)
- Extensor tendon gliding exercises
- Shoulder and elbow ROM

Transitional, Mobilization Phase (Weeks 2 to 6)

- Orthosis is continued and may need to be remolded to maintain appropriate fit.
- Scar management
- Continue thumb and finger ROM exercises.
- AROM and active-assistive range of motion (AAROM) exercises in volar flexion, dorsiflexion, and radial and ulnar deviation (Figure 33.4)
- Shoulder and elbow ROM
- Initiate light nonresistive and nonrepetitive ADLs.

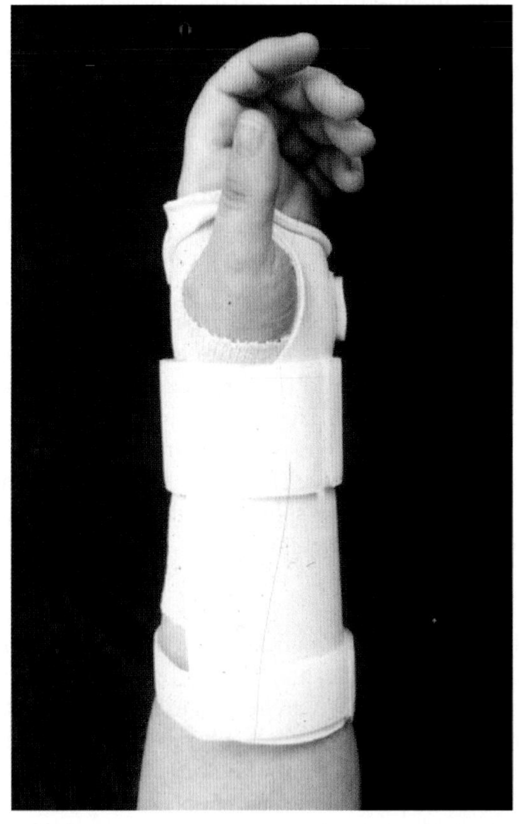

Figure 33.3 Photograph of a custom-fabricated volar wrist orthosis.

© 2018 American Academy of Orthopaedic Surgeons

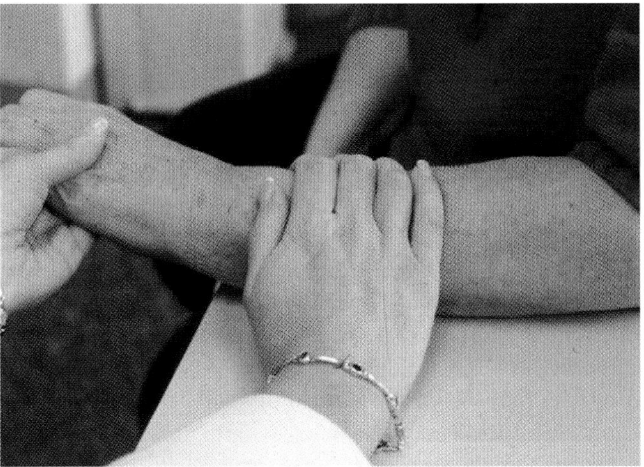

Figure 33.4 Photograph of active-assistive range of motion.

Strengthening Phase (Weeks 6 to 8)

- Wean from wrist orthosis, may use flexible support (e.g., neoprene wrist wrap) as needed (Figure 33.5)
- Continue thumb and finger range of motion exercises
- Continue active and active assisted wrist range of motion
- Initiate isometric wrist strengthening exercises (Figure 33.6)
- Initiate light grip strengthening exercises using resistive putty
- Activities of daily living tasks as tolerated

Functional Restoration (Weeks 8 to 12)

- Address wrist stiffness with dynamic progressive (Figure 33.7, A) or static progressive (Figure 33.7, B) stretching orthoses.
- Use assistive devices and/or modified techniques to assist ADL tasks, as needed.
- Continue thumb, finger, and wrist exercises, as needed, to maximize functional outcome.
- Progressive return to ADLs, as tolerated
- Impact activities (e.g., hammering) or activities that load the wrist in extreme positions (e.g., push-ups) should be avoided after TWA.

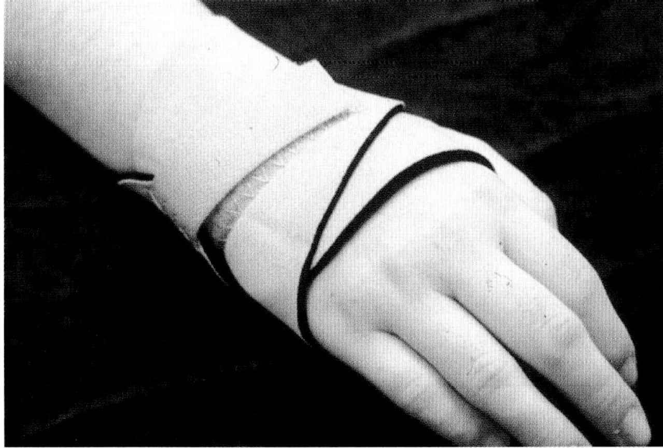

Figure 33.5 Photograph of a flexible neoprene wrist support.

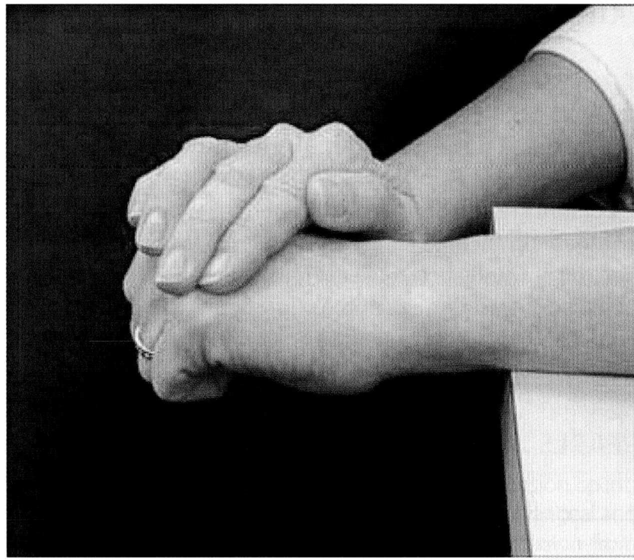

Figure 33.6 Photograph of isometric wrist strengthening exercise.

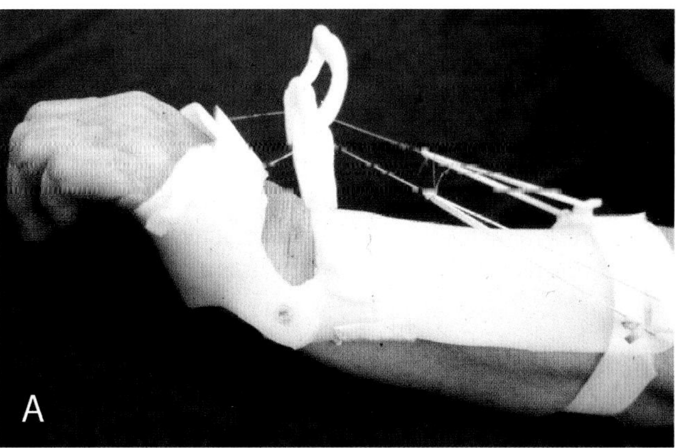

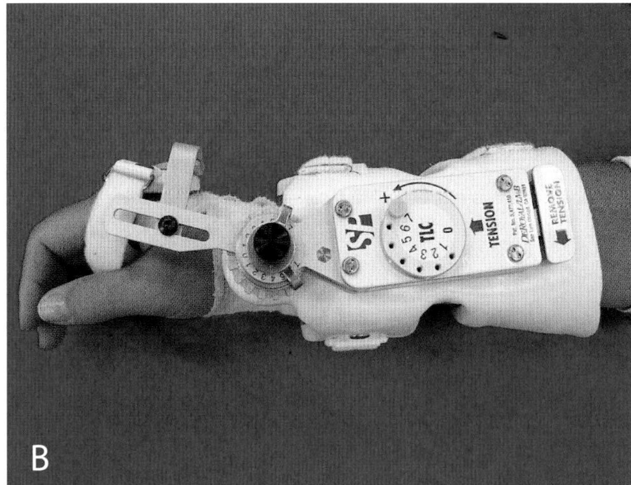

Figure 33.7 Photographs of assistive devices used to improve range of motion for goal activities of daily living. **A**, Dynamic extension wrist orthosis. **B**, Static progressive wrist orthosis.

© 2018 American Academy of Orthopaedic Surgeons

OUTCOMES

Outcomes after TWA are difficult to assess, as implant systems continue to be altered and revised. Therefore, the literature on this topic often lags behind the currently available systems. Studying currently available implants, Nydick et al reported 7 complications with 1 implant removal in 23 wrists at 28 months. Functional outcomes were reasonable, with reduction in pain, and an average flexion extension arc of 90°. Similarly, in 20 cases at 32 months, loosening of 2 components occurred, but did not require revision in a study of another wrist arthroplasty system.

PEARLS

- Carefully select patients when considering TWA to ensure that expectations are to maintain motion for ADLs as opposed to anticipation of resumption of impact activities.
- Carefully perform bony resections to ensure proper tensioning when performing TWA.

SUMMARY

TWA continues to evolve as a salvage procedure to preserve wrist motion. It is a technically demanding procedure that requires careful patient selection. The procedure has the potential to substantially improve the patient's quality of life by reducing pain and improving function. In the future, continued improvements in design and techniques are anticipated. Long-term studies are needed to define clinical outcomes and survivorship.

BIBLIOGRAPHY

Beer TA, Turner RH: Wrist arthrodesis for failed wrist implant arthroplasty. *J Hand Surg Am* 1997;22:685–693.

Brumfeld RH, Champoux JA: A biomechanical study of normal functional wrist motion. *Clin Orthop Relat Res* 1984;(187):23–25.

Carroll RE, Dick HM: Arthrodesis of the wrist for rheumatoid arthritis. *J Bone Joint Surg Am* 1971;53:1365–1369.

Crisco JJ, Heard WM, Rich RR, Paller DJ, Wolfe SW: The mechanical axes of the wrist are oriented obliquely to the anatomical axes. *J Bone Joint Surg Am* 2011;93(2):169–177.

Hamalainen M, Kammonen M, Lehtimaki M: Epidemiology of wrist involvement in rheumatoid arthritis. *Rheumatol* 1992;17:1–7.

Hastings H 2nd: Total wrist arthrodesis for post-traumatic conditions. *Indiana Hand Center Newsletter* 1993;1:14.

Herzberg G: Prospective study of a new total wrist replacement: Short term results. *Chir Main* 2011;30(1):20–25.

Ilan DI, Rettig ME: Rheumatoid arthritis of the wrist. *Bull Hosp Jt Dis* 61(3–4):179–185.

Landsmeer JM: Studies in the anatomy of articulation, 1 and 2. *Acta Morphol Neerl Scand* 1961;3:287–303.

Lorei MP, Figgie MP, Ranawat CS, Inglis AE: Failed total wrist arthroplasty: analysis of failures and results of operative management. *Clin Orthop Rel Res* 1997;(342):84–93.

MacConaill MA: The mechanical anatomy of the carpus and its bearings on some surgical problems. *J Anat* 1941;75:166–175.

McBeath R, Osterman AL: Total wrist arthroplasty. *Hand Clin* 2012;28(4):595–609.

Millender LH, Nalebuff EA: Arthrodesis of the rheumatoid wrist. An evaluation of sixty patients and a description of a different surgical technique. *J Bone Joint Surg Am* 1973;55:1026–1034.

Nydick JA, Greenberg SM, Stone JD, Williams B, Polikandriotis JA, Hess AV: Clinical outcomes of total wrist arthroplasty. *J Hand Surg Am* 2012;37:1580–1584.

Palmer AK, Werner FW, Murphy D, Glisson R: Functional wrist motion: a biomechanical study. *J Hand Surg Am* 1985;10(1):39–46.

Rizzo M, Ackerman DB, Rodrigues RL, Beckenbaugh RD: Wrist arthrodesis as a salvage procedure for failed implant arthroplasty. *J Hand Surg Eur* 2011;36:29–33.

Ryu JY, Cooney WP 3rd, Askew LJ, An KN, Chao EY: Functional ranges of motion of the wrist joint. *J Hand Surg Am* 1991;16(3):409–419.

Trieb K: Treatment of the wrist in rheumatoid arthritis. *J Hand Surg Am* 2008;33A:113–123.

© 2018 American Academy of Orthopaedic Surgeons

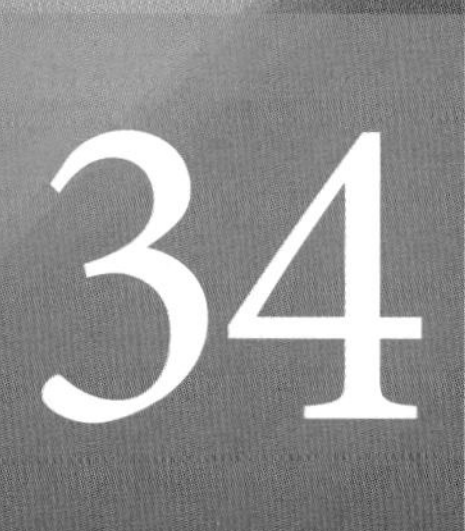

34 Wrist Arthrodesis: Limited and Complete

Nicole S. Schroeder, MD, and Karen Pitbladdo, MS, OTR/L, CHT

INTRODUCTION

Untreated carpal malalignment can result in abnormal stresses across the radiocarpal joint and eventually produce arthritis in the wrist. Limited and complete wrist arthrodeses are regarded as final salvage procedures for symptomatic posttraumatic, degenerative, postinfectious or inflammatory arthritis of the wrist. The goal of any type of wrist arthrodesis is to provide a functionally stable wrist that allows painless performance of activities of daily living (ADLs). Although fusion reduces pain at the expense of diminished range of motion (ROM), the goal of postoperative rehabilitation is to maximize allowable motion, limit pain, and ultimately restore and preserve hand function.

Several authors have demonstrated that normal wrist motion far exceeds what is needed to perform ADLs. Palmer and colleagues showed that only 5° of flexion, 30° of extension, 10° of radial deviation, and 15° of ulnar deviation are required to perform most standard tasks. Therefore, while arthodeses may restrict some motion, the elimination of pain and preservation of some motion that the procedures provide may not be detrimental to daily tasks.

This chapter reviews the surgical procedure and postoperative rehabilitation protocols for the following types of arthrodesis: scaphotrapezial-trapezoidal (STT), intercarpal fusion (ICF), four-corner fusion (FCF), and total wrist (Figure 34.1). In addition, the indications and surgical techniques for proximal row carpectomy (PRC) will be discussed. The choice of treatment depends on the findings of a complete evaluation of the patient, including an assessment of the patient's functional needs and goals. Given that arthritic findings on plain radiographs do not always correlate with clinical symptoms, it is critical to use the clinical examination to identify the precise location that generates pain. In the setting of diffuse arthritis, isolated scaphotrapezial trapezoid or radiocarpal injections with lidocaine 1% can help to localize the pain as well as give a patient an idea of the degree of pain relief to expect after surgery. While there are general principles of postoperative rehabilitation, there are some aspects that relate to the specific surgical procedures.

REHABILITATION

Postoperative care varies depending on the exact procedure, but all protocols share three common phases: (1) protection, (2) ROM, and (3) strengthening. Progression from one phase to the next depends on radiographic evidence of fusion as well as surgeon's preference. A clear understanding of the physician's postoperative goals and expectations should be discussed at the initiation of any therapy. Most limited wrist arthrodeses are expected to reduce the preoperative wrist arc of motion by 40%.

Phase 1: Protection Phase (0–6 Weeks)

- A postoperative splint is applied following the surgical procedure.
- Splint (operative dressing) is removed at 2 weeks and a short arm or thumb spica cast is applied.
- Casting should allow full finger motion through the metacarpophalangeal joints.
- Immediate active finger ROM immediately with tendon gliding (Figure 34.2).
- Arm elevation to minimize swelling and edema
- Patients demonstrating substantial edema or those unable to comply with postoperative digital motion should be referred to hand rehabilitation early.
- Shoulder and elbow ROM.

Phase 2: Range of Motion Phase (6–10 Weeks)

Postoperative goal is pain-free, functional arc of wrist motion.

- ROM phase typically begins when the physician notes a solid fusion mass on radiographs.
- Avoid maximizing ROM at the expense of stability and/or pain.
- Cast is removed. Continue with edema management.

Neither of the following authors nor any immediate family member has received anything of value from or has stock or stock options held in a commercial company or institution related directly or indirectly to the subject of this article: Dr. Pitbladdo and Dr. Schroeder.

© 2018 American Academy of Orthopaedic Surgeons

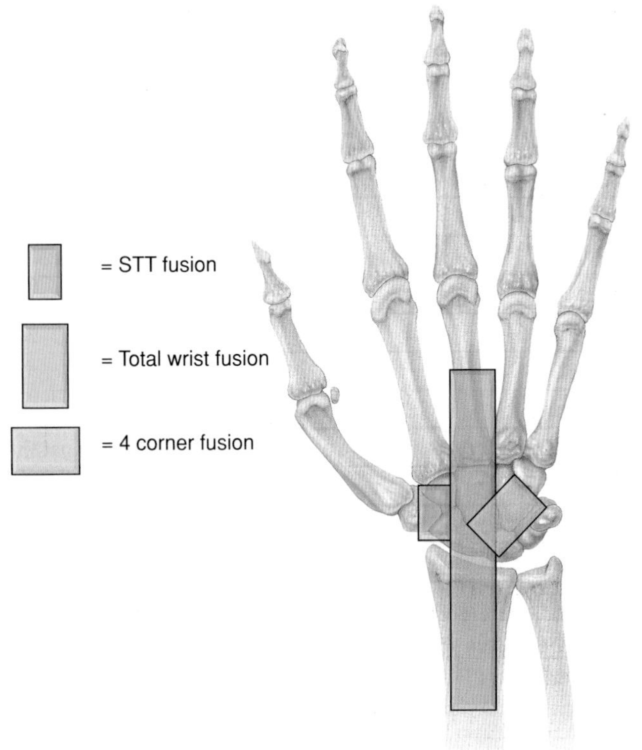

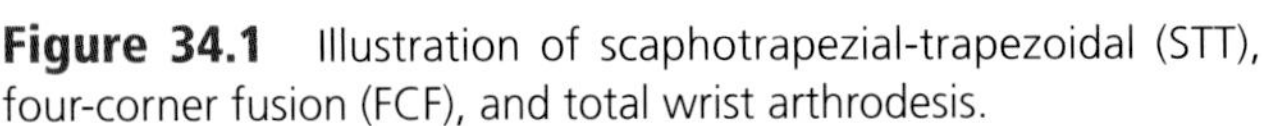

Figure 34.1 Illustration of scaphotrapezial-trapezoidal (STT), four-corner fusion (FCF), and total wrist arthrodesis.

- Custom-made or prefabricated splint is used and is selected based on comfort, fit, and extent of support needed.
- Begin scar desensitization. Silicone gel sheets and scar massage are the cornerstones of desensitization (Figure 34.3, A and B).
- Active ROM exercises should focus on synergistic motion of finger flexion with wrist extension
- Passive stretching toward terminal degrees assisted in part by the surgeon's expectation for maximal motion recovery
- Patients are encouraged to use their hand in light bilateral activity and basic hygiene to allow incorporation of the operated hand in ADLs.

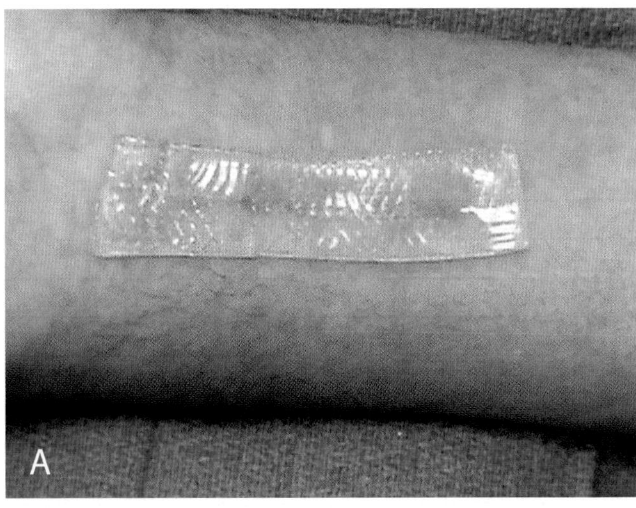

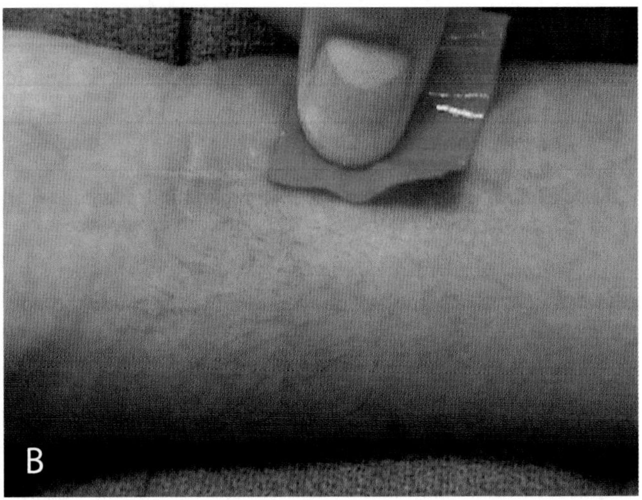

Figure 34.3 **A**, Silicone scar pad applied directly over the healing surgical scar. **B**, Desensitization of the scar and surrounding soft tissues using an abrasive surface.

Phase 3: Strengthening Phase (10+ Weeks)

- At 10 to 12 weeks, patients begin to gradually increase the load across the joint with a combination of grasping activity and isometric, concentric, and eccentric wrist exercises.

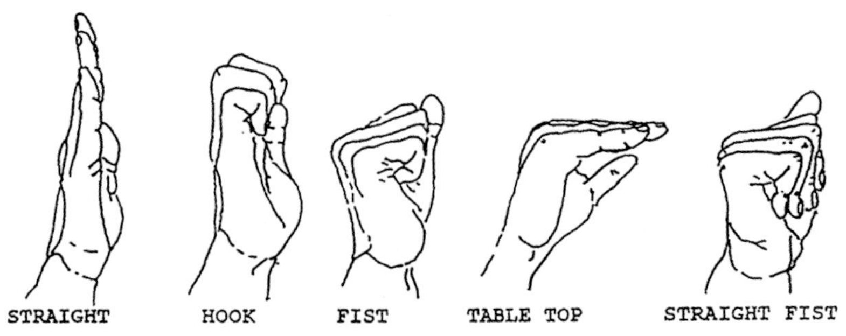

Figure 34.2 Illustration of active tendon gliding exercises.

 © 2018 American Academy of Orthopaedic Surgeons

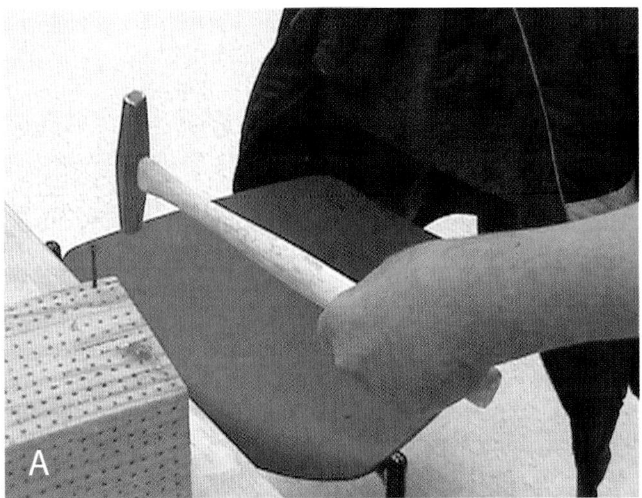

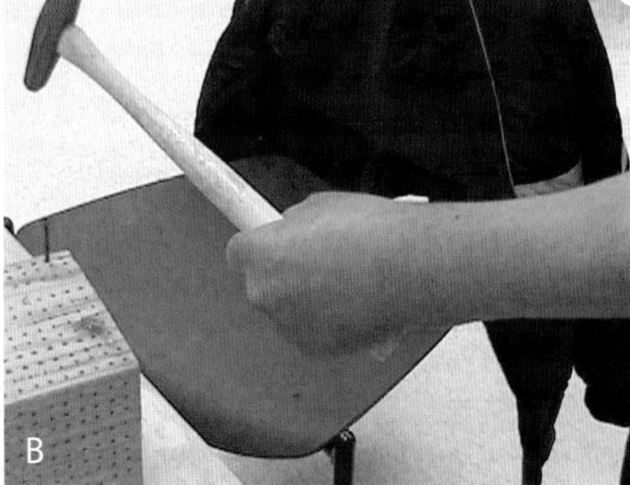

Figure 34.4 Active exercising of the wrist in the dart thrower's path from radial extension to ulnar flexion. **A**, With flexion and ulnar deviation. **B**, With extension and radial deviation.

- Continue to address limitations in ROM while transitioning to strengthening.
- Dart thrower's motion (DTM) allows a patient to perform exercises in radial deviation/extension and ulnar deviation/flexion patterns that best duplicate many ADLs (Figure 34.4, A and B).
- With evidence of complete fusion (typically around 12 weeks), grip strengthening and job simulation is initiated.
- Strengthening can be done with the use of therapy putty or the incorporation of light free weights in ROM exercises.

SURGICAL PROCEDURES

Scaphotrapezial Trapezoidal (STT) Arthrodesis

Indications

STT arthrodesis is indicated for the treatment of symptomatic osteoarthritis of the STT joint. It can also be used in select cases of midcarpal instability, static or dynamic rotatory subluxation of the scaphoid, chronic scapholunate dissociation, and avascular necrosis of the lunate. It has been shown to preserve pinch-and-grip strength without compromising functional ROM.

Contraindications

STT arthrodesis is contraindicated in pancarpal arthritis or associated radioscaphoid arthritis. While it has been advocated as a treatment of chronic scapholunate instability, there is a significant complication rate and it is rarely performed for isolated scapholunate ligament incompetence.

Procedure

The STT joint can be approached through either a transverse or oblique dorsoradial incision. Typically, a radial styloidectomy is performed through the same incision. The dorsal wrist capsule is incised and the articular surfaces of the distal scaphoid and proximal trapezium and trapezoid are denuded of articular cartilage and subchondral bone. The joint is fused with the scaphoid in approximately 50° to 55° of flexion to optimally center functional wrist motion. Fusion methods include variable pitch headless screws, fusion plates, or Kirschner wires. Ipsilateral distal radius bone graft is harvested and packed into the fusion site prior to fixation (Figure 34.5). A bulky thumb

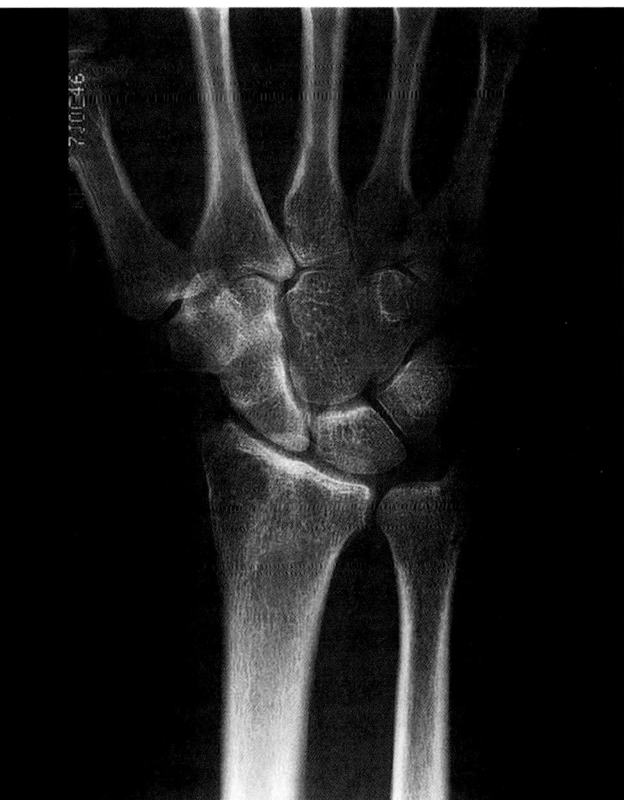

Figure 34.5 Anteroposterior plain radiograph of a right wrist after scaphotrapezial-trapezoidal (SST) fusion. (Reproduced with permission from Watson HK, Wollstein R, Joseph E, et al: Scaphotrapeziotrapezoid arthrodesis: a follow-up study. *J Hand Surg Am* 2003;28(3):397–404.)

© 2018 American Academy of Orthopaedic Surgeons

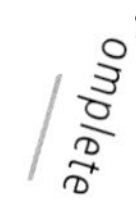

applied immediately postoperatively. After ›oved at 2 weeks, a thumb spica cast is applied ›al 4 weeks.

Comp... ›s

Postoperative wrist flexion may be limited if the scaphoid is fixed in excessive extension. Postoperative complications include radiographic evidence of radioscaphoid or trapeziometacarpal arthritis, nerve injury, and nonunion.

Postoperative Rehabilitation

We recommend placement of a short-arm thumb spica cast during the protective phase to limit rotational torque on the fusion mass. In the ROM phase, patients are weaned out of a thumb spica splint as wrist motion improves. A wrist flexion–extension arc of approximately 100° is expected after STT fusion.

Four-corner Arthrodesis (Lunate-Capitate-Triquetrum-Hamate)

Indications

A scaphoid excision and four-corner arthrodesis (lunate-capitate-triquetrum-hamate arthrodesis) is indicated for the treatment of wrist arthritis caused by scaphoid nonunion advance collapse (SNAC) or scapholunate advanced collapse (SLAC). In both instances, the fusion prevents further carpal collapse and proximal migration of the capitate.

Contraindications

Four-corner fusion is contraindicated in wrists that demonstrate arthritis of the radiolunate articulation.

Procedure

A dorsal longitudinal incision is made over the wrist. The third extensor compartment is opened and the second through fourth compartments elevated off the radius. The radiocarpal and midcarpal joints are exposed through a ligament-sparing approach. The scaphoid is excised in its entirety and the articular surfaces and subchondral bone of the capitolunate, lunotriquetral, and hamate-triquetrum joints are débrided to cancellous bone. To maximize wrist extension, the lunate should be fused in a neutral or slightly flexed position. Arthrodesis techniques include headless screws, staples, or fusion plates and typically require harvesting local distal radius bone graft (Figure 34.6). A bulky short-arm thumb spica splint is applied immediately postoperatively.

Complications

Complications may include delayed union, nonunion, and progression to radiographic radiocarpal arthritis. Risk of incomplete fusion or nonunion greatly increases in smokers. Therefore, we require our patients to quit smoking for 2 months prior to fusion. If the lunate is fused in extension, postoperative wrist extension is limited.

Rehabilitation

Given that the method of fixation varies widely for this procedure, the length of the protective phase is also highly variable. We typically use headless compression screws and immobilize in a thumb spica cast for 8 weeks or until evidence of fusion. Finger ROM and edema control are essential during this period. Once a solid fusion is observed, the ROM

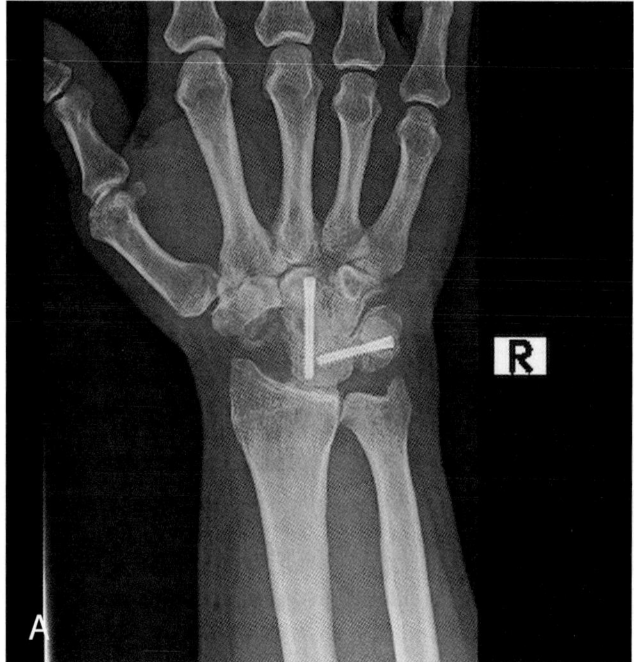

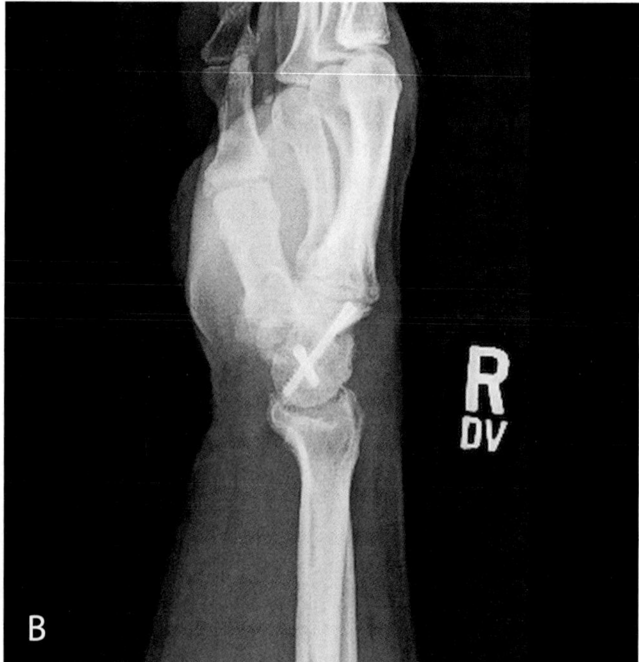

Figure 34.6 Anteroposterior (**A**) and lateral (**B**) plain radiographs of a right wrist after scaphoid excision and four-corner fusion: lunate-capitate-triquetrum-hamate arthrodesis. (Courtesy of Christopher Got, MD)

© 2018 American Academy of Orthopaedic Surgeons

phase is begun and the patient is weaned out of a thumb spica splint.

Functional Goals and Restrictions

Patients should expect approximately an 80° arc of flexion–extension or 60% of preoperative motion. Grip strength has been shown to equal 80% of the contralateral wrist.

Total Wrist Arthrodesis

Indications

Total wrist arthrodesis is a salvage procedure for pancarpal inflammatory or osteoarthritis, osteonecrosis, posttraumatic arthritis, or failed prior limited arthrodesis. It may also be used following bone loss from infection, tumor resection, or trauma. There are numerous methods for fusion, but the ultimate goal is stable fixation to allow early digit mobilization. Prior to total wrist arthrodesis, a period of wrist immobilization in an orthosis is used to (1) determine the ideal wrist fusion position and (2) demonstrate to the patient the functional limitations that may be incurred with the planned surgical intervention.

Contraindications

Total wrist arthrodesis is contraindicated in patients who have inflammatory osteoarthritis and poor bone stock. In a patient with a prior contralateral total wrist arthrodesis, one may discuss performing a wrist arthroplasty, but we have found that bilateral wrist arthrodesis may be well tolerated.

Procedure

A dorsal longitudinal incision is made and the extensor retinaculum is incised in a step-cut fashion. The extensor tendons (2nd–4th compartments) are retracted and a posterior interosseous neurectomy is performed. The wrist capsule is incised longitudinally. The articular surfaces and subchondral bone are removed from radioscaphoid, radiolunate, scapholunate, lunotriquetral, capitolunate, and capitate–third metacarpal joints. A proximal row carpectomy may be performed to minimize the joint surfaces required for fusion and possible risk of nonunion. If needed, fusion may be enhanced with autograft from the PRC or distal radius. A contoured, low-profile, dorsal, limited-contact, dynamic compression plate is then applied and secured with screws to the radius, capitate, and third metacarpal (Figure 34.7). The wrist is fused in neutral to slight extension to allow for improved grip strength. The extensor pollicis longus tendon is left transposed radially in the subcutaneous tissues to avoid contact with the plate. A bulky short-arm splint is applied immediately postoperatively for 2 weeks.

Complications

Short-term complications include wound complications, extensor lag, transient paresthesias, infection, and pain.

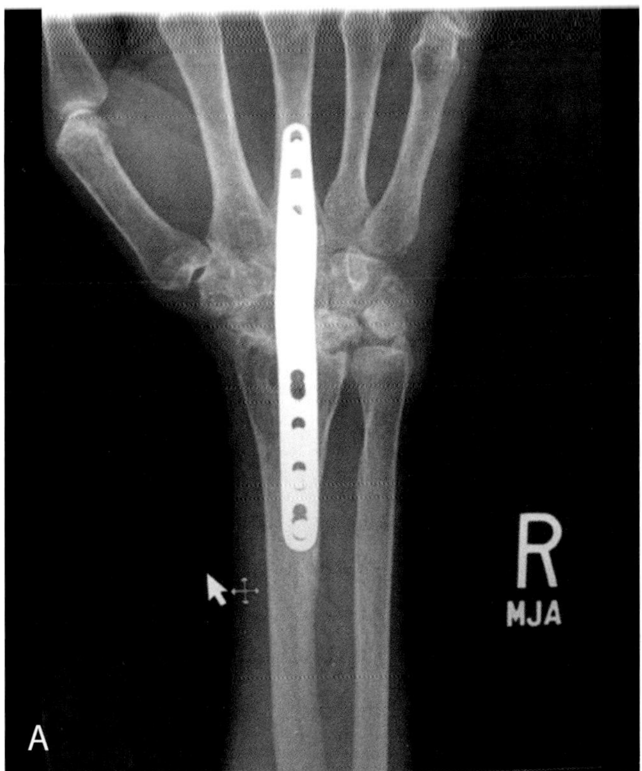

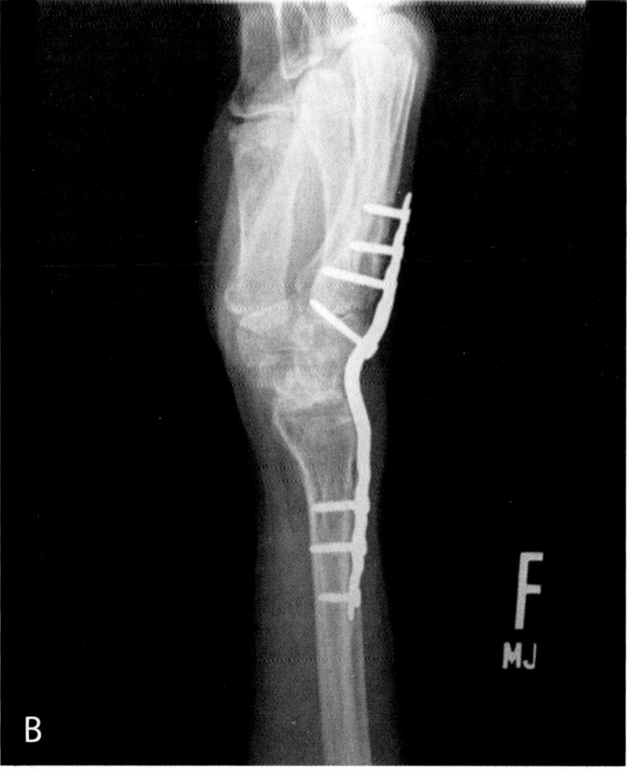

Figure 34.7 Anteroposterior (**A**) and lateral (**B**) plain radiographs of a right wrist after total wrist arthrodesis. Note the dorsal plate with fixation to the distal radius, capitate, and the base of the third metacarpal as well as the slight extension of the wrist, which optimizes grip strength.

© 2018 American Academy of Orthopaedic Surgeons

Long-term complications include persistent pain, metacarpophalangeal stiffness, STT arthritis, fracture, need for plate removal, and symptomatic ulnocarpal abutment. Risk of incomplete fusion or nonunion greatly increases in smokers. Therefore, we require our patients to quit smoking for 2 months prior to fusion.

Rehabilitation

Unlike the partial wrist arthrodesis procedures, there is no preservation of wrist flexion–extension motion following total wrist arthrodesis. Therefore, ADLs may need to be modified with use of adaptive equipment. Grip strength does not plateau until 1 year and maximal improvement in function requires between 6 and 14 months. Perineal care is noted to be one of the more difficult tasks following wrist fusion.

Functional Goals and Restrictions

Functional outcome following wrist fusion is typically determined by the amount of pain relief, patient satisfaction, and ability to return to ADLs or prior occupational and recreational activities. Reports on patient satisfaction and pain have varied widely in the literature but overall show that most patients have good pain relief at rest and are satisfied with the procedure. Studies have demonstrated that most patients retain the ability to return to heavy manual labor following wrist arthrodesis.

Proximal Row Carpectomy

PRC is a motion-preserving option that is indicated for the treatment of the degenerated wrist resulting from SLAC and SNAC, carpal osteonecrosis (Kienböck or Preisser), and chronic perilunate dislocations. PRC may also be considered as definitive management in the setting of acute perilunate dislocation in the elderly or for those with preexisting wrist arthritis. PRC appears to be optimal in patients older than 35 years of age and those with a preserved articular cartilage at the radiocapitate articulation.

Contraindications

Patients younger than 35 years of age and those with evidence of arthritic changes at the proximal capitate or lunate facet of the radius are not indicated for PRC.

Procedure

A dorsal longitudinal incision is made over the third compartment and full-thickness flaps are elevated over the extensor retinaculum, with care taken to preserve dorsal sensory nerve branches. The retinaculum is divided longitudinally, the EPL is transposed radially, and a posterior interosseous neurectomy is performed. The wrist capsule is incised longitudinally and subperiosteal elevation of the fourth compartment is performed in an ulnar direction. Care must be taken to preserve the ulnocarpal ligaments to prevent postoperative ulnar translocation. The base of the capitate and the lunate facet of the radius are examined for evidence of arthrosis. If significant arthrosis is noted, a wrist arthrodesis or PRC with soft tissue interposition should be considered. Once adequate exposure is obtained, the bones of the proximal row are removed (Figure 34.8). Visualization may be enhanced with the use of a large Knowles pin acting as a joystick. When excising the scaphoid, care is taken to preserve the volar radioscaphocapitate ligament and protect the volar radial artery. Following scaphoid resection, the lunate and triquetrum are excised. Radiographs are taken to confirm excision and alignment

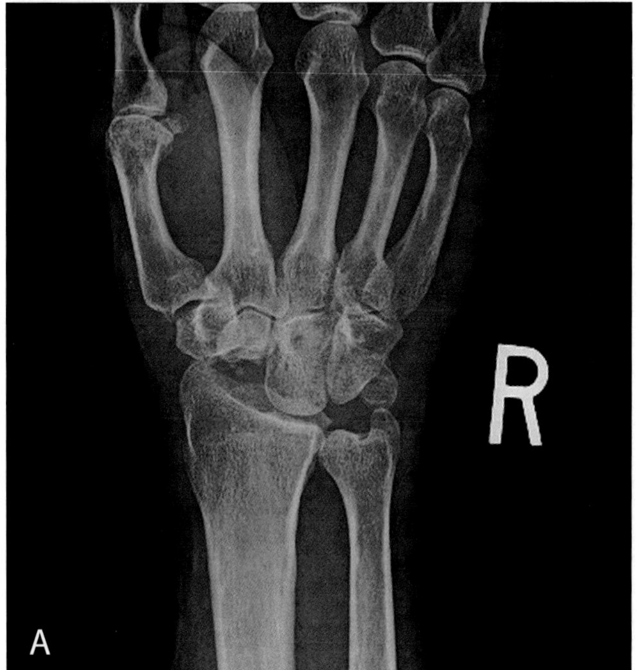

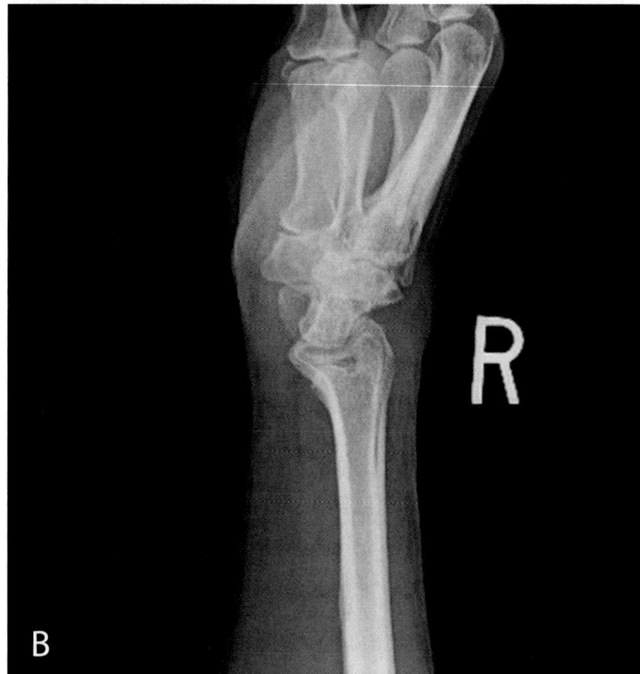

Figure 34.8 Anteroposterior (**A**) and lateral (**B**) plain radiographs of a right wrist after proximal row carpectomy performed to treat a patient with a painful scaphoid nonunion. (Courtesy of Christopher Got, MD)

 © 2018 American Academy of Orthopaedic Surgeons

of the capitate in the lunate facet of the radius. The capsule is closed with 2–0 nonabsorbable sutures, the retinaculum closed, and the extensor pollicis longus is left transposed in the subcutaneous tissue.

In the presence of mild radiocapitate arthritis, some surgeons elect to perform an interposition arthroplasty instead of a wrist fusion. This can be done with a proximally based capsular interposition flap. Once the PRC is performed, the flap is interposed between the lunate fossa and capitate and is sutured to the volar capsule.

Of note, a PRC may be performed as an arthroscopic procedure using the 3–4, 4–5, 6R, 6U, and midcarpal portals. Weiss and colleagues reported their technique using resection with a 4.0-mm burr through the midcarpal portal.

Complications

Short-term complications include postoperative swelling or hematoma, infection, transient neurapraxia, and finger stiffness. Long-term complications primarily include persistant pain, limited motion, finger stiffness, and progression of radiocapitate arthrosis. While arthrosis is frequently documented on postoperative radiographs, it has not been shown to predict a poor outcome.

Rehabilitation

At the first follow-up visit, the wound is inspected, a removable wrist splint is applied, and finger motion encouraged. We advise patients to keep the splint on for 4 weeks. At 4 weeks after surgery, gentle wrist motion is begun under the guidance of a hand therapist. Full activity is resumed at 3 months.

Functional Goals and Restrictions

Long-term follow-up of PRC shows satisfactory results. Two long-term studies have shown that wrist motion is between 63% and 71% of the contralateral side, while grip strength is between 83% and 91%.

PEARLS

General

- Clinical evaluation is used to determine the location of pain; local anesthetic injection can be helpful.

Surgical for Any Type of Wrist Fusion

- Performing a posterior interosseous neurectomy can diminish postoperative pain.
- Preservation of volar radiocarpal and ulnocarpal ligaments is essential to maintaining radiocarpal stability.
- Complete removal of cortical bone at the arthrodesis site is essential to ensure fusion.
- Releasing the tourniquet prior to closure will allow for adequate hemostasis and can limit postoperative swelling.
- Postoperative prevention and management of swelling and edema is essential.
- Early finger ROM helps to prevent stiffness and promotes faster functional recovery.

SUMMARY

Treatment of wrist arthritis is aimed at relieving pain while simultaneously preserving any motion possible and maximizing wrist function. When considering treatment options, the surgeon must consider the patient's functional goals, expectations, and potential compliance with postoperative rehabilitation. Preoperative injections and/or splinting can help set patient's expectations for postoperative pain control and functional limitations. In general, long-term functional results show good to excellent functional outcome and patient satisfaction for all wrist fusions.

BIBLIOGRAPHY

Adey L, Ring D, Jupiter JB: Health status after total wrist arthrodesis for posttraumatic arthritis. *J Hand Surg Am* 2005;30(5): 932–936.

Brigstocke GH, et al: In-vivo confirmation of the use of the dart thrower's motion during activities of daily living. *J Hand Surg Eur Vol* 2014;39(4):373–378.

DiDonna ML, Kiefhaber TR, Stern PJ: Proximal row carpectomy: study with a minimum of ten years of follow-up. *J Bone Joint Surg Am* 2004;86-A(11):2359–2365.

Jebson PJ, Hayes EP, Engber WD: Proximal row carpectomy: a minimum 10-year follow-up study. *J Hand Surg Am* 2003; 28(4):561–569.

Rechnagel K: Arthrodesis of the wrist joint. A follow-up study of sixty cases. *Scand J Plast Reconstr Surg* 1971;5(2):120–123.

Salenius P: Arthrodesis of the carpal joint. *Acta Orthop Scand* 1966;37(3):288–296.

Wagner ER, Elhassan BT, Kakar S: Long-term functional outcomes after bilateral total wrist arthrodesis. *J Hand Surg Am* 2015;40(2):224–228 e1.

Weiss AC, Wiedeman G Jr, Quenzer D, Hanington KR, Hastings H 2nd, Strickland JW: Upper extremity function after wrist arthrodesis. *J Hand Surg Am* 1995;20(5):813–817.

Weiss ND, Molina RA, Gwin S: Arthroscopic proximal row carpectomy. *J Hand Surg Am* 2011;36(4):577–582.

Zachary SV, Stern PJ: Complications following AO/ASIF wrist arthrodesis. *J Hand Surg Am* 1995;20(2):339–344.

© 2018 American Academy of Orthopaedic Surgeons

Hip 4

35 Functional HIP Anatomy for Rehabilitation

Scott K. Siverling, PT, OCS, and Alejandro Della Valle, MD

INTRODUCTION

The hip joint comprises the ball of the femoral head and the socket of the acetabular cup. This articulation serves the functioning musculoskeletal system as an important shock attenuator and force generator through most weight-bearing movements. When considering the forces that traverse the joint with the appreciable mobility of the hip, it is easy to understand why this joint is a frequent source for arthritic pain.

Draovitch et al introduced the concept of viewing the hip joint in terms of anatomic layers, in order to guide examination and treatment of painful conditions. This perspective is useful in its simplicity as well as leading the clinician toward appropriate rehabilitation methods. The layer concept presents the hip joint in four layers: (1) osteochondral, (2) inert, (3) contractile, and (4) neuromechanical. The functional anatomy of the hip joint will be presented in this format.

The hip is a ball-and-socket type joint with six degrees of movement. Often, the dialogue regarding hip motion is presented from the perspective of the ball of the femoral head moving within the acetabular cup. However, because most human motion is performed in weight-bearing positions, the clinician should consider the motion of the hip joint as the free pelvis moving over a fixed femoral head. This can be designated as acetabulofemoral movement, rather than femoroacetabular motion. Neuromuscular stability and control of the pelvis is imperative for proper functioning of the hip joint.

LAYER I

The osteochondral layer is comprised of the femur, acetabulum, and the pelvis and associated cartilaginous layers. The pelvis is the entire conjoined unit of the two innominate bones. The acetabular socket is the convergence of the three bones of each innominate: the ilium, ischium, and pubic bones each with its own degree of variability. These variances can alter the congruency of the joint. It is valuable for the clinician to understand the variability, deformities, and limits of the bony structure of the hip joint in order to individualize a rehabilitation program. These irregularities of the hip joint can involve one or both hips asymmetrically and vary from established norms, making examination and treatment challenging even for the most astute clinician.

The position and depth of the acetabulum are variable. The acetabulum may be oriented anteriorly or posteriorly in the transverse plane, which is termed acetabular anteversion or retroversion, respectively. Additionally, it can face superiorly or inferiorly in the sagittal plane. The depth of the socket can vary, leading to a shallow or deep acetabulum.

- An abnormally shallow socket is called acetabular dysplasia, while a deep socket can be labeled acetabular protrusion or coxa profunda.
- A measurement of the lateral center edge angle (LCEA) can diagnose and quantify a dysplastic acetabulum. Normative values of LCEA of 25° to 39° have been defined, with less than 25° objectifying hip dysplasia and more than 39° characterizing coxa profunda or protrusion.
  - Commonly, a dysplastic hip can be referred to as being "undercovered," while a profunda hip may be termed "overcovered."
- It is important to note the tilt of the pelvis, which can greatly affect the appearance of acetabular version. An anteriorly tilted pelvis will cause the acetabulum to seem excessively retroverted, while a posteriorly tilted pelvis may

Dr. Gonzalez Della Valle or an immediate family member serves as a paid consultant to Link Orthopaedics, Merz Pharmaceuticals, Orthodevelopment, and Orthosensor. Neither Dr. Siverling nor any immediate family member has received anything of value from or has stock or stock options held in a commercial company or institution related directly or indirectly to the subject of this article.

© 2018 American Academy of Orthopaedic Surgeons

make the acetabulum seem anteverted. This can influence hip joint mechanics and stability, as well as cause microtraumas that may lead to injury.

The femoral head is spherically shaped and protrudes from the femoral neck. The sphericity of the femoral head can differ and affect the congruency of the femoroacetabular joint. Abnormal sphericity may cause instability of the hip joint with limited motion. When the sphericity, in relation to the head–neck junction, exceeds normative values in the head–neck offset measurement, a CAM deformity exists.

The angle at which the neck courses between the femoral head and shaft is known as the angle of inclination. A steeper neck, with an increased angle of inclination, is known as coxa valga. Coxa vara is the term used to describe a decreased angle of inclination.

The neck can possess variable-angle torsion, labeled femoral torsion. This "twist" of the femoral shaft, in relation to the femoral neck, is measured by comparing an imaginary line drawn transversely through the femoral neck and shaft, and a line drawn through the epicondylar axis. Excessive femoral torsion—anything greater or less than 15° to 20°—can be biased anteriorly or posteriorly. Femoral torsion can be measured radiographically or by use of the Craig test in the clinic. Abnormal femoral torsion has been extensively related to several other orthopaedic injuries and problems.

- Femoral anteversion is characterized by femoral torsion of more than 20° and has been associated with an increased incidence of slipped capital femoral epiphysis (SCFE). Those with femoral anteversion are more likely to display excessive or increased internal rotation of the hip joint.
- Femoral retroversion is objectified by a femoral torsion of less than 10°, and has been linked to an increased incidence of degenerative joint disease (DJD) and osteoarthritis (OA) of the hip joint. As well, femoral retroversion has been associated with an increased incidence of tears of the labral complex of the hip joint.
    - Those with femoral retroversion may have less internal rotation of the hip joint and excessive external rotation, with evidence of acetabular anteversion.

Bony incongruences will affect the kinematics of the joint. Deformities, whether congenital or acquired, may lead to tears of the acetabular labral complex. Labral tears are frequently present in arthritic joints. The cartilage of the hip joint is subject to wear and degradation. The cartilage of the acetabulum covers the lunate surface in an upside-down "U-shaped" manner, and is meant to attenuate the forces travelling from the lower extremity up through the femur and femoral head, and into the pelvis and torso. Highest compression forces during the gait cycle have been shown to occur during midstance, when the entire lunate surface is in contact with the femoral head.

The hip joint functions as a traditional ball-and-socket joint. The axis of rotation is centered through the femoral head. In the classical description of hip kinematics, motion is described in relation to the femur's movement within the acetabulum, or femoral-on-pelvic movement. However, as previously stated, most locomotion requires the pelvis to move over a fixed femur, or as pelvic-on-femoral motion.

- All hip motion must be considered as pelvic motion, as well. For example, hip flexion may occur in the fixed femur by way of an anterior pelvic tilt, as a posterior pelvic tilt will effectively cause hip extension. This concept complicates rehabilitation, as the dysfunctional or recovering hip joint must be examined as an open-chain or closed-chain medium. The hip can be dysfunctional in an open-chain situation as femoral-on-pelvic motion, during the swing phase of gait. Also, during the stance phase of gait, the pelvic-on-femoral motion must be assessed.
- Along with bony restraints, ligamentous and muscular restraints may exist that may influence the kinematics of the hip joint. The extensibility and tone of all soft tissue surrounding the hip joint and pelvis must be considered when assessing the joint's motion.
    - For example, in mid-stance of gait on the fixed femur, pelvic lateral tilt will occur to allow adduction of the hip joint. This may be limited by a tight iliotibial band, gluteus medius, tensor fascia latae (TFL) or a contralateral quadratus lumborum.

LAYER II: INERT

The second layer of the hip joint's anatomy is the inert layer, comprised of the labral complex, the joint capsule, the surrounding ligaments, and the ligamentum teres. All of these structures assist in providing and extending stability of the hip joint.

The labrum's proposed purpose is to increase the depth of the acetabular socket and provide increased contact area for the femur during movement. This increased surface area of the acetabular socket helps to decrease contact forces on the intra-articular cartilage. The labrum acts as a gasket and, along with the synovial fluid, creates negative intra-articular pressure. This negative pressure is an effective suction seal effect that gives the femoroacetabular joint further stability. In cadaveric subjects, Ferguson compromised the suction-seal effect on hip joints, and applied distraction forces. The joint capsule complex was either vented or a labral tear was created. The forces required to distract the joint decreased by 43% and 60%, respectively, in the two simulated situations.

Tears of the labrum can occur due to repetitive increased stress or an acute macrotrauma to the labral complex. Labral tears have been associated with primary OA of the hip joint. Femoroacetabular impingement (FAI) is one of the chief causes of gradual labral injuries.

- FAI can be caused by joint incongruences that have led to suboptimal joint biomechanics.
    - A CAM lesion may lead to impingement of the labrum and capsule by the aspherical head with hip motion. Repetitive impingement may lead to labral tearing.

© 2018 American Academy of Orthopaedic Surgeons

- An acetabulum that has been quantified as dysplastic may exhibit undercoverage in one or multiple regions of the joint. This lack of coverage and stability may increase joint intra-articular movement. More important, the dysplastic hip has a reduced contact area. This will lead to excessive ground reaction forces during gait over small areas where the contact occurs. Over time, these excessive contact forces may lead to premature onset OA of the joint.

The ligaments of the hip joint form the external joint capsule.

- Anteriorly, the joint is reinforced by the iliofemoral ligament, or Y-ligament. This ligament is considered the strongest of the hip. The iliofemoral ligament becomes taut with full hip extension, and some fibers may help to resist excessive external rotation.
- The ischiofemoral ligament originates from the posteroinferior borders of the acetabulum and attaches antero superior on the femoral neck. This ligament becomes taut during internal rotation, extension, and adduction.
- The pubofemoral ligament courses along the inferior portion of the hip joint and becomes taut during end-range hip abduction and extension.
- The medial and anterior portion of the femoral head is exposed and unprotected. This area may be covered by a bursa, and the iliopsoas muscle and tendon course just anteriorly to the joint.

LAYER III: CONTRACTILE

The contractile tissues of the hip consist of the muscles that surround and control the joint. In considering the muscles that influence hip motion, the muscles that control the pelvis must be included. The muscles will be presented according to function.

HIP FLEXORS

The primary flexors of the hip include the iliopsoas, TFL, sartorius, rectus femoris, pectineus, and adductor longus.

- The iliopsoas serves as the most powerful hip flexor and consists of two muscles: the iliacus and psoas muscles. The iliacus originates in the iliac fossa, while the psoas major originates from the lower thoracic and upper lumbar region. A conjoined tendon of the two muscles attaches at the lesser trochanter of the femur.
  - Because of the origin of the psoas major, this muscle can greatly influence lumbar spinal positioning. It has been postulated that the psoas may provide compressive stability to the lumbar spine.
  - An appropriate force from the abdominal musculature to stabilize the pelvis must be present to counteract a contraction of the iliopsoas. If not, this may increase the lordosis of the lumbar spine, or the energy is misspent on anteriorly tilting the pelvis rather than flexing the hip.
- The rectus femoris also serves as a knee extensor, along with the rest of the quadriceps musculature.
- The TFL is a short muscle that blends into the iliotibial band. Along with the gluteus maximus, this iliotibial tract reinforces the hip joint laterally. The TFL also performs abduction and functions as a secondary internal rotator of the hip.
- The sartorius is the longest muscle in the body performing flexion, abduction, and external rotation of the hip.
- From the hip angles of 40° or less, the adductor longus may act as a flexor.

HIP EXTENSORS

The hip extensor muscle group includes the gluteus maximus and the hamstring muscles as the primary movers. Secondary extensors are the adductors and the posterior fibers of the gluteus medius.

- The gluteus maximus has multiple origins at the ilium, sacrum, coccyx, sacrotuberous ligament, and posterior sacroiliac ligaments. The muscle then blends into the iliotibial band, along with the TFL, and also attaches to the gluteal tuberosity on the femur.
  - The gluteus maximus is also a primary extensor.
  - As described earlier, the ligaments of the hip muscle all, in varying ways, resist end-range extension. Flexion of the hip will relax these ligaments, and the posterior capsule will be stretched along with the gluteus maximus. A tight maximus may impede hip flexion during the squatting motion.
  - Decreased gluteal activity and force has been associated with excessive anterior femoral head translation within the joint and low back pain. Those exhibiting inhibited gluteal activity have been shown to overuse the hamstrings and erectors of the trunk to perform hip extension.
- The hamstring attachment into the tibia and fibula makes it an effective knee flexor, as well as a hip extensor.
  - While bending over, if the knees are straight, motion at the hip will be heavily influenced by the length of the hamstrings. As well, the moment arm of the gluteus maximus is actually decreased and decreases the ability of the maximus to assist with balance and stabilization.
  - The posterior fibers and head of the adductor magnus function as almost a "third" hamstring muscle, and assist in hip extension.
- From the angles of 70° of hip flexion, the adductors can act as a powerful extensor of the hip. This is important for climbing hills or stairs.
- The hip extensors can also act as posterior tilters of the pelvis on a fixed femur.

© 2018 American Academy of Orthopaedic Surgeons

HIP ABDUCTORS

The gluteus medius has the most efficient moment arm and the largest cross-sectional area of any of the abductors. The gluteus minimus and TFL contribute to abduction forces as well.

- The gluteus medius is comprised of three sets of fibers: anterior, middle, and posterior. The anterior fibers will also internally rotate the hip joint, while the posterior fibers can perform external rotation. The muscle as a whole stabilizes the pelvis over the femur during the single-leg stance phase of gait. As well, the gluteus medius will compress the femoral head into the acetabulum to create midstance stability of the joint.
  - Weakness or injury to this muscle may cause a Trendelenberg gait, in which the pelvis may shift, causing aberrations of the center of gravity and inefficient locomotion.
  - In instances of cartilage loss and OA within the hip joint, compression of the femur into the acetabulum may be painful. The pain can be alleviated by a compensatory Trendelenberg gait in which the subject shifts the trunk over the affected leg, eliminating the need of the gluteus medius to stabilize the pelvis.
  - Evidence exists to suggest atrophy and loss of muscle force in those presenting with FAI or OA of the hip joint.
- Fibers of the gluteus minimus insert into the superior portion capsule.

HIP ADDUCTORS

The adductors of the hip occupy the medial side of the thigh. These include the adductor magnus, longus, brevis, pectineus, and gracilis. The primary role of the adductors is adduction of the hip joint. However, the adductor magnus and longus are multifaceted.

- Because of the orientation of the adductor magnus, it can influence the hip in the sagittal, frontal, and coronal planes. The most obvious function of the magnus is adduction. The contralateral adductors may assist in pelvic stability during single-limb tasks.
  - In a flexed hip, the magnus and longus may assist in hip extension.
  - In a neutrally aligned hip, the longus may act as a secondary hip flexor.

HIP INTERNAL ROTATORS

No muscles exist that perform hip internal rotation as their primary role. All the muscles that perform internal rotation at the hip do so as a secondary function. These internal rotators include the anterior fibers of the gluteus minimus and medius, TFL, adductor longus and brevis, and pectineus.

- As the hip flexes, it is theorized that the moment arm internal rotators of the hip increase greatly. As well, it is possible that some of the external rotators of the hip actually change their purpose and begin to assist with internal rotation.

HIP EXTERNAL ROTATORS

The gluteus maximus and the short external rotator muscle group of the hip serve as the primary external rotators. The short external rotators include the obturator internus and externus, superior and inferior gemellus, piriformis, and quadratus femoris.

- The piriformis also acts as a secondary hip abductor.
- Contraction of the obturator internus on a fixed femur compresses the joint, effecting further stability.

The relevance of the primary and secondary functions of these muscles is the idea of compensation. Due to injury, chronic disuse, poor postural habits, or atrophy, the body can adopt compensatory strategies. These adaptations may not be ideal and may interfere with proper biomechanics of the hip joint or peripheral joints in the kinetic chain. The clinician should take care to observe all weaknesses and insufficiencies of the muscles that control the hip joint and the possible implications of those weaknesses.

LAYER IV: NEUROMECHANICAL

The final layer that Draovitch et al described is a theorized anatomic layer that is comprised of "physiological events and kinematic changes throughout the chain which drive proprioception and pain within the hip." It is felt that due to the anatomic organization of nerve types and endings in the hip, the joint is more apt to undergo improper adaptations in response to injury. Loss of proprioceptive capabilities of the hip joint may greatly influence the knee and ankle joints adversely.

The hip joint may suffer secondarily to peripheral pathologies. Disc degeneration and nerve root compression in the lower lumbar spine may affect motor recruitment of several muscles innervated by the L5 and S1 nerve roots.

SUMMARY

- The hip joint is subjected to and generates large forces, and is capable of motion in all three planes.
- The several permutations of the osteology of the hip joint may have a profound impact on the potential motion of the joint and moment arms of the contributing muscles.
- The hip joint should not be thought of simply as the ball of the femoral head moving within the acetabulum. Instead, because a large portion of the gait cycle occurs on a fixed leg and femur, the motion of the hip occurs as pelvis-on-femoral movement.

© 2018 American Academy of Orthopaedic Surgeons

- The muscles that control the hip joint can have multiple functions. The implications are that during rehabilitation following injury or surgery, suboptimal adaptations may occur and negatively affect the joint mechanics.

BIBLIOGRAPHY

Cibulka MT: Determination and significance of femoral neck anteversion. *Phys Ther* 2004;84(6):550–558.

Draovitch P, Edelstein J, Kelly BT: The layer concept: utilization in determining the pain generators, pathology and how structure determines treatment. *Curr Rev Musculoskelet Med* 2012; 5(1):1–8.

Ferguson SJ, Bryant JT, Ganz R, Ito K: An in vitro investigation of the acetabular labral seal in hip joint mechanics. *J Biomech* 2003;36(2):171–178.

Ganz R, Leunig M, Leunig-Ganz K, Harris WH: The etiology of osteoarthritis of the hip: an integrated mechanical concept. *Clin Orthop Relat Res* 2008;466:264–272.

Gelberman RH, Cohen MS, Shaw BA, Kasser JR, Griffin PP, Wilkinson RH: The association of femoral retroversion with slipped capital femoral epiphysis. *J Bone Joint Surg Am* 1986;68:1000–1007.

Ito K, Minka MA 2nd, Leunig M, Werlen S, Ganz R: Femoroacetabular impingement and the CAM-effect: a MRI-based quantitative anatomical study of the femoral head-neck offset. *J Bone Joint Surg Br* 2001;83:171–176.

Lewis CL, Sahrmann SA, Moran DA: Anterior hip joint force increases with hip extension, decreased gluteal force, or decreased iliopsoas force. *J Biomech* 2007;40(16):3725–3731.

Mavcic B, Antolic V, Brand R, Iglic A, Kralj-Iglic V, Pederson DR: Peak contact stress in human hip during gait. *Pflugers Arch* 2000;440(5 Suppl):R177–R178.

Neumann, D: *Kinesiology of the Musculoskeletal System: Foundations for Rehabilitation*, ed 2. New York, NY, CV Mosby Co, 2012.

Pohtilla JF: Kinesiology of hip extension at selected angles of pelvifemoral extension. *Arch Phys Med Rehabil* 1969;50(5): 241–250.

Tonnis D, Heinecke A: Diminished femoral antetorsion syndrome: a cause of pain and osteoarthritis. *J Pediatr Orthop* 1991; 11:419–431.

Werner CM, Copeland CE, Ruckstuhl T, Stromberg J, Turen CH, Bouaicha S: The relationship between Wiberg's lateral center edge angle, Lequesne's acetabular index, and medial acetabular bone stock. *Skeletal Radiol* 2011;40(11): 1435–1439.

© 2018 American Academy of Orthopaedic Surgeons

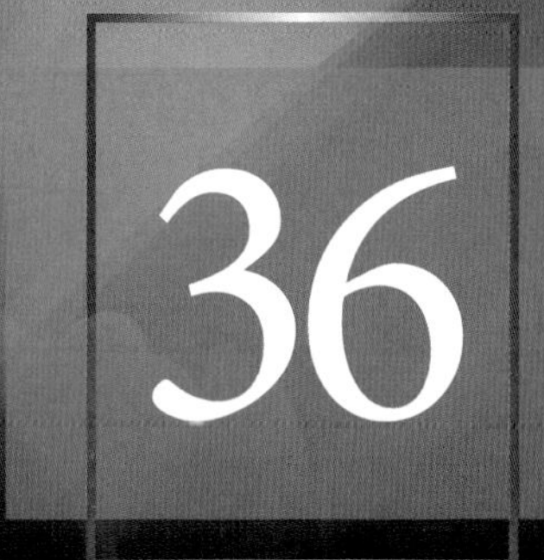

36 Total Hip Arthroplasty

Maya C. Manning, PT, DPT, CSCS, Matthew P. Titmuss, PT, DPT, Jessica Bloch, MS, OTR/L, and Alejandro Gonzalez Della Valle, MD

OVERVIEW OF TOTAL HIP ARTHROPLASTY

Modern total hip arthroplasty (THA), perfected by the pioneering work of Sir John Charley, has revolutionized the treatment of end-stage arthritis of the hip, and has relieved the pain and restored function of millions of patients worldwide. The Agency for Healthcare Research and Quality reported that over 420,000 THAs were performed in the United States during 2012. The number of THAs is expected to increase six times by the year 2030.

The majority of THAs in the United States are performed on patients with idiopathic arthritis or hip fractures. Other indications include rheumatoid arthritis, avascular necrosis, posttraumatic arthritis, psoriatic arthritis, systemic lupus erythematosus, and tumor resection.

Patients considering elective THA surgery usually present with progressive severe hip pain and limitation of motion associated with extensive cartilage loss. Patients usually complain of difficulty performing activities of daily living (ADLs) including standing, walking, sitting, negotiating stairs, and sleeping. With the progression of arthritis, contractures (often in flexion and external rotation) develop, as well as limitation of range of motion (ROM). The ideal patients for elective THA have usually tried a period of conservative measures aimed at relieving pain and maintaining function.

Contraindications to THA include unexplained hip pain in the absence of pathology, acute or chronic hip infection, Charcot arthropathy, inability to follow postoperative recommendations and precautions, a well-functioning, painless hip arthrodesis or resection arthroplasty, and chronic medical conditions (uncontrolled diabetes; or severe heart, lung, neurologic, vascular, or systemic diseases).

Careful preoperative patient assessment and meticulous surgical planning are important to increase the likelihood of success. During history taking and physical examination, the patient's complaints and expectations for function and activity following surgery are assessed and discussed to ensure that they are realistic and attainable by the surgeon. Assessment of abnormal gait patterns, neurovascular condition, functional and actual leg length discrepancy, ROM and the presence of fixed or correctable pelvic obliquity are necessary. Preoperative planning consists of generating a surgical plan utilizing the information obtained during the physical examination along with standardized radiographs with known magnification. The plan allows for the anticipation of implant sizes, position, and fixation. In addition, it determines the position of the bone cuts that will restore leg length, offset, and other features of a biomechanically sound reconstruction. A precise reconstitution of hip biomechanics is essential to ensure a stable and durable reconstruction. Malposition of prosthetic components or failure to restore offset and/or leg length can result in postoperative hip instability (including dislocation), premature wear, and patient dissatisfaction.

Different surgical approaches have been used, including anterior, anterolateral, posterolateral, and transtrochanteric. Despite careful surgical technique, each of the surgical approaches will cause a controlled amount of soft-tissue damage. The type of approach will dictate the type of postoperative precautions that the patient needs to follow. The surgical approach used for each individual patient should be well documented and taken into consideration by the surgical team (including physical therapists, nurses, physician assistants, and so on).

The characteristics of each surgical approach are described here.

- *Posterolateral:* The incision is located in the posterior aspect of the greater trochanter and divides the fibers of the gluteus maximus muscle. A detachment and subsequent repair of the external rotators (conjoined tendon, quadratus femoris), and posterior capsule is necessary, and creates a relative weak posterior soft-tissue envelope. The anterior capsule remains intact.

Dr. Gonzalez Della Valle or an immediate family member serves as a paid consultant to Link Orthopaedics, Merz Pharmaceuticals, Orthodevelopment, and Orthosensor. None of the following authors or any immediate family member has received anything of value from or has stock or stock options held in a commercial company or institution related directly or indirectly to the subject of this article: Dr. Bloch, Dr. Caspi, and Dr. Titmuss.

© 2018 American Academy of Orthopaedic Surgeons

- *Anterolateral:* The incision is located in the anterior aspect of the greater trochanter and divides the fibers of the gluteus medius muscle. A detachment and subsequent repair of the anterior capsule is necessary, and creates a relative weak anterior soft-tissue envelope. The division of the gluteus medius fibers can create transient postoperative abductor weakness. The posterior capsule remains intact.
- *Anterior:* The incision is made distal and lateral to the anterosuperior iliac spine. The dissection is carried out between the tensor fascia lata and rectus femoris. The limited working space and reduced visualization of structures may require resection of the anterior joint capsule and release of the piriformis tendon, the use of intraoperative fluoroscopy, and specially designed traction surgical tables. The approach compromises the anterior soft-tissue envelope of the hip.
- *Transtrochanteric (rarely used):* The incision is made centered on the trochanter and a trochanteric osteotomy is performed for wide access to the joint. The approach requires an additional anterior capsulotomy. Reattachment and subsequent healing of the greater trochanteric osteotomy are necessary for a successful outcome. If nonunion of the trochanteric osteotomy develops, patients may experience pain, abductor lurch, and hip instability.

The socket and stem of the THA can be fixed with acrylic cement or relying on cementless press-fit (Figure 36.1). Today, the majority of sockets are fixed without cement. This requires reaming the acetabular cavity to a diameter 1 to 2 mm smaller than the socket to be implanted. The socket has a porous surface onto which the native acetabular bone will grow. Acetabular screws are used when the bone quality is poor or in some acetabuli with bony anomalies. The femoral components can be fixed with or without acrylic cement. When cement fixation is used, there is immediate, stable fixation of the implant to the bone. The patients can bear weight as tolerated immediately following surgery. When cementless femoral fixation is used, the amount of weight that the patient can bear following surgery will be determined by the fit achieved during final stem insertion. Some patients with poor bone quality or less than perfect stem fit may benefit from a period of protected weight bearing.

Wound closure usually includes careful repair of the soft-tissue envelope disrupted by the surgical approach, thus the need to apply dislocation precautions that are specific to the surgical approach utilized (e.g., posterior dislocation precautions for a posterolateral approach and anterior dislocation precautions for an anterior and anterolateral approach.

The risk of medical and local complications of surgery is multifactorial and depends on surgeon and patient factors. They include infection, fracture, dislocation, loosening, neurologic and vascular damage, and thromboembolic disease. Gentle postoperative rehabilitation plays a crucial role in preventing pain, dislocation, thromboembolism, and wound complications.

In the last two decades, emphasis has been placed on reducing hospital stay and overall hospital costs associated with the procedure. Consequently, in-hospital rehabilitation guidelines for recovery following THA have evolved. Therapy after surgery focuses on early mobilization and preparation for a prompt and safe discharge. Postdischarge rehabilitation programs have been developed to achieve a full recovery. Preoperative surgical rehabilitation can also be used.

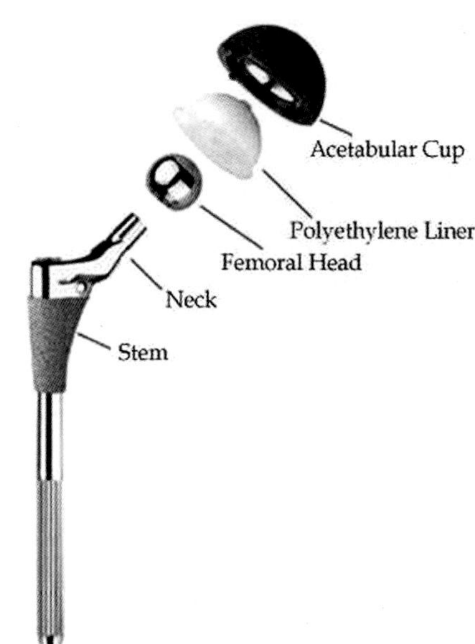

Figure 36.1 Illustration of a generic total hip replacement.

Acute Phase (First Several Days–2 Weeks)

The initial phase of rehabilitation includes the patient's immediate recovery from surgery and discharge from hospital to home or a rehabilitation facility. In this phase, there is a strong emphasis on patient and family education, ADL training, transfer training and gait training, and initiation of a therapeutic exercise program.

Patient Education

Prior to surgery, patients are often instructed in a classroom setting regarding what to do in the days before surgery, what to expect on the day of their surgery and the days following while in the hospital, and discharge planning. A physical therapist or nurse may give a presentation, during which postoperative hip precautions, basic exercises, basic postoperative mobility, and expected changes in ADLs are reviewed. Online resources may complement this process. This preoperative class addresses patients' concerns prior to surgery and teaches them how to set up their homes to accommodate their recovery appropriately before coming to the hospital. Equipment may be recommended by an occupational therapist to assist with ADLs.

Total Hip Precautions

Posterolateral Approach

Patients whose hip replacement is performed through a posterolateral approach are instructed to follow posterolateral hip precautions for 6 to 8 weeks postoperatively in order to allow for the hip capsule to heal, and to reduce the chance of hip dislocation.

 © 2018 American Academy of Orthopaedic Surgeons

The postoperative precautions include:

- No hip flexion greater than 90°
- No hip adduction past midline
- No hip internal rotation past neutral

Anterior Approach

For the patients that undergo THA through an anterior approach, the postoperative precautions include:

- No hip external rotation past neutral
- No excessive hip extension

Transfer and Gait Training

In the days immediately following surgery, patients are instructed to transfer in and out of bed on the same side as the operated limb in order to avoid hip internal rotation. If the patient is able to do so with adequate control while maintaining hip precautions, he can be instructed on exiting and entering on either side. For patients with bilateral THA, they are instructed to use the same side of the bed that they will use at home.

With length of stay (LOS) decreasing, early mobility is greatly encouraged. It has been shown that early mobilization following THA decreases hospital LOS. Patients who are medically stable to participate with the physical therapist are often able to have their first session on the day of surgery, several hours after coming out of the operating room. Ambulation is initiated with a rolling walker to allow for upper extremity weight bearing, to support the surgical lower extremity, and provide increased stability and patient confidence. Following an uncomplicated THA, the majority of patients are allowed to bear weight as tolerated (WBAT). Activity level on the day of surgery ranges from dangling at the bedside to walking up to approximately 100 feet with a rolling walker.

On the day of surgery prior to getting up for the first time, the postoperative radiograph is reviewed to confirm that no fracture or dislocation has occurred after surgery. The goal on postoperative day (POD) #0 is for the physical therapist to evaluate the strength and sensation in the lower extremities, educate the patient on his exercises and precautions and, if appropriate, ambulate a short distance. On POD #1, the patient may have several sessions of physical therapy, spaced throughout the day and designed to progress independence with transfers, ambulation, therapeutic exercises, and overall tolerance for activity. If the patient is able to demonstrate a nonantalgic, step-through gait pattern with good balance, he will be progressed to walking with a cane or crutches by the afternoon of POD #1 or as early as the morning of POD #1. When the patient is able to ambulate with equal step length bilaterally using a cane, he will progress to ascending and descending stairs with use of a cane and handrail, following a step-to pattern. This usually occurs in the afternoon of POD #1.

On POD #2, patients work on developing safe and independent ADL. This includes transferring, ambulation with an appropriate assistive device, ascending/descending stairs (nonreciprocal), and independence with a home exercise program. Some patients may require further reinforcement and education in order to ensure a safe home discharge. Once they are able to perform all activities safely and independently, they are discharged by the physical therapist and considered safe to go home. Some patients will be discharged home on POD #1, but most patients are ready to be discharged home on POD #2. Few patients are discharged to rehabilitation facilities.

Patients are encouraged to sit in a chair several times per day, at least for all meals. However, sitting is limited to less than 1 hour each time in order to avoid increased pain, swelling, and stiffness. Hospital staff play an important role in assisting patients out of bed at their meal times, and provide additional opportunities for patients to ambulate, helping to reduce stiffness that may occur with reduced mobility.

Therapeutic Exercise

During the first session of physical therapy following surgery, patients are instructed on basic bed exercises to perform on an hourly basis. Initial exercises aim to promote circulation in the lower extremities, reducing the chance of a blood clot and promoting reactivation of the lower extremity (LE) muscles disturbed during the surgery. A note card with written instructions that include pictures of all exercises, how often to perform them, and any precautions is a useful aid for patients.

Supine Exercise

Patients are instructed to perform these exercises 10 times an hour every hour while in bed.

- Ankle pumps (Figure 36.2)
- Quadriceps sets (Figure 36.3)
- Gluteal sets (Figure 36.4)
- Heel slides to 45° of hip flexion (Figure 36.5)
- Hip rotation to neutral (posterior lateral only) (Figure 36.6)

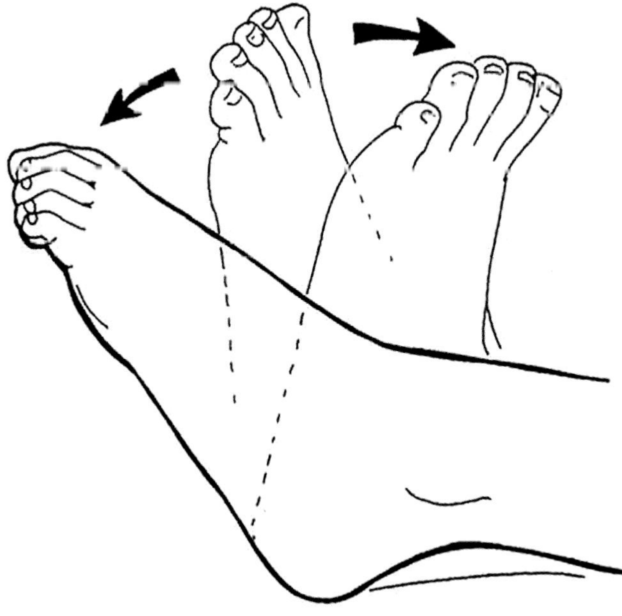

Figure 36.2 Illustration of ankle pump.

© 2018 American Academy of Orthopaedic Surgeons

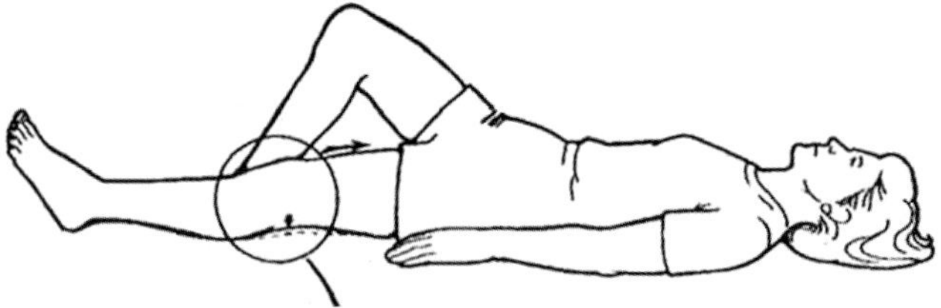

Figure 36.3 Illustration of quadricep sets.

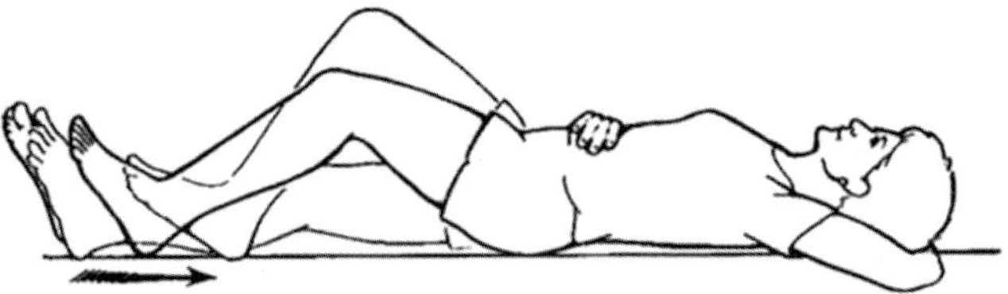

Figure 36.5 Illustration of heel slides/supine hip flexion.

Seated Exercise

When the patient is able to tolerate a comfortable seated position, either at the edge of the bed or in a chair, the therapist instructs him on:

- Open-chain knee extension (Figure 36.7)
- Hip flexion (<90° degrees for the posterolateral approach) (Figure 36.8)

Standing Exercise

- Hip abduction (Figure 36.9)
- Knee flexion (Figure 36.10)
- Hip extension (posterolateral approach only) with the operative lower extremity only (Figure 36.11)
- Emphasis is placed on ensuring that the patient moves the femur on the pelvis and does not flex or side bend at the trunk during standing exercises.

Cryotherapy and Elevation

Edema is normal and expected after a total hip replacement. Controlling early swelling is important in alleviating pain and reducing stiffness. Cryotherapy is used along with analgesics to help manage pain and swelling. Patients are advised to use ice for 20 to 30 minutes, at least 5 or 6 times per day, particularly after exercise or walking. Dependent positioning of the leg can result in increased swelling; therefore, elevation is encouraged to help counteract excessive swelling in the lower limb.

Activities of Daily Living Training

During the hospital stay, an occupational therapist may evaluate patients. The occupational therapist reviews the postoperative restrictions of the hip precautions, instructs patients in basic ADLs and provides them with equipment to allow them to function as independently as possible upon discharge.

Lower body dressing will need to be modified if the patient cannot bend past 90°. For safety, it is recommended that the patient get dressed seated on the edge of the bed or while seated on a high chair. In order to don pants and underwear, the patient will need to use a reacher (Figure 36.12) to pull the garment

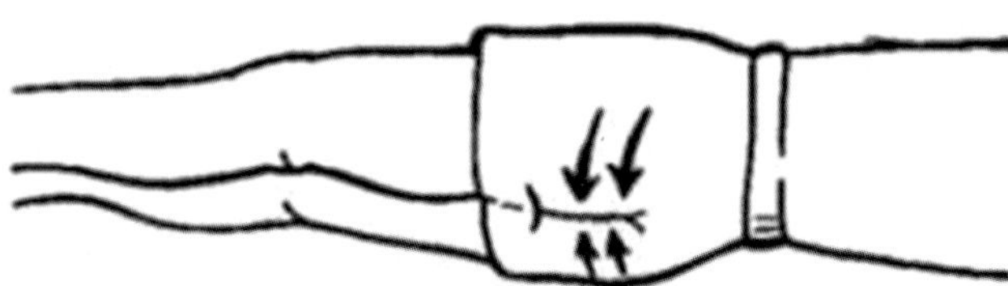

Figure 36.4 Illustration of gluteal sets.

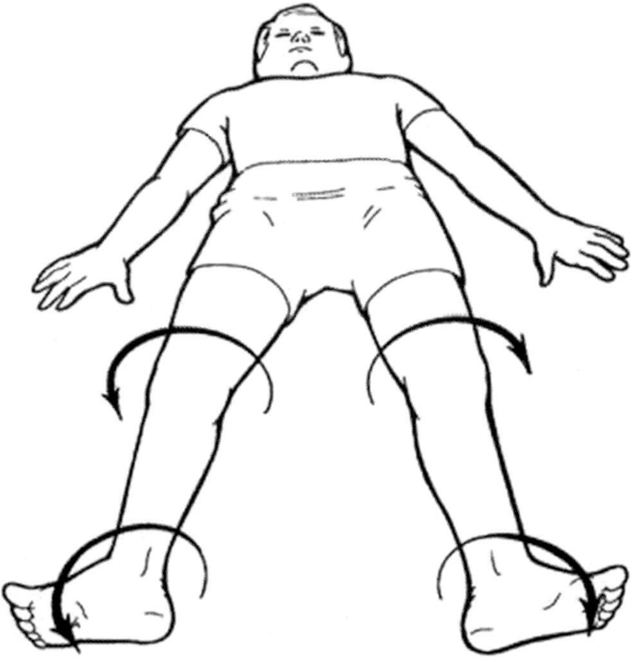

Figure 36.6 Illustration of hip external rotation.

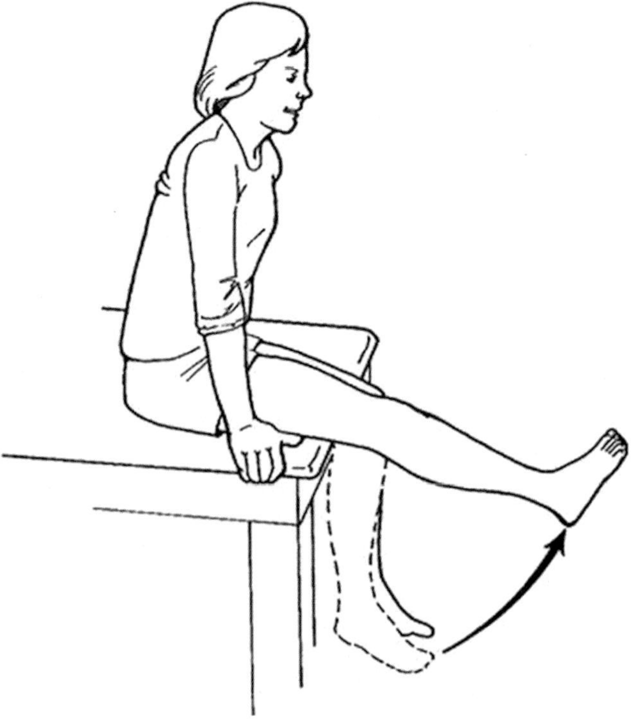

Figure 36.7 Illustration of seated knee extension.

© 2018 American Academy of Orthopaedic Surgeons

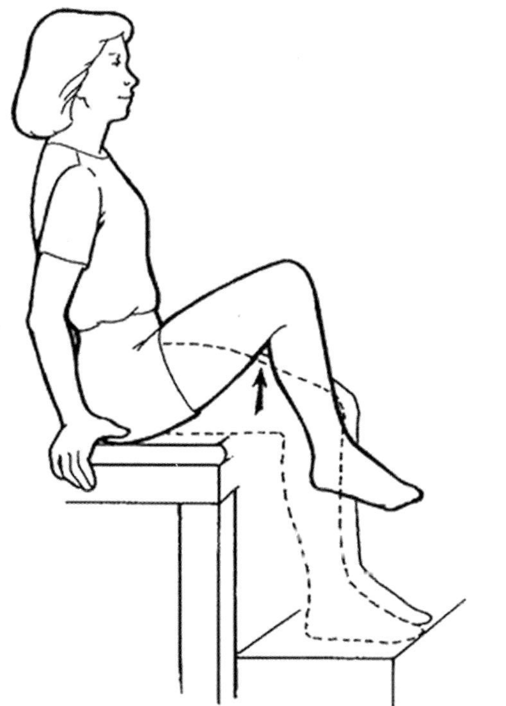

Figure 36.8 Illustration of seated hip flexion (for posterolateral approach, the knee should not be lifted beyond the line).

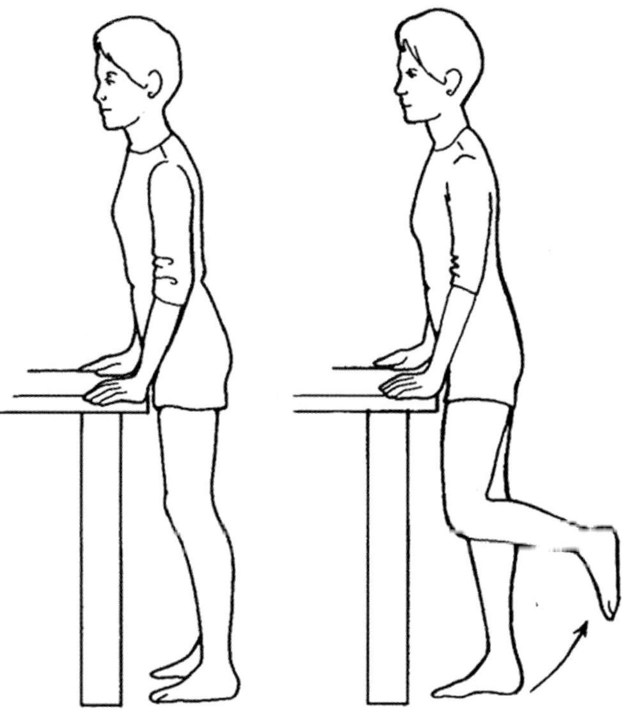

Figure 36.10 Illustration of standing knee flexion.

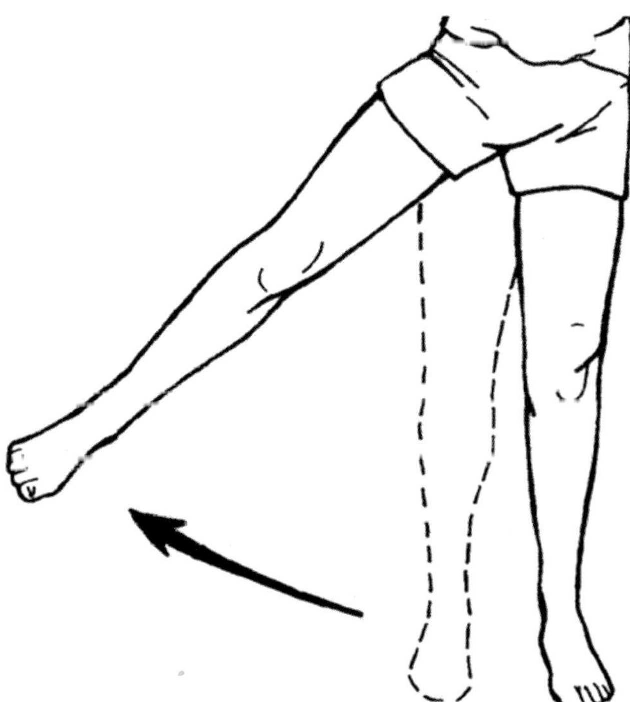

Figure 36.9 Illustration of standing hip abduction.

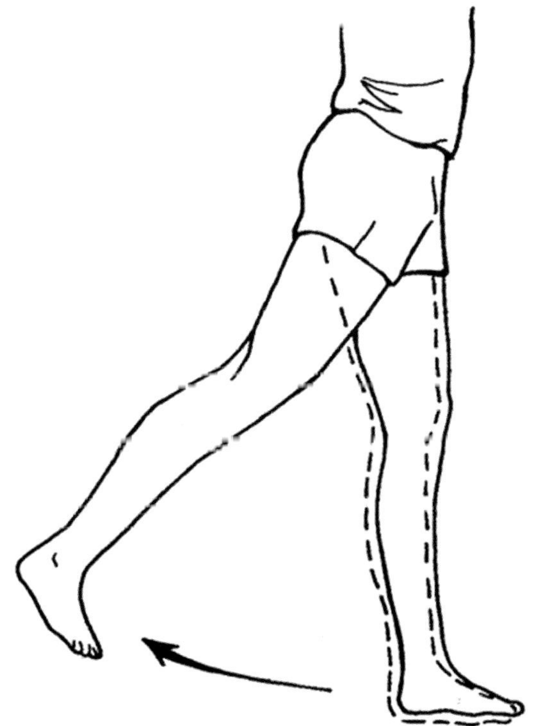

Figure 36.11 Illustration of standing hip extension (contraindicated for anterior approach).

© 2018 American Academy of Orthopaedic Surgeons

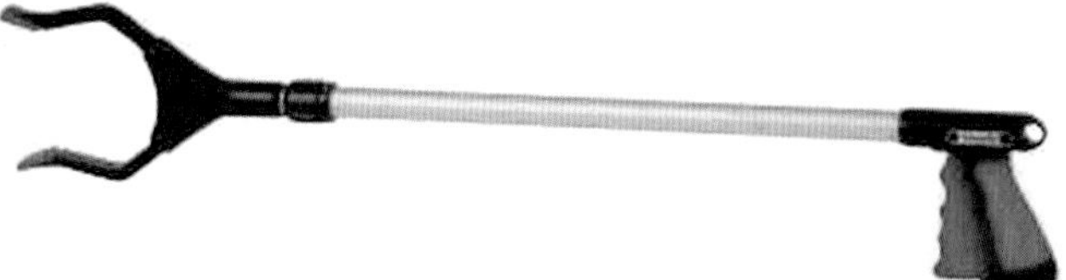

Figure 36.12 Photograph of a reacher.

up without violating the precautions. Patients are advised to dress their operated leg first, followed by their nonoperative leg. Finally, the patient will stand and pull the pants up to the waist.

A device called a sock aide (Figure 36.13) assists the patient with donning socks without bending over, lifting the leg, or crossing the leg. A long-handled shoehorn is recommended to prevent internally rotating the hip while sliding a shoe on (Figure 36.14). Elastic laces are recommended for patients since they cannot bend over to tie their sneakers.

Patients' bathrooms often need several modifications. For approximately 6 weeks after surgery, while the posterolateral precautions are in place, the patient will need to install a raised toilet seat (Figure 36.15). Patients with a bathtub will be educated to side step into the tub, and extend the leg behind them from the knee so that the hip joint does not move. Using a hand-held shower or a long-handled sponge will protect the patient from bending too far forward while bathing (Figure 36.16). Patients who are not full weight bearing after surgery (PWB, TTWB) will not be able to step into a bathtub. For these patients, a transfer tub bench will necessary to ensure that they do not weight bear through their lower extremity.

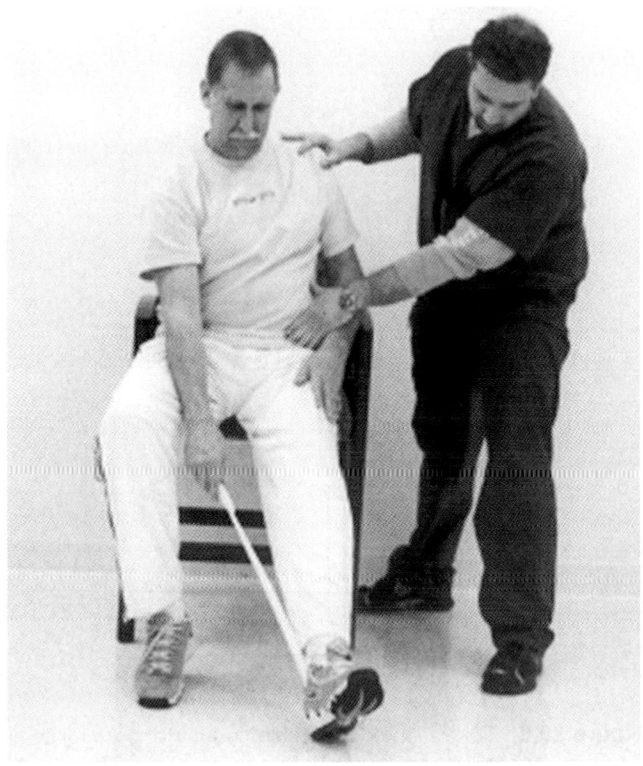

Figure 36.14 Long handled shoe horn. (Reprinted from Radomski MV, Trombly CA. *Occupational Therapy for Physical Dysfunction*. Philadelphia, PA: Wolters Kluwer; 2014.)

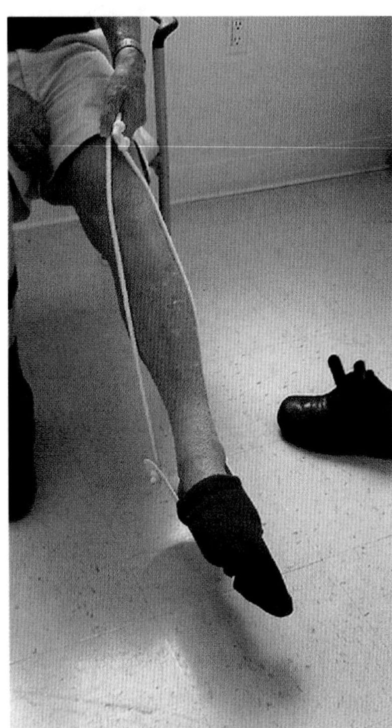

Figure 36.13 Sock/stocking aid. (Reprinted from Wagenfeld A. *Foundations of Theory and Practice for the Occupational Therapy Assistant*. Philadelphia, PA: Wolters Kluwer; 2015.)

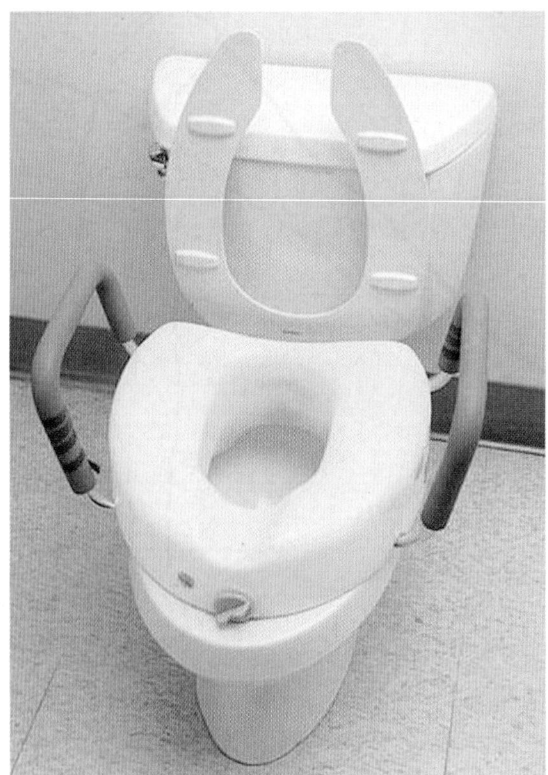

Figure 36.15 Raised toilet seat. (Reprinted from Rosdahk CB, Kowalski MT. *Textbook of Basic Nursing*. 10th ed. Philadelphia, PA: Wolters Kluwer Health; 2012.)

© 2018 American Academy of Orthopaedic Surgeons

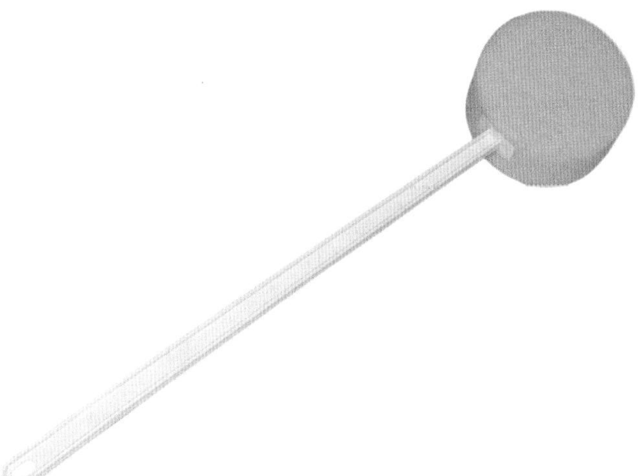

Figure 36.16 Photograph of a long-handled bath sponge.

Home seating will also need to be modified. Patients will need to sit on a high sturdy chair with armrests. Some options include renting a high chair from a local medical supply store or building up a chair with a firm cushion or two pillows. For patients with posterolateral precautions, the patient's knee should be below the level of their hip.

Patients should also be educated on the safe way to enter a car. The front passenger seat best accommodates patient limitations. The front seat should be pushed all the way back and slightly reclined. A firm cushion or two pillows should be placed on the front passenger seat as well. Patients are educated to back into the car seat and, once seated, swing their lower extremities in.

It is important to review with patients any upcoming plans that they have to either return to work or travel for the first 6 weeks following their surgery. Work modifications include adding a sturdy chair and making sure that they have a raised toilet seat for work. If a patient usually drives to work, a ride will need to set up until the surgeon clears him to drive. Patients who have clearance from the surgeon to travel will need to make sure that they sit in a seat with plenty of legroom and also bring a firm cushion to sit on. Whether at home, at work, or while travelling, the patient should walk once an hour to help with circulation and decrease stiffness.

Following the occupational therapy session, the patient should feel comfortable following/adhering to the hip precautions in ADLs. Popular adaptive devices include the reacher, sock aide, long-handled shoehorn, long-handled sponge, a firm cushion, and a raised toilet seat, all of which can be ordered in advance.

Discharge Expectations

With major changes occurring in health care, and improved surgical techniques and anesthesia, the majority of THA patients are discharged home (on POD #2) rather than to a rehabilitation facility. Once home, patients receive homecare services consisting of a nurse's visit and 3 to 5 physical therapy sessions per week designed to progress the therapy started in the hospital. After 10 to 14 days, the patient usually begins an outpatient physical therapy program, often based on the surgeon's preference or the physical therapist's recommendation if gait deviations or strength deficits are still noted. The patient will continue with the home exercise program initiated in the hospital following the guidelines for progression set up by the physical therapist. In some instances, patients who are otherwise healthy may not require further physical therapy.

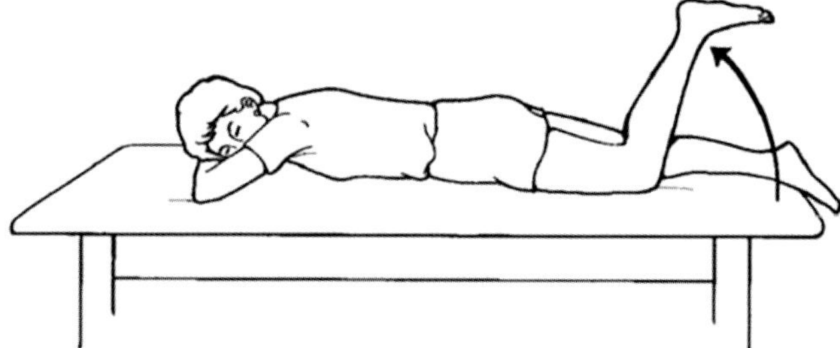

Figure 36.17 Illustration of the prone quadriceps stretch.

Subacute Phase (Weeks 2–6)

A recent systematic review of postoperative exercise programs after THA indicates that programs consisting of hip ROM, isometric exercises, and weight-bearing eccentric strengthening exercises help to increase muscle strength and walking speed. The subacute phase of rehabilitation begins with the foundation of the advanced exercises given to the patient in the acute care setting. In this phase, the focus is on monitoring swelling and pain, normalizing the gait pattern with or without an assistive device, and improving flexibility. Active range of motion (AROM) and strengthening exercises are progressed while adhering to hip precautions. Balance exercises are added and progressed at this point as well.

At approximately 6 weeks postoperatively, patients return to the surgeon for a follow-up appointment. At this point, gait is observed, a radiograph is taken, and the overall quality of the recovery process is assessed. Usually, the surgeon will discontinue any precautions at this point.

Flexibility, Strengthening, and Functional Training

It is important to recognize limitations in flexibility and strength early in the patient's recovery in order to obtain maximal gains. Quite often, tightness of the quadriceps, iliopsoas, and internal rotators is seen when the posterolateral approach is used. These patients are instructed in the prone quad stretch (Figure 35.17), Thomas test position stretch (Figure 36.18)

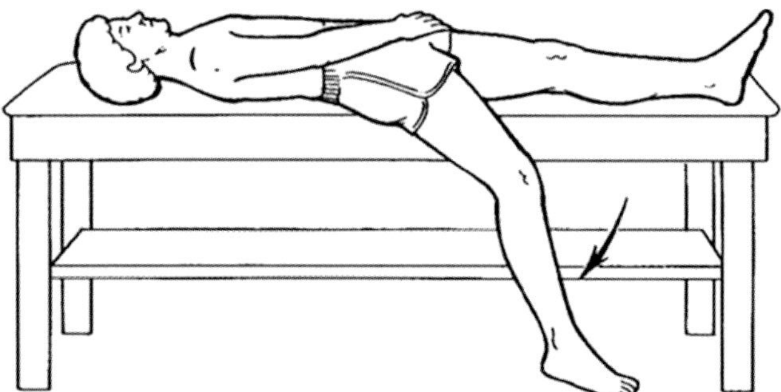

Figure 36.18 Illustration of the supine hip flexor stretch or the Thomas test position stretch.

© 2018 American Academy of Orthopaedic Surgeons

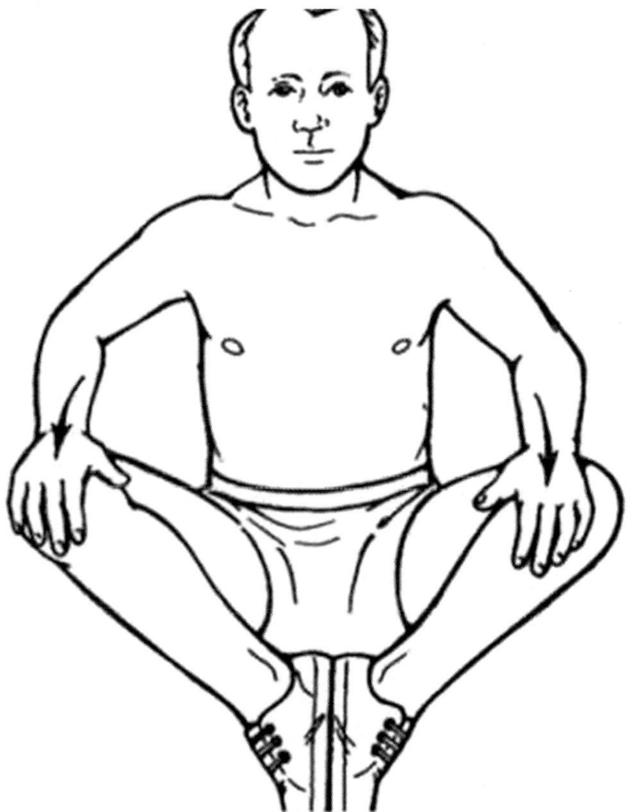

Figure 36.19 Illustration of the supine "butterfly" stretch.

and supine butterfly stretch (Figure 36.19). Gentle hamstring stretching is also recommended and with less restriction for the anterior approach patients (Figure 36.20).

The short-crank stationary bike limits hip flexion and is initiated when the patient is able to get on and off the bike safely. This allows the patient to achieve gentle ROM while maintaining total hip precautions. Increasing the resistance can facilitate muscle strengthening and maintenance of cardiovascular endurance. When the patient demonstrates good balance and coordination, retrograde treadmill walking at low speeds will be incorporated into the program. This activity encourages quadriceps, hamstring, and gluteal muscle activity

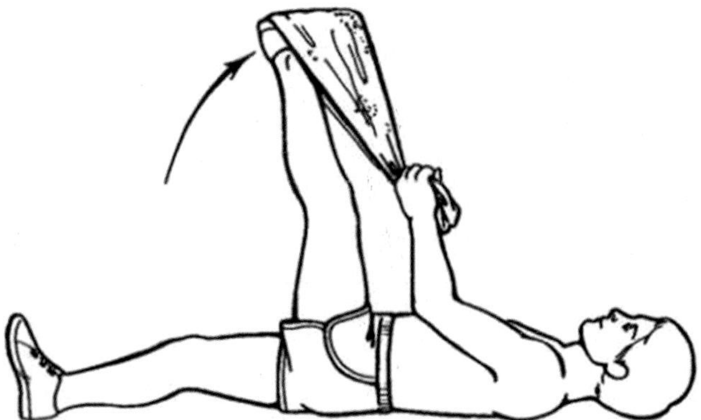

Figure 36.20 Illustration of the supine hamstring stretch.

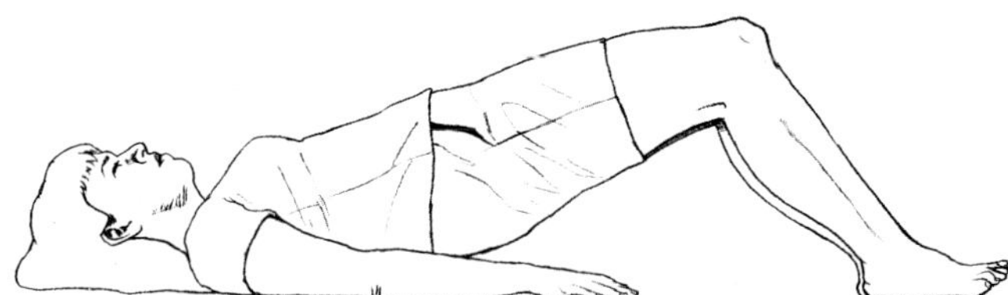

Figure 36.21 Supine bridging. (*ACC Trigger Points FlipBook*. Philadelphia, PA: Wolters Kluwer; 2007.)

while promoting hip extension ROM and challenging coordination and balance.

Strengthening exercises are progressed based on the patient's deficits. Hip muscle strength is significantly decreased in the first week after surgery and progressive strengthening for hip flexors, abductors, adductors, and extensors is recommended. Bridging exercises starting from both feet on the floor (Figure 36.21) and progressing to more challenging single-leg bridging emphasizes the development of hip extensor strength (Figure 36.22). Eventually, the use of an exercise ball can be incorporated for core strengthening and balance training. Side-lying clam shells (Figure 36.23) will allow strengthening of the hip abductors and extensors, and can be progressed to the use of exercise with a resistance band around the patient's

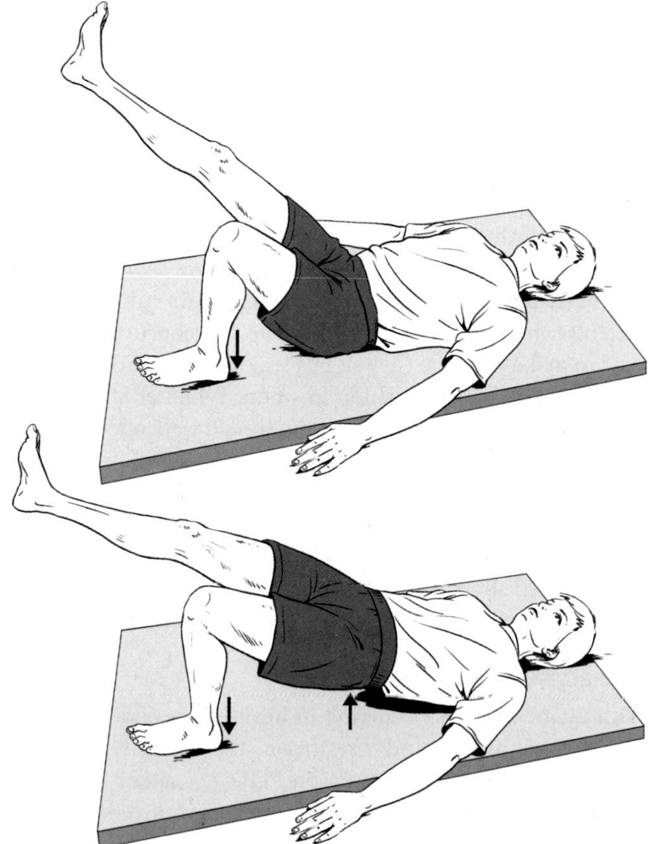

Figure 36.22 Single-leg bridging. (Reprinted from Liebenson C. *Functional Training Handbook*. Philadelphia, PA: Wolters Kluwer Health; 2014.)

 © 2018 American Academy of Orthopaedic Surgeons

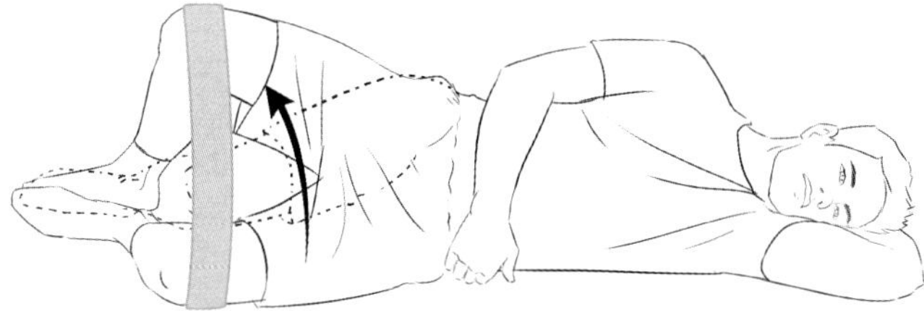

Figure 36.23 Illustration of the side-lying external rotation, with resistance band.

knees or an ankle weight attached to the knee (Figure 36.23). To further strengthen the hip and knee extensors, patients can initiate bilateral leg press with modified range of hip motion (<90° with posterolateral precautions) with progression to unilateral leg press when the patient is able to demonstrate adequate control.

When the patient is able to demonstrate a reciprocal gait pattern without deviation, the standing exercises from the acute phase of recovery can be progressed to the nonsurgical limb to further develop balance and strength, particularly of the abductors on the involved side. Additionally, when the patient is able to ambulate without a device, the forward step-up is introduced, starting with the 4-inch, and progressing to the 6-inch and 8-inch step when the patient is able to ascend with good control and no pain (Figure 36.24). Eccentric

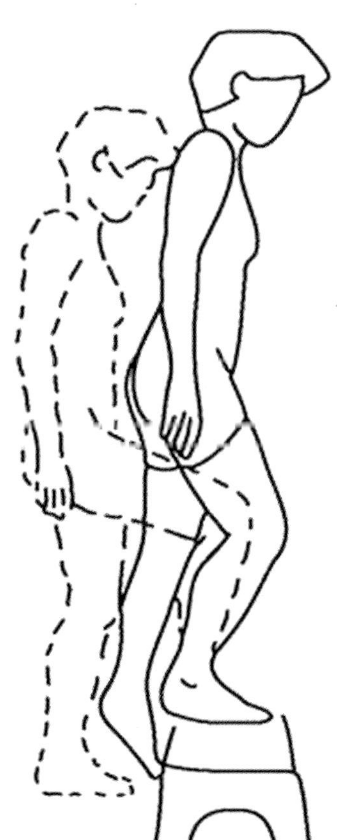

Figure 36.24 Illustration of the forward step-up exercise.

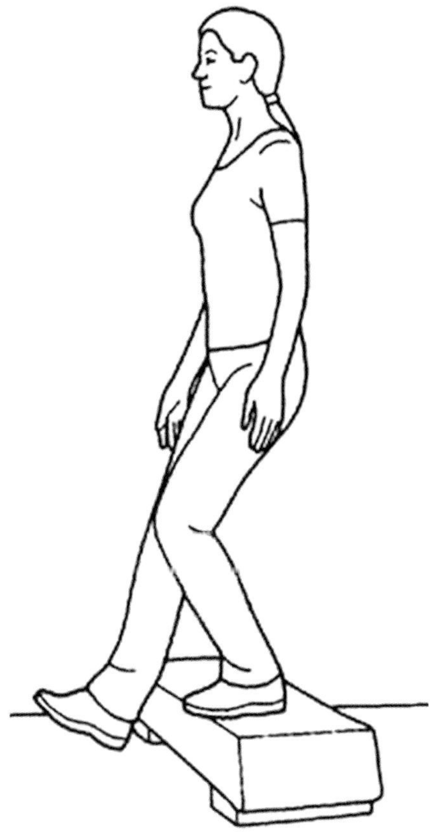

Figure 36.25 Illustration of the forward step-down exercise.

control of the quadriceps muscles is initiated at this point as well. Exercises will begin with forward stepping down off of a small (2-inch) step using a handrail for support and will progress to stepping down from a 6-inch step with no handrail (Figure 36.25).

Balance and Outcome Measures

Part of the outpatient visit will include balance assessment. Several tools are available for physical therapists to use, such as the single leg stance (SLS) test or the timed up and go (TUG) test. Regular retesting will be completed during the physical therapy sessions and used to monitor improvements in balance. As the patient's balance improves, balance exercises will be progressed to challenge the patient further. Exercises for balance include SLS after stepping up a 6-inch step, deliberate perturbing of the patient while he stands on one leg, and having the patient perform upper extremity exercises or catch an object while standing on an uneven or soft surface.

Return to Driving and Work

One of the most common questions from patients is: "When can I start driving again?" The answer depends on various factors. Since most patients do take some pain medication for postoperative pain, they are advised against driving at least until these medications are discontinued. The patient must also be able to perform active hip flexion in order to

© 2018 American Academy of Orthopaedic Surgeons

move his foot from one pedal to the next. In studies looking at braking reaction time (BRT), patients were deemed safe to drive between 4 and 8 weeks following right total hip replacement. Patients are advised to obtain clearance form their surgeon before they return to driving. For at least the first 6 weeks, they must consider that the type of car they travel in, even as a passenger, must enable them to maintain their precautions.

Advanced Strengthening, Return to Function (Week 6 and Onward)

The pace of rehabilitation programs for postoperative patients is also being driven by changes in the number of physical therapy visits reimbursed by insurance companies. Therefore, the typical postoperative exercise program is accelerated. After hip precautions are lifted, patients can begin to resume higher levels of activity. In order to achieve optimal function, patients will be progressed to a higher level of flexibility, ROM, and strength, as well as addressing gait pattern and more advanced ADLs. Many patients express a desire to return to some form of athletics, thus sport-specific training may become part of the patient's program. Advancement to sport activity is at the discretion and direction of the operating surgeon in concert with the therapist. The physical therapist will give consideration to the patient's prior level of activity when developing a more advanced program and tailor the program to suit the patient's goals, his current medical condition, and his sport-specific exercises.

Complications During the Recovery Period

The development of a proximal deep venous thrombosis or pulmonary embolism is rare with modern regimens of prophylaxis. However, if the diagnosis is made, there is a general consensus that postoperative physical therapy should be reinitiated as soon as the patient is medically stable and anticoagulated. Other complications, such as early dislocation and periprosthetic fracture, are likely to delay recovery and alter the guidelines of rehabilitation discussed in this chapter. Their therapy regimen—to include bracing, weight-bearing restrictions, and progression of exercises—is determined on a case-by-case basis under the direction of the surgeon. It is determined by the stability of the implants and patient factors, such as compliance and patient goals.

ACKNOWLEDGMENTS

The authors would like to thank Janine Pelegano, BA, BS/RN, for her editorial input for this contribution and helping us to bring the information together into a concise chapter. This work was partially funded by Mr. Glen Bergenfield and The Sidney Milton and Leoma Simon Foundation.

BIBLIOGRAPHY

American Academy of Orthopedic Surgeons: *Primary Total Hip and Total Knee Arthroplasty Projections to 2030 (Appendix C).*

Coulter CL, Scarvell JM, Neeman TM, Smith PN: Physiotherapist-directed rehabilitation exercises in the outpatient or home setting improve strength, gait speed and cadence after elective total hip replacement: a systematic review. *J Physiother* 2013;59(4): 219–226.

González Della Valle A, Padgett D, Salvati EA: Preoperative planning for primary total hip arthroplasty. *J Am Acad Orthop Surg* 2005;13(7):455–462.

Holm B, Thorborg K, Husted H, Kehlet H, Bandholm T: Surgery-induced changes and early recovery of hip-muscle strength, leg press power, and functional performance after fast-track total hip arthroplasty: a prospective cohort study. *PLoS One* 2013;8(4):e62109.

Hurvitz EA, Richardson JK, Werner RA, Ruhl AM, Dixon MR: Unipedal stance testing as an indicator of fall risk among older outpatients. *Arch Phys Med Rehabil* 2000;81(5):587–591.

Jonsson E, Seiger A, Hirschfeld H: One-leg stance in healthy young and elderly adults: a measure of postural steadiness? *Clin Biomech (Bristol, Avon)* 2004;19(7):688–694.

Lin MR, Hwang HF, Hu MH, Wu HD, Wang YW, Huang FC: Psychometric comparisons of the timed up and go, one-leg stand, functional reach, and Tinetti Balance Measures in Community-Dwelling Older People. *J Am Geriatr Soc* 2004; 52(8):1343–1348.

Marecek GF, Schafter MF: Driving after orthopedic surgery. *J Am Acad Orthop Surg* 2013;21:696–706.

Nankaku M, Tsuboyama T, Kakinoki R, Akiyama H, Nakamura T: Prediction of ambulation ability following total hip arthroplasty. *J Orthop Sci* 2011;16(4):359–363.

Tayrose G, Newman D, Slover J, et al: Rapid mobilization decreases length-of-stay in joint replacement patients. *Bull Hosp Jt Dis* 2013;71(3):222–226.

© 2018 American Academy of Orthopaedic Surgeons

37 Hip Resurfacing

Scott K. Siverling, PT, OCS, and Edwin P. Su, MD

INTRODUCTION

Hip resurfacing (HR) is a joint replacement procedure and alternative surgical option to total hip replacement (THA). HR allows conservation of bone in comparison to the traditional THA. Recent advancements in surgical technique, instrumentation, and prosthetic design of HR have improved the durability of HR prostheses and allowed increased motion and activity for those patients seeking surgical treatment of end-stage hip osteoarthritis (OA) when compared to contemporary posterior-approach THA.

The HR components involve a metal femoral cap with a short stem being inserted into the femoral head, once diseased and arthritic bone is eliminated surgically. Healthy bone of the femoral head and neck are preserved. The acetabular component is similar to the traditional THA acetabular prosthesis, utilizing the placement of a metal cup into the manually formed acetabular socket (Figure 37.1).

In addition to bone conservation, the appeal of HR is an increased postoperative activity level as compared to THA. Current thought and protocol regarding THA advises lower-level activity and a cessation of running and high-impact sports in order to preserve the prosthesis and avoid dislocation. The larger femoral component utilized in HR decreases the risk of dislocation and enables increased range of motion (ROM). The inherent stability and mobility of the HR prosthesis allows higher-level daily and recreational activity.

Guidelines for postoperative rehabilitation following HR have been proposed by the authors. The rehabilitation is divided into three phases. The first phase is considered the maximum protection phase, the second phase is the functional strengthening phase, and the third phase is the return to activity and/or sport phase. These guidelines are meant to assist in decision making for the practicing rehabilitation clinician in treating a patient who has undergone HR via the posterior approach. Other approaches, such as the anterolateral or anterior, may also be used and may require some modifications of the rehabilitation protocol, which should be discussed with the surgeon.

INDICATIONS

The ideal patient to undergo an HR is a male under the age of 65 years or a female under the age of 60 who has exhausted conservative care for a symptomatic arthritic hip joint.

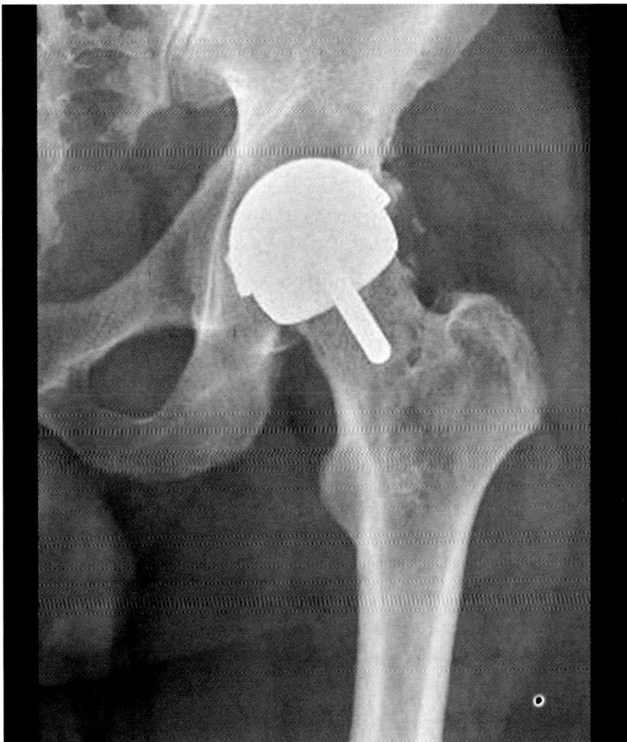

Figure 37.1 Radiograph of a hip resurfacing arthroplasty.

Dr. Su or an immediate family member serves as a paid consultant to Smith & Nephew; has stock or stock options held in Orthoalign; has received research or institutional support from Smith & Nephew; and serves as a board member, owner, officer, or committee member of the American Journal of Orthopedics *and* Techniques in Orthopedics. *Neither Dr. Siverling nor any immediate family member has received anything of value from or has stock or stock options held in a commercial company or institution related directly or indirectly to the subject of this article.*

Candidates must have normal bone stock, as determined by plain radiographs, in order to support the femoral cap and stem. Subjects with evidence of large or numerous cysts and pitting within the bone may be at a greater risk for postoperative fracture.

CONTRAINDICATIONS

Contraindications to undergoing HR include females of childbearing age, severe obesity, renal insufficiency, and patients with known metal allergy or metal sensitivity. Osteoporosis may weaken existing bone, providing inadequate support, and may decrease the stability of the prosthetic components, increasing the risk of fracture.

SURGICAL TECHNIQUE

The patient is positioned laterally for the posterior surgical approach, and the arthritic hip joint is exposed. For proper exposure and insertion of the acetabular component, a complete capsulotomy is necessary. The acetabular socket must be positioned ideally in order to avoid edge loading and erosion of the prosthesis. The socket is placed more horizontally, at approximately 40° of abduction, for protection against edge wearing.

The femoral head is sculpted, eliminating the diseased bone, and a metal cap with a short stem is placed into the underlying healthy bone. The femoral neck remains intact and is preserved. When aligning the femoral cap and stem, it is important to ignore the parameters of the femoral head—often, the femoral head is congenitally misshapen and can guide the surgeon toward improper femoral cap placement. The femoral component is instead inserted aligning to the center of the femoral neck.

Although a majority of the femoral head is retained during HR surgery, the preserved bone is briefly compromised by the surgical procedure. Excision of the arthritic bone and placement of the prosthetic cap and stem temporarily weakens the bone, increasing the risk of a postoperative fracture involving the femoral head or neck.

Metal ion dispersal into the bloodstream is a concern and risk following HR. To date, the authors have no knowledge of a predictive test for metal allergy or sensitivity. The current generation of metal-on-metal prostheses minimizes surface wear; however, metal ion dispersal has been observed in a small percentage of patients. Carrothers reported a 0.3% incidence of aseptic lymphocytic vascular and associated lesions (ALVAL) over a 5,000-subject sample. Those patients with normally functioning kidney and execratory systems are able to eliminate the cobalt and chromium metal ions through the urine. Metal ion blood levels are monitored on a regular basis following HR.

It is inferred that the increased exertion and activity of the younger demographic that have undergone HR may lead to a higher risk for heterotopic ossification (HO). The prophylactic use of aspirin or nonsteroidal anti-inflammatory drugs (NSAIDs) may be used to prevent ankylosing or severe HO.

REHABILITATION

Rehabilitation following HR surgery is divided into three basic phases. These phases have temporal properties, but the advancement between phases should be judged by the achievement of the milestones and goals outlined in each phase.

Entering into surgery, many patients suffering from end-stage hip OA complain of debilitating pain and exhibit compensatory gait patterns, a loss of hip joint motion in multiple directions, and muscle atrophy with weakness in the surrounding musculature. All of this can lead to altered neuromuscular patterns that may be suboptimal for efficient and pain-free movement. The correction of substitution patterns is emphasized during rehabilitation, and proper movement is instilled. Neuromuscular reeducation is imperative to achieve full recovery and to attain the patient's goals.

Initially, ROM, healing, and advancement of independence with gait are the emphasis of the maximum protection phase. Strength of the specific muscles that control hip motion is the focus of the functional strengthening phase; however, ROM should not be neglected during the second phase. In the final phase, the clinician should focus on neuromuscular strengthening and sport-specific demands. While each phase emphasizes a different objective, each patient and his or her goals, physiologic deficits, and weaknesses vary. The clinician is reminded to individualize each rehabilitation program according to the deficits, inadequacies, and goals of the patient.

Maximum Protection Phase

- *Healing and Gait Training:* The goal of the first phase is to allow the natural healing of the involved tissues. Cryotherapy and relative rest are employed to moderate edema. Gentle soft-tissue mobilization may assist in mitigating edema within the myofascial structures. Because of the compromise to bone strength immediately following surgery, patients are asked to ambulate with crutches bilaterally. Often, patients complain only of muscle soreness that does not inhibit their motion or activity. Despite the lack of pain, these patients are encouraged to continue use of the crutches for at least 2 weeks following the HR procedure in order to guard against the risk of fracture. Those patients who feel comfortable and demonstrate a reciprocal and symmetrical gait using two crutches can be weaned to using one crutch. Males who exhibit good strength, do not report pain, and have evidence of strong bone stock may use a cane. Eventually, weaning from all assistive devices is encouraged. This occurs, most often, within 2 to 4 weeks following HR surgery.
- *No Motion Restrictions:* It is believed that the large femoral ball component fortifies the stability of the prosthetic joint. Because of this, the only restrictions following HR are concerning weight bearing.

© 2018 American Academy of Orthopaedic Surgeons

- Early and pain-free motion and stretching are heavily encouraged, beginning in non–weight bearing positions.
- Many patients will present with a loss of hip ROM, especially with rotational movements and hip flexion. Active external rotation of the hip is encouraged in a supine position, to tolerance. Hip flexion is promoted by performing a "rocking" motion from the quadruped position. This is commonly called the "child's pose" by practitioners of yoga. The Thomas test and stretch position—typically used to assess the resting length of the hip flexors—is taught to the patient to stretch the anterior soft tissues surrounding the hip joint, increasing hip extension ROM.

- *Strengthening:* Initially, strengthening of the muscles controlling the hip joint is initiated in a non–weight bearing position. The abductors, external rotators, and extensors of the hip are engaged early, with little or no resistance. The patient is educated in eliciting contractions of these muscles without substitution patterns or pain. Core strengthening can begin in a non–weight bearing position. Once the incision has healed properly, aquatic therapy becomes an option, if available. Use of a stationary upright bike is encouraged to begin cardiovascular strengthening and promote gentle ROM.
- *Goals*
  - Normalize gait pattern and wean from assistive devices.
  - Promote healing and minimize edema and pain.
  - Increase hip ROM in all tolerated directions with stretching.
  - Independence with a home exercise program emphasizing motion and ambulation.
  - Begin non–weight bearing and pain-free strengthening of the muscles that control hip motion.

Functional Strengthening Phase

The second phase of rehabilitation following HR surgery can begin as early as 2 weeks postoperatively, but normally at 4 weeks after surgery. The functional strengthening phase is meant to provide the strength needed for the patient to complete activities of daily living (ADLs), regular ambulation, and light exercise without pain or assistance. This phase usually lasts 4 to 8 weeks.

- *Advance Motion:* Entering the second phase of rehabilitation, the surgical incision should be completely healed. The primary goal at this stage of recovery should continue to be increasing ROM and mobility.
  - Manual mobilizations may be utilized. The clinician should communicate properly with the operating surgeon to ensure that manual mobilizations are appropriate, and that the surface implant can tolerate manual stretching.
  - While the loss of hip flexion and rotational movements are most common with hip OA, the clinician should use expertise and instinct, as well as communication with the patient, while stretching the patient to avoid injury.
- *Specific Strengthening:* Exercises meant to isolate specific key muscles are practiced in order to build strength and endurance of the muscles that control the hip joint. Preliminary exercises are performed in a non–weight bearing position and gradually progressed to weight bearing and closed-chain exercises. Example exercises include the "clamshell" exercise, side-lying hip abduction with the knee bent (short-lever arm) and knee straight (long-lever arm), supine hip flexion with the knee bent, and the straight-leg raise. Emphasis is placed on the abductors, extensors, and flexors of the hip joint.
  - Once gait is normalized without use of an assistive device, the patient can begin to use an elliptical machine without resistance or incline. Gradual increases in resistance and incline are introduced slowly.
- *Functional Strengthening and Neuromuscular Control:* As ROM is restored, strength must be instilled in the affected joints in order to exert controlled motion. Compensatory patterns have often been observed in patients with end-stage OA. Postoperatively, these suboptimal movement habits need to be diminished or abolished entirely, and replaced with proper movement patterns.
  - Gross movement without subtle and foundational control leads to an inefficient transfer of forces throughout, putting joints at risk for injury. While flexibility and motion are regained, the clinician must initiate strengthening throughout the hip joint's available range.
  - In weight bearing, this should begin in the double-limb stance position and gradually progress to single-limb. Squats and lunges will prepare the patient for rising from a seated position, getting up from the floor, or climbing stairs and hills. Single-leg balance tasks are begun at this stage as well: first in static positions, then perturbations on unstable surfaces are introduced. Reaching while standing on the single leg challenges strength and balance.
  - The ROM of the hip should always be considered during any activity. For example, without full hip flexion and control, the patient may flex the lumbar spine during a simple squat task. This microtrauma to posterior lumbar tissues may lead to a peripheral injury.
- *Lumbopelvic mobility and stability:* It is not uncommon for the patient to have difficulty performing anterior and posterior tilting of the pelvis. On a fixed lower extremity, the gluteus maximus will posteriorly tilt the pelvis during the stance phase to propel the trunk forward. Limited ability to tilt the pelvis will directly affect the potential action of the gluteal muscles and their ability to stabilize the hip joint. Patients are educated in how to properly dissociate the pelvis from the femoro-acetabular joint. Strengthening of the lumbopelvic unit then enhances proximal stability for distal control.
  - Lumbopelvic dissociation is begun in the supine position by tilting the pelvis anteriorly and posteriorly. The ability to tilt to the pelvis in the sagittal plane can be integrated to weight-bearing positions.
  - Educating the patient on the anatomy and elicitation of the deeper lumbar stabilizers will enhance facilitation of

© 2018 American Academy of Orthopaedic Surgeons

lumbopelvic stability. These muscles are then engaged while moving the limbs; for example, a "bird-dog" exercise in the quadruped position, or a "dying bug" exercise in the supine position. Eventually, the patient is trained to engage the deep stabilizers in weight-bearing positions.

- *Goals*
  - Ambulation for approximately 2 miles or more without use of an assistive device, demonstrating a symmetric and reciprocal gait pattern.
  - Ipsilateral single-leg stance for 5 seconds, demonstrating control.
  - Pain-free dressing and ADLs.
  - Functional hip flexion, extension, internal and external ROM.
  - Negotiate an 8-inch step with proper control.
  - Able to perform 4/5 hip abductor muscle strength hold against resistance for five consecutive manual muscle tests.

Return-To-Sport Phase and Advanced Strengthening

During the advanced stage of rehabilitation (Phase III), strengthening and neuromuscular facilitation are enhanced with a gradual escalation in the difficulty of exercises. Elicitation of the hip abductor, hip extensor, and hip flexor muscles is a primary goal. Neuromuscular reeducation and observation of movement patterns is continually employed, as well. The patient's balance system is challenged with unstable surfaces in double-limb and single-limb stance positions.

Part of the allure of undergoing HR is the possibility of returning to an active lifestyle. In the authors' experience, it is possible to perform noncontact sports after surgery. Multiple studies have confirmed a return to higher-level activity following HR surgery.

- Once permission is granted from the surgeon and the patient has expressed a desire to return to a particular sport or activity, rehabilitation should be focused on control of movements that are activity-specific.
  - Control of movement, facilitated by the proximal and core muscles, is reinforced. During the running motion, hamstring and gluteal strength is imperative for late stance propulsion. However, the deep lumbopelvic stabilizers must regulate pelvic motion over the femur. This will allow pure movement without risk of microtrauma and injury to the HR prostheses or peripheral tissues and joints.
  - Muscle endurance must be reinforced. Muscle fatigue leads to dysfunctional biomechanics and injury. The clinician should take care at each phase of rehabilitation to reinforce activity of the proper muscles needed to complete each movement. Repetition is paramount, as it will reinforce the neuromuscular preference for a particular task and create muscle endurance.

Patients most commonly report and request a return to running as a form of regular exercise. Fouilleron reported that 33 out of 40 (91.6%) patients that ran prior to undergoing HR returned to running safely postoperatively. The mean time from surgery to resumption of running was 16.4 weeks, and 23 subjects reported running up to 4 hours per week. Multiple subjects reported returning to competitive running successfully.

- A return to running activities can be approved once full strength and motion have been restored. It is advised to wait approximately 6 months following surgery to avoid placing inordinate risk on the femur and femoral component of the HR and allow full healing.
- Our recommendations, in regard to a return to running, are to regain full ROM in all planes (as compared to preoperative measures), adequate hip abduction and extension strength, and a gradual recommencement of a running regimen.
  - Patients wishing to return to a running lifestyle should be able to exhibit proper control with a side-plank exercise for 60 seconds and perform 10 single-leg squats ideally, without aberrations through the kinetic chain, on each side.
  - We advise beginning to run first on softer surfaces, such as grass, artificial turf, packed dirt, or a rubberized track, for short distances. Once this is tolerated, distance per run and frequency of runs can be slowly increased. Firmer surfaces, such as a treadmill or asphalt road, can be gradually introduced eventually, after 2–6 weeks of running on softer surfaces without negative consequences. Muscle soreness following running should be respected, and rest imparted, if necessary, to allow proper healing.

PEARLS

- *Femoral Neck Fractures:* As previously stated, placement of the femoral component of the HR prostheses may weaken the femoral neck and increase the risk for femoral neck fracture. According to Shimmin, in a literature review, risk of femoral neck fracture is significant for 18 weeks following HR surgery.
  - To decrease the risk of fracture, it is advised to avoid carrying weight of more than 20 pounds for 1 month following surgery, and 30 pounds for 3 months postoperatively. After 3 months, carrying weight may gradually increase to tolerance, but should not exceed 50 pounds before 6 months postoperatively.
  - Patients with possible femoral neck fracture may complain of extreme and inordinate groin and hip pain with weight bearing. If a femoral neck fracture is suspected, the patient should be placed on immediate weight bearing restrictions and the operating surgeon should be notified.
- *Iliopsoas Tendinopathy:* It is our experience that patients may acquire symptoms of hip flexor and iliopsoas

© 2018 American Academy of Orthopaedic Surgeons

tendinopathies. The etiology is unknown; however, many patients exhibit poor strength and a lack of ROM prior to surgery. When motion of the hip and tilt of the pelvis are regained postoperatively, the iliopsoas muscle may have to work through and control a larger amount of motion than prior to surgery.

- Patients may complain of anterior hip and groin pain with exertion and movement. Tenderness at the tendinous insertion on the lesser trochanter of the femur and pain with resisted hip flexion are hallmark objective signs of iliopsoas tendinopathy.
- As motion through the hip and lumbopelvic region are regained, strength and control of the proximal regions must be attained in order to avoid unnecessary stress to the iliopsoas muscle and tendon.

- *Gluteus Medius Tendinopathy (GMT) and Greater Trochanter Bursitis (TB):* It can be difficult to distinguish between these two common and often interrelated pathologies. It is our experience that GMT and TB may arise during the rehabilitative process following HR.
    - In cases of GMT, the patient may complain of pain just posterior to the greater trochanter, and pain with palpation to the superior portion of gluteus medius muscle belly, just distal to the iliac ridge. As well, pain with resisted hip abduction will be present.
    - In those affected by TB, pain is elicited from direct palpation to the greater trochanter.
- *Proper Progression to Avoid Injury:* If the rehabilitation program is individualized according to the needs and limits of the patient, an ideal outcome can be expected. To achieve this, the clinician must be devoted to a process of constant reassessment of the current status and ability of the patient.
    - A key principle of rehabilitation is to promote proximal stability for distal mobility and control. Without adequate motion of the lumbar spine and pelvis and control of that motion, the potential strength and control of the limb is limited. The initiation of core stability can begin in Phase I and is gradually increased in difficulty and repetition, to tolerance of the patient, throughout all three phases.
    - Weight-bearing exercises should begin in double limb stance and appropriately progress to a single limb stance position. At first, exercises should be performed in one plane of motion. Eventually, the patient can perform multiplanar exercises and tasks. The clinician must place detail on the activity and facilitation of the apposite muscles for optimal movement and strengthening.
    - Special emphasis must be placed on gaining open-chain and closed-chain strength of the hip flexors, abductors, and extensors. These muscle groups are often very weak prior to surgery. Habitual movement patterns that avoid using these muscles may persist following surgery. These faulty patterns should be corrected through the recovery process.

BIBLIOGRAPHY

Carrothers AD, Glibert RE, Jaiswal A, Richardson JB: Birmingham hip resurfacing: prevalence of failure. *J Bone Joint Surg Br* 2010;92(10):1344–1350.

Fouilleron N, Wavreille G, Endjah N, Girard J: Running activity after hip resurfacing arthroplasty: a prospective study. *Am J Sports Med* 2012;40(4):889–894.

Girard J, Miletec B, Deny A, Migaud H, Fouilleron N: Can patients return to high-impact physical activities after hip resurfacing? A prospective study. *Int Orthop* 2013;37(6):1019–1024.

Neumann D: Kinesiology of the musculoskeletal system: *Foundations for Rehabilitation,* ed 2. New York, NY, CV Mosby Co., 2012.

Rahman WA, Greidanus NV, Siegmuth A, Masri BA, Duncan CP, Garbuz DS: Patients report improvement in quality of life and satisfaction after hip resurfacing arthroplasty. *Clin Orthop Relat Res* 2013;471(2):444–453.

Rydevik K, Fernandes L, Nordsletten L, Risberg MA: Functioning and disability in patients with hip osteoarthritis and mild to moderate pain. *J Orthop Sports Phys Ther* 2010;40(10):616–624.

Shimmin AJ, Back D: Femoral neck fractures following Birmingham hip resurfacing: a national review of 50 cases. *J Bone Joint Surg Br* 2005;87(4):463–464.

Siverling S, Felix I, Chow SB, Niedbala E, Su EP: Hip resurfacing: not your average hip replacement. *Curr Rev Musculoskelet Med* 2012;5(1):32–38.

38 Total Hip Arthroplasty for Hip Fracture

David J. Mayman, MD

INTRODUCTION

Hip arthroplasty for treatment of hip fracture can be an excellent treatment option that can allow for a very fast recovery to prefracture level of activity.

Historically, total hip arthroplasty (THA) has been used in a limited amount for hip fractures because of risk of dislocation, infection, and periprosthetic fracture. Hemiarthroplasty is commonly performed in elderly patients for displaced fractures as a reliable means of maintaining mobility. Fixation is commonly performed in younger patients or in nondisplaced fractures in the elderly to preserve the native hip. However, the challenges of reduction, fixation, and healing of femoral neck fractures have made total hip replacement a good option for the active older patient while avoiding the problem of acetabular wear with hemiarthroplasty. The increasing success of modern THA for degenerative conditions in younger patients has led to its growing popularity for hip fractures in the middle-aged or older active patient. Hemiarthroplasty is still more commonly performed in elderly patients, although pain relief has been shown to be better with total hip replacement.

ANATOMY

Hip fractures come in many forms. The definition of the fracture is based on the anatomic location. The more proximal in the femur the fracture is, the simpler THA becomes.

Femoral Neck Fracture

Femoral neck fractures occur between the femoral head and the trochanters. This fracture is typically at or above the level at which the femoral neck would be cut for a standard total hip replacement.

Basicervical Fracture

Basicervical fractures occur just above the intertrochanteric ridge. They do not involve either the lesser or greater trochanter and typically below the level of where a neck cut would be made for a THA. Revision hip implants may be required in these cases given the lack of supporting bone remaining in the femoral calcar to support a primary hip prosthesis.

Intertrochanteric Fracture

Intertrochanteric fractures involve the lesser trochanter, the greater trochanter, or both. THA for this fracture pattern is performed uncommonly—these fractures are most commonly fixed with an intramedullary nail or a plate and screws, and tend to heal. If a THA is performed in this case, usually after failure of fixation, revision femoral implants need to be used.

The large majority of total hip replacements done for hip fractures are done for displaced femoral neck fractures (Figure 38.1).

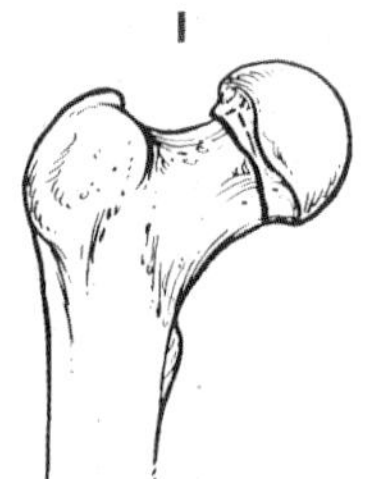

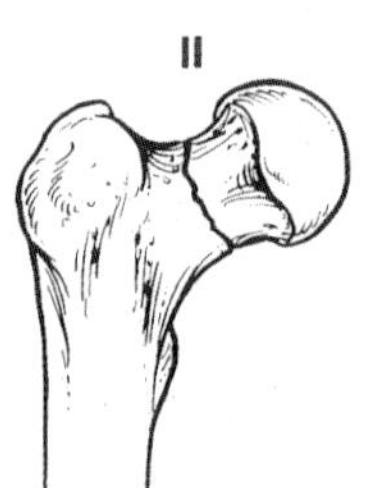

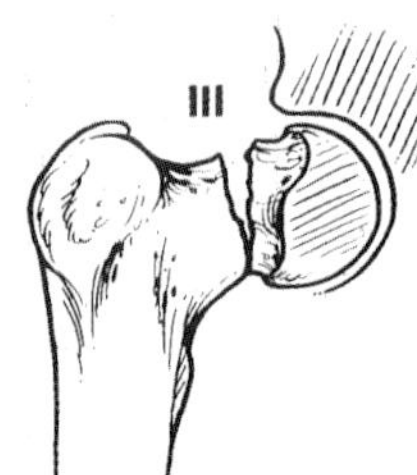

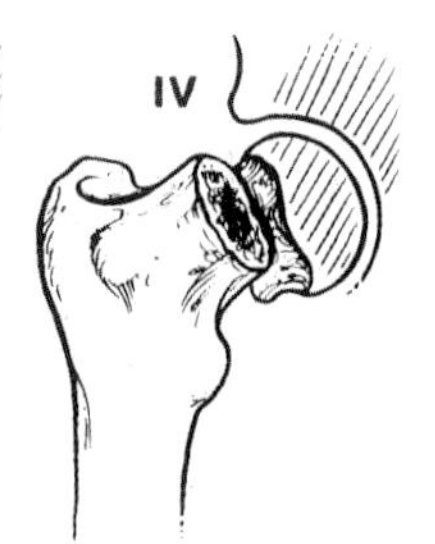

Figure 38.1 Illustration of the types of hip fractures. The large majority of total hip replacements done for hip fractures are done for displaced femoral neck fractures (type III and IV). (Reproduced with permission from Koval KJ, Zuckerman JD: *Atlas of Orthopaedic Surgery: A Multimedia Reference*. Philadelphia, Lippincott Williams & Wilkins, 2004.)

Dr. Mayman or an immediate family member is a member of a speakers' bureau or has made paid presentations on behalf of Smith & Nephew; serves as a paid consultant to Smith & Nephew; has stock or stock options held in OrthAlign; and serves as a board member, owner, officer, or committee member of the Knee Society.

 © 2018 American Academy of Orthopaedic Surgeons

SURGICAL PROCEDURES

THA resurfaces the acetabulum with a socket and puts a stem into the canal of the femur. A liner is placed in the socket and a ball is placed on a stem that fits into the canal of the proximal femur. Today, the majority of acetabular components are titanium implants with a porous ingrowth surface. Cemented femoral implants are still used commonly in elderly patients or patients with questionable femoral bone quality. The socket then has a modular liner inserted into it. These liners are usually made of cross-linked polyethylene.

The femoral implant is either made of titanium with a porous ingrowth surface or is cemented into the femur for fixation. The decision of whether to use a cemented or uncemented femoral implant is based on bone quality and surgeon preference.

The surgery can be done through a number of surgical approaches. The approach used for surgery and surgeon preferences will affect the limitations or precautions in the early postoperative period.

Direct Anterior Approach

The direct anterior approach utilizes the intramuscular plane between the tensor fascia lata and the rectus femorus muscle. Exposure to the acetabulum is relatively simple, but exposure of the femur is more difficult. Posterior structures are left intact. The risk of posterior instability is low, but the risk of anterior instability is higher.

Anterolateral Approach

The anterolateral approach has a low risk of dislocation, but the anterior portion of the gluteus minimus and gluteus medius are taken off of the trochanter for the procedure, and have to heal back to the trochanter after surgery.

Direct Lateral Approach

The direct lateral approach incorporates an osteotomy of the greater trochanter. This approach is not commonly used today; it requires time for the osteotomy to heal.

Posterolateral Approach

The posterolateral approach is the most common approach used for hip arthroplasty in the United States today. The abductors are left intact, but the posterior capsule, piriformis tendon, and conjoined tendon are released from the posterior aspect of the femur, necessitating posterior hip precautions during the healing period.

EARLY POSTOPERATIVE REHABILITATION

Early postoperative rehabilitation is highly dependent on the surgical approach used. Early ambulation is encouraged to minimize postoperative medical risks such as deep vein thrombosis (DVT), pulmonary embolism, and pneumonia.

Most patients will be weight bearing as tolerated immediately after surgery unless a complication such as fracture is noted.

Direct Anterior Approach

- Weight bearing, as tolerated.
- Avoid hyperextension and external rotation.
- Progress from a walker to a cane to no ambulatory aids, as tolerated.

Anterolateral Approach

- Weight bearing, as tolerated.
- Avoid hyperextension and external rotation.
- Progress from a walker to a cane, but a cane should be used, and avoid active abduction to protect the abductor repair for the first 6 weeks.

Direct Lateral Approach

- Weight bearing, as tolerated.
- Avoid flexion, adduction, and internal rotation.
- Progress from a walker to a cane; a cane should be used to protect the osteotomy for the first 6 weeks.

Posterolateral Approach

- Weight bearing, as tolerated.
- Avoid flexion, adduction, and internal rotation.
- Progress from a walker to a cane to no ambulatory aids, as tolerated.

Posterior Hip Precautions

Hip replacement done through a posterior approach leaves the abductors fully intact, but releases the piriformis tendon and the conjoined tendon from the back of the femur. The posterior capsule is then released. The hip is dislocated by a combination of hip flexion, adduction, and internal rotation.

Posterior hip precautions are designed to avoid harming the repair of the posterior structures or dislocation of the hip joint.

- No hip flexion past 90°.
- No adduction past neutral.
- No internal rotation of the hip (Figure 38.2).

EARLY POSTOPERATIVE REHABILITATION EXERCISES

Ankle Pumps

Slowly push the foot up and down. Do this exercise several times as often as every 5 or 10 minutes. This exercise can begin immediately after surgery (Figure 38.3).

Ankle Rotations

Move the ankle inward toward your other foot, then outward away from your other foot.

© 2018 American Academy of Orthopaedic Surgeons

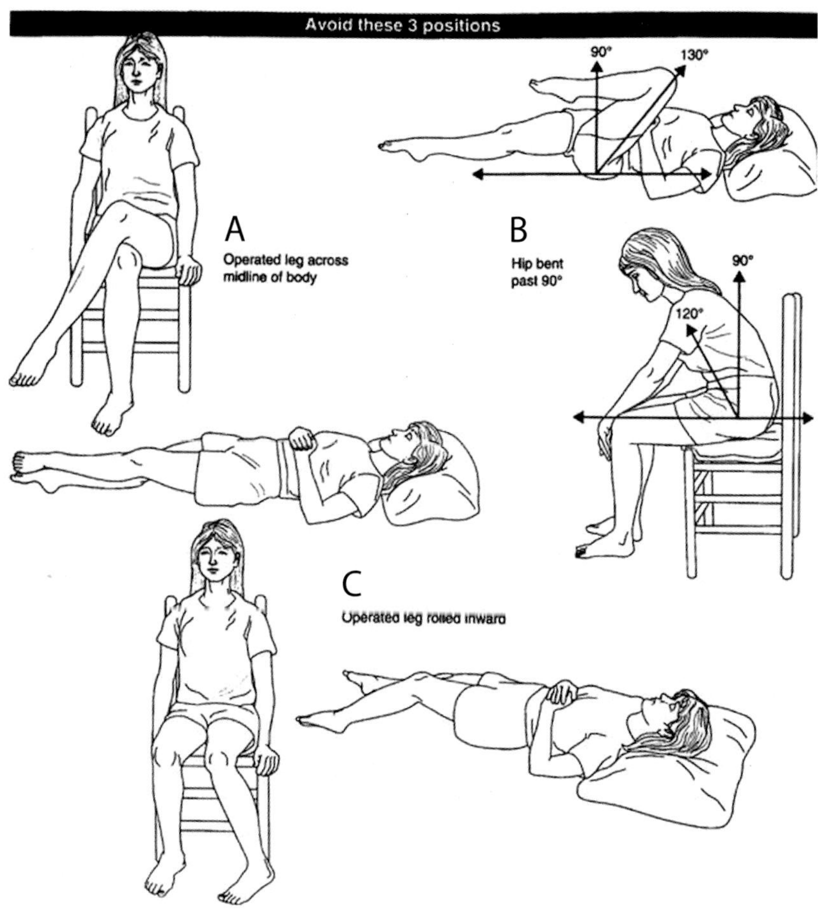

Figure 38.2 Illustrations of standard posterior hip precautions: **A**, no adduction past neutral; **B**, no hip flexion past 90 degrees; **C**, no internal rotation of the hip for the first six weeks. (Reproduced with permission from Sculco TP, Lim MR, Pearle AD, Ranawat AS: *Hospital for Special Surgery Orthopaedics Manual*. Philadelphia, Lippincott Williams & Wilkins, 2014.)

Repeat five times in each direction three or four times a day (Figure 38.4). These exercises will begin reactivating lower extremity muscles and will help with venous return using the lower extremity muscles to pump blood through the venous system, lowering the risk of DVT.

Bed-Supported Knee Bends

Slide the heel toward the buttocks, bend the knee and keep the heel on the bed. Do not let the knee roll inward (Figure 38.5). Repeat 10 times three or four times a day. This exercise begins reactivating the hip flexor muscles after surgery.

Buttock Contractions

Tighten buttock muscles and hold to a count of five (Figure 38.6). Repeat 10 times three or four times a day. This exercise will help reactivate the gluteal muscles required for ambulation.

Abduction Exercise

Slide the leg out to the side as far as possible, and then back (Figure 38.7). Repeat 10 times three or four times a day.

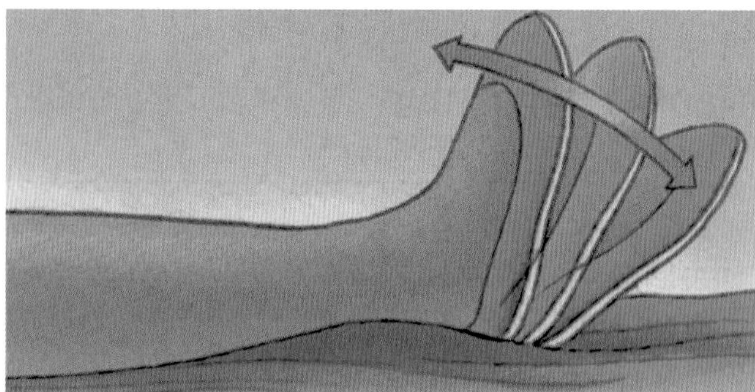

Figure 38.3 Illustration of ankle pumps. (Reproduced with permission from OrthoInfo. © American Academy of Orthopaedic Surgeons. Available at: http://orthoinfo.aaos.org.)

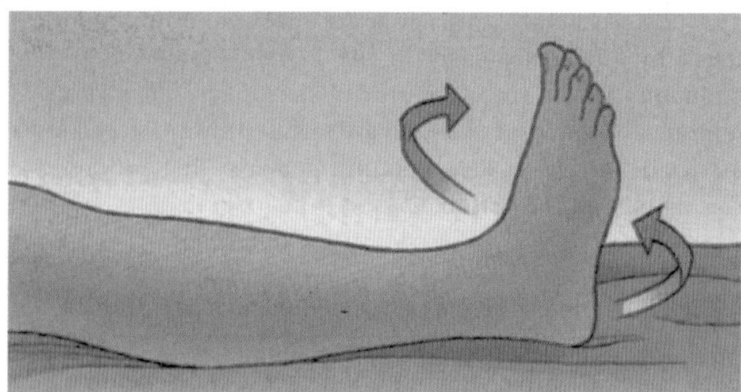

Figure 38.4 Illustration of ankle rotations. (Reproduced with permission from OrthoInfo. © American Academy of Orthopaedic Surgeons. Available at: http://orthoinfo.aaos.org.)

© 2018 American Academy of Orthopaedic Surgeons

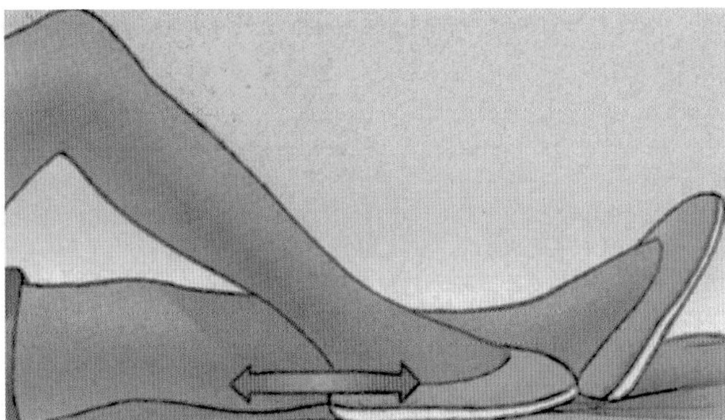

Figure 38.5 Illustration of bed-supported knee bends. (Reproduced with permission from OrthoInfo. © American Academy of Orthopaedic Surgeons. Available at: http://orthoinfo.aaos.org.)

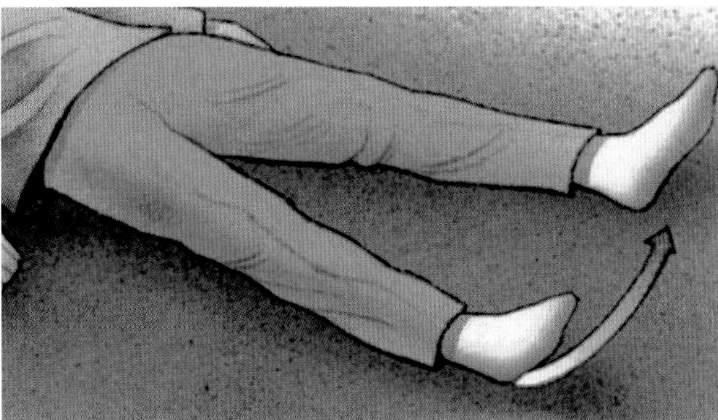

Figure 38.7 Illustration of abduction exercise. (Reproduced with permission from OrthoInfo. © American Academy of Orthopaedic Surgeons. Available at: http://orthoinfo.aaos.org.)

Abduction exercises will be the most important exercises to continue in order to regain normal gait mechanics without a limp.

Quadriceps Set

Tighten the thigh muscle. Try to straighten the knee. Hold for 5 to 10 seconds (Figure 38.8). Repeat this exercise 10 times during a 10-minute period. Continue until the thigh feels fatigued.

Straight Leg Raises

Tighten the thigh muscle with the knee fully straightened on the bed. As the thigh muscle tightens, lift the leg several inches off the bed. Hold for 5 to 10 seconds. Slowly lower (Figure 38.9). Repeat until the thigh feels fatigued. This exercise will work the hip flexors as well as the quadriceps mechanism.

Standing Exercises

Standing Knee Raises

Lift the operated leg toward the chest. Do not lift the knee higher than the waist. Hold for two or three counts and put the leg down (Figure 38.10). Repeat 10 times three or four times a day.

This exercise will also help strengthen the hip flexors required for gait.

Standing Hip Abduction

Be sure that the hip, knee, and foot are pointing straightforward. Keep the body straight. With the knee straight, lift the leg out to the side. Slowly lower the leg so that the foot is back on the floor (Figure 38.11). Repeat 10 times three or four times a day.

This exercise is a midlevel exercise that will continue to improve abductor strength and will lead to the next level, which is lying on the nonoperative side and performing the same exercise. This exercise should not be performed in the first 6 weeks to allow healing of abductors in cases done through anterolateral and direct lateral approaches.

Standing Hip Extensions

Lift the operated leg backward slowly. Try to keep the back straight. Hold for two or three counts. Return the foot to the floor (Figure 38.12). Repeat 10 times three or four times a day.

Things to Watch for

After discharge from the hospital, the therapist often sees the patient more frequently than does the physician. Therapists need to be aware of potential early complications.

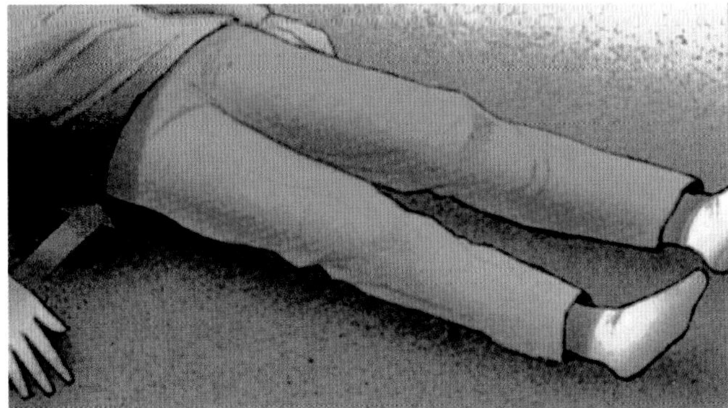

Figure 38.6 Illustration of buttock contractions. (Reproduced with permission from OrthoInfo. © American Academy of Orthopaedic Surgeons. Available at: http://orthoinfo.aaos.org.)

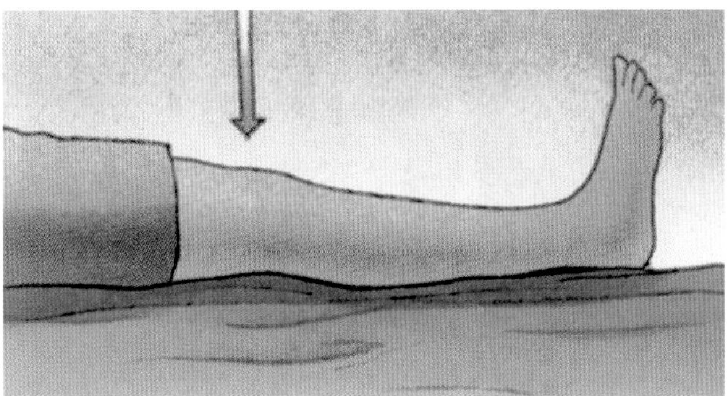

Figure 38.8 Illustration of quadriceps set. (Reproduced with permission from OrthoInfo. © American Academy of Orthopaedic Surgeons. Available at: http://orthoinfo.aaos.org.)

© 2018 American Academy of Orthopaedic Surgeons

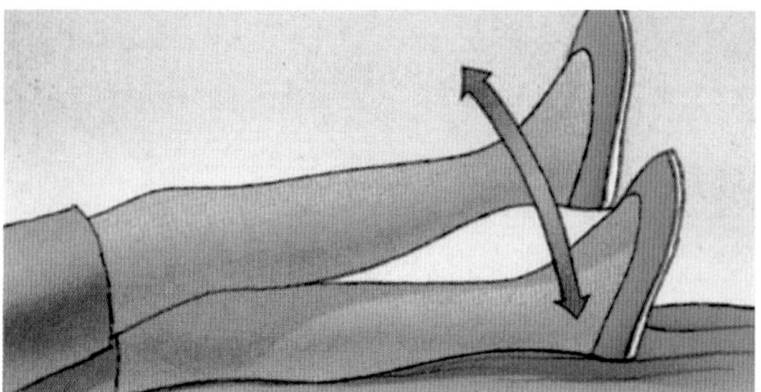

Figure 38.9 Illustration of straight leg raises. (Reproduced with permission from OrthoInfo. © American Academy of Orthopaedic Surgeons. Available at: http://orthoinfo.aaos.org.)

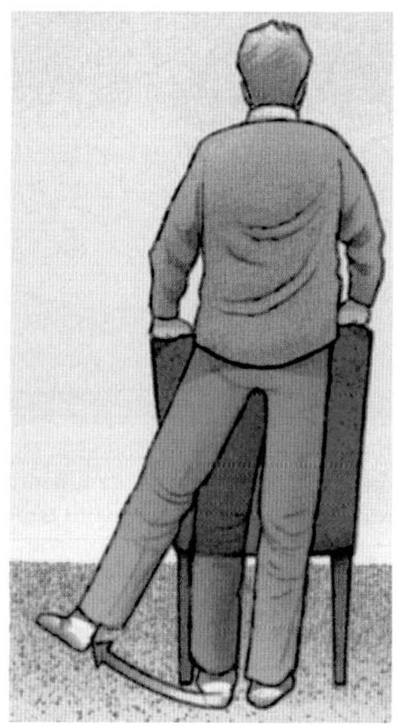

Figure 38.11 Illustration of standing hip abduction. (Reproduced with permission from OrthoInfo. © American Academy of Orthopaedic Surgeons. Available at: http://orthoinfo.aaos.org.)

Wound Infection

Redness around the incision or drainage from the incision are concerning for infection. The physician needs to be made aware of either of these findings.

Deep Vein Thrombosis

Most patients have swelling in the operative leg for at least 6 weeks after surgery. This swelling should improve in the morning, but will get worse through the day. Having the leg in a dependent position through the day increases the amount of the swelling. Swelling that does not improve with leg elevation or overnight is concerning and needs to be evaluated for the possibility of DVT.

Dislocation

Dislocation is an obvious complication, which generally happens when the hip is inadvertently placed in a provocative position with a sudden sense of instability. Patients will not be able to weight bear on a dislocated hip, and the position of the leg will be abnormal. Patients with a posterior hip dislocation will have the leg flexed and internally rotated. Patients with an anterior dislocation will be externally rotated and the leg will be shortened.

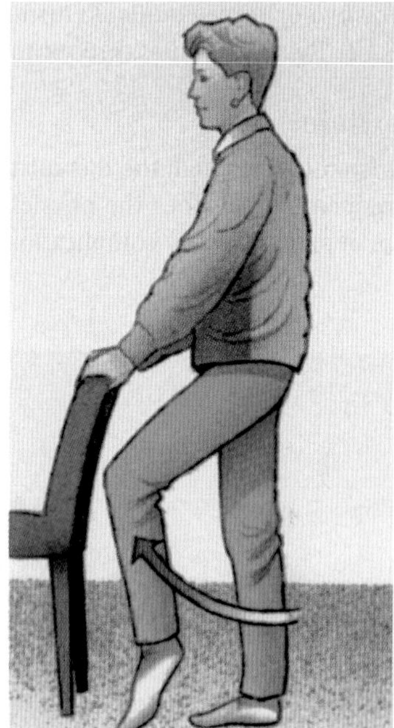

Figure 38.10 Illustration of standing knee raises. (Reproduced with permission from OrthoInfo. © American Academy of Orthopaedic Surgeons. Available at: http://orthoinfo.aaos.org.)

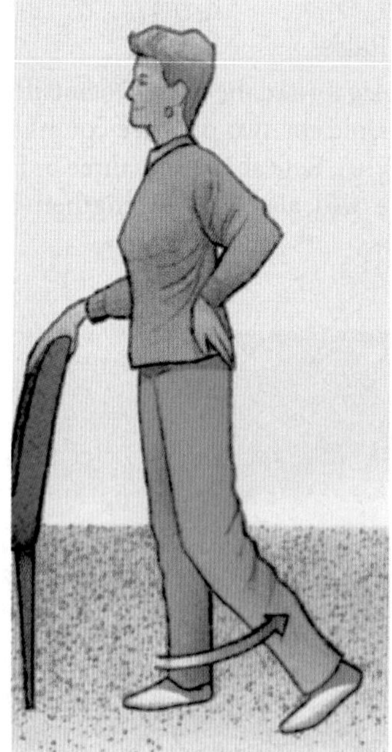

Figure 38.12 Illustration of standing hip extensions. (Reproduced with permission from OrthoInfo. © American Academy of Orthopaedic Surgeons. Available at: http://orthoinfo.aaos.org.)

© 2018 American Academy of Orthopaedic Surgeons

Periprosthetic Fracture

Fracture after surgery can be obvious, with inability to weight bear, but can also be more subtle, with only an increase in pain. It may occur as a result of a fall or without trauma. In the latter case, the fracture may have occurred during surgery but was not noticed.

ADVANCED POSTOPERATIVE REHABILITATION (6 WEEKS POSTOPERATIVELY)

Elastic Tube Exercises

Resistive Hip Flexion

Stand with the feet slightly apart. Bring the operated leg forward, keeping the knee straight. Allow the leg to return to its previous position (Figure 38.13).

Resistive Hip Abduction

Stand sideways from the door and extend the operated leg out to the side. Allow the leg to return to its previous position (Figure 38.14).

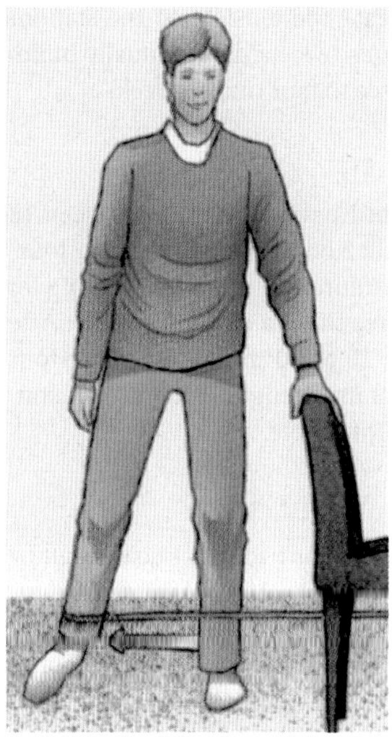

Figure 38.14 Illustration of resistive hip abduction. (Reproduced with permission from OrthoInfo. © American Academy of Orthopaedic Surgeons. Available at: http://orthoinfo.aaos.org.)

Resistive Hip Extensions

Face the door or heavy object to which the tubing is attached and pull the leg straight back. Allow the leg to return to its previous position (Figure 38.15).

Stationary Bike

A stationary bike is an excellent activity to regain muscle strength and hip mobility. Patients may begin using a stationary bike postoperatively as soon as they can get on and off comfortably. Adjust the seat height so that the bottom of the foot just touches the pedal, with the knee almost straight. Pedal backward at first. Pedal forward only after comfortable cycling motion is possible backward. After becoming

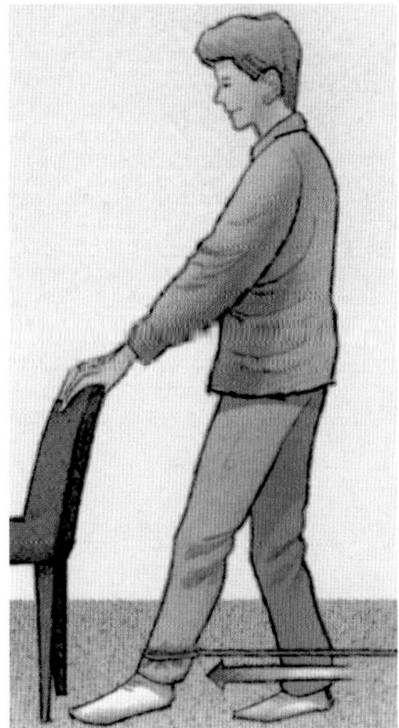

Figure 38.13 Illustration of resistive hip flexion with an elastic band. (Reproduced with permission from OrthoInfo. © American Academy of Orthopaedic Surgeons. Available at: http://orthoinfo.aaos.org.)

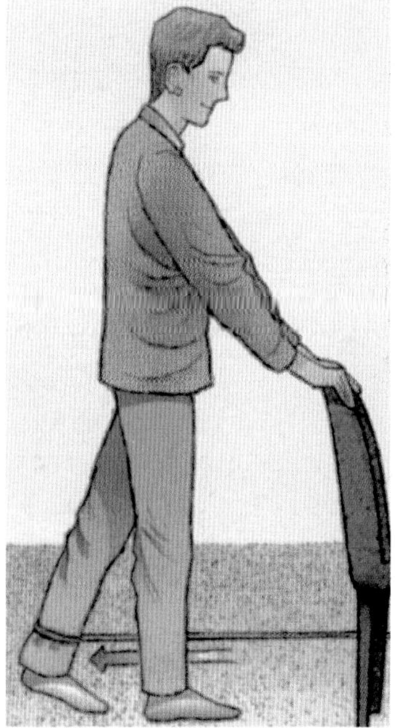

Figure 38.15 Illustration of resistive hip extensions. (Reproduced with permission from OrthoInfo. © American Academy of Orthopaedic Surgeons. Available at: http://orthoinfo.aaos.org.)

© 2018 American Academy of Orthopaedic Surgeons

stronger, increase the tension on the stationary bike. Cycle 10 to 15 minutes twice a day, gradually building up to 20 to 30 minutes three to four times a week.

Walking

Use a cane until balance skills have been regained. In the beginning, walk 5 or 10 minutes three or four times a day. As strength and endurance improves, walking for 20 or 30 minutes two or three times a day is advisable. After full recovery, regular walks, 20 or 30 minutes three or four times a week, will help maintain strength. Patients can start stairs as soon as they feel comfortable.

Return to Normal Activity

Return to all prefracture activity is usually allowed by 3 months postoperatively as long as strength and balance has returned to normal.

As with THA for osteoarthritis, patients should be cautioned against high impact activities such as running. In general, lower-impact activities—such as swimming, cycling, walking, or working on an elliptical trainer—are suggested for aerobic exercise.

Many patients with hip replacements do return to activities such as golf, tennis, skiing, and other moderate impact activities, as tolerated. Modern-day implants do appear to be able to tolerate these activities, but all patients should be counselled to routinely follow up with their surgeon to monitor any potential wear of the implant.

BIBLIOGRAPHY

Berry DJ, von Knoch M, Schleck CD, Harmsen WS: The cumulative long-term risk of dislocation after primary Charnley total hip arthroplasty. *J Bone Joint Surg Am* 2004;86-A:9–14.

Talbot N, Brown J, Treble N: Early dislocation after total hip arthroplasty: are postoperative restrictions necessary? *J Arthroplasty* 2002;17:1006–1008.

van der Weegen W, Kornuijt A, Das D: Do lifestyle restrictions and precautions prevent dislocation after total hip arthroplasty? A systematic review and meta-analysis of the literature. *Clin Rehabil* 2016;30(4):329–339.

Woolson ST, Pouliot MA, Huddleston JI: Primary total hip arthroplasty using an anterior approach and a fracture table: short-term results from a community hospital. *J Arthroplasty* 2009;24:999–1005.

© 2018 American Academy of Orthopaedic Surgeons

39 Revision Total Hip Arthroplasty

David Mayman, MD

INTRODUCTION

Revision total hip arthroplasty (THA) can mean many different things, thus rehabilitation protocols will be different depending on the type of revision. It is critically important to work directly with the surgeon on a specific rehabilitation protocol for each patient following revision THA. While primary THA is a successful surgery, revision THA is more complex and often challenging. The most common reason for failure after primary THA is instability, with mechanical loosening as the second most reported complication. Loosening can develop early or late after a primary THA that causes pain and poor clinical outcomes. Infection is another reason for revision arthroplasty. Patients requiring a revision THA can present for a variety of reasons, as described with each case assessed individually based on symptoms, clinical examination, and radiographs.

General categories of revision THA are:

- Femoral head and acetabular liner exchange
- Isolated acetabular revision
- Isolated femoral revision
- Both-component revision

Questions that need to be answered before developing a rehabilitation protocol include:

- Weight-bearing status
- Status of the abductors and greater trochanter
- Precautions necessary

A case example of a chronically infected primary total hip replacement requiring a two-stage revision is seen in Figure 39.1.

SURGICAL APPROACHES

Hip replacement can be done through a number of surgical approaches. The approach used for surgery will affect the limitations or precautions in the early postoperative period.

Direct Anterior Approach

The direct anterior approach utilizes the intramuscular plane between the tensor fascia lata and the rectus femoris muscle. Exposure to the acetabulum is relatively simple, but exposure of the femur is more difficult. Posterior structures are left intact. The risk of posterior instability is low, but the risk of anterior instability is higher. The direct anterior approach can be used for acetabular revisions, but is rarely used for femoral revision.

Anterolateral Approach

The anterolateral approach has a low risk of dislocation, but the anterior portion of the gluteus minimus and gluteus medius are taken off of the trochanter for the procedure and have to heal back to the trochanter after surgery. This approach can be used for revisions but is not commonly used for femoral revisions.

Direct Lateral Approach

The direct lateral approach incorporates an osteotomy of the greater trochanter. This approach is commonly used if a well-fixed, uncemented femoral implant needs to be removed. If this approach is used, then the trochanteric fragment must be protected during rehabilitation until bony healing has occurred.

Posterolateral Approach

The posterolateral approach is the most common approach used for revision THA in the United States today. The abductors are left intact, but the posterior capsule, piriformis tendon, and conjoined tendon are released from the posterior aspect of the femur, necessitating posterior hip precautions during the healing period.

EARLY POSTOPERATIVE REHABILITATION

Early postoperative rehabilitation is highly dependent on the surgical approach and weight bearing status. Early ambulation

Dr. Mayman or an immediate family member is a member of a speakers' bureau or has made paid presentations on behalf of Smith & Nephew; serves as a paid consultant to Smith & Nephew; has stock or stock options held in OrthAlign; and serves as a board member, owner, officer, or committee member of the Knee Society.

© 2018 American Academy of Orthopaedic Surgeons

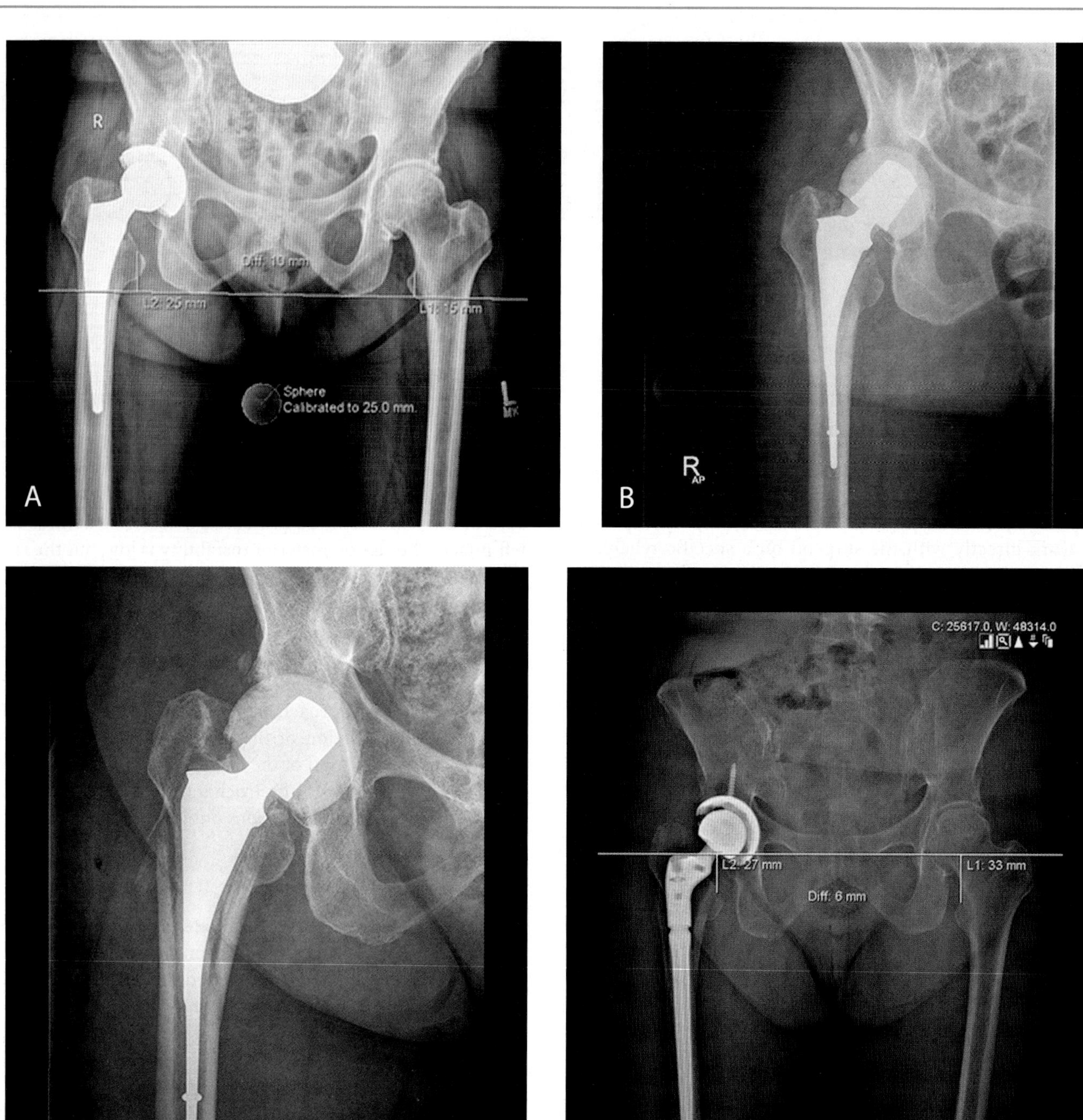

Figure 39.1 Radiographs of a case example of a chronically infected primary total hip replacement requiring a two-stage revision. **A**, Preoperative radiograph shows a total hip replacement with implants in good position, but the right hip is 10 mm shorter than the left. Bone quality is good around the acetabular and femoral implants. **B**, The implant is removed and an antibiotic-impregnated cement spacer is inserted. This spacer resembles a hip replacement but is not solidly fixed to the femur or acetabulum. The implants were removed through a posterior approach; thus, posterior hip precautions (no internal rotation, no flexion >90°, no internal rotation) were required and the patient was kept partial weight bearing because the implant is not fixed into the bone. **C**, The patient fell at home 3 weeks later, sustaining a greater trochanteric fracture, and the implant subsided approximately 6 mm. Abductor precautions and toe-touch weight bearing were instituted. Ambulation required a walker, but all other lower extremity exercises continued. **D**, At 10 weeks following completion of antibiotics with repeat hip aspiration negative, revision surgery was performed. The greater trochanteric fracture was healed. Revision was done through a posterior approach and, although the trochanter appeared healed, the healing was not robust at that time. The patient began standard postoperative early rehabilitation exercises, but followed trochanteric or abduction precautions and posterior hip precautions for 6 weeks. At 6 weeks, the patient progressed to weight bearing as tolerated and hip precautions were lifted. Leg length was restored and the infection cleared.

© 2018 American Academy of Orthopaedic Surgeons

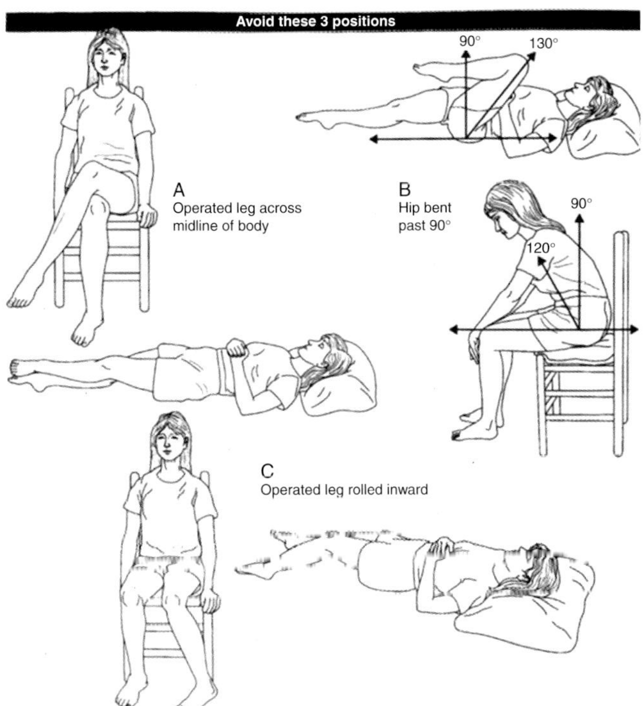

Figure 39.2 Illustration of standard posterior hip precautions. (Reproduced with permission from Sculco TP: *Hospital for Special Surgery Orthopaedic Manual*. Philadelphia, PA, Wolters Kluwer/Lippincott Williams & Wilkins, 2013.)

is encouraged to minimize postoperative medical risks, such as deep vein thrombosis (DVT), pulmonary embolism, and pneumonia.

Direct Anterior Approach

Avoid hyperextension and external rotation (ER). These precautions decrease the risk of anterior dislocation.

Anterolateral Approach

Avoid hyperextension and ER. These precautions decrease the risk of anterior dislocation.

The abductor repair is protected for the first 6 weeks.

Direct Lateral Approach

Avoid flexion, adduction, and internal rotation (IR). Limitations to abduction will depend on the quality of the greater trochanteric fragment and the quality of the repair. The bony fragment can be a very solid piece of bone requiring minimal precautions or a very tenuous piece of bone requiring strict abductor precautions until healing is complete. This must be reviewed with the surgeon on a case-by-case basis.

Posterolateral Approach

Avoid flexion, adduction, and internal rotation. Take the following posterior hip precautions: Hip replacement done through a posterior approach leaves the abductors fully intact, but releases the piriformis tendon and the conjoined tendon from the back of the femur. The posterior capsule is then released. The hip is dislocated by a combination of hip flexion, adduction, and IR. Posterior hip precautions are designed to avoid harming the repair of the posterior structures or dislocation of the hip joint.

Standard Posterior Hip Precautions Are:

No hip flexion past 90°
No adduction past neutral
No IR of the hip (Figure 39.2)

Early Postoperative Rehabilitation Exercises

Ankle Pumps

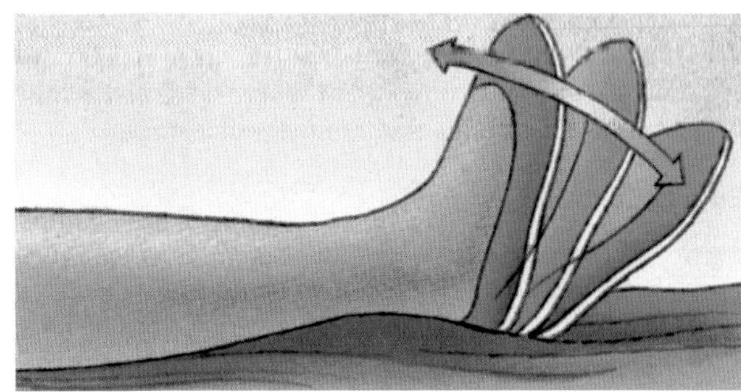

Figure 39.3

Slowly push the foot up and down. Do this exercise several times, as often as every 5 or 10 minutes. This exercise can begin immediately after surgery (Figure 39.3).

Ankle Rotations

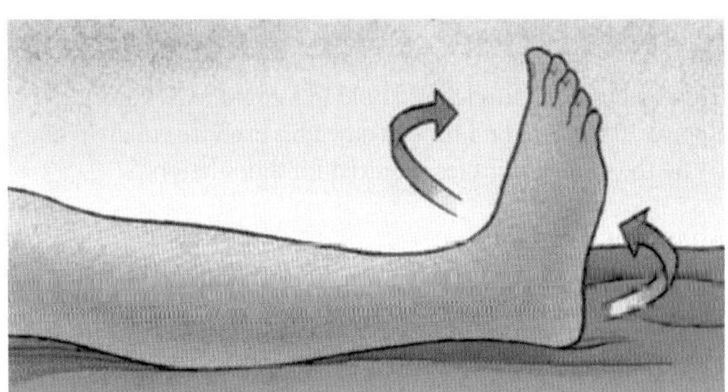

Figure 39.4

Move the ankle inward toward your other foot, then outward away from your other foot (Figure 39.4). Repeat 5 times in each direction, 3 or 4 times a day.

These exercises will begin reactivating lower extremity muscles and will help with venous return using the lower extremity muscles to pump blood through the venous system, lowering the risk of DVT.

© 2018 American Academy of Orthopaedic Surgeons

Bed-Supported Knee Bends

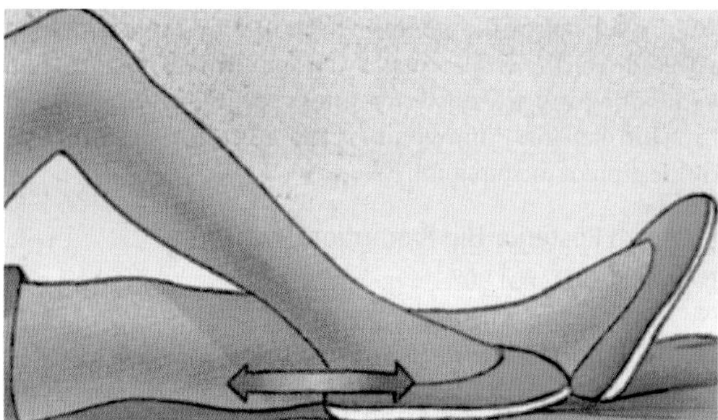

Figure 39.5

Slide the heel toward the buttocks, bend the knee, and keep the heel on the bed. Do not let the knee roll inward (Figure 39.5). Repeat 10 times, 3 or 4 times a day. This exercise begins reactivating the hip flexor muscles after surgery.

Buttock Contractions

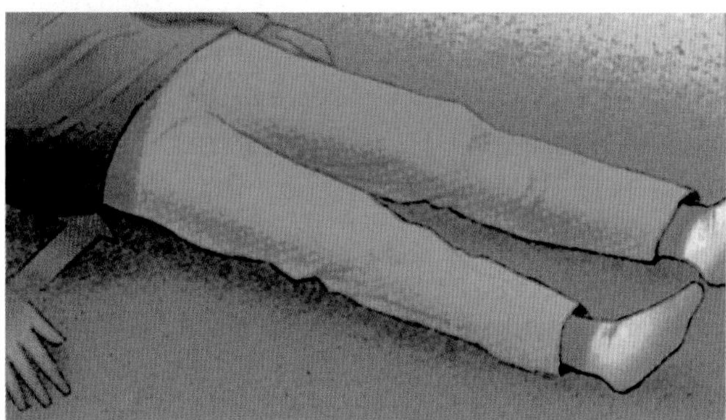

Figure 39.6

Tighten buttock muscles and hold to a count of 5 (Figure 39.6). Repeat 10 times, 3 or 4 times a day. This exercise will help reactivate the gluteal muscles required for ambulation.

Abduction Exercise

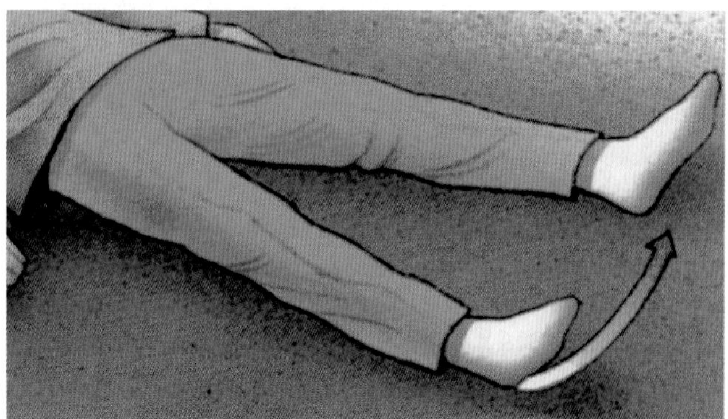

Figure 39.7

Slide the leg out to the side as far as possible, then back (Figure 39.7). Repeat 10 times, 3 or 4 times a day. Abduction exercises will be the most important exercises to continue in order to regain normal gait mechanics without a limp.

Quadriceps Set

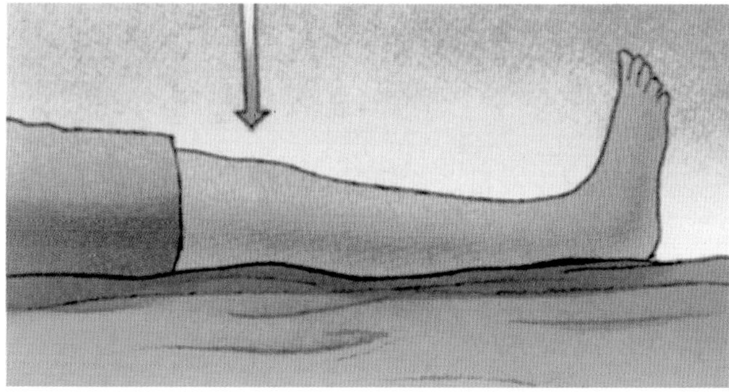

Figure 39.8

Tighten the thigh muscle. Try to straighten the knee. Hold for 5 to 10 seconds (Figure 39.8). Repeat this exercise 10 times during a 10-minute period. Continue until the thigh feels fatigued.

Straight-Leg Raises

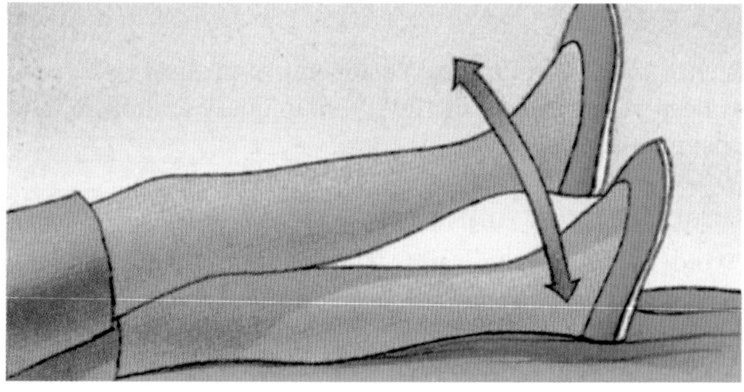

Figure 39.9

Tighten the thigh muscle with the knee fully straightened on the bed. As the thigh muscle tightens, lift the leg several inches off the bed. Hold for 5 to 10 seconds. Slowly lower (Figure 39.9). Repeat until the thigh feels fatigued. This exercise will work the hip flexors as well as the quadriceps mechanism.

© 2018 American Academy of Orthopaedic Surgeons

Standing Exercises

Standing Knee Raises

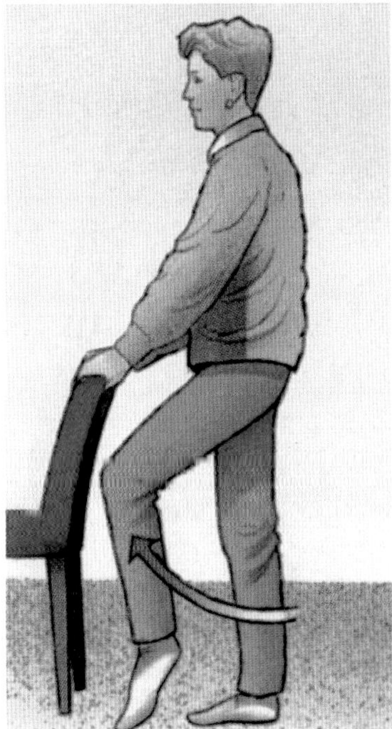

Figure 39.10

Lift the operated leg toward the chest. Do not lift the knee higher than the waist. Hold for 2 or 3 counts and put the leg down (Figure 39.10). Repeat 10 times, 3 or 4 times a day. This exercise will also help strengthen the hip flexors required for gait.

Standing Hip Abduction

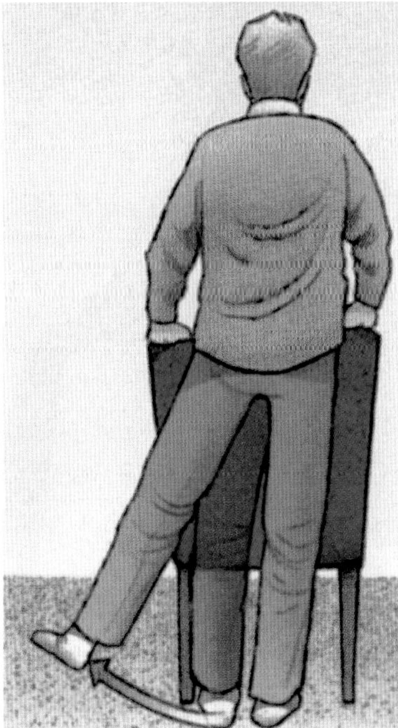

Figure 39.11

Be sure that the hip, knee, and foot are pointing straight forward. Keep the body straight. With the knee straight, lift the leg out to the side. Slowly lower the leg so that the foot is back on the floor (Figure 39.11). Repeat 10 times, 3 or 4 times a day.

This exercise is a mid-level exercise that will continue to improve abductor strength and will lead to the next level, which is lying on the nonoperative side and performing the same exercise.

Standing Hip Extensions

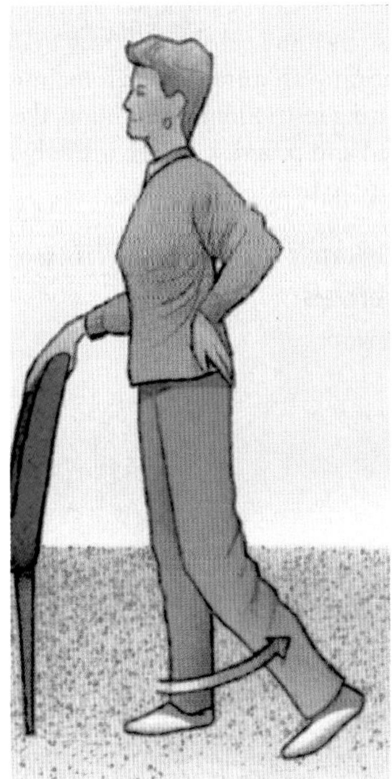

Figure 39.12

Lift the operated leg backward slowly. Try to keep the back straight. Hold for 2 or 3 counts. Return the foot to the floor (Figure 39.12). Repeat 10 times, 3 or 4 times a day.

Things to Watch for

After discharge from the hospital, the therapist often sees the patient more frequently than does the physician. Therapists need to be aware of potential early complications.

Wound Infection

Redness around the incision or drainage from the incision are signs of infection. The physician needs to be made aware if there are either of these findings.

Deep Vein Thrombosis

Most patients have swelling in the operative leg for at least 6 weeks after surgery. This swelling should be improved in the morning and will get worse throughout the day. Having the leg in a dependent position throughout the day increases the amount of the swelling. Swelling that does not improve with leg elevation or overnight is concerning and needs to be evaluated for the possibility of DVT.

© 2018 American Academy of Orthopaedic Surgeons

Dislocation

Dislocation is an obvious complication. Patients will not be able to weight bear on a dislocated hip and the position of the leg will be abnormal. Patients with a posterior hip dislocation will have the leg flexed and internally rotated. Patients with an anterior dislocation will be externally rotated and the leg will be shortened. The risk of dislocation is increased following revision THA, and hip precautions should be followed for the first six weeks.

Periprosthetic Fracture

Fracture after surgery can be obvious, with inability to weight bear, but can also be more subtle, with just an increase in pain. Patients presenting with a fracture will maintain precautions with weight-bearing restrictions. In addition, these patients may use a walking aid and progress slower with physical therapy to allow the fracture to heal.

Advanced Postoperative Rehabilitation

Elastic Tube Exercises

Resistive Hip Flexion

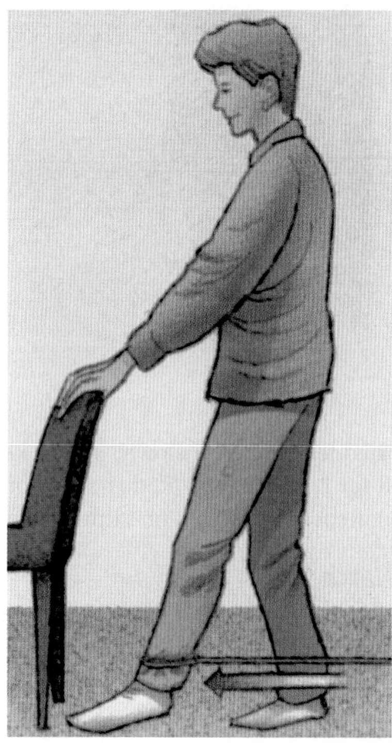

Figure 39.13

Stand with the feet slightly apart. Bring the operated leg forward, keeping the knee straight. Allow the leg to return to its previous position (Figure 39.13).

Resistive Hip Abduction

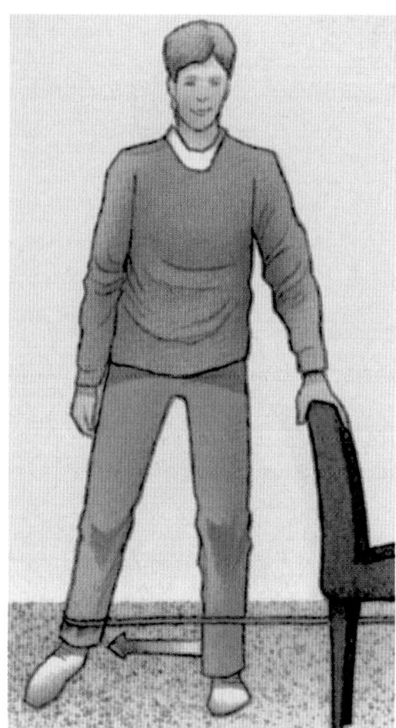

Figure 39.14

Stand sideways from the chair and extend the operated leg out to the side. Allow the leg to return to its previous position (Figure 39.14).

Resistive Hip Extensions

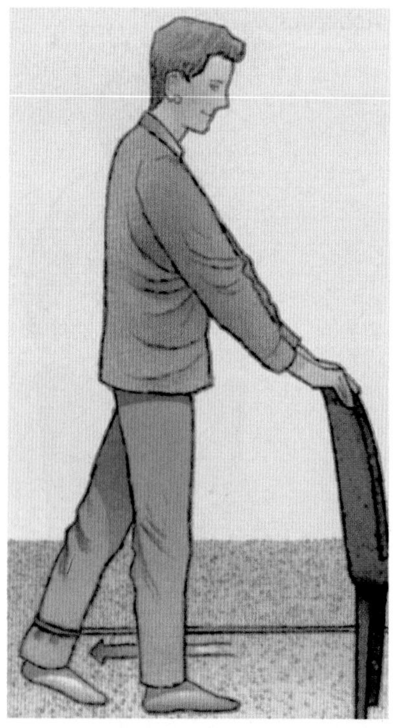

Figure 39.15

© 2018 American Academy of Orthopaedic Surgeons

Face the chair or heavy object to which the tubing is attached and pull the leg straight back. Allow the leg to return to its previous position (Figure 39.15).

Stationary Bike

Use of a stationary bike is an excellent activity to regain muscle strength and hip mobility. Adjust the seat height so that the bottom of the foot just touches the pedal with the knee almost straight. Pedal backwards at first. Pedal forward only after comfortable cycling motion is possible backwards. After becoming stronger, increase the tension on the exercycle. Exercycle forward 10 to 15 minutes twice a day, gradually building up to 20 to 30 minutes 3 to 4 times a week.

Walking

Use a cane until balance skills have been regained. In the beginning, walk 5 or 10 minutes 3 or 4 times a day. As strength and endurance improves, walking for 20 or 30 minutes 2 or 3 times a day is advisable. After full recovery, regular walks, 20 or 30 minutes 3 or 4 times a week, will help maintain strength.

Return to Normal Activity

Return to normal activity is usually allowed by 3 months postoperatively as long as strength and balance have returned to normal. This is variable depending on the patient, the reason for revision, and the implants used. Some patients will have permanent limitation in activity following revision THA. All patients should be told to ask their surgeon about return to more vigorous activities.

As with primary total hip arthroplasty, patients should be cautioned against high-impact activities, such as running. In general, lower-impact activities—such as swimming, cycling, walking, or working on an elliptical trainer—are suggested for aerobic exercise.

Many patients with hip replacements do return to activities such as golf, tennis, skiing, and other moderate-impact activities as tolerated. Modern day implants do appear to be able to tolerate these activities, but all patients should be counselled to routinely follow up with their surgeon to monitor any potential wear of the implant. Ultimately, the complexity of the revision and the patient's overall state of health and fitness determine the overall function of the limb.

© 2018 American Academy of Orthopaedic Surgeons

40 Hip Arthroscopy: Femoroacetabular Impingement and Labral Tears

Eilish O'Sullivan, PT, DPT, OCS, SCS, and Bryan T. Kelly, MD

INTRODUCTION

Femoroacetabular impingement is a relatively new diagnosis in the field of orthopaedic surgery that poses specific challenges to the rehabilitation specialist. The concept consists of abnormal contact between the femur and the acetabulum that restricts hip mobility, creates pain, and leads to degeneration of the hip joint. This may occur on the femoral side (cam impingement) or the acetabular side (pincer impingement), but most often occurs on both sides of the joint (mixed impingement). Cam impingement damages the labrum and cartilage when the deformity enters the joint (inclusion injury). Pincer impingement injures the labrum where the excess rim impacts the femoral head or femoral neck.

The acetabular labrum is a fibrocartilagenous structure that surrounds the acetabulum and increases the depth of the acetabulum. It creates a suction seal effect, resisting distraction of the femur from the acetabulum. It may act as a secondary stabilizer of the hip joint, and with a primary restraint being the iliofemoral ligament, resisting anterior translation of the femoral head and external rotation. The hip capsular ligaments act as static stabilizers of the hip, and are dynamically supported by the surrounding musculature. Crossing the hip joint and aiding in stability are 27 different muscles that work in a coordinated sequence to decrease joint loading with movement.

Pain elicited by impingement may cause weakness with impaired abdominal activation and motor patterning. The hip abductors and external rotators stabilize the hip, holding the femoral head within the acetabulum. The extensors create the most torque across the hip joint, and are paramount in athletic function. The tilt of the pelvis will either create more or less coverage of the femoral head. Challenges in making the diagnosis often lead to delays of up to several years. This delay in diagnosis generates compensatory strategies that must be addressed for recovery. Therefore, examining the entire kinematic chain is imperative throughout the rehabilitative process in order to eradicate dysfunctional patterns that may have developed. The diagnosis is established by clinical examination and diagnostic imaging, including plain radiographs, magnetic resonance imaging (MRI), and three-dimensional computed tomography (CT) scans.

The correct diagnosis allows for appropriate preoperative planning and the required operation. The next step is a structured rehabilitation program, which is an integral part of a successful outcome. Each rehabilitation program is tailored to the patient's specific needs. As many of these patients are young, active individuals with high-level athletic aspirations, the return-to-sport phase is an important culmination of the rehabilitative process. This phase requires constant vigilance in order to avoid soft-tissue irritation and delayed return.

HIP ARTHROSCOPY FOR FEMOROACETABULAR IMPINGEMENT AND LABRAL TEARS

Hip arthroscopy is indicated for the treatment of cam lesions, pincer lesions, labral débridement, labral refixation, loose bodies, and ligamentum teres tears. In order to maximize the likelihood of a successful outcome, the patient should demonstrate positive impingement testing, radiographic evidence of impingement, failure of conservative measures (physical therapy, activity modification, nonsteroidal anti-inflammatory drugs [NSAIDs], soft-tissue massage), and a positive result from an intra-articular injection. The most common reasons for failure of an arthroscopic hip surgery are osteoarthritis, residual impingement, and acetabular dysplasia. The success of the surgery is dependent on the amount of cartilage damage and whether or not adequate bony correction of impingement is achieved.

Contraindications

Hip arthroscopy is contraindicated in the setting of advanced arthritis. If there is a question as to the status of the cartilage, appropriate imaging should be completed prior to surgery. Those with developmental dysplasia of the hip that demonstrate a hypertrophic labrum due to static overload are not candidates for a solely arthroscopic surgery, and may require

Dr. Kelly or an immediate family member serves as a paid consultant to Arthrex; serves as an unpaid consultant to A3 Surgical; and has stock or stock options held in A3 Surgical. Neither Dr. O'Sullivan nor any immediate family member has received anything of value from or has stock or stock options held in a commercial company or institution related directly or indirectly to the subject of this article.

© 2018 American Academy of Orthopaedic Surgeons

a concomitant open procedure (periacetabular osteotomy). Complex deformities, such as a previous slipped capital femoral epiphysis or Perthes disease, may require open surgery.

Arthroscopic Femoroacetabular Impingement Surgery

Set-up

The patient is placed in the supine position on a fracture table. Traction distracts the joint, allowing instrumentation to enter the joint without damaging the cartilage. It should be kept to less than 2 hours to minimize the risk of nerve injury. Traction is released to address the peripheral compartment.

Relevance to Rehabilitation

Patients should be assessed at the postoperative visit for neuropraxia. Those with lumbar and sacroiliac pathology may experience discomfort following surgery because of traction. There may be foot and ankle discomfort as a result of traction as well. The nerves commonly affected include the lateral femoral cutaneous nerve (due to portal placement), pudendal nerve (from compression against the perineal post), and common peroneal nerve (due to traction).

Access

A safe zone for portal placement to minimize the risk of injury to the surrounding neurovascular structures is limited by the sciatic nerve posteriorly, the femoral nerve anteriorly, and proximally by the superior gluteal nerve. The two structures that remain vulnerable within this area are the lateral femoral cutaneous nerve (LFCN) and the lateral circumflex femoral artery (LCFA). The most commonly used portals are the lateral, mid-anterior, and distal anterolateral accessory portal. The anterolateral portal is in close proximity to the LFCN. This portal passes through the junction between the iliotibial and gluteal fascia. It then passes through the interval between the gluteus minimus and rectus femoris into the joint capsule. The mid-anterior portal passes through the tensor fascia lata and the interval between the gluteus minimus and the rectus femoris close to the LCFA. The distal anterolateral accessory portal passes through the fascia anterior to the iliotibial band. The anterior portal passes through the tensor fascia lata muscle and the gluteus minimus–rectus femoris interval. This portal poses the greatest risk to the LFCN. Once the portals have been established, an initial survey is conducted of the joint.

Relevance to Rehabilitation

LFCN paresthesias may occur; therefore, assessment should be conducted and symptoms should be monitored. These usually resolve. Scar tissue may form around portal sites and fascial restrictions often occur; therefore, these should be mobilized after adequate soft-tissue healing has occurred.

Capsule Cut/Intra-articular Assessment

An intraportal capsulotomy connects the mid-anterior portal to the anterolateral portal in order to be able to fully visualize the pathology. The joint is examined to determine the injury pattern on the femoral and acetabular sides. Frayed labral tissue may be débrided.

Rim Preparation/Resection

The acetabular rim is prepared with a burr down to bleeding bone. If needed, a resection of the rim may be completed at this point to restore the relationship between the anterior and posterior walls of the acetabulum.

Labral Refixation

If the labral tissue is amenable to repair, suture anchors are placed along the acetabular rim in an attempt to restore normal labral mechanics.

Relevance to Rehabilitation

To avoid stressing the labral repair, weight bearing is restricted for the initial 2 weeks, and forced end range motion is avoided. Impact activities and cutting are not initiated prior to 12 weeks, when the labrum has healed. If the labrum is débrided instead, the patient may move more quickly through the phases, but the same functional milestones must be achieved prior to advancing.

Cam Decompression

Traction is released, and the peripheral compartment is entered. A T cut in the capsule is created through the plane between the gluteus minimus and iliocapsularis. With a large capsulotomy, there is full exposure of the deformity as well as the ability to visualize the retinacular vessels.

Relevance to Rehabilitation

Weight bearing is restricted initially due to bony decompression, as risk of femoral neck fracture is associated with decompression of the femoral neck greater than 30%. Weight bearing may be restricted for 4 to 6 weeks following surgery.

Capsular Repair

The T-capsulotomy is repaired with sutures to restore native anatomy and stability. In the setting of instability, a capsular plication may be done in order to increase static stability of the hip.

Relevance to Rehabilitation

The anterior capsule should be protected in the initial phase in order to allow healing of the repair, namely, in extension and external rotation (for 6 weeks). Following this phase, range of motion (ROM) is gradually increased as per patient tolerance. Soft-tissue restrictions (fascial and muscular) should be cleared prior to the initiation of joint mobilization techniques.

Complications

Rates of complications from hip arthroscopy surgery vary significantly. Most recently, overall complication rates have been reported at 6.9%, which is greater than reported previously. LFCN irritation is the most likely issue encountered by patients postoperatively, and most often resolves. Other complications may include iatrogenic chondral or labral injury, superficial

© 2018 American Academy of Orthopaedic Surgeons

portal infections, superficial peroneal neuropraxia, deep vein thrombosis (DVT), pudendal neuropraxia, and heterotopic ossification.

The patient should be assessed for sensory disturbances and monitored for changes if there are deficits. Wounds should be monitored for erythema or drainage, notifying the physician if present. The incidence of heterotopic ossification has decreased dramatically with the use of prophylactic measures consisting of NSAID use for 4 weeks.

Preoperative Rehabilitation

Patients should be assessed preoperatively to initiate a strengthening program prior to surgery. The preoperative assessment may highlight the other compensatory movement patterns that have developed and will require reeducation. Lower abdominal and gluteal exercises are emphasized in the pain-free range. Education on appropriate exercises, such as avoiding deep squats and lunges, should occur. Patients are also educated on the immediate postoperative rehabilitation exercises.

Postoperative Rehabilitation

Rate of progression will be based on a number of factors. The greater the duration of symptoms, the longer there has likely been dysfunction and muscle inhibition due to pain. Chondral defects will extend the period of decreased weight bearing. The exact surgical procedures will also impact the rate of progression, such as with a capsular shift. Those with pelvic floor muscle dysfunction/pelvic pain will also progress at a more cautious rate due to the risk of causing a flare of these symptoms. The rehabilitation specialist should be mindful of active external rotation and careful with the stationary bicycle, as both these interventions may cause a pelvic pain flare. Lower back pain and dysfunction is another common disorder in these patients, which will likely have to be addressed during the postoperative course.

GENERAL REHABILITATION PRINCIPLES

First and foremost, one must be cognizant of tissue healing time frames. Overloading tissue structures prematurely may lead to disruption of the surgical repair. The therapist should have an open line of communication with the surgeon's team to understand the exact procedure carried out. If multiple procedures are done, as often occurs, the most conservative guidelines will prevail. With surgery for femoroacetabular impingement, new motion will be gained with a bony decompression. This new motion must be reeducated or it will not be utilized during functional activities.

Multiple compensatory patterns frequently arise during the often lengthy diagnostic and treatment process. Through the rehabilitation phases, these patterns must be identified and reeducated. This may involve treating the patient's thoracic spine or foot and ankle complex to maximize the patient's function. Impaired motor patterning often results from pain in the lower back or groin. Proper sequencing of muscle activation during exercises must be emphasized to ensure optimal stability. An example of this sequence is the following: while bridging, the patient should consciously contract the lower abdominals, followed by gluteals, and then extend the hips. Soft-tissue dysfunction is a frequent issue for these patients, which should be assessed and appropriately addressed as well.

Monitoring a patient's progress throughout the postoperative course is important to determine appropriate interventions. This should be done with a systematic approach, utilizing certain functional tasks (such as normalized gait or a step down) to determine whether the patient is ready to progress to the next phase of rehabilitation. Patients' achievement of functional milestones is monitored in preparation for their return to activity—whether activities of daily living (ADLs) or high level sporting activity. Patients often need to be counseled to limit their ADLs at the inception of their postoperative hip rehabilitation course, as these activities will frequently be the cause of increased pain. Many of these patients are young athletes looking to return to sport, some at an elite level. Patients should be educated from early on (preferably preoperatively) about what is entailed in the postoperative rehabilitative course and approximate time frames for recovery.

All phases indicated are approximate and advances are based on a functional criterion-based progression and soft-tissue healing. Those with compensatory disorders will be on the longer end of the spectrum; those who had little compensation will progress more quickly. As the hip is a weight-bearing joint, it is important to see how the patient responds to loading following intervention.

Phase 1: Protection Phase (4–8 Weeks)

The primary goal of the incipient phase of rehabilitation is to protect the surgical rehabilitation in order to ensure appropriate healing. The rehabilitation specialist should aim to reduce pain and inflammation through manual therapy and modalities, as needed. By the completion of this phase, the patient should demonstrate normal gait and should be able to complete basic ADLs. This phase will generally last from 4 to 8 weeks.

Patients are usually evaluated on postoperative day one to assess the patient's basic functional mobility (transfers and gait) as well as to begin passive range of motion (PROM) and isometric strengthening. Patients ambulate 20% weight-bearing with the foot flat for 2 weeks, then transition to weight bearing as tolerated. It is important to emphasize the placement of the operative foot on the ground to avoid hip flexor irritation. For the initial period following surgery (2 weeks), hip extension during gait should be limited in order to protect the capsular repair. A hip brace is utilized when patients are outside of their home for the first 2 weeks following surgery in order to increase stability. A cryotherapy unit with pneumatic compression is utilized to decrease inflammation and decrease pain for the first 3 weeks following surgery. A Continuous passive motion (CPM) machine is also utilized for 3 to 4 weeks following the surgery in order to reduce adhesion formation and increase nutrition to the joint. If tolerated, the patient may substitute use of a stationary bicycle for the CPM machine. Pivoting while standing or walking should be avoided as well in the

© 2018 American Academy of Orthopaedic Surgeons

initial stages. Comorbidities, such as soft-tissue laxity, should be taken into consideration when progressing these patients.

Gentle soft-tissue mobilization is an important portion of the initial phases of postoperative hip rehabilitation. This may begin at the initial visit with gentle effleurage through the thigh to decrease edema, if required. The incisional mobility should be assessed once the portals are healed, as scar tissue may form. Once one begins to address the musculature, it is important to differentiate between muscle tightness and muscle tone. The fascial complexes surrounding the hip—especially the thoracolumbar fascia and the adductor fascia—should be assessed as well. The most common muscles that require attention are the psoas, adductor longus, adductor magnus, hamstrings, tensor fascia lata, gluteals, external rotators, and rectus femoris. Following soft-tissue work, neuromuscular reeducation must occur immediately to ensure appropriate motor patterning. Function and/or ROM should be reassessed to determine the efficacy of the intervention. Lower abdominal strengthening is paramount in order to maintain pelvic stability and decrease load through the operative hip. Hip adductor strengthening is done with caution in the early phases, as the adductors tend to be hypertonic initially. Hip flexor activation is avoided in the incipient phase, as flexor irritation is likely.

The patient is weaned from crutches in a gradual manner, transitioning from weight bearing on two crutches, as tolerated, to one crutch before finally discontinuing them. Patients will often have to decrease their stride length initially because of anterior tightness and decreased gluteal control. The patient may discontinue use of an assistive device when able to ambulate with a normal stride length without a pelvic "wink." This involves maintaining adequate mobility through the rectus femoris as well as gluteus maximus and gluteus medius control through the operative hip.

Precautions

- Symptom provocation with therapeutic exercise, ADLs, or ambulation
- ROM within pain-free range
- Active hip flexion with a long lever arm (straight-leg raise)

Interventions

- PROM in flexion, circumduction, abduction, internal rotation (IR) and external rotation (ER) in flexion, prone IR
- Prone rectus femoris stretch: Begin with pillows underneath the hips
- Stationary bicycle: Initiate with a short crank bike
- Isometrics strengthening: Transversus abdominis, quadriceps, gluteals
- Neuromuscular training of core musculature
- Active assistive range of motion (AAROM): Quadruped rocking, stool rotations
- Core and pelvic stability: Begin in hook lying (supine, back flat, knees bent) and progress to standing (Figures 40.1 to 40.5)
- Proprioception and balance exercises
- Hydrotherapy

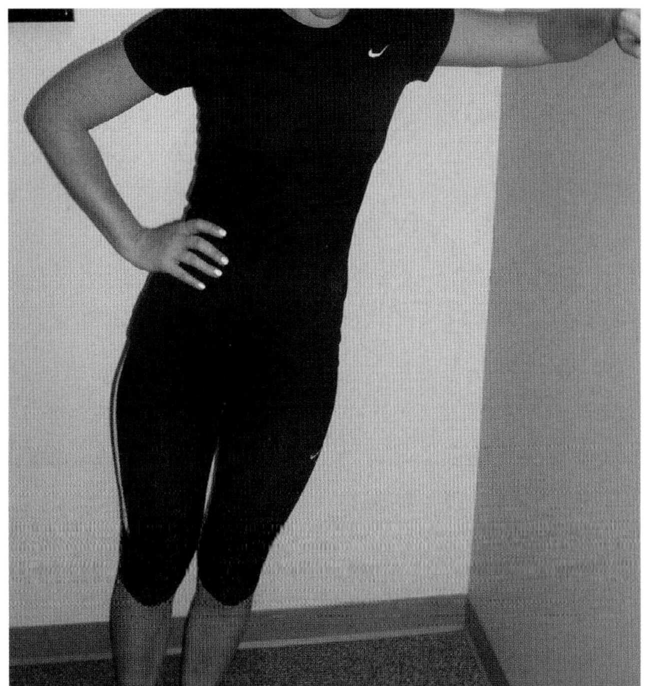

Figure 40.1 Photograph of side plank on wall exercise.

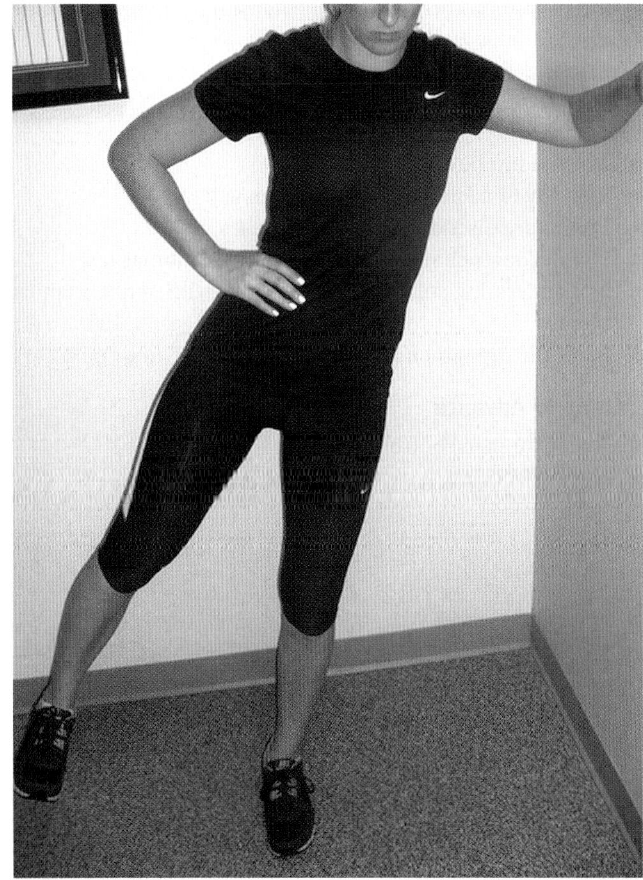

Figure 40.2 Photograph of side plank on wall exercise with hip abduction.

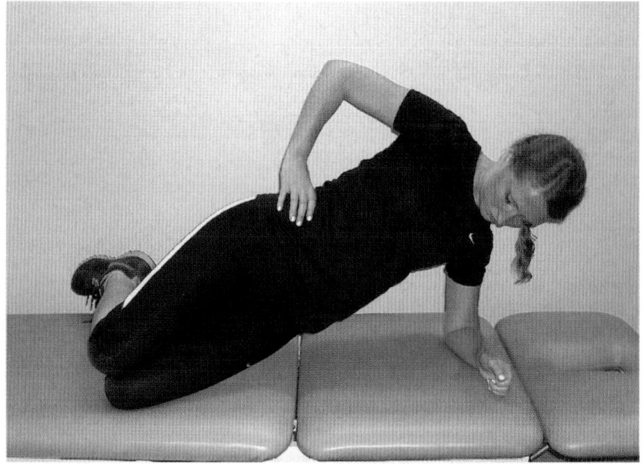

Figure 40.3 Photograph of modified side plank exercise.

- Pilates reformer (footwork) or ball squat to initiate functional gluteal control when appropriate lumbopelvic stability exists
- Gentle soft-tissue mobilization

Special Considerations

- *Capsular Shift:* With this procedure, extension is limited to 0°, and ER is limited to 30° for 6 weeks. Crutches are utilized for 4 weeks with limited stride length on the operative side. Derotation boots or pillows may be utilized for sleeping to prevent ER in extension. The brace will be utilized for 4 weeks.
- *Microfracture:* Weight bearing is restricted for up to 6 weeks.

Potential Errors

- Isolated hip flexor strengthening
- Inability to achieve hip extension in gait
- Premature discontinuation of crutches
- Hip flexor stretching without a positive Thomas test
- Not addressing soft-tissue restrictions with gentle manual therapy
- Early ER strengthening in those with pelvic floor pain

Criteria to Advance

- Adequate pain control
- Normalized gait

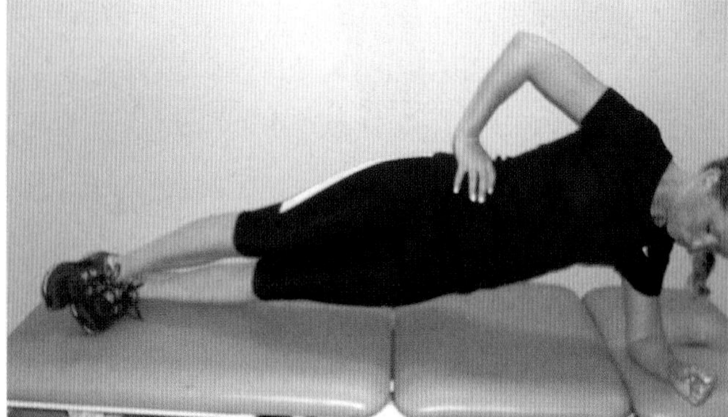

Figure 40.4 Photograph of side plank exercise.

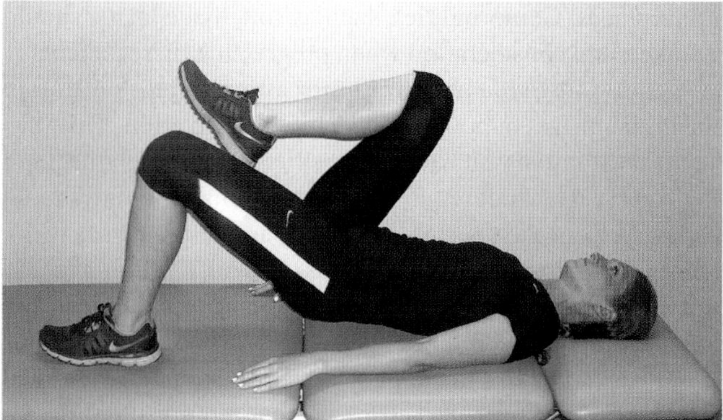

Figure 40.5 Photograph of short lever single-leg bridge exercise.

- 90° of passive hip flexion, able to achieve neutral hip extension
- Good lumbopelvic control in single-limb stance

Phase 2: Functional Phase (Weeks 4–8 to Weeks 10–20)

During the second phase of the rehabilitation process, the patient moves toward increasing function. The patient works to regain good lumbopelvic control in single-limb stance. During this phase, it is important to identify and address possible compensatory kinematic chain impairments. This phase of the rehabilitative process generally lasts 6 to 9 weeks.

In this phase, the patient will begin to strengthen the hip and surrounding musculature in a more functional manner. The early portion of this phase may lead to some inflammation and irritation of the surrounding soft-tissue structures if the progression of exercises is not specifically tailored to the patient and the patient's specific surgical procedure. Patients must be educated on the importance of graded increases in activity and function. During this phase, the patient's functional movements—single-leg stance, squat (within pain-free range), and step down—should be assessed for aberrant movement up and down the kinematic chain. Deficits, such as decreased talocrural mobility or decreased thoracic rotation, should be addressed during this period in preparation for the following phase. Appropriate motor control and sequencing continue to be emphasized in order to eradicate dysfunctional movement and patterning. The patient's response to increased volume and intensity must be carefully monitored in order to avoid soft-tissue inflammation. Soft-tissue mobilization should be continued through this phase. ROM should be checked before and after interventions to determine the patient's reaction to joint loading, and addressed accordingly.

Precautions

- Symptom provocation secondary to rapid increases in activity
- Hip flexor tendonitis
- Trochanteric bursitis

© 2018 American Academy of Orthopaedic Surgeons

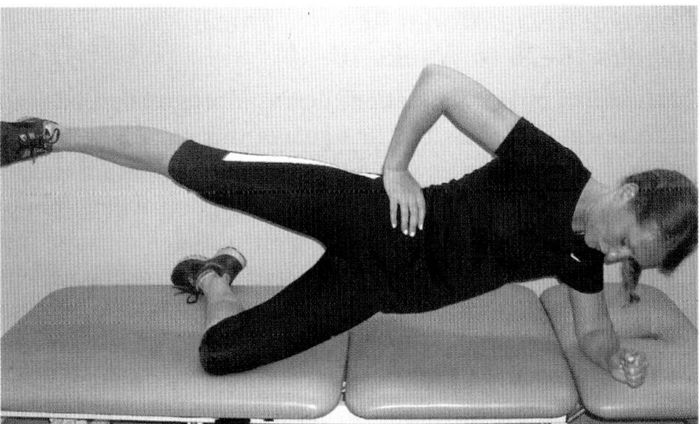

Figure 40.6 Photograph of modified side plank exercise with hip abduction.

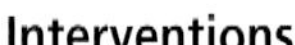

Interventions

- Manual therapy to decrease soft-tissue impairments
- Neuromuscular reeducation, especially within the increased soft-tissue envelope
- Progress core control (planks; Figures 40.6 and 40.7)
- Soft-tissue mobilization
- Functional strengthening with hip extensor and hip abductor focus
  - Leg press progression bilateral to unilateral
  - Frontal plane work with resistance band
- Balance
  - Progressing single-limb exercises (Figures 40.8–40.11)
- Flexibility
  - Hip flexor if need is demonstrated
  - Hamstrings, hip rotators, latissimus dorsi

Potential Errors

- Premature progression to sport or vigorous ADLs or work without full ROM or adequate strength

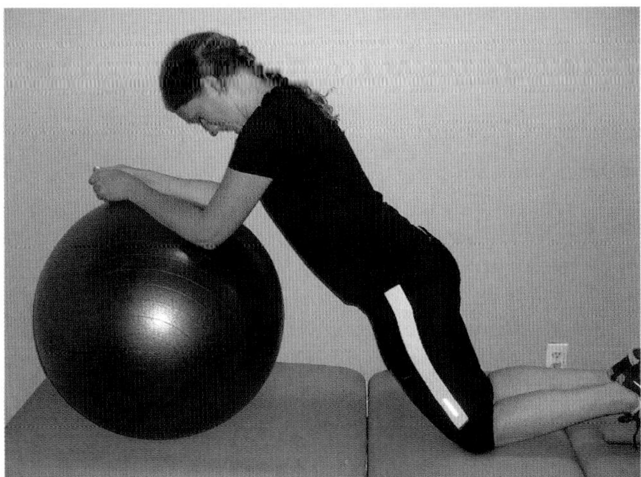

Figure 40.7 Photograph of modified stir-the-pot exercise.

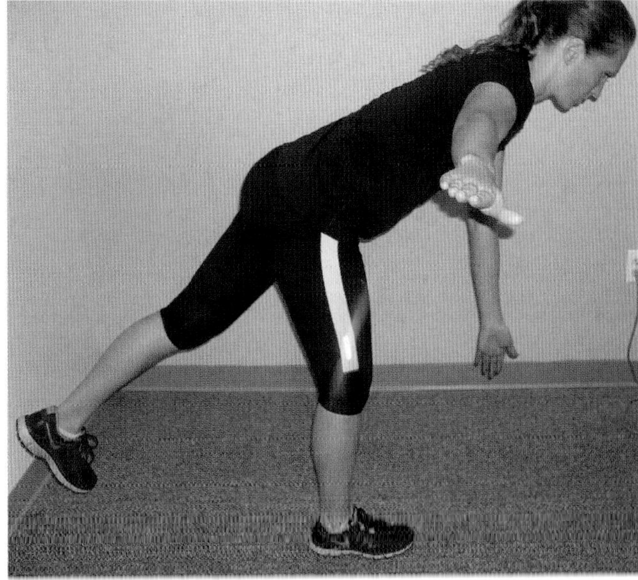

Figure 40.8 Photograph of windmill exercise (A).

Criteria for Advancement

- ROM within functional limits
- Able to ascend and descend 8-inch step with good control
- Good lumbopelvic control with single-limb squat

Special Considerations

- *Labral refixation:* With this procedure, impact and cutting activities should be held until 12 weeks (unless surgeon directed) due to labral healing.
- *Capsular plication:* Gentle restoration of ROM within patient tolerance. Joint mobilizations are not appropriate.

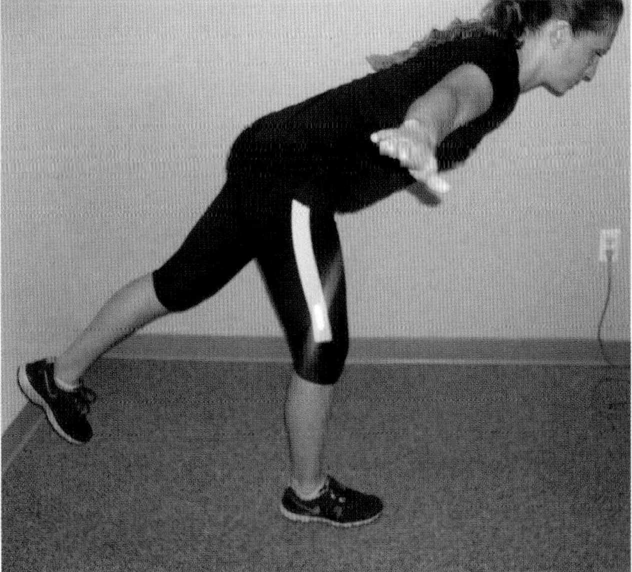

Figure 40.9 Photograph of windmill exercise (B).

© 2018 American Academy of Orthopaedic Surgeons

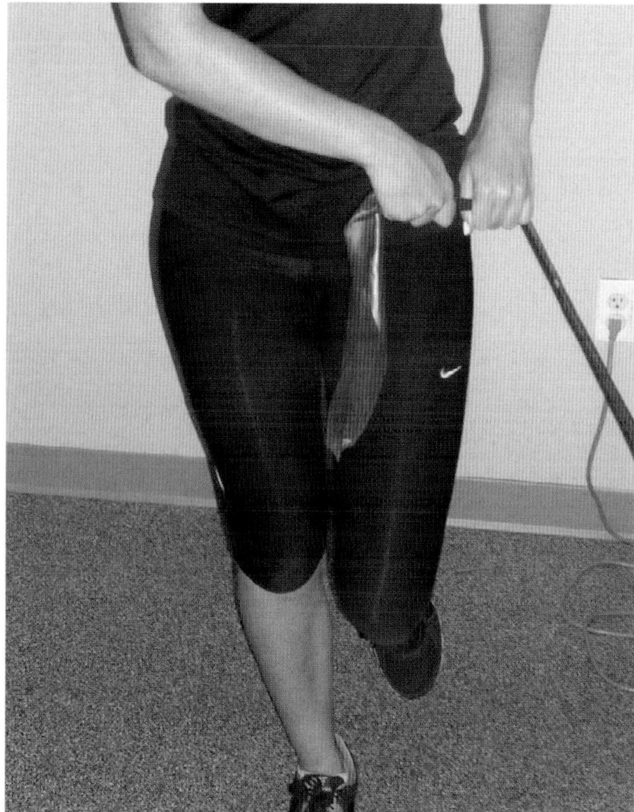

Figure 40.10 Photograph of double-arm D2 in single-leg stance 1 exercise.

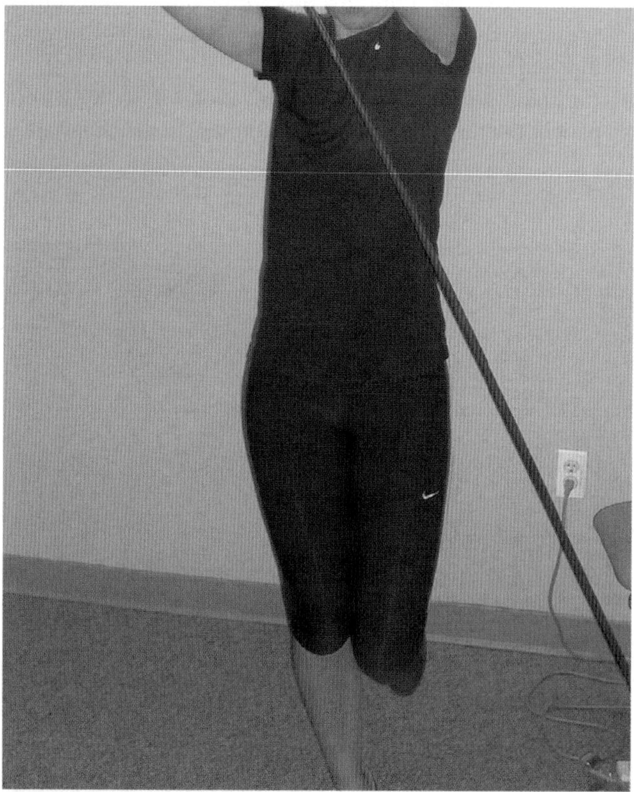

Figure 40.11 Photograph of double-arm D2 in single-leg stance 2 exercise.

Phase 3: Recreational Activity Phase (Weeks 10–20 to Weeks 16–30)

In the third phase, the patient begins a progression back to recreational activities. The first goal of this phase of rehabilitation is independence with a home exercise program (HEP) to supplement, and/or a gym-based program when appropriate. The second goal is for the patient to demonstrate full ROM and good core control. The third goal is for the patient to demonstrate 5/5 lower extremity strength. This phase generally lasts 6 to 9 weeks.

The transition between phase 2 and phase 3 may lead to irritation of the soft-tissue structures and development of tendonitis if functional progression is not implemented as scheduled. The patient must be counseled on the gradual progression of activity. At this point in time, deep tissue work may be an appropriate adjunct to advanced exercises. Before impact activity is initiated, adequate strength and stability must be demonstrated through a series of tests. The first task is 10 repetitions of resisted side-lying hip abduction with a manual muscle test score of greater than or equal to 4+/5. The second test is 10 repetitions of an 8-inch step-down with good stability throughout the trunk, hip, and knee, and no deviations or compensations. The third test is 10 single-leg squats with good control and no deviations. Patients should also demonstrate the ability to maintain a side plank for 1 minute with good stability. Once the patient has successfully completed these tasks, the patient may begin with short runs on a treadmill, progressing in a graded fashion. The exercise program should encompass not only pure sagittal plane, frontal plane, and transverse plane activity, but also combined motions in preparation for return to the athletic environment. Endurance of the gluteus medius is one of the last things to develop following hip arthroscopy. This is a key component of athletic function and must be trained accordingly, or patients will develop pain and irritation.

Interventions

- Endurance activities
- Initiate plyometrics
- Initiate treadmill running progression
- Dynamic balance activities
- Advanced core exercises
- Medicine ball exercises (squats, chops)
- Kinetic-chain exercises (squat press)
- Deep tissue massage

Precautions

- Symptom provocation
- Not following functional progression schedule
- Progressing volume of exercise too quickly

Criteria for Advancement

- Good dynamic balance
- Good core control
- 5/5 gluteus medius and maximus strength for 10 repetitions
- Pain-free with high-level exercises

© 2018 American Academy of Orthopaedic Surgeons

Phase 4: Return to Sport

The final phase of hip rehabilitation takes the patient back to sport, with the goal being full sport participation. The decision to return the athlete to sport is multifactorial. The patient must demonstrate adequate strength, flexibility, endurance, and power. A functional test battery should be administered, including components assessing each of these areas. Sport-specific training should be initiated and evaluated for pain or compensation. This includes drills or warm-ups that are native to the patient's sport. These are also utilized to assess the patient's readiness to return to formal sport participation. The patient should perform a basic routine of core and gluteal activation exercises as part of the warm-up. Without regular completion of their maintenance program, patients will frequently develop pain and tightness, which will lead to impaired performance. This phase lasts approximately 6 weeks.

Precautions

- Symptom provocation
- Not following functional progression schedule
- Maintaining core and gluteal strength base

Interventions

- Advanced plyometrics
- Cutting and agility activities
- Endurance exercises
- Sport-specific drills

Table 40.1 CLINICAL COMMENTARIES ON POSTOPERATIVE GUIDELINES

Author	ROM	Weight Bearing	CPM	Brace
Spencer-Gardner	Flexion 0°–90° for 4 weeks, ER to 20° Capsular repair: ER and extension if capsulectomy Labral repair: Avoid hyperextension, passive ER > 20°	Labral Repair: FFWB × 4 weeks Labral débridement: FFWB × 2 wk	Microfracture: 4 h for 2–4 wk 30°–70°, AAT	n/a
Edelstein	Labral repair + osteochondroplasty: no restrictions	Labral repair + osteochondroplasty: FFWB 20% × 2 wk Microfracture: FFWB 20% × 6 wk	3 wk	0°–90° × 10 d
Tyler	90° flexion for 2 wk	FFWB with 20 lb for 2–4 wk	Initiate at 30°–70°, advance to 0°–90°, for 2 wk	Brace for daytime use 0°–90°
Enseki	Derotation boots for 1–2 wk. Avoid end-range motion for 2–3 wk. Capsular plication: Gentle ER, 10° extension. Osteoplasty: Avoid forced IR in flexion.	FFWB 30 pounds × 10–14 d. Microfracture: 4 wk FFWB 30 lb. Osteoplasty: 4 wk FFWB 30 lb.	High-seat stationary bike 10–20 min 1–2×/d	1–2 wk 0°–80°
Stalzer 2006	Labral repair: 25° abduction and gentle extension and ER for 3 wk, 90° flexion for 10 d. Osteoplasty: 90° flexion for 10 d. Microfracture: 90° flexion for 10 d. Capsular plication/ capsulorrhaphy: Extension and ER to neutral for 3 wk, progressed to gentle motion for the next 3 wk. Derotation boots for 3 wk while supine. 90° of flexion for 10 d.	Labral repair: FFWB 20 lb for 2 wk. Osteoplasty: FFWB 20 lb for 4 wk. Microfracture: FFWB 20 lb for 6–8 wk. Capsular plication: FFWB 20 lb for 4 wk, neutral rotation emphasized during gait.	Labral repair: 4 wk 8–12 h/d. Osteoplasty: 4 wk. Microfracture: 6–8 wk. Capsular plication: 4 wk	×10 days
Stalzer 2005	Labral repair: 90° flexion for 10 d, gentle extension and ER for 3 wk, 25° of abduction for 3 wk, IR unlimited. Chondroplasty: 90° flexion for 10 d, other motions unlimited.	Labral repair: FFWB 20 lb for 2 wk. Chondroplasty: FFWB 20 lb for 4 wk.	Labral Repair: 4 wk. Chondroplasty: 4 wk.	Labral repair: Bledsoe brace 0°–90° for 10 d. Chondroplasty: Brace 0°–90° for 10 d.
Griffin	Labral Debridement: Pain-free range	Labral débridement: Weight bearing as tolerated × 1–2 wk	n/a	n/a

AAT = advance as tolerated, CPM = continuous passive motion, ER = external rotation, FFWB = foot flat weight bearing, IR = internal rotation, ROM = range of motion.

© 2018 American Academy of Orthopaedic Surgeons

Criteria for Return to Sport

- Manual muscle test of gluteus medius and maximus 5/5 for 10 repetitions
- Pain-free
- Full ROM
- Single-leg hop test with good limb symmetry (≤10% side-to-side discrepancy)
- Side plank isometric hold within normative range
- Demonstrate good control and endurance with squatting, single-leg squatting, lunging, and lateral bounding.
- No pain or compensation with sport-specific activity

Review of Evidence

There is a dearth of literature exploring the efficacy of postoperative rehabilitation guidelines or protocols following hip arthroscopy. There are many clinical commentaries on a myriad of postoperative guidelines, which are outlined in Table 40.1. There has been one report of clinical outcomes following a phased rehabilitation process in 52 patients. Of the patients, 61% demonstrated good or excellent results on the modified Harris hip score at 1 year postoperatively, which was found to be comparable to other studies at 1 year. All guidelines are based on the specific surgical procedure, and have slight variations in the immediate postoperative course. One caveat when examining these changes in guidelines is that the surgical procedure carried out in 2001 is vastly different from the procedure done today, and the rehabilitation course has been altered appropriately to reflect this change. Further research is required in the field as both the surgical and rehabilitative processes continue to evolve.

A recent meta-analysis demonstrates that 88% of patients achieve the acceptable symptomatic state for the modified Harris Hip Score (mHHS), and 90% of patients achieve the minimal clinically important difference for the mHHS and Hip Outcome Score. Of the 9,317 hips, 5.8% included required revision hip arthroscopy, and 5.5% were converted to hip arthroplasty. The likelihood of conversion to arthroplasty is significantly greater in the presence of cartilage deterioration. At an average of 4 years follow-up, patients demonstrated excellent results, and there was a conversion to total arthroplasty at a mean time of 3.9 years in 7% of patients. Return-to-sport rates following hip arthroscopy average 87%, with 82% returning to the same level of sport as prior to surgery. Diffuse degeneration of cartilage was found to limit ability to return to sport according to a systematic review.

PEARLS

- Hip arthroscopy rehabilitation is a dynamic process that involves constant vigilance and assessment, in which no two patients are alike.
- There should be communication between the surgeon's team and the rehabilitation specialist to guide the patient's recovery.
- Every patient must be evaluated and treated based on the impairments that the patient presents with and progressed based on attainment of functional milestones, not just time frames.
- Manual therapy is a key component of hip rehabilitation, and restoration of gluteus medius endurance is essential for successful return to sport.
- Due to the long duration of symptoms that typically exist, the entire kinematic chain must be addressed in order to maximize the patient's outcome following surgery.

BIBLIOGRAPHY

Bogunovic L, Gottlieb M, Pashos G, Baca G, Clohisy JC: Why do hip arthroscopy procedures fail? *Clin Ortho Relat Res* 2013;471(8):2523–2529.

Casartelli NC, Leunig M, Item-Glatthorn JF, Lepers R, Maffiuletti NA, et al: Hip muscle weakness in patients with symptomatic femoroacetabular impingement. *Osteoarthritis Cartilage* 2011;19:816–821.

Casartelli NC, Leunig M, Maffiuletti NA, Bizzini M: Return to sport after hip surgery for femoroacetabular impingement: a systematic review. *Br J Sports Med* 2015;49:819–824.

Edelstein J, Ranawat A, Enseki KR, Yun RJ, Draovitch P: Postoperative guidelines following hip arthroscopy. *Curr Rev Musculoskelet Med* 2012;5(1):15–23.

Enseki KR, Martin R, Kelly BT: Rehabilitation after arthroscopic decompression for femoroacetabular impingement. *Clin Sports Med* 2010;29(2):247–255, viii.

Freeman S, Mascia A, McGill S: Arthrogenic neuromuscular inhibition: a foundational investigation of existence in the hip joint. *Clin Biomech (Bristol, Avon)* 2013;28:171–177.

Ganz R, Parvizi J, Beck M, Leunig M, Notzli H, Siebenrock KA: Femoroacetabular impingement: a cause for osteoarthritis of the hip. *Clin Orthop Relat Res* 2003;(417):112–120.

Garrison JC, Osler MT, Singleton SB: Rehabilitation after arthroscopy of an acetabular labral tear. *N Am J Sports Phys Ther* 2007;2(4):241–250.

Griffin KM: Rehabilitation of the hip. *Clin Sports Med* 2001; 20(4):837–850, viii.

Harris JD, McCormick FM, Abrams GD, Gupta AK, Ellis TJ, Bach BR Jr, Bush-Joseph CA, Nho SJ: Complications and reoperations during and after hip arthroscopy: a systematic review of 92 studies and more than 6,000 patients. *Arthroscopy* 2013;29(3):589–595.

Levy DM, Kuhns BD, Chahal J, Philippon MJ, Kelly BT, Nho SJ: Hip arthroscopy outcomes with respect to patient acceptable symptomatic state and minimal clinically important difference. *Arthroscopy* 2016;32(9):1877–1886.

Mardones RM, Gonzalez C, Chen Q, Zobitz M, Kaufman KR, Trousdale RT: Surgical treatment of femoroacetabular impingement: evaluation of the effect of the size of the resection. *J Bone Joint Surg Am* 87(2):273–279.

Moreside JM, McGill SM: Improvements in hip flexibility do not transfer to mobility in functional movement patterns. *J Strength Cond Res* 2013;27:2635–2643.

© 2018 American Academy of Orthopaedic Surgeons

Myers CA, Register BC, Lertwanich P, et al: Role of the acetabular labrum and the iliofemoral ligament in hip stability: an in vitro biplane fluoroscopy study. *Am J Sports Med* 2011;39S:85S–91S.

Neumann DA: Kinesiology of the hip: a focus on muscular actions. *J Orthop Sports Phys Ther* 2010;40:82–94.

Nwachukwu BU, Rebolledo BJ, McCormick F, Rosas S, Harris JD, Kelly BT: Arthroscopic versus open treatment of femoroacetabular impingement a systematic review of medium-to long-term outcomes. *Am J Sports Med* 2015;44:1062–1068.

Robertson WJ, Kelly BT: The safe zone for hip arthroscopy: a cadaveric assessment of central, peripheral, and lateral compartment portal placement. *Arthroscopy* 2008;24(9): 1019–1026.

Spencer-Gardner L, Eischen JJ, Levy BA, Sierra RJ, Engasser W, Krych AJ: A comprehensive five-phase rehabilitation programme after hip arthroscopy for femoroacetabular impingement. *Knee Surg Sports Traumatol Arthrosc* 2014;22(4): 848–859.

Stalzer S, Wahoff M, Scanlan M: Rehabilitation following hip arthroscopy. *Clin Sports Med* 2006;25(2):337–357, x.

Stalzer S, Wahoff M, Scanlan M, Draovitch P: Rehabilitation after hip arthroscopy. *Operative Techniques in Orthopaedics* 2005;15(3):280–289.

Tyler TF, Slattery AA: Rehabilitation of the hip following sports injury. *Clin Sports Med* 2010;29(1):107–126.

Voight ML, Robinson K, Gill L, Griffin K: Postoperative rehabilitation guidelines for hip arthroscopy in an active population. *Sports Health* 2010;2(3):222–230.

Wahoff M, Ryan M: Rehabilitation after hip femoroacetabular impingement arthroscopy. *Clin Sports Med* 2011;30(2): 463–482.

© 2018 American Academy of Orthopaedic Surgeons

41 Periacetabular Osteotomy

Ernest L. Sink, MD, and Maureen Suhr, PT, DPT, PCS

INTRODUCTION

The goal of any acetabular osteotomy is to change the pathologic mechanics of the abnormal hip that lead to intra-articular damage, pain, and osteoarthritis. The orientation of the acetabulum is altered, improving the bony coverage of the femoral head. Reorientation of a dysplastic acetabulum increases the load-bearing surface area of the joint while maintaining or improving joint stability. The Bernese periacetabular osteotomy (PAO) was developed by Reinhold Ganz and colleagues in 1983. Compared with other surgical techniques for acetabular reorientation, it involves a series of reproducible cuts around the acetabulum that leave the posterior column of the pelvis intact. Since the original description, the technique of the bony cuts has remained constant, although the understanding of the biomechanics has continued to evolve, such that Ganz wrote in 2001, "Our understanding of what is an optimal correction has improved considerably over time. It is a balancing of the maloriented horseshoe-shaped acetabular cartilage over the femoral head, which leads to an optimal use of a limited area of hyaline cartilage for weight-bearing."

The Bernese PAO has several advantages compared to other acetabular reorientation osteotomies. Specifically, the posterior column of the pelvis remains intact, which maintains the stability of the pelvis and allows early patient mobility. Because the osteotomy is relatively close to the joint, there is no change in the dimensions of the true pelvis. As a result, vaginal childbirth is still safe for these patients, which is not the case for adult patients who have had double or triple pelvic osteotomies. The proximity of the osteotomy to the joint also allows for potentially significant correction of the bony morphology. The acetabulum is medialized; therefore, the lever arm of the abductors improves and the joint reactive forces decrease. Finally, because all of the osteotomy cuts are made from the inner aspect of the pelvis, the abductors can be preserved. Unlike other curved or spherical periacetabular osteotomies that are very close to the acetabulum, the cuts of the Bernese PAO allow the osteotomized fragment to be well vascularized and less susceptible to osteonecrosis. The Bernese PAO is technically complex, and there is a substantial surgical learning curve to the procedure. Rehabilitation following PAO is crucial to successful outcome. Due to the nature of the procedure and resultant change in mechanical forces about the hip and pelvis, a comprehensive rehabilitation program is imperative to strengthen and train the musculature in its new position to optimize patient function and satisfaction.

PERIACETABULAR OSTEOTOMY (PAO)

Indications and Contraindications

The most accepted indication for acetabular reorientation is mild to moderate symptomatic hip dysplasia (Figure 41.1). Initially, there was controversy about the degree of dysplasia and concomitant femoral head deformity that can be adequately addressed with a PAO; it was felt that severely subluxed hips would not be candidates for a PAO. Subsequently, good outcomes have been published for more severe deformities, and the indications have been expanded as long as a concentric hip joint is possible. Thus, dysplasia secondary to Legg-Calvé-Perthes disease and dysplasia secondary to flaccid and spastic neuromuscular disorders can be considered appropriate indications for PAO. Global acetabular retroversion causing impingement is also considered an indication for PAO, particularly if the retroversion is associated with posterior wall deficiency or posterior instability.

There may also be a role for acetabular reorientation in patients with borderline dysplasia (center edge angle of 20°–25°) and clinically symptomatic instability. This occurs most often in the setting of increased femoral and/or acetabular anteversion, and primarily manifests as iliopsoas or abductor fatigue symptoms.

Mid- and long-term follow-up have established that the most predictable outcomes are in patients less than 35 years

Dr. Sink or an immediate family member serves as a board member, owner, officer, or committee member of the Pediatric Orthopaedic Society of North America. Neither Dr. Suhr nor any immediate family member has received anything of value from or has stock or stock options held in a commercial company or institution related directly or indirectly to the subject of this article.

© 2018 American Academy of Orthopaedic Surgeons

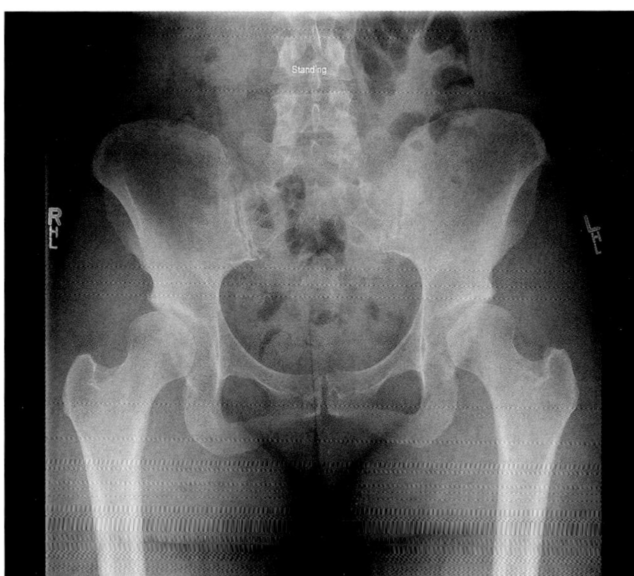

Figure 41.1 Anteroposterior pelvis radiograph of a 21-year-old female with bilateral symptomatic acetabular dysplasia who was indicated for a periacetabular osteotomy (PAO).

old at the time of surgery with little to no arthritis (Tönnis Grade 0 or 1) on plain radiographs. Good results have, however, been reported for patients over 35 or 40, even in early series, with the caveat that there is minimal arthrosis and the hip is concentric on preoperative imaging.

Study results of PAO in patients with preoperative arthrosis reveal that Tönnis Grades 2 and 3 are greater predictors of failure. Although the presence of Tönnis Grade 2 or 3 arthrosis is a predictor of failure, some patients with this degree of arthrosis show improved outcomes scores and relatively preserved joint space in midterm follow-up. Thus, although arthrosis is a relative contraindication to PAO, PAO may be preferable to total hip arthroplasty in certain younger patients.

Contraindications to PAO include incongruence on functional radiographs (abduction and internal rotation images or flexion false profile images), which indicates potentially worse congruency after acetabular reorientation and is thus a predictor of worse outcomes. This can occur in nonspherical femoral heads or when the acetabular radius is smaller than the femoral head radius. PAO is also contraindicated in very young patients (less than 10 or 11 years of age) because of the risk of injury to the triradiate cartilage.

Procedure

The PAO can be performed with adjuvant arthroscopy, which is performed for labral repair or débridement and cartilage assessment; the arthroscopy is performed first with the patient on a traction table using a standard technique. Most patients with hip dysplasia also have some form of intra-articular pathology and labral injury; concurrent hip arthroscopy allows intra-articular injury to be addressed concomitant with the PAO. The combination of arthroscopy and PAO in the same setting has been previously described, but outcomes data are not yet available.

For the PAO, the incision is slightly curved lateral to the anterior superior iliac spine (ASIS) and the tensor-sartorius interval. The ASIS is osteotomized and reflected medially, preserving the sartorius attachment on the osteotomized fragment. Care is taken near the ASIS because the lateral femoral cutaneous nerve emerges proximally within 5 cm of and medial to the ASIS, and can be injured during the approach. Proximally, the external oblique aponeurosis is sharply incised and the iliacus is elevated subperiosteally and medially off the iliac wing. Because of reports of prolonged hip flexor weakness after PAO, the direct and indirect head of the rectus can be left attached (rectus-sparing modification) and retracted laterally during the capsular exposure. A retractor is placed deep to the iliopsoas tendon to allow retraction of the tendon. Once the lateral aspect of the superior pubic ramus is visualized, the subperiosteal dissection of the ilium can be extended to the quadrilateral plate. This allows a blunt Hohmann to be placed on the ischial spine near the sciatic nerve, and enables visualization of the inner table of the pelvis. EMG studies indicate that nerve irritation does occur intraoperatively; thus, it is critical that care be taken with retractor placement.

The interval between the iliopsoas tendon and the joint capsule is developed medially, allowing access to the ischium for the first osteotomy. A specially curved or angled chisel is then passed into the interval and used to make the first cut (Figure 41.2). The osteotomy is performed using fluoroscopic visualization and begins just inferior to the infracotyloid notch, extending posteriorly towards the base of the ischial spine (Figure 41.3). The lateral portion of the ischial osteotomy is very close to the sciatic nerve; the nerve is at risk if the osteotome slips laterally. The nerve can be protected to a certain extent by placing the leg in abduction and knee flexion, and directing the osteotome medially.

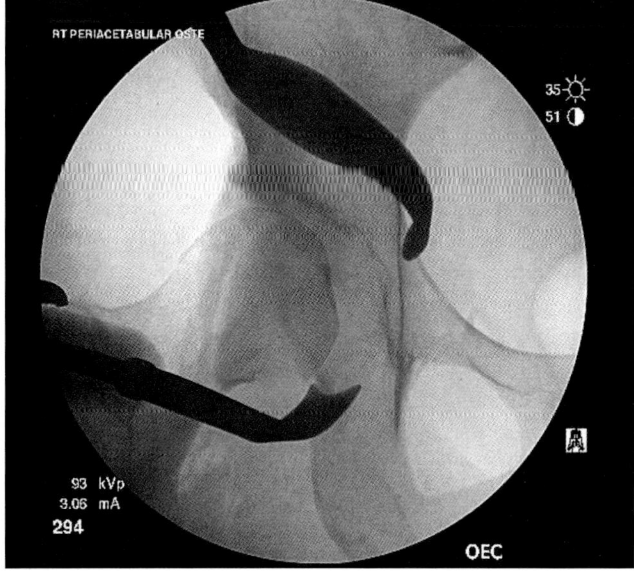

Figure 41.2 Intraoperative fluoroscopy confirming the position of the chisel on the ischium on the anteroposterior view.

© 2018 American Academy of Orthopaedic Surgeons

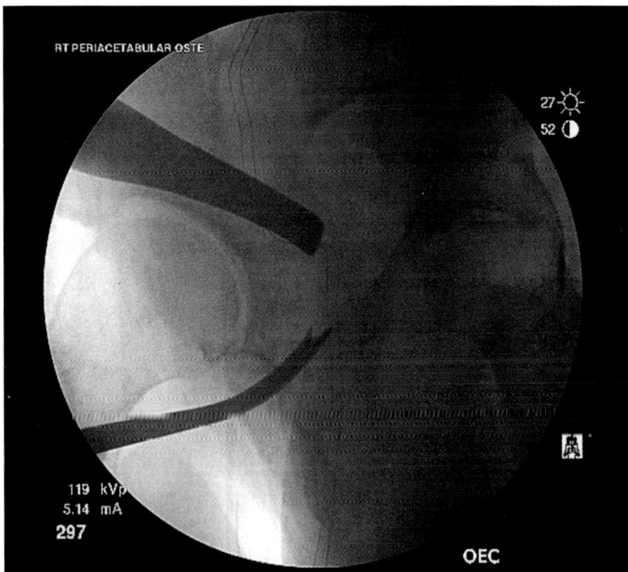

Figure 41.3 Intraoperative fluoroscopy confirming the orientation of the chisel on the false profile view. The chisel, which enters the bone in the infracotyloid notch, is directed towards the base of the ischial spine.

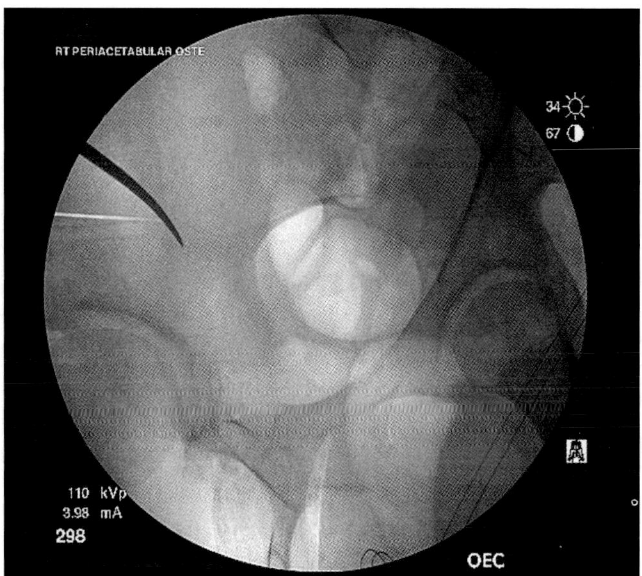

Figure 41.4 Intraoperative fasle profile view with a curved chisel starting the posterior column cut. There is sufficient supra-acetabular bone, and the posterior column cut starts in a position to allow the osteotomy to be directed toward the base of the ischial spine and the ischial osteotomy.

Attention is then directed to the pubic osteotomy. The superior pubic ramus is dissected subperiosteally. Blunt retractors are placed around the bone to protect the obturator nerve, which runs on the inferior aspect of the ramus. The cut is made just medial to the iliopectineal eminence and perpendicular to the bone, which is generally about 45° to the plane of the table. This osteotomy is deep to the retracted Iliopsoas tendon; therefore, the iliopsoas will be weak in the postoperative period.

Attention is turned to the supra-acetabular osteotomy. The abductors are tunneled only at the level of the osteotomy, and a blunt Hohman retractor is placed laterally near the greater sciatic notch. Additional soft tissue is elevated off the quadrilateral surface. There are two portions to the supra-acetabular cuts; the first passes through the iliac wing and the second is retroacetabular, meeting up with the ischial osteotomy. Both are often performed under direct and fluoroscopic visualization, and can be made with either an oscillating saw or osteotome. The retroacetabular cut angles 120° from the supra-acetabular cut and is directed toward the first ischial cut (Figure 41.4).

Depending on the patient's anatomy, the retroacetabular osteotomy is performed with either a straight or curved osteotome. This extends along the posterior column to meet the ischial osteotomy. The cut should be just posterior to the midpoint of the width of the posterior column, defined as the area between the hip joint and the sciatic notch. The osteotome is angled slightly from anterior to posterior to avoid the posterior part of the joint (Figure 41.5). A useful fluoroscopic technique is to see a perfect lateral image of the osteotome on false profile view when beginning the osteotomy. Once the osteotomy is completed medially, the lateral cortex is osteotomized as a controlled fracture. This is undertaken to protect the sciatic nerve, which is directly inferior to the lateral cortex and would be at risk if the osteotomes were used to complete the lateral osteotomy. Fluoroscopy is used to ensure that the retroacetabular osteotomy meets the ischial osteotomy. Once the medial aspects of the osteotomy are performed, the posterolatereral cortex where the iliac and the posterior column osteotomies meet can be cut with an angled osteotome, which also allows more fragment mobilization (Figure 41.5). At this

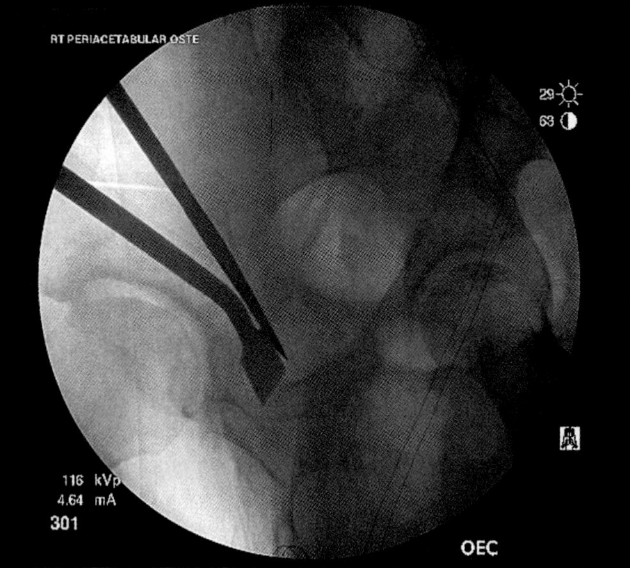

Figure 41.5 Intraoperative fluoroscopic false profile confirming the path of the chisel down the posterior column directed toward the region of the ischial osteotomy. The angled chisel is utilized to connect the posterior column osteotomy with the ischial osteotomy.

© 2018 American Academy of Orthopaedic Surgeons

point, there is some risk of the osteotomy propagating into the sciatic notch, with subsequent discontinuity of the posterior column. Although this may ultimately be of little consequence, it does compromise the stability of the healing fragment; thus, the patient must remain non–weight-bearing until evidence of fragment healing is seen.

When all of the cuts have been made, a Schanz pin is placed in the acetabular fragment at the anterior inferior iliac spine (AIIS), angled posterior between the inner and outer tables of the pelvis. This facilitates fragment mobilization and control of the fragment during correction. At this time, the fragment should move freely (Figure 41.6). This is important because, if it does not, the soft tissue or bony hinging hinders the correction and limits medialization of the joint. For "classic dysplasia," lateral and anterior correction is essential; thus, the fragment should be adducted and flexed. Nonetheless, the correction should be individualized for each patient and based on the anatomy and information from the preoperative radiographs. Once a preliminary correction has been obtained, the fragment is fixed with 2.4-mm Kirschner wires (K-wires) and evaluated fluoroscopically. There are five parameters to assess intraoperatively:

1. The sourcil and acetabular index: This should be horizontal, but not negative. The sourcil should balance over the femoral head.
2. Lateral coverage and center edge angle
3. Medial translation of the hip center: The hip center should be slightly medialized to improve joint reactive forces. However, excessive medialization can lead to iatrogenic protrusio.
4. Position of the teardrop and ilioischial line
5. Acetabular version: The anterior and posterior walls should meet at the lateral edge of the joint. A cross-over sign indicates that the fragment has been flexed too far forward, which results in acetabular retroversion and can contribute to postoperative femoroacetabular impingement (FAI).

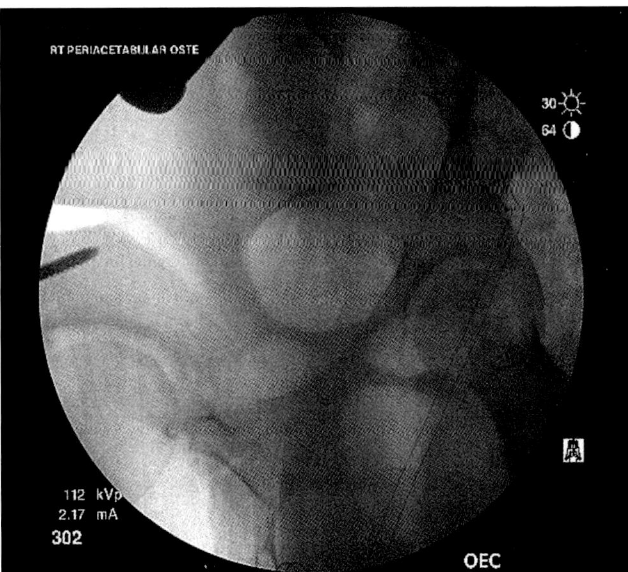

Figure 41.6 A Shanz screw is placed in the supra-acetabular bone, and the fragment is mobilized.

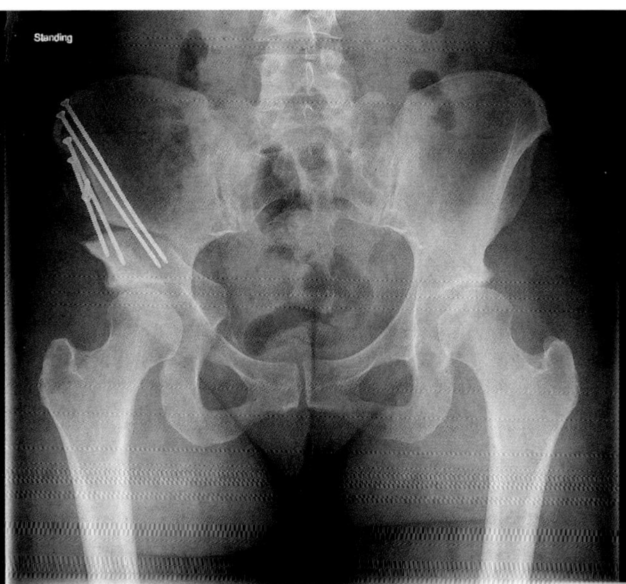

Figure 41.7 A postoperative anteroposterior pelvis radiograph showing improved coverage of the femoral head. The weight-bearing zone of the acetabulum (sourcil) is now balanced over the femoral head. The acetabular version is correct and the hip center is medialized.

Once a satisfactory correction has been obtained, 3.5-mm or 4.5-mm cortical screws can be placed for definitive fixation (Figure 41.7).

Once the correction is obtained and stable, any potential impingement is addressed. Hip range of motion (ROM) in flexion and internal and external rotation are evaluated. An anterior capsulotomy to evaluate for impingement is routinely performed to evaluate any potential impingement. Depending on the proximal femoral anatomy, a femoral neck osteoplasty can be performed, particularly if there are any limits to motion. In addition, any restrictions in motion or impingement from the AIIS can be assessed and bone from the AIIS can be resected if it is causing impingement. The capsule is then repaired with absorbable suture. The ASIS osteotomy is fixed with a 3.5-mm cortical screw and the remainder of the wound is closed in a layered fashion.

Complications

Postoperatively, patients remain in the hospital for 3 to 6 days for pain control and mobilization. Weight bearing is limited to 20% the first 4 to 6 weeks because load-to-failure testing of the screw constructs found that ultimate failure can occur with loads as low as 1.27 times body weight. In addition, loss of correction and stress fractures of the intact pelvis have occurred in patients who began weight bearing too soon after surgery. Aspirin is used for routine thrombosis prophylaxis. The overall incidence of venous thrombosis following PAO is low (0.94%). In otherwise low-risk patients, the complications

© 2018 American Academy of Orthopaedic Surgeons

of enoxaparin (Lovenox) or other chemoprophylaxis include prolonged wound drainage, hematoma, and bleeding, which largely outweigh the risk of deep vein thrombosis (DVT) or pulmonary embolus.

POSTOPERATIVE REHABILITATION

Rehabilitation following a PAO must take into account the nature of the pathology of developmental hip dysplasia, the preoperative and postoperative orientation and topography of the hip joint, as well as the underlying healing constraints of osseous and soft-tissue structures.

Dysplasia is, by definition, a developmental abnormality. In the case of hip dysplasia, it is an undercoverage of the femoral head by the acetabulum, which may lead to subluxation or frank dislocation. The femur is inherently unstable within the acetabulum; therefore, it relies on support and stability from soft-tissue structures. This leads to abductor and flexor fatigue, as well as pain with prolonged standing or activity. Additionally, because of this undercoverage, the significant normal forces through the hip are distributed over a smaller area, leading to asymmetrical wear or breakdown, particularly of the articular cartilage, possibly resulting in a hypertrophied labrum, labral tears, or chondral lesions. These injuries and their repairs must be taken into account when designing a rehabilitation program. Rehabilitation following PAO must respect the significant healing that must occur at the osteochondral and muscular levels, while gently restoring hip ROM and promoting muscular balance and stability in the core, pelvic floor, and hip.

Rehabilitation following PAO is a significant undertaking, both physically and emotionally. The patient should be prepared to commit an average of 12 months to rehabilitation to return to full function. This timeline may be variable based on patient goals and comorbidities. The following description is meant to serve as a guideline for rehabilitation with the understanding that the program needs to be tailored to the individual and progression through these guidelines is gated by specific criteria.

REHABILITATION GUIDELINES

Phase I, Protection: Day 1–Week 6

Postoperatively, patients remain in the hospital for 3 to 6 days for pain control and mobilization. The primary goal of this phase is healing and pain control. Patient education emphasizes protection of the surgical site and compliance with activity modification to minimize pain and inflammation. Weight bearing (WB) is limited to 20% of body weight to protect the healing osteotomy (Figure 41.8). It is important to note that non-weight bearing (NWB) should be avoided, as this will place undue stress on the hip flexors, which will be working to hold the lower extremity from contacting the floor—this action will result in pain. Patients are encouraged to ambulate with a foot flat progression to establish a more natural walking pattern. Home exercise instruction focuses on isometric contraction and establishment of core stability.

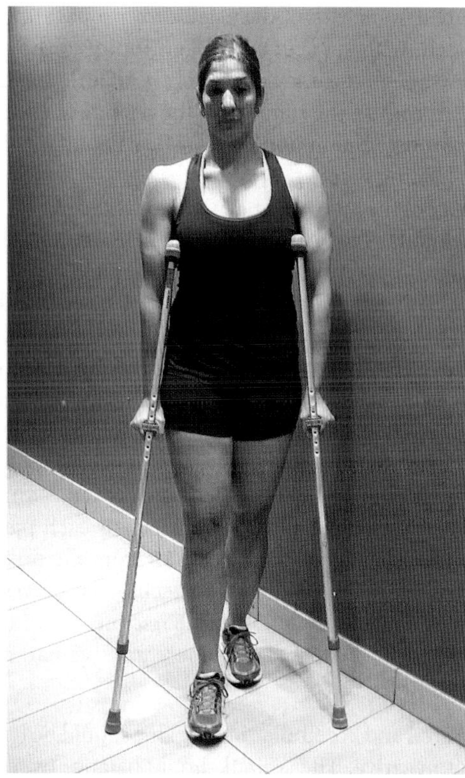

Figure 41.8 Weight bearing (WB) is limited to 20% of body weight to protect the healing osteotomy. Patients are encouraged to ambulate with a foot flat progression to establish a natural walking pattern, as seen in this photograph.

Although activity is limited during the first phase of rehabilitation, it is important that the patient be comfortable moving. The patient should avoid prolonged periods in one position and should be comfortable lying prone by 2 weeks postoperatively (although he or she may require assistance to achieve this position). The other focus of activity during this time is to build the foundation of anticipatory postural control. Utilizing the home exercise program, the patient should be focusing on developing a "feed-forward" mechanism of postural control, performing abdominal activation prior to motion, establishing proximal stability for distal mobility. It is often easiest to begin this training supine, preparing the patient for more challenging positions when beginning Phase II.

Precautions

- 20% foot flat weight bearing with assistive device
- Avoid sitting with hips flexed to 90° or greater for prolonged periods of time.
- Avoid open-chain hip exercise, for example, straight leg raise (SLR).
- Avoid symptom provocation during ambulation, activities of daily living (ADLs), therapeutic exercise.
- Avoid ambulation to fatigue.
- Avoid capsular irritation.

© 2018 American Academy of Orthopaedic Surgeons

Table 41.1 PHASE I TREATMENT RECOMMENDATIONS

Exercise/Modality	Rationale for Use	Special Cues
CPM	Provide gentle range of motion (ROM) to lubricate the joint, mobilize synovial fluid, and prevent muscle and joint stiffness.	Set motion 0–30° Slow, constant, rate Patient may sit with head of bed elevated 1.5- to 2-hrs intervals 3–4 times/day. **In hospital only**
Ankle pumps	Improve circulation, flush out swelling.	
Quadriceps set	Strengthen quadriceps in preparation for ambulation and functional activity.	Place towel roll beneath extended knee. Maintain quadriceps contraction 10 seconds. Rest 10 seconds.
Abdominal set	Activate transversus abdominis to stabilize trunk and pelvis	In supine position, lie with [illegible] extended. Perform transversus abdominis contraction. Cue patient to draw in lower abdominals while maintaining pelvis in neutral position. Maintain contraction 10 seconds. Rest 10 seconds between contractions.
Abdominal set with upper extremity motion	Maintain core stabilization during dynamic upper extremity exercise; engage transversus abdominis and obliques	In supine position, hold 2 to 5-lb dumbbell or weighted ball in two hands with upper extremities extended in front of pelvis. Perform transversus abdominis contraction as outlined earlier. Slowly raise weight above head and return to starting position, maintaining ribcage and back in neutral position. Repeat motion in diagonal direction from one hip to opposite shoulder. Repeat on other side.
Gluteal Set	Strengthen gluteus maximus in preparation for functional activities and to aid in core stability and trunk and pelvic control.	In prone position, place pillow under pelvis. Maintain gluteal contraction 10 seconds. Rest 10 seconds between contractions.
Rectus femoris stretch with abdominal control	Improve rectus femoris length and activate abdominals for pelvic stabilization.	In prone position, with bilateral lower extremities extended, perform abdominal set, maintaining neutral spine. Gently flex knee on operative side until patient achieves a gentle stretch. Cue patient to maintain hip in neutral rotation.
Knee ROM	Maintain full knee motion postoperatively to minimize stiffness and facilitate normal gait pattern.	Sitting in a slightly reclined position with upper extremities providing support posterior to pelvis. Gently flex knee on operated side, assisting with nonoperated limb as necessary. Hold 3–5 seconds. Extend operated knee. Hold 3–5 seconds [Figure 41.9, A and B].
Upright stationary bicycle	Promote motion in operated hip.	Begin at postoperative week 4. Start cycling for 5–10 minutes/day. Progress slowly to 20 or 25 minutes over the course of a week. Adjust seat height to allow a 15°–20° bend in the knee when it is extended on the down side of the pedal stroke to prevent too much hip flexion or pinching at the anterior joint. Begin with light and progress to moderate resistance, as tolerated.

© 2018 American Academy of Orthopaedic Surgeons

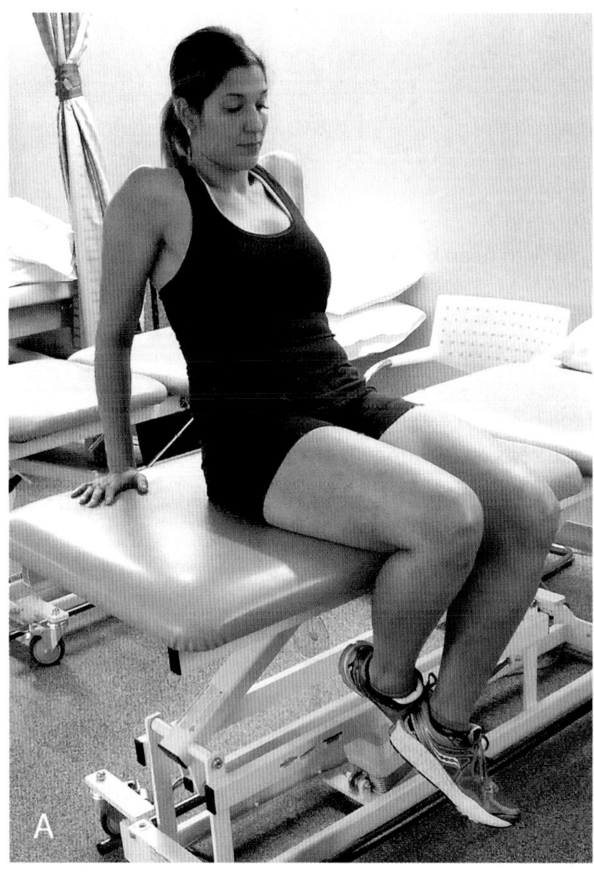

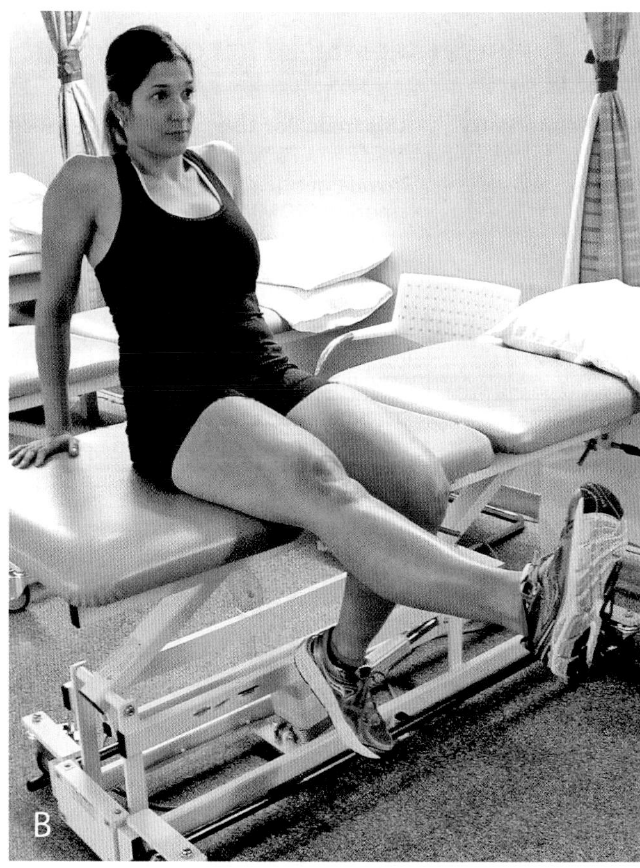

Figure 41.9 Photographs of knee ROM exercises: Patient is seated in a slightly reclined position with upper extremities providing support posterior to pelvis. She gently flexes the knee on the operated side, assisting with the nonoperated limb as necessary (**A**). Patient then extends the operated knee (**B**).

Treatment Recommendations (Table 41.1)

- Continuous Passive Motion (CPM) machine during hospital stay to limit adhesion formation and to allow the patient to acclimate to gentle motion in the sagittal plane.
- Home exercise program for isometric and co-contraction exercises for core and hip stability
- Ambulation in pool with water chest high may begin at 4 weeks postoperatively, once the incision is well healed.
- Upright stationary bicycle may begin at 4 weeks postoperatively.

Criteria for Advancement

- Controlled pain
- Normalized gait with appropriate assistive device
- Healed osteotomy site on radiograph

Phase II, Strengthening: Week 6–Week 12

Phase II generally begins approximately 6 weeks postoperatively. Advancement of weight bearing depends on physician recommendation based on radiographic findings and patient comorbidities. In some cases, patients may be allowed to begin weight bearing as tolerated (WBAT) with crutches as early as 4 weeks postoperatively. However, the majority of patients begin around 6 to 8 weeks. Once radiographic evidence supports sufficient healing, a patient may be advanced to WBAT and begin a course of outpatient physical therapy. Physical therapy at this stage focuses on gait quality and progressing off an assistive device as tolerated, strengthening of core and hip musculature to allow for adequate pelvic stability during ADLs and functional tasks, and continued pain control as functional demand increases. Quality of movement is essential, and the therapist is cautioned about premature discharge of the assistive device. Too rapid a progression may result in compensatory gait mechanics and injury. Outpatient physical therapy visits average twice per week based on patient need. It is imperative that the patient also commit to a home exercise program for core and gluteal strength.

Precautions

- Avoid premature discontinuation of assistive device. Bone healing on radiograph does *not* indicate discontinuation of an assistive device. Once sufficient osseous healing has taken place, the patient should continue to use an assistive device until able to consistently demonstrate a nonantalgic gait pattern (Table 41.2)
- Avoid symptom provocation during ADLs or therapeutic exercise.
- Continually monitor for faulty movement patterns or posture.

 © 2018 American Academy of Orthopaedic Surgeons

Table 41.2 PROGRESSION OF GAIT/DISCONTINUATION OF ASSISTIVE DEVICE

Acute Postoperative Period (~4–6 wks)	Radiographic Evidence of Healing (~6–8 wks)	Nonantalgic Gait with Bilateral Crutches, WBAT (~8–10 wks)	Nonantalgic Gait with One Crutch, WBAT (~10–12 wks)
20% WB with bilateral crutches	WBAT with bilateral crutches	Progress to one crutch on nonoperative side	Progress to ambulation without assistive device

WB = weight bearing, WBAT = weight bearing as tolerated.

- Avoid active hip flexion if symptomatic, particularly with a long lever arm, as with the SLR.
- Avoid premature use of gym equipment for hip strengthening.

Treatment Recommendations (Table 41.3)

- Active range of motion/active assistive range of motion (AROM/AAROM)
- Soft-tissue mobilization (Figure 41.10)
- Core stability and neuromuscular control work utilizing upper extremity movement patterns and functional, closed-chain movements.
- Hip strengthening
  - Closed chain for stability
  - Open-chain hip extension and abduction for mobility (Figure 41.12, A and B)
- Proprioception/balance work

Criteria for Advancement

- ROM within functional limits
- Normalized gait without an assistive device
- Good pelvic control during single-limb stance
- Able to ascend and descend an 8-inch step with good pelvic control (Figure 41.13)

Phase III, Single Limb Stability and Coordination: 3 Months–6 Months

Phase III generally begins approximately 12 weeks postsurgery. At this point. the patient should be ambulating without an assistive device without deviation. Treatment focus should be on optimizing strength and core control to achieve pain-free ADLs, optimal ROM, and good dynamic balance for functional activities.

Precautions

- Avoid symptom provocation.
- Be mindful of functional progressions.
- Do not sacrifice quality of movement for quantity of exercise repetitions or distance covered.

Table 41.3 PHASE II TREATMENT RECOMMENDATIONS

Exercise/Modality	Rationale	Special Cues	Progression
Heel slides	Increase range of motion (ROM) actively	Avoid hip flexor irritation. Cue patient for abdominal contraction to maintain a stable pelvis.	May progress to gentle heel–hand quadruped rock as tolerated (Figure 41.11, A and B)
Soft Tissue Mobilization (STM)	Improve tissue mobility Decrease muscular tension. Improve circulation to healing tissues. Provide pain relief	Scar mobilization Assess tension and provide intervention as needed to hip flexors, adductors, abductors, extensors, and rotators.	May progress to Active Release Treatment (ART) as needed/tolerated.
Bilateral bridges	Promote gluteal strengthening and core stability.	Loop resistance band proximal to knee to promote gluteus medius contraction to enhance proximal stability. Cue patient for abdominal contraction prior to hip extension to promote pelvic stabilization.	May progress to bilateral feet on unstable surface (e.g., ball) to address proprioception.

Continued on following page

© 2018 American Academy of Orthopaedic Surgeons

Table 41.3 PHASE II TREATMENT RECOMMENDATIONS *(Continued)*

Exercise/Modality	Rationale	Special Cues	Progression
Bent-knee fall out	Promote core and gluteal strengthening and stabilization on operative limb.	Cue patient to rotate nonoperative leg and keep the operative leg still. Cue patient for abdominal contraction prior to hip rotation to promote pelvic stabilization.	Loop resistance band proximal to knee to increase difficulty of stability exercise.
Hip extension with abduction in prone position (Figure 41.12, A and B)	Promote anticipatory core stabilization for distal movement and gluteal strengthening.	Focus on neuromuscular timing and control. Cue patient to contract abdominals, followed by gluteals, then hip extension and abduction.	Initially in Phase II, the patient may only be able to perform isometric contractions. Once the patient can maintain pelvic stability, he may be progressed to open-chain extension and abduction within pain-free ROM.
Standing Abduction	Facilitate weight shifting. Promote core stability with closed- and open-chain exercise in functional position.	Perform exercise abducting operative limb for open-chain strengthening. Perform exercise abducting nonoperative leg to promote stance leg stability on operative limb.	Progress to standing abduction and extension with resistance bands or machines.
Standing core stability	Strengthen abdominals and gluteals to improve stability with dynamic upper extremity work.	Perform standing exercise with resisted upper extremity bilateral or alternating flexion/extension. Perform exercises in sagittal and transverse planes.	Increase resistance. Progress to standing on dynamic surface.
Squats/leg press/ step progression	Promote gluteal strengthening and core stability in function.	Limit squat depth to comfortable ROM. May use exercise ball behind patient's back, against a wall for stability. Cue patient to push through heels on ascent from squat to recruit gluteals. Monitor patient movement pattern with step up/down Cue for level pelvis and avoid valgus moment at knee (Figure 41.13).	Leg press may also be used for strength progression (limiting hip flexion to comfortable ROM). Progress from bilateral leg press to bilateral concentric extension with single-limb eccentric flexion. Progress step height as patient demonstrates improved pelvic control and eccentric strength.
Proprioception/ recruitment/ balance activities	Improve body awareness, and proprioceptive and kinesthetic sense in operative hip.	May be performed in various positions, including quadruped, side-lying, or quadruped with operative limb in extension rolling a small ball on the wall, supine bridges on ball, bilateral stance on dynamic surfaces, and so on. Utilize visual, auditory, and proprioceptive feedback. Provide Proprioceptive Neuromuscular Facilitation (PNF) techniques: Rhythmic Stabilization for rotators.	Progress positions adding more degrees of freedom and progress from double limb to single limb support as stability improves

 © 2018 American Academy of Orthopaedic Surgeons

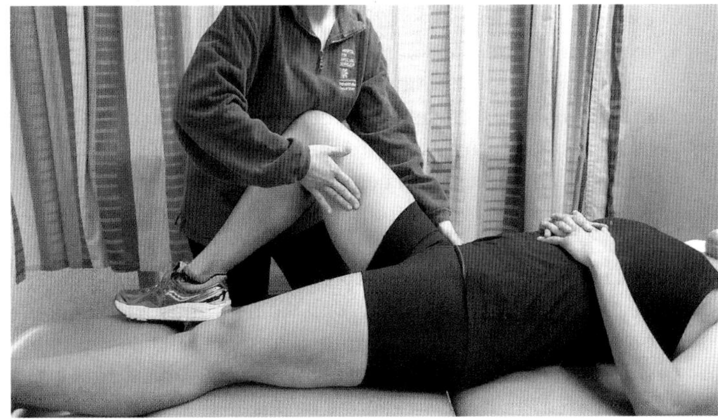

Figure 41.10 Photograph of soft-tissue mobilization: Assess tension and provide intervention as needed to hip flexors, adductors, abductors, extensors, and rotators.

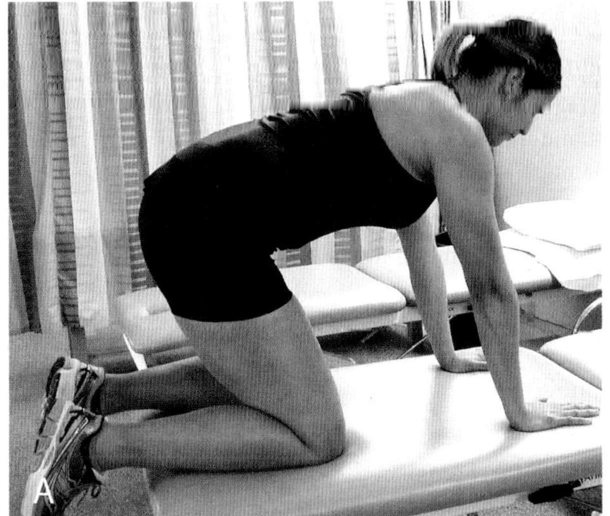

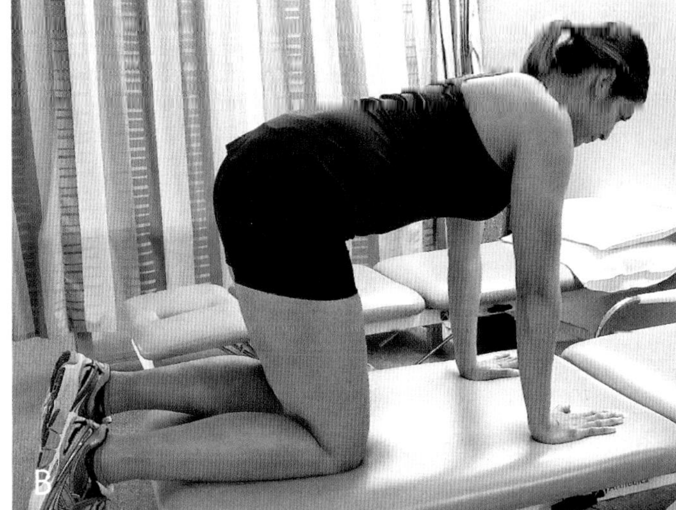

Figure 41.11 **A**, **B**, Photographs of patient performing gentle ROM progression: the heel–hand quadruped rock.

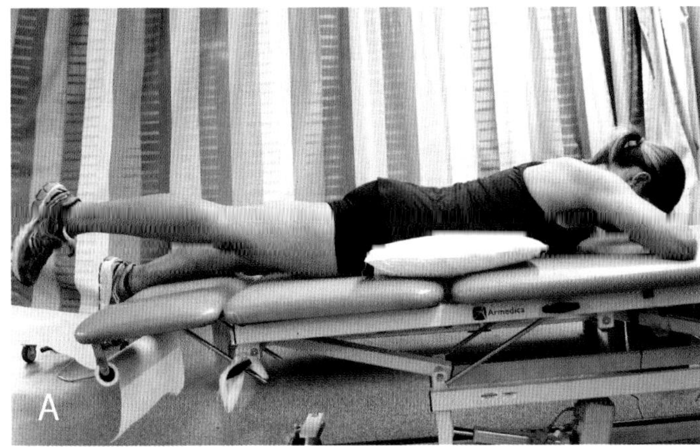

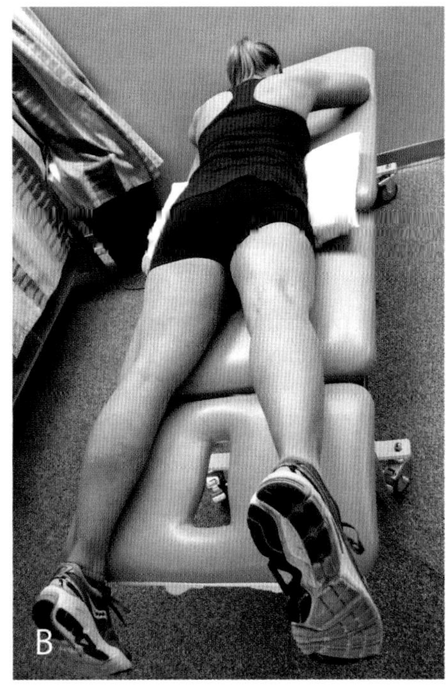

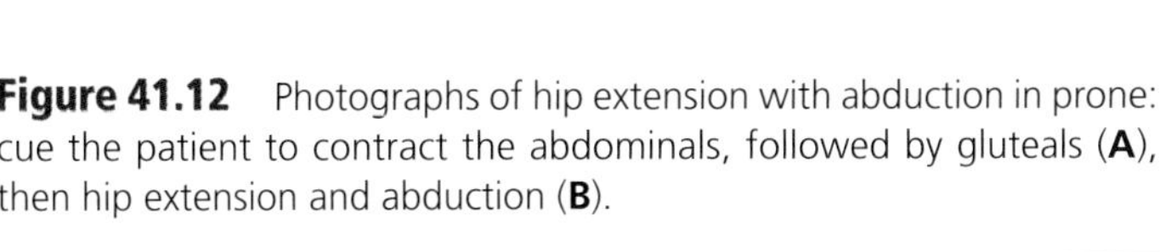

Figure 41.12 Photographs of hip extension with abduction in prone: cue the patient to contract the abdominals, followed by gluteals (**A**), then hip extension and abduction (**B**).

© 2018 American Academy of Orthopaedic Surgeons

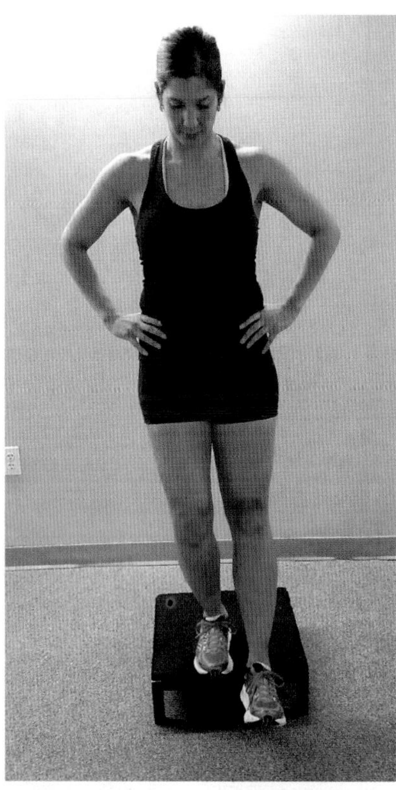

Figure 41.13 Photograph of the forward step down: Progress step height when the patient is able to maintain level pelvis and control valgus moment at the knee.

Treatment Recommendations (Table 41.4)

- Moderate-level core exercises in functional patterns of movement, for example, quadruped, standing diagonals
- Cross-training, for example, stationary bike, elliptical, aquatics, and so on
- Initiate plyometrics

Criteria for Advancement

- Adequate core muscle recruitment and control to consistently maintain a stable pelvis during Phase III exercise and closed-chain, single-limb activities.
- Good dynamic balance, 5/5 lower extremity strength
- Sufficient ROM to meet demands of desired activities

Phase IV, Return to Play: 6 Months–12 Months

This phase is not necessarily a component of rehabilitation for all patients. Phase III may be the final phase for those who are socially or moderately active, who wish to return to a gym program or mild to moderate recreational activities. Phase IV is specific to athletes and those wishing to return to competitive or moderate to high-intensity activities or occupations. This phase of rehabilitation should be catered to the individual's needs. The timing and duration of this phase varies widely based on individual fitness levels and task demands. Special attention and training should be given to sport-specific movements and body mechanics. Functional and dynamic exercise should mimic the demands placed on the body by the particular sport or task. For example, is the patient a golfer who needs particular attention in the transverse plane or a dancer who requires significant core stability while preserving flexibility and ROM? Does the throwing athlete have sufficient power in extension and rotation? The therapist needs to make sure the patient has adequate ROM, strength, endurance, and neuromuscular control and timing to meet the demands of his or her chosen sport. Quality of movement is essential to safe and pain-free return to play.

During Phase IV of therapy, the therapist and patient may begin working more closely with trainers and coaches as the patient prepares to transition back to sport. The nature of the surgery and the goals of rehabilitation should be clearly communicated, as well as cautions of possible pitfalls. The relationship between patient, therapist, and trainer is extremely important to make sure that the patient is adequately prepared to return to play.

Precautions

- Avoid symptom provocation.
- Be mindful of functional progressions.
- Maintain an adequate strength base.
- Do not compromise quality of movement.

Treatment Recommendations

- Advance core strength and endurance.
- Dynamic balance activities
- Advance plyometric training.
- Cutting and agility skills
- Initiate running program with interval training.

Criteria for Discharge

- Core and hip strength and stability adequate to maintain pelvic control during dynamic activities
- Performance of advanced activities without symptom provocation
- Optimal ROM
- Ability to maintain appropriate body mechanics during demands of sport, for example, jump mechanics

PEARLS

While PAO improves osseous alignment and femoral coverage with the goal to stabilize the hip, the pelvis undergoes significant trauma during surgery, and must be allowed adequate healing time. In addition, the patient has significant emotional needs when managing the pain and psychological challenges of temporarily reduced function and socialization. It is essential for the physical therapist to recognize and validate these issues during the course of treatment. Rehabilitation following PAO is a delicate balance of restoring strength, ROM, and function within the patient's physical and emotional healing constraints. One needs to see the global perspective of the patient, rather than isolating the view to the hip. Evaluate and continuously assess posture, circulation, the integumentary system, muscle recruitment, timing, control, endurance, and biomechanics of the entire kinematic chain.

© 2018 American Academy of Orthopaedic Surgeons

Table 41.4 PHASE III TREATMENT RECOMMENDATIONS

Exercise/Modality	Rationale	Special Cues	Progression
Unilateral bridge	Promote gluteal strengthening and core stability.	Cue patient for abdominal contraction prior to movement to promote pelvic stabilization.	Pelvic stability may be challenged by changing nonoperative limb from resting in open-chain knee flexion to open-chain knee extension.
Functional squat/lunges/forward step down/monster walks/three-point step/lawnmower	Promote gluteal strengthening and core stability during functional positions.	Limit squat/lunge depth to comfortable and equal ROM bilaterally. Cue patient to push through heels on ascent from squat to recruit gluteals. Cue patient to maintain level upper body while performing side stepping exercise.	Progress to standing on dynamic surfaces. Vary platform height for lunges. Progress step height when patient is able to maintain level pelvis and control valgus moment at knee. Progress squat to single limb support when patient is able to maintain level pelvis and control valgus moment at knee. Advance resistance during monster walks by moving the resistance band distally from above knee to ankles to toes.
Rotational activities: standing trunk rotation/windmills/hip external rotation	Promote controlled movement in the transverse plane.	Work both acetabulum rotating over stable femur (Figure 41.14, A and B) and femur rotating beneath stable acetabulum (Figure 41.14C). Vary patient stance to address different functional movement patterns/arcs of motion while working acetabulum over femur. Utilize swivel stool and/or rotary discs for closed-chain femur rotating beneath acetabulum (Figure 41.14C).	Progress from bilateral closed chain activities to single limb stance (e.g., standing trunk rotation with cable column to windmills with trunk rotation) Add PNF patterns
Forward plank/side plank	Promote core stability.	Cue patient to elongate body through head and heels. Monitor patient performance, avoiding excessive recruitment of hip flexors during forward plank, which may cause increased pain.	Progress forward plank to dynamic surface. Progress side plank to include hip and/or shoulder abduction.
Eccentric hip flexor strengthening (Figure 41.15)	Strengthen hip flexors without causing irritation.	Begin working eccentrically. For example: have patient seated with feet supported. Patient performs controlled lowering of upper body to reclined position; therapist passively returns patient to starting position.	Progress isometrics and gentle concentric work cautiously, as tolerated.
Continue STM as outlined earlier, as needed			
Continue proprioception activities, as needed			

© 2018 American Academy of Orthopaedic Surgeons

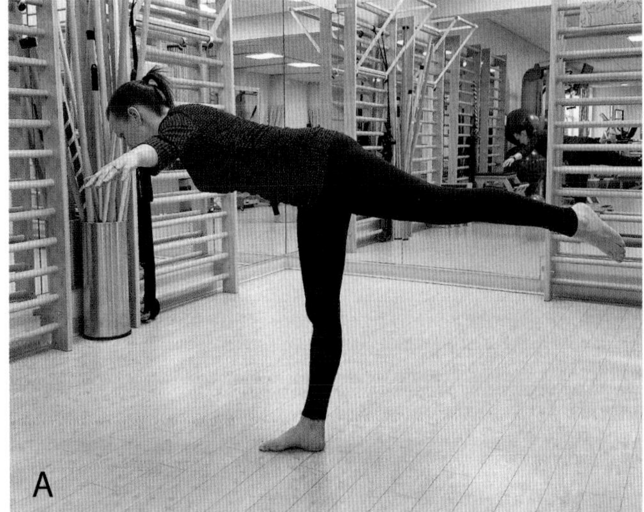

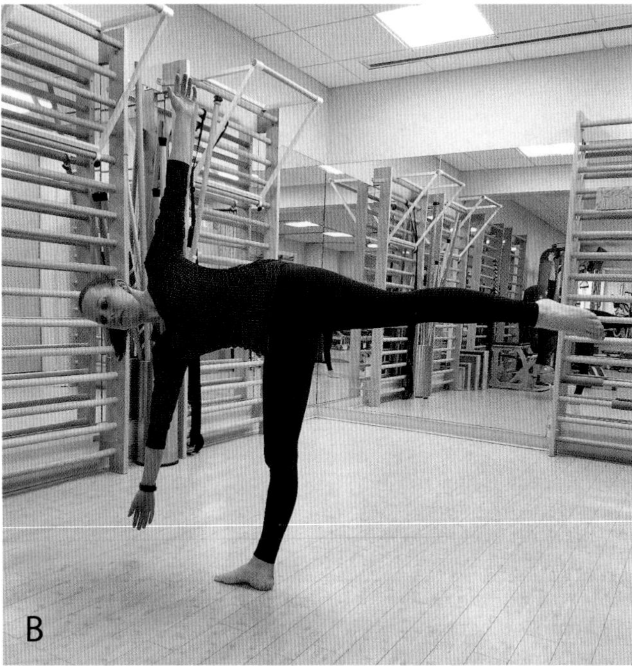

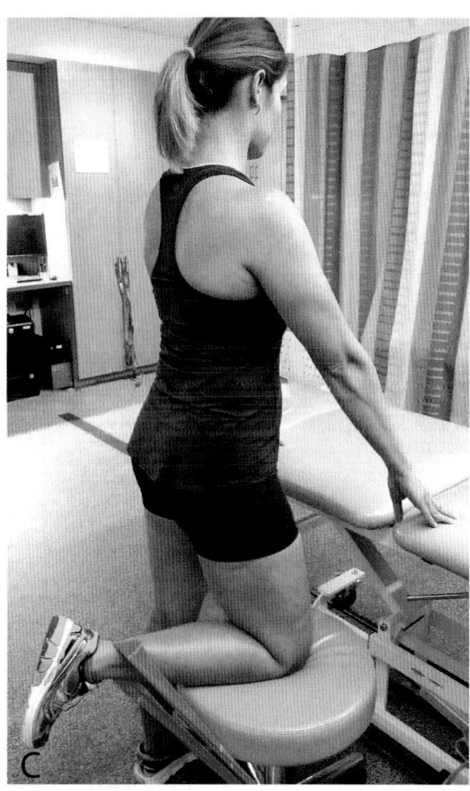

Figure 41.14 Photographs of rotational activities: The therapist should have the patient work both the acetabulum rotating over a stable femur (**A**, **B**) and the femur rotating beneath a stable acetabulum (**C**).

Ideally, the patient should undergo preoperative physical therapy. This helps the patient optimize strength and learn proper engagement and recruitment of muscles prior to surgery. Additionally, the therapist should evaluate the spine, knee, and ankle, ruling out or addressing any restrictions or pathology that may contribute to pain. Preoperative physical therapy helps establish a healthy foundation for postoperative rehabilitation.

Core and gluteal activation are essential to restoring (and, in many cases, initiating) healthy biomechanics about the hip and pelvis. Stabilization and anticipatory postural control allow the patient to function in proper alignment, permitting muscles to work as intended and minimizing stress across the joint. Pilates-based exercises are helpful in addressing this. A patient with difficulty achieving adequate core stabilization or gluteal activation may be aided by the use of electrical stimulation (e-stim) to multifidi or gluteals to promote contraction. The therapist may mimic a functional position such as step stance while using e-stim in prone or side-lying positions with the use of pillows.

A frequent complaint of patients postoperatively is deep pain near the ischial tuberosity. This is the site of one of the pelvic cuts used to reorient the acetabulum. Occasionally, the deep rotators near the area may spasm. Soft-tissue mobilization to the area and particularly release of the obturator internus often provide relief. Soft-tissue mobilization in general is particularly important during rehabilitation after PAO. Muscle imbalance produces stress and pain about the hip joint and thigh. Soft-tissue mobilization to the rectus femoris, psoas, adductors, tensor fascia latae (TFL), and quadratus lumborum (QL) may relieve pain and promote optimal alignment for proper muscle activation. That said, it is important

© 2018 American Academy of Orthopaedic Surgeons

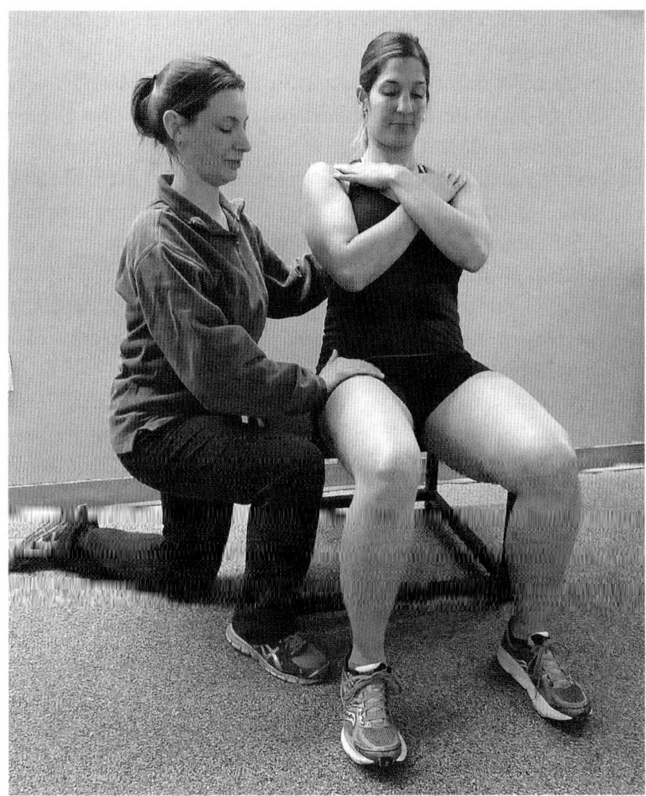

Figure 41.15 Photographs of eccentric hip flexor strengthening: The patient is seated with feet supported. She controls the lowering of the upper body to a reclined position; the therapist then passively returns the patient to the starting position.

that the therapist perform a proper assessment to determine the cause of pain, spasm, or tightness. Is the muscle being overused? For example, the QL may become overused to achieve hip abduction if a patient lacks adequate core stabilization from the transversus abdominus or sufficient gluteus medius strength. Are postural changes forcing muscles to act outside of their intended action or line of pull? Are postural changes inhibiting muscle activation? For example, increased anterior pelvic tilt alters the length–tension relationship and limits gluteal activation. The therapist must also be mindful not to stretch or release an already loose muscle, as it may increase instability.

Hip flexor strength is traditionally the slowest to return following PAO. Recently, changes in operative technique allow the rectus femoris to remain intact rather than implementing the convention of resecting the rectus to improve visualization of the pubic cut during the osteotomy. Clinical evidence supports more rapid return of strength when the rectus is left intact, allowing improved ease of transfers and ambulation. This is currently under investigation to seek scientific validation of this finding. In either case, however, it is important not to irritate the rectus or psoas during rehabilitation. This may be avoided by focusing attention on pelvic position, soft-tissue mobilization, and gluteal and core activation. Begin hip flexor strengthening eccentrically and progress isometrics and concentrics cautiously as tolerated by the patient.

Aquatic therapy is an excellent adjunct to land-based treatment. Patients may begin ambulating forward and backward in chest-high water as early as 4 weeks postoperatively as part of a home exercise program. True aquatic therapy may begin when the patient initiates Phase II outpatient therapy. In the water, a patient may work on gently restoring ROM and strength with limited ground reaction and gravitational forces, thus limiting stress and pain on the healing pelvis. Moreover, the dynamic aquatic environment provides a great opportunity to work on stabilization exercises and quality of movement.

It is imperative that the therapist examine the entire kinetic chain. The mechanics of the ankle, knee, lumbar spine, and thoracic spine, in addition to the hip and pelvis, should be examined. Perhaps what seems to be poor control during a forward step down is actually due to a limitation in ankle dorsiflexion. Perhaps a patient is not achieving adequate weight shift during ambulation or early running because he lacks thoracic rotation.

For those patients returning to sports or physically demanding occupations, Quality of Movement Assessment (QMA) is recommended during Phase IV. If possible, this assessment should be interdisciplinary, including input from physical therapist, trainer, and physician. The QMA may include physical examination and video analysis of functional movement strategies to home in on areas of weakness or breaks in the kinetic chain. Repeated movements are examined to anticipate the effects of fatigue on the patient. The goal of the QMA is to direct the final weeks of rehabilitation to optimize functional strength and quality of movement to maximize performance and prevent injury.

SUMMARY

Rehabilitation following PAO requires patience and respect for healing constraints, acute attention to quality of movement and neuromuscular connection, and excellent communication between the patient, therapist, and physician. The duration of rehabilitation varies by patient age, fitness level, comorbidities, and ultimate functional goals. Communication, anticipation of needs, and clear expectations of the surgery help to make rehabilitation smooth and effective. A PAO with adequate and appropriate rehabilitation will help preserve the hip, improve stability, and optimize patient function and participation in society.

BIBLIOGRAPHY

Clohisy JC, Barrett SE, Gordon JE, Delgado ED, Schoenecker PL: Periacetabular osteotomy for the treatment of severe acetabular dysplasia. *J Bone Joint Surg Am* 2005;87-A:254–259.

Clohisy JC, Barrett SE, Gordon JE, Delgado ED, Schoenecker PL: Periacetabular osteotomy in the treatment of severe acetabular dysplasia. Surgical Technique. *J Bone Joint Surg Am* 2006;88 Suppl 1:65–83.

Ganz R, Klaue K, Vinh TS, Mast JW: A new periacetabular osteotomy for the treatment of hip dysplasias. *Clin Orthop Relat Res* 1988;232:26–36.

© 2018 American Academy of Orthopaedic Surgeons

Hussell JG, Rodriguez JA, Ganz R: Technical complications of the Bernese periacetabular osteotomy. *Clin Orthop Relat Res* 1999;363:81–92.

Leunig M, Siebenrock KA, Ganz R: Instructional Course Lecture, American Academy of Orthopaedic Surgeons. Rationale of periacetabular osteotomy and background work. *J Bone Joint Surg Am* 2001;83-A:437–447.

Matheney T, Kim YJ, Zurakowski D, Matero C, Millis M: Intermediate to long-term results following the Bernese periacetabular osteotomy and predictors of clinical outcome. *J Bone Joint Surg Am* 2009;91-A:2113–2123.

Millis MB, Kain M, Sierra R, et al: Periacetabular osteotomy for acetabular dysplasia in patients older than 40 years. *Clin Orthop Relat Res* 2009;467:2228–2234.

Siebenrock KA, Leunig M, Ganz R: Instructional Course Lecture, American Academy of Orthopaedic Surgeons. Periacetabular osteotomy: The Bernese experience. *J Bone Joint Surg Am* 2001; 83A:449–455.

Steppacher SD, Tannast M, Ganz R, Siebenrock KA: Mean 20-year follow-up of Bernese periacetabular osteotomy. *Clin Orthop Relat Res* 2008;466:1633–1644.

Sucato DJ, Tulchin K, Shrader MW, DeLaRocha A, Gist T, Sheu G: Gait, hip strength and functional outcomes after a Ganz periacetabular osteotomy for adolescent hip dysplasia. *J Pediatr Orthop* 2010;30:344–350.

Thawrani D, Sucato DJ, Podeszwa DA, DeLaRocha A: Complications associated with the Bernese periacetabular osteotomy for hip dysplasia in adolescents. *J Bone Joint Surg Am* 2010;92-A: 1707–1714.

Turner R, O'Sullivan E, Edelstein J: Hip dysplasia and the performing arts: is there a correlation? *Curr Rev Musculoskelet Med* 2012;5:39–45.

© 2018 American Academy of Orthopaedic Surgeons

SECTION 5

Knee

42 Knee Anatomy

Steven Haas, MD, Davis V. Reyes, PT, DPT, OCS, and Benjamin F. Ricciardi, MD

INTRODUCTION

The knee is a modified hinge-type synovial joint. It consists of four bones: the tibia, femur, fibula, and patella. There are three articulations: the tibiofemoral joint, patellofemoral joint, and the tibiofibular joint.

BONY ANATOMY

The distal femur forms the proximal aspect of the tibiofemoral joint. It consists of the medial and lateral condyles, which serve as attachment sites for many soft-tissue stabilizing structures around the knee. The medial condyle is larger, more symmetrical in the sagittal plane, and extends farther distal relative to the lateral condyle. Anteriorly, the femoral trochlea separates the medial and lateral condyles, and contains the patellofemoral articulation. Distally, the intercondylar notch separates the two condyles and contains the origins of the anterior cruciate ligament (ACL) and posterior cruciate ligament (PCL). The lateral epicondyle and medial epicondyle are bony prominences of the lateral and medial condyles, respectively, that serve as attachment sites for the lateral collateral ligament (LCL) and medial collateral ligament (MCL). The epicondyles are important anatomic structures in total knee arthroplasty (TKA) because a line drawn connecting these two structures in the axial plane helps identify the appropriate plane for rotation of the femoral component. Malrotation of the femoral component can contribute to poor patellofemoral joint tracking and soft-tissue imbalance after TKA.

The proximal tibia forms the distal aspect of the tibiofemoral joint. It contains soft-tissue insertions for structures such as the MCL and patellar tendon, which inserts anteriorly onto the tibial tuberosity. The medial tibial plateau has a relatively concave articular surface, while the lateral tibial plateau is not concave and has a posterior slope. This bony structure allows for a rotational moment to occur between the tibia and femur through the flexion-extension axis, which is centered on the medial side of the knee. The intercondylar eminence separates the medial and lateral tibial plateau and serves as an attachment site for the menisci and cruciate ligaments. The fibula articulates with the tibia at the tibiofibular joint. It serves as an attachment site for soft-tissue structures such as the LCL, biceps femoris muscle, and ligaments of the posterolateral corner. There is a synovial aspect to the tibiofibular joint proximally; however, the distal part of the joint is a syndesmosis with little motion, secured together by a strong interosseous ligament.

The patella is the largest sesamoid bone (a bone embedded within a tendon or muscle) in the body, and it has the thickest articular cartilage of any joint. Its posterior aspect contains hyaline cartilage and consists of medial, lateral, and odd facets, which articulate with the femoral trochlea forming the patellofemoral joint. It serves as the insertion point for the quadriceps tendon, and increases its functional lever arm during active knee extension.

Dr. Haas or an immediate family member has received royalties from Innovative Medical Products and Smith & Nephew; is a member of a speakers' bureau or has made paid presentations on behalf of Smith & Nephew; serves as a paid consultant to Smith & Nephew; has stock or stock options held in Ortho Secure; has received research or institutional support from Smith & Nephew; and has received nonincome support (such as equipment or services), commercially derived honoraria, or other non-research–related funding (such as paid travel) from APOS Medical & Sports Technologies. Neither Dr. Reyes nor any immediate family member has received anything of value from or has stock or stock options held in a commercial company or institution related directly or indirectly to the subject of this article.

© 2018 American Academy of Orthopaedic Surgeons

SOFT-TISSUE ANATOMY

Intra-articular and extra-articular soft tissue structures contribute a significant portion of the inherent stability of the knee joint. Two important intra-articular structures in the native knee are the medial and lateral menisci. The menisci are fibrocartilaginous structures that help deepen and improve the conformity of the articular surfaces of the medial and lateral tibiofemoral joint, distributing forces across the articular surface. The lateral meniscus covers a greater proportion of its tibial articular surface (75%–93%) relative to the medial meniscus (51%–74%). Loss of the meniscus from injury or meniscectomy results in increased peak loads across the articular cartilage. The lateral meniscus has weaker attachments to the tibia and is more mobile than the medial meniscus, making it less likely to tear than the medial meniscus, which has more firm attachments to the tibia and MCL. The outer periphery of the meniscus has good vascularity, while the inner aspect of the meniscus is avascular, which has important implications in the decision to repair the meniscus or excise the torn aspect of the meniscus (meniscectomy) during surgery.

Two intra-articular, extrasynovial cruciate ligaments (ACL and PCL) connect the distal femur and proximal tibia centrally. The ACL inserts anterior to the intercondylar eminence and originates on the posteromedial aspect of the lateral femoral condyle. It has two bundles: the anteromedial bundle, which tightens as the knee flexes, and the posterolateral bundle, which tightens as the knee extends. The primary role of the ACL is resistance to anterior tibial translation, while also providing resistance to tibial rotation. Reconstruction of the ACL to its proper anatomic location is critical to restoring these functions; improper tunnel placement during ACL reconstruction is a major cause of failure. The ACL has a variety of nerve endings, suggesting that it also plays a significant proprioceptive role in the knee. The PCL inserts posterior to the intercondylar eminence, approximately 1 cm distal to the posterior tibial joint line, and originates from the posterolateral aspect of the medial femoral condyle. It displays maximal tension at 90° of knee flexion and serves as the primary resistance to posterior translation of the tibia.

The medial side of the knee has three layers. Layer I lies under the subcutaneous tissues and consists of the crural fascia, including the sartorius muscle. In between layer I and layer II lie the gracilis and semitendinosus tendons, forming part of the pes anserinus. Layer II contains the superficial MCL, medial patellofemoral ligament, and posterior oblique ligaments. Layer III contains the deep MCL, knee joint capsule, and coronary ligaments anchoring the meniscus. In a varus knee, these medial-sided structures can become contracted; sequential releases of some of these structures have been described to aid in balancing the knee during TKA.

The lateral soft-tissue structures of the knee are also divided into layers. The first layer contains the iliotibial band and biceps femoris. The iliotibial band attaches anterolaterally to the patella, patellar ligament, and the anterolateral aspect of the proximal tibia (Gerdy's tubercle), providing some anterolateral knee stability. The biceps femoris attaches to both the proximal fibula and tibia, and is an important stabilizer to the lateral aspect of the knee. Layer II contains the patellar retinaculum and patellofemoral ligament. Layer III contains the LCL and lateral joint capsule, arcuate ligament, and fabellofibular ligament. The popliteus muscle originates on the lateral femoral condyle, and its tendon has an intra-articular portion with attachments to the lateral meniscus. Taken together, the LCL and popliteal-arcuate ligament complex help stabilize the posterolateral aspect of the knee.

Muscles crossing the knee joint serve as important dynamic stabilizers. Proper rehabilitation of these muscles after injury is crucial to restore appropriate joint function and reduce stress on static stabilizers. The knee flexors consist of the hamstrings (biceps femoris, semitendinosus, semimembranosus), gastrocnemius, gracilis, and sartorius muscles. Muscles with proximal insertions also act as hip joint extensors (hamstrings) or hip joint flexors (sartorius), while muscles with distal insertions act across the ankle joint (gastrocnemius). The sciatic nerve innervates the hamstrings, the femoral nerve innervates the sartorius, the obturator nerve innervates the gracilis, and the tibial nerve innervates the gastrocnemius. Knee joint extensors are the quadriceps (rectus femoris, vastus medialis, lateralis, intermedius). Only the rectus femoris crosses a second joint (the rectus femoris originates on the anterior inferior iliac spine and is a hip flexor). The femoral nerve provides innervation to the knee extensors. The vastus medialis oblique (VMO) is an important anatomic structure in TKA. Traditional approaches to TKA typically include a quadriceps tendon–splitting medial parapatellar arthrotomy to access the knee joint. This approach violates the medial aspect of the quadriceps tendon. In order to reduce trauma to the tendon and improve rehabilitation post-TKA, alternative approaches have been described. These include the midvastus approach (which splits the VMO along its muscle fibers, avoiding an arthrotomy through the quadriceps tendon) and the subvastus approach (which involves elevating underneath the VMO to gain exposure, avoiding an incision through the quadriceps tendon).

ALIGNMENT AND MECHANICS

The weight-bearing axis through the knee joint in the frontal plane extends along a line from the center of the ankle joint to the center of the hip joint (Figure 42.1, A). In the general population, this line most commonly passes just medial to the tibial spine. In valgus knee alignment, the weight-bearing axis passes through the lateral compartment of the knee, resulting in increased force through the lateral articular surface (Figure 42.1, B). Patients with a valgus knee typically present with lateral compartment joint space narrowing and arthritis prior to medial-sided disease. In addition, the lateral-sided soft-tissue structures become contracted. In varus knee alignment, the weight-bearing axis passes through the medial compartment of the knee, resulting in increased force through the medial articular surface (Figure 42.1, C). This results in

 © 2018 American Academy of Orthopaedic Surgeons

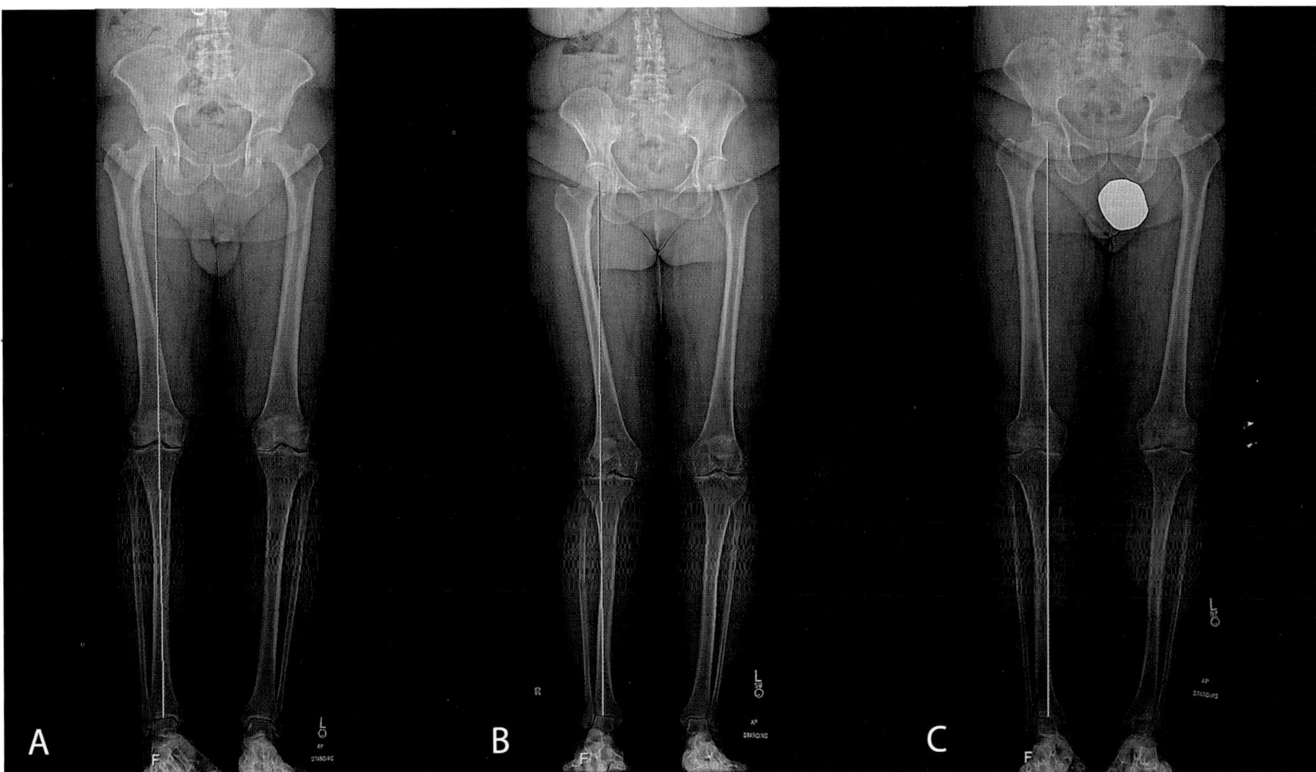

Figure 42.1 **A**, Radiograph showing a weight-bearing axis passing from the center of the ankle to the center of the hip joint. This line should pass just medial to the tibial spine in the center of the knee joint. **B**, In valgus knee alignment, the weight-bearing axis passes through the lateral compartment of the knee in this radiograph. **C**, In varus knee alignment, the weight-bearing axis passes through the medial compartment of the knee in this radiograph.

earlier medial compartment osteoarthritis and medial soft-tissue contractures. Two other important axes in the frontal plane include the anatomic axis and the mechanical axis. The mechanical axis of the femur passes from the center of the femoral head to the center of the intercondylar notch, and the mechanical axis of the tibia passes from the center of the ankle to the center of the tibial plateau (Figure 42.2, A). The anatomic axis of the femur bisects the intramedullary canal of the femur (Figure 42.2, B). It typically lies between 5° and 7° from the mechanical axis of the femur. The anatomic axis of the tibia bisects the intramedullary canal of the tibia, and in a neutral alignment, lies parallel to the mechanical axis (Figure 42.2, B). Frontal plane alignment is critical to the outcomes of both TKA and soft-tissue ligamentous reconstructions in the knee. In TKA, the most common goal is to resect the bone of the distal femur and proximal tibia at 90° to their respective mechanical axes. Failure to restore a neutral alignment of the knee in the frontal plane after TKA may result in increased loosening and need for revision surgery. Additionally, realignment of the tibia in the frontal plane is an important secondary procedure in cases of multiligamentous knee injury undergoing reconstruction to avoid abnormal stresses on the ligament repair or grafts. Another useful measurement in the frontal plane is the Q angle, which is represented by the angle between a line from the anterior superior iliac spine (ASIS) to the center of the patella and from the center of the patella to the tibial tubercle (normal 11° ± 6°). An increased Q angle can result in patellar maltracking. In the sagittal plane, the tibia slopes anterior to posterior, and posterior slope averages approximately 9°.

The joint reactive force across the tibiofemoral articulation averages three times body weight during normal walking. The motion of the tibiofemoral joint is primarily in the flexion-extension plane with a small degree of rotation. The motion of the knee joint differs from a true hinge because the axis of motion changes with the degree of flexion and extension, allowing some rotation, particularly of the lateral compartment, and gliding, or rollback, in the sagittal plane of the femur on the tibia as the knee approaches deeper flexion. The joint reactive force across the patellofemoral articulation averages 0.5 body weight with normal walking; however, this can increase to over seven times body weight with deep knee bending. In full extension, the patella lies proximal and lateral to the trochlea and is not in contact with its articular surface. Exercise involving straight-leg raise with the knee in full extension minimizes force across the patellofemoral joint because the patella has not engaged the trochlea. In early flexion, the patella engages within the trochlear groove. Maximal surface area contact between the patella and trochlea occurs at 45° of knee flexion. Patellar tracking can be affected by many factors, including Q angle, soft-tissue laxity, dysplasia of the trochlear groove, lateral femoral condyle hypoplasia, and muscular or soft-tissue imbalances. Achieving appropriate amounts of external rotation and

© 2018 American Academy of Orthopaedic Surgeons

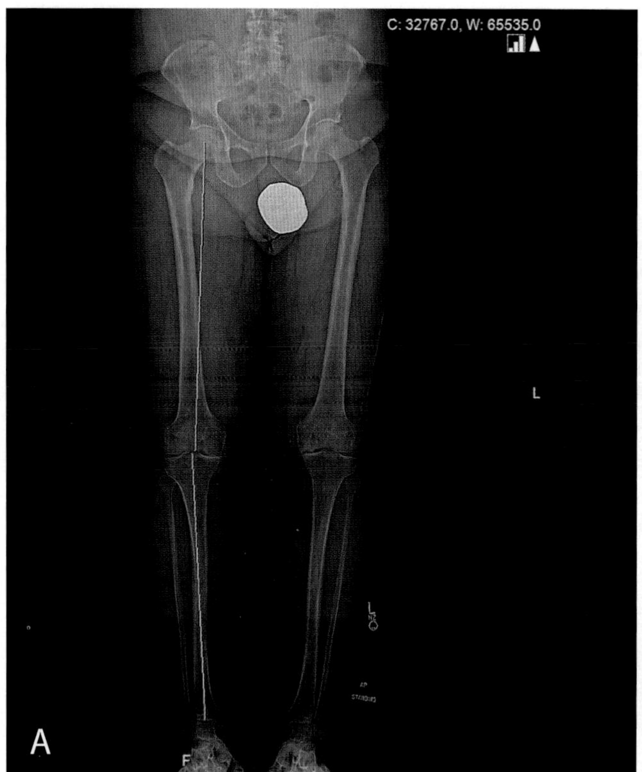

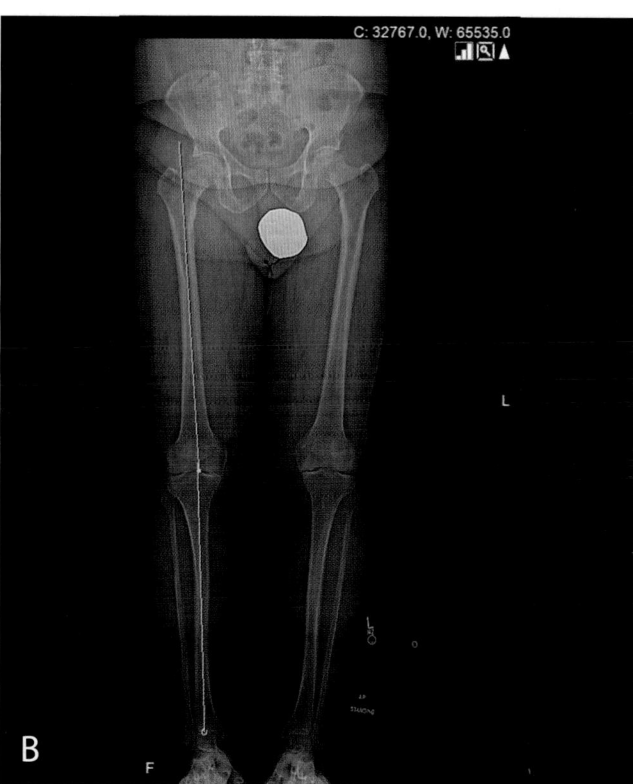

Figure 42.2 **A**, Radiograph showing a mechanical axis of the femur passing from the center of the femoral head to the center of the intercondylar notch. The mechanical axis of the tibia passes from the center of the ankle to the center of the tibial plateau. **B**, The anatomic axis of the femur bisects the intramedullary canal of the femur in this radiograph. The anatomic axis of the tibia bisects the intramedullary canal of the tibia.

lateralization of the tibial and femoral components in TKA helps optimize patellar tracking within the groove of the implant.

BIBLIOGRAPHY

Cantin O, Magnussen RA, Corbi F, Servien E, Neyret P, Lustig S: The role of high tibial osteotomy in the treatment of knee laxity: a comprehensive review. *Knee Surg Sports Traumatol Arthrosc* 2015;23(10):3026–3037.

Fang DM, Ritter MA, Davis KE: Coronal alignment in total knee arthroplasty: just how important is it? *J Arthroplasty* 2009;24(6 Suppl):39–43.

Hsu RW, Himeno S, Coventry MB, Chao EY: Normal axial alignment of the lower extremity and load bearing distribution at the knee. *Clin Orthop Relat Res* 1990;(255):215–227.

Luo CF: Reference axes for reconstruction of the knee. *Knee* 2004;11:251–257.

Makris EA, Hadidi P, Athanasiou KA: The knee meniscus: structure-function, pathophysiology, current repair techniques, and prospects for regeneration. *Biomaterials* 2011;32(30): 7411–7431.

Warren LF, Marshall JL: The supporting structures and layers on the medial side of the knee: an anatomical analysis. *J Bone Joint Surg Am* 1979;61:56–62.

© 2018 American Academy of Orthopaedic Surgeons

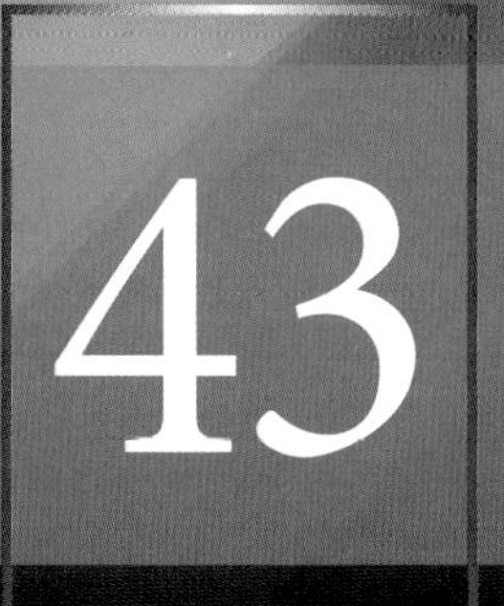

43 Total Knee Arthroplasty

Steven Haas, MD, Benjamin F. Ricciardi, MD, and Davis V. Reyes, PT, DPT, OCS

INTRODUCTION

With the increasing number of total knee arthroplasties (TKAs) being performed in the United States each year, it is more important than ever that clear rehabilitation guidelines and principles be instituted in order to ensure success of the surgery. Such guidelines and principles should be based on stages of healing, objective measurements, best-practice therapeutic exercise progressions, clinical research, and typical time frames for the resolution of major impairments and achievement of functional milestones. Utilization of such guidelines and principles will allow for more effective management of the initial phases postoperatively and throughout the continuum of care. Physical therapists are challenged in today's healthcare climate, in which progressive limitations in rehabilitation coverage each year require physical therapists to address a wide range of postsurgical impairments with fewer visits. The following is an overview of updated best-practice postoperative rehabilitation guidelines and principles.

TKA is a resurfacing procedure. The femur is resurfaced with a metal implant 8 to 10 mm thick. The tibia in resurfaced with a metal implant that accepts a polyethylene inset. The patella in resurfaced with a 7- to 9-mm polyethylene implant in most cases. The collateral ligaments are left in place to support the knee in most cases. The anterior cruciate ligament (ACL) is often absent or attenuated from the arthritis, and the remnant is excised. The posterior cruciate ligament (PCL) can be retained or substituted by the implant with equal success.

The indications for TKA are pain and/or dysfunction caused by cartilage damage to the knee. The most common reason is osteoarthritis, but other causes include rheumatoid arthritis, posttraumatic arthritis, and osteonecrosis. While the average age for a TKA patient is approximately 65 years old, patients in their 50s are more often undergoing TKA. This is likely due to increases in sports-related injuries and obesity rates in the United States. While there is no absolute age-related contraindication, TKA in patients under 40 is uncommon. Patients in their 80s and even 90s have been shown to benefit from TKA, but they must be medically cleared for the procedure.

Contraindications for conventional arthroplasty include active infection, poor bone stock (including acute fracture), and patients unable to comply with rehabilitation.

SURGICAL PROCEDURE

Knee arthroplasty is performed through a midline approach, but may be modified based on preexisting incisions. The joint is opened by incising the extensor mechanism medially around the patella, starting in the quadriceps tendon. Alternatively, an incision is made into the vastus medialis, allowing lateral mobilization of the patella. With this access, the menisci are excised as well as the ACL. Depending on implant design, the PCL may be excised or retained. The collateral ligaments must be retained but may be mobilized, especially in the case of varus or valgus deformity. Cutting jigs then create precise cuts in the femur and tibia to ensure accurate alignment and good motion. The metal femoral and tibial component is fixed into place with cement. Soft tissue and collateral ligament balance is a critical component in ensuring stability. The modular plastic trays assist in adjusting soft-tissue tension. The patella may be resurfaced. The tracking of the patella is checked and may require a lateral release. Secure layered closure is critical to infection-free healing.

POSTOPERATIVE REHABILITATION

Rehabilitation of knee arthroplasty is critical to a successful outcome. It allows the patient to overcome mobility, strength, and motion defects that have developed over time.

Dr. Haas or an immediate family member has received royalties from Innovative Medical Products and Smith & Nephew; is a member of a speakers' bureau or has made paid presentations on behalf of Smith & Nephew; serves as a paid consultant to Smith & Nephew; has stock or stock options held in Ortho Secure; has received research or institutional support from Smith & Nephew; and has received nonincome support (such as equipment or services), commercially derived honoraria, or other non-research–related funding (such as paid travel) from APOS Medical & Sports Technologies. Neither Dr. Reyes nor any immediate family member has received anything of value from or has stock or stock options held in a commercial company or institution related directly or indirectly to the subject of this article.

© 2018 American Academy of Orthopaedic Surgeons

Acute Phase (First 3 Days–2 Weeks)

In the initial days after surgery, the goal is to functionally prepare the patient for a safe discharge home or to an inpatient rehabilitation center. The primary emphasis during this phase is on patient education, transfer training, gait training, stair training, initiation of knee range of motion (ROM), remedial strengthening of the involved lower extremity, and adaptive functional mobility. Preoperative "prehabilitation" can improve strength and ROM and aid in postoperative rehabilitation, especially in the acute phase. Preoperative therapy can also educate patients, allowing them to achieve their therapy landmarks more quickly and discharge from hospital sooner.

Patient Education

In the acute phase, patients are advised to be as active as tolerated in order to minimize deconditioning, improve upright activity tolerance, initiate functional ROM, and to regain general mobility. Patients are typically advised against sitting for extensive periods of time to avoid static positions that could foster stiffening of the involved knee. Patients should alternate between walking, sitting, and bed rest with leg elevation, with decreasing bed rest as time after surgery passes. Patients are also advised against excessive standing or walking. Although regular upright activity can maintain healthy functioning of peripheral vasculature, too much activity can exacerbate swelling, overwhelm peripheral vasculature, and be counterproductive to the healing process. A balance between activity and rest is necessary. The therapist will need to monitor individualized responses to activity and modify activity accordingly.

In addition to general activity guidelines, patients are instructed on elevation of the involved lower extremity and regular use of cold modalities in order to manage postoperative swelling and pain. When this is performed concomitantly with the intake of prescribed anti-inflammatory drugs and the optional use of compression stockings, postoperative swelling can be managed appropriately. There are a variety of cold mediums available, such as gel and ice packs, that simply provide cryotherapy, whereas some commercial devices combine cryotherapy with pneumatic compression for the intention of mobilizing edema. While there are advantages and disadvantages to both, there is currently no evidence that one form is superior in managing postoperative swelling in the initial phases or throughout the duration of recovery. The modality of cryotherapy itself, however, has been demonstrated to control generalized swelling, decrease muscle hypertonicity, and provide analgesic effects, which patients and therapists have found beneficial in efforts to recover ROM and manage pain throughout rehabilitation.

Another component of patient education in the acute phase of rehabilitation is advising the patient in the use of adaptive equipment for activities of daily living (ADLs) such as reachers, long-handled shoe-horns, and long-handled bath sponges, as well as sock aides that facilitate modified function. The use of such devices can be phased out as the patient increases ROM of the involved knee and regains strength, endurance, balance, and independent mobility.

In the acute phase and throughout all phases of postoperative rehabilitation, one of the hallmarks of physical therapy is teaching patients various functional movement strategies through transfer and gait training. Education is provided on proper mechanics of transferring into and out of bed as well as transferring into and out of chairs, car seats, and toilets with the use of adaptive equipment. If necessary, equipment such as raised seat cushions and raised toilet seats can be provided to facilitate sit-to-stand movement. Education is also provided on appropriate mechanics to initially negotiate stairs nonreciprocally and then reciprocally when adequate strength and ROM are achieved. Finally, educational instruction is provided on proper mechanics to reestablish normalized gait. A patient's ability to execute these activities will be commensurate with the patient's progress in knee ROM as well as level of strength and balance. Full independence and complete proficiency can be attained in 1 to 2 months in a motivated patient with a straightforward arthroplasty or can take upward of 3 to 4 months of intensive rehabilitation.

Range of Motion

Initiation of ROM in the acute phase is vital to the success of this surgery. Based on the literature, the following knee flexion ROMs are necessary to perform the associated functional activities:

Walking	65°
Ascend stairs	65°
Descend stairs	90°–100°
Sitting and rising from a standard chair	95°–100°
Biking	105°
Kneeling	125°
Squatting	>130°

It is important to remember that the single best predictor of postoperative ROM is preoperative motion. The providers must know patients' pre- preoperative condition to accurately assess their postoperative progress and counsel appropriately for outcomes.

Attaining more than 130° of knee flexion after TKA will allow patients to perform the more difficult activities of kneeling and squatting. However, if a patient regains a minimum of 110° to 120° of knee flexion, one should be able to perform the more essential ADLs without difficulty. In terms of knee extension ROM, there are no studies currently that establish how much range is necessary to be fully functional and reflect a successful outcome. Ideally, patients should achieve 0° of knee extension because maintenance of a flexion contracture, especially one that is greater than 15°, has been shown to increase energy expenditure and increase the patient's likelihood of developing clinical issues in both the involved and noninvolved knee. Patients can also develop clinical issues in the lumbar spine, hip, and ankle from compensatory movement. Initiation of knee ROM in the acute phase can be accomplished by employing a continuous passive motion (CPM) machine multiple times a day for various durations. Some postoperative protocols utilize such devices. Although

© 2018 American Academy of Orthopaedic Surgeons

the efficacy of such machines in expediting ROM and improving functional outcome scores is questionable in the literature, they can provide the advantage of promoting early knee flexion and moderating pain through continuous reciprocal movement. The disadvantages are that such devices may increase blood loss and wound complications. They may even increase pain, undermine knee extension, and foster dependency on the device in regaining motion passively rather than doing so actively. Such devices are used in conjunction with assistive and active range of motion (AROM) exercises. Further improvements in ROM can be obtained by the patient stretching independently and by the therapist's utilization of a wide spectrum of skilled manual techniques. Techniques such as passive light manual stretching of the quadriceps and hamstrings can help patients flex and extend beyond what they are willing to achieve independently and elongate immature fibrous tissue. In this author's clinical opinion, performance of passive knee flexion stretching supine or sitting is recommended, as these positions allow the therapist to maintain visual as well as verbal communication with the patient. When knee flexion stretching is performed prone, the benefit of visual communication is lost and the position itself puts unnecessary pressure on the knee. Other beneficial techniques include patellar mobilizations and soft-tissue massage, which can help break down adhesions, improve muscle extensibility, minimize pain, and mobilize swelling. All of these, when combined, can help progress ROM.

Strengthening

In the acute phase, remedial strengthening of the lower extremity is often initiated. It is accomplished with primarily open-chain exercises to moderate excessive weight bearing through the involved knee. Exercises in this stage of recovery are intended to activate and reeducate muscles that have been inhibited prior to and compounded as a result of surgery. The muscle group primarily affected is the quadriceps. Reeducation and strengthening can be accomplished through a progression of a combination of isometric, concentric, and eccentric exercises. A simple example of this is to position a patient sitting on a chair or at the edge of a bed with an ankle weight around the ankle for introduction of progressive resistance, if necessary. The patient is instructed to straighten the knee, which concentrically activates the quadriceps. The patient then holds the contraction isometrically at end range for several seconds (Figure 43.1). Finally, the patient lowers the leg twice as slow to eccentrically activate the quadriceps. Incorporating neuromuscular electrical stimulation via an electrical stimulation device, primarily when the patient presents with knee extensor lag, may assist in regaining quadriceps activation. Reeducation and strengthening of core, hip, and ankle musculature

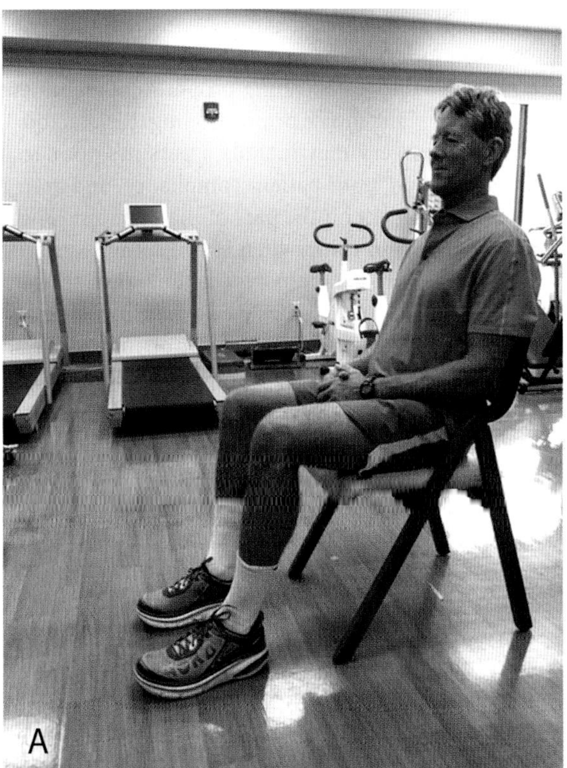

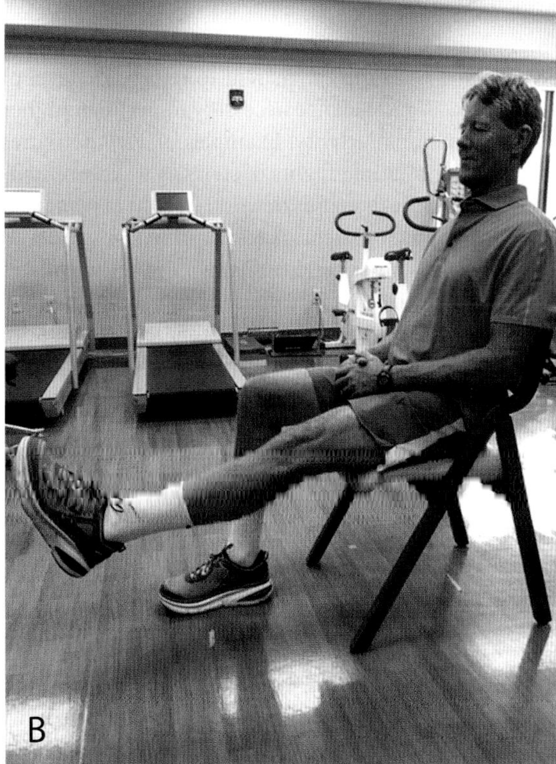

Figure 43.1 **A**, **B**, Photographs of seated active range of motion knee extension. Movement: The patient is seated and actively extends involved knee. Purpose: Remedial quadriceps strengthening by utilizing weight of lower limb as resistance. The movement/strengthening exercise can also used as an assessment tool by therapists to assess degree of quadriceps strength in early stages of recovery. If patients are unable to straighten the knee fully with full engagement of the quadriceps muscle, this indicates use of electrical stimulation to facilitate greater activation and recruitment. This approach has been proven by research to help in the recovery of quadriceps strength.

© 2018 American Academy of Orthopaedic Surgeons

simultaneously can ensure reintegration of complementary muscle activity and provide a more complete exercise program.

Pain Management

One of the main hindrances in progressing through all phases of rehabilitation is pain. Many patients are aware that they will experience varying degrees of postoperative pain despite the provision of pain medication. Many will assume that the level of pain they are experiencing is the level they will have to endure for the duration of their recovery. This should not be the case. During the formative stages of recovery, it is important for physical therapists to establish open communication with the patient to continually explore whether the patient's pain medication regimen is adequate enough to allow toleration of not only daily activity but also the rigors of physical therapy. If it is not, encouraging the patient to consult with the surgeon and/or pain management team again is indicated. A recuperative pain service may be consulted to assist in managing postoperative pain after discharge from the hospital. Once pain is adequately managed, use of palliative soft-tissue techniques can assist even further with pain management. If the pain is not well controlled, the patient will have difficulty improving ROM, achieving functional milestones, and experiencing a successful outcome.

Subacute Phase: Postoperative Phase II (Weeks 2–8) and Postoperative Phase III (Weeks 9–16)

The primary emphasis during this stage is continuing to improve ROM and assisting the patient to regain the level of strength, endurance, and balance necessary to perform higher levels of daily functional activity. Examples of such activities include negotiating multiple flights of stairs as well as returning to and tolerating the demands of work. In light of projected trends, in which younger patients (<65 years old) will undergo arthroplasty as well as older patients being more active in later decades of life, the scope of this phase of rehabilitation has expanded. The goals can include assisting patients to achieve the foundation of strength, endurance, and balance in order to promote desired recreational activity.

Patient Education

Instructions are provided on modifying activity based on the patient's progress with rehabilitation. Some patients who are highly motivated may be advised to scale back activity to allow adequate rest and to foster healing while others may need to be encouraged to actively participate in exercises to facilitate overall progress. Patients are advised to continue edema management with elevation of the affected leg in conjunction with the use of cryotherapy. If a significant amount of edema develops below the knee, patients may be encouraged to discuss with their medical doctor or surgeon whether compression stockings can be used as an adjunct to control swelling. As more ROM, strength, and balance are recovered, the use of assistive devices can be phased out and transfer and gait training is fine-tuned for normalized movement.

Range of Motion

Based on stages of healing, by the fifth week and beyond is a critical window in which to take advantage of the presence of immature scar tissue and improve ROM. Although scar tissue typically does not mature until after the fifth and sixth weeks, there are patients who inherently develop dense scar tissue earlier, making the critical window shorter. The typical time frames that provide a general guide in achieving milestones for knee flexion ROM are:

By the end of 4 weeks postoperatively: Between 90°–100°
By the end of 4–8 weeks postoperatively: Between 100°–110°
By the end of 8–12 weeks postoperatively: Between 110°–120° or greater

A discussion with the surgeon is critical if a patient's ROM is not advancing with therapy. Although there are no general time frames for recovering knee extension, achieving full knee extension before discharge from formal rehabilitation will be an ongoing goal.

In this phase, the patient and therapist can encounter the most difficulty in the recovery process. A patient's success in progressing will be dependent on a multitude of risk factors that may occur preoperatively, intraoperatively, and/or postoperatively. Preoperative factors—such as a history of knee surgeries, the presence of a long-standing knee flexion contracture, and those who are on disability—have been shown to contribute to increased difficulty in regaining knee flexion ROM. Intraoperatively, some of the risk factors include, but are not limited to, establishing proper joint alignment and/or improper implant choice or positioning. Risk factors that may occur after surgery may include a patient's poor response to pain medication, poor patient compliance, and poor rehabilitation management on the part of the therapist. These factors need to be kept in mind when establishing realistic goals for ROM. To address the many risk factors, the term "aggressive rehabilitation" is often employed when high-intensity overstretching that "exceeds the weight of the patient's limb" is used. However, a cultural shift in clinical practice needs to be made away from aggressive approaches and to moderate rehabilitation techniques, and differs from motivating a disengaged patient. Aggressive approaches—such as intense manual overstretching, especially within the first several weeks of recovery, as well as utilization of a standard stationary bike to introduce repetitive revolutions to move a stiff knee into greater knee flexion—can increase shear and patellofemoral joint force and exacerbate existing pain and inflammation. This will inevitably undermine healing, cause progress to plateau or even regress, and will be counterproductive overall. It may even foster the development of compensatory movements in the back, hip, and ankle to avoid further knee pain. A stationary bike can aid in rehabilitation, but we have found that initiating before patients achieve 100° of motion can irritate the newly operated knee. Therefore, we do not initiate the use of the bike until a patient will need to achieve between 100° and 110° of ROM. The use of the bike at this point can promote further gains in ROM.

© 2018 American Academy of Orthopaedic Surgeons

Clinicians need to address all of the underlying components properly that contribute to lack of ROM such as the intensity of pain, severity of swelling, and degree of hamstring and gastrocnemius/soleus tightness. Utilizing short-crank bikes, in which the length of the pedal crank arm is shorter than standard large-crank stationary bikes, can allow for proper revolutions with knee flexion angles of 90° or less. In general, bike therapy after TKA should employ relatively lower resistance settings. Increasing the amount of spin is preferable to increasing resistance. This type of bike can help foster ROM without placing additional stress on the surgical knee.

Employing more palliative soft-tissue techniques in combination with moderated stretching and active ROM exercises would also better assist in the recovery of ROM. Finally, planning days of rest between sessions to allow the joint to recover and prepare it for subsequent rehabilitation sessions can better optimize progress as well.

Some patients will have difficulty achieving adequate ROM after surgery. Inadequate pain control is often the problem, and should be addressed by the surgeon. Utilization of low-load stretching devices, such as dynamic knee splints, may be used as an adjunct, which may prove to be beneficial in improving ROM. These braces are especially helpful for achieving full extension but can be helpful for flexion as well. If stiffness and lack of progress with ROM continues despite such approaches, then a conversation with the surgeon will need to take place to discuss further options, such as manipulation under anesthesia.

Strengthening, Functional Training, and Functional Outcome Measures

Modified progressive resistance training that target muscles of the core—as well as bilateral hips, ankles, and knees—will provide a comprehensive program to foster recovery of functional strength. All programs will be individually designed based on prior level of function, ROM, flexibility, levels of balance, influence of existing comorbidities, postoperative complications, and the patient's short- and long-term goals. Utilizing functional outcome measures, such as the Chair Stand Test, in which a patient repeatedly stands and sits from a standard chair without the use of one's arms for 30 seconds, can help establish baseline measures of lower extremity strength and endurance. Much of the strengthening during this phase will be beyond isometric and open-chain movements and will focus primarily on a combination of both concentric and eccentric movements in more closed-chain positions for functional carryover. An example of this would be a wall squat (Figure 43.2). In this

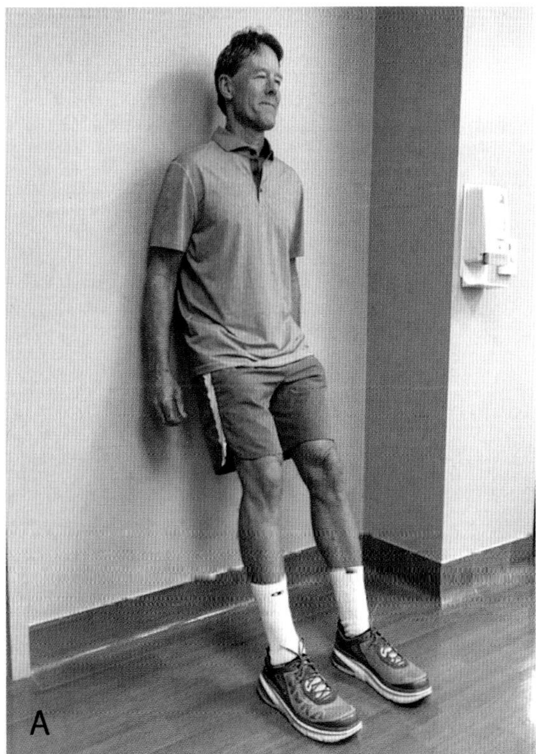

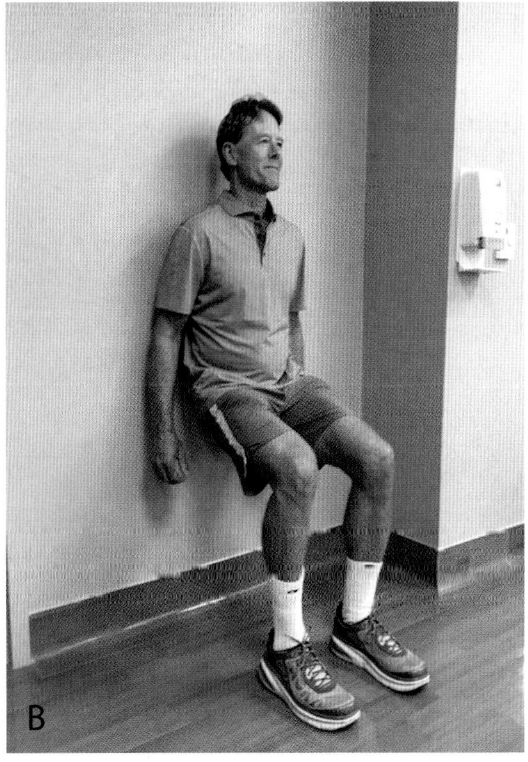

Figure 43.2 **A**, **B**, Photographs of wall squat. Movement: The patient stands with back against a wall, feet shoulder width apart, and feet forward far enough to ensure proper knee angles with squat movement. The patient is instructed to slowly slide the body down the wall until the knees are bent between 100° and 110° to not place excessive pressure on the patellar tendon and irritate peripatellar structures with knee angles that are less. Patient is then instructed to hold the position for several seconds. Finally, the patient is instructed to slide upward to return to the starting position. Modification: A ball can be placed between the lower back and the wall to decrease friction and allow for easier movement. Purpose: General lower extremity strengthening that targets quadriceps in particular in several ways: eccentrically, isometrically, and concentrically. This motion can be performed in conjunction with or as a progression to the functional exercise of standing to and from a sitting position.

© 2018 American Academy of Orthopaedic Surgeons

exercise a patient places the back against a wall and performs a controlled squat eccentrically, holds the position isometrically for a couple of seconds, then concentrically returns to the starting position while maintaining the back against the wall. Special instruction is given for maintaining proper foot and knee alignment and avoiding knee flexion angles less than 90° to minimize excessive patellofemoral pressures. Another example would be to have the patient perform forward lunges (Figure 43.3). These exercises, when combined into a program with other quadriceps-intensive exercises, has shown to result in superior quadriceps strength, 6-minute walk distances, timed up and go times, and stair climb test times. Frequency parameters will be based on therapeutic exercise progression principles. Performance of such general strengthening exercises will be done in concert with the performance of function-specific exercises for the achievement of higher-level functional strength. Functional exercises, such as sidestepping over an 8-inch-high object, will activate and develop muscles that help entry into and exit from a bathtub (Figure 43.4). Practicing step-ups and step-downs from graded height steps help recruit and develop muscles necessary to ultimately negotiate flights of stairs (Figure 43.5). Achievement of comprehensive lower extremity strength that allows for the performance of controlled, unilateral eccentric knee flexion, such as when descending stairs, is often considered the pinnacle of functional strength achievements after TKA.

Balance and Outcome Measures

Addressing balance and proprioception issues simultaneously in this phase of rehabilitation complements assisting the

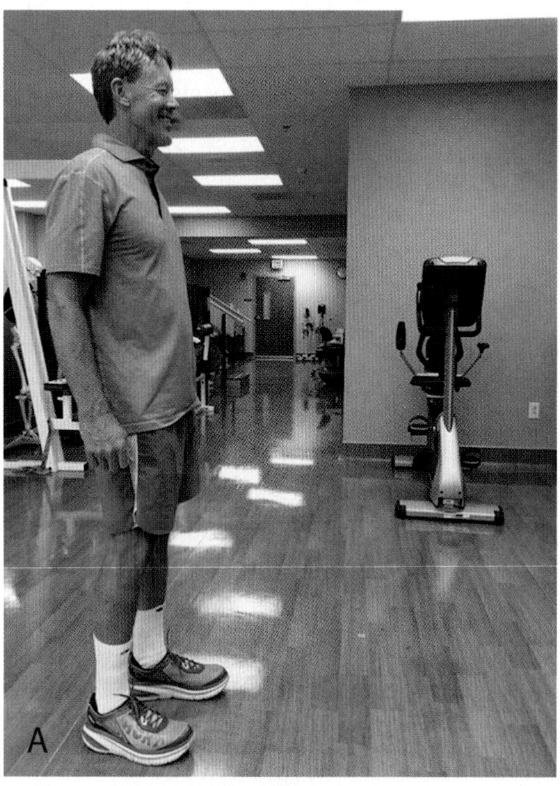

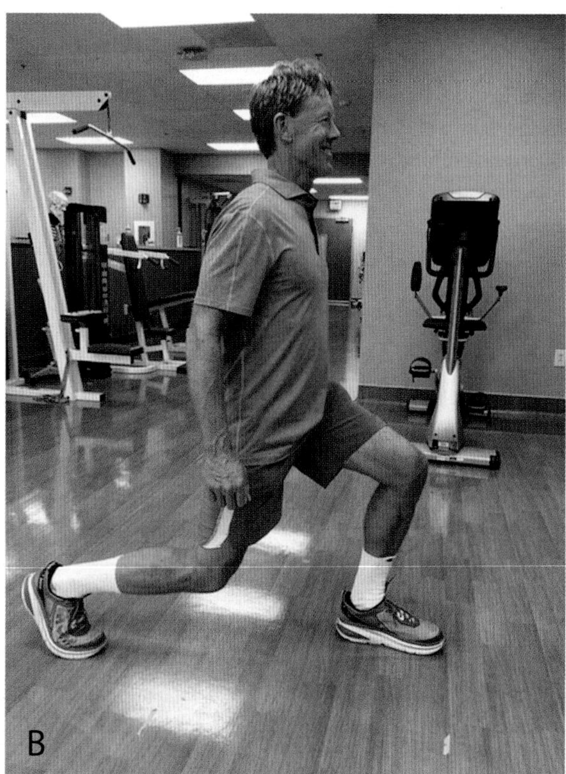

Figure 43.3 **A**, **B**, Photographs of static or dynamic lunge. Movement: *Static lunge:* Mid to late stages of recovery. The patient positions the involved lower extremity forward and noninvolved lower extremity behind with the heel raised; feet are maintained shoulder width apart. The patient then bends both knees to lower the waist and body downward and limits the bend of the forward knee to 100° to 110° to not place excessive pressure on the patellar tendon and irritate peripatellar structures with knee angles that are less. The patient then straightens both knees to return to the starting position. Modification: The patient can hold onto a cane or place the contralateral hand of the involved lower extremity on a stable object for balance and support. *Dynamic lunge:* Late stages of recovery. The patient stands with feet shoulder width apart. The patient takes a step forward while maintaining feet shoulder width apart. The patient then bends both knees to lower the waist and body downward and limits the bend of the forward knee to 100° to 110° to not place excessive pressure on the patellar tendon and irritate peripatellar structures. The patient then brings the leg that is behind forward. The patient then lunges forward with the noninvolved lower extremity and progresses forward; the process is then repeated. Forward lunge steps are alternated between extremities. Modifications: The patient can hold light weights for added resistance. Once in the squat position, the patient can extend arms forward and turn shoulders and arms to one side, back to the center, and then to the opposite side to add more focus to postural/core musculature. Purpose: This exercise is multipurpose. It facilitates general lower extremity strengthening that targets the quadriceps of forward lower extremity in particular in several ways: eccentrically, isometrically, and concentrically. It is also a balance exercise, as well as core and postural exercise. It is for functional movement as well, since it reflects the initial movement of kneeling down onto both knees, which may be a patient goal.

© 2018 American Academy of Orthopaedic Surgeons

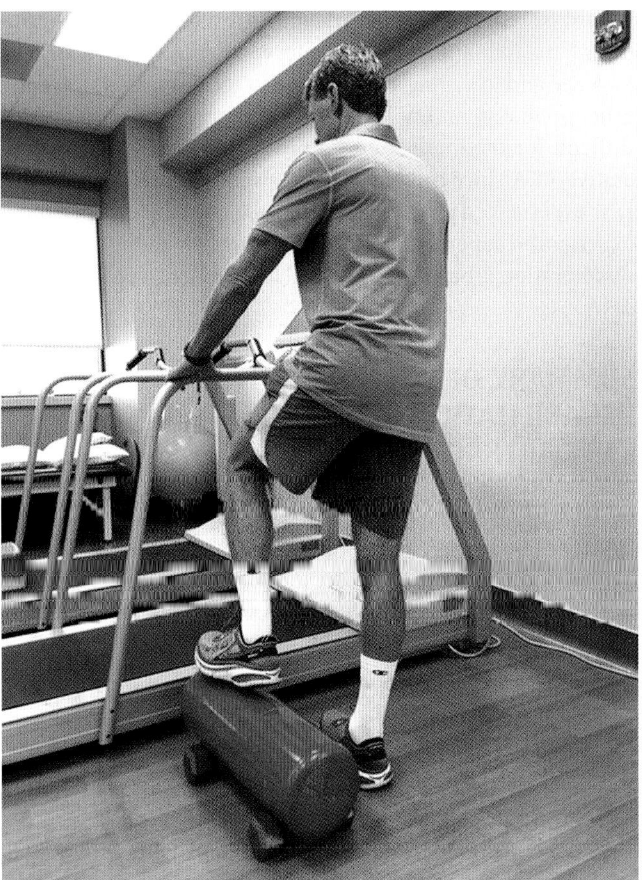

Figure 43.4 Photograph of side-step over. Movement: The patient stands to the side of an object approximately 6 inches to 8 inches in height while holding onto a stable object in front of the patient. The patient flexes both hip and knee and dorsiflexes the foot in order to side-step over the object. The patient is instructed to side-step far enough over the object in order to follow with and allow space for the contralateral lower extremity. The patient repeats this motion over the object again to return to the starting position. Purpose: The exercise is multipurpose. It increases range of motion actively of the involved knee as well as the ipsilateral hip and ankle. It strengthens the lower extremity by activating all muscles associated with each joint to accomplish movement. At the hip, this movement facilitates activation of hip abductors; at the ankle, this movement facilitates activation of dorsiflexors and plantar flexors—all of which are equally as weak as the quadriceps. If the patient is able to be challenged, then the patient should be encouraged to not use hands on a stable object for support. This would promote improvement of general balance and single-leg stability. The exercise introduces lateral movement into the knee to acclimate it to such motions. The exercise promotes functional movement since it mimics getting into and out of a bathtub.

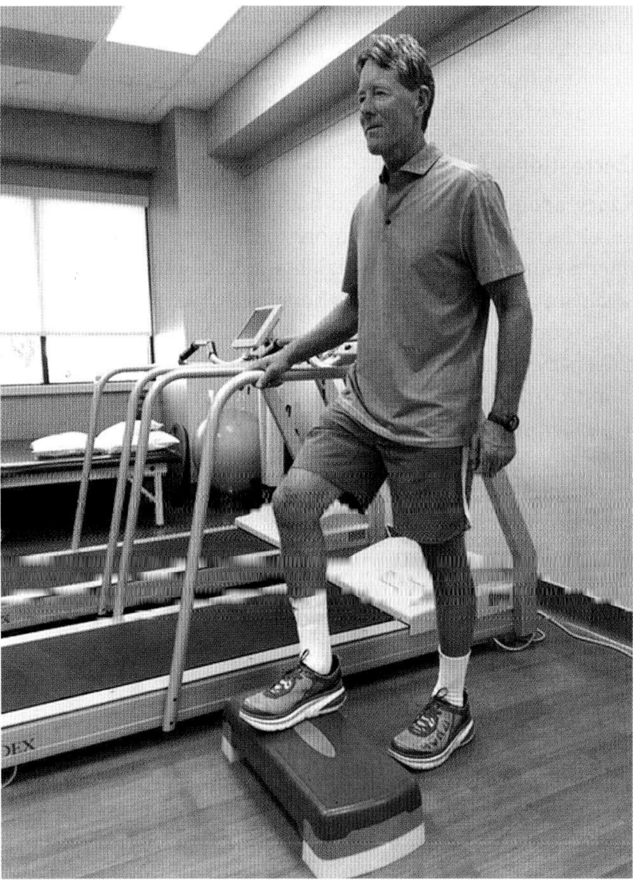

Figure 43.5 Photograph of step progression. Movement: The patient holds onto a stable object while stepping up onto a 2-inch rise step with the involved lower extremity only. The patient then steps backward and downward with the noninvolved lower extremity. Motion is alternated between the extremities. Once the patient is able to accomplish the task easily without pain and good knee stability and control, the patient is progressed to a 4-inch step, then to a 6-inch step, and finally to an 8-inch step. Modification: The patient is encouraged once on the step to balance on single leg for 5 to 10 seconds. This progression could also be used for stepping forward and downward. Purpose: This exercise is multipurpose: for general lower extremity strengthening, single stability and balance, and to promote functional movement that helps the patient to regain the ability to negotiate stairs.

progression of strength and fostering the coordination and integration of muscle activity throughout the lower extremity. Balance and proprioceptive exercises will typically progress from static and dynamic *bilateral* lower extremity movements to static and dynamic *unilateral* lower extremity movements. The ultimate balance goal is to achieve age-appropriate norms reflected by balance outcome measurements such as the single-leg stance and timed up and go tests. In doing so, patients can demonstrate a decreased risk for falls. Another commonly used balance outcome measure is the Berg Balance Scale. Utilization of these and other functional outcome measures—such as the disease-specific Western Ontario and McMasters Universities Arthritis Index, the global health SF-36, and functional capacity tests such as the 6-minute walk, stair climb test, Knee Injury and Osteoarthritis Outcome Score (KOOS) and Lower Extremity Function Scale—can help demonstrate progress, help guide and modify plans of care, and help establish criteria for discharge.

Return to Driving and Work

Clearance for return to driving and return to work come from the surgeon based on the rehabilitation progress of the patient.

© 2018 American Academy of Orthopaedic Surgeons

Generally, patients return to driving after a right TKA at 4 to 6 weeks postoperatively. The patient must be able to transfer the foot from the gas to brake rapidly and be able to apply adequate force. The patient should not be on narcotics as well.

Recreational Activity

Once adequate strength and balance are achieved for high-level functional activities, more recreational specific movements can be the focus of rehabilitation. Patients are cautioned against participating in recreational activities, such as running and jumping, that introduce high impact. Such movements can adversely affect the fixation of the knee implant and cause early failure. Patients are advised to consult with their surgeon for a list of approved activities. Since the majority of insurances will typically not cover rehabilitation beyond the achievement of functional milestones, transitioning the patient to well-skilled athletic or personal trainers who are knowledgeable about the precautions associated with the procedure should be a consideration. Supervised wellness and community recreational programs may also be an avenue of referral for patients.

Peripatellar Pain

Peripatellar pain is common after TKA. Most patients enter surgery with quadriceps atrophy due to prolonged dysfunction from arthritis, and surgery itself initially promotes further muscle atrophy. Forces at the patellofemoral joint are also quite high during activities such as climbing stairs, arising from a low chair/toilet, and squatting, generating up to five times body weight through the patella. Therapy should be directed to strengthening the quadriceps, especially focusing on the vastus medialis. For patients with persistent patellar pain beyond 6 months, we prefer to perform the quadriceps-strengthening exercise in limited flexion (<45°) to avoid overloading and irritating the patella. Persistent peripatellar pain in present in 5% to 15% of TKA patients. These patients should be evaluated by their surgeon for alignment, peripatellar scarring, or other treatable conditions; however, in most cases, the primary cause is persistent quadriceps atrophy.

Some patients undergoing knee arthroplasty require an additional procedure to treat the patella and extensor mechanism. The simplest is a lateral retinacular release. No change in therapy is necessary, but the therapist and patient should be aware that prominent lateral swelling is often persistent for many months after lateral release. Less commonly, patients will have other extensor mechanism procedures, such as quadriceps lengthening, vastus advancement, or tibial tubercle osteotomy. These are more common in revision arthroplasty; the therapist should communicate with the surgeon for specific instructions in these cases.

Thromboembolic and Wound Issues

All patients undergoing TKA should have some form of prophylaxis for deep vein thrombosis (DVT) and pulmonary embolism. Prophylactic modalities include anticoagulants, such as warfarin, enoxaparin, rivaroxaban, and aspirin. While knee and leg ecchymosis is common, any wound drainage should be reported to the surgeon since alterations in postoperative rehabilitation or other intervention may be necessary.

Knee and lower leg swelling is also common after TKA and is not predictive on DVT in the postoperative period. It is often difficult for the inexperienced provider to assess the postoperative TKA since most have pain, swelling, and discoloration. Less experienced providers should seek assistance from a more experienced supervisor or the surgeon when pain, swelling, or discoloration is beyond the typical level seen in a postoperative TKA.

SUMMARY OF POSTOPERATIVE REHABILITATION FOR TOTAL KNEE ARTHROPLASTY

Postoperative Phase I: Acute Care (First 3 Days–2 Weeks)

Goals

- Control postoperative swelling
- Monitor pain levels
- Active Assistive/Active Range of Motion: flexion >80°; extension 0°
- Unassisted bed mobility
- Unassisted transfers, ambulation, and stair negotiation (nonreciprocal) with appropriate assistive device
- Independent or Modified Independent with activities of daily living (ADLs) with assistive devices
- Independent or modified independent with home exercise program

Precautions

- Avoid prolonged sitting, standing, walking
- Severe pain with daily activities and ROM exercises

Treatment Strategies

- Edema management: cryotherapy, elevation, manual techniques to mobilize edema
- Pain management: palliative manual techniques
- Range of motion
  - Passive
    - Use of CPM, initiate 0–60 and advance as tolerated for knee flexion (KF), rolled towel under ankle in supine and sitting for knee extension (KE)
  - Active Assistive
    - Use of contralateral lower extremity (LE) for KF/KE in sitting, use of stretch strap for KF/KE in supine, light manual assist for KF/KE
  - Active
    - Sitting KF/KE or stair stretch for KF/KE
- Bed mobility training
- Transfer, gait, and stair negotiation (nonreciprocal) training with appropriate assistive device
- ADL training with assistive devices
- Increase upright activity tolerance with progressive ambulation distances

© 2018 American Academy of Orthopaedic Surgeons

- Home exercise program (HEP): focus on reactivation and remedial strengthening of quadriceps, core, hip, and ankle musculature

Criteria for Advancement

- Discharge home within 3 to 4 days from hospital or from inpatient rehabilitation when safe with modified mobility
- Gait progression from rolling walker or crutches to cane when able to demonstrate symmetrical weight bearing and step through gait pattern

Postoperative Phase II: Subacute Care (2–8 Weeks)

Goals

- Ongoing edema management and monitoring of pain levels
- Active Assistive/Active Range of Motion: flexion >105°; extension 0°
- Progress weight-bearing status, if necessary
- Begin normalizing gait mechanics with or without assistive device
- Able to ascend and descend 4-inch step with handrail assist and assistive device
- Modified independence or independence with ADLs
- Independent with home exercise program
- Initiate functional outcome measures for baseline levels

Precautions

- Contact MD if ROM plateauing or regressing
- Avoid ambulation without assistive device if gait deviations present.
- Avoid reciprocal stair negotiation without adequate strength/control of involved limb.
- Avoid prolonged sitting, standing, and walking if upright activity exacerbates swelling.
- Avoid severe pain with daily activities and ROM exercises.
- Avoid use of standard upright bike for ROM unless AROM is 110° or greater.
- Avoid consecutive days of intensive ROM.
- Avoid aqua therapy until incision is fully healed and approved by surgeon.

Treatment Strategies

- Edema management: Cryotherapy, elevation, and manual techniques to mobilize edema
- Pain management: Palliative manual techniques
- Range of motion
  - Passive:
    - Discharge CPM, light to moderate manual assist KF/KE, patellar and integumentary mobilizations
  - Active assistive
    - Use of contralateral LE for KF/KE in sitting, supine KF wall slides, supine KF/KE with physioball, use of stretch strap for KF & hamstring/gastroc-soleus flexibility supine, light to moderate manual assist for KF/KE
  - Active
    - For example, sitting KF/KE, stair stretch for KF/KE
- Modalities: Cryotherapy, neuromuscular electrical stimulation for quadriceps
- Therapeutic exercise
  - Open- and closed-chain movements to target core, hip, knee, and ankle muscles
  - Short-crank cycle ergometry for ROM 105° or less
  - Long-crank cycle ergometry for ROM 110° or greater
- Aqua therapy
- Balance and proprioception training: progress bilateral to unilateral when appropriate
- ADL training with assistive devices
- Functional training: Step-up/step-down progression 2 inches to 4 inches

Criteria for Advancement

- Knee flexion >105°
- Absence of quadriceps lag
- Normalized gait pattern with/without assistive device
- Ascend/descend 4 inch step with/without assistive device

Postoperative Phase III: Subacute Care (9–16 Weeks)

Goals

- Ongoing edema management and monitoring of pain levels
- AROM: flexion > 115°; extension 0°
- Transfers and performs upright activity with equal limb symmetry and equal weight bearing independently or with least restrictive assistive device
- Independence with ADLs
- Maximize lower extremity strength, control, and flexibility to meet the demands of high-level ADLs
- Reciprocal stair negotiation: able to ascend and descend 6- to 8-inch step with handrail assist and assistive device, if necessary.
- Functional outcome measures nearing normal levels for chronological age

Precautions

- Contact MD if ROM plateauing or regressing
- Avoid ambulation without assistive device if gait deviations present.
- Avoid reciprocal stair negotiation without adequate strength/control of involved limb
- Avoid running, jumping, or plyometric activity unless allowed by MD.
- Avoid prone position for ROM
- Avoid use of standard upright bike for ROM unless AROM is 110° or greater.
- Avoid consecutive days of intensive ROM.

Treatment Strategies

- Edema management: Cryotherapy, elevation, and manual techniques to mobilize edema
- Pain management: Palliative manual techniques
- Range of motion
  - Passive

© 2018 American Academy of Orthopaedic Surgeons

- Light to moderate manual assist KF/KE, patellar and integumentary mobilizations
  - Active assistive
    - Use of contralateral LE for KF/KE in sitting, supine KF wall slides, supine KF/KE with physioball, use of stretch strap for KF and hamstring/gastrocnemius-soleus flexibility, light to moderate manual assist)
  - Active
    - For example, sitting KF/KE, stair stretch for KF/KE
- Modalities: Cryotherapy, neuromuscular electrical stimulation for quadriceps
- Manual: Patellar and integumentary mobilizations when incision is stable
- Therapeutic exercise
  - Closed-chain, dynamic movements to target core, hip, knee, and ankle musculature
  - Short-crank cycle ergometry for ROM 105° or less
  - Large-crank cycle ergometry for ROM 110° or greater
- Aqua therapy
- Cardiovascular: Bike, elliptical, treadmill
  - Balance and proprioception training: Progress bilateral to unilateral when appropriate, incorporate unstable surfaces when appropriate
- Functional training: Step-up/step-down progression 6 inches to 8 inches

Criteria for Discharge

- Achieved all realistic goals and functional outcomes
- Functional outcome measures within age-appropriate norms
  - Negotiate stairs reciprocally with handrail assist with minimal pain

BIBLIOGRAPHY

Bade MJ, Stevens-Lapsley JE: Restoration of physical function in patients following total knee arthroplasty: an update on rehabilitation practices. *Rehab Med in Rheum Dis* 2012; 24(2):208–214.

Bass S, Cox CE, Salud CJ, Lyman GH, McCann C, Dupont E, Berman C, Reintgen DS. The effects of postinjection massage on the sensitivity of lymphatic mapping in breast cancer. *J Am Coll Surg* 2001;192(1):9–16.

Binkley JM, Stratford PW, Lott SA, Riddle DL: The Lower Extremity Functional Scale (LEFS): scale development, measurement properties, and clinical application. North American Orthopaedic Rehabilitation Research Network. *Phys Ther* 1999;79(4):371–383.

Brotzman S, Manske R: *Clinical Orthopedic Rehabilitation,* ed 3. Philadelphia, PA, Elsevier-Mosby, 2011.

Chen LH, Chen CH, Lin SY, et al: Aggressive continuous passive motion exercise does not improve knee range of motion after total knee arthroplasty. *J Clin Nurs* 2013;22(3–4):389–394.

Cioppa-Mosca J, Cahill J, Cavanaugh J, Corradi-Scalise D, Rudnick H, Wolf A: Post-surgical Rehabilitation Guidelines for the Orthopedic Clinician. St. Louis, MO, Mosby Elsevier, 2006.

Kettelkamp DB: Clinical implications of knee biomechanics. *Arch Surg* 1973;107(3):406–410.

Kittelson AJ, Stackhouse SK, Stevens-Lapsley JE: Neuromuscular electrical stimulation after total joint arthroplasty: a critical review of recent controlled studies. *Eur J Phys Rehabil Med* 2013;28:1–12.

Nelson CL, Kim J, Lotke PA: Stiffness after total knee arthroplasty: surgical technique. *J Bone Joint Surg Am* 2005; 87(Suppl 1 Part 2):264–270.

Papotto B, Mills T: Treatment of severe flexion deficits following total knee arthroplasty: a randomized control trial. *Orthop Nurs* 2012;31(1):29–34.

Stevens-Lapsley JE, Balter JE, Wolfe P, Eckhoff DG, Schwartz RS, Schenkman M, Kohrt WM: Relationship between intensity of quadriceps muscle neuromuscular electrical stimulation and strength recovery after total knee arthroplasty. *Phys Ther* 2012;92(9):1187–1196.

Yashar AA, Venn-Watson E, Welsh T, Colwell CW Jr, Lotke P: Continuous passive motion with accelerate flexion after total knee arthroplasty. *Clin Orth Relat Res* 1997;345:38–43.

© 2018 American Academy of Orthopaedic Surgeons

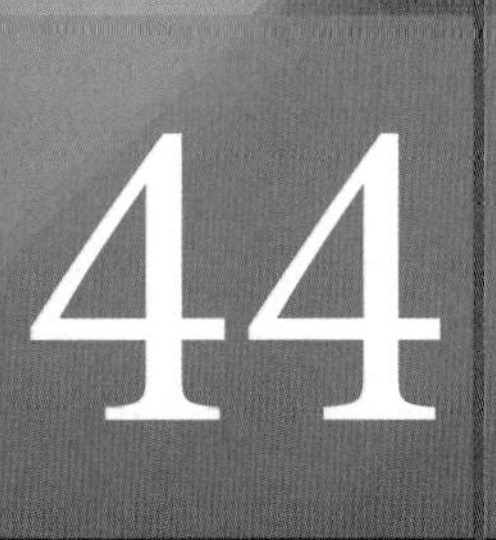

Unicompartmental Knee Arthroplasty

Friedrich Boettner, MD, and Tom Schmidt-Braekling, MD

INTRODUCTION

Unicompartmental knee arthroplasty (UKA) is indicated if degenerative changes are limited to one compartment of the knee. The surgical procedure replaces only the affected compartment, differentiating a medial and lateral unicompartmental knee replacement and the patellofemoral knee replacement (Figure 44.1). The medial unicompartmental knee replacement is the most common of these. Currently, there are 45,000 UKAs and 600,000 primary total knee arthroplasties (TKAs) performed in the United States annually. While the number of TKAs is growing at a rate of 9.4% per year, the number of UKAs is increasing at a rate of 32.5%.

The benefits of a UKA include less blood loss, quicker recovery, shorter hospital stay, increased range of motion (ROM), higher postoperative activity levels, and earlier return to work. UKAs have decreased infection rates and lower perioperative complication rates.

The main disadvantage of UKA compared to TKA is lower long-term survival rates at 15 years compared to TKA. However, more recent studies have shown excellent long-term survival rates of UKA in selected patients.

With improved implant designs and more careful patient selection, the overall results of unicompartmental knee replacement have improved; currently, 10-year survival rates reported by experienced surgeons are better than 95% and quite similar to TKA.

SURGICAL PROCEDURE

Because the UKA replaces only one compartment, the other compartments have to be relatively unaffected by osteoarthritis. It is well known from the literature that the progression of the arthritis in the adjacent compartment remains the main failure mechanism of UKA.

Indication Criteria for Medial and Lateral UKA

- Unicompartmental arthritis (medial or lateral compartment)
- Weight: <200 pounds
- Activity: no heavy labor or high-impact sport (e.g., long-distance running)
- Pain: Be able to pinpoint the pain to the correspondent joint line (the "one finger sign")
- ROM: preoperative flexion >90°
- Flexion contracture <10°
- Varus and valgus deformity <10°

Contraindications

- Inflammatory diseases (e.g., rheumatoid arthritis, crystalline arthropathy)
- Anterior cruciate ligament (ACL) deficiency
- Patellofemoral arthritis (lateral patella facet)
- Severe anterior knee pain

Surgical Technique

The surgical technique for different implants can vary based on the individual implant. However, all medial unicompartmental knee replacements have some similar features:

- The incision is smaller and dissection into the quadriceps tendon is avoided.
- Before implanting a medial unicompartmental knee replacement, the surgeon needs to be certain of the integrity of the ACL and the cartilage in the lateral and patellofemoral compartment using radiographs or MRI.

Dr. Boettner or an immediate family member has received royalties from OrthoDevelopment; is a member of a speakers' bureau or has made paid presentations on behalf of DJO Surgical; serves as a paid consultant to DePuy, A Johnson & Johnson Company, OrthoDevelopment, and Smith & Nephew; has received research or institutional support from Smith & Nephew; and serves as a board member, owner, officer, or committee member of the OrthoForum GmbH. Neither Dr. Schmidt-Braekling nor any immediate family member has received anything of value from or has stock or stock options held in a commercial company or institution related directly or indirectly to the subject of this article.

© 2018 American Academy of Orthopaedic Surgeons

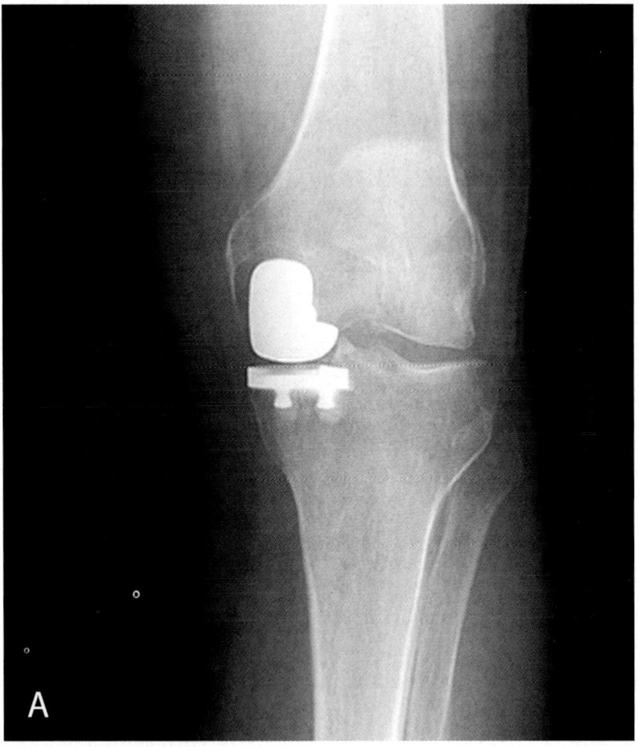

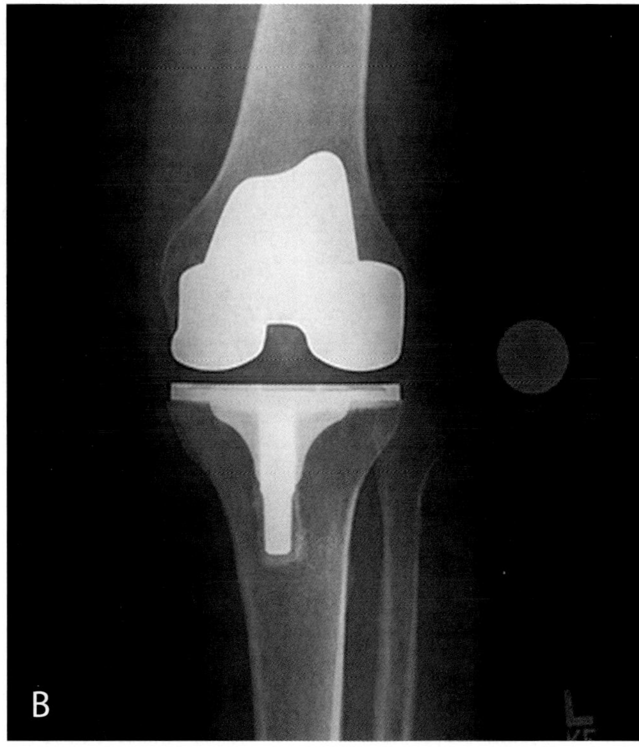

Figure 44.1 Radiograph of a unicompartmental knee replacement (**A**) and a total knee replacement (**B**).

- The medial release around the tibia is limited, and surgical correction of the varus deformity by means of a medial soft-tissue release is not attempted.
- The femoral component should be lined up in order to center the femoral component on the tibial component throughout the ROM from extension to flexion.
- Tibial component rotation is crucial, especially for mobile-bearing unicompartmental knee replacements. Usually, the center of the femoral head is used to align the tibial component.
- The thickness of the plastic insert should be selected to allow for some minimal laxity of the medial joint space. Overstuffing the medial compartment and pushing the knee into valgus alignment should be avoided to decrease the risk of progressive lateral compartment arthritis. A preoperative valgus stress view can help to judge the degree of medial laxity.
- Remove posterior condyle osteophytes and the meniscus to minimize impingement in flexion.
- At the end of the procedure, evaluate the patella tracking to avoid patella lateralization. A lateral release can be considered in cases of maltracking.

Perioperative Complications

In general, the risk of perioperative complications—including deep implant infection, deep venous thrombosis (DVT), and pulmonary emboli—is reduced with UKA compared to TKA. Complications after UKA include:

- DVT and pulmonary emboli: Prophylaxis with coated aspirin is recommended in combination with regional anesthesia.
- The risk for perioperative blood transfusion is minimal; thus, routine preoperative autologous blood donations is not recommended.
- Deep implant infection: Routine 24-hour antibiotic prophylaxis is enforced.
- Instability and mechanical malalignment predispose to early progression of the arthritis in the lateral or patellofemoral compartment.
- Postoperative stiffness is a rare complication.
- Perioperative fractures have been described in the past, but are less common with modern instruments.

POSTOPERATIVE REHABILITATION

In most cases, patients undergoing unicompartmental knee replacement are considered candidates for accelerated rehabilitation and early discharge. Preoperative education classes and prehabilitation can prepare the patient for the early postoperative rehabilitation. As part of these protocols, postoperative exercises and walking with a cane should be reviewed prior to surgery. The patient needs to be familiar with the desired postoperative exercises if the procedure is performed on an outpatient basis or a discharge is planned for postoperative day 1. The patient should develop a clear understanding of postoperative goals and the timeline for rehabilitation prior to surgery. This includes realistic planning of return to work and driving. In general, patients should be able to return to low-demand work, such as office-type jobs, within 1 to 3 weeks and can return to driving a car once they are off all narcotic

 © 2018 American Academy of Orthopaedic Surgeons

pain medications and have pain-free ROM and command over their knee. This is usually the case after 2 to 4 weeks. Communicating realistic expectations is crucial and of special importance for less-invasive procedures such as UKA since patients might be misguided by information presented on the Internet and other media.

Preoperative Exercises

Preoperative conditioning and strengthening is important for patients that plan to benefit from an accelerated postoperative rehabilitation. These exercises include:

- General conditioning on a stationary bike or elliptical machine for 30 minutes as tolerated three to four times a week
- ROM exercises to improve preoperative ROM
- Quadriceps strengthening exercises: Closed-chain exercises: wall sits and mini-squats (0°–45°), as tolerated

Days 1 to 7

Pain Management

- Multimodal pain management is crucial in the first week. It combines regional anesthesia, antiemetic medications, oral and intravenous nonsteroidal anti-inflammatory drugs (NSAIDs) and narcotic pain medications. During the first 7 days, narcotic pain medications should be utilized every 4 to 8 hours as needed.

Activities of Daily Living (ADLs)

- Patients are encouraged to spend the first week in-house or participate in outpatient physical therapy, minimizing the commute to therapy. We do not encourage return to work or driving within the first 7 days. In addition, walking longer distance (>1 block) should be avoided until active range of motion (AROM) 0° to 100° is achieved and swelling of the knee is controlled.
- The patient should be able to achieve independence from external help within the first week after surgery.

Reduce Swelling

After the surgery, it is crucial to minimize swelling in order to avoid the quadriceps inhibition phenomenon and facilitate early ROM.

- Icing the knee multiple times a day or utilizing commercial cold-therapy compression devices, such as Game Ready (Game Ready®, Concord, CA) is recommended.
- An elastic bandage can help to reduce the swelling. The bandage should be applied from the foot toward the knee to minimize the risk of calf and foot swelling.
- NSAIDs can be considered as part of multimodal postoperative pain management.
- Reduce walking in the first 3 days. The goal is not to return to unlimited walking in the first 7 days. The priority during the first 3 to 7 days is to reduce the swelling and regain ROM. Both are the requirement for more aggressive work on strength and increased walking.

Range of Motion

- Regaining full extension is of crucial importance during the early rehabilitation. Therefore, the leg should be positioned in extension with a towel under the ankle to facilitate full extension, especially in beds with a soft mattress. Routine use of a knee immobilizer is not necessary in patients undergoing unicompartmental knee replacements; however, knee immobilizers can be utilized during the night in patients who struggle to regain full extension.
- The patient should be instructed to activate the quadriceps and push the knee into the bed until full extension is achieved (active quadriceps isometrics). Extension exercises should be performed 15 minutes six times a day during the first 7 days. The therapist can support this early phase by passive hamstring and gastrocnemius soleus stretches, pushing the knee into full extension with a towel under the ankle
- Postoperative flexion exercises can incorporate passive range of motion (PROM) exercises on a continuous passive motion (CPM) machine during the first 7 days after surgery. Because most patients progress relatively fast to 100° of flexion, long-term utilization of a CPM machine is rarely indicated.
- Active patient-controlled flexion exercises as well as therapist-guided PROM exercises are initiated within days of surgery. The patient should spend 15 to 30 minutes six times a day working on flexion.
  Goals: 90° by Postoperative Day (POD) 2, 110° by POD 7
- Once the patient achieves flexion beyond 90°, active flexion exercises in a seated position are the mainstay of home therapy.

Strength Training

- We limit early strength training to gait training and isometric exercises involving the quadriceps, gluteal muscles, and the core muscles.
- Too aggressive early strength training, including weights or squatting exercises, should be avoided until full ROM is achieved, which is usually by 7 days after surgery.
- Basic strength training in the first week includes straight leg raises and isometric quadriceps and hamstring exercises.

Gait Training and Proprioceptive Exercises

- Within the first 7 days, focus is on basic gait training utilizing a cane for support, achieving full weight bearing. The patient should focus on full extension during heel strike.
- Stair climbing can be initiated the day after surgery utilizing one step at a time holding on to the railing. The patient will go up the stairs with the nonoperated leg and down the stairs with the operated leg first.
- Basic proprioceptive exercises involve standing on the operated leg and balancing the body. Once the patient has good control on a hard surface, balance exercises can incorporate foam cushions. Balance training can also incorporate weight shifting from side to side and forward to back.

© 2018 American Academy of Orthopaedic Surgeons

Adjuvant Treatments

- Local ice (commercial ice and compression device)
- Elevation and compression (ACE bandage) to reduce swelling.
- Electrical muscle stimulation (EMS) can be utilized to augment ice, elevation and compression.

Days 8 to 21

Pain Management

- During the second and third week, the patient should reduce exposure to narcotic pain medication. Usually, more potent narcotics should be utilized prior to physical therapy and at night. The patient can be moved to less aggressive pain medication. Tramadol and acetaminophen are good alternatives to narcotic pain medication during this phase of rehabilitation.

Activities of Daily Living

- Once the swelling is controlled and the patient has achieved AROM 0° to 110°, walking distance can be increased.
- The patient should now participate in outpatient physical therapy.
- Return to work can often be achieved within 2 weeks after surgery. However, this is only a realistic goal if the patient has achieved good AROM and full extension.
- The patient has to be off narcotic pain medication and has to have full control over the operated leg to return to driving. Driving is usually possible within 2 weeks after left UKA and 3 to 4 weeks after right UKA.

Adjuvant Treatments

- Local ice (commercial ice and compression device) utilized after physical therapy and after longer walks
- Elevation and compression (elastic bandage) to reduce swelling: During the second and third week, the patient should utilize elevation and compression if swelling is encountered as a result of increasing activities.

Range of Motion

- Active quadriceps isometrics to achieve full extension are continued 15 minutes six times a day. The patient should be able to achieve full extension during active extension exercises. Patients who have not achieved full active extension usually need to slow down their daily activities and focus on regaining full extension. Passive hamstring and gastrocnemius-soleus stretches pushing the knee into full extension with a towel under the ankle remain an important part of every physical therapy session.
- Active patient-controlled flexion exercises as well as therapist-guided PROM exercises are continued. The patient should spend 15 to 30 minutes four to six times a day working on flexion.
  Goals: 120° by 2 weeks, 130° by 3 weeks after surgery
- Caution: Patients who have not achieved full extension and flexion beyond 110° cannot return to work or advance strength training.

Strength Training

- Once AROM 0° to 110° is achieved, more aggressive strength training exercises can be initiated.
- Starting with straight leg raises and isometric quadriceps and hamstring exercises, the patient is advanced during the second and third week to the following:
  - Stationary Bike: with increasing resistance 20 to 30 minutes a day
  - Closed-chain exercises: wall sits and mini-squats (0°–30°)
  - Heel raise, toe raise

Gait Training and Proprioceptive Exercises

- Gait training with and without a cane. The focus is on full extension during heel strike and establishing a balanced gait pattern.
- Stair climbing can be advanced to alternating steps as tolerated. During the first 2 to 3 weeks, the hand railing is utilized for support.
- Proprioceptive exercises, including heel raise and toe raise standing on a hard surface, balance exercises on foam cushions or balance boards. Weight shifting exercises from side to side and forward to back.

Days 21 to 35

Pain Management

- The patient should now be off narcotic pain medications. Pain management is achieved using NSAIDs once the patient has stopped DVT prophylaxis with coated aspirin. In addition, acetaminophen and tramadol are the mainstay of pain management after 3 weeks.

Activities of Daily Living

- Outpatient physical therapy is continued one to three times a week.
- In coordination with the physical therapist, the patient can now return to the gym to increase ability to work on strength and conditioning.
- The patient can now return to more vigorous work schedules, including traveling.
- Return to driving can be anticipated by 3 weeks after surgery.

Adjuvant Treatments

- Local ice is now only utilized after physical therapy or gym exercises.
- Swelling should be minimal by 3 weeks after surgery.

Range of Motion

- Active quadriceps isometrics to achieve full extension are continued 15 minutes three times a day. The patient should now easily achieve full extension during active extension exercises. The patient should display full extension while walking during heel strike. Passive hamstring and gastrocnemius-soleus stretches pushing the knee into full extension are continued during the warm-up phase in physical therapy.
- Active patient-controlled flexion exercises as well as therapist-guided PROM exercises are continued. The patient should

© 2018 American Academy of Orthopaedic Surgeons

spend 15 minutes four times a day working on flexion. Flexion exercises now incorporate squatting down to reach the floor and getting up from a low chair.
Goals: >130° of ROM

Strength Training

- Stationary bike or elliptical machine: increasing resistance 30 minutes
- Closed-chain exercises: wall sits and tquads (0°–45°)
- Leg presses (0°–45°)

Gait Training and Proprioceptive Exercises

- Patient should have a balanced gait without a cane. Continued focus is on full extension during heel strike and on a balanced gait pattern.
- Stair climbing with alternating steps is continued. Independent stair climbing should be achieved by 5 weeks after surgery.
- Proprioceptive exercises, including heel raise and toe raise standing on a hard surface, and more complex balance exercises on balance boards. More dynamic weight-shifting exercises from side to side and forward to back.

Beyond 35 Days after Surgery

Pain Management

- NSAIDs or acetaminophen are utilized as needed.

Activities of Daily Living

- Outpatient physical therapy is continued once a week to address functional, ROM, and strength deficits.
- The patient is encouraged to return to his gym routine. Supervision by a physical therapist is encouraged, and the once-a-week therapy session can be utilized to review gym exercises.

Adjuvant Treatments

- Local ice is utilized, primarily after exercises.

Range of Motion

- Active quadriceps isometrics to achieve full extension, passive hamstring and gastrocnemius-soleus stretches pushing the knee into full extension, and active flexion exercises are continued as part of the daily exercise routine and during the warm-up prior to gym and physical therapy exercises.
- Patients should achieve 0° to 130° ROM by 5 weeks after surgery.

Strength Training

- Stationary bike or elliptical machine: increasing resistance 30 to 60 minutes
- Closed-chain exercises: wall sits and mini-squats (0°–60°)
- Leg presses (0°–45°) with increasing resistance

Gait Training and Proprioceptive Exercises

- Patient should have a balanced gait without a cane.
- Patient should achieve independent stair climbing by 3 to 5 weeks after surgery.
- Proprioceptive exercises, including balance boards and dynamic weight-shifting exercises, should be incorporated into the gym and physical therapy routine.

By 2 months after the surgery, the patient should have achieved all milestones and should be able to discontinue physical therapy. Beginning 6 weeks after surgery, sport-specific exercises can be incorporated into the physical therapy session to prepare the patient to return to sport.

Sport after Unicompartmental Knee Arthroplasty

Patients should be encouraged to remain physically active after unicompartmental knee replacement, although technically more demanding activities (skiing, tennis) should be delayed until 3 months after surgery. Appropriate sport activities after UKA are guided by the 1999 Knee Society recommendations. The authors recommend the following activities for patients with knee replacement: aerobics (low impact), bicycling (stationary), bowling, croquet, ballroom dancing, jazz dancing, walking, square dancing, golf, shooting, shuffle boarding and swimming. For patients with previous experience in the sport, the authors recommend: bicycling, canoeing, hiking, rowing, speed walking, skiing (cross-country and alpine), tennis (doubles) and weight lifting. Although not recommended by the Knee Society guidelines for patients undergoing total knee replacement, patients might return to lower impact: baseball, softball, squash, tennis (singles), racquetball, gymnastic and medium-impact aerobics.

SUMMARY

Unicompartmental knee replacement allows for fast progression through physical therapy, and many patients are able to return to work and driving within 1 to 3 weeks after surgery. However, patients should only be advanced to increased activities and strength training once 0° to 110° ROM is achieved. It is of outmost importance that the patient has achieved full active extension by 1 week after surgery. Patients need to be informed that postoperative rehabilitation can vary from patient to patient and not all patients return to work within 3 weeks after surgery. Supervision by a knowledgeable therapist as well as earlier follow-ups (1–2 weeks after surgery) with the surgeon allow evaluation of whether a patient can continue a more accelerated rehabilitation, including return to work, or whether special attention is necessary to address functional limitations.

BIBLIOGRAPHY

Berger RA, Nedeff DD, Barden RM, Sheinkop MM, Jacobs JJ, Rosenberg AG, Galante JO: Unicompartmental knee arthroplasty. Clinical experience at 6- to 10-year followup. *Clin Orthop Relat Res* 1999;(367):50–60.

Fuchs S, Frisse D, Laass H, Thorwesten L, Tibesku CO: Muscle strength in patients with unicompartmental arthroplasty. *Am J Phys Med Rehabil* 2004;83(8):650–654; quiz 5–7, 62.

© 2018 American Academy of Orthopaedic Surgeons

Goodfellow J, O'Connor J. The anterior cruciate ligament in knee arthroplasty. A risk-factor with unconstrained meniscal prostheses. *Clin Orthop Relat Res* 1992;(276):245–252.

Healy WL, Iorio R, Lemos MJ: Athletic activity after total knee arthroplasty. *Clin Orthop Relat Res* 2000;(380):65–71.

Koskinen E, Eskelinen A, Paavolainen P, Pulkkinen P, Remes V: Comparison of survival and cost-effectiveness between unicondylar arthroplasty and total knee arthroplasty in patients with primary osteoarthritis: a follow-up study of 50,493 knee replacements from the Finnish Arthroplasty Register. *Acta Orthop* 2008;79(4):499–507.

Kozinn SC, Scott R: Unicondylar knee arthroplasty. *J Bone Joint Surg Am* 1989;71(1):145–150.

Murray DW, Goodfellow JW, O'Connor JJ: The Oxford medial unicompartmental arthroplasty: a ten-year survival study. *J Bone Joint Surg Br* 1998;80(6):983–989.

Riddle DL, Jiranek WA, McGlynn FJ: Yearly incidence of unicompartmental knee arthroplasty in the United States. *J Arthroplasty* 2008;23(3):408–412.

Swank ML, Alkire M, Conditt M, Lonner JH: Technology and cost-effectiveness in knee arthroplasty: computer navigation and robotics. *Am J Orthop (Belle Mead NJ)* 2009;38(2 Suppl):32–36.

Yang KY, Wang MC, Yeo SJ, Lo NN: Minimally invasive unicondylar versus total condylar knee arthroplasty–early results of a matched-pair comparison. *Singapore Med J* 2003;44(11):559–562.

 © 2018 American Academy of Orthopaedic Surgeons

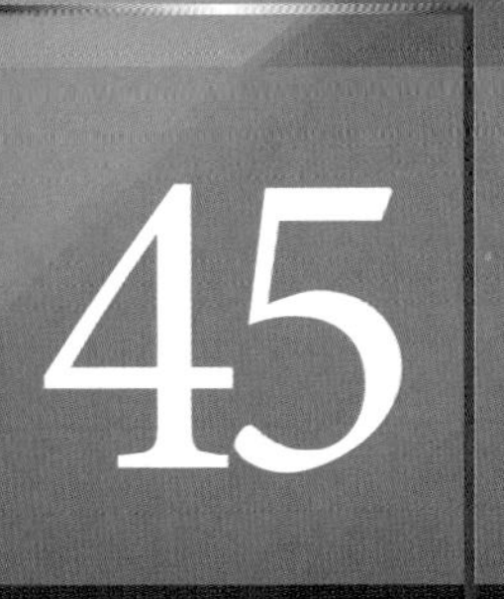

Tibial and Femoral Osteotomy

S. Robert Rozbruch, MD, and Austin T. Fragomen, MD

INTRODUCTION

Osteotomy is a reconstructive surgery that involves cutting the bone to obtain limb deformity correction and/or limb length equalization. In this chapter, we focus on the long bones of the lower extremity: the femur and tibia. Osteotomy of the femur and tibia may be indicated for both children and adults. In most cases, the goal of rehabilitation is simply to maintain adjacent joint range of motion (ROM) and muscle strengthening as well as progressing gait within certain weight-bearing limitations. There are a variety of treatment variations that include location of osteotomy, acute or gradual deformity correction, bone lengthening, and choice of hardware. The etiologies of deformity include congenital, posttraumatic, and developmental. The etiology, location of the osteotomy, use of internal or external fixation, postoperative immobilization, and the amount of limb lengthening or shortening will affect the rehabilitation needs and challenges (Table 45.1).

SURGICAL PROCEDURE

Osteotomy is indicated for correction of deformity and/or limb lengthening. When analyzing a deformity, the proximal and distal bone axes are drawn to form an angle at the apex of deformity. In most cases, the osteotomy is performed at the apex of deformity; the bone is straightened and then stabilized. Deformity correction may be done acutely with an open, closed, or neutral wedge, and stabilized with plate and screws, an intramedullary (IM) rod, or an external fixator. The indications for gradual correction are large deformity, compromised soft tissue envelope, and the need for bone lengthening. These are done with external fixation or an internal lengthening IM rod.

Distraction osteogenesis is used for gradual bone lengthening and deformity correction. Ilizarov showed that bone could successfully regenerate if a low-energy osteotomy was performed, proper stability was accomplished, and distraction was done with a proper rate and rhythm (usually 1 mm per day divided into 3–4 adjustments per day).

Osteotomy Technique Variations

Acute Deformity Correction and Insertion of Plate

This technique is indicated for moderate deformity in the proximal or distal femur. A common use of this technique is for correction of a distal femur valgus deformity with an open wedge correction and insertion of a locked plate. Other indications include varus deformity of the distal femur and proximal femur malunion. In the tibia, acute correction is used to correct moderate varus deformity of the proximal tibia with an open wedge correction and insertion of a locked plate. Other indications include angular deformity correction of the distal tibia and realignment of the ankle.

Acute Deformity Correction and Insertion of Intramedullary Rod

This approach is indicated for correction of rotational and/or angular deformity in the diaphysis of the femur. This is indicated for a patient with congenital femur malrotation or for a malunion after trauma. While this can be done in the tibia, it carries a greater risk of compartment syndrome and nerve injury.

Limb Lengthening with Internal Lengthening Intramedullary Rod

This approach is indicated for leg length discrepancy (LLD) and can be done in the femur or tibia. Acute correction of moderate deformity may be done followed by gradual lengthening. In the femur, the IM rod can be inserted antegrade or retrograde.

Dr. Fragomen or an immediate family member has received royalties from Stryker; is a member of a speakers' bureau or has made paid presentations on behalf of Nuvasive and Smith & Nephew; serves as a paid consultant to Nuvasive, Smith & Nephew, and Synthes; and serves as a board member, owner, officer, or committee member of the Limb Lengthening Research Society. Dr. Rozbruch or an immediate family member has received royalties from Small Bone Innovations and Smith & Nephew; is a member of a speakers' bureau or has made paid presentations on behalf of Ellipse Technologies, Smith & Nephew, and Stryker; serves as a paid consultant to Ellipse Technologies, Small Bone Innovations, Smith & Nephew, and Stryker; has received nonincome support (such as equipment or services), commercially derived honoraria, or other non-research–related funding (such as paid travel) from Informa and Springer; and serves as a board member, owner, officer, or committee member of the Limb Lengthening Reconstruction Society.

© 2018 American Academy of Orthopaedic Surgeons

Table 45.1 OSTEOTOMY TYPES WITH SURGICAL AND REHABILITATION NOTES

Location	Fixation	Acute/Gradual Correction	Diagnosis/ Etiology	Goal of Surgery	Surgical Notes	Rehabilitation Guidelines
Proximal femur	Plate	Acute	Malunion	Rotational and angular deformity correction	Use blade plate	PWB for 6 wk; hip ROM
Femur diaphysis	IM rod	Acute	Malunion, congenital	Rotational and angular deformity correction	Percutaneous osteotomy and rod insertion	WBAT; hip and knee ROM
Distal femur (DFO)	Plate	Acute	Arthrosis, knee deformity	Angular deformity correction	Use locked plate	PWB for 6 wk; knee ROM
Middle to distal femur	Internal lengthening rod	Gradual	LLD, deformity Malunion, congenital	Equalization of leg lengths and correction of deformity	Can do acute correction of angular and rotational deformity	PWB for 3–4 mo, hip extension, knee ROM
Middle to distal femur	External fixation	Gradual	LLD, large deformity Malunion, congenital	Equalization of leg lengths and correction of deformity	Can do acute correction of angular and rotational deformity	WBAT; hip extension, knee ROM
Proximal tibia (PTO)	Plate	Acute	Arthrosis, knee deformity	Correction of deformity	Correct varus deformity <10°	PWB for 6 wk; knee ROM
Proximal and middle tibia	External fixation	Gradual	Tibial deformity and LLD, arthrosis, knee deformity	Equalization of leg lengths and correction of deformity	Used for complex or large deformity	WBAT, knee and ankle ROM, especially knee extension, ankle DF
Middle tibia	Internal lengthening rod	Gradual	LLD	Equalization of leg lengths		PWB for 3–4 mo, knee and ankle ROM, especially knee extension, ankle DF
Distal tibia (SMO)	Plate	Acute	Ankle deformity Malunion, congenital	Correction of deformity	Correct varus or valgus of <10°	PWB for 6 weeks, ankle ROM
Distal tibia	External fixation	Gradual	Ankle deformity Malunion, congenital LLD	Equalization of leg lengths and correction of deformity	Used for complex or large deformity	WBAT, ankle ROM, especially DF

DF = dorsiflexion of ankle, DFO = distal femoral osteotomy, IM = intramedullary, LLD = leg length discrepancy, PTO = proximal tibial osteotomy, PWB = partial weight bearing, ROM = range of motion (active and passive), SMO = supramalleolar osteotomy, WBAT = weight bearing as tolerated.

Lengthening and/or Gradual Deformity Correction with External Fixation

This approach is indicated in children with open growth plates and for patients who have narrow IM canals or deformity, for whom an IM rod is contraindicated. This is also indicated for patients with large deformity for whom acute correction would be dangerous. Patients with infection, or poor soft-tissue envelope, are indicated for external fixation. The external fixator also allows fine-tuning of deformity correction after surgery is complete. This can be helpful in complex situations in which the goal is to achieve a plantigrade foot. Patient feedback regarding the position of the foot while the patient is standing can be very reliable.

Bone Transport with External Fixation

When there is bone loss from infection, trauma, or tumor, limb salvage reconstruction can be accomplished with bone transport. The bone defect is closed by apposing the adjacent bone ends. The limb shortening is treated with lengthening of the bone in a different location (Table 45.1).

REHABILITATION CHALLENGES

Femur

After reconstruction of the femur, the main focus is on knee motion. Patients will lose terminal extension and flexion without a diligent exercise program. Exercise to maintain hip motion is also important. The rehabilitation goal is to maintain hip and knee ROM and to strengthen the muscles around the hip and knee (Figures 45.1 and 45.2). Both active (AROM) and passive ROM (PROM) are needed (Figure 45.3).

Partial weight bearing is allowed until there is adequate consolidation of bone radiographically. Passive extension of the hip is achieved with manual stretching and by spending time in the prone position (5 minutes, four times per day) (Figure 45.4). PROM of the knee to maximize extension and flexion (Figure 45.5) is prescribed (15 repetitions four times per day). Passive stretches are held for a count of 5 seconds.

Tibia

After reconstruction of the tibia, the main focus is on knee and ankle motion. Patients will lose terminal motion of knee and ankle, especially knee extension and ankle dorsiflexion, without a focused exercise program. The rehabilitation goal is to maintain knee and ankle ROM (AROM and PROM) and to strengthen the muscles around the knee and ankle.

Partial weight bearing is allowed until there is adequate consolidation of the bone. AROM and PROM of the knee and ankle are prescribed. The focus is on passive ankle dorsiflexion and knee extension (15 repetitions four times per day) (Figures 45.6 and 45.7). Splinting the knee in extension and the ankle in dorsiflexion may be needed when risk of contracture is high.

External Fixation

External fixation pins pierce skin and other soft-tissue structures. This increases the difficulty of maintaining adjacent joint

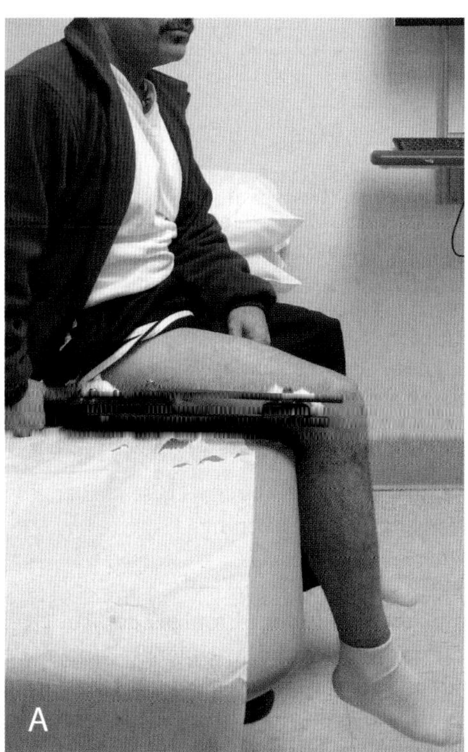

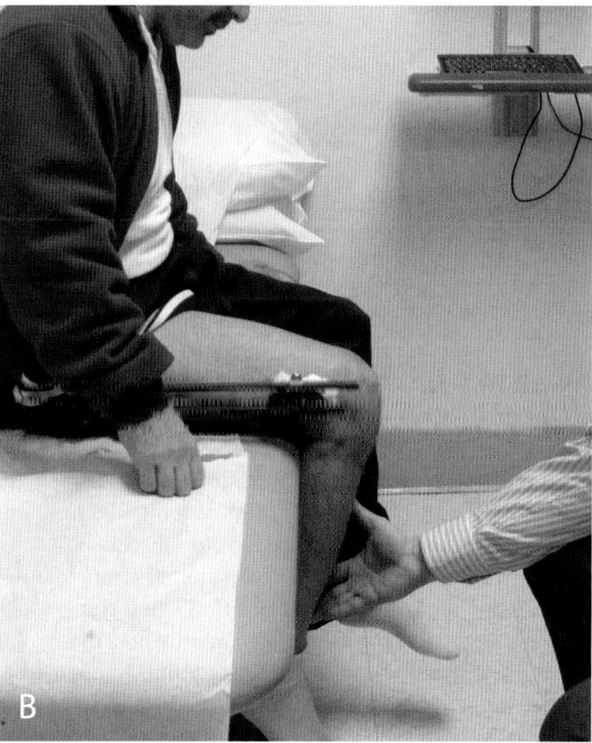

Figure 45.1 **A**, Photograph of desirable resting position after femur osteotomy with knee at 90° of flexion and foot dangling. This helps the patient maintain knee flexion. **B**, Photograph of passive flexion greater than 90° by therapist after femoral osteotomy.

© 2018 American Academy of Orthopaedic Surgeons

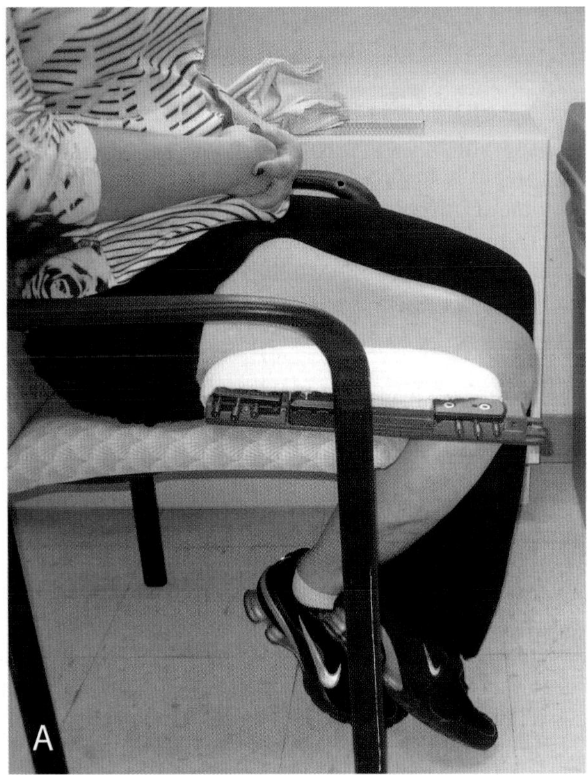

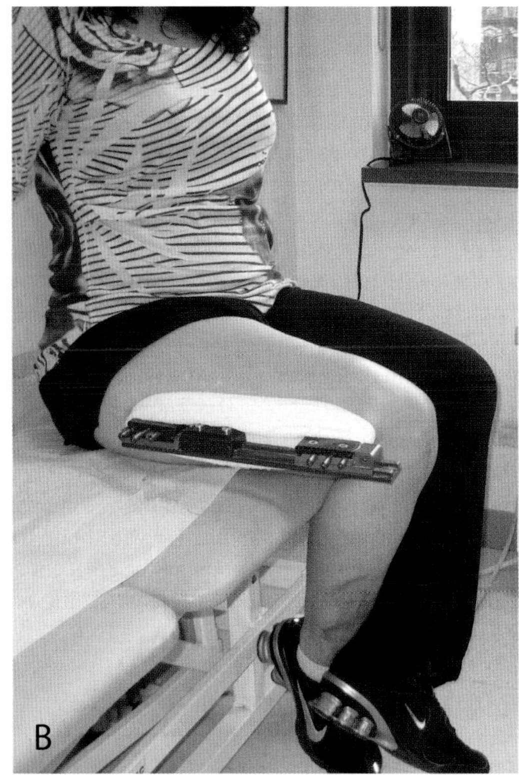

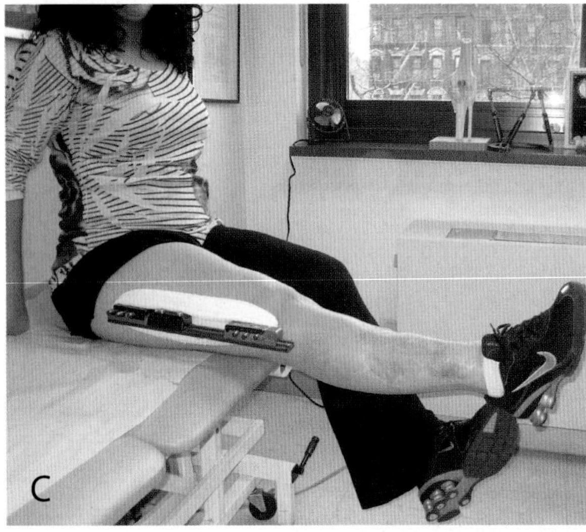

Figure 45.2 **A**, Photograph of passive knee flexion using the other leg while seated in a chair after femoral osteotomy. The foot is resting on the floor. **B**, Photograph of passive knee flexion using the contralateral leg after femoral osteotomy with the leg dangling over the side of the bed. **C**, Photograph of passive extension of the knee using the contralateral leg after femoral osteotomy.

ROM. Upon completion of the surgical procedure, it is ascertained that there is full unencumbered ROM of joints. Pain and a hesitancy to move the joints is what leads to subsequent joint stiffness. Furthermore, the shape of the external fixator may naturally put the joint into a flexed position when resting. For example, a circular frame on the leg naturally puts the knee into flexion when resting supine. Pacing a bump under the foot is needed to maintain the knee in full extension. With low-profile internal fixation, this problem is less challenging. In general, patients are allowed to be weight bearing as tolerated (WBAT) after external fixation. This is not the case for plate fixation where weight bearing is usually protected for the first several weeks after surgery. These challenges are further increased with limb lengthening.

Limb Lengthening

Distraction is typically done 1 mm per day. The challenges outlined earlier are increased when lengthening is done. While muscle does have the ability to stretch and grow, typical patterns of stiffness are expected. During tibia/fibula lengthening, the gastrocnemius-soleus complex becomes increasingly tight, leading to a loss of knee extension and a loss of ankle dorsiflexion (DF). Exercise aimed to extend the knee and dorsiflex the ankle is mandatory. Both AROM and PROM are needed.

 © 2018 American Academy of Orthopaedic Surgeons

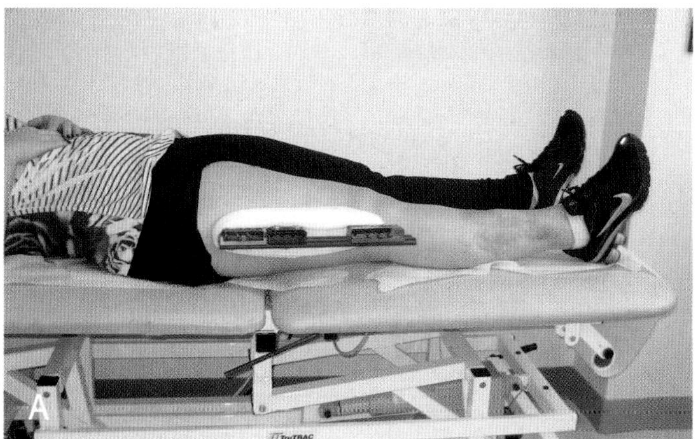

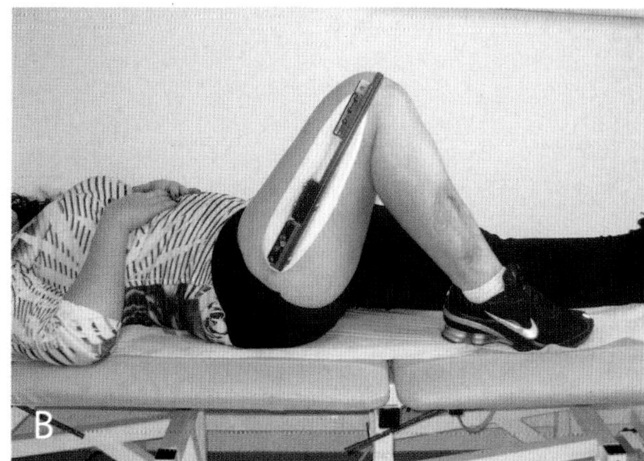

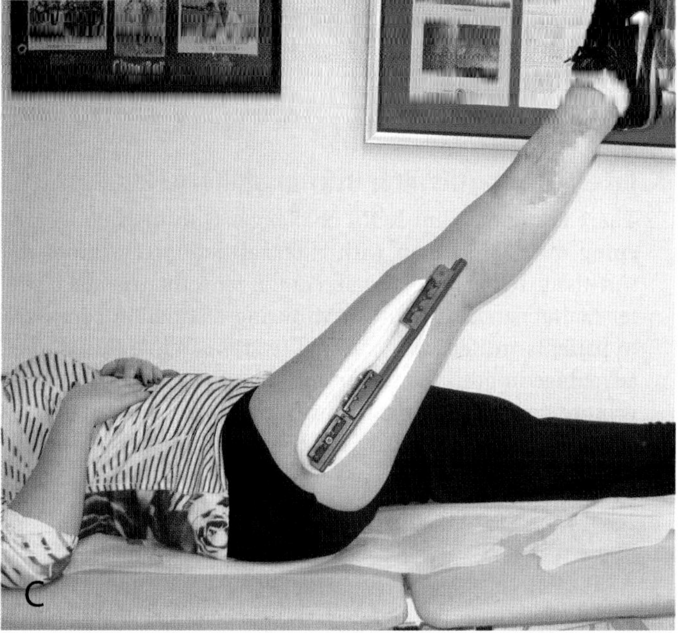

Figure 45.3 **A**, Photograph of the knee in full extension after femoral osteotomy is the supine position. **B**, Photograph of the heel slide actively done by the patient. This works on active hip flexion and active knee flexion. This is an exercise done 2 to 3 weeks after femoral osteotomy. **C**, Photograph of the leg lift. This works on active hip flexion and isometric quadriceps. This is an exercise done 3 to 4 weeks after surgery.

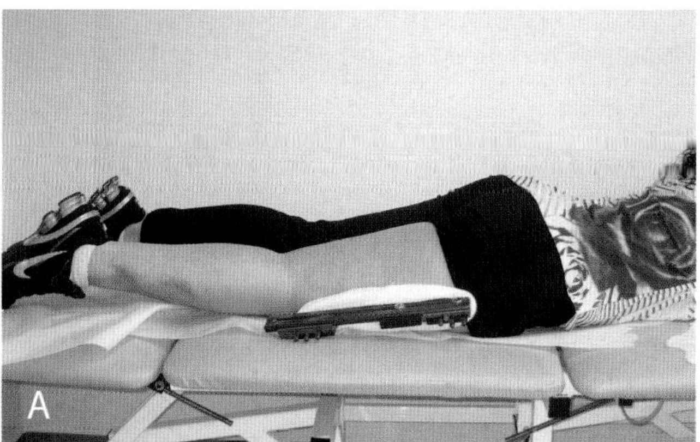

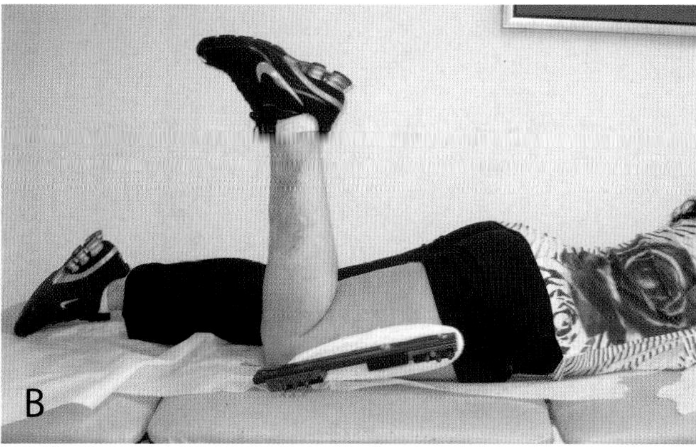

Figure 45.4 **A** and **B**, Photographs of prone knee flexion after femoral osteotomy. This can be done both passively at first and then actively. This stretches the rectus femoris and the hip flexors.

© 2018 American Academy of Orthopaedic Surgeons

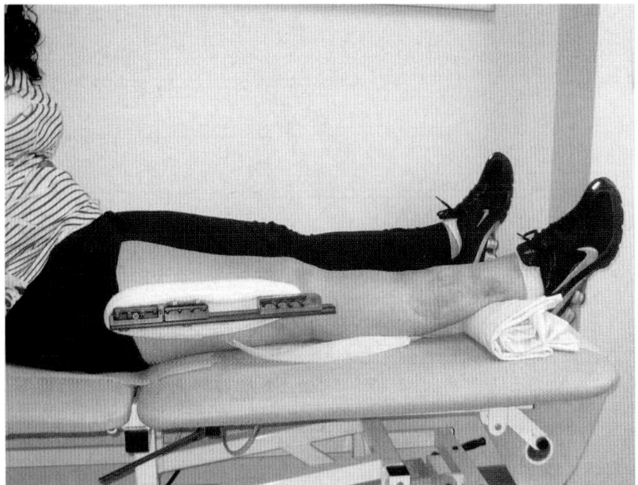

Figure 45.5 Photograph of the resting position of the knee in maximum extension by placing a bump under the ankle after femoral osteotomy. The bump under the ankle elevates the knee and calf from the table, encouraging full extension at the knee.

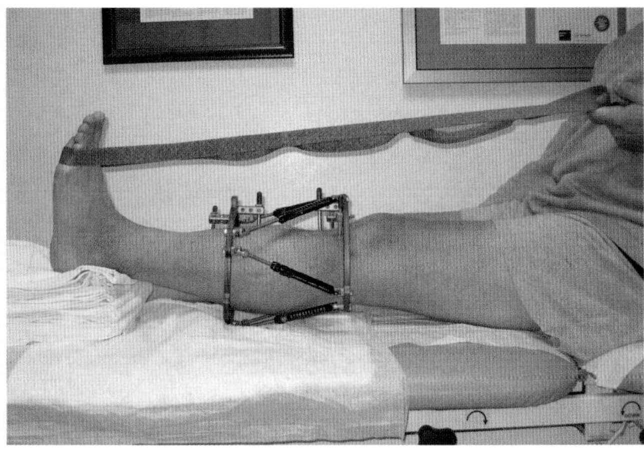

Figure 45.6 Photograph of passive dorsiflexion of the ankle with a strap after tibial osteotomy. A bump is under the ankle, lifting the rings off the table to keep the knee in extension, which is desirable resting as well.

During femur lengthening, the hamstrings, quadriceps, iliotibial band (ITB), and rectus femoris become increasingly tight. Exercises to maintain knee extension, knee flexion, and hip extension are mandatory. If there is knee instability, such as in a congenital case, loss of knee extension can lead to posterior subluxation. Excessive ITB tightness can lead to valgus deformation at the knee. Excessive tightness of the rectus femoris and quadriceps can lead to extension contracture of the knee and flexion contracture of the hip. These challenges are further increased with external fixation.

Internal Lengthening Intramedullary Rod

There are fewer joint ROM challenges with internal lengthening over a rod than with external fixation. Without the soft-tissue tethers of external fixation pins, there is much better maintenance of joint ROM during distraction compared to patients treated with external fixation. While this is a big advantage in both the femur and the tibia, the improvement is more significant in the femur. Weight bearing must be protected until there is sufficient consolidation of the bone to

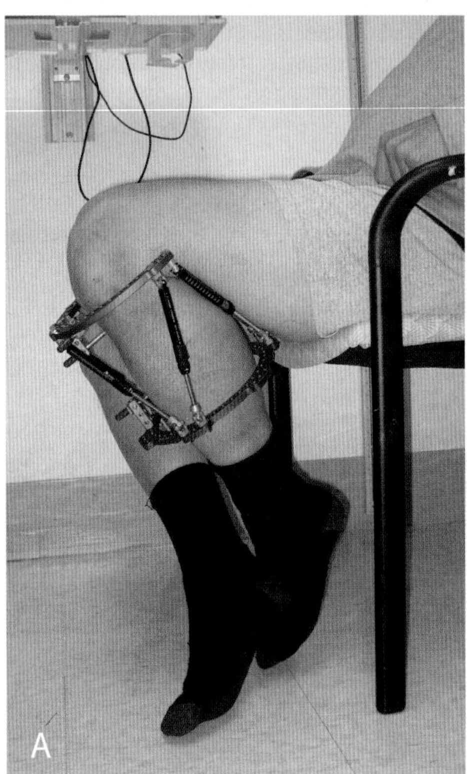

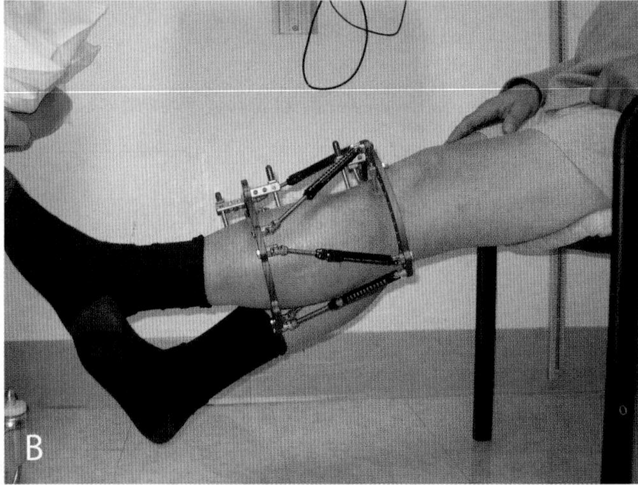

Figure 45.7 **A** and **B**, Photographs of passive knee flexion and extension after tibial osteotomy using the contralateral leg.

 © 2018 American Academy of Orthopaedic Surgeons

Table 45.2 REHABILITATION CHALLENGES AFTER OSTEOTOMY

Osteotomy Surgery	Rehabilitation Challenges
Femur	Knee and hip ROM, especially knee flexion and hip extension
Tibia	Knee and ankle ROM, especially knee extension and ankle dorsiflexion
External fixation	Soft-tissue tethering and pain from pins increases the likelihood of stiffness
Limb lengthening	Stretching of muscles increase likelihood of stiffness patterns noted above
Internal lengthening IM rod	Joint ROM less of a challenge compared to external fixation. Protected weight bearing needed for longer time than with external fixation

IM = intramedullary, ROM = range of motion (active and passive).

avoid implant failure. AROM and PROM of the adjacent joints is necessary (Table 45.2).

ADJUVANT SOFT-TISSUE PROCEDURES

Quadricepsplasty

When patients lose knee flexion to less than 60° despite rehabilitation, we perform quadricepsplasty to increase knee flexion. This would be done at the end of the distraction phase of lengthening via a limited quadricepsplasty, in which only the ITB and the vastus intermedius tendon are released. Weight bearing and the AROM and PROM knee regimen are not limited by this surgical intervention.

Iliotibial Band Release

We routinely perform an ITB release for femoral lengthening of greater than 1 inch at the time of the initial surgery. While this is most helpful in cases of congenital etiology, we also find it helpful in posttraumatic conditions. This is a tight band of tissue that resists distraction, and we have found that it lengthens as the bone lengthens. No defect in the ITB results from this intervention. This procedure does not affect the rehabilitation program.

Gastrocnemius-soleus Recession (GSR)

When patients lose critical ankle DF, we perform a gastrocnemius-soleus recession (GSR). This is often needed if tibia lengthening is greater than 4.2 cm and/or lengthening is greater than 13% of the original tibial length. Congenital etiology is also a factor that increases likelihood of needing GSR. GSR is performed through a posterior approach at the mid-distal third of the leg, during which the gastrocnemius and soleus fascia as well as the median raphe are transversely incised. This does not affect the weight-bearing status or the rehabilitation program. This can be done at the index surgery in a preventive manner or at the end of the distraction once a contracture develops.

SUMMARY

While there are specifics to each bone and technique used (Table 45.2), there are some general themes that can be summarized. After surgery, the early goals are ambulation within the safe range. This usually starts as partial weight bearing and progresses to WBAT once there is adequate bony consolidation. ROM of the adjacent joints is an important early focus; we prescribe AROM and PROM. Passive stretching to avoid predictable contractures is especially important during the distraction phase of bone lengthening when muscle tendon units will become tight. PROM is done early and progress is made to AROM typically a few weeks later. As the patient moves into the consolidation phase, weight bearing is advanced and strengthening programs are added to optimize recovery.

BIBLIOGRAPHY

Ilizarov GA: The tension-stress effect on the genesis and growth of tissues: Part II. The influence of the rate and frequency of distraction. *Clin Orthop Relat Res* 1989;(239):263–285.

Khakharia S, Fragomen AT, Rozbruch SR: Limited Quadricepsplasty for contracture during femoral lengthening. *Clin Orthop Relat Res* 2009;467(11):2911–2917.

Rozbruch SR, Birch JG, Dahl MT, Herzenberg JE: Motorized intramedullary nail for treatment of limb length discrepancy and deformity. *J Am Acad Orthop Surg* 2014;22:403–409.

Rozbruch SR, Fragomen A, Ilizarov S: Correction of tibial deformity using the Ilizarov/Taylor spatial frame. *J Bone Joint Surg Am* 2006;88 Suppl 4:156–174.

Rozbruch SR, Fragomen AT: Hybrid lengthening techniques: lengthening and then nailing (LATN), lengthening and then plating (LAP), in Tsuchiya, Kocaoglu, Eralp, eds: *Advanced Techniques in Limb Reconstruction Surgery*, Springer, 2015.

Rozbruch SR, Hamdy R: *Limb Lengthening and Reconstruction Surgery Case Atlas, Major Reference Work*. Switzerland, Springer International Publishing, 2015, Online reference and Textbook (3 volumes)

Rozbruch SR, Pugsley JS, Fragomen AT, Ilizarov S: Repair of tibial nonunions and bone defects with the taylor spatial frame. *J Orthop Trauma* 2008;22(2):88–95.

Rozbruch SR, Segal K, Ilizarov S, Fragomen AT, Ilizarov G: Does the Taylor spatial frame accurately correct tibial deformities? *Clin Orthop Rel Res*2010;468(5):1352–1361.

Rozbruch SR, Zonshayn S, Muthusamy S, Borst EW, Nguyen JT: What risk factors predict usage of gastrocsoleus recession during tibial lengthening? *Clin Orthop Relat Res* 2014;472(12):3842–3851.

Seah KT, Shafi R, Fragomen AT, Rozbruch SR: Distal femoral osteotomy: is internal fixation better than external? *Clin Orthop Rel Res* 2011;469:2003–2011.

© 2018 American Academy of Orthopaedic Surgeons

46 Partial Meniscectomy/ Chondroplasty

Seth Jerabek, MD

INTRODUCTION

Articular cartilage covers the articulating portions of the knee, including the distal femur, proximal tibia, and patella. Articular cartilage is composed of hyaline cartilage, which is the smoothest form of cartilage, allowing for low-friction joint motion. This layer of cartilage has no direct blood supply and is susceptible to injury with little regenerative potential. More advanced cartilage lesions can lead to degenerative joint disease or arthritis.

The medial and lateral menisci are composed of fibrocartilage, and play an important role in the articulation between the femur and tibia. The menisci contribute significantly to the knee's natural function and motion. They fill the void between the joint and the surrounding synovium and capsule, which prevent the synovium and capsule from being drawn into the joint during motion. Additionally, the menisci increase the weight-bearing surface of the knee, thus distributing the load and decreasing the contact pressure between the femur and tibia. They also play a role in joint stability, as they are cup-shaped structures, which increases the joint's congruence with the femur, contributing to the stability of the knee. Last, they are believed to be responsible for joint fluid movement and lubrication. The menisci have a variable blood supply. The blood vessels enter from the periphery, thus the peripheral portion of the meniscus has the most pronounced blood supply, while the inner portion has the least blood supply and is essentially avascular. Zones of vascular supply have been described that help guide treatment in the setting of meniscus tears (Figure 46.1). The most peripheral zone is the red-red zone, which is approximately the peripheral 25% of the meniscus, where the blood supply is the best. The red-white zone is at the junction of the vascular peripheral meniscus and the inner avascular portion of the meniscus. The white-white zone is the avascular peripheral meniscus. Injuries in the red-red zone are most likely to heal, as that is where the blood supply is best. Injuries in the red-white zone have the potential to heal, while injuries in the white-white zone are unlikely to heal.

Both the articular cartilage and menisci are susceptible to injury and degeneration. This can be thought of as a spectrum of disease. Younger patients typically sustain a trauma to the knee, which results in an articular cartilage injury or meniscus tear, and are often seen in the setting of a concomitant ligament injury. Older patients, who may have thinner, weaker, and less pliable cartilage and menisci, may sustain an injury with relatively little trauma.

Lesions or damage to the articular cartilage surface leave rough areas on the joint surfaces, potentially leading to pain, swelling, and mechanical symptoms, such as locking or catching of the knee joint. In some cases, articular cartilage can be completely dislodged and float around the joint, which is called a loose body. These may also lead to mechanical symptoms, particularly locking or catching of the joint. The treatment of a cartilage lesion depends on the patient's symptoms, age, location, and size of the defect. This chapter focuses primarily on chondroplasty, which is performed primarily in the setting of another procedure, such as partial meniscectomy, loose body removal, or ligament reconstruction. It is uncommon to perform chondroplasty alone. In younger patients with cartilage injuries, advanced cartilage reconstructive or regenerative procedures, such as autologous chondrocyte implantation, may be preferred. In older patients, with degenerative articular cartilage thinning or a full-thickness lesion, chondroplasty alone does not generally provide durable pain relief and improved function. Therefore, joint replacement may be considered for these patients.

Similarly, meniscus tears can be degenerative or acute/traumatic. The symptoms are similar to those of articular cartilage injury, including pain, swelling, locking, and catching. Displaced meniscus tears should be suspected in the setting of knee locking. The patient's age and activity level, as well as location of the meniscus tear, go into the medical decision on what may be the best treatment option for the patient. Typically, knee arthroscopy and partial meniscectomy are indicated in the settings of persistent pain that has failed conservative treatments, meniscus tears in the avascular zone (white-white)

Dr. Jerabek or an immediate family member is a member of a speakers' bureau or has made paid presentations on behalf of Stryker, and serves as a paid consultant to Stryker.

© 2018 American Academy of Orthopaedic Surgeons

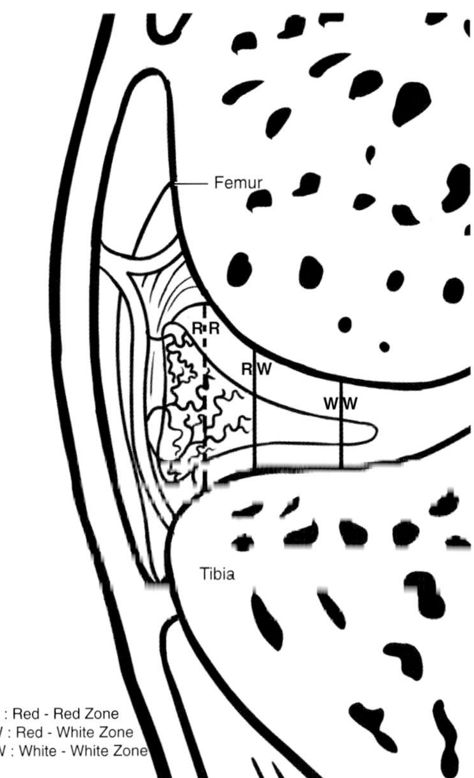

Figure 46.1 Illustration of meniscus vasculature.

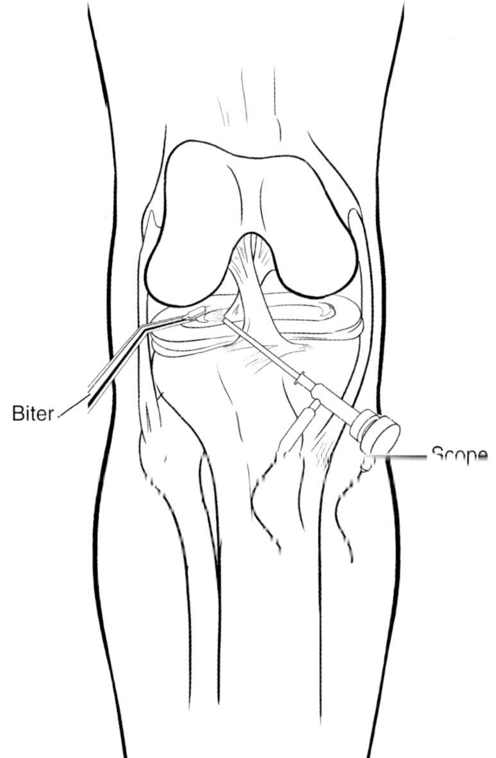

Figure 46.2 Illustration of the set-up for knee arthroscopy.

zone, and for displaced meniscus tears causing mechanical symptoms. Chondroplasty is often performed during the same surgery to smooth any rough or displaced articular cartilage lesions.

SURGICAL PROCEDURE: KNEE ARTHROSCOPY, PARTIAL MENISCECTOMY, AND CHONDROPLASTY

Indications

- Articular cartilage lesion causing mechanical symptoms
- Meniscus tears causing mechanical symptoms
- Meniscus tears causing persistent pain and swelling

Contraindications

- Young patient for whom a cartilage regenerative procedure is indicated
- Young patient for whom a meniscal repair is indicated
- Severely arthritis knee for which joint replacement is indicated
- Active skin infection at the surgical site

Procedure

Both partial meniscectomy and chondroplasty can be performed using knee arthroscopy (rather than open surgery). In knee arthroscopy, the knee is typically accessed through 2 to 3 portals. The two most common portals are the anterolateral (lateral to the patellar tendon at the joint line) and anteromedial (medial to the patellar tendon at the joint line) with an optional superolateral (superior and lateral to the patella) outflow portal. Chondroplasty is performed using an arthroscopic shaving device. Surgeons typically remove any loose cartilage flaps or smooth rough transitions between the cartilage and the bone. Partial meniscectomy is performed using a combination of arthroscopy bitters and shavers (Figure 46.2). The meniscus is typically débrided or trimmed down to a stable rim of remaining meniscus. After arthroscopic solution is evacuated from the knee, closure can be performed with simple subcutaneous reabsorbable stitches or with simple external nonreabsorbable sutures.

POSTOPERATIVE REHABILITATION

Introduction

Compared to most knee procedures, the rehabilitation after knee arthroscopy with partial meniscectomy and/or chondroplasty progresses rather quickly. Since the pain-generating lesion has been addressed and there is no repair or reconstruction to protect, recovery is only limited by the surrounding soft tissue and joint swelling.

Functional Goals and Restrictions

Goals for the first 2 weeks after surgery include controlling pain and swelling, maintaining knee motion, and regaining quadriceps activation. From weeks 2 to 6, the goals change to regaining full muscle strength and transitioning back to all preoperative activities.

© 2018 American Academy of Orthopaedic Surgeons

Table 46.1 EXERCISES FOR WEEKS 0 TO 2

Exercise Type	Goal for Exercise	Number of Repetitions/Sets	Number of Days per Week
Supine heel slides	Regain flexion	20 reps/3 sets	7
Seated heel slides	Regain flexion	20 reps/3 sets	7
Heel prop	Regain extension	10 min/3 sets (can do with quadriceps sets)	7
Quadriceps sets	Regain extension and reactivate quadriceps	20 reps/3 sets	7
Ankle pumps	Maintain circulation	10–20 reps per h	7

Weeks 0 to 2

- Control swelling with ice and compression
- Full weight bearing
- Full motion
- Quadriceps activation
- Gait training

Weeks 2 to 6

- Full weight bearing
- Full motion
- Full strengthening
- Transition back to preoperative activities when swelling and pain are minimal and strength is full.

Author's Preferred Protocol

Weeks 0 to 2 (Table 46.1)

- Ice or a cooling device should be used for 20 minutes per hour for the first 48 to 72 hours (while awake). Thereafter, ice should be used at least three times per day for 20 minutes per treatment.
- Full weight bearing is encouraged.
- Bracing is not needed.
- Supine heel slides: Have the patient lying supine; use the patient's contralateral leg or towel to assist in knee flexion. Hold the maximal bent position until tightness or stretching is perceived and hold for 5 seconds. Straighten the knee and repeat 20 times; perform three sets per day (Figure 46.3).
- Sitting heel slides: Sitting in a chair, the patient should slide the heel underneath the chair until maximum flexion is gained. The patient can slide the body forward in the chair while keeping the foot planted firmly on the floor to enhance flexion. Hold for 5 seconds and straighten the leg. Repeat 20 times and perform three sets per day (Figure 46.4).
- Heel prop: With the patient in the sitting position, prop the foot on a foot stool or low table and allow for passive extension. This exercise can be enhanced by adding quadriceps sets to the exercise, which would provide active extension. Hold the stretch for 10 minutes, three times daily, until full extension is gained (Figure 46.5).
- Quadriceps sets: With the patient supine or sitting, the patient should activate the quadriceps and forcefully extend the knee for a 5-second hold. A rolled towel underneath the heel may allow for more aggressive extension and quadriceps firing. This should be performed 20 times, 3 sets per day (Figure 46.6).
- Ankle pumps: This should be performed as much as possible to maintain circulation.

Weeks 2 to 6 (Table 46.2)

- The exercises for weeks 2 to 6 should be continued until full extension and flexion are attained.
- Once full flexion is gained, heel slides may be discontinued.
- Once full extension is gained, heel prop may be discontinued, but quadriceps sets should be continued.
- Quadriceps sets: With the patient supine or sitting, the patient should activate the quadriceps and forcefully extend

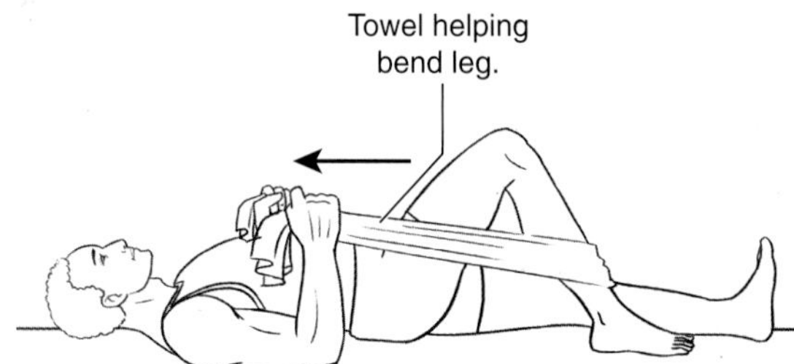

Figure 46.3 Illustration of the supine heel slide.

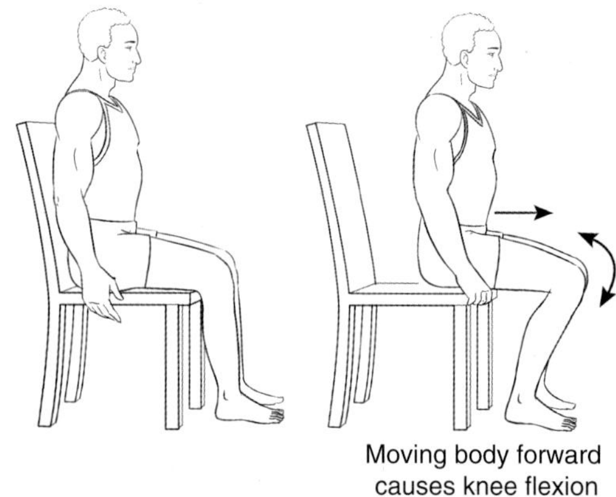

Figure 46.4 Illustration of the sitting heel slide.

© 2018 American Academy of Orthopaedic Surgeons

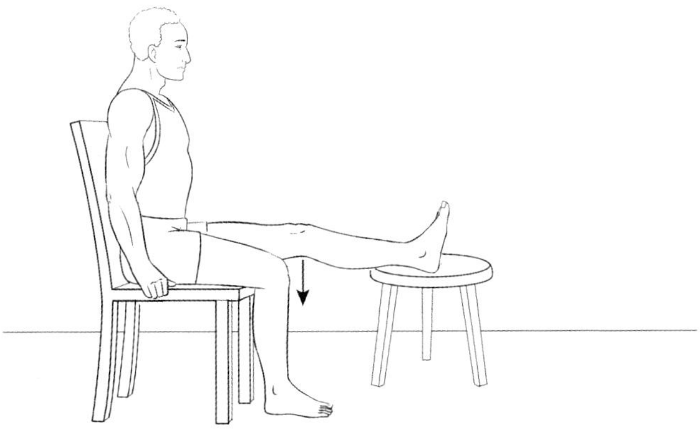

Figure 46.5 Illustration of the heel prop.

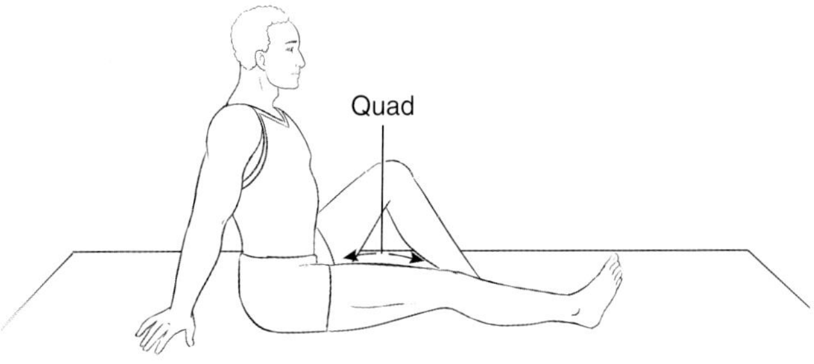

Figure 46.6 Illustration of the quadriceps set.

the knee for a 5-second hold. A rolled towel under the heel may allow for more aggressive extension and quadriceps firing. This should be performed 20 times, 3 sets per day (see Figure 46.6).

- Stationary bicycle: This can help with motion and strength. Set the seat so that the operative leg is at full extension at the bottom of the pedal cycle. Start at low resistance and increase slowly over 4 weeks, 20 to 30 minutes per day for 4 weeks (Figure 46.7).
- Straight leg lift: With the patient supine, have the patient fire the quadriceps to keep the leg straight and raise the entire leg off the ground. Hold at 45° for 1 to 2 seconds, then lower slowly. Perform 20 times, 3 sets per day. This works on the quadriceps, as well as on hip flexors and core. If not ready for this exercise, the patient will inadvertently flex the knee when performing the exercise. The patient will likely need to work up to the 20 repetitions with 3 sets daily (Figure 46.8).

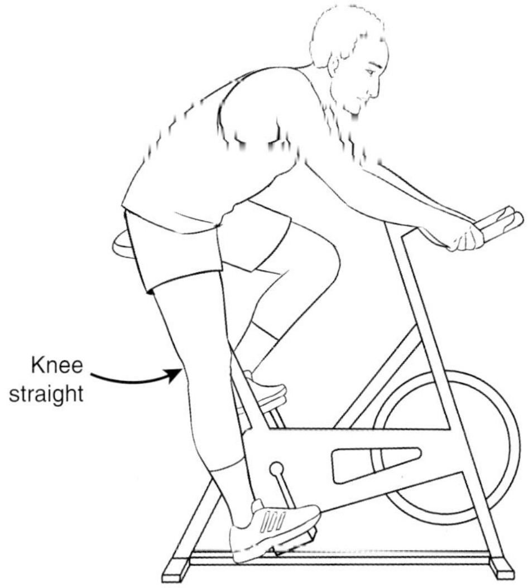

Figure 46.7 Illustration of riding a stationary bicycle.

Table 46.2 EXERCISES FOR WEEKS 2 TO 6

Exercise Type	Goal for Exercise	Number of Repetitions/Sets	Duration
Supine heel slides	Regain flexion	20 reps/3 sets	Continue until full flexion gained
Seated heel slides	Regain flexion	20 reps/3 sets	Continue until full flexion gained
Heel prop	Regain extension	10 min/3 sets (can do with quadriceps sets)	Continue until full extension gained
Quadriceps sets	Regain extension and reactivate quadriceps	20 reps/3 sets	Continue until full extension gained
Straight leg lift	Reactivate and strengthen quadriceps	20 reps/3 sets	Start only when the knee can be held straight during exercise
Short arc lift	Quadriceps strengthening and reactivation	20 reps/3 sets	2–6 wk
Standing hamstring curl	Hamstrings strengthening	20 reps/3 sets	2–6 wk
Standing toe raise	Quadriceps and balance	20 reps/3 sets	2–6 wk
Stationary bike	Range of motion, strength	20–30 min per day	2–6 wk

© 2018 American Academy of Orthopaedic Surgeons

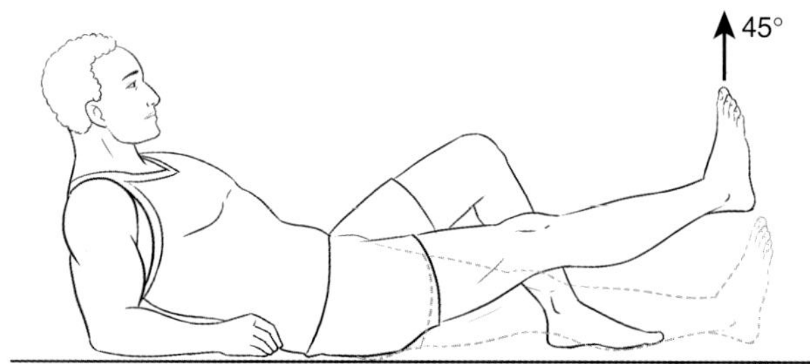

Figure 46.8 Illustration of the straight leg lift.

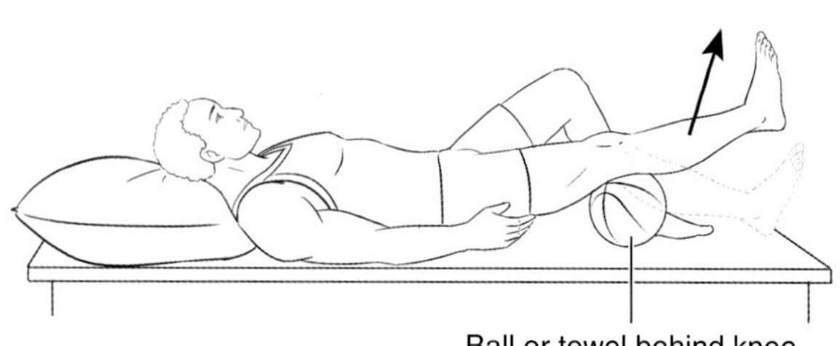

Figure 46.9 Illustration of the short arc lift.

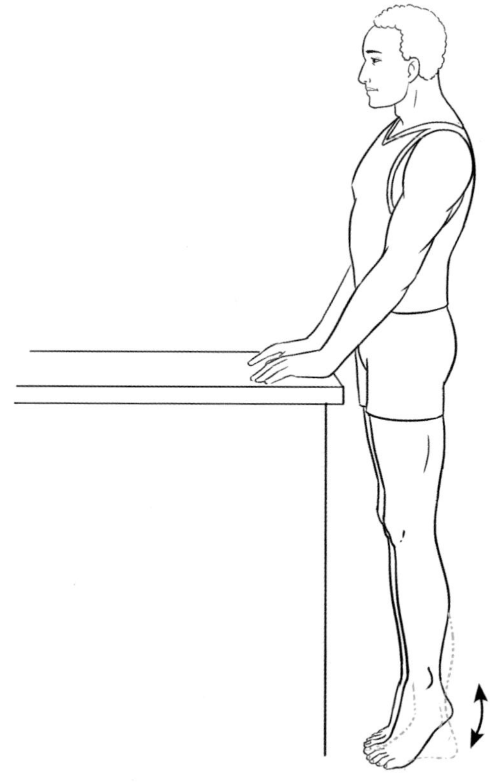

Figure 46.11 Illustration of the standing toe raise.

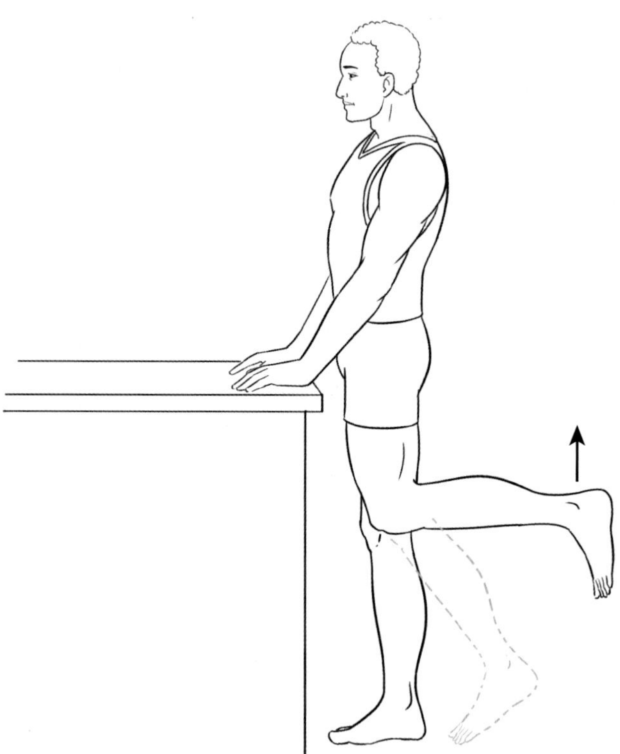

Figure 46.10 Illustration of the standing hamstring curl.

- Short arc lift: With the patient supine, slightly flex the operative knee over a ball or rolled-up blanket to flex the knee to approximately 30° to 45°. The patient should straighten the knee and hold for a 5-second count, then lower slowly. Perform 20 times, 3 sets per day (Figure 46.9).
- Standing hamstring curl: The patient should be standing and holding onto a balance bar or wall for support. The patient should slowly bend the operative knee so that the heel approaches the buttock. Perform 20 times, 3 sets per day (Figure 46.10).
- Standing toe raise: Standing and facing the wall, fire both quadriceps to make the knee straight and raise up on the toes for 1 second, then lower slowly. Have the patient use the wall as little as possible to work on balance. Perform 20 times, 3 sets per day (Figure 46.11).
- When full motion and strength have been regained, gradually transition to all activities.

PEARLS

- Control swelling early.
- Early quadriceps activation will help with extension and eventual strength.
- Regain motion during the first 2 weeks.
- Regain strength from weeks 2 to 6.

© 2018 American Academy of Orthopaedic Surgeons

BIBLIOGRAPHY

Bin SI, Lee SH, Kim CW, Kim TH, Lee DH: Results of arthroscopic medial meniscectomy in patients with grade IV osteoarthritis of the medial compartment. *Arthroscopy* 2008;24(3): 264–268.

Dias JM, Mazuquin BF, Mostagi FQ, Lima TB, Silva MA, Resende BN, Borges da Silva RM, Lavado EL, Cardoso JR: The effectiveness of postoperative physical therapy treatment in patients who have undergone arthroscopic partial meniscectomy: systematic review with meta-analysis. *J Orthop Sports Phys Ther* 2013;43(8):560–576.

Kelin BM, Ingersoll CD, Saliba S, Miller MD, Hertel J: Effect of early active range of motion rehabilitation on outcome measures after partial meniscectomy. *Knee Surg Sports Traumatol Arthrosc* 2009;17(6):607–616.

© 2018 American Academy of Orthopaedic Surgeons

47 Meniscal Repair

Seth Jerabek, MD

INTRODUCTION

Meniscal injury is one of the most common knee injuries seen by orthopaedic surgeons. Meniscal tears can cause persistent pain, swelling, mechanical symptoms, and disability. As mentioned in the prior chapter (Meniscectomy/Chondroplasty), the menisci contribute significantly to the knee's natural function, motion, and stability.

Often the decision to repair a meniscus is complex. The age and activity level of the patient—as well as the chronicity, location, and type of tear—all must be considered prior to indicating a patient for repair. Classically, the meniscus has been divided into three zones (red-red, red-white, and white-white) based on the vascularity of the meniscus. Given that the meniscus has a variable blood supply where the blood vessels enter from the periphery, the peripheral portion of the meniscus has the most pronounced blood supply, while the inner portion has the least blood supply and is essentially avascular (Figure 47.1). Tears in the red-red zone have the best blood supply, thus the best potential to heal a repair. Tears in the white-white zone have very little blood supply, thus are unlikely to heal with repair and are best treated with partial meniscectomy. Tears in the red-white zone are more controversial; the decision to repair depends on the age and demands of the patient as well as the type and location of the tear. For example, a young patient with an acute vertical tear has a better chance of healing than an older patient with a chronic, degenerative, horizontal tear. Associated injury and surgery may also affect the propensity to heal. Meniscal tears treated in conjunction with tibial plateau fracture fixation or reconstruction of cruciate ligaments are also felt to have a better prognosis for healing compared to isolated repairs.

SURGICAL PROCEDURE: MENISCAL REPAIR

Indications

- Acute meniscus tear in the red-red or red-white zones
- Full-thickness tear of at least 5 to 10 mm
- Relatively young and active patient

Contraindications

- Tears in the white-white zone
- Advanced osteoarthritis
- Chronic, degenerative tears
- Older, inactive patients

Procedure

There are several techniques used to repair menisci, depending on the location of the tear and the surgeon's preference. They can be repaired arthroscopically using an all-inside technique with suture passer with anchors, open surgery using an arthrotomy, or a combination of arthroscopy with an open approach. The last approach is done to visualize the joint capsule near the tear, and sutures are passed from the inside of the knee through the meniscus and capsule (inside-out technique) or from the outside of the knee through the capsule and meniscus (outside-in technique), facilitating repair (Figure 47.2). Most repairs are either all inside or inside-out with the exception of the less common anterior tears, in which an outside-in approach facilitates suture passage.

POSTOPERATIVE REHABILITATION

Introduction

Rehabilitation after meniscal repair will be variable depending on the type and location of the repair. For example, a patient with a relatively stable, peripheral vertical tear repair may be advanced faster than a patient with an unstable, radial tear repair. The surgeon often determines the patient's weight bearing and early motion restrictions during surgery. Flexion beyond 90° puts increased stress on a meniscal repair and is often limited for up to 6 weeks after surgery. Thus, it is critical for the surgeon and therapist to have specific recommendations and open communication with each patient with a meniscal repair. To follow is a "typical" rehabilitation strategy for meniscal repair, which may be modified based on the characteristics of each repair.

Dr. Jerabek or an immediate family member is a member of a speakers' bureau or has made paid presentations on behalf of Stryker, and serves as a paid consultant to Stryker.

© 2018 American Academy of Orthopaedic Surgeons

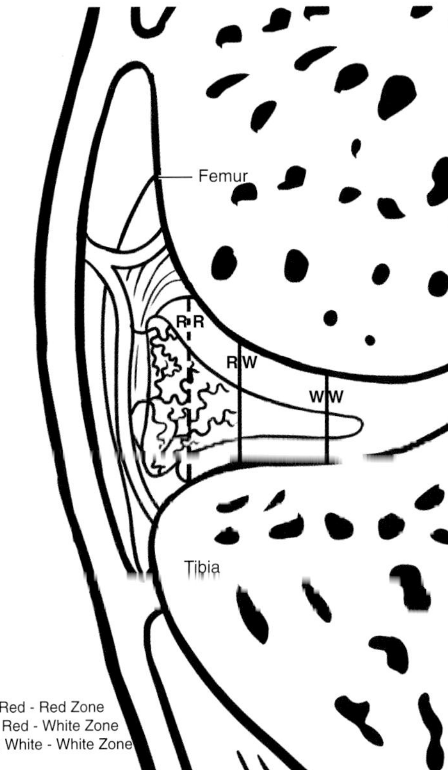

Figure 47.1 Illustration of the meniscis vasculature.

Functional Goals and Restrictions

Goals for the first 2 weeks after surgery include controlling pain and swelling, initiating knee motion, and regaining quadriceps activation. From weeks 2 to 6, the patient is still in a hinged knee brace, but can work on gaining motion to 90°, and can start muscle strengthening. At 6 weeks and onward, the patient comes out of the brace and works on regaining full motion and strength. Generally, patients can return to in-line sports such as bicycling and running at 3 months and pivoting sports at 6 months. The rehabilitation goals can be subdivided as follows.

Phase 1: Swelling and Symptom Control (Weeks 0–2)

- Control swelling with ice and compression
- Weight bearing as tolerated, with hinged knee brace locked in full extension and crutches (consider limited weight bearing depending on tear)
- Gentle early motion when seated with maximum flexion between 60° to 90° depending on tear
- Quadriceps activation

Phase 2: Early Motion and Strengthening (Weeks 2–6)

- Weight bearing as tolerated, with hinged knee brace locked in full extension and crutches (consider limited weight bearing depending on tear)
- Full extension and flexion to 90°
- Begin muscle strengthening

Phase 3: Functional Return (Weeks 6–12)

- Transition out of brace
- Regain full motion
- Muscle strengthening

Phase 4: Early Sports Training (Weeks 12–24)

- Regain full muscle strength
- Cardiovascular conditioning
- In-line sports
- Sport-specific training (speed and agility training)

Phase 5: Advanced Sport Activity (Week 24 Onward)

- Return to pivoting sports

Author's Preferred Protocol

Phase 1 (Weeks 0–2)

- Ice or a cooling device should be used for 20 minutes per hour for the first 48 to 72 hours (while awake). Thereafter, ice should be used at least three times per day for 20 minutes per treatment.
- Weight bearing as tolerated with hinged knee brace locked in full extension and crutches (consider limited weight bearing depending on tear). If the patient has pain, limit weight bearing until pain free.
- Sitting heel slides: Sitting in a chair with the brace unlocked, the patient should slide the heel toward the chair until 60° to 90° degrees of flexion is gained. *Do not exceed 90°*. Hold for 5 seconds, straighten leg, and repeat 20 times. Perform three sets per day (Figure 47.3).
- Heel prop: With the patient in the sitting position, prop the foot on a [illegible] table and allow for passive

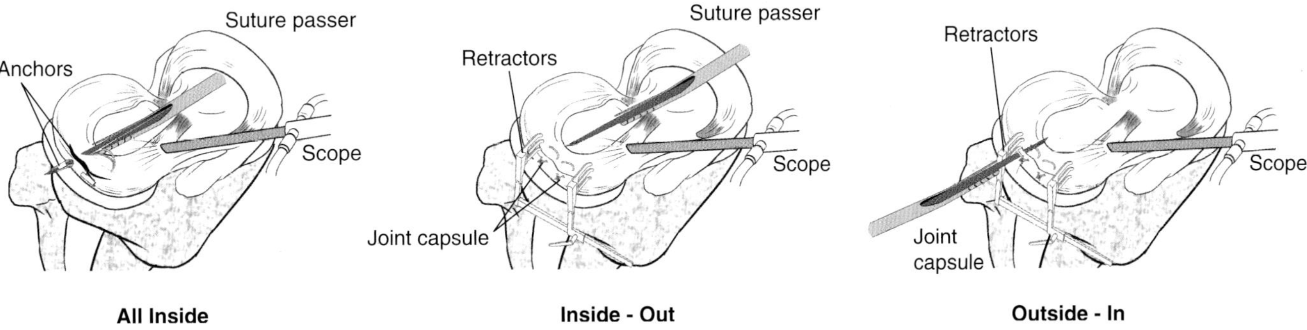

Figure 47.2 Illustration of meniscal repair.

© 2018 American Academy of Orthopaedic Surgeons

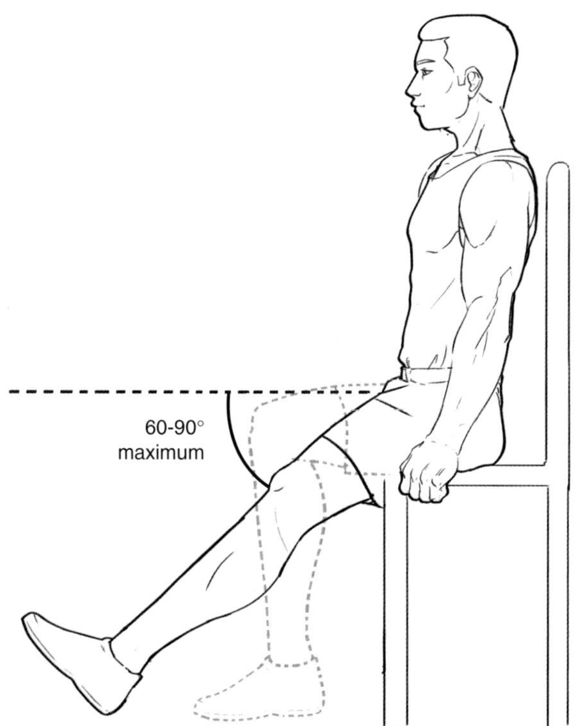

Figure 47.3 Illustration of sitting heel slide.

extension. This exercise can be enhanced by adding quadriceps sets to the exercise, which would provide active extension. Hold the stretch for 10 minutes, three times daily, until full extension is gained (Figure 47.4).

- Quadriceps setting: With the patient supine or sitting, the patient should activate the quadriceps and forcefully extend the knee for a 5-second hold. A rolled towel underneath the heel may allow for more aggressive extension and quadriceps firing. This should be performed 20 times, 3 sets per day (Figure 47.5).
- Ankle pumps: This should be performed as much as possible to maintain circulation.

Phase 2 (Weeks 2–6)

- Weight bearing as tolerated with hinged knee brace locked in full extension and crutches (consider limited weight bearing depending on tear). If the patient has pain, limit weight bearing until pain free.
- Sitting heel slides: Sitting in a chair with the brace unlocked, the patient should slide the heel toward the chair until 90° of flexion is gained. *Do not exceed 90°*. Hold for 5 seconds, straighten leg, and repeat 20 times. Perform three sets per day (see Figure 47.3).
- Once full extension is gained, heel prop may be discontinued, but quadriceps sets should be continued.
- Quadriceps sets: With the patient supine or sitting, activate the quadriceps and forcefully extend the knee for a 5-second hold. A rolled towel underneath the heel may allow for more aggressive extension and quadriceps firing. This should be performed 20 times, 3 sets per day (Figure 47.5).
- Straight leg lift: With the patient supine, have the patient fire the quadriceps to keep the leg straight and raise the entire leg off the ground. Hold at 45° for 1 to 2 seconds, then lower slowly. Repeat 20 times, and perform 3 sets per day. This works on the quadriceps, as well as on hip flexors and the core. If the patient is not ready for this exercise because of weak quadriceps activation, the knee bend will flex. The patient will likely need to work up to the 20 repetitions with 3 sets daily (Figure 47.6).
- Short arc lift: With the patient supine, slightly flex the operative knee over a ball or rolled up blanket to flex the knee to approximately 30° to 45°. The patient should straighten the knee and hold for 5 seconds, then lower slowly. Repeat 20 times, 3 sets per day (Figure 47.7).
- Standing toe raise: Standing and facing the wall, fire both quadriceps to keep the knee straight, and raise up on toes one second, then lower slowly. Have the patient use the wall

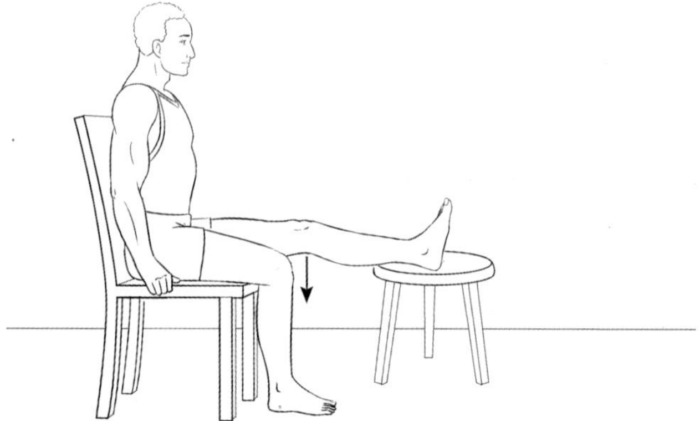

Figure 47.4 Illustration of heel prop.

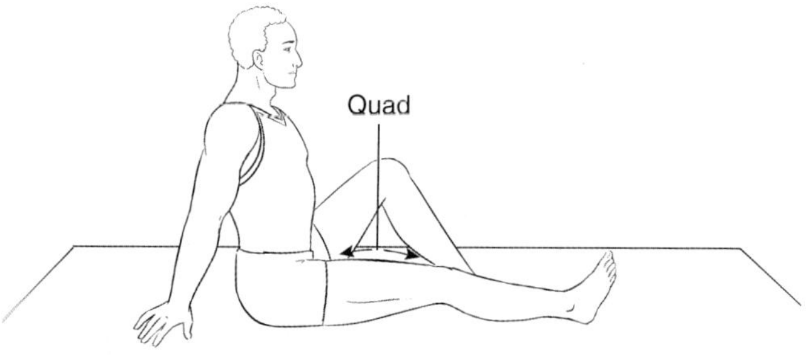

Figure 47.5 Illustration of quadriceps set exercise.

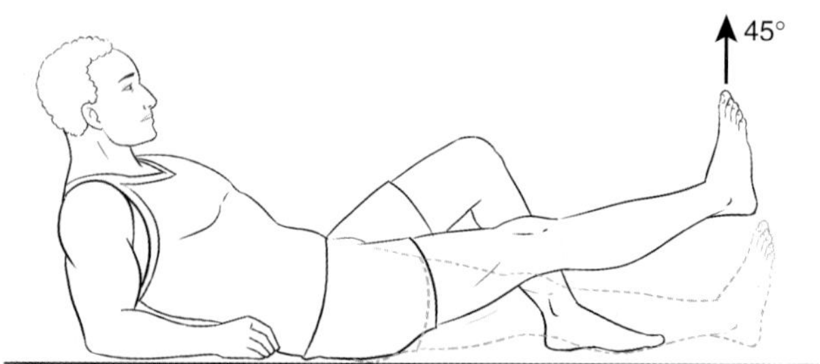

Figure 47.6 Illustration of straight-leg lift exercise.

© 2018 American Academy of Orthopaedic Surgeons

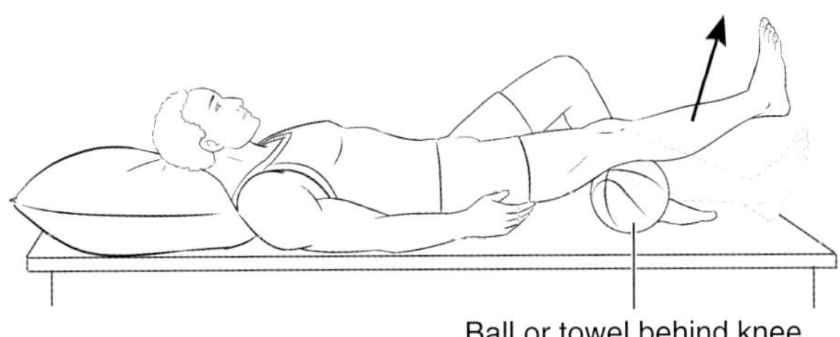

Figure 47.7 Illustration of short arc lift exercise.

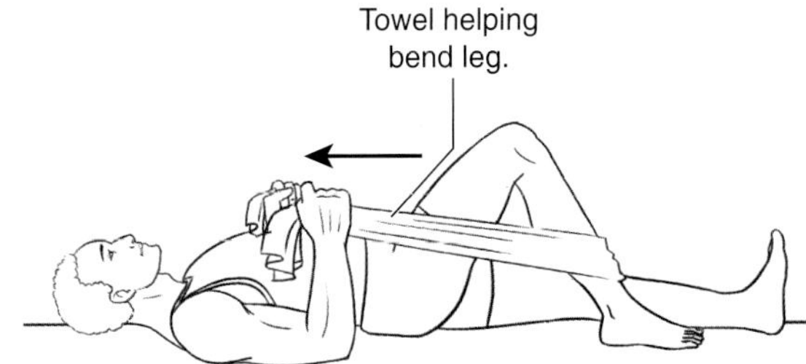

Figure 47.9 Illustration of supine heel slide exercise.

as little as possible to work on balance. Repeat 20 times, 3 sets per day (Figure 47.8).

Phase 3 (Weeks 6–12)

- Discontinue brace and transition to full weight bearing.
- Supine heel slides: With the patient lying supine, have the patient use the contralateral leg or towel to assist in knee flexion. Hold the maximal bent position until tightness or stretching is perceived and hold for 5 seconds, then straighten the knee and repeat. Three sets of 20 repetitions (Figure 47.9).
- Sitting heel slides: Sitting in a chair, the patient should slide the heel underneath the chair until maximum flexion is gained (may go beyond 90° of flexion). The patient can slide the body forward in the chair while keeping the foot planted firmly on the floor to enhance flexion. Hold for 5 seconds, straighten the leg, and repeat. Three sets of 20 repetitions (Figure 47.10).
- Quadriceps sets: With the patient supine or sitting, the patient should activate the quadriceps and forcefully extend the knee for a 5-second hold. A rolled towel underneath the heel may allow for more aggressive extension and quadriceps firing. Three sets of 20 repetitions (Figure 47.5).
- Straight leg lift: With the patient supine, have the patient fire the quadriceps to keep the leg straight and raise the entire leg off the ground. Hold at 45° for 1 to 2 seconds, then lower slowly. Repeat 20 times, and perform 3 sets per day. This works on the quadriceps, as well as on hip flexors and core. If not ready for this exercise, the patient will start to flex the knee when bending. The patient will likely need to work up to the 20 repetitions with 3 sets daily (Figure 47.6).
- Short arc lift: With the patient supine, slightly flex the operative knee over a ball or rolled up blanket to approximately 30° to 45°. The patient should straighten the knee and hold for a 5-second count, then lower slowly. Perform 3 sets of 20 repetitions (Figure 47.7).
- Standing toe raise: Standing and facing the wall, fire both quadriceps to keep the knee straight, raise up on the toes for 1 second, and lower slowly. Have the patient use the wall as little as possible to work on balance. Perform 3 sets of 20 repetitions (Figure 47.8).
- Standing hamstring curl: The patient should be standing and holding onto a balance bar or wall for support. The patient should slowly bend the operative knee so that the heel approaches the buttock. Perform 3 sets of 20 repetitions (Figure 47.11).

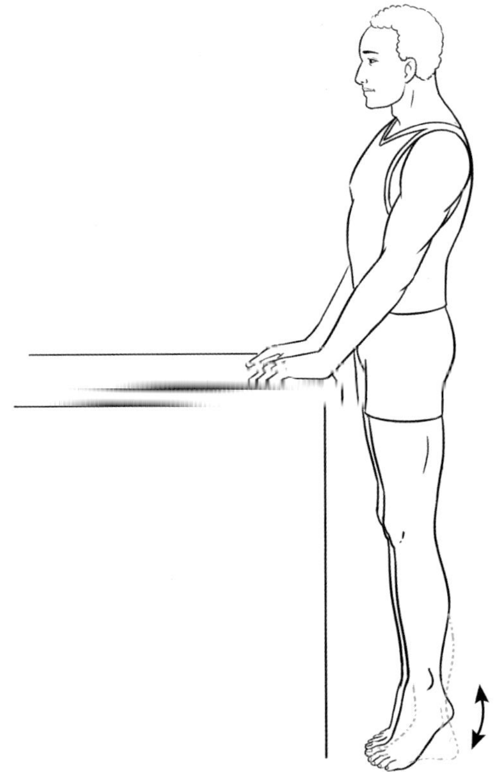

Figure 47.8 Illustration of standing toe raise exercise.

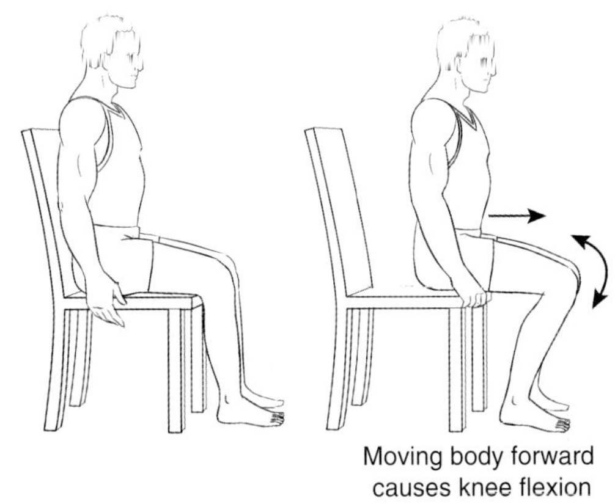

Figure 47.10 Illustration of sitting heel slide exercise.

© 2018 American Academy of Orthopaedic Surgeons

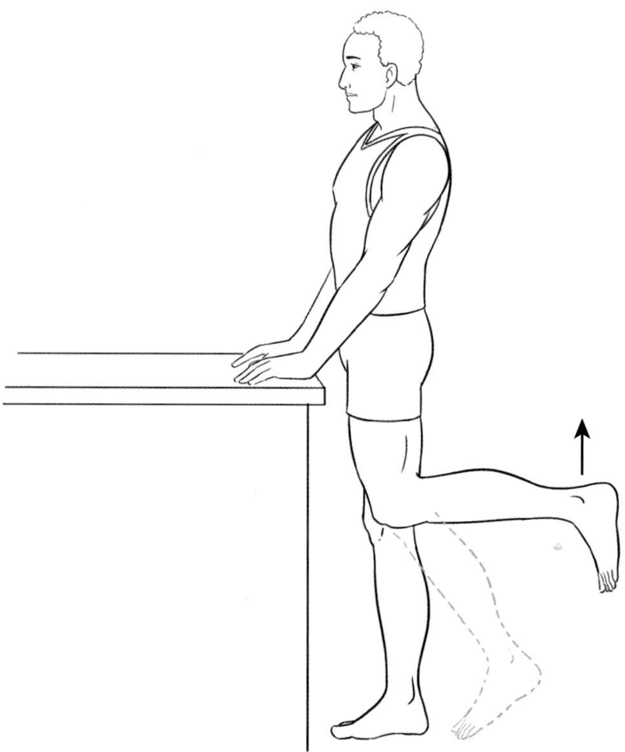

Figure 47.11 Illustration of standing hamstring curl exercise.

- Stationary bicycle: This can help with motion and strength. Set the seat so that the operative leg is at full extension at the bottom of the pedal cycle. Start at low resistance and increase slowly over 4 weeks. Do 20 to 30 minutes per day (Figure 47.12).
- Hip abduction: Lie on the unoperated side. With the knee held straight, raise the operated leg to the side 45°. Hold for 1 second, and lower slowly. Repeat 20 times per day (Figure 47.13).

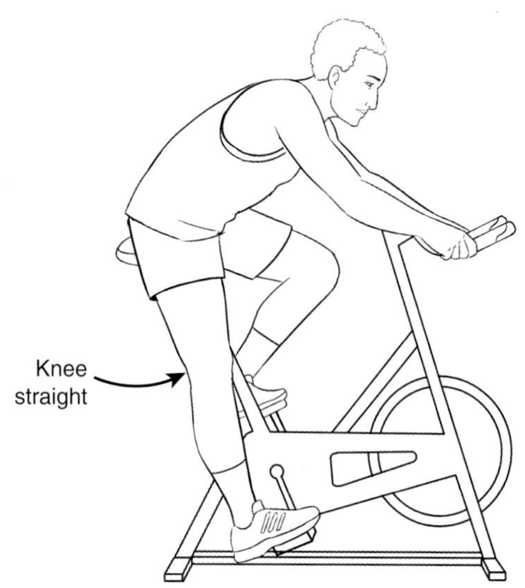

Figure 47.12 Illustration of stationary bicycle exercise.

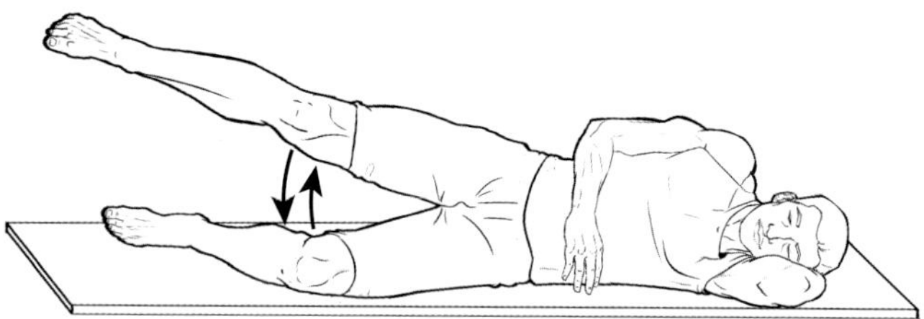

Figure 47.13 Illustration of hip abduction exercise.

- Wall slides: Have the patient stand with the back touching the wall. Have the patient's feet facing forward and about 6 to 12 inches from the wall. The patient should lower the body by flexing through both the hips and knees until the knees are flexed to 45°. Pause for 5 seconds at 45°, then slide up the wall to the original position. Perform 3 sets of 20 repetitions (Figure 47.14).
- Squat to chair: Have the patient stand above a chair, then slowly squat down to the chair until the buttocks touch the chair, then immediately return to the starting standing position. Do not allow the patient to sit on the chair. Hand weights can be added as strength improves. Perform 3 sets of 20 repetitions (Figure 47.15).
- Seated leg press: Builds quadriceps strength. Start with an easily lifted weight and progress weekly as the patient makes progress. Do not exceed the patient's own body weight. Do not allow flexion beyond 90°. Perform 3 sets of 20 repetitions (Figure 47.16).

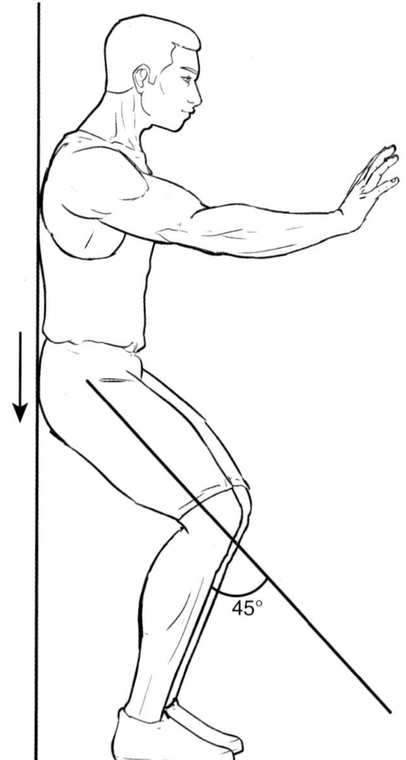

Figure 47.14 Illustration of wall slide exercise.

© 2018 American Academy of Orthopaedic Surgeons

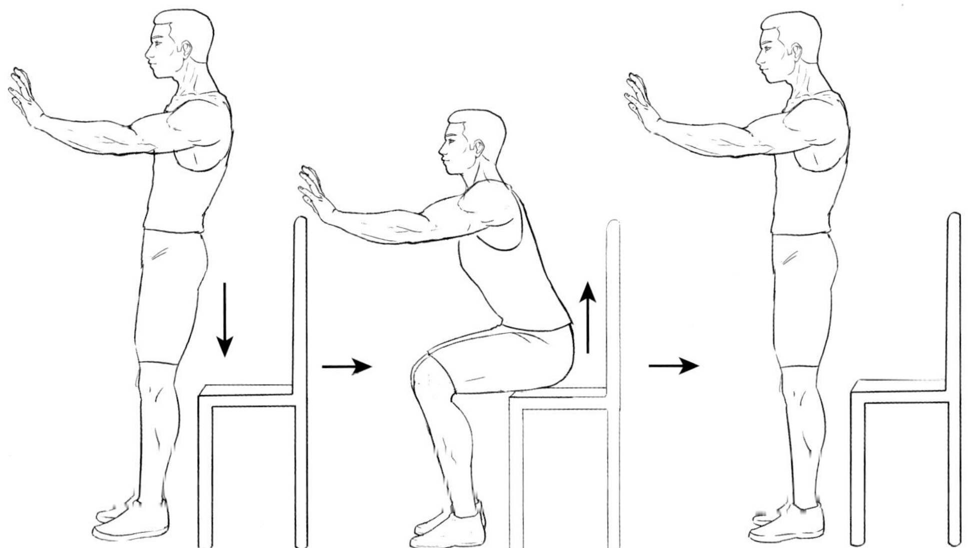

Figure 47.15 Illustration of squat-to-chair exercise.

- Step-up/step-down: Builds strength, balance, and proprioception. Place the operated leg on a low, flat, stable stool. Have the unoperated leg off the ground and slowly bend the operated leg so that the unoperated leg just touches the ground. Straighten the operated leg to go back to the original position. Maintain a balanced upright posture during the exercise. Keep the thigh, knee, and foot all pointed forward and do not allow rotation. The stool height can be increased from 3, 6, and 9 inches as the patient progresses. Perform 3 sets of 10 to 20 repetitions depending on conditioning and balance (Figure 47.17).
- Stretching exercises: It is important to work on stretching in addition to strengthening. The three main stretches are the prone quadriceps, hamstrings, and calf. Each should be done twice per day, 5 repetitions, holding for 15 to 20 seconds (Figure 47.18).

Phase 4 (Weeks 12–24)

- The phase 3 exercises should be continued, but the number of sets and repetitions will have to be decreased (2 sets of 10–15 reps) to allow more time for advanced muscular strengthening, cardiovascular conditioning, and sport-specific training.
- Strength training should alternate every other day with cardiovascular/sport-specific training.
- Strength training days (3 days per week)
  - Phase 3 exercises (2 sets of 10–15 repetitions). Add light weights if more resistance is needed.
  - Single-leg wall slides: Have the patient stand with the back touching the wall. Have the feet facing forward and about 6 to 12 inches from the wall. Holding the nonoperative leg off the ground, have the patient lower the body by flexing the operative hip and knee until the knee is flexed to 45°. Pause for 5 seconds at 45°, then slide up the walk to the original position. Perform 3 sets of 5 to 10 repetitions per day.
  - Single-leg squat to chair: Have the patient stand above a chair, then slowly squat down to the chair using only the operative leg until the buttock touches the chair, then return to the starting standing position. Do not allow the

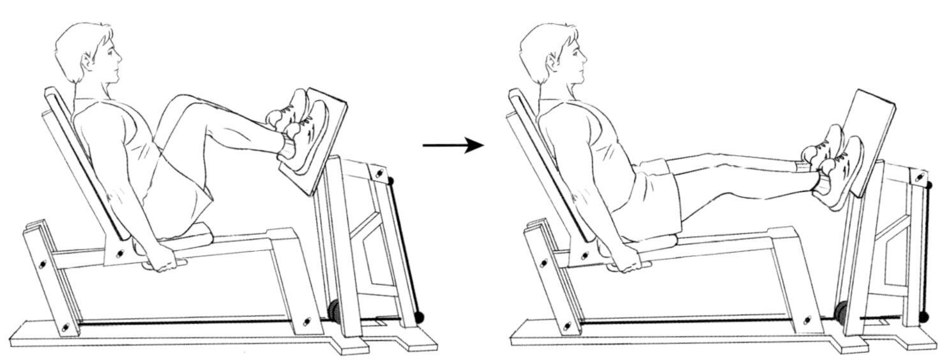

Figure 47.16 Illustration of leg press exercise.

© 2018 American Academy of Orthopaedic Surgeons

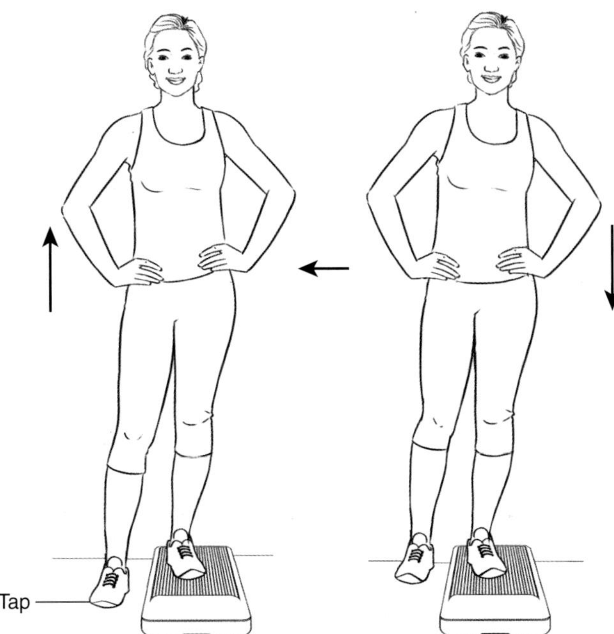

Figure 47.17 Illustration of step-up/step-down exercise.

patient to sit on the chair. Hand weights can be added as strength improves. Perform 3 sets of 5 to 10 repetitions.

- Cardiovascular/sport-specific training days (3 days per week)
  - Stationary bicycle or elliptical machine: Increase resistance as tolerated; 30 minutes per session.
  - Light running on a soft, level surface: Start running for 5 minutes and increase to 30 minutes over a 4-week period. This should be alternated with strengthening every other day.
- Speed and agility training: When running in line for 30 minutes is relatively easy and does not cause pain or swelling, consider starting speed and agility training. This portion of rehabilitation will have to be individualized to the patient. Progression typically follows the following pattern:
  - In-line sprinting starting half speed for 100 yards for 10 repetitions
  - Advance in-line sprinting to full speed, 100 yards for 10 repetitions
  - Add cones or zig-zag running
  - Add forward and backward running
  - Add figure-of-eight running
  - Add carioca running
  - Add shuttle run

Phase 5 (Weeks 24 and Beyond)

- Return to unrestricted pivoting sports when motion and strength have returned without swelling during advanced rehabilitation.

OUTCOMES

Meniscal repair is a highly successful procedure, with most patients free of symptoms and able to return to sport similar to meniscectomy results. However, a fraction of these patients may re-tear or not heal their meniscal repair, evidenced by recurring symptoms. These patients may then require repeat surgery, although the tear is often not as large.

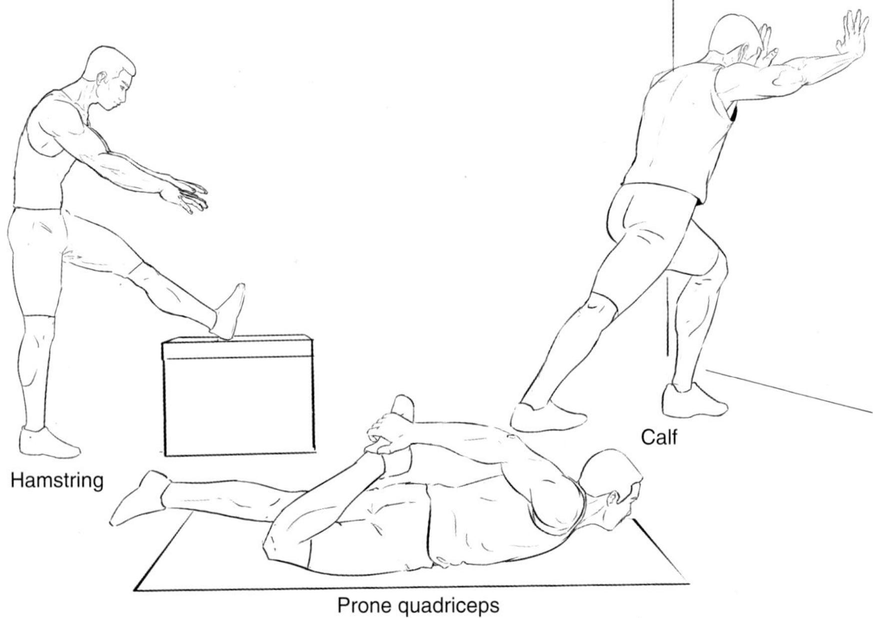

Figure 47.18 Illustration of stretching exercises.

© 2018 American Academy of Orthopaedic Surgeons

PEARLS

- Protect the repair. Surgeons will determine the duration of bracing, weight-bearing status, and ROM restrictions based on patient factors, type of tear, and stability of repair.
- Pain and swelling are normal after surgery. However, if the patient develops worsening pain and/or swelling, contact the surgeon and do not advance the rehabilitation program.
- Strength and motion should be normal prior to advancing to running.
- Meniscus repair is often done in the setting of ligament reconstruction, which generally dictates the rehabilitation plan.

BIBLIOGRAPHY

Cavanaugh JT, Killian SE: Rehabilitation following meniscal repair. *Curr Rev Musculoskelet Med* 2012;5(1):46–58.

Henning CE, Lynch MA, Clark JR: Vascularity for healing of meniscus repairs. *Arthroscopy* 1987;3(1):13–18.

Miller MD, Warner JJP, Harner CD: Meniscal Repair, in Fu FH, Harner CD, Vince KG, eds: *Knee Surgery.* Baltimore, MD, Williams & Wilkins, 1994.

Starke C, Kopf S, Peterson W, Becker R: Meniscal repair. *Arthroscopy* 2009;25(9):1033–1044.

© 2018 American Academy of Orthopaedic Surgeons

48 ACL Reconstruction

Seth Jerabek, MD

INTRODUCTION

The anterior cruciate ligament (ACL) is the most commonly injured and reconstructed knee ligament. More than 100,000 ACL reconstructions are performed annually in the United States.

The ACL is located in the intercondylar notch originating from the posteromedial wall of the lateral femoral condyle and inserting on the central tibial plateau. It is comprised of two bundles, anteromedial and posterolateral, which have different orientations that allow the ACL to resist both anterior translation and internal rotation of the tibia (Figure 48.1).

The ACL is most commonly injured in sporting activities without contact; ACL injuries are often seen when athletes are attempting to decelerate and change direction or pivot. The menisci and medial collateral ligament (MCL) may be injured at the same time. Many report an audible "pop" at the time of injury. Immediately after injury, the patient will typically have pain with weight bearing and motion. An effusion develops shortly after injury. The examiner can often detect instability on physical examination by performing the anterior drawer, Lachman, and Pivot shift tests. Magnetic resonance imaging (MRI) is performed to confirm the injury and to evaluate for concomitant injuries.

An ACL-deficient knee can lead to instability, particularly with pivoting activities, meniscus tears, and possibly arthritis. Thus, young, active patients are typically reconstructed. There is no age limit for ACL reconstruction, but older patients with lower demands may not require ACL reconstruction, as they may not participate in activities that would cause instability, while stiffness following surgery in these patients may be more problematic.

Graft choice remains controversial and depends most heavily on surgeon experience. The two most popular autologous grafts are the hamstrings and the patellar tendon. Allograft is also an option, but is typically used in older patients who are lower demand. There is concern that allografts may have higher failure rates in young, active patients. However, there is no donor site morbidity when using an allograft; thus, the recovery may be easier.

SURGICAL PROCEDURE—ACL RECONSTRUCTION

Indications

- ACL rupture in a young, active patient
- ACL rupture and symptomatic instability in a patient of any age

Contraindications

- Stiffness/lack of full knee motion
- Older, low-demand patients
- Significant knee deformity
- Advanced and symptomatic osteoarthritis
- Inability or unwillingness to perform requisite rehabilitation

Procedure

In general, the goal is to place the graft in its anatomic location to reproduce the kinematics and stability of the knee joint. At the start of the surgical procedure, the knee is examined to evaluate its motion and stability followed by a thorough arthroscopic examination to confirm the preoperative diagnoses and rule out other pathology.

The ligament reconstruction can then commence. There are multiple different techniques and graft types for reconstruction. There are potential benefits and risks of each, but ultimately the technique is dictated by surgeon preference and experience. In some cases, previous or associated injury, previous surgery, or deformity may alter the approach. A number of different landmarks and tools are used to determine the precise location of the origin and insertion to bone of the ligament and to create the tunnels visualized arthroscopically. The stump of the ruptured ACL is débrided with an arthroscopic shaver and serves as the principal landmark for tunnel location. The graft, whether autograft or allograft, bone tendon bone, or tendon alone, is passed into the tunnels. One end is secured, the graft tensioned, and the free end is secured with screws or other devices. The restoration of stability is confirmed and the wounds closed unless there are concomitant procedures, such as meniscal repair.

Dr. Jerabek or an immediate family member is a member of a speakers' bureau or has made paid presentations on behalf of Stryker, and serves as a paid consultant to Stryker.

© 2018 American Academy of Orthopaedic Surgeons

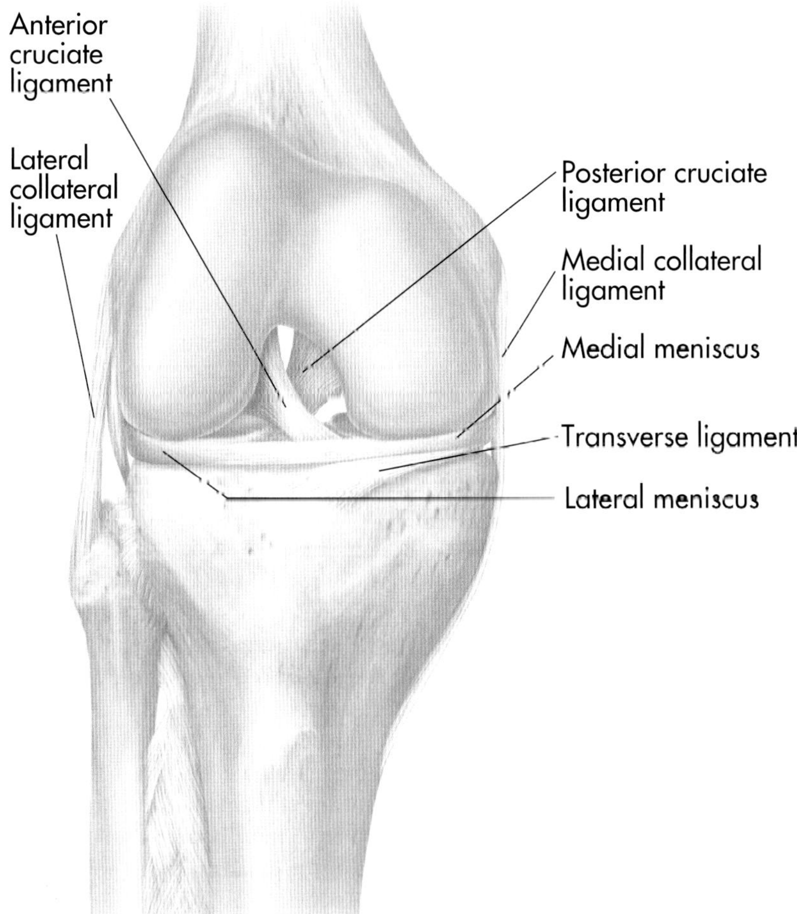

Figure 48.1 Illustration of ligaments of the knee. (Anatomical Chart Company. Hip and Knee Inflammations Anatomical Chart. Philadelphia, PA, Wolters Kluwer, 2007.)

Complications

In the postoperative period, the patient, surgeon, and therapist must be vigilant for potential complications. Wound healing problems, infection, and thromboembolic events are uncommon but possible. Similarly, fracture of the patella in the case of bone tendon bone reconstruction, femur or tibia fracture have been reported, but are also uncommon. Stiffness, especially loss of knee extension and knee pain, are more frequent, but can be addressed with rehabilitation.

POSTOPERATIVE REHABILITATION

Introduction

Rehabilitation after ACL reconstruction will vary from surgeon to surgeon. It will be based on graft choice, fixation choice, patient-specific factors, and surgeon preference. Thus, it is critical for the surgeon and therapist to have specific recommendations and open communication regarding bracing, weight bearing, and motion.

Functional Goals and Restrictions

Goals for the first 2 weeks after surgery include control of pain and swelling, initiating knee motion, and regaining quadriceps activation. From 2 weeks to 6 weeks, the patient is working on ambulation with a goal to transition off crutches. Emphasis is on regaining motion, and starting muscle strengthening. At 6 weeks and onward, the patient comes out of the brace and works on regaining full motion and strength. Generally, patients can return to in-line sports such as bicycling and light running at 3 months, and pivoting sports between 6 and 9 months. The rehabilitation goals can be subdivided into phases with progression to the next phase determined by meeting objectives of each phase.

Phase 1 (Swelling Control and Early Motion): Weeks 0 to 2

- Control swelling with ice and compression
- Weight bearing as tolerated with hinged knee brace unlocked and crutches
- Gentle early motion, work on regaining full extension
- Quadriceps activation

Phase 2 (Establishing Functional Motion and Quadriceps Control): Weeks 2 to 6

- Weight bearing as tolerated with hinged knee brace unlocked
- Discontinue crutches when comfortable doing so
- Maintain full extension and flexion to 120°
- Begin quadriceps strengthening

Phase 3 (Normal Gait and Strengthening): Weeks 6 to 12

- Transition out of brace
- Regain full flexion
- Walk with normal heel-toe gait
- Muscle strengthening

Phase 4 (Early Sport Training): Weeks 12 to 24

- Regain full muscle strength
- Cardiovascular conditioning
- In-line running
- Sport-specific training (speed and agility training)

Phase 5 (Advanced Sports Training): Week 24 Onward

- Return to pivoting sports (consider using an ACL brace)

Preferred Protocol

Phase 1: Weeks 0–2

- Ice or a cooling device should be used for 20 minutes per hour for the first 48 to 72 hours (while awake). Thereafter, ice should be used at least three times per day for 20 minutes per treatment.
- Weight bearing as tolerated with hinged knee brace unlocked and crutches
- *Continuous passive motion (CPM) machine:* There is debate regarding its benefit. Potential merits may be discussed with patients. Regardless, regaining motion is a critical component of recovery.
- *Supine heel slides:* With the patient lying supine, have the patient use the contralateral leg or towel to assist in knee flexion. Hold the maximal bent position until tightness or stretching is perceived and hold for 5 seconds. Then, straighten the knee and repeat, with the goal to get to 90° by 2 weeks. Two sets of 10 repetitions (Figure 48.2).
- *Sitting heel slides:* Sitting in a chair, the patient should slide his or her heel underneath the chair until maximum flexion is gained, with the goal to get to 90° by 2 weeks. However, if the patient has a concomitant meniscus repair, the motion may be limited to 90° and not beyond. The patient can slide the body forward in the chair while keeping the foot planted firmly on the floor to enhance flexion. Hold for 5 seconds and straighten leg and repeat. Two sets of 10 repetitions (Figure 48.3).
- *Quadriceps setting:* With the patient supine or sitting, the patient should activate the quadriceps and forcefully extend the knee for a 5-second hold. A rolled towel underneath the heel may allow for more aggressive extension and quadriceps firing. Two sets of 10 repetitions (Figure 48.4).
- *Straight leg lift:* With the patient supine, have the patient fire the quadriceps to keep the leg straight and raise the entire leg off the ground. Hold at 45° for 1 to 2 seconds, then lower slowly. This works on the quadriceps, as well as on hip flexors and core. If the patient is not ready for this exercise because of poor quadriceps activation, the knee will flex when the leg is raised. The patient will likely need to work up to the 10 repetitions with 2 sets daily (Figure 48.5).
- *Prone ankle hang:* Passively work on knee extension. Perform this exercise on a bed. Lie face down with the leg dangling off the mattress. The edge of the mattress should be just above the level of the patella. If the knee does not come fully straight, the exercise can be augmented with an ankle weight ranging from 1 to 5 pounds. Three sets for 3 to 5 minutes (Figure 48.6).
- *Ankle pumps:* This should be performed as much as possible to maintain circulation.

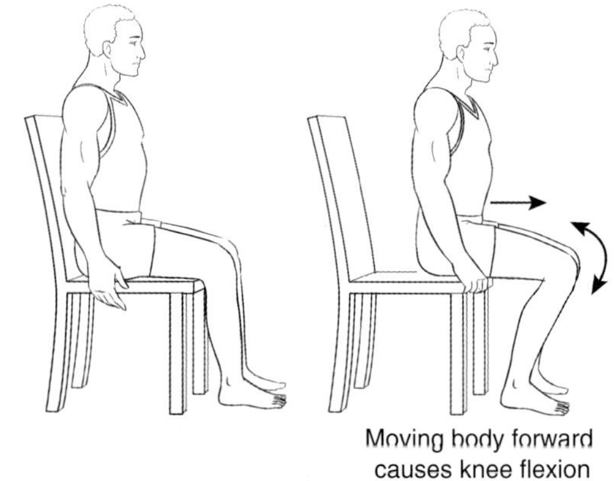

Figure 48.3 Illustration of the sitting heel slide.

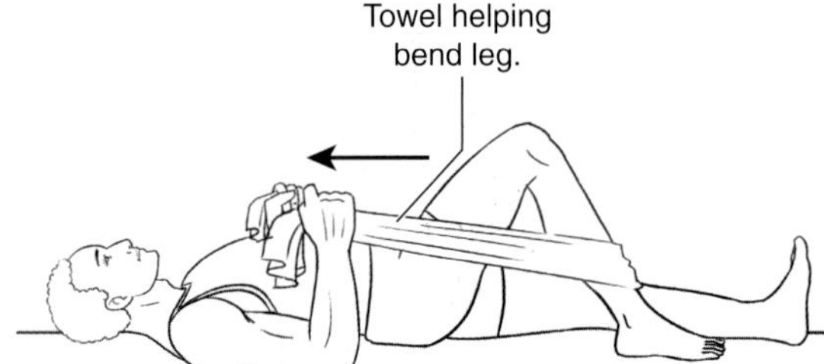

Figure 48.2 Illustration of the supine heel slide exercise.

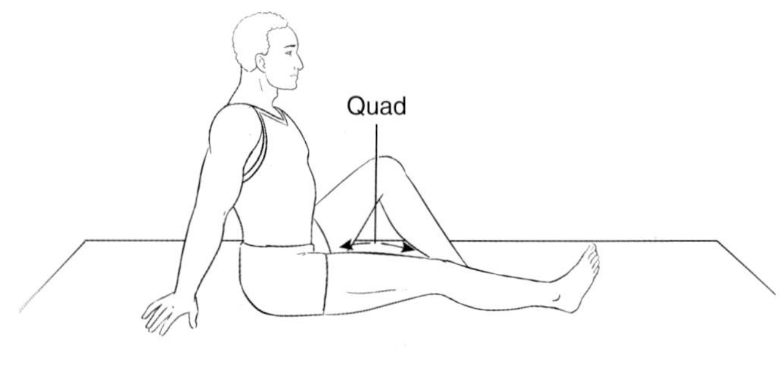

Figure 48.4 Illustration of the quadriceps setting exercise.

© 2018 American Academy of Orthopaedic Surgeons

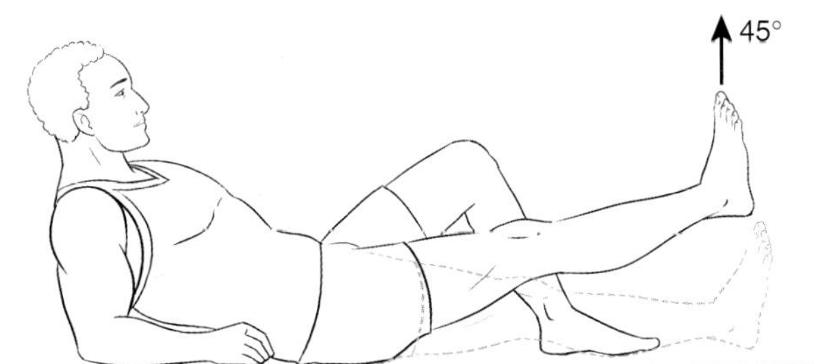

Figure 48.5 Illustration of the straight leg lift exercise.

Phase 2: Weeks 2 to 6

- Weight bearing as tolerated with hinged knee brace unlocked. Wean off crutches.
- Exercises may be performed without brace.
- *Supine heel slides:* With the patient lying supine, have the patient use the contralateral leg or towel to assist in knee flexion. Hold the maximal bent position until tightness or stretching is perceived and hold for 5 seconds. Then, straighten the knee and repeat, with the goal to get to 120° by 6 weeks. Three sets of 20 repetitions (Figure 48.2).
- *Sitting heel slides:* Sitting in a chair, the patient should slide the heel underneath the chair until maximum flexion is gained, with the goal to get to 120° by 6 weeks. However, if the patient has a concomitant meniscus repair, the motion may be limited to 90° and not beyond. The patient can slide the body forward in the chair while keeping the foot planted firmly on the floor to enhance flexion. Hold for 5 seconds and straighten leg and repeat. Three sets of 20 repetitions (Figure 48.3).
- *Quadriceps setting:* With the patient supine or sitting, the patient should activate the quadriceps and forcefully extend the knee for a 5-second hold. A rolled towel underneath the heel may allow for more aggressive extension and quadriceps firing. Three sets of 20 repetitions (Figure 48.4).
- *Straight leg lift:* With the patient supine, have the patient fire the quadriceps to keep the leg straight and raise the entire leg off the ground. Hold at 45° degrees for 1 to 2 seconds, then lower slowly. This works on the quadriceps, as well as on hip flexors and core. The patient will likely need to work up to the 10 repetitions with 3 sets daily (Figure 48.5).
- *Prone ankle hang:* Passively work on knee extension. Perform this exercise on a bed. Lie face down with the leg dangling off the mattress. The edge of the mattress should be just above the level of the patella. If the knee does not come fully straight, the exercise can be augmented with an ankle weight ranging from 1 to 5 pounds. Three sets for 3 to 5 minutes (Figure 48.6).

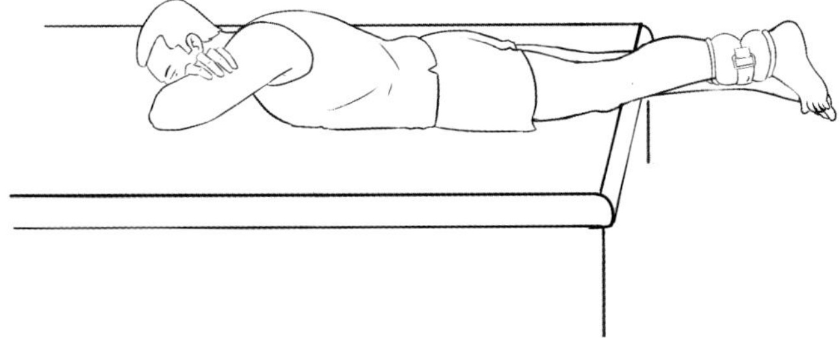

Figure 48.6 Illustration of the prone ankle hang exercise.

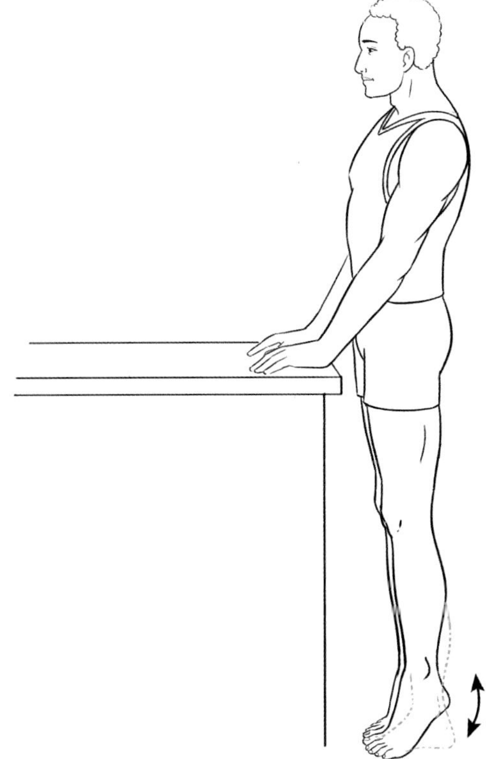

Figure 48.7 Illustration of the standing toe raise exercise.

- *Standing toe raise:* Standing and facing the wall, fire both the quadriceps to keep the knee straight and raise up on the toes for one 1 second, and then lower slowly. Have the patient use the wall as little as possible to work on balance. Repeat 20 times for 3 sets per day (Figure 48.7).
- *Standing hamstring curl:* The patient should be standing and holding onto a balance bar or wall for support. The patient should slowly bend the operative knee so that the heel approaches the buttock. Three sets of 20 repetitions (Figure 48.8).
- *Hip abduction:* Lie on the unoperated side. With the knee held straight, raise the operated leg to the side 45°. Hold for 1 second and lower slowly. Repeat 20 times daily (Figure 48.9).
- *Wall slides:* Stand with the patient's back touching the wall. Have the patient's feet facing forward and about 6 to 12 inches from the wall. Have the patient lower the body by flexing through both the hips and knees until the knees are flexed to 45°. Pause for 5 seconds at 45°, then slide up the walk to the original position. Three sets of 20 repetitions (Figure 48.10).

Phase 3: Weeks 6–12

- Discontinue brace
- *Supine heel slides:* With the patient lying supine, have the patient use the contralateral leg or towel to assist in knee flexion. Hold the maximal bent position until tightness

© 2018 American Academy of Orthopaedic Surgeons

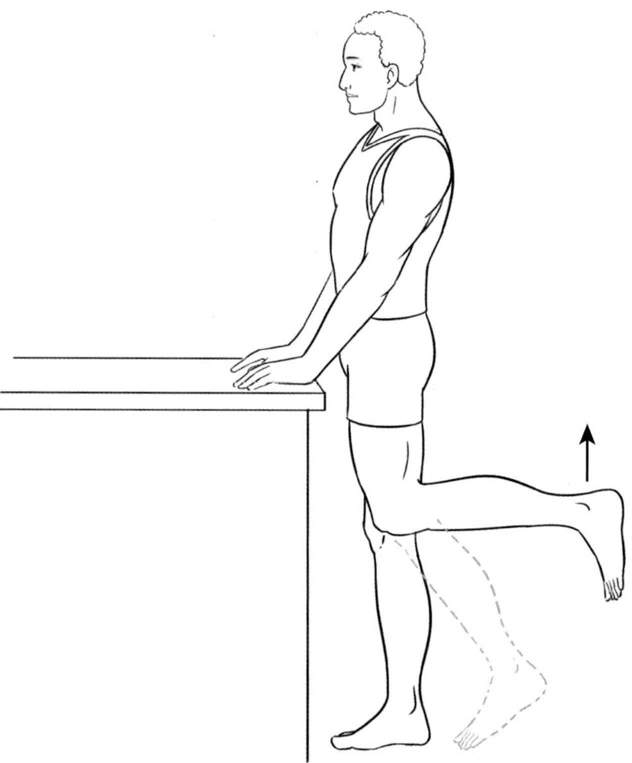

Figure 48.8 Illustration of the standing hamstring curl.

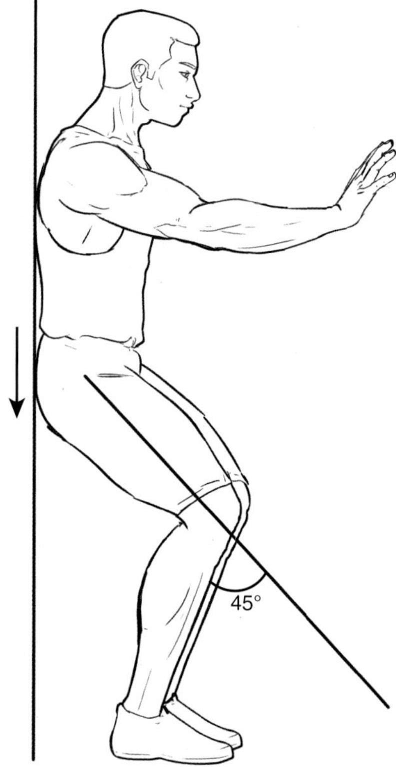

Figure 48.10 Illustration of the wall slide exercise.

or stretching is perceived and hold for 5 seconds. Then, straighten the knee and repeat, with the goal to get to full flexion by 12 weeks. Three sets of 20 repetitions (Figure 48.2).

- *Sitting heel slides:* Sitting in a chair, the patient should slide the heel underneath the chair until maximum flexion is gained, with the goal to get to full flexion by 12 weeks. The patient can slide the body forward in the chair while keeping the foot planted firmly on the floor to enhance flexion. Hold for 5 seconds and straighten leg and repeat. Three sets of 20 repetitions (Figure 48.3).
- *Quadriceps setting:* With the patient supine or sitting, the patient should activate the quadriceps and forcefully extend the knee for a 5-second hold. A rolled towel underneath the heel may allow for more aggressive extension and quadriceps firing. Three sets of 20 repetitions (Figure 48.4).
- *Straight leg lift:* With the patient supine, have the patient fire the quadriceps to keep the leg straight and raise the entire leg off the ground. Hold at 45° for 1 to 2 seconds, then lower slowly. This works on the quadriceps, as well as on hip flexors and core. The patient will likely need to work up to the 10 repetitions with 3 sets daily (Figure 48.5).

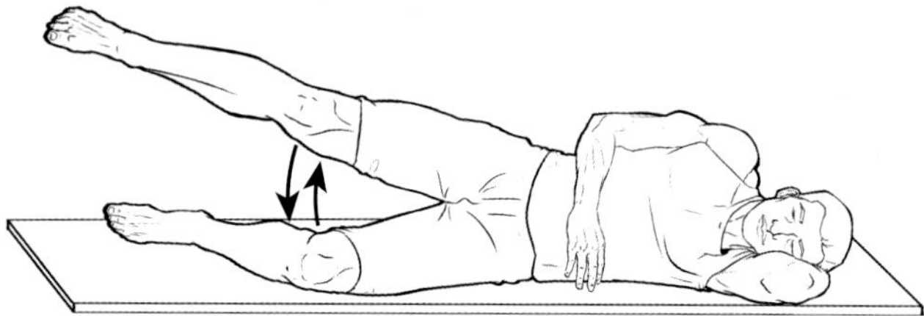

Figure 48.9 Illustration of the hip abduction exercise.

- *Prone ankle hang:* Passively work on knee extension. Perform this exercise on a bed. Lie face down with the leg dangling off the mattress. The edge of the mattress should be just above the level of the patella. If the knee does not come fully straight, the exercise can be augmented with an ankle weight ranging from 1 to 5 pounds. Three sets for 3 to 5 minutes (Figure 48.6).
- *Standing toe raise:* Standing and facing the wall, fire both the quadriceps to keep the knee straight and raise up on the toes for 1 second, then lower slowly. Have the patient use the wall as little as possible to work on balance. Repeat 20 times for 3 sets per day (Figure 48.7).
- *Standing hamstring curl:* The patient should be standing and holding onto a balance bar or wall for support. The patient should slowly bend the operative knee so that the heel approaches the buttock. Three sets of 20 repetitions (Figure 48.8).
- Hip abduction: Lie on the unoperated side. With the knee held straight, raise the operated leg to the side 45°. Hold for 1 second and lower slowly. Repeat 20 times daily (Figure 48.9).
- Wall slides: Stand with the patient's back touching the wall. Have the feet facing forward and about 6 to 12 inches from the wall. Have the patient lower the body by flexing through both the hips and knees until the knees are flexed to 45°. Pause for 5 seconds at 45° degrees, then slide up the walk to the original position. Three sets of 20 repetitions (Figure 48.10).
- *Squat to chair:* Have the patient stand above a chair, then slowly squat down to the chair until the buttock touches the

© 2018 American Academy of Orthopaedic Surgeons

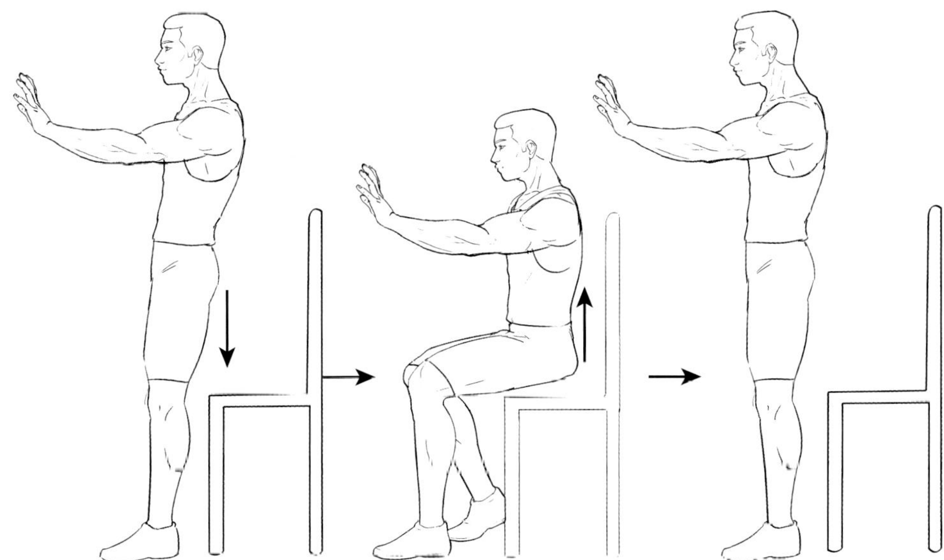

Figure 48.11 Illustration of the squat to chair exercise.

chair, and then immediately return to the starting standing position. Do not allow the patient to sit on the chair. Hand weights can be added as strength improves. Three sets of 20 repetitions (Figure 48.11).

- *Seated leg press:* Build quadriceps strength. Start with an easily lifted weight and progress weekly as the patient makes progress. Do not exceed the patient's own body weight. Do not allow flexion beyond 90°. Three sets of 20 repetitions (Figure 48.12).
- *Stationary bicycle:* This can help with motion and strength. Set the seat so that the operative leg is at full extension at the bottom of the pedal cycle. Start at low resistance and increase slowly over 4 weeks. Do 20 to 30 minutes per day (Figure 48.13).
- *Stretching exercises:* It is important to work on stretching in addition to strengthening. The three main stretches are the prone quadriceps, hamstrings, and calf. Each should be done twice per day, 5 repetitions, holding for 15 to 20 seconds (Figure 48.14).

Phase 4: Weeks 12–24

- The Phase 3 exercises should be continued, but the number of sets and repetitions will have to be decreased (2 sets of 10–15 repetitions) to allow more time for advanced muscular strengthening, cardiovascular conditioning, and sport-specific training.
- Strength training should alternate every other day cardiovascular/sport-specific training.
- Strength training days (3 days per week)
    - Phase 3 exercises (2 sets of 10–15 repetitions). Add light weights if more resistance is needed.
    - *Step-up/Step-down:* Builds strength, balance, and proprioception. Place the operated leg on a low, flat, stable stool. Have the unoperated leg off the ground and slowly bend the operated leg so that the unoperated leg just touches the ground. Straighten the operated leg to go back to the original position. Maintain a balanced upright posture during the exercise. Keep the thigh, knee, and foot all pointed forward and do not allow rotation. The stool height can be increased from 3, 6, and 9 inches as the patient progresses. 2 sets of 10 to 15 repetitions depending on conditioning and balance (Figure 48.15).
    - *Single leg wall slides:* Stand with the patient's back touching the wall. Have the patient's feet facing forward and about 6 to 12 inches from the wall. Holding the nonoperative leg off the ground, have the patient lower the body by flexing the operative hip and knee until the knee is

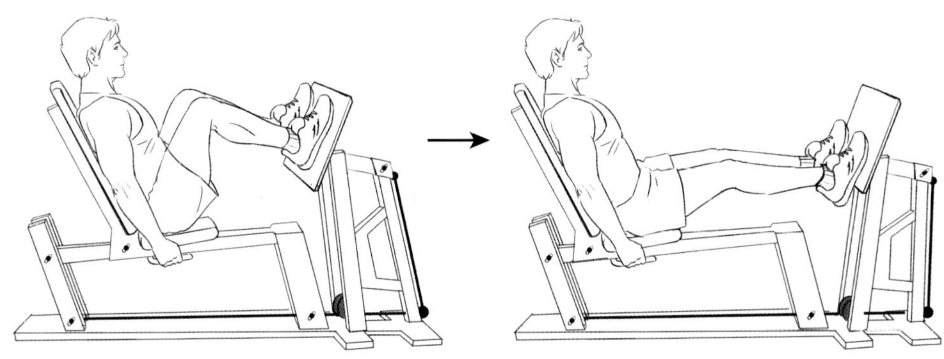

Figure 48.12 Seated leg press.

© 2018 American Academy of Orthopaedic Surgeons

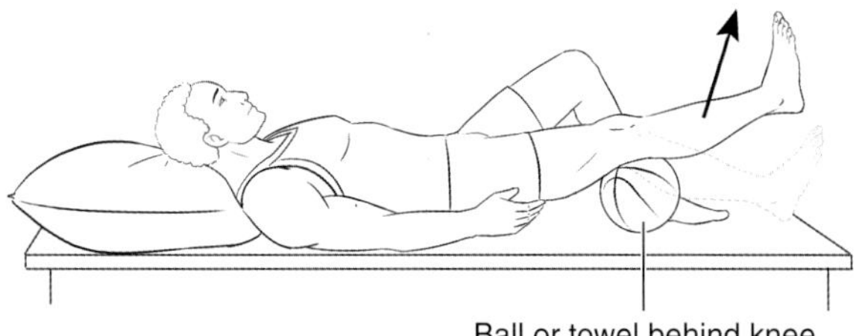

Figure 48.13 Illustration of the stationary bicycle exercise.

flexed to 45° degrees. Pause for 5 seconds at 45 degrees, then slide up the wall to the original position. Three sets of 5 to 10 repetitions.

- Single leg squat to chair: Have the patient stand above a chair, then slowly squat down to the chair using only the operative leg until the buttock touches the chair, and then return to the starting standing position. Do not allow the patient to sit on the chair. Hand weights can be added as strength improves. Three sets of 5 to 10 repetitions.

- Cardiovascular/sport-specific training days (3 days per week)
  - *Stationary bicycle or elliptical machine:* Increase resistance as tolerated. Do 30 minutes per session.
  - Light running on a soft, level surface. Start running for 5 minutes and increase to 30 minutes over a 4-week period. This should be alternated with strengthening every other day.
  - *Speed and agility training:* When running in line for 30 minutes is relatively easy and does not cause pain or swelling, consider starting speed and agility training. This portion of rehabilitation will have to be individualized to the specific patient. Progression typically follows the following pattern:
    - In-line sprinting starting at half speed for 100 yards for 10 repetitions

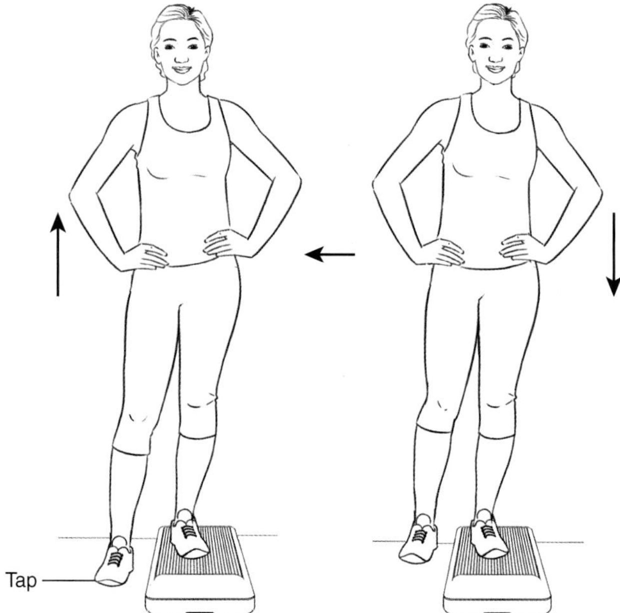

Figure 48.15 Illustration of the step-up/step-down exercise.

    - Advance in-line sprinting to full speed, 100 yards for 10 repetitions
    - Add cones or zig-zag running
    - Add forward and backward running
    - Add figure-of-eight running
    - Add carioca running
    - Add shuttle run
    - Jumping and plyometric training

Phase 5: Weeks 24 and Beyond

- Return to unrestricted pivoting sports (ACL brace recommended)

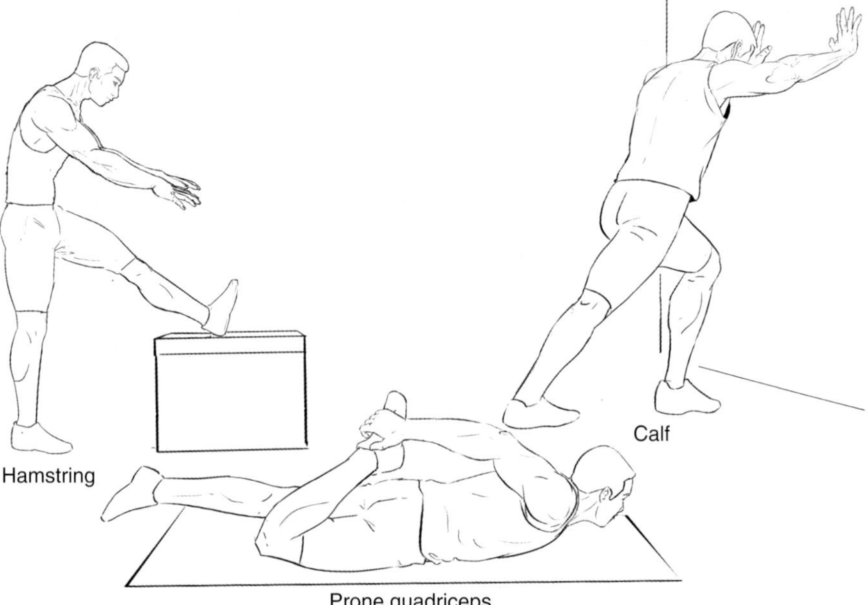

Figure 48.14 Illustration of stretching exercises.

© 2018 American Academy of Orthopaedic Surgeons

OUTCOMES

ACL reconstruction surgery is a common and highly successful procedure that is able to restore stability of the knee following appropriate rehabilitation. However, full recovery may take up to a year to resume high-level sport. Not all patients are able to do so for a variety of reasons. Although a majority can return to their preinjury level of activity, some can only return to a lower level. Long-term, many reconstructed patients may still develop arthritis. Clinicians are working on techniques to optimize results, limit complications, and predict those at risk for arthritis and re-rupture.

PEARLS

- Protect the reconstruction early. Surgeons will determine the duration of bracing, weight-bearing status, and ROM restrictions based on patient factors, graft selection, and fixation.
- Quadriceps reactivation and strengthening are critical to recovery.
- Pain and swelling are normal after surgery. However, if the patient develops worsening pain and/or swelling, contact the surgeon and do not advance the rehabilitation program.
- Strength and motion should be normal prior to advancing to running.
- If there are concomitant injuries, such as meniscal, cartilage, or other ligaments, the rehabilitation may have to be significantly altered.

BIBLIOGRAPHY

Beynnon BD, Johnson RJ, Fleming BC, Kannus P, Kaplan M, Samani J, Renström P: Anterior cruciate ligament reconstruction: Comparison of bone-patellar tendon-bone grafts with two strand hamstring graft. A prospective, randomized study. *J Bone Joint Surg Am* 2002;84-A(9):1503–1513.

Czuppon S, Racette BA, Klein SE, Harris-Hayes M: Variables associated with return to sport following anterior cruciate ligament reconstruction: a systematic review. *Br J Sports Med* 2014;48(5):356–364.

Mariscalco MW, Magnussen RA, Mehta D, Hewett TE, Flanigan DC, Kaeding CC: Autograft versus nonirradiated allograft tissue for anterior cruciate ligament reconstruction: A systematic review. *Am J Sports Med* 2014;42(2):492–499.

© 2018 American Academy of Orthopaedic Surgeons

49 Patellar Realignment

Seth Jerabek, MD

INTRODUCTION

Patellofemoral dislocation is estimated to account for 2% to 3% of all knee injuries. Females between the ages of 10 to 17 years are the highest risk group. Those who participate in pivoting sports, have patella alta, a high Q angle, a high tibial tubercle to tibial groove (TT-TG) distance, and/or a dysplastic trochlea are at higher risk for instability and dislocation (Figure 49.1). The Q angle is formed by a line bisecting the axis of the patella and the patellar tendon and a line along the shaft of the femur, which determines the vector of pull of the quadriceps. When treated nonsurgically, recurrent dislocations occur at an estimated rate of 15% to 50% depending on activity-level underlying risk factors.

Lateral dislocations occur when the medial patellofemoral ligament (MPFL) ruptures, which is the primary medial patellar stabilizer (Figure 49.2). If the MPFL becomes incompetent, the patella will track laterally and may tilt. This likely increases the risk of dislocation and increases pressure of the lateral patellar facet and lateral trochlea, which could lead to arthritis. Additionally, the bony alignment, including the Q angle and TT-TG distance, affect patellar tracking and stability.

Patients with patellar instability often have chondral or osteochondral injuries leading to crepitus or even locking or catching of the knee. After the acute injury, patients may experience a vague sense of instability of the knee, particularly in sports that requiring pivoting. On examination, the patella is often hypermobile and tracks laterally. Manual lateral subluxation of the patella causes apprehension.

Patients with chronic instability and multiple dislocations often benefit from surgery. However, patients with a single, acute dislocation may be indicated for surgery depending on the presence of a loose body requiring surgery, limb alignment, and underlying risk of further dislocations. Carefully selected patients without dislocation but chronic pain around the patella and distinct clinical evidence of maltracking may also be candidates for surgical realignment if nonoperative measures fail to provide adequate relief.

SURGICAL PROCEDURE—PATELLAR REALIGNMENT

Indications

- Patella dislocation in a young, active patient with abnormal patellar tracking
- Loose body requiring surgery
- Recurrent instability

Contraindications

- Single dislocation with a normal tracking patella and normal bony alignment
- Skeletal immaturity

Procedure

Treating patellar instability has been divided into proximal and distal realignment procedures. In both procedures, a knee arthroscopy is often performed to treat a loose body, evaluate the cartilage surfaces, and to assess patellar tracking during knee motion. In proximal realignment, the repair is soft-tissue based, and is often a combination of an MPFL repair, reconstruction, or medial reefing with or without a lateral retinacular release. Distal realignment procedures focus on correcting underlying bony malalignment by using an osteotomy to translate the tibial tubercle in the medial or anteromedial direction to decrease the Q angle, TT-TG distance, and contact pressure at the lateral patellar facet. Distal realignment procedures often incorporate a proximal soft-tissue procedure, such as an MPFL reconstruction and/or lateral release during the procedure. The decision on the best procedure for the patient is dependent on patient anatomy, alignment, activity level, and surgeon preference.

POSTOPERATIVE REHABILITATION

Introduction

Rehabilitation after patellar realignment will vary from patient to patient and from surgeon to surgeon. It will be based on the reconstruction performed and surgeon preference. It is critical

Dr. Jerabek or an immediate family member is a member of a speakers' bureau or has made paid presentations on behalf of Stryker, and serves as a paid consultant to Stryker.

© 2018 American Academy of Orthopaedic Surgeons

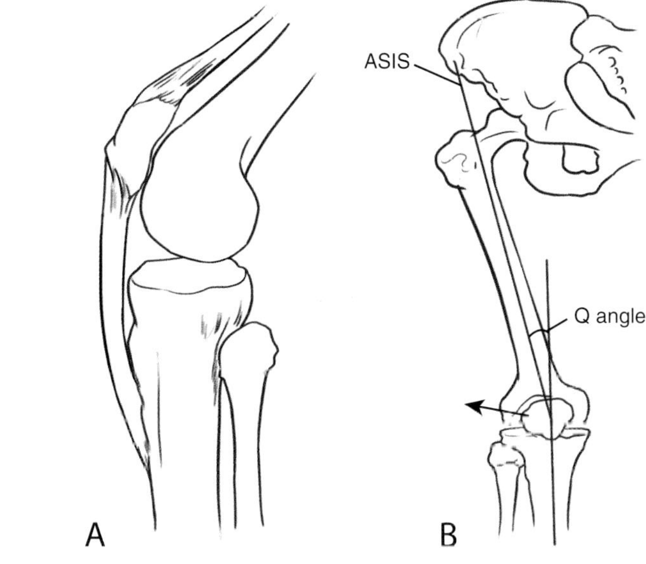

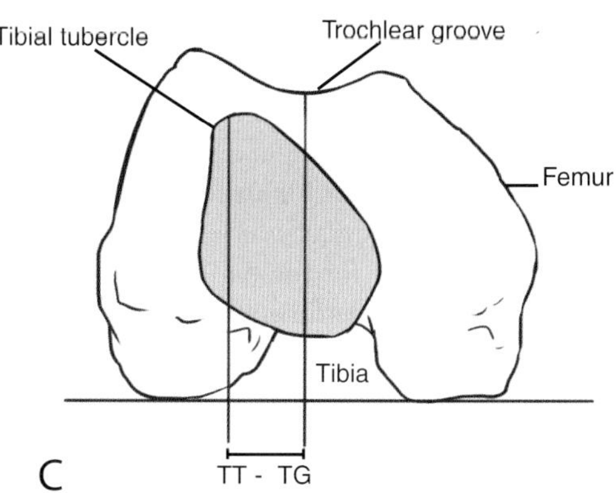

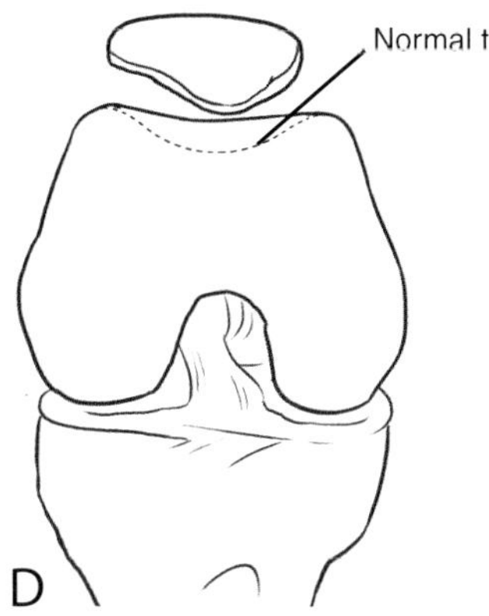

Figure 49.1 Illustrations of risk factors for dislocation. **A**, Patella alta: High patella relative to joint line. **B**, Q-angle: The higher the Q-angle the more lateral force with quadriceps contraction. **C**, Tibial tubercle to trochlear grove distance. The higher the distance, the more lateral force on the patella. **D**, Trocheal dysplasia: The trocheal groove is shallow leading to instability.

for the surgeon and therapist to have specific recommendations and open communication regarding bracing, weight bearing, and motion. The following outline is a standard protocol and progression that may be used for both proximal and distal realignments.

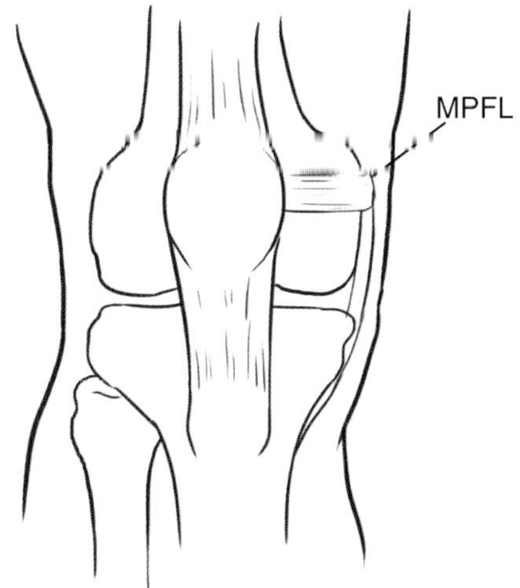

Figure 49.2 Illustration of medial patellofemoral ligament.

Functional Goals and Restrictions

Goals for the first 2 weeks after surgery include controlling pain and swelling, initiating knee motion, and regaining quadriceps activation. From weeks 2 to 6, the patient is typically in a hinged knee brace locked in extension for weight bearing, but can transition off crutches. The patient can work on regaining motion, and can start muscle activation. At 6 weeks and onward, the patient comes out of the brace and works on regaining full motion and strength. Generally, patients can return to in-line sports such as bicycling and light running at 3 months, and pivoting sports between 6 and 9 months. However, patients who undergo an osteotomy may have an altered rehabilitation protocol depending on the surgeon's assessment of fixation and degree of bone healing, especially in the first 2 to 3 months. The rehabilitation goals can be subdivided as below.

Phase 1 (Swelling Control): Weeks 0 to 2

- Control swelling with ice and compression
- Weight bearing as tolerated with hinged knee brace locked in extension and crutches
- Gentle early motion, work on regaining full extension
- Quadriceps activation

© 2018 American Academy of Orthopaedic Surgeons

Phase 2 (Motion and Early Strengthening): Weeks 2 to 6

- Weight bearing as tolerated with hinged knee brace locked in extension
- Discontinue crutches when comfortable doing so
- Maintain full extension and flexion to 120°
- Begin quadriceps strengthening

Phase 3 (Normal Gait and Motion): Weeks 6 to 12

- Transition out of brace
- Regain full flexion
- Walk with normal heel-toe gait
- Muscle strengthening

Phase 4 (Early Sport Activity): Weeks 12 to 20

- Regain full muscle strength
- Cardiovascular conditioning
- In-line running
- Sport-specific training (speed and agility training)

Phase 5 (Full Sport Activity): Week 20 Onward

- Return to pivoting sports

Preferred Protocol

Phase 1: Weeks 0–2

- Ice or a cooling device should be used for 20 minutes per hour for the first 48 to 72 hours (while awake). Thereafter, ice should be used at least three times per day for 20 minutes per treatment.
- Weight bearing as tolerated with hinged knee brace locked in extension and crutches
- *Supine heel slides:* With the patient lying supine, have the patient use the contralateral leg or towel to assist in knee flexion. Hold the maximal bent position until tightness or stretching is perceived and hold for 5 seconds. Then, straighten the knee and repeat, with the goal to get to 90° by 2 weeks. Two sets of 10 repetitions (Figure 49.3)
- *Sitting heel slides:* Sitting in a chair, the patient should slide the heel underneath the chair until maximum flexion is gained, with the goal to get to 90° by 2 weeks. The patient can slide the body forward in the chair while keeping the foot planted firmly on the floor to enhance flexion. Hold for 5 seconds and straighten leg, and repeat. Two sets of 10 repetitions (Figure 49.4).

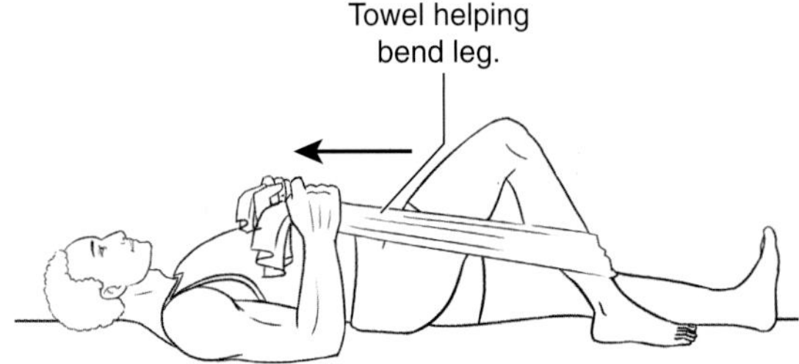

Figure 49.3 Illustration of supine heel slide exercise.

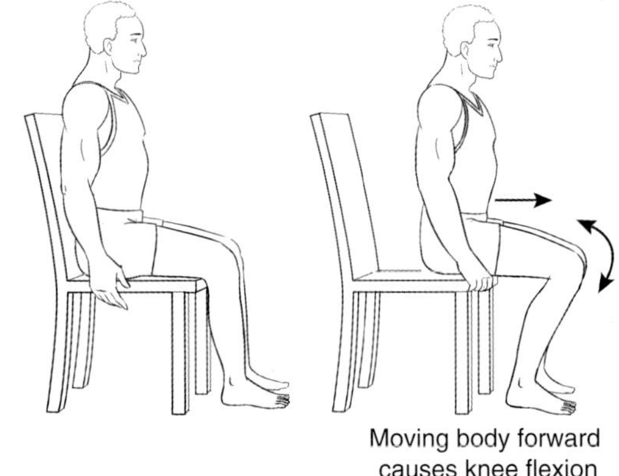

Figure 49.4 Illustration of sitting heel slide exercise.

- *Quadriceps setting:* With the patient supine or sitting, the patient should activate the quadriceps and forcefully extend the knee for a 5-second hold. A rolled towel underneath the heel may allow for more aggressive extension and quadriceps firing. Two sets of 10 repetitions (Figure 49.5).
- *Straight leg lift:* With the patient supine, have the patient fire the quadriceps to keep the leg straight and raise the entire leg off the ground. Hold at 45° for 1 to 2 seconds, then lower slowly. This works on the quadriceps, as well as on hip flexors and core. It is important for the patient to be able to maintain full extension while performing this exercise. The patient will likely need to work up to the 10 repetitions with 2 sets daily (Figure 49.6).
- *Prone ankle hang:* Passively work on knee extension. Perform this exercise on a bed. Lie face down with the leg dangling off the mattress. The edge of the mattress should be just above the level of the patella. If the knee does not come fully straight, the exercise can be augmented with an ankle weight ranging from 1 to 5 pounds. Three sets for 3 to 5 minutes (Figure 49.7).
- *Ankle pumps:* This should be performed as much as possible to maintain circulation.

Phase 2: Weeks 2–6

- Weight bearing as tolerated with hinged knee brace locked in extension. Wean off crutches.
- Exercises may be performed without brace.

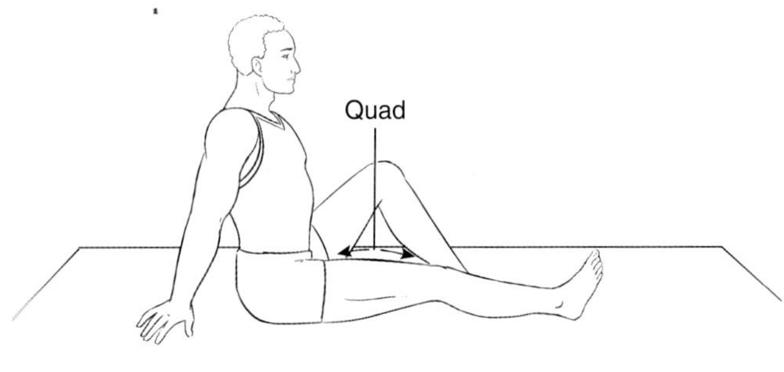

Figure 49.5 Illustration of quadriceps sitting exercise.

 © 2018 American Academy of Orthopaedic Surgeons

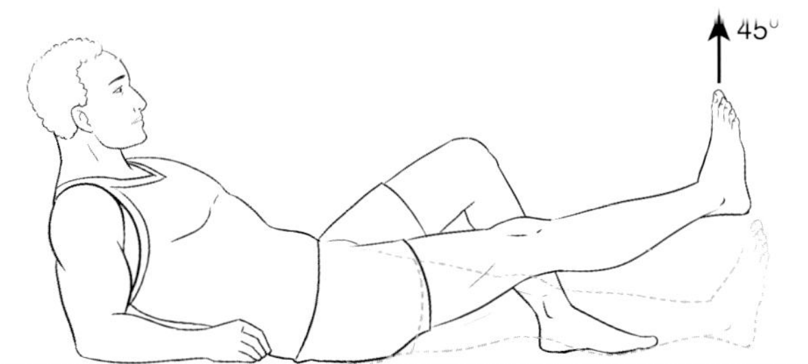

Figure 49.6 Illustration of straight leg lift exercise.

- *Supine heel slides:* Goal is to get to 120° by six weeks. Three sets of 20 repetitions.
- *Sitting heel slides:* Goal is to get to 120° by 6 weeks. Three sets of 20 repetitions.
- *Quadriceps setting:* Three sets of 20 repetitions.
- *Straight leg lift:* Three sets of 10 repetitions.
- *Prone ankle hang:* If the knee does not come fully straight, the exercise can be augmented with an ankle weight ranging from 1 to 5 pounds. Three sets for 3 to 5 minutes.
- *Standing toe raise:* Standing and facing the wall, fire both the quadriceps to keep the knee straight and raise up on toes for 1 second, then lower slowly. Have the patient use the wall as little as possible to work on balance. Repeat 20 times for 3 sets per day (Figure 49.8).
- *Standing hamstring curl:* The patient should be standing and holding onto a balance bar or wall for support. The patient should slowly bend the operative knee so that the heel approaches the buttock. Three sets of 20 repetitions (Figure 49.9).
- *Hip abduction:* Lie on the unoperated side. With the knee held straight, raise the operated leg to the side 45°. Hold for 1 second and lower slowly. Repeat 20 times daily (Figure 49.10).

Phase 3: Weeks 6–12

- Discontinue brace
- *Supine heel slides:* May discontinue when full flexion is reached. Three sets of 20 repetitions.
- *Sitting heel slides:* May discontinue when full flexion reached. Three sets of 20 repetitions.
- *Quadriceps setting:* Three sets of 20 repetitions.
- *Straight leg lift:* May add 1- to 5-pound ankle weights. Three sets of 10 repetitions.
- *Prone ankle hang:* Three sets for 3 to 5 minutes.
- *Standing toe raise:* Three sets of 20 repetitions.

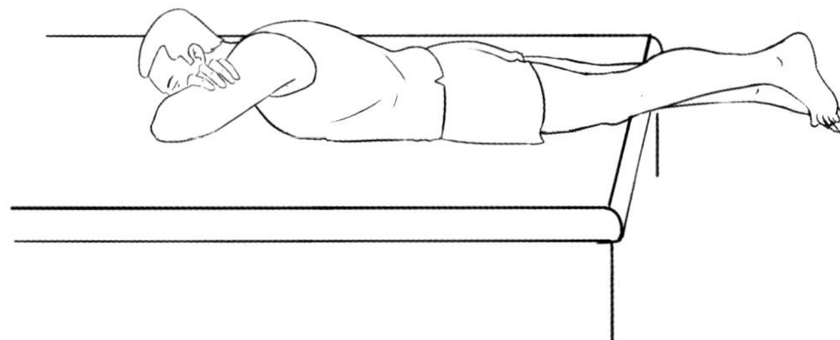

Figure 49.7 Illustration of prone ankle hang exercise.

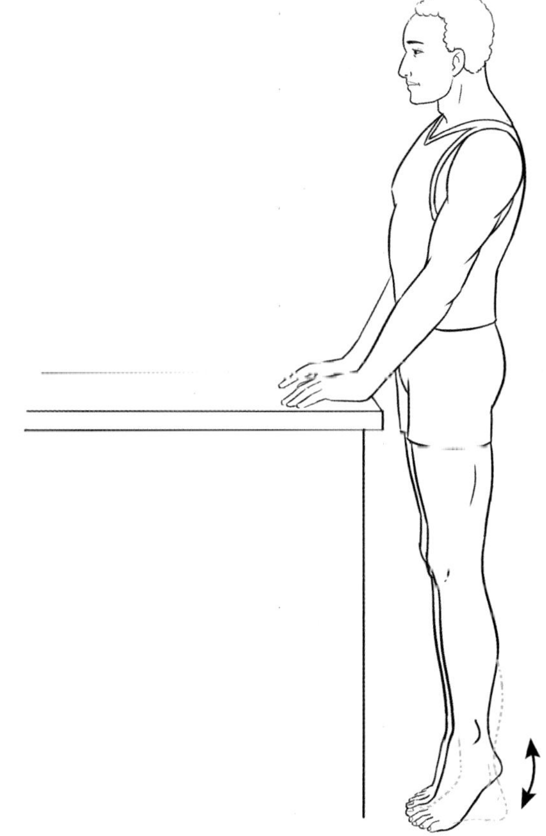

Figure 49.8 Illustration of standing toe raise exercise.

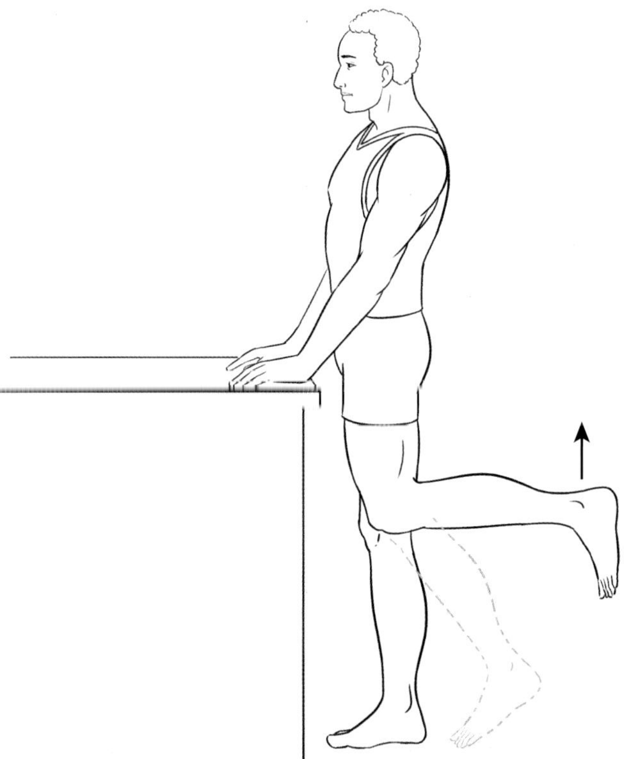

Figure 49.9 Illustration of standing hamstring curl exercise.

© 2018 American Academy of Orthopaedic Surgeons

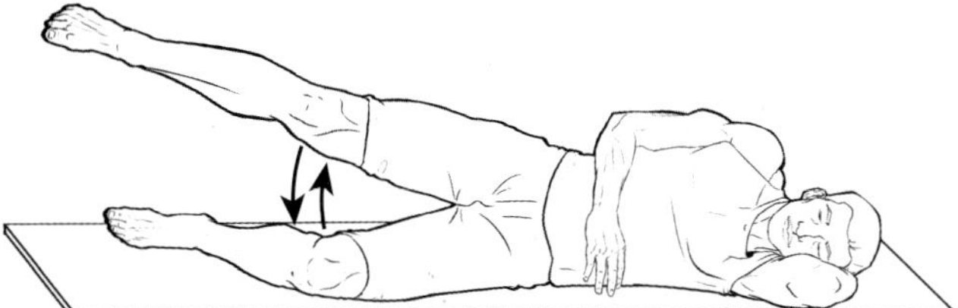

Figure 49.10 Illustration of the hip abduction exercise.

- *Standing hamstring curl:* May incorporate hamstring curl machine if more resistance needed. Three sets of 20 repetitions.
- *Hip abduction:* Twenty repetitions daily.
- *Wall slides:* Stand with the patient's back touching the wall. Have the patient's feet facing forward and about 6 to 12 inches from the wall. Have the patient lower the body by flexing through both the hips and knees until the knees are flexed to 45°. Pause for 5 seconds at 45°, then slide up the wall to the original position. Three sets of 20 repetitions (Figure 49.11).
- *Stationary bicycle:* This can help with motion and strength. Set the seat so that the operative leg is at full extension at the bottom of the pedal cycle. Start at low resistance and increase slowly over 4 weeks. Do 20 to 30 minutes per day (Figure 49.12).
- *Stretching exercises:* It is important to work on stretching in addition to strengthening. The three main stretches are the prone quadriceps, hamstrings, and calf. Each should be done twice per day, 5 repetitions, holding for 15 to 20 seconds (Figure 49.13).

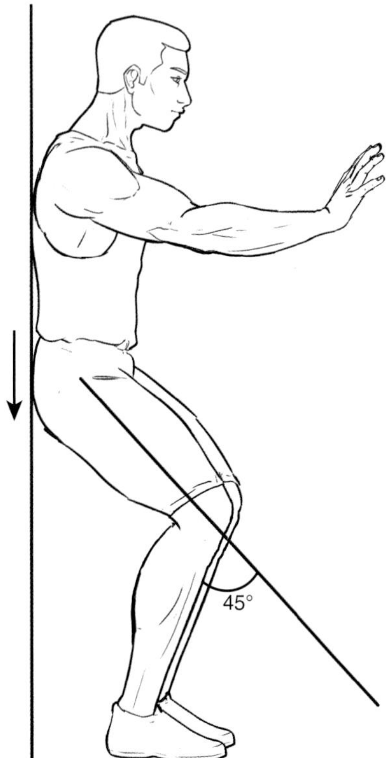

Figure 49.11 Illustration of wall slide exercise.

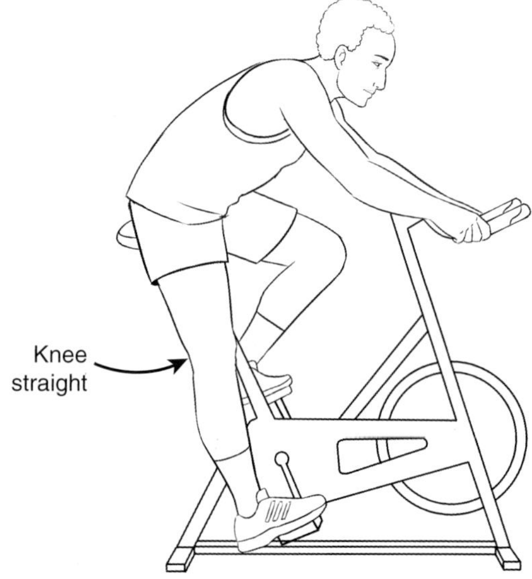

Figure 49.12 Illustration of stationary bicycle exercise.

Phase 4: Weeks 12–20

- The Phase 3 exercises should be continued, but the number of sets and repetitions will have to be decreased (2 sets of 10–15 reps) to allow more time for advanced muscular strengthening, cardiovascular conditioning, and sport-specific training.
- Strength training should alternate every other day with cardiovascular/sport-specific training.
- Strength training days (3 days per week)
    - Phase 3 exercises (2 sets of 10–15 repetitions). Add light weights if more resistance is needed.
    - *Squat to chair:* Have the patient stand above a chair and then slowly squat down to the chair until the buttock touches the chair, then immediately return to the starting standing position. Do not allow the patient to sit on the chair. Hand weights can be added as strength improves. Three sets of 20 repetitions (Figure 49.14).
    - *Seated leg press:* Build quadriceps strength. Start with an easily lifted weight and progress weekly as the patient makes progress. Do not exceed the patient's own body weight. Patients with osteotomies also perform this exercise when the bone has healed. Do not allow flexion beyond 90°. Three sets of 20 repetitions (Figure 49.15).
    - *Step-up/step-down:* Builds strength, balance, and proprioception. Place the operated leg on a low, flat, stable stool. Have the unoperated leg off the ground and slowly bend the operated leg so that the unoperated leg just touches the ground. Straighten the operated leg to go back to the original position. Maintain a balanced upright posture during the exercise. Keep the thigh, knee, and foot all pointed forward and do not allow rotation. The stool height can be increased from 3, 6, and 9 inches as the patient progresses. Two sets of 10 to 15 repetitions depending on conditioning and balance (Figure 49.16).

 © 2018 American Academy of Orthopaedic Surgeons

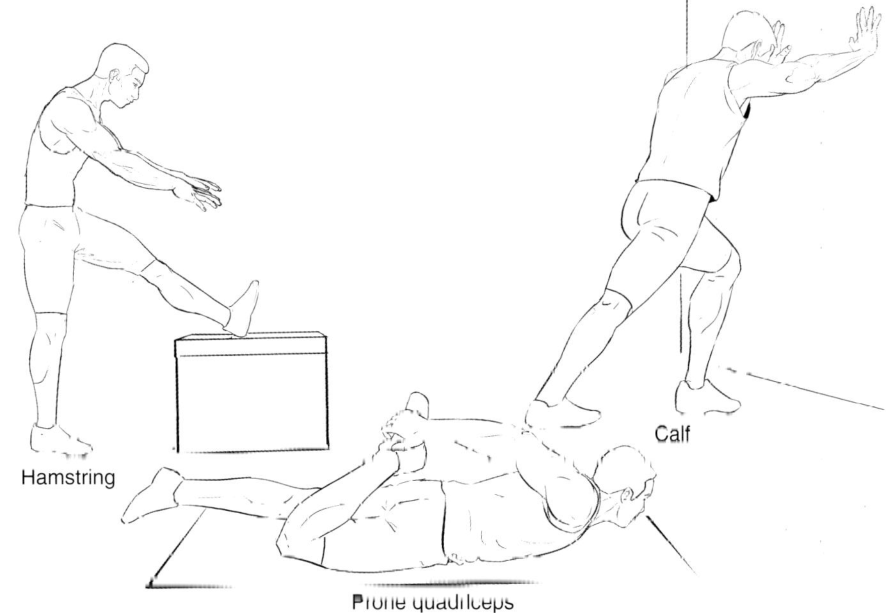

Figure 49.13 Illustration of stretching exercises.

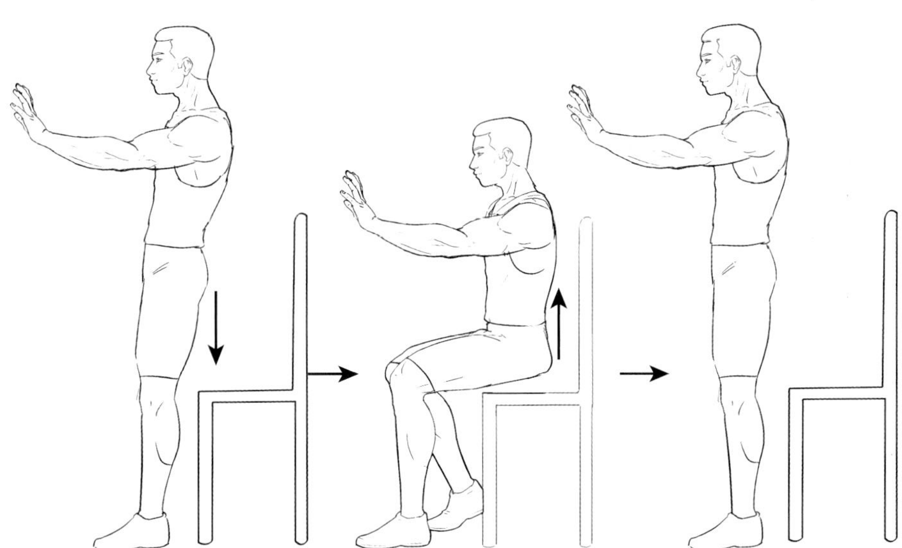

Figure 49.14 Illustration of squat to chair exercise.

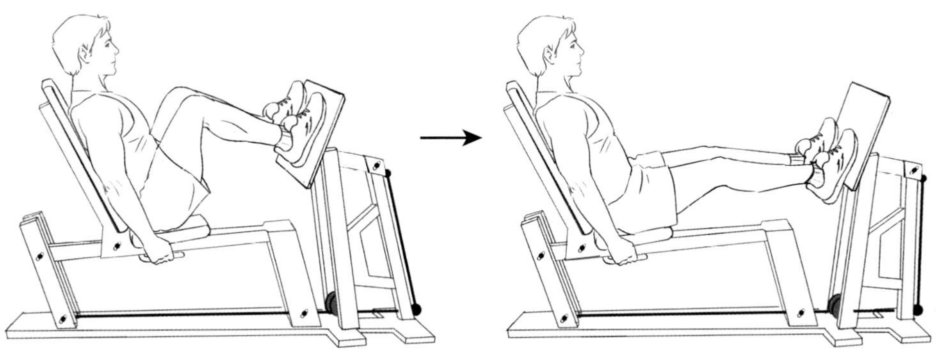

Figure 49.15 Illustration of seated leg press exercise.

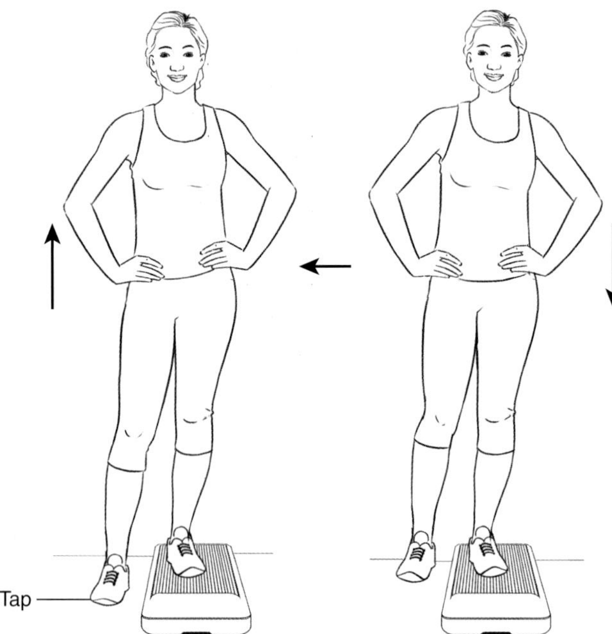

Figure 49.16 Illustration of step-up/Step-down exercise.

- *Single leg wall slides:* Stand with the patient's back touching the wall. Have the patient's feet facing forward and about 6 to 12 inches from the wall. Holding the nonoperative leg off the ground, have the patient lower the body by flexing the operative hip and knee until the knee is flexed to 45°. Pause for 5 seconds at 45°, then slide up the walk to the original position. Three sets of 5 to 10 repetitions.
- *Single leg squat to chair:* Have the patient stand above a chair and then slowly squat down to the chair using only the operative leg until the buttock touches the chair, then return to the starting standing position. Do not allow the patient to sit on the chair. Hand weights can be added as strength improves. Do not start this exercise until standard squat to chair is effortless. Three sets of 5 to 10 repetitions.

- Cardiovascular/sport-specific training days (3 days per week)
  - *Stationary bicycle or elliptical machine:* Increase resistance as tolerated. Do 30 minutes per session.
  - Light running on a soft, level surface. Start running for 5 minutes, increasing to 30 minutes over a 4-week period. This should be alternated with strengthening every other day.
  - *Speed and agility training:* When running in line for 30 minutes is relatively easy and does not cause pain or swelling, consider starting speed and agility training. This portion of rehabilitation will have to be individualized to the specific patient. Progression typically follows the following pattern:
    - In-line sprinting starting at half speed for 100 yards for 10 repetitions
    - Advance in-line sprinting to full speed, 100 yards for 10 repetitions
    - Add cones or zig-zag running
    - Add forward and backward running
    - Add figure-of-eight running
    - Add carioca running
    - Add shuttle run
    - Jumping and plyometric training

Phase 5: Weeks 20 and Beyond

- Return to unrestricted pivoting sports

OUTCOMES

The various patellar realignment procedures are successful in preventing recurrent instability and reducing pain. These improvements are durable, but residual symptoms are common. Pain with stair climbing and kneeling often persists and may limit vigorous activity. Pain related to prominent hardware from distal realignment procedures is reliably relieved with removal.

PEARLS

- The surgical procedure can vary greatly depending on the patient's underlying soft-tissue injury and mechanical alignment.
- Protect the realignment early. Surgeons will determine the duration of bracing, weight-bearing status, and range of motion restrictions based on patient factors and procedure performed.
- Quadriceps reactivation is critical to recovery.
- Regain full motion by 6 to 8 weeks after surgery.
- Strength and motion should be normal prior to advancing to running.

BIBLIOGRAPHY

Arendt EA, Fithian DC, Cohen E: Current concepts of lateral patella dislocation. *Clin Sports Med* 2002;21(3):499–519.

Boddula MR, Adamson GJ, Pink MM: Medial reefing without lateral release for recurrent patellar instability: midterm and long-term outcomes. *Am J Sports Med* 2014;42(1):216–224.

Colvin AC, West RV: Patellar instability. *J Bone Joint Surg Am* 2008;90(12):2751–2762.

Fulkerson JP, Becker GJ, Meaney JA, Miranda M, Folcik MA: Anteromedial tibial tubercle transfer without bone graft. *Am J Sports Med* 1990;18(5):490–496; discussion 496–497.

 © 2018 American Academy of Orthopaedic Surgeons

50 Patellar and Quadriceps Tendon Repairs

Andrea Tychanski, PT, DPT, SCS, ATC, CSCS, John Cavanaugh, PT, ATC, SCS, and Anil S. Ranawat, MD

INTRODUCTION

Patellar and quadriceps tendon ruptures are debilitating injuries that usually require surgical repair and physical therapy. The patellar and quadriceps tendons are crucial components of the extensor mechanism of the knee. Knee extension plays an important role in one's ability to perform basic activities of daily living (ADLs). Most quadriceps tendon injuries occur in individuals around 50 years of age, while the majority of patellar tendon injuries occur in patients around 40 years of age.

Complete patellar or quadriceps ruptures typically present with a palpable infrapatellar or suprapatellar defect and a noticeable effusion. With a patellar tendon rupture, the patella is high riding, while with a quadriceps rupture it may be masked by the swelling. In both cases, assessment of the extensor mechanism will demonstrate an inability to straight leg raise or an extension lag.

INDICATIONS AND CONTRAINDICATIONS

For optimal results, a complete patellar or quadriceps tendon disruption requires surgical repair. Ideal timing for surgical intervention is within 3 weeks following the acute episode. Nonambulators, patients who possess severe comorbidities or have compromised soft tissues in the area secondary to prior trauma, are not candidates for surgery. Patients who have a known history of noncompliance with rehabilitation or have a partial tear without a knee extensor lag during a straight leg raise are best treated conservatively. Some partial quadriceps tendon ruptures may also be treated nonoperatively.

SURGICAL PROCEDURE

The surgical technique utilized for patellar and quadriceps tendon tears occurring at or near the osteotendinous junction involves a patellar drill hole technique. An anterior incision is made, exposing the extensor mechanism. Interlocking nonabsorbable sutures are passed through the tendonous portion of the torn tendon. Interlocking sutures are then passed through longitudinal transosseous patellar drill holes and tied over a patellar bone bridge. Midsubstance tears are repaired via an end-to-end primary repair utilizing interrupted nonabsorbable sutures. The final step of a surgical repair involves attention to the medial and lateral retinaculum. Tears to either retinaculum are identified and repaired with sutures using a figure-of-eight technique. Following repair, the knee is taken through a gentle range of motion (ROM) from 0° to 60° to assess the tension on the repair.

POSTOPERATIVE REHABILITATION

Rehabilitation following a quadriceps or patellar tendon repair should be initiated immediately following surgery, although full tensile strength is not achieved until 9 to 12 months from injury. Communication between the physical therapist and surgeon is important to discuss surgical procedure, including the quality of the repaired tissue and any concomitant injuries. In addition, postoperative ROM progression and weight-bearing status is clarified. The surgeon and physical therapist will counsel the patient to expect a gradual and lengthy progression with therapy. The patient is continuously educated regarding the importance of following precautions in order to protect the

Dr. Ranawat or an immediate family member has received royalties from Conformis; is a member of a speakers' bureau or has made paid presentations on behalf of Arthrex, CONMED Linvatec, DePuy Mitek, and Stryker MAKO; serves as a paid consultant to Arthrex, CONMED Linvatec, DePuy Mitek, and Stryker MAKO; has stock or stock options held in Conformis; has received nonincome support (such as equipment or services), commercially derived honoraria, or other non-research–related funding (such as paid travel) from Saunders/Mosby-Elsevier and Springer; and serves as a board member, owner, officer, or committee member of Current Trends in Musculoskeletal Medicine and the EOA. Neither of the following authors nor any immediate family member has received anything of value from or has stock or stock options held in a commercial company or institution related directly or indirectly to the subject of this article: Dr. Cavanaugh and Dr. Tychanski.

© 2018 American Academy of Orthopaedic Surgeons

repair throughout rehabilitation. A criteria-based functional progression is followed in order to safely advance through postsurgical rehabilitation, and goals are individualized for each patient. Active discussion between the physical therapist, surgeon, and patient is imperative.

Phase 1: Initial Mobilization and Protection of Repair (Weeks 0–4)

- Immobilizer or brace in extension
- Protected weight bearing with crutches/walker
- Quadriceps activation

During the initial phase (0–4 weeks) protection of the repair is essential. The patient is educated regarding proper use of the brace and crutches. The brace is locked in 0° of extension at all times for the first 4 weeks. Ambulation is initially permitted up to 50% weight bearing with a locked brace and crutches; weight bearing is then gradually progressed, as tolerated. The patient is educated to frequently elevate the extremity and apply ice for pain and inflammation management. Use of a combined cryotherapy and compression unit three to five times per day for 20 to 30 minutes at a time is advised for the first 4 weeks postoperatively. Any signs of atypical healing—including signs of infection, repair failure, as well as patient's degree of compliance to prescribed exercises and activity modifications—should be communicated with the surgeon immediately. Once the surgical incision is completely healed, scar tissue and patellar mobilizations are encouraged. These interventions will aide the mobility of the patella along the trochlear groove, minimize scar-tissue adhesions, and assist with the progression of knee ROM.

Early activation of the quadriceps muscle is important and is initiated via isometric quadriceps sets with a small towel roll under the knee multiple times per day (Figure 50.1). If the patient demonstrates inhibition of the quadriceps muscle, a neuromuscular electrical stimulation (NMES) unit is utilized to facilitate quadriceps activation. Once the patient demonstrates adequate quadriceps activation, supine straight leg raises with the brace locked at 0° extension are initiated (Figure 50.2). Straight leg raises in all other planes are performed to maintain hip strength. Distal lower extremity strength and flexibility is introduced during this phase. Typical exercises would include ankle plantarflexion with a resistance band and seated calf stretching with a strap (Figure 50.3). Hamstring flexibility

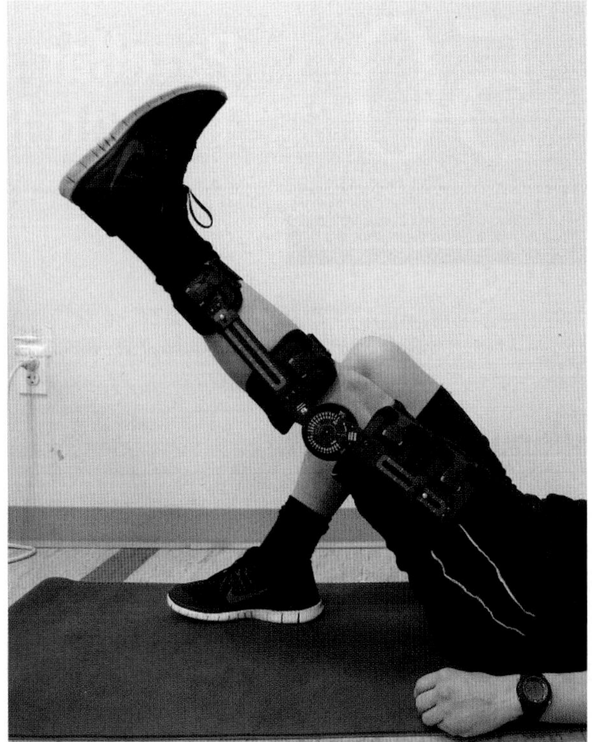

Figure 50.2 Photograph of supine straight leg raises with brace locked at 0° of knee extension.

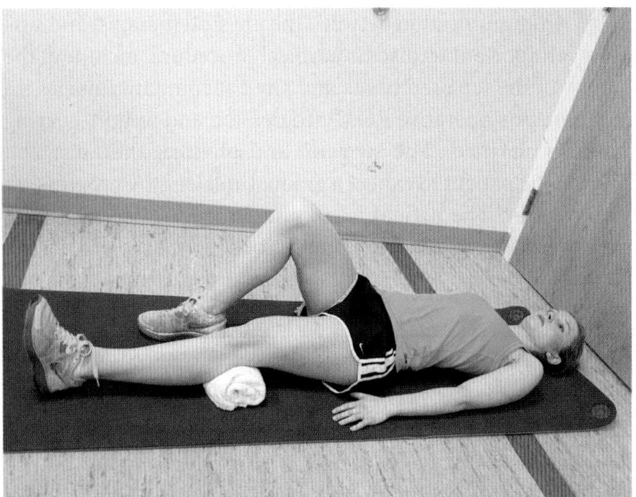

Figure 50.1 Photograph of isometric quadriceps activation with a towel roll under the ankle. Hold each contraction for 10 seconds for 10 repetitions, five or more times per day.

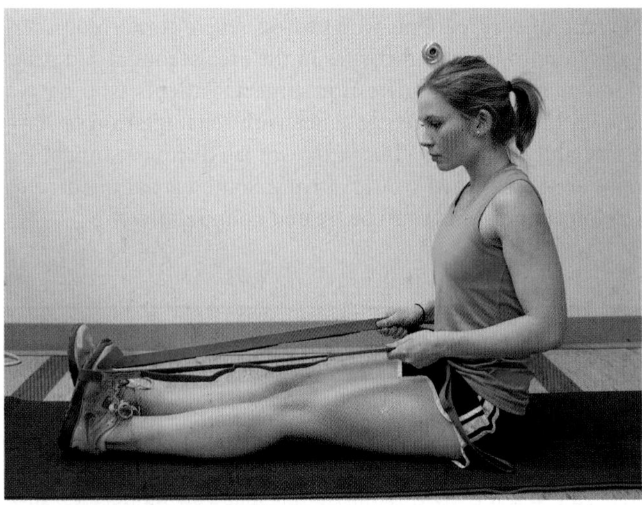

Figure 50.3 Photograph of seated calf stretching with a strap. Hold each stretch 20 to 30 seconds.

© 2018 American Academy of Orthopaedic Surgeons

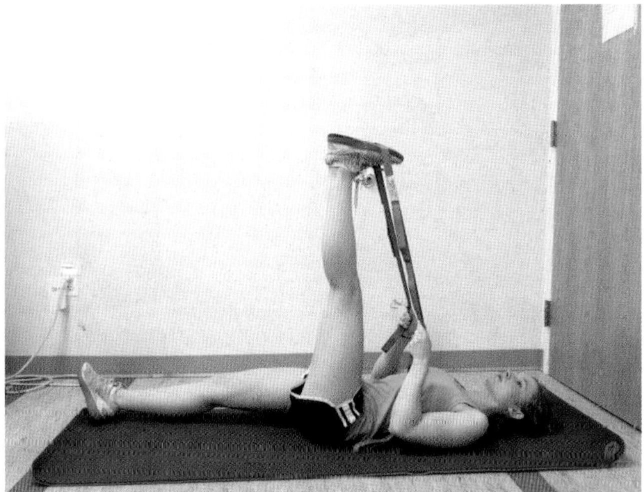

Figure 50.4 Photograph of supine hamstring stretch. Hold each stretch 20 to 30 seconds.

is addressed in the supine position (Figure 50.4). Bilateral weight shifting with upper extremity support on a uniplanar rocker can be initiated in cardinal planes for proprioceptive stimulation.

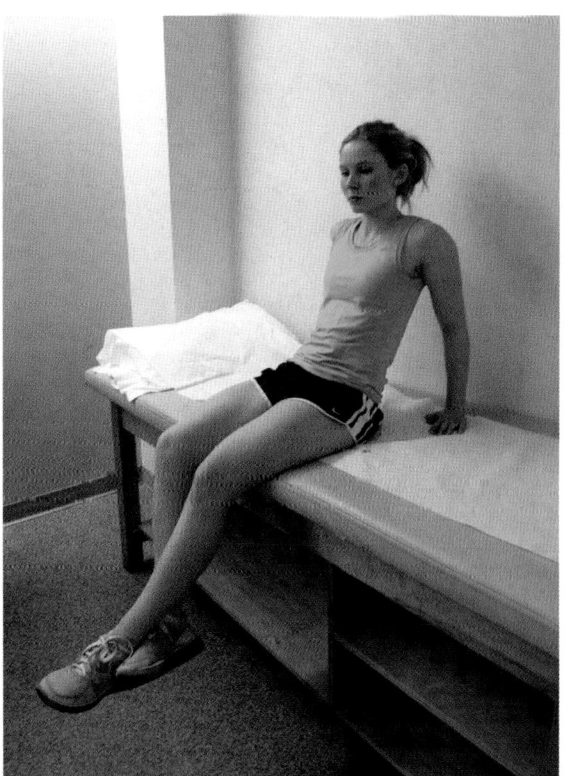

Figure 50.5 Photograph of seated active assistive ROM knee flexion utilizing the contralateral leg for assistance.

Phase 2: Restoration of Motion and Progression of Weight Bearing (Weeks 4–12)

- Progressive ROM
- Progression to full weight bearing with a brace and wean as quadriceps control is regained
- Proprioception and closed kinetic chain exercise

The second phase of rehabilitation (4–12 weeks) permits gradual increases in ROM, increased use and function of the limb, and progressive weight bearing. Gentle active assistive range of motion (AAROM) is initiated and progressed gradually. Knee flexion ROM is performed in a seated position using the nonsurgical leg for support (Figure 50.5). The patient is educated regarding the fact that ROM should not be forced and should not cause pain. As the patient reaches approximately 90° of knee flexion, gentle overpressure into knee flexion with the nonsurgical leg is applied to further progress ROM. Knee flexion AAROM may also be advanced via supine wall slides, knee flexion stretching on a step (Figure 50.6) and half-moon motion on a low-seated stationary bicycle. When the patient achieves 85° of knee flexion, a stationary short-crank bicycle may be utilized to encourage movement and lubrication of the knee joint (Figure 50.7). The patient can begin cycling on a full-crank bicycle upon achieving 110° to 115° of knee flexion. As the patient approaches 120° of knee flexion, gentle quadriceps flexibility stretching in the supine position may be introduced (Figure 50.8).

Once the patient demonstrates adequate quadriceps activation and control, the brace is unlocked and then weaned. Utilization of crutches is continued until the patient demonstrates a nonantalgic gait. Retrograde ambulation on a treadmill with upper extremity support for balance may be

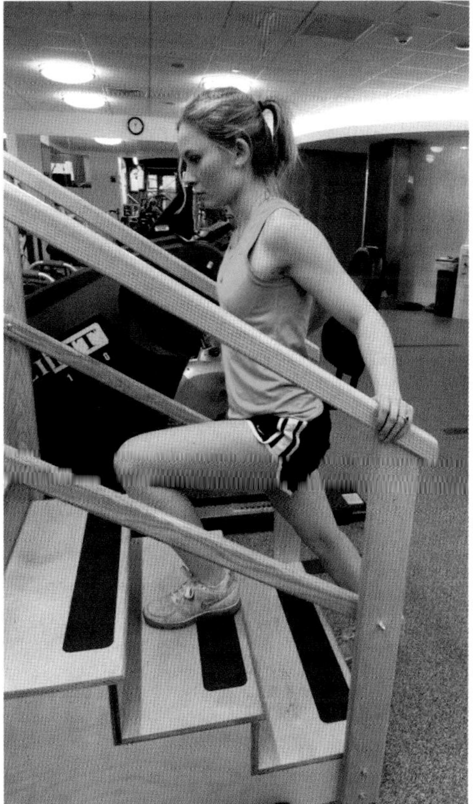

Figure 50.6 Photograph of forward knee flexion bends on a step.

© 2018 American Academy of Orthopaedic Surgeons

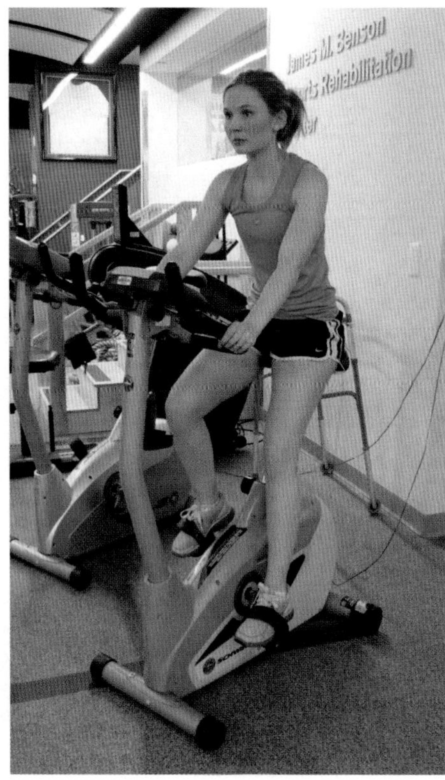

Figure 50.7 Photograph of short-crank bicycle, which may be utilized once 85° to 90° of knee flexion is demonstrated.

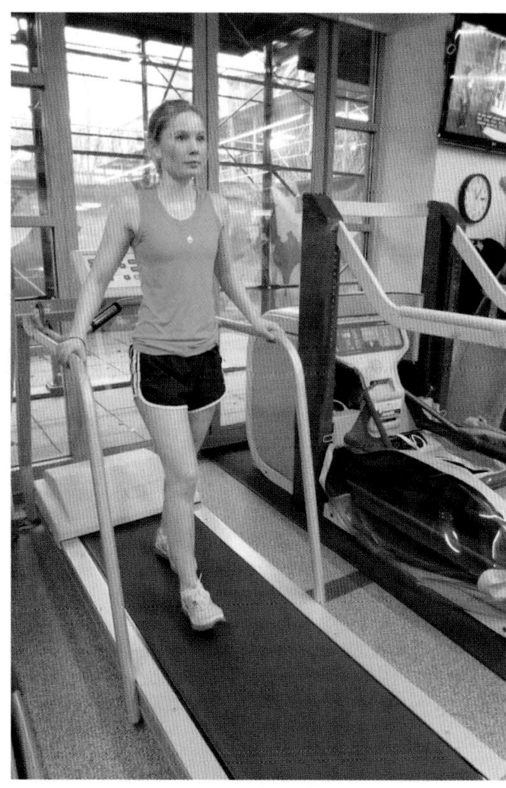

Figure 50.9 Photograph of retrograde ambulation on a treadmill at 0% incline at a slow speed to encourage lower extremity control.

performed to assist in normalizing gait (Figure 50.9). Gait re-education may also be facilitated via ambulation in water in a pool (Figure 50.10) or with an underwater treadmill. Aquatic therapy is useful through the phases of rehabilitation as water aids support of body weight and decreases loads on the lower extremities to facilitate normalization of various movement patterns. Proprioceptive training is continued and progressed to a multiplanar balance device (Figure 50.11).

A two-legged leg press for closed-chain lower extremity strengthening is performed as long as the patient demonstrates

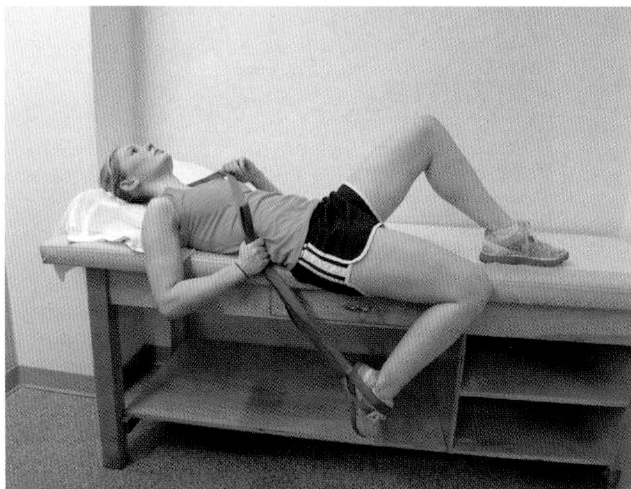

Figure 50.8 Photograph of quadriceps stretch with a strap in supine position. With the surgical leg hanging off the edge of a table, hip in full extension, and a strap around the ankle to gently flex, the knee. This will stretch the quadriceps muscle while minimizing forces under the patellofemoral joint.

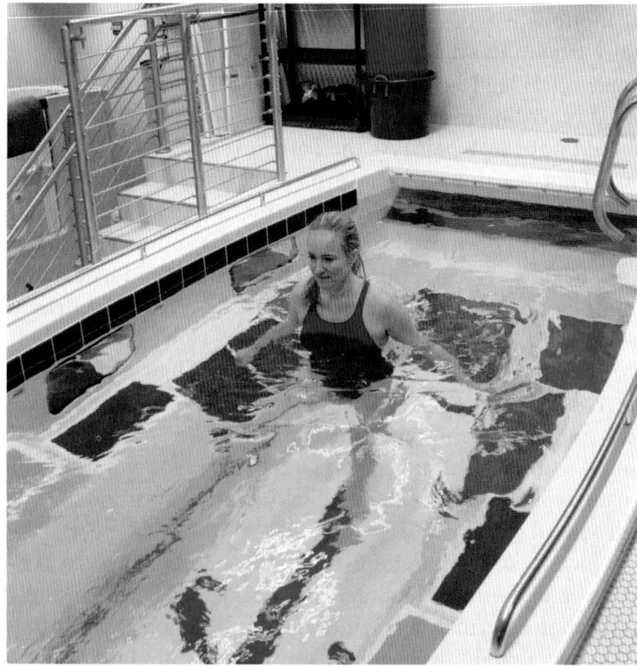

Figure 50.10 Photograph of aquatic therapy for gait re-education.

© 2018 American Academy of Orthopaedic Surgeons

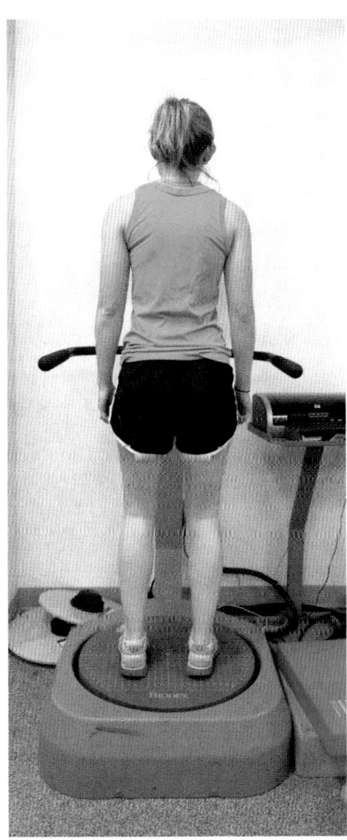

Figure 50.11 Photograph of bilateral proprioceptive training on a Biodex Balance System™.

at least 90° of knee flexion. It is imperative to encourage muscle control through the ROM and symmetrical pressure through the lower extremities. Bilateral standing heel raises are also performed to further strengthen the gastrocnemius-soleus complex. Heel raises are gradually advanced to eccentric and then single-leg heel raises as strength progresses.

Phase 3: Progression to Functional Activity (Weeks 12–18)

- Progressive strengthening and proprioception with single-limb exercise

The third phase (weeks 12–16) following quadriceps or patellar tendon repair emphasizes quadriceps strengthening and progressive functional movement patterns. As the patient continues to display improved motor control of the operative leg, the leg press may be progressed to eccentric and then single-leg press (Figure 50.12). The patient may advance to wall-assisted squats (Figure 50.13) within a limited ROM to start (0°–45°). The physical therapist should carefully monitor for pain, alignment, symmetry, and technique while squatting. Wall-assisted squats may be progressed to chair squats and then free squats.

Single-leg balancing on a stable surface is initiated to further stimulate proprioceptive feedback (Figure 50.14). As the patient demonstrates improved balance on a stable surface, unstable surfaces and dynamic movements with single-leg balancing are introduced (Figures 50.15 and 50.16). Forward step-up exercises are introduced if the patient has achieved 120° of knee flexion and demonstrates the ability to load full weight on the surgical leg with control. Step-ups are initiated on a 4-inch step and gradually advanced in step height. Step-down exercises (Figure 50.17) are then later introduced as the patient continues to demonstrate improved quadriceps strength. When the patient demonstrates the ability to ascend a 6-inch step without compensations or pain, the patient may begin using an elliptical machine. Progressive resistive exercises for

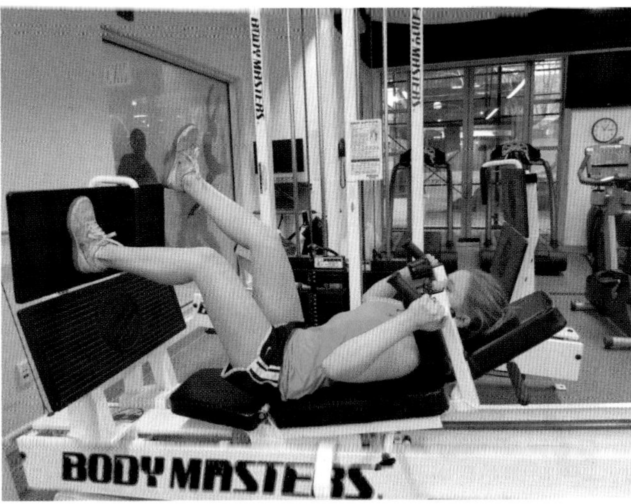

Figure 50.12 Photograph of single-legged leg press. Apply 60% of the weight utilized during the eccentric leg press.

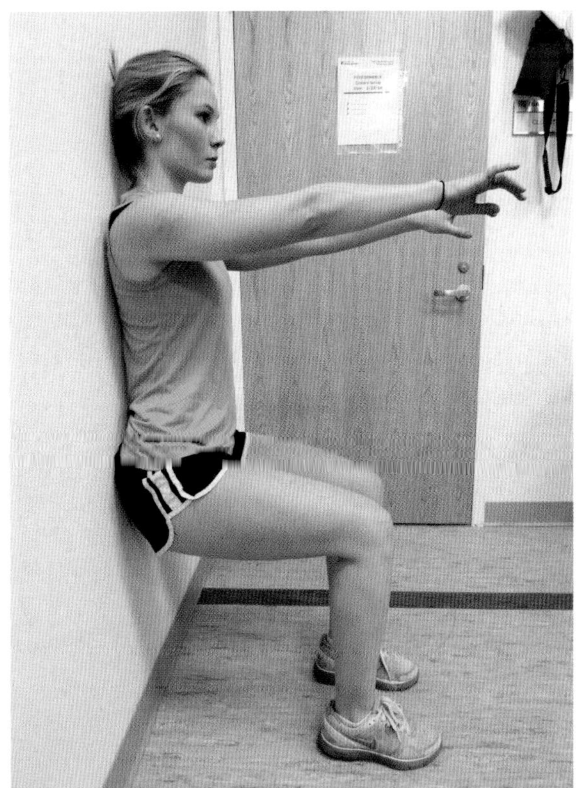

Figure 50.13 Photograph of wall-assisted squats. Initiate at a limited ROM of 0° to 45°, gradually progressing ROM, as tolerated.

© 2018 American Academy of Orthopaedic Surgeons

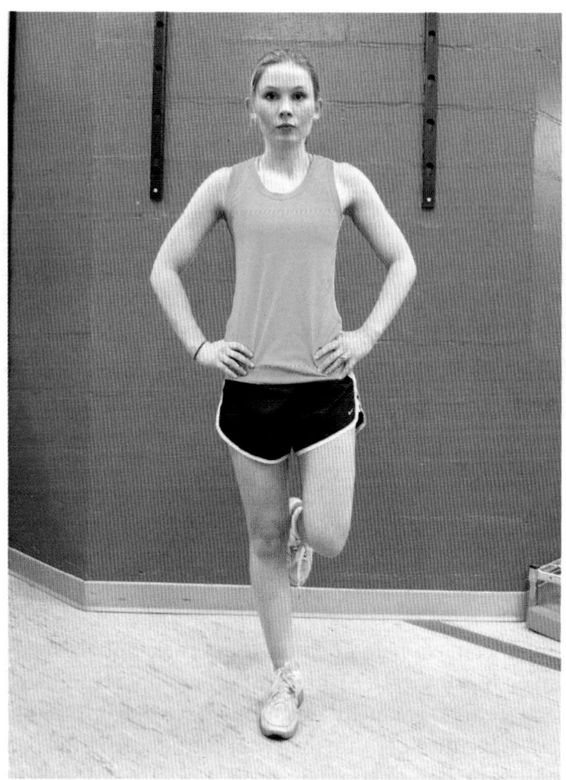

Figure 50.14 Photograph of single-leg balance on a stable surface.

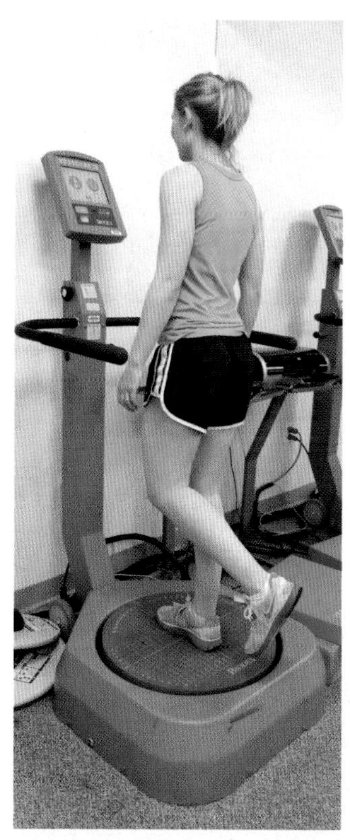

Figure 50.16 Photograph of unilateral proprioceptive training on a Biodex Balance System™.

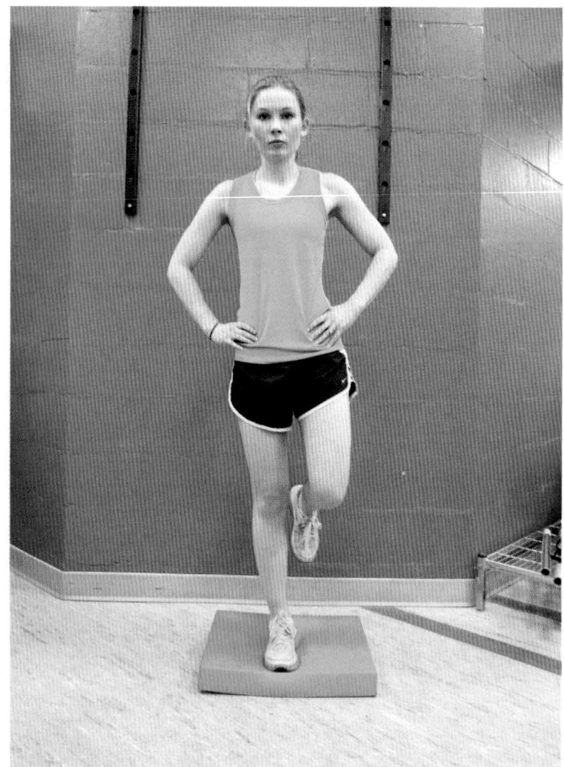

Figure 50.15 Photograph of single-leg balance on foam. Careful monitoring for compensations throughout the chain—including the trunk, pelvis, and hips—is important.

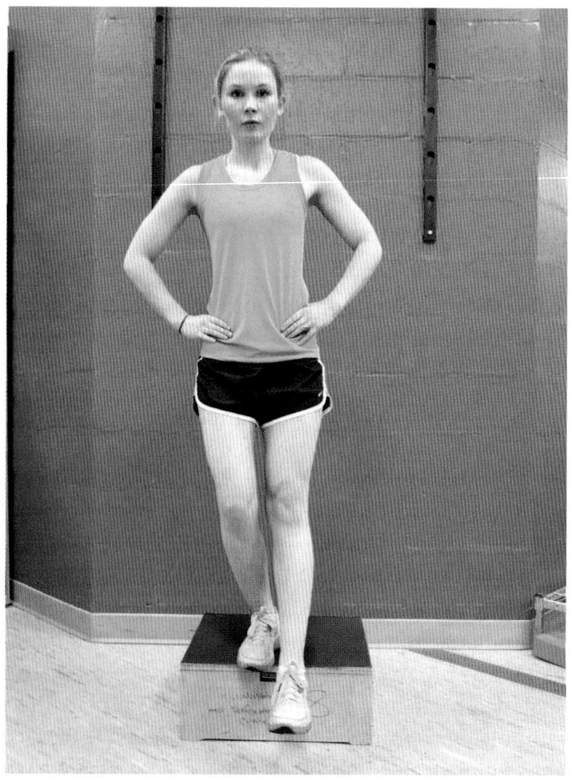

Figure 50.17 Photograph of step-down on an 8-inch step. Begin step-downs with a 4-inch step, then gradually progress to 6 inches and then 8 inches.

© 2018 American Academy of Orthopaedic Surgeons

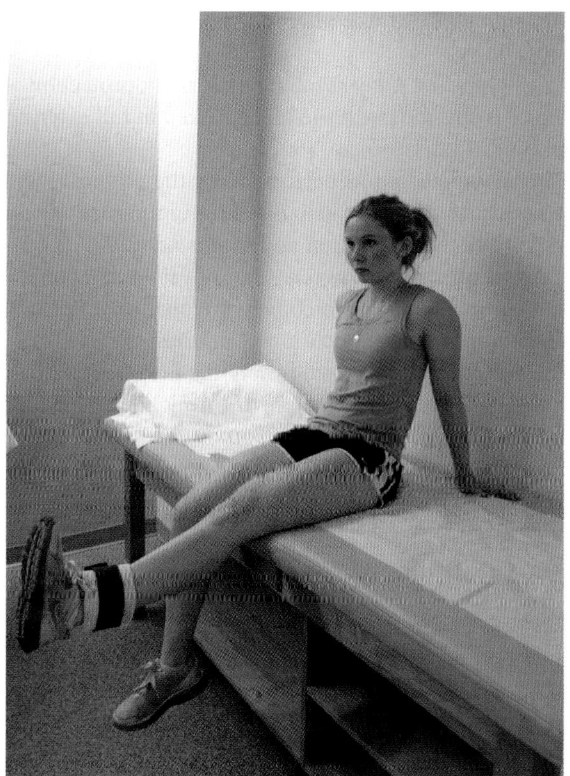

Figure 50.18 Photograph of seated progressive resistive exercises for open kinetic chain knee extension.

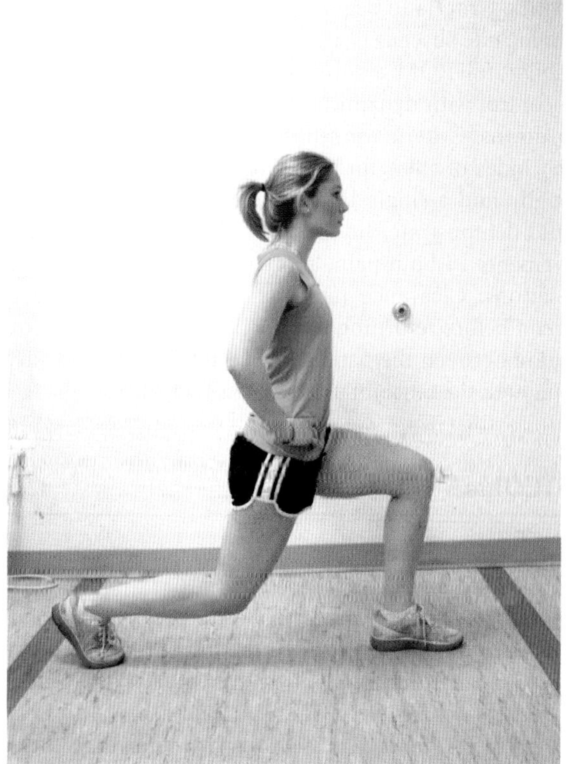

Figure 50.19 Photograph of lunges.

knee extension in an open kinetic chain (OKC) may be initiated in a limited arc of 90° to 30° (Figure 50.18). The physical therapist should carefully monitor for pain, crepitus, and maltracking of the patella. If the patient tolerates a limited arc, the arc may gradually be increased to 90° to 0° of knee extension. Lunges (Figure 50.19) and single-leg squats (Figure 50.20) are later introduced as the patient displays increased ROM, adequate quadriceps control, and single-leg balance with functional exercises. As exercises are advanced, exercise volume should be monitored for muscle fatigue and development of edema at the knee. Muscle fatigue will become evident when the patient is no longer able to perform the exercise with proper form and may compensate with other musculature. This may also be accompanied by pain. The physical therapist should monitor for alignment and compensations throughout the kinetic chain as the patient performs more complex exercises.

Phase 4: Advanced Activities (18+ Weeks)

- Progression to advanced functional goals
  - Dynamic activity: running, sprinting, jumping and sport-specific activity

During the final phase (Phase 4) of rehabilitation, postpatellar or postquadriceps repair advanced movement patterns and physical demands related to individual functional goals, including return to sport, are addressed. These include agility exercises, plyometrics, running, and other sport-specific

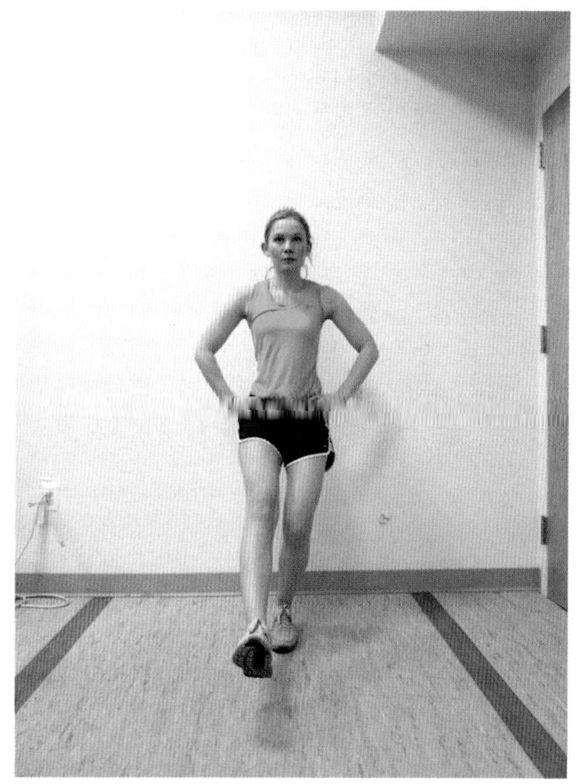

Figure 50.20 Photograph of single-leg squats.

© 2018 American Academy of Orthopaedic Surgeons

activities. Criteria to begin a plyometric and/or running program include absence of edema or pain with ADLs, adequate flexibility, full ROM, a symmetrical squat >90° of knee flexion, and control with dynamic single-leg activities such as 8-inch step-downs. Criteria for return to sport include a limb symmetry index of >90% for isokinetic quadriceps and hamstring strength, and a single-leg hop test. In addition, the patient should demonstrate the ability to perform all sport-specific movements without pain, apprehension or movement compensations. Clearance must be obtained by the referring surgeon before returning to sport; thus, continuous communication between the patient, physical therapist, and surgeon throughout the rehabilitation process is critical.

OUTCOMES

Repair of quadriceps and patellar tendon ruptures generally lead to excellent results with restoration of not only ambulatory capacity but also most recreational activities. Particularly with well-executed therapy, a motivated patient recovers near full motion, strength, and activity. Generally, full recovery is achieved at 9 to 12 months. Mild anterior knee symptoms may persist along with some difficulty with eccentric loads, such as descending stairs and high-intensity sport.

PEARLS

- Early recognition and repair of a patellar or quadriceps tendon rupture is critical for optimal outcomes.
- Key clinical signs of a patellar or quadriceps tendon rupture include inability to straight leg raise with an extension lag, palpable infrapatellar or suprapatellar defect, and effusion.
- During the first 4 weeks following surgery, protection of the repair is stressed, with the brace locked in full extension at all times.
- Patellar mobilizations performed by the physical therapist are crucial to restore patellar mobility, minimize adhesions, and promote knee flexion and extension ROM.
- Communication between the physical therapist and surgeon is important to convey the quality of the surgical procedure and any concomitant injuries.
- Following a criteria-based functional progression, it is critical to ensure safe advancement throughout rehabilitation while minimizing pain and edema.

BIBLIOGRAPHY

Bhargava SP, Hynes MC, Dowell JK: Traumatic patella tendon rupture: early mobilization following surgical repair. *Injury* 2004;35:76–79.

Boublik M, Schlegel TF, Koonce RC, Genuario JW, Kinkartz JD: Quadriceps tendon injuries in National Football League players. *Am J Sports Med* 2013;41:1841–1846.

Marder RA, Timmerman LA: Primary repair of patellar tendon rupture without augmentation. *Am J of Sports Medicine* 1999;27:304–307.

Roudet A, Boudissa M, Chaussard C, Rubens-Duval B, Saragaglia D: Acute traumatic patellar tendon rupture: Early and late results of surgical treatment of 38 cases. *Orthop Traumatol Surg Res* 2015;101:307–311.

Tejwani NC, Lekic N, Bechtel C, Montero N, Egol KA: Outcomes after knee joint extensor mechanism disruptions: Is it better to fracture the patella or rupture the tendon? *J Orthop Trauma* 2012:26(11):648–651.

© 2018 American Academy of Orthopaedic Surgeons

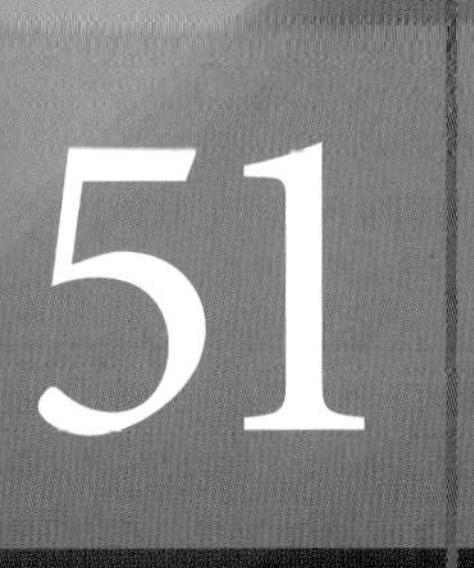

51 Collateral Ligament and Multiple Ligament Injury

Andrea Tychanski, PT, DPT, SCS, ATC, CSCS, John Cavanaugh, PT, ATC, SCS, and Anil S. Ranawat, MD

INTRODUCTION

Stable motion of the knee requires the coordinated function of the ligaments, menisci, muscles and bone structure. The knee has four major ligaments: the 2 cruciates controlling anterior posterior motion and the 2 collaterals, which control varus and valgus stability. Detailed biomechanical evaluation has shown a more complex function in controlling rotational movement by these ligaments and other structures, especially in the posterolateral corner. Injuries to these ligaments occur as a result of sports activities, falls, and motor vehicle crashes. They mostly occur as single-ligament injuries, but also occur in combination with one another. The medial collateral ligament (MCL) is often injured with the anterior cruciate ligament (ACL) while the lateral collateral ligament (LCL) in combination with the posterior cruciate ligament (PCL) and posterolateral corner (PLC).

COLLATERAL LIGAMENT INJURIES

Collateral ligament injuries can range from a minor isolated grade 1 sprain to a complete grade 3 tear, often in the setting of multiple ligament knee injuries (MLKIs). Isolated collateral ligament sprains are commonly managed nonoperatively with a progressive rehabilitation program. Initial treatment for an isolated grade 1, 2, or 3 collateral injury includes rest, ice, and compression to limit edema and permit healing of the injured ligament. Grades 2 and 3 collateral ligament injuries are initially managed with the protection of a hinged brace. Weight bearing will be restricted for 2 to 4 weeks for grade 2 injuries and 4 to 6 weeks for grade 3 injuries. Typically, the higher the grade of ligament damage, the longer the recovery period, ranging from days to multiple weeks. Rehabilitation for an isolated collateral ligament injury follows a symptom-based range of motion (ROM) and lower extremity strengthening progression. In the early phases of rehabilitation, the clinician should be cautious when incorporating exercises in the frontal and transverse planes in order to protect the collateral ligaments from excess stress. Proprioceptive training exercises are incorporated throughout the rehabilitation program. Following a criteria-based rehabilitation program, the injured ligament is then reevaluated and the final decision to return to play is determined.

Collateral injuries are often combined with ACL injuries. Should the healing response not be effective in the preoperative phase, the collateral ligament is often surgically augmented concomitantly with an ACL reconstruction.

MULTILIGAMENT KNEE INJURY

With larger traumatic forces, such as those occurring in motor vehicle accidents and sporting event collisions, MLKIs inclusive of the cruciate ligaments are common. Knowing the mechanism of injury is often helpful to the examiner to determine what side of the knee was in tension versus compression. Evaluation of an MLKI begins with a thorough neurovascular examination followed by a physical examination, including assessment of ligaments and the extensor mechanism. Arterial compromise and nerve disruptions are known to occur with these injuries. Radiographs and MRI can assist in assessing the degree and location of soft-tissue damage. Aside from assessment of ligamentous structures, MRI permits assessment of other structures, including menisci, articular cartilage, and bone.

More extensive injuries involving multiple ligaments commonly require surgical intervention. The goal of treatment is to anatomically repair and/or reconstruct all necessary ligamentous and other associated injuries. In low-demand patients,

Dr. Ranawat or an immediate family member has received royalties from Conformis; is a member of a speakers' bureau or has made paid presentations on behalf of Arthrex, CONMED Linvatec, DePuy Mitek, and Stryker MAKO; serves as a paid consultant to Arthrex, CONMED Linvatec, DePuy Mitek, and Stryker MAKO; has stock or stock options held in Conformis; has received nonincome support (such as equipment or services), commercially derived honoraria, or other non-research–related funding (such as paid travel) from Saunders/Mosby-Elsevier and Springer; and serves as a board member, owner, officer, or committee member of Current Trends in Musculoskeletal Medicine and the EOA. Neither of the following authors nor any immediate family member has received anything of value from or has stock or stock options held in a commercial company or institution related directly or indirectly to the subject of this article: Dr. Cavanaugh and Dr. Tychanski.

© 2018 American Academy of Orthopaedic Surgeons

there is a role for nonsurgical treatment for MLKI. Excluding neurovascular injury, initial treatment for an MLKI is brace immobilization in extension. If there is more extensive injury, such as a knee dislocation, prompt imaging and reduction is paramount. Emergency surgery is usually not necessary unless there is vascular injury, irreducible knee, or traumatic arthrotomy. In most cases, surgery is delayed 1 to 3 weeks to permit reduction of effusion, capsular healing, establishment of ROM, and time for surgical planning. There is debate regarding the optimal time to proceed with surgery. Early surgery affords the best chance for primary repairs, but increases chances for postoperative stiffness. The decision to operate with MLKI is usually dependent on multiple factors, including the patient, affected structures, and surgeon preference.

Early surgery allows primary repair of some injuries, but may use augmentation procedures. Early surgery is commonly indicated for cruciate injuries with repairable PLC injuries. With lateral side involvement, surgery is performed at 2 weeks post-injury. The cruciate ligaments are usually reconstructed and the lateral structures are primarily repaired with or without augmentation. However, in certain cases, these surgeries may be delayed if the risk of stiffness is felt to be too high. With injury on the medial side of the knee, there is a tendency to be more conservative and delay surgery. Likewise, many low-grade MCL sprains with bicruciate injuries are often rehabilitated first to restore knee motion and then undergo delayed surgical reconstructions. Certain high-grade medial injuries that are tibial sided benefit from early surgery. The cruciates can be reconstructed simultaneously or staged depending on the risk of stiffness.

SURGICAL TECHNIQUE

There are numerous surgical techniques for these injuries. For the most part, cruciates are reconstructed and collateral ligaments are repaired if the injury is acute. However, they are reconstructed (vs. repaired) when the injury is chronic or the quality of the tissue is too compromised for repair. There are numerous cruciate reconstruction techniques utilizing a single- or double-bundle ACL, but a single-bundle ACL and PCL is the gold standard with multiligament knee. These involve drilling bone tunnels in the femur and tibia, and passage of the graft, as described in the ACL Reconstruction chapter (Chapter 48). Given the number of tunnels, attention must be paid to their trajectory to limit the risk of fracture. For collateral reconstruction, there exists multiple techniques as well, such as Larson, LaPrade, Bosworth, and others, but no technique has been found to be superior; therefore; the surgeon uses one's preferred technique. Stability is restored through accurate graft placement and secure fixation.

Optimal order for tissue repair takes an inside out approach, which includes open meniscal repair, capsular repair followed by collateral ligament repair/augmentation. Cruciate reconstruction or repairs are also performed. Grafts are chosen based on preference and availability; however, with an MLKI, allograft tissue is commonly used. Autograft choices include ipsilateral or contralateral bone–patellar tendon–bone, hamstrings, and quadriceps tendon. Allograft options include Achilles tendon, bone–patellar tendon–bone, hamstrings and tibialis anterior. Optimal order for tissue repair includes open meniscal repair, cruciate ligament reconstruction, capsular repair, and, last, collateral ligament repair or reconstruction.

Following surgery, achieving a balance between motion and protection is important in healing and recovery. Although a hinged brace is often sufficient, in certain cases, some surgeons use a hinged external fixator during the initial postoperative phase.

REHABILITATION

The pace and intensity of rehabilitation is governed by many factors, but particularly the degree of injury and patient goals. More complex injury and higher patient goals require greater involvement of the patient, therapist, and surgeon. The rehabilitation is consequently tailored to each individual.

Collateral and Cruciate Rehabilitation

Phase 1: Early Protection Period

Rehabilitation of a cruciate reconstruction with a collateral ligament injury is similar to isolated cruciate reconstruction. Postoperative weight bearing is protected for 6 weeks utilizing a long-leg brace locked in extension. Restoring knee extension is an important early postoperative goal. Knee extension is best restored by placing a towel roll under the patient's ankle and allowing gravity to passively stretch the knee into extension (Figure 51.1). To encourage quadriceps re-education, the patient is encouraged to perform isometric quadriceps sets with a towel roll under the knee multiple times per day (Figure 51.2). If the patient demonstrates inhibition of the quadriceps muscle, a neuromuscular electrical stimulation (NMES) unit is utilized to facilitate quadriceps activation. Once the patient demonstrates adequate quadriceps activation, supine straight leg raises are initiated with the brace locked

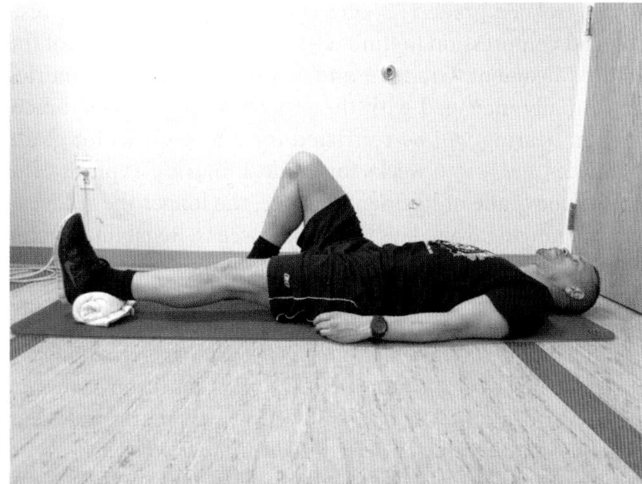

Figure 51.1 Photograph of passive knee extension with a towel roll under the ankle.

 © 2018 American Academy of Orthopaedic Surgeons

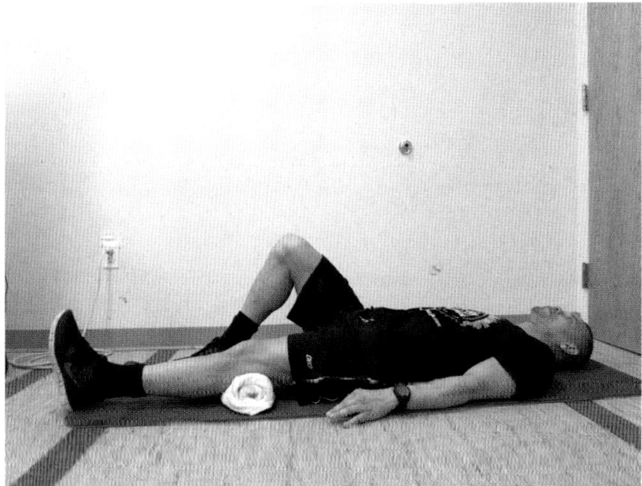

Figure 51.2 Photograph of isometric quadriceps activation with a towel roll under the ankle. Hold each contraction for 10 seconds for 10 repetitions, 5 or more times per day.

in extension. Straight leg raises in all other planes are also performed to strengthen the hip musculature. Distal lower extremity strengthening and flexibility begins in the first phase; this typically includes ankle plantarflexion with a resistance band (Figure 51.3) and seated calf stretching with a strap. In addition, the hamstring muscles are stretched in the supine position with a strap; caution is advised if the hamstring tendon was harvested for ligament reconstruction.

Phase 2: Gait Restoration

Following the immediate protection phase, the brace may be unlocked as the patient demonstrates the ability to perform a straight leg raise without a lag. Gait re-education with crutches is emphasized to facilitate a normal gait pattern. The patient is then gradually weaned from two crutches to one crutch or cane, then eventually to no assistive device. Criteria for advancement include a nonantalgic gait, the ability to perform straight leg raises without a lag, and no pain with ambulation. Retrograde ambulation on a treadmill with 0% incline and upper extremity support may be performed to assist in normalizing gait (Figure 51.4). Ambulation in a therapeutic pool or underwater treadmill (Figure 51.5) can also assist with gait re-education. Water aids with support of body weight and decreases loads on the lower extremities to facilitate normalization of movement patterns. With demonstration of a normalized gait, the patient will transition to use an off-the-shelf functional brace to protect the injured ligaments.

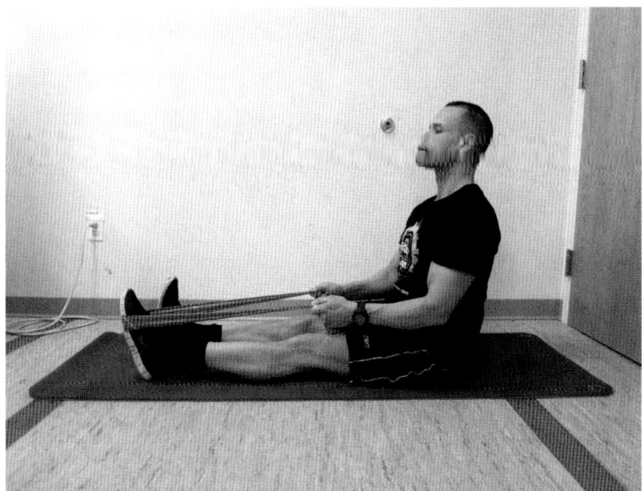

Figure 51.3 Photograph of ankle plantarflexion with a resistance band.

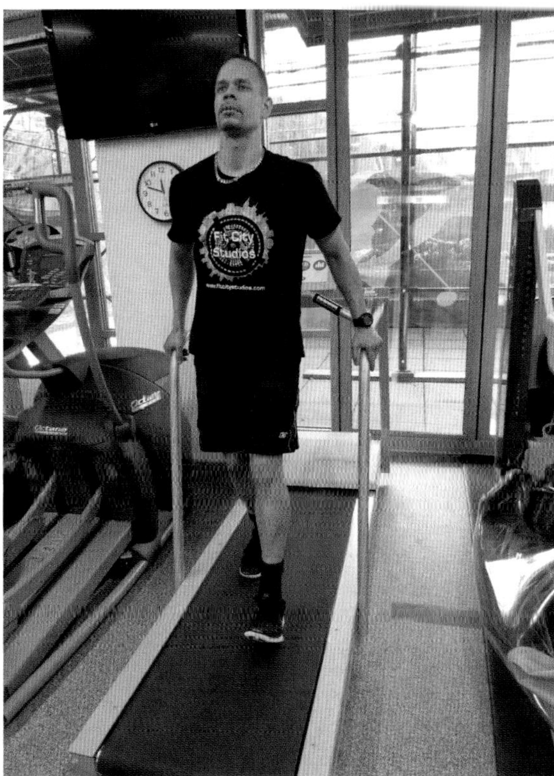

Figure 51.4 Photograph of retrograde ambulation on a treadmill, initiated at 0% incline and performed at a slow speed to encourage lower extremity control.

Gradual restoration of flexion is best initiated via seated active assistive range of motion (AAROM) (Figure 51.6). To further progress ROM, supine wall slides (Figure 51.7), forward knee flexion bends on a staircase and half-moons while seated low on a stationary bicycle are performed. When the patient achieves 85° of knee flexion, a stationary short-crank bicycle (90 mm) is utilized to encourage movement and lubrication of the knee joint (Figure 51.8). The patient will begin cycling on a standard bicycle (170 mm) upon achieving approximately 115° of knee flexion. As the patient continues to advance, a criteria-based functional progression should be implemented throughout the rehabilitation program, as discussed later in this chapter.

Multiligament Rehabilitation

Rehabilitation following MLKI reconstruction is expected to be a long and lengthy recovery. Return to full activity is seldom demonstrated less than 1 year after surgery. Ongoing

© 2018 American Academy of Orthopaedic Surgeons

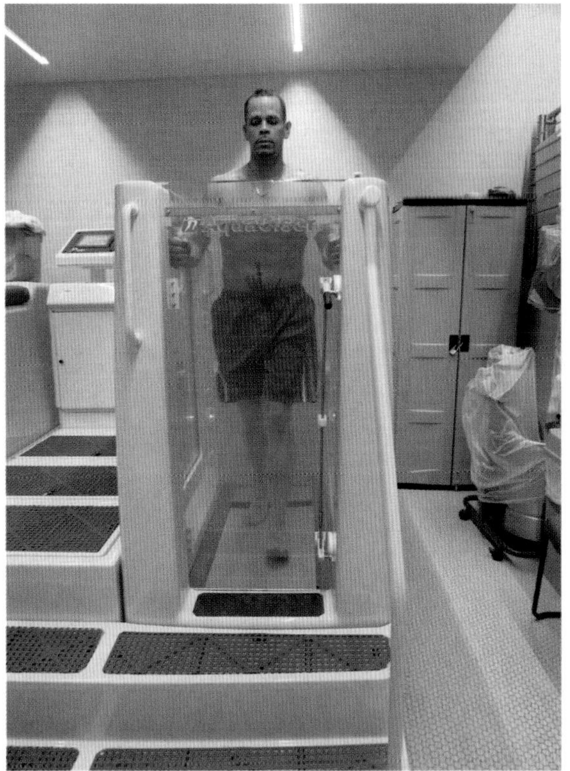

Figure 51.5 Photograph of aquatic ambulation on an underwater treadmill to facilitate with gait re-education.

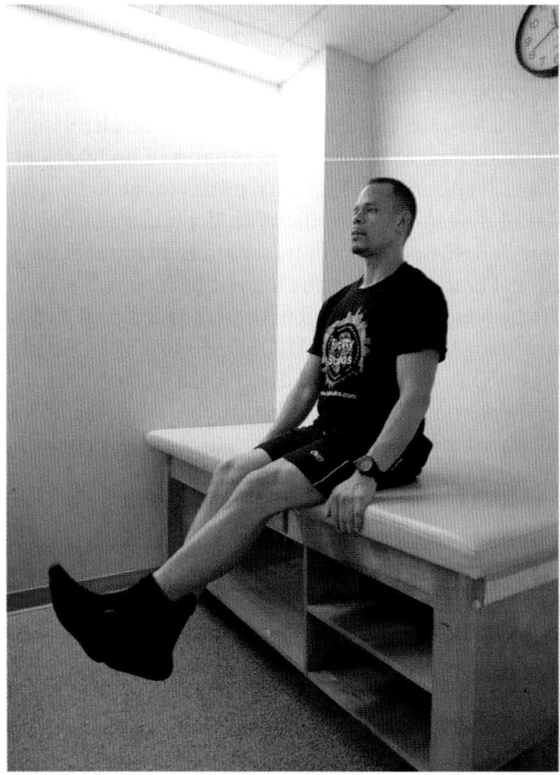

Figure 51.6 Photograph of seated active assistive knee flexion/extension ROM utilizing the contralateral leg for assistance.

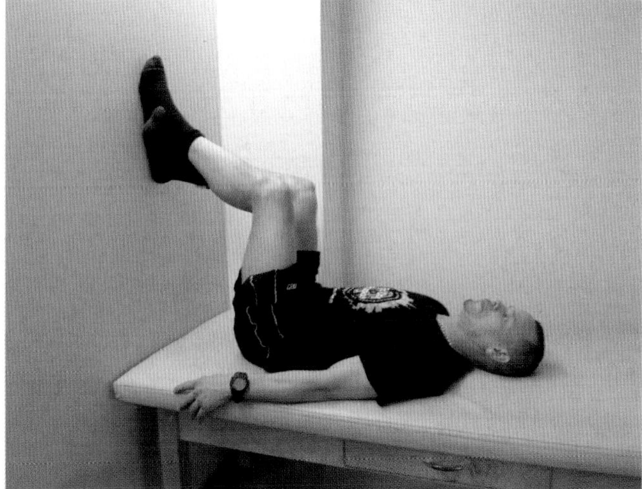

Figure 51.7 Photograph of supine active assistive knee ROM wall slides utilizing the contralateral leg for assistance.

conversation between the patient, physical therapist, and surgeon is recommended.

Preoperative Rehabilitation

A preoperative discussion between the surgeon and the patient includes the surgical procedure recommended—including the injured and reconstructed structures, type(s) of grafts (i.e., autograft vs. allograft), and concomitant injuries (i.e., neurovasculature, menisci, articular cartilage, fracture, and so on). In addition, postoperative ROM progression, weight-bearing status, weight-bearing progression, and any other relevant precautions are defined. Every rehabilitation program is customized to the patient based on the affected structures and personal goals of the patient to ensure optimal outcomes. The

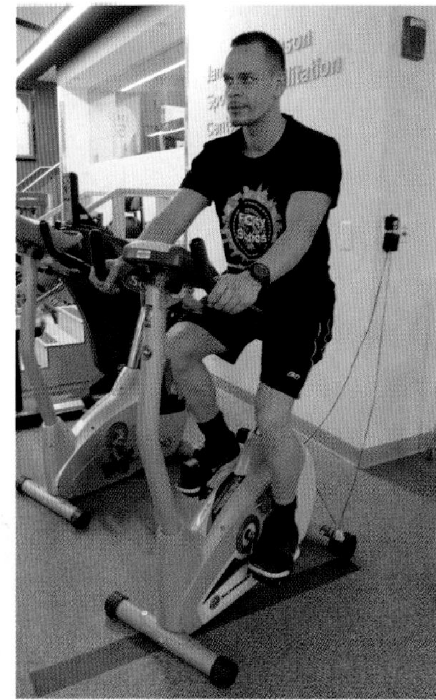

Figure 51.8 Photograph of a short-crank bicycle, which may be utilized once 85° to 90° of knee flexion is demonstrated.

© 2018 American Academy of Orthopaedic Surgeons

physical therapist should guide the patient through a criteria-based functional progression to ensure a safe rehabilitation process. The surgeon and physical therapist should counsel and educate the patient regarding the importance of respecting precautions in order to protect the reconstructed structures throughout rehabilitation. The biggest rehabilitation challenge following MLKI reconstruction is balancing the protection of the reconstructed tissue while preventing stiffness to maximize postoperative mobility and return to preinjury function.

Phase 1: Initial Recovery

Protection of the repaired tissues is most essential during the first 6 weeks following surgery. The patient is educated regarding proper use of the brace and crutches. The brace will be locked in 0° of extension for crutch ambulation and while sleeping for up to 4 to 6 weeks. Weight bearing is initially limited to toe-touch weight bearing to partial weight bearing with crutches based on surgeon instruction. In the initial protection phase, the patient is also educated regarding frequent elevation of the extremity and application of ice for pain control and reduction of inflammation. Use of a combined cryotherapy and compression unit 3 to 5 times per day for 20 to 30 minutes at a time is advised for the first 4 to 6 weeks postoperatively. Any signs of atypical healing, including signs of infection, should be communicated to the surgeon immediately. Patellar mobilizations are performed immediately postsurgery to encourage mobility of the patella along the trochlear groove, prevent development of arthrofibrosis, and aide with the progression of knee ROM. Once the incisions are healed, scar-tissue massage is performed to minimize scar-tissue adhesions.

It is crucial to ensure restoration of full knee extension as soon as possible postsurgery. Knee extension at the surgical knee should be symmetrical to knee extension at the nonsurgical knee. With involvement of the PCL reconstruction, a pillow is placed under the tibia to protect the graft with an anterior-directed force while avoiding hyperextension (Figure 51.9). To encourage early controlled motion, a continuous passive motion (CPM) machine may be utilized at home beginning with ROM specified by the surgeon, and then gradually progressed. Gentle AAROM is initiated early and limited to 90° during the first 6 weeks. Active knee flexion ROM for patients with PCL reconstruction is contraindicated to minimize hamstring firing and tension on the graft. The patient is educated regarding the fact that ROM should not be forced and should not cause pain.

Quadriceps re-education is performed as described earlier, and an NMES unit is applied, as needed. Once the patient demonstrates adequate quadriceps activation, supine straight leg raises with the brace locked at 0° of extension are initiated. Prone straight leg raises for hip extension are also performed to strengthen the hip musculature. Side-lying hip adduction or abduction is contraindicated for 6 weeks following reconstruction or repair of medial or lateral structures, respectively. Distal lower extremity strengthening and flexibility is initiated, as described earlier in this chapter. Hamstring stretching is initiated with caution if the hamstring tendon was harvested or if a PCL and/or PLC repair/reconstruction was performed. With 50% weight bearing permitted, weight shifting on a uniplanar rocker is initiated in the sagittal plane for proprioceptive stimulation.

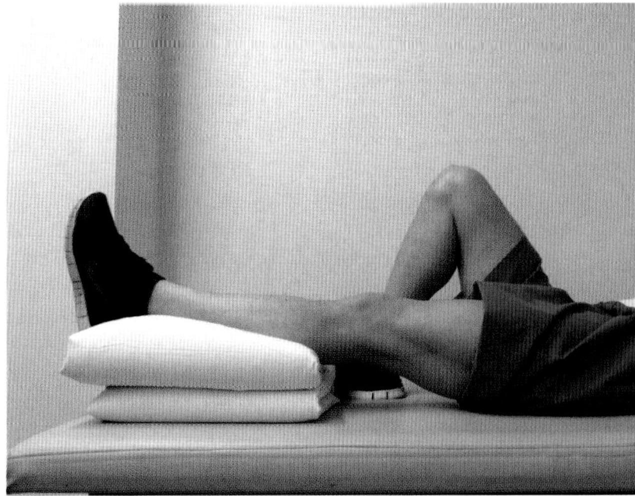

Figure 51.9 Photograph of passive knee extension with a towel roll under the mid-tibia to protect the posterior cruciate ligament (PCL) post–PCL reconstruction.

Phase 2: Gait Restoration and Strengthening

The second phase following MLKI surgery (6–12 weeks) emphasizes restoration of normal gait, ROM, and gradually introducing additional lower extremity strengthening, flexibility, and balance exercises. Techniques for gait re-education and restoration of flexion ROM are performed, as described earlier in this chapter. ROM is expected to continue to gradually progress and full symmetrical ROM should be achieved by the completion of this phase. A common complication following MLKI surgery is the development of arthrofibrosis. Should the patient cease to advance ROM over a period of time, manipulation may be necessary. When manipulation is indicated, it is best done within 12 weeks after surgery.

Once adequate ROM is restored, cycling on a stationary bicycle is initiated. Upon achieving 90° of knee flexion, the patient will begin performing a two-legged leg press for closed-chain lower extremity strengthening. Initially, ROM with the leg press is limited from 0° to 60°, notably if the PCL was reconstructed. It is imperative to encourage muscle control through the ROM and symmetrical pressure through the lower extremities. Strengthening on the leg press is advanced as the patient continues to display improved motor control of the operative leg. The leg press is progressed to eccentric (Figure 51.10) and then eventually a single-leg press. Proximal strengthening is continued with progressive resistance for straight leg raises in all directions. Bilateral standing heel raises are also performed to further strengthen the gastrocnemius-soleus complex. As the patient is progressed to full weight bearing, single-leg balance exercises on a stable surface are initiated for balance training and proprioceptive stimulation.

Upon demonstration of ≥100° of knee flexion, forward step-up exercises are progressively introduced, beginning with

© 2018 American Academy of Orthopaedic Surgeons

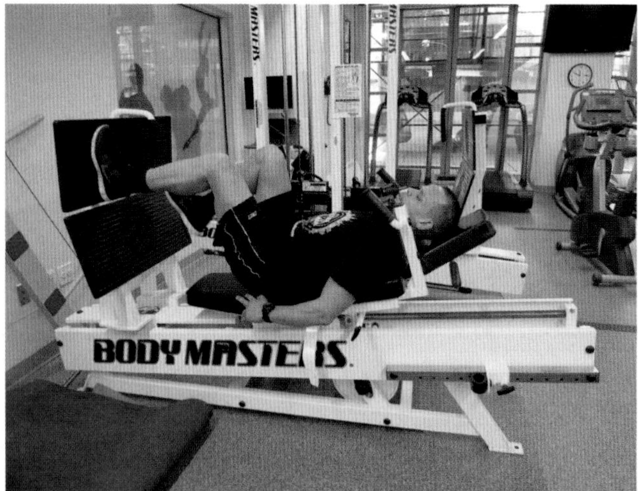

Figure 51.10 Photograph of eccentric leg press. Apply 60% of the weight utilized during a two-legged leg press.

a 4-inch step (Figure 51.11). Step-down exercises (Figure 51.12) are initiated upon demonstration of ≥120° of knee flexion and improved quadriceps strength and control, beginning with a 4-inch step and advanced based on patient tolerance and performance. The physical therapist should monitor for alignment and compensations as the patient progresses with step-up and step-down exercises. Upon demonstration of step-ups on a 6-inch step without compensations or pain, the patient will begin utilization of an elliptical machine (Figure 51.13). At approximately 8 weeks postsurgery and upon demonstrating ≥120° of knee flexion, gentle quadriceps flexibility stretching is introduced (Figure 51.14). Following a PCL and post-PLC repair/reconstruction, open kinetic chain (OKC) knee flexion is contraindicated for 12 weeks.

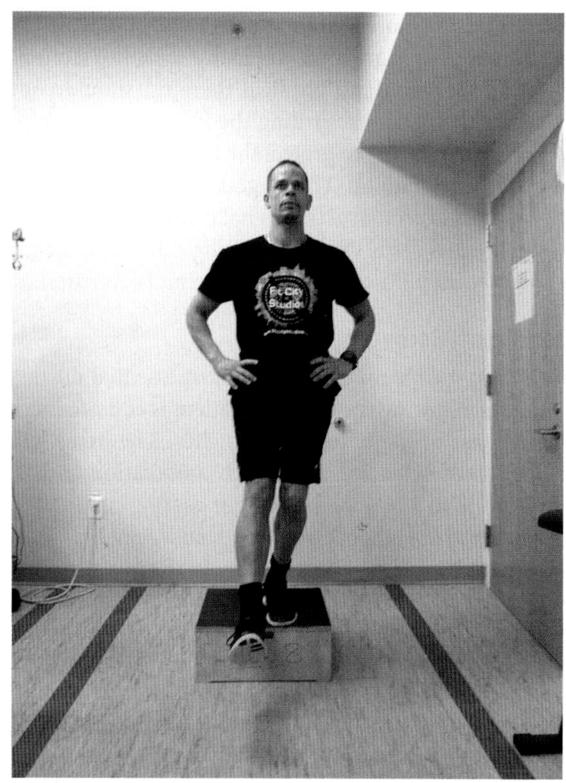

Figure 51.12 Photograph of step-down on an 8-inch step. Begin step-downs with a 4-inch step, gradually progressing to 6 inches and then 8 inches.

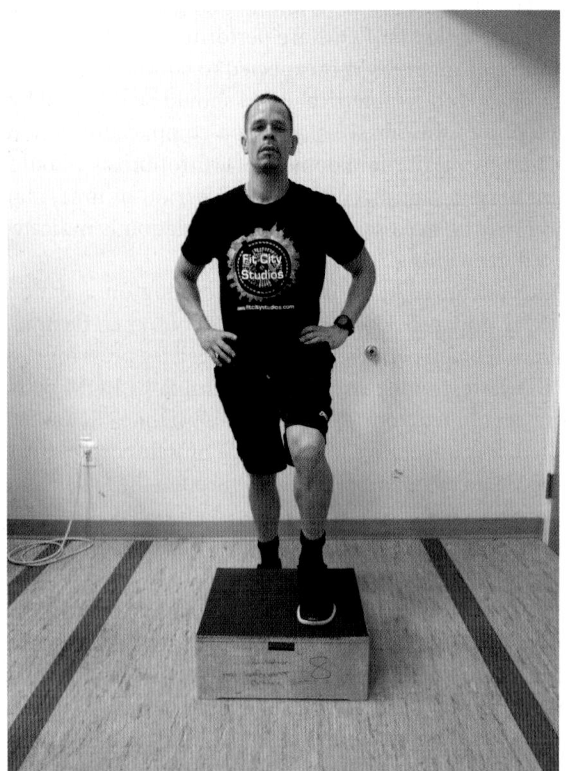

Figure 51.11 Photograph of step-up on an 8-inch step. Begin step-ups with a 4-inch step, gradually progressing to 6 inches and then 8 inches.

Phase 3: Preparation for Advanced Activity

The third phase (weeks 12–20) involves continued gradual advancement of lower extremity strengthening, flexibility, and balance to prepare for return to previous activities. The patient will perform wall-assisted squats (Figure 51.15) within a limited ROM to start (0°–45°), then gradually progress squat ROM. Wall-assisted squats are gradually advanced to chair squats and then free squats, constantly monitoring the patient for compensations. OKC knee extension exercises with progressive resistance are initiated for isolated quadriceps muscle strengthening upon achieving ≥130° of knee flexion at 12 weeks postsurgery. The arc is initially limited to 90° to 30° of knee extension, then gradually progressed to full motion. The physical therapist should monitor for pain, crepitus, and maltracking of the patella. Isolated hamstring exercises are introduced in this phase and gradually advanced. Neuromuscular training exercises are essential for recovery following ligamentous injury, with or without repair or reconstruction, to stimulate proprioceptive receptors about the knee and lower extremity. Balance exercises will continue to be advanced to unstable surfaces and

© 2018 American Academy of Orthopaedic Surgeons

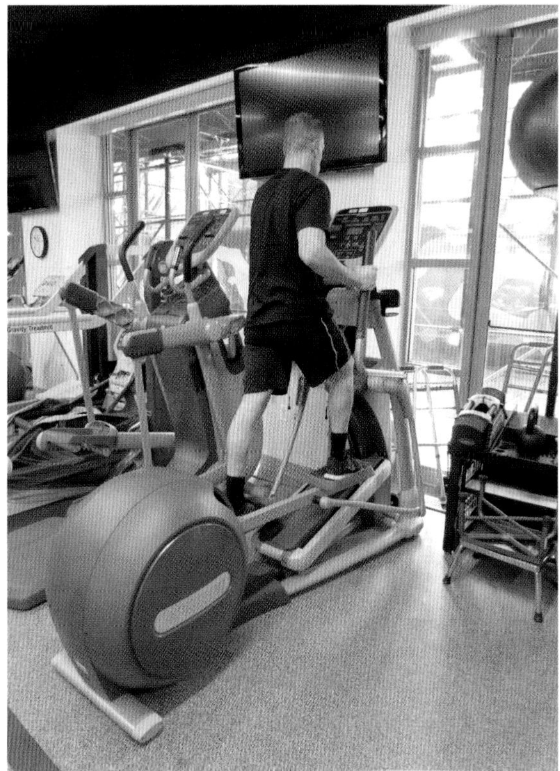

Figure 51.13 Photograph of an elliptical machine.

performing dynamic activities. Examples include balancing on a half drum (Figure 51.16) and single-leg balancing while tossing a weighted medicine ball in various planes. Careful observation and correction for compensations throughout the kinetic chain—including the trunk, pelvis and hips—is important. As exercises are progressed, volume must also be monitored for muscle fatigue and development of edema at the knee.

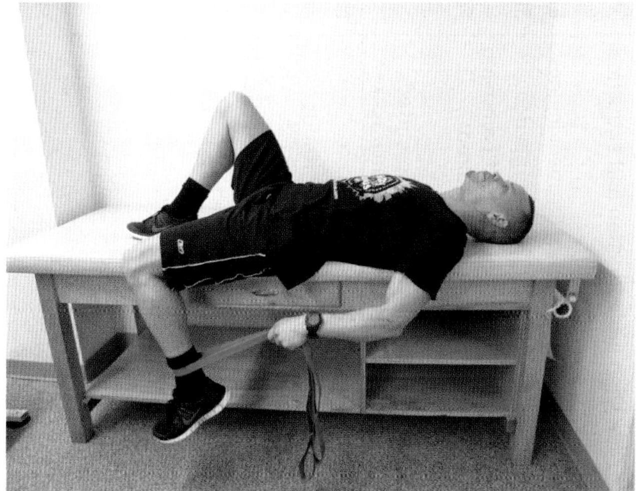

Figure 51.14 Photograph of the quadriceps stretch in the supine position performed with the surgical leg hanging off the edge of a table, hip in full extension, and a strap around the ankle, as the knee is gently pulled into further flexion. This will minimize compressive forces at the patellofemoral joint. Hold each stretch 20 to 30 seconds.

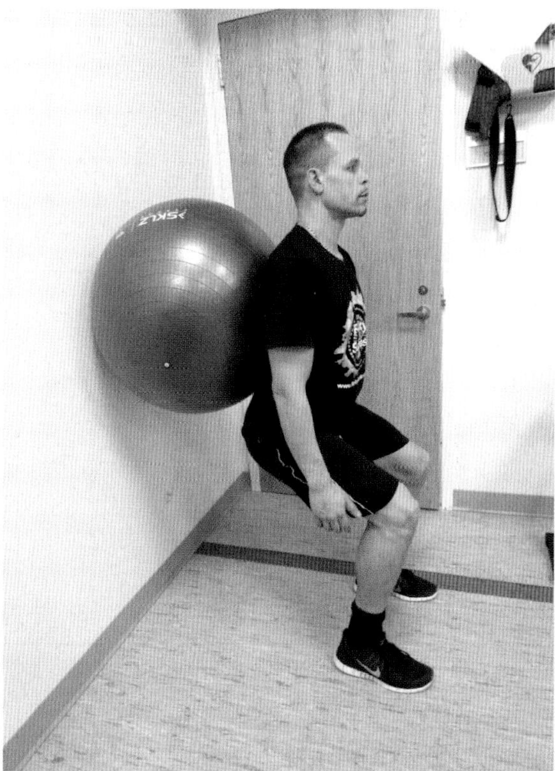

Figure 51.15 Photograph of wall-assisted ball squats. Initiate at a limited ROM of 0° to 45°, gradually progressing ROM. The physical therapist carefully monitors for pain, alignment, symmetry, and technique while squatting.

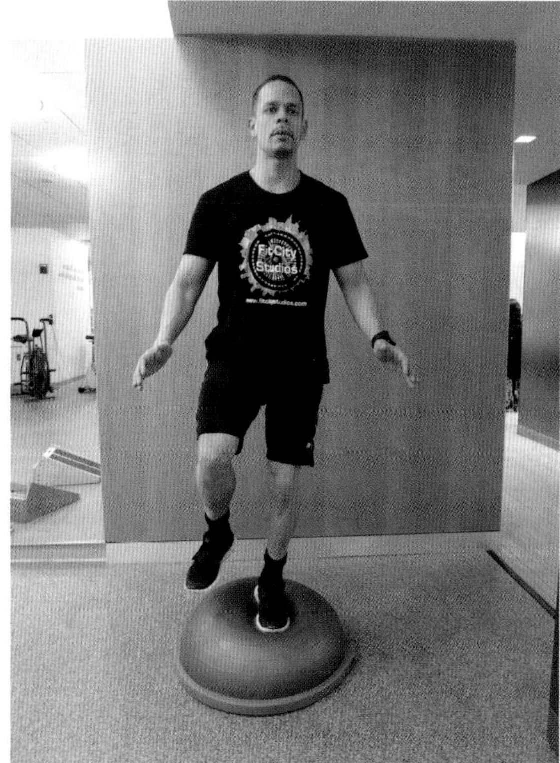

Figure 51.16 Photograph of single-leg balance on a half drum.

© 2018 American Academy of Orthopaedic Surgeons

Table 51.1 POST-OPERATIVE REHABILITATION GUIDELINES

	Phase 1	Phase 2	Phase 3	Phase 4
Precautions	Protection of the repaired tissues. PCL: Flexion to 90° for the first 6 wk. No active knee flexion for the first 12 wk. Avoid hyperextension.	Protection of the repaired tissues. PCL: No active knee flexion for the first 12 wk.	None.	None.
Goals	Full knee extension (0°). Knee flexion to 90°. Good quadriceps activation. Able to supine SLR without support.	Normalize gait without support. Restore full normal knee ROM. Able to single-leg balance on a stable surface >30 s with good alignment and control. Able to step up an 8-inch step with good alignment and control. Able to step down an 8-inch step with good alignment and control. Able to squat on two legs symmetrically with good alignment and control.	Continue to progress strengthening and flexibility exercises. Introduce more functional movement patterns.	Gradually progress the patient to return to more advanced functional activities as appropriate.
Activities	Isometric quadriceps activation. Supine SLRs. Prone SLRs. Side-lying hip adduction and abduction SLRs. (Caution with collateral ligament injuries). NMES for the quadriceps as needed. Hamstring stretching (hold if hamstring was harvested or PCL repaired/ reconstructed). Once 50% weight bearing permitted, weight shifting on a uniplanar rocker.	Stationary bicycle Add ankle weights to supine/prone/side-lying SLR Leg press: double leg/eccentric/single leg. Forward step up 4-inch step → 8-inch step. Elliptical machine Single-leg balance activities on stable and unstable surfaces. Forward step down 4-inch step → 8-inch step.	Stationary bicycle Elliptical OKC knee extension with progressive resistance. Isolated hamstring strengthening Dynamic single-leg balance activities on unstable surfaces. Squats Forward step-up Forward step down. Lunges	Squats. Single-leg squats Running Cutting Agility drills Plyometrics Sport-specific skills
Criteria for Advancement	Good quadriceps activation. Able to SLR without a lag without support. Knee flexion to 90°. Pain-free with all activities.	Normalize gait without support. Restore full normal knee ROM. Able to single-leg balance on a stable surface >30 s with good alignment and control. Able to step up an 8-inch step with good alignment and control. Able to step down an 8-inch step with good alignment and control. Able to squat on two legs symmetrically with good alignment and control. Pain-free with all activities.	Symmetrical squat >90° with good alignment and control. Able to single-leg balance on unstable surfaces >30 s with good alignment and control. Pain-free with all activities	Pain-free with all activities

NMES = neuromuscular electrical stimulation, OKC = open kinetic chain, PCL = posterior cruciate ligament, SLR = single leg raise.

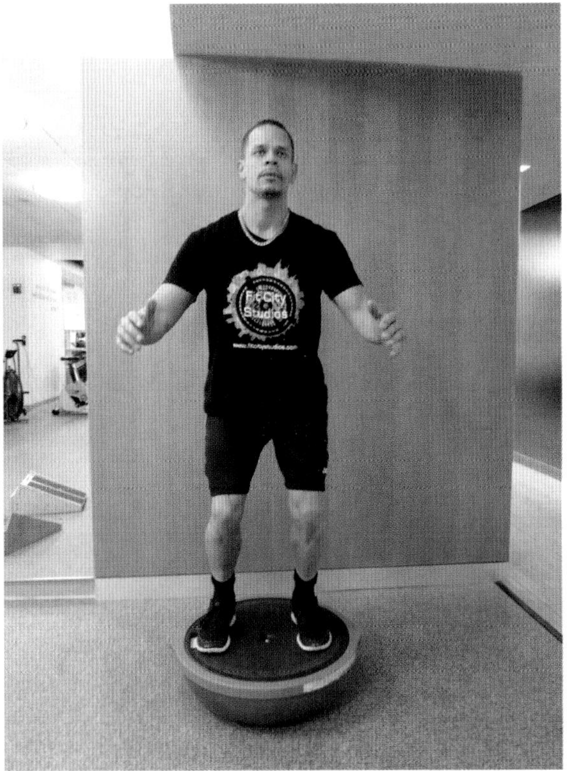

Figure 51.17 Photograph of squats on a half drum for complex proprioceptive stimulation.

Phase 4: Advanced Activities

The fourth and final phase of rehabilitation (weeks 20+) post–MLKI reconstruction guides the patient through advanced movement patterns and physical demands related to individual functional goals. These include complex lower extremity exercises on various surfaces (Figure 51.17), agility exercises, plyometrics, jogging, running, and other sport-specific activities. Criteria to begin a plyometric and/or running program include absence of edema or pain with activities, adequate flexibility and ROM, symmetrical squat >90° of knee flexion, and control with dynamic single-leg activities, including an 8-inch forward step-down. Criteria for return to sport include a limb symmetry index of >90% for isokinetic quadriceps and hamstring strength, single-leg hop test, and the ability to demonstrate all sport-specific movements without pain, compensations, or edema. The physical therapist should communicate the results of objective testing and subjective observations with the surgeon for final clearance to return to play (Table 51.1).

Outcomes

Prognosis following multiligament surgery is at best guarded. The patient should be counselled preoperatively in this regard. Loss of end ROM, residual stiffness, decreased strength, and varying degrees of function loss are common. Engebretsen et al. found that high-energy knee dislocations had significantly inferior outcomes versus low-energy knee dislocations. They also determined that individuals who injured two or three ligaments displayed more favorable outcomes versus those who sustained injury to all four knee ligaments. Radiographic examination revealed significant evidence of knee osteoarthritis in 87% of injured knees.

Jenkins et al. found that, out of 20 patients who sustained a multiligament injury, 95% returned to work at 2 years postinjury. Four of the patients changed occupation due to the injury. All 20 patients participated in sports preinjury, but only 30% were able to return to their preinjury sport level at 2-year follow-up. Of the patients, 10% failed to return to sport. A meta-analysis by Peskun et al. found a lower return to work rate at 80.9% and a higher return to previous level of competition at 50%. A multiligament injury can lead to long-term disability, thus proper management from the onset of injury is imperative to maximize long-term function of the injured knee.

PEARLS

- A careful preoperative assessment is critical for these injuries, including a thorough neurovascular examination.
- MRI is critical to complete the soft-tissue evaluation of the knee following traumatic MLKI.
- Communication regarding all affected tissues, including nonsurgical and surgically repaired/reconstructed structures, is crucial and will guide the progression of rehabilitation.
- Patellar mobilizations and scar massage will help minimize adhesions and promote knee mobility, but recognize that these injuries have high manipulation rates.
- A criteria-based functional progression is applied throughout the rehabilitation process to ensure a safe and complication-free recovery.

BIBLIOGRAPHY

Engebretsen L, Risberg MA, Robertson B, Ludvigsen TC, Johansen S: Outcome after knee dislocations: a 2–9 years follow-up of 85 consecutive patients. *Knee Surg Sports Traumatol Arthrosc* 2009;17:1013–1026.

Jenkins PJ, Clifton R, Gillespie GN, Will EM, Keating JF: Strength and function recovery after multiple-ligament reconstruction of the knee. *Injury* 2011;42:1426–1429.

Middleton KK, Hamilton T, Irrgang JJ, Karlsson J, Harner CD, Fu FH: Anatomic anterior cruciate ligament (ACL) reconstruction: a global perspective. Part 1. *Knee Surg Sports Traumatol Arthrosc* 2014;22:1467–1482.

Peskun CJ, Whelan DB: Outcomes of operative and nonoperative treatment of multiligament knee injuries. *Sports Med Arthrosc Rev* 2011;19(2):167–173.

Pierce CM, O'Brien L, Griffin LW, LaPrade RF: Posterior cruciate ligament tears: functional and postoperative rehabilitation. *Knee Surg Sports Traumatol Arthrosc* 2012;21:1071–1084.

Ranawat A, Baker CL 3rd, Henry S, Harner, CD: Posterolateral corner injury of the knee: evaluation and management. *J Am Acad Orthop Surg* 2008;16:506–518.

Smyth MP, Koh JL: A review of surgical and nonsurgical outcomes of medial knee injuries. *Sports Med Arthrosc Rev* 2015;23:15–22.

© 2018 American Academy of Orthopaedic Surgeons

Foot and Ankle 6

52 Introduction to Rehabilitation of the Foot and Ankle

Justin K. Greisberg, MD, and Jenna Baynes, MD

INTRODUCTION

The human foot is one of the few anatomic structures that separates us from other primates. While one could argue that other parts of the limbs, such as the hand or shoulder, are just modifications of the basic primate design, the foot has evolved from a position of mobility to one of stability. The basic primate foot is adapted for grasping, while the human foot is meant for prolonged weight bearing.

In simplest terms, the foot provides a stable foundation, with a "universal joint" (ankle/hindfoot) that can keep the leg vertical while the foot accommodates any uneven terrain. The rigid arch provides a lever arm to amplify contractions of the Achilles tendon.

FOOT AND ANKLE ANATOMY

Bone Morphology

The talus is the center of the ankle/hindfoot complex. A large part of the bone is covered with articular cartilage, and there are no tendon insertions on the bone. With little soft-tissue coverage, the blood supply to the talus is tenuous, and injuries can result in avascular necrosis and collapse.

The anterior process of the calcaneus is just below the talus, but the body of the calcaneus sits a bit more laterally, to give some valgus to the hindfoot. The Achilles tendon inserts on the large tuberosity, which is also the sole hindfoot point of contact with the ground.

The navicular, cuboid, and cuneiforms pack in together tightly (Figure 52.1). The first metatarsal is much larger in diameter than the other metatarsals. While it is quite mobile in other primates, in the human, the first metatarsal is tucked in tightly alongside the second in a position of stability. In the ideal human foot, the first metatarsal should take about 40% of normal weight-bearing forces.

Joints

The distal tibia and fibula come together to form the ankle mortise, a highly constrained socket for the talus. The talus rotates in the mortise to provide the majority of plantarflexion and dorsiflexion motion.

The talus also articulates with the navicular (talonavicular joint) and the calcaneus (subtalar joint). Although these joints are generally separate, the two joints form the hindfoot complex. Together, they provide most of the inversion and eversion. These joints actually make a three-dimensional screw motion, so that inversion is accompanied by some plantarflexion and forward translation of the foot, and eversion is accompanied by dorsiflexion and some posterior translation. Fusion of either joint eliminates most of the motion in the other.

Although there are three joints around the talus, in reality, the ankle and hindfoot joints act together as a universal joint, to allow the foot to accommodate any terrain while the leg remains vertical.

The calcaneocuboid provides a small amount of additional hindfoot motion. Together with the talonavicular joint, these

Dr. Greisberg or an immediate family member serves as a paid consultant to Extremity Medical; has received research or institutional support from Extremity Medical; has received nonincome support (such as equipment or services), commercially derived honoraria, or other non-research–related funding (such as paid travel) from Saunders/Mosby-Elsevier; and serves as a board member, owner, officer, or committee member of the American Orthopaedic Foot and Ankle Society. Neither Dr. Baynes nor any immediate family member has received anything of value from or has stock or stock options held in a commercial company or institution related directly or indirectly to the subject of this article.

 © 2018 American Academy of Orthopaedic Surgeons

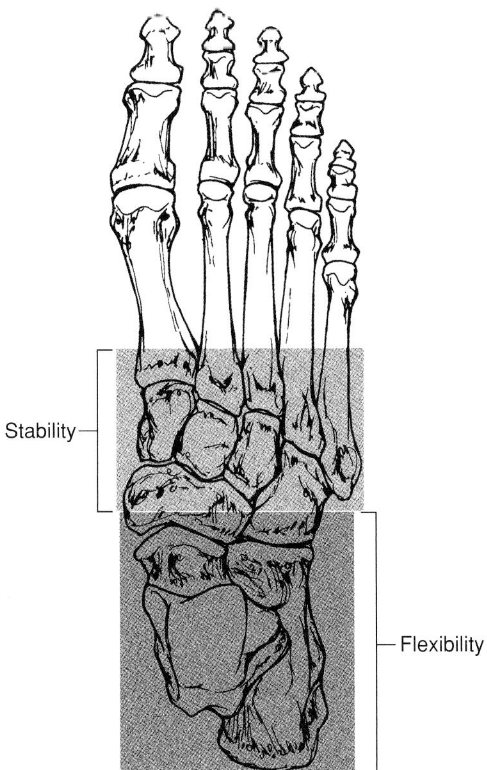

Figure 52.1 Illustration of fhe hindfoot, which contains the subtalar and talonavicular joints, where most inversion/eversion occurs. The midfoot provides very little motion, and actually is more important for rigidity than flexibility. (Modified from Oatis CA: *Kinesiology—The Mechanics and Pathomechanics of Human Movement*. Baltimore, Lippincott Williams & Wilkins, 2004.)

two joints, also called the Chopart joints, can provide a moderate amount of plantar/dorsiflexion when the ankle is stiff or fused.

The articulations between the navicular, the cuneiforms, and the medial three metatarsals are relatively rigid. These joints have evolved in the human for stability, not mobility. Insufficient stability of these midfoot joints can result in foot deformities, such as a collapsed arch or hallux valgus.

Motion at the metatarsophalangeal (MTP) joints is helpful during the gait cycle, especially extension/dorsiflexion during heel rise, but stiffness/fusion of the first MTP joint is surprisingly well tolerated (as long as there is no pain). The interphalangeal joints are not essential to normal human locomotion.

Muscles

The Achilles tendon is the culmination of the two heads of the gastrocnemius and the soleus. The gastrocnemius origin is on the posterior distal femur; thus, it crosses the knee and the ankle. In quadrupeds (e.g., the horse or cheetah), a contracture of the Achilles tendon holds the calcaneus off the ground; the heel never touches the ground. Active extension of the knee automatically causes a passive plantarflexion of the ankle, which leads to efficiency when running. In humans, some of this evolutionary Achilles tightness is still present, such that gastrocnemius tightness is a common problem in many patients.

Furthermore, the gastrocnemius-soleus complex is so much larger than any other leg muscles that there is a constant imbalance, with a tendency to develop an equinus contracture, especially with prolonged nonweight bearing. Achilles stretching, especially of the gastrocnemius, is an important part of rehabilitation from most ankle injuries or surgeries.

Active contraction of the Achilles tendon results in plantarflexion through the ankle joint. This rotation is amplified across the rigid midfoot joints to the metatarsal heads, acting as a lever. (In other words, a centimeter of contraction in the Achilles tendon leads to several centimeters of plantarflexion at the metatarsal heads.) This is the key to efficient propulsion in human gait (Figure 52.2).

In the normal gait cycle, the posterior tibial tendon fires just before heel rise, inverting and locking the hindfoot and midfoot joints in a stable position, thus creating the rigid lever across the midfoot. If the posterior tibial tendon fails to lock the arch (as in posterior tibial tendon dysfunction), the midfoot remains flexible, and the Achilles contraction leads to progressive breakdown of the arch ligaments, with a progressive flatfoot deformity. Thus, a healthy posterior tibial tendon is essential to normal gait.

As the human foot accommodates uneven terrain, intermittent firing of the leg muscles keeps the leg vertical. In particular, the peroneal tendons, especially the peroneus brevis, prevents accidental inversion that might lead to a sprain. The peroneal tendons constantly work in response to input from the position sense receptors in the ankle joint, so that ankle stability is controlled somewhere below the level of the cerebral cortex.

If the peroneal tendons and their balance reflexes are not functioning properly (such as when recovering from an injury or following a long period of immobilization), inversion injuries will occur. Rehabilitation of the ankle will require

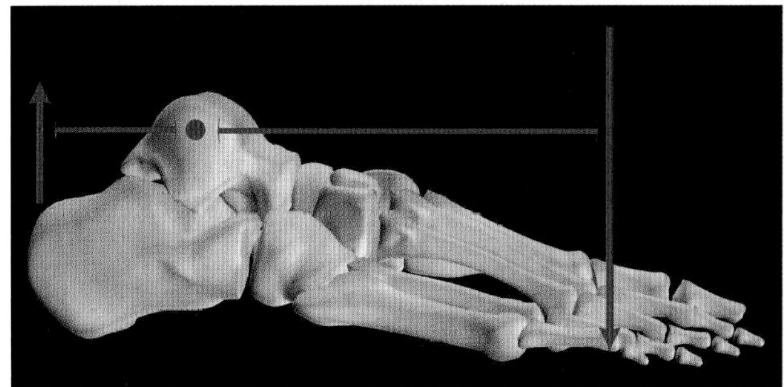

Figure 52.2 Illustration of the midfoot. When the midfoot is rigid, the medial column acts as a rigid lever from the talus to the first metatarsal head. A relatively small magnitude of Achilles contraction is amplified to make a large amount of plantar flexion at the metatarsal head, through a "lever" effect. (Modified from LifeART image copyright (c) 2016, Lippincott Williams & Wilkins. All rights reserved.)

© 2018 American Academy of Orthopaedic Surgeons

strengthening of the peroneals and recovery of the position sense reflexes.

PRINCIPLES OF REHABILITATION

Immediately following an injury or surgery, the body reacts by initiating the inflammatory response. The first phase is the acute inflammatory phase, which usually lasts about 48 to 72 hours, but can be as long as 7 to 10 days. Damage to small blood and lymph vessels initiates a temporary vasoconstriction that lasts a couple of seconds to minutes. This is quickly followed by vasodilation and increased permeability, with an influx of blood, serum proteins, clotting factors, and platelets that make up the inflammatory exudate. What we see clinically is localized swelling, redness, pain, increased temperature, and loss of normal function.

The second phase of soft-tissue healing is the subacute migratory and proliferative phase, which typically lasts 10 days to about 6 weeks and overlaps the inflammation phase. The transition from debris removal to granulation tissue formation is a marker of proliferation and is necessary for scar tissue formation. Initially, the tensile strength of the wound matrix is low and is made up of type III collagen, but soon the weaker type III collagen begins to be replaced by a stronger type I collagen. Clinically, there is reduced erythema and swelling.

The third and final phase of soft-tissue healing is the remodeling phase, which can last anywhere from 6 weeks to 1 year depending on the degree of injury. During remodeling, the initial healing tissue converts to dense scar tissue, whereby the injured area becomes stabilized and restored. Clinically, this phase may initially be characterized by pain or soreness occurring after activity, but progresses toward pain-free function.

Although tendons, ligaments, muscles, articular cartilage, and bones show some variation in sequence and duration of events, all tissues follow the same general phases of soft-tissue healing. Thus, the same general intervention principles can be applied to most soft-tissue injuries of the foot and ankle. However, specific rehabilitation protocols must be followed after certain injuries and surgical procedures.

The timing of treatment after a foot and ankle injury is crucial, and should coincide directly with the various stages of healing and principles of weight-bearing progression. Just as the phases of soft-tissue healing overlap, the stages of rehabilitation should as well. Immediately after trauma to an injured body part, the primary goal is controlling pain and inflammation. Although some inflammation is necessary for healing, if not controlled, secondary injury can occur and lead to chronic inflammation. Initial treatment includes rest, protection, ice, compression, elevation, early motion, gentle manual therapy, medication, and therapeutic modalities.

A period of rest does not mean that the patient must be completely inactive. Rather, in order to avoid the harmful effects of immobilization, a period of "relative" rest is typically recommended. Most foot and ankle surgeons will rest and even immobilize the leg for a few days up to as long as 6 weeks following surgery. Once the tissues are rested and the wounds are healed, a patient can begin to initiate controlled activity. Be mindful that pain is a subjective response to injury and all people have a different pain threshold. It can be an extremely useful warning signal in most situations; therefore, use it to guide progression.

Cryotherapy, or cold therapy, is used in the management of acute trauma based on physiologic responses to a decrease in tissue temperature. Cryotherapy reduces bleeding; decreases metabolism and vasoactive agents, reducing inflammation and decreasing vessel permeability; limits swelling and edema; and increases the pain threshold, allowing the patient more comfort. Because of the irregular shape of the foot and ankle, a cold whirlpool or cold immersion bath is often the modality of choice. However, these two types of cold therapy place the foot and ankle in a gravity-dependent position; furthermore, following foot and ankle surgery, the extremity is often immobilized and not accessible to cryotherapy. Of course, whirlpool or bath immersion cannot begin until surgical wounds are healed; thus, cryotherapy is less commonly used after surgery than after injury.

In conjunction with cryotherapy, compression and elevation of the foot and ankle are used to aid in venous return and pump edema fluid from the extremity. Although compression may be difficult to achieve immediately after surgery, elevation is an essential part of the first few weeks. While elevating, patients can work on frequent active motion exercises in the leg (knee and toes if in a splint/cast). Isometric contractions of the Achilles also are helpful at increasing venous return, diminishing the chance for deep vein thrombosis (DVT), and decreasing edema.

Motion

There is a conflict during the early postoperative period; the desire for early mobilization to prevent stiffness must be balanced against the need for immobilization to facilitate wound healing. Furthermore, pain will often lead to equinus and lack of ankle dorsiflexion; thus, there is a propensity to develop an Achilles contracture. Larger foot and ankle surgeries will begin with about 2 weeks of immobilization in an ankle neutral splint to maintain some stretch of the Achilles and allow wound healing.

Once wounds are healed, the surgeon may allow the patient to begin motion exercises with a therapist. Early range of motion (ROM) exercises can be active range of motion (AROM) or passive range of motion (PROM) and performed as open kinetic chain (OKC) or closed kinetic chain (CKC) exercise. The most basic form of ROM exercise is the OKC AROM exercises, in which the distal segment is free in space. Examples of foot and ankle OKC AROM exercises include ankle "pumping," or active plantarflexion (PF) and dorsiflexion (DF) active inversion and eversion; ankle "alphabets," or circumduction; toe "crunches," or flexion and extension of the MTP and interphalangeal (IP) joints of the foot; and paper pickups using intrinsic toe flexors to move a small piece of

© 2018 American Academy of Orthopaedic Surgeons

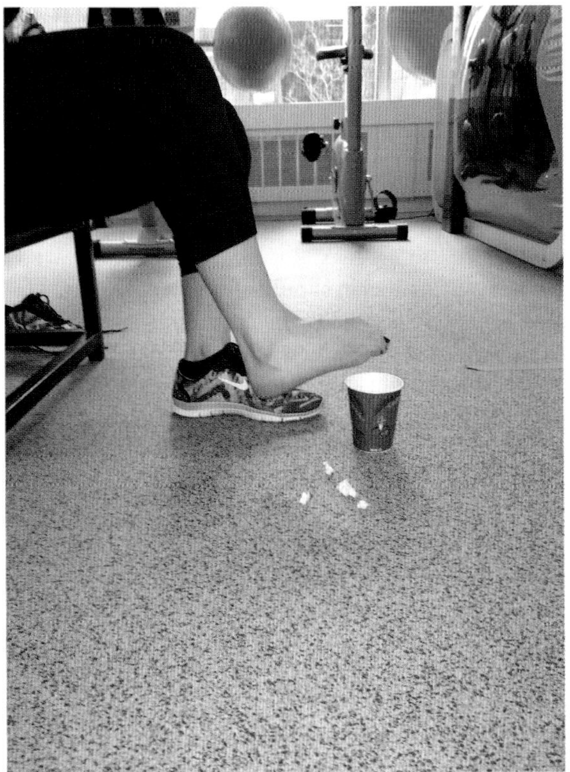

Figure 52.3 Photograph of patient performing paper pick-ups. Pick up the small pieces of paper with your toes and place them in the cup.

paper or marbles (Figure 52.3). These exercises are appropriate if the patient has non–weight bearing precautions and is cleared to do AROM of the foot and ankle. Early CKC AROM exercises, in which the distal segment is fixed, include seated heel raises (Figure 52.4, A) and toe raises (Figure 52.4, B), seated BAPS board for triplanar motion, seated balance board for PF/DF and inversion/eversion and seated arch raises. Light stretching of the gastrocnemius, soleus and Achilles tendon can be performed on the treatment table using a resistance band or towel, or it can be done in a weight-bearing (and more functional) position on the ground (Figure 52.5).

Gentle manual therapy should be initiated as early as possible after injury. Gentle massage and effleurage techniques increase blood flow and decrease swelling, joint mobilizations and gentle distraction aid in reduction of swelling and pain, gentle PROM increases joint mobility, and gentle stretching maintains soft -issue extensibility. At the talocrural joint, distraction of the talus on the ankle mortise and oscillations of the talus posteriorly or anteriorly are used to increase general joint play. At the subtalar joint, gentle distraction of the calcaneus on the talus and medial and lateral calcaneal glides are used to increase general joint play. The midtarsal joint can be mobilized along the longitudinal or oblique axis, via DF/PF and abduction/eversion and adduction/inversion, respectively. Anterior to posterior (A/P) glides of the intermetatarsal joints can increase intermetatarsal mobility. At the tarsometatarsal, MTP, and distal IP joints, distraction of the distal joint on

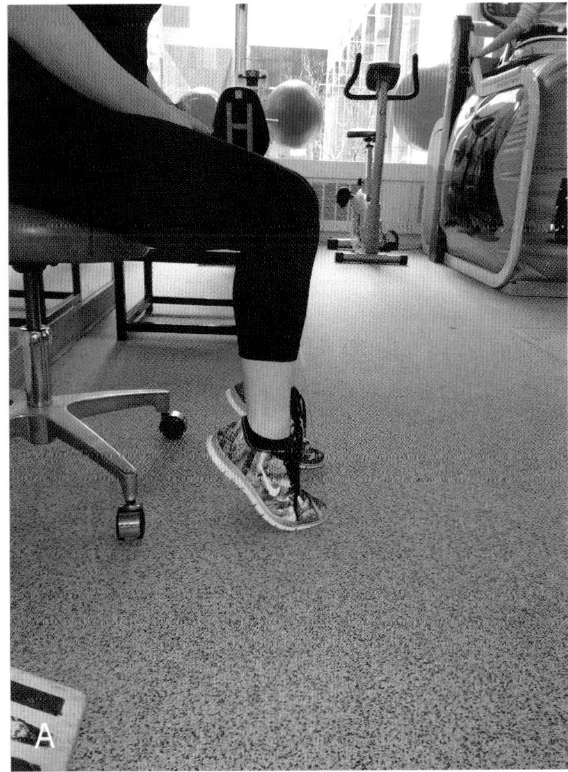

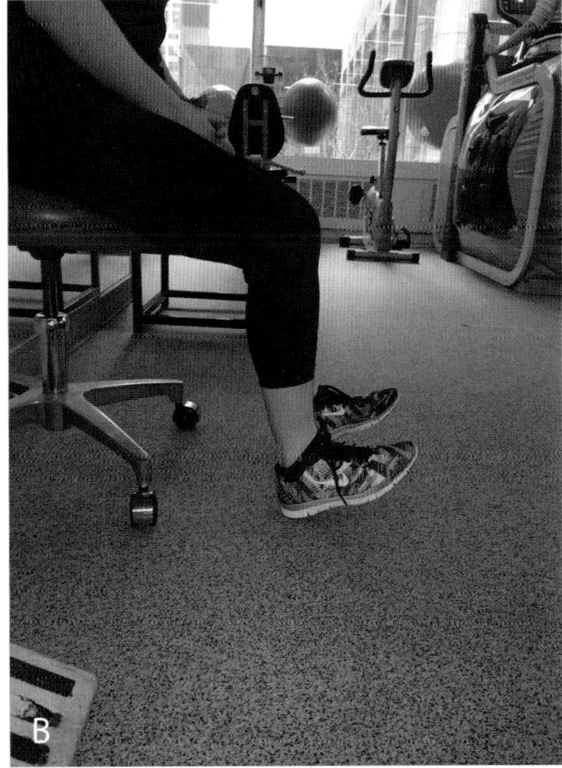

Figure 52.4 **A**, Photograph of seated plantarflexion, or seated heel raises. **B**, Photograph of seated dorsiflexion, or seated toe raises.

© 2018 American Academy of Orthopaedic Surgeons

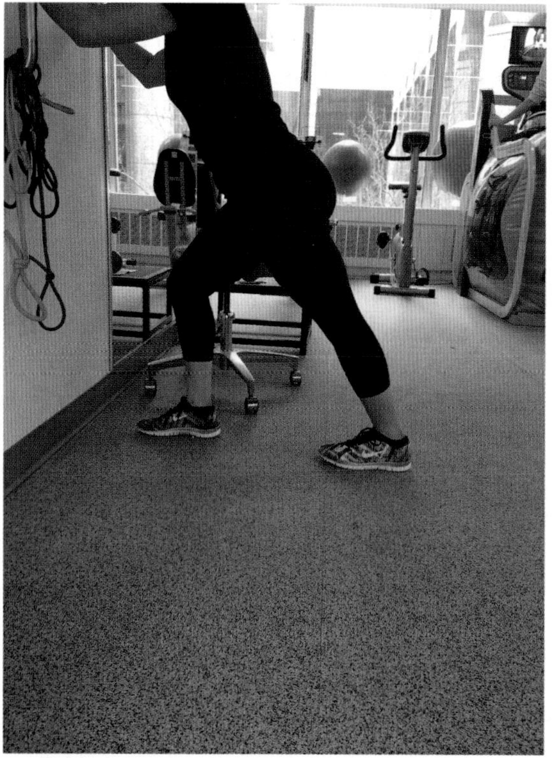

Figure 52.5 Photograph of standing calf stretch. Keep the heel on the ground and the knee straight. Position the toes so that they are perpendicular with the wall.

the proximal joint or A/P glides can be performed to increase general forefoot joint play.

Weight Bearing

Foot and ankle procedures often require prolonged periods of non–weight bearing. Progression may begin with partial weight for a week or so, then progression to weight bearing as tolerated over 1 to 2 weeks. Regardless of the weight-bearing precautions, the clinician should always emphasize a heel-to-toe gait pattern so that faulty mechanics are avoided.

Early weight-bearing exercises include, but are not limited to, (a) standing weight shifts or shifting weight to the affected side, as tolerated or prescribed by the clinician; (b) postural sways, in which the patient sways forward to the point just before the heels rise, mimicking the midstance phase of gait (this exercise is quite effective at targeting the peroneus longus muscle as it everts the ankle and drives the base of the first MT toward the ground during midstance, supporting the arch of the foot; Figure 52.6, A and B); (c) standing arch raises targeting the intrinsic foot muscles and, more important, the posterior tibialis muscle; (d) step-throughs, in which the patient works through the entire stance phase of gait, holding on to external support if needed for balance; (e) gait training over cones, emphasizing heel-to-toe gait pattern anteriorly, side-stepping, or walking backward to increase

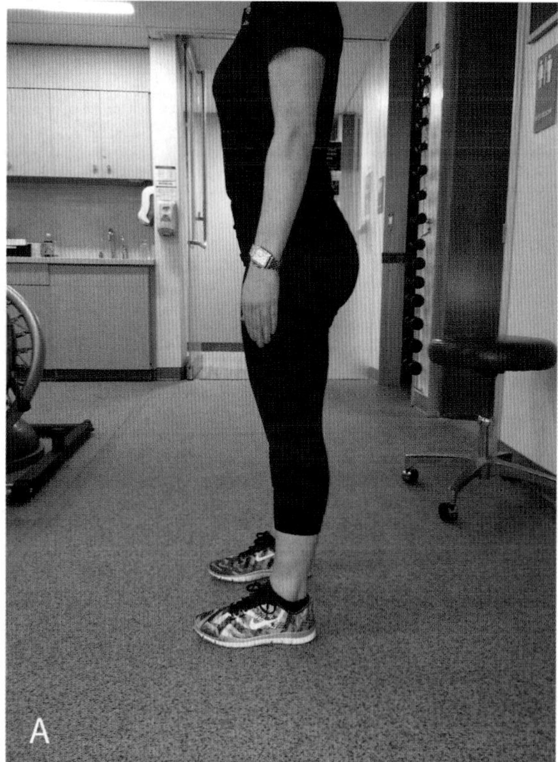

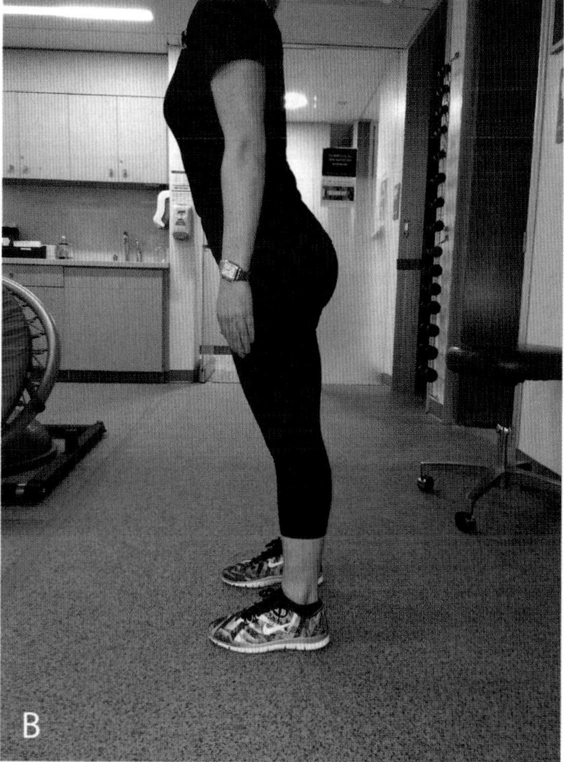

Figure 52.6 **A**, Photograph of postural sways, start position. Stand upright with feet shoulder width apart. **B**, Photograph of postural sways. Sway your entire body forward, maintaining erect position of the trunk, to the point just before your heels leave the ground. You will feel your toes flex. Return to start position.

© 2018 American Academy of Orthopaedic Surgeons

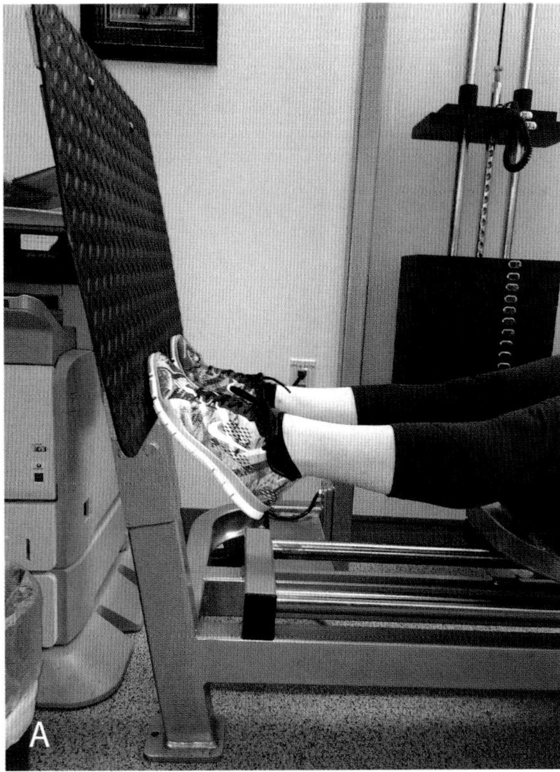

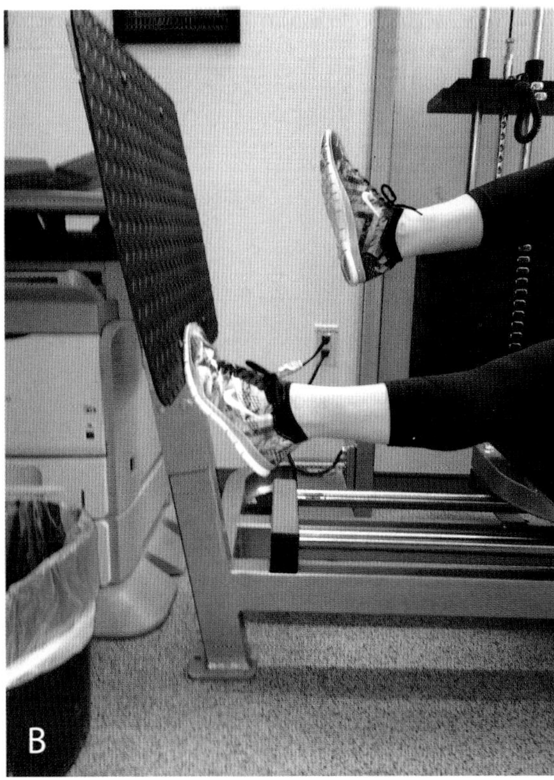

Figure 52.7 A, Photograph of bilateral plantarflexion (heel raises) on the leg press. B, Photograph of unilateral plantarflexion (heel raises) on the leg press.

weight through the forefoot and initiate functional balance; (f) using a leg press machine for heel raises (initially bilateral—Figure 52.7, A, then progress to unilateral—Figure 52.7, B) or total leg strengthening; (g) standing BAPS board for foot and ankle proprioception, ROM and strength (Figure 52.8). If available, use of a body weight–assisted treadmill, such as the anti-gravity machine, is an excellent way to practice gait training at a preadjusted body weight percentage, that is, if allowed to partially weight bear, the patient can ambulate on the anti-gravity treadmill at 50% of one's body weight. Aquatherapy is another avenue for foot and ankle patients to take since the buoyancy of the water unloads body weight, making it easier to walk.

Over the next couple of weeks after injury, the patient should show gradual progression of muscle strength and endurance. The muscles of the foot and ankle are generally endurance muscles, meaning that they need to be able to contract repeatedly and for long periods of time, thus, have low fatigability. Endurance muscles to target during this phase of rehabilitation include the peroneus longus, tibialis posterior, and tibialis anterior. High repetition, low resistance for the following CKC exercises are recommended: standing BAPS board, standing heel raises, standing toe raises, standing arch raises, and heel raises on the leg press. If the patient shows signs of specific muscle weakness or is not ready to bear weight through the affected limb, the patient may use OKC resistance band exercises to isolate any of the muscles of the foot/ankle (Figure 52.9, A and B).

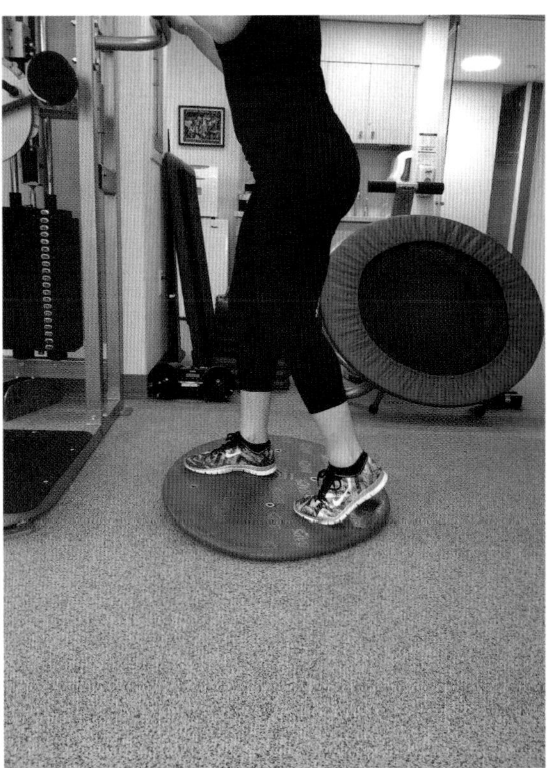

Figure 52.8 Photograph of BAPS board. Place affected foot on the board. Use contralateral foot to guide motion and try to have all borders of the board contact the ground in a circular motion. Turn clockwise and counterclockwise.

© 2018 American Academy of Orthopaedic Surgeons

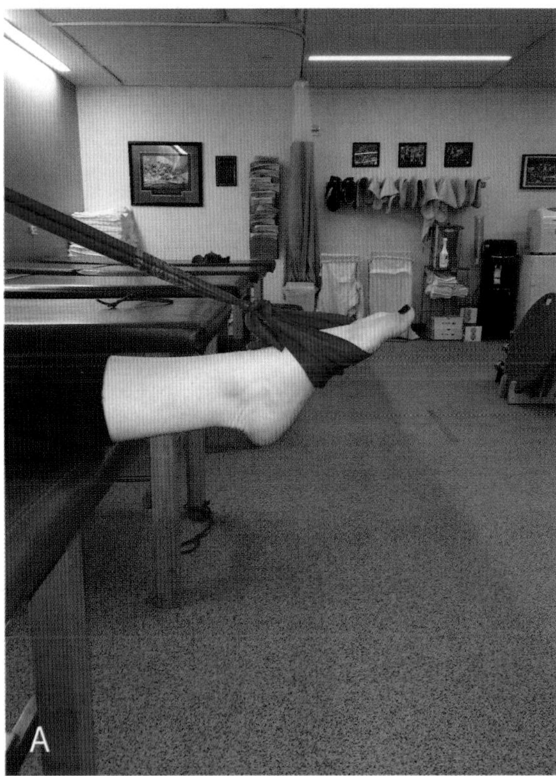

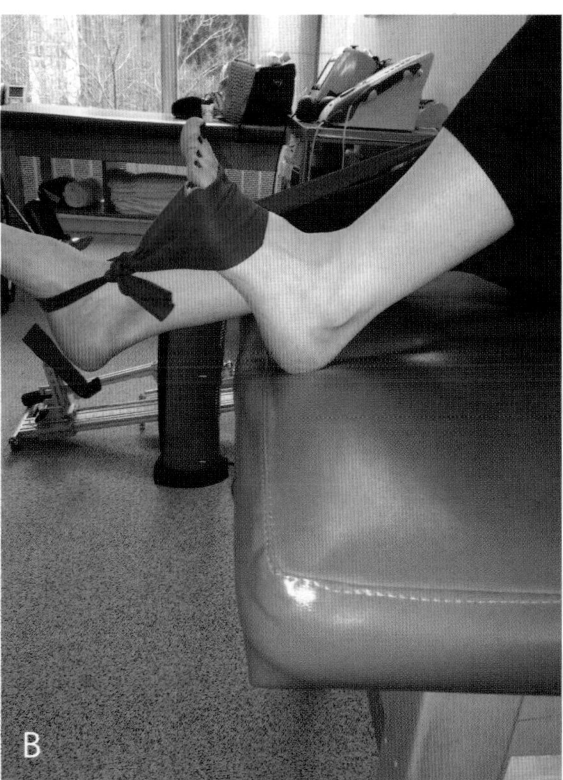

Figure 52.9 **A**, Photograph of open kinetic chain resistance band plantarflexion. **B**, Photograph of open kinetic chain resistance band dorsiflexion.

Balance, proprioception, and functional exercises should also be incorporated at this point. Following injury to the foot/ankle, especially injuries involving the lateral ligaments and peroneal muscles, stability is compromised. The ligaments are the static stabilizers and the muscles are the dynamic stabilizers; both must be rehabilitated for optimal function. Examples of proprioceptive exercises to be used in this phase include tandem stance, tandem walking (forward or backward), and standing on an unstable surface, that is, a balance board (Figure 52.10, A and B), soft foam pad, or trampoline, progressing from bilateral to unilateral stance. Start with static stability and progress into the next phase with dynamic stability exercises. The following functional, total lower extremity strengthening activities can be added as tolerated: sit to stand or squats, step-ups and step-downs and hip and core strengthening.

During the final, remodeling phase of soft-tissue healing, the goals are to achieve full pain-free ROM and strength, and allow safe return to functional and recreational activities at the preinjury level. All of the principles of rehabilitation from the prior phases of healing should be carried over into this last phase. In order for optimal remodeling of the healing tissue to occur, there must be a continuum of controlled stress application throughout the recovery process. Cartilage, bones, ligaments, tendons, and muscles respond favorably to these controlled stresses based on the Specific Adaptation to Imposed Demands (SAID) principle. SAID means that the body will respond and adapt directly to specific demands placed on it. For example, to increase endurance of the posterior tibialis muscle, high-repetition and low-resistance supination exercises should be used. To increase strength of the gastrocnemius muscle, high-resistance and low-repetition ankle plantarflexion exercises should be performed. The SAID principle should be applied throughout the healing process. However, it is particularly important in this final phase when greater loads and stresses can be placed through the healing tissue and the patient is getting ready to return to recreational activity. The SAID principle pertains to all forms of exercise that include flexibility, strength, endurance, balance, proprioception, plyometrics, and agility.

The patient will transition from bilateral to unilateral exercises and from static stability exercises to dynamic stability exercises in order to challenge the static and dynamic stabilizers of the foot and ankle. Unilateral stance can be performed statically on the floor with progression to a foam pad, trampoline, or balance board. Dynamic stability exercises include unilateral stance with active ball rotation (Figure 52.11, A and B), ball toss off of a rebounder, ball catch with the clinician, manual perturbations from the clinician, resistance band exercises on one leg (Figure 52.12, A and B), and single-leg squats, among many more.

Return to Sport

The SAID principle is especially pertinent in determining which exercises the patient should perform when preparing to return to activity. At first, light, general plyometric exercises

 © 2018 American Academy of Orthopaedic Surgeons

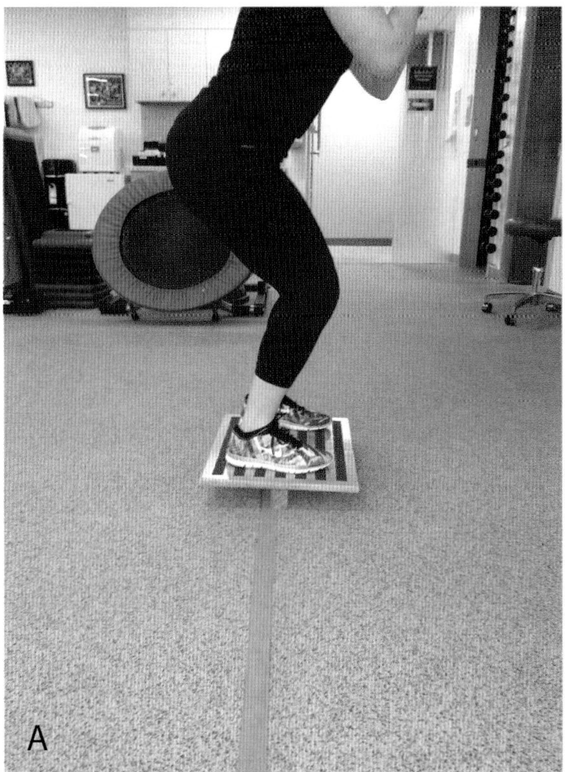

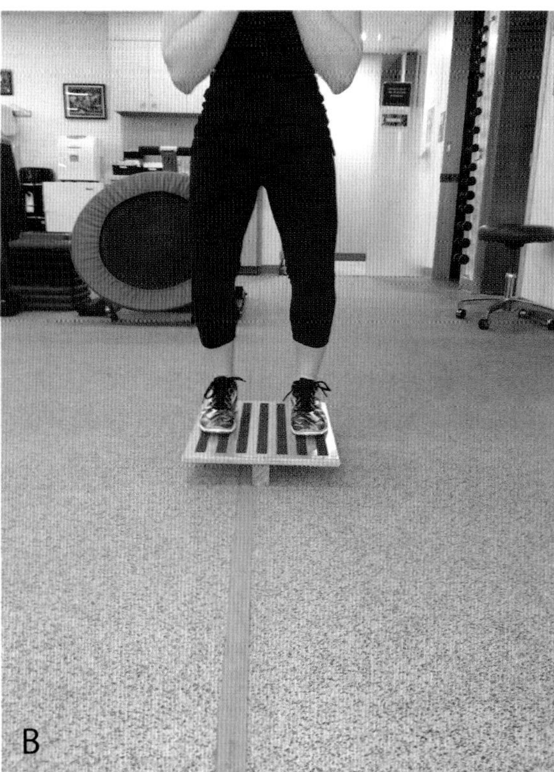

Figure 52.10 **A**, Photograph of balance board used for sagittal plane stability. **B**, Photograph of balance board used for frontal plane stability.

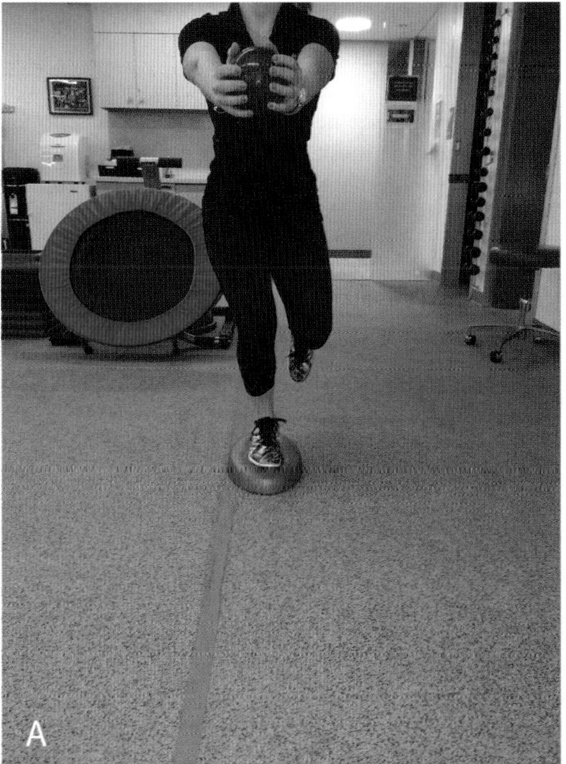

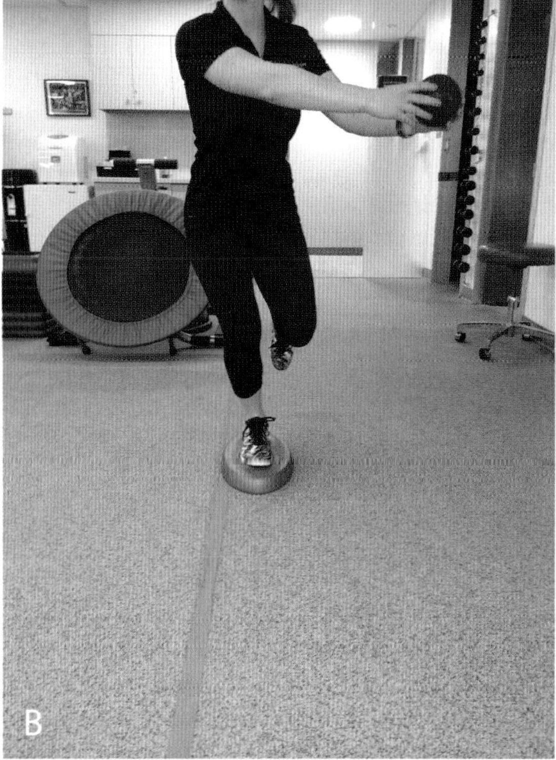

Figure 52.11 **A**, Photograph of unilateral stance on foam with ball rotation, start position. **B**, Photograph of unilateral stance on foam with ball rotation. Rotate ball up, down, left, right, and on a diagonal to challenge stability in all planes of motion.

© 2018 American Academy of Orthopaedic Surgeons

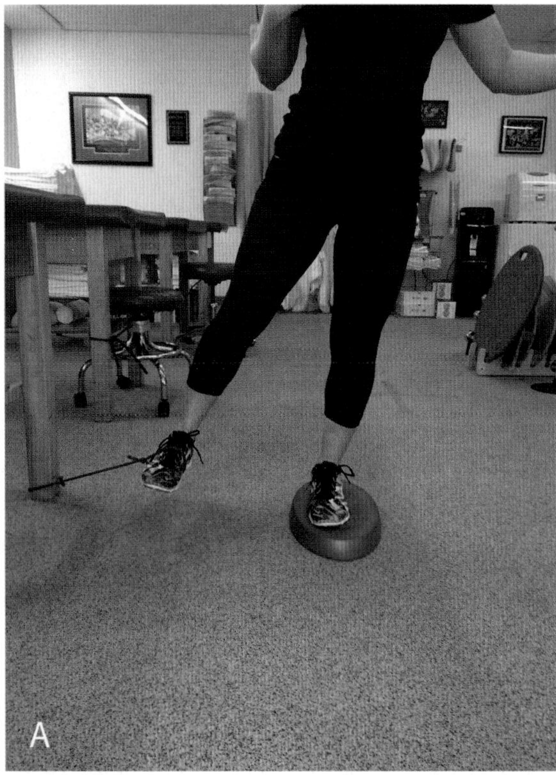

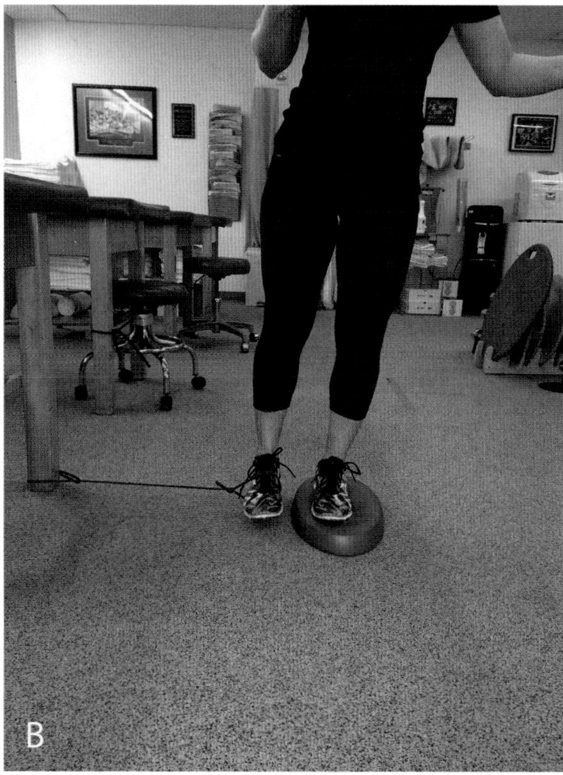

Figure 52.12 **A**, Photograph of resistance band adduction, start position. Affected foot is on the foam. **B**, Photograph of resistance band adduction. Adduct the contralateral lower extremity. Increase speed and increase distance to challenge stability.

like bilateral hops or plyometric lunges should be performed to assess how the patient will respond and to provide a transition to more challenging activities. Initially, the plyometric program design should begin with low intensity, volume and frequency, and a longer recovery time between sets and days performed. If power is the goal, then a longer recovery time is warranted; if endurance is the goal, then a shorter recovery time is necessary. The advanced activities should mimic those required for the sport-specific activity. For example, a soccer player returning to sport after an ankle procedure needs to be able to sprint, cut, and plant, and the lateral ligaments need to be able to withstand these forces. See how the patient tolerates exercise in the sagittal plane first, such as forward/backward running and A/P hops and lunges. Then, progress to frontal plane exercises, such as lateral lunges, hopping, and side shuffles. If the initial injury occurred while the patient was planting and cutting, then a goal for rehabilitation and a requirement for return to sport should be the ability to cut and plant with good control and tolerance.

Before advancing the patient back to high-level athletics, certain prerequisites must be met in order to ensure safe rehabilitation progression and to avoid reinjury. The patient should present with full or close to full ROM and flexibility. Pain level should be well controlled and there should be minimal soreness after activity. Watch out for antalgic gait and faulty body mechanics; these are signs that the patient may feel apprehensive, unstable or weak, experiencing pain, or utilizing faulty movement patterns to compensate for strength deficits.

"Soft signs" of adequate preparation include symmetric ability to single-leg heel rise, and the ability to sprint for 100 yards without hesitation. If an athlete returns to cutting sports before the leg is adequately rehabilitated, inversion injury is likely.

COMPLICATIONS OF FOOT AND ANKLE SURGERY

Any surgery can be complicated by postoperative infection. Motion at the surgical site may lead to shearing of the wound edges, with delayed healing. Dependent edema is especially likely in the foot, which always is "down" relative to other parts of the leg. Thus, during the initial weeks of wound healing, immobilization in a splint and elevation to chest-height are especially important for larger surgeries.

Unfortunately, immobilization can increase the rate of DVT; thus, early motion exercises are helpful. Even when a splint or cast is in place, patients can actively flex their toes, firing the foot and leg intrinsic muscles. Contractions compress the venous plexi in the foot and leg, increasing venous outflow and decreasing the chance for DVT. This motion also promotes gliding of tendons in the tight confines of the foot and ankle, reducing contracture.

 © 2018 American Academy of Orthopaedic Surgeons

Postoperatove pain may decrease a patient's desire to move the extremity, and excessive immobilization may contribute to the development of regional pain syndrome (reflex sympathetic dystrophy) in rare cases. Those early toe flexion exercises are important to lessen this risk, as well as aggressive mobilization once the soft tissues are healed. Scar massage/mobilization may be helpful in addition to active and passive motion exercises whenever the postoperative plan permits it.

SUMMARY

The following guidelines should be adhered to as the patient moves through the various stages of recovery:

- Any sign of acute inflammation warrants reassessment and temporary suspension of progression.
- AROM should be performed before PROM.
- CKC strengthening exercises are preferred over OKC unless there is a weight-bearing restriction.
- Exercises should generally progress from bilateral support to unilateral support, isometric to isotonic, concentric to eccentric, static to dynamic, slow to fast, simple to complex, general skills to specific skills.
- Allow for adequate recovery time between sets and days performed.
- Strength, endurance, flexibility, coordination, and proprioception must be achieved before initiating plyometric, agility and sport-specific exercises.
- Follow the SAID (Specific Adaptation to Imposed Demands) and overload principles when prescribing exercises in order to individualize treatment based on patient-specific needs.

BIBLIOGRAPHY

Dutton M: *Orthopaedic Examination, Evaluation, and Intervention,* ed 2. Pittsburgh, The McGraw-Hill Companies, Inc, 2008, pp 127–130, 319, 348–351.

Houglum P: *Therapeutic Exercise for Musculoskeletal Injuries,* ed 2. Pittsburgh, Peggy A. Houglum, 2005, pp 37–42, 128, 211–212, 249–251, 268.

Michlovitz SL, Nolan TP: *Modalities for Therapeutic Intervention,* ed 4. Philadelphia, FA, Davis, 2005, pp 43, 46, 56.

© 2018 American Academy of Orthopaedic Surgeons

53 Hallux Valgus

J. Turner Vosseller, MD, and Joseph L. Ciccone, PT, DPT, SCS, CIMT, CSCS

INTRODUCTION

Hallux valgus deformity, colloquially known as a bunion, is a result of medial deviation of the first metatarsal with a resultant increase in the intermetatarsal angle between the first and second metatarsals. In patients who have pain associated with this deformity that precludes normal activity or becomes a limiting problem, surgery is a reasonable option in an effort to correct the bony deformity and thereby decrease the related pain.

Hallux valgus is one of the most common foot deformities seen in orthopaedic clinical practice. This pathology can cause a cascade of events affecting the foot as well as more proximal joints in the lower extremity. It has been linked to foot pain, impaired gait patterns, poor balance, and falls in older adults. It is more common in females, and the incidence increases with age.

A full understanding of foot anatomy, kinesiology and biomechanics is pivotal when treating this patient population. An array of factors can influence the foot and have the potential to compound the deformity. Deficits in talocrural dorsiflexion, increased pronation of the foot, and narrow shoe wear are all factors to consider. Although less common in adolescents, it can be a cause of impairment related to structural defects that predispose to the condition.

An altered plantar pressure pattern is typically seen in bunion patients, with decreased loading of the hallux and increased loading under the second and third metatarsal heads. With surgical intervention and physical therapy, these plantar pressures can be restored close to normal values, and symptoms can be eliminated. Given the multifactorial nature of this problem, it is important for the therapist to assess and address these concerns in the postoperative patient.

In general, bunion operations, of which there are quite literally over a hundred variations, all essentially consist of either cutting bones (metatarsal, phalangeal osteotomies) or fusing joints (tarsometatarsal [TMT], metatarsophalangeal [MTP]) to straighten out the first ray.

Depending on what type of operation is performed, the postoperative protocol can vary significantly. In general, metatarsal osteotomies and phalangeal osteotomies require less time non–weight bearing (NWB) than fusion operations. For the purposes of this chapter, we will talk about one specific type of metatarsal osteotomy, the scarf osteotomy, for which postoperative rehabilitation can be generalized for all metatarsal osteotomies. In addition, we will review one specific type of fusion operation, the Lapidus procedure, or first TMT fusion. Both procedures are typically accompanied by a lateral release and a medial plication of the MTP joint. The lateral release, often called a modified McBride procedure, consists of the release of the tight lateral structures (the adductor hallucis tendon, lateral joint capsule, and transverse metatarsal ligament). This lateral release and medial plication allows for appropriate realignment of the proximal phalanx on the metatarsal head. It is important to note that although rehabilitation protocols are often generalized, there should be an open communication with the surgeon and therapist to customize each individual's progressions based on age, comorbidities, surgical procedure, tissue quality, expectation, and physical fitness levels. We will not review rehabilitation after MTP fusion, which has a more limited role in bunion treatment.

In general, metatarsal osteotomies are done for less severe deformity, whereas first TMT fusions are done for severe deformity that may include looseness at the metatarsal-cuneiform joint. While the debate over which operation is more appropriate for different types of bunions has existed for many years and has been contentious at times, most would not argue that a Lapidus provides the greatest capacity to correct deformity and keeps the bones straight, whereas a metatarsal osteotomy makes the bone crooked to make it appear straight. However, metatarsal osteotomies typically heal more readily than a first TMT fusion; thus, they usually require NWB for about half the time or less than a Lapidus would, which is not an insignificant consideration.

From a rehabilitation perspective, concerns include regaining full motion at the metatarsophalangeal joint, gait retraining, and

Dr. Vosseller or an immediate family member serves as a paid consultant to DJ Orthopaedics; and serves as a board member, owner, officer, or committee member of the American Academy of Orthopaedic Surgeons, the American Orthopaedic Association, and the American Orthopaedic Foot and Ankle Society. Neither Dr. Ciccone nor any immediate family member has received anything of value from or has stock or stock options held in a commercial company or institution related directly or indirectly to the subject of this article.

© 2018 American Academy of Orthopaedic Surgeons

regaining/maintaining full strength. Most of these concerns are frankly secondary to the healing of the osteotomy/fusion. Motion can typically be regained once healing of the bones is assured.

SURGICAL PROCEDURES

General Overview

The principle indication for bunion surgery is pain associated with the bunion deformity. Many surgeons will hesitate to operate on anyone who does not have pain. Interestingly, the deformity and pain do not necessarily correspond in a linear fashion, meaning that sometimes people with severe deformity have little or no pain, while people with mild deformity have significant pain. It is not always logical in this sense. Once again, generally speaking, a scarf osteotomy is performed for mild and moderate-to-severe deformity, while a Lapidus procedure is for moderate-to-severe deformity.

Scarf Osteotomy

Indications

Indications for a scarf osteotomy are pain, as well as mild and moderate-to-severe deformity.

Contraindications

Contraindications to a scarf osteotomy are uncontrolled diabetes mellitus, open wounds, active infection, and anything that stands as a contraindication for an elective procedure.

Procedure

The patient typically has some form of regional anesthesia prior to the procedure. The patient is placed supine on the operating room table. The modified McBride is performed first: through an incision is made in the first web space and carried down to the lateral aspect of the MTP joint. The adductor and transverse metatarsal ligament are incised sharply off the sesamoid, with the adductor often incised off the phalanx as well.

Attention is then turned to the medial aspect of the MTP joint. A longitudinal incision is made medially, exposing the medial joint capsule, which is incised longitudinally in line with the skin incision. The median eminence is then resected in line with the metatarsal shaft. The scarf osteotomy is performed; care is taken to cut in a dorsomedial to plantarlateral direction to relatively plantarflex, or at least not dorsiflex, the metatarsal head. Once the cuts have been completed, the osteotomy is rotated and translated to correct the deformity. If the deformity correction is sufficient, then it is fixed with a minimum of two partially threaded screws. The medial capsular closure is then performed, taking care to pull the sesamoids medially and try to pull the phalanx and toe out of valgus. Often, this can be accomplished simply by the capsular closure. If it cannot be accomplished by the capsular closure, then an Akin osteotomy of the phalanx can be added to straighten the toe. The skin is then closed in layers, and a bunion dressing is applied, with the patient placed into a postoperative shoe. The wrap is applied so that it pulls the toe out of valgus.

The patient is often made NWB for a period of 2 weeks, after which the patient is allowed foot flat weight bearing in a postoperative shoe, although some surgeons allow earlier weight bearing. At the 4-week mark, the patient is allowed to weight bear as tolerated in the postoperative shoe, and the patient comes out of the postoperative shoe once swelling allows wearing a regular shoe. Swelling after bunion surgery can take some time to completely recede, with some degree of swelling often present for up to 6 months, sometimes longer. In general, patients are walking normally by 2 months out from surgery and can begin to return to sports at 3 months out from surgery.

Complications

The complications of this procedure include undercorrection, overcorrection (hallux varus), recurrence, nonunion, malunion, and loss of MTP range of motion (ROM). A circumspect surgeon should be able to avoid undercorrection, as the surgeon should not leave the operating room until sure that the deformity is adequately corrected. This adequacy is assessed in a few ways, but most notably by the position of the sesamoids under the first metatarsal head. Recurrence certainly does occur, although the rate at which it happens is not well defined, nor is its temporal occurrence clear; that is, the rate of recurrence presumably increases with time from correction, although long-term data related to this question is lacking. Nonunion is uncommon. Malunion can occur if the osteotomy shifts, although adequate fixation can largely obviate this risk. Metatarsophalangeal motion can be lost with this operation, although it can often be regained with aggressive joint mobilization once the osteotomy is healed.

Lapidus Procedure

Indications

Indications for a Lapidus procedure are pain, as well as moderate-to-severe bunion deformity.

Contraindications

Contraindications to a Lapidus procedure are uncontrolled diabetes mellitus, open wounds, active infection, and medical contraindications for elective surgery.

Procedure

The first half of the procedure proceeds much as with the scarf osteotomy in terms of anesthesia and positioning. The modified McBride is performed as described under the previous section "scarf osteotomy". The medial incision is then made, and the median eminence resected. Once that is done, attention is turned to the dorsal foot overlying the first TMT joint. An incision is made in this area and carried down to the extensor hallucis longus tendon (EHL), which is then retracted. Once directly over the TMT joint, the capsule and periosteum over the first metatarsal and medial cuneiform are incised sharply and confluently to expose the joint. The joint is then denuded of cartilage, and a saw is used to remove a minimal amount of bone in a superiorly based wedge (inferior closing wedge) so that the ray is relatively plantarflexed. A pointed reduction

© 2018 American Academy of Orthopaedic Surgeons

clamp can be placed distally between the first and second metatarsals to reduce the intermetatarsal angle and hold the first ray in position. It is stabilized with two 3.5- or 4.0-mm lag screws placed across the joint. Alternatively, a lag screw with a neutralization plate can be used or any of a multitude of proprietary plates that allow for a lag screw through the plate. If placing lag screws outside of a plate, a small area must often be burred out for the screw head, which helps to gain extra compression and avoids prominence of the screw head. Burr holes are often placed at the fusion sites and filled with calcaneal autograft, which can be obtained through a small incision on the lateral heel. Closure then proceeds as with the scarf osteotomy. After a Lapidus, a patient is NWB for 2 weeks in a splint. At 2 weeks, the splint and sutures are removed, and the patient is placed into a boot to remain NWB out to 6 weeks from surgery. Physical therapy usually starts once the patient has begun bearing full weight in the boot at 6 weeks. Patients wean out of the boot typically between 9 and 12 weeks out from surgery. Maximal recovery is between 3 and 6 months, with most patients walking normally at 3 to 4 months out from surgery and returning to sport between 4 to 6 months out from surgery.

Complications

Many of the same complications can occur after a Lapidus procedure; thus, the earlier discussion is germane. However, the risk of nonunion is greater than that from metatarsal osteotomy. MTP stiffness can be a concern as well, although near full ROM can typically be attained.

REHABILITATION

In general, there is one consideration that is present for any bunion operation: swelling. Swelling is often an issue in any foot surgery, and can take a frustratingly long time to dissipate even in young, healthy people. Perhaps one of the biggest advantages of utilizing physical therapy after bunion surgery is in trying to mitigate this ubiquitous issue. The surgeon and therapist must educate the patient regarding swelling control. The therapist can then work to address the swelling with elevation and compression, and can also perform manual lymph drainage to help encourage fluid out of this area. Although this is surgery of the foot, it is important to also pay attention to the leg and hip. Addressing strength, mobility, soft-tissue extensibility and balance are essential in a patient's recovery. This approach addresses deficits that the patient might have been dealing with prior to surgery and facilitates the return to desired activities.

Scarf Osteotomy

Rehabilitation following a metatarsal osteotomy typically begins about 3 to 4 weeks following surgery. During that time, the patient has been in a postoperative shoe that decreases the amount of stress in the forefoot. This type of surgery requires less overall physical therapy sessions than a fusion due to the fact that the patient started weight bearing 2 weeks after surgery. As a result, deconditioning of the lower leg is significantly less.

Close attention should be paid to the amount of hallux dorsiflexion present, as a deficit will alter how the patient can ambulate, especially when returning to normal shoe wear. The therapist should be aware of the amount of weight bearing through the first metatarsal during midstance and terminal stance. It is during these two phases when active push-off by the first ray plantarflexors occurs. The first ray should be the most heavily loaded structure during gait. Restoring this through gait training is essential and has been proven to be effective in postoperative treatment.

The first ray contacts the ground, allowing for push-off as the rearfoot starts to supinate. Strengthening the peroneus longus is crucial to allow proper foot mechanics to occur so that inappropriate compensation, such as overpronation and stressing the hallux into an abducted position, is minimized. Exercises such as sways and step-throughs can help strengthen and restore correct contact pressure to avoid pathologic gait patterns (Figures 53.1 and 53.2).

A multimodal rehabilitation program is implemented to restore normal kinematics in the foot, especially the first ray's ability to dorsiflex. In addition, the talocrural joint must have sufficient mobility to allow the tibia to travel over the foot during normal gait. Manual techniques consisting of mobilization and oscillations to restore talocrural and hallux mobility are paramount to a successful recovery.

Manual techniques performed during the recovery process should include mobilization of the first MTP joint and dorsiflexion of MTP joints 2 to 5. Additionally, the other joints in the foot should be restored with mobilization to encourage acceptable movement patterns. Scar mobilization and soft-tissue releases of the foot intrinsics are performed to avoid pathologic tissue interconnection. This mobilization allows increased blood flow to the area and decreases the amount of soft-tissue tension.

Strengthening is implemented after the initial session to focus on the foot intrinsics, as well as peroneus longus. The intrinsics help the foot support itself, and the peroneus longus depresses the first ray into the ground for push-off. Balance exercises in single-limb stance can also help with proprioception and strengthening of the foot and ankle, which is needed to have a support system from which push-off can occur (Figure 53.3). Depending on how the patient is progressing, any part of gait, mobility, strengthening, or proprioception training can be repeated or advanced as per therapist discretion.

Lapidus Procedure

A patient following a fusion will have been NWB for 6 weeks. This inactivity typically results in hypomobility in the neighboring joints in the foot as well as weakness and deconditioning of the musculature in the leg and foot. Overall lower extremity strength, balance, joint mobility, and soft-tissue restrictions must be evaluated so that a baseline can be created to restore symmetry.

The therapist typically sees a patient once the surgeon allows the patient to bear weight. The therapist must factor in the patient's overall health as well as postoperative status. Close attention is placed on ROM, as well as strength and balance of

© 2018 American Academy of Orthopaedic Surgeons

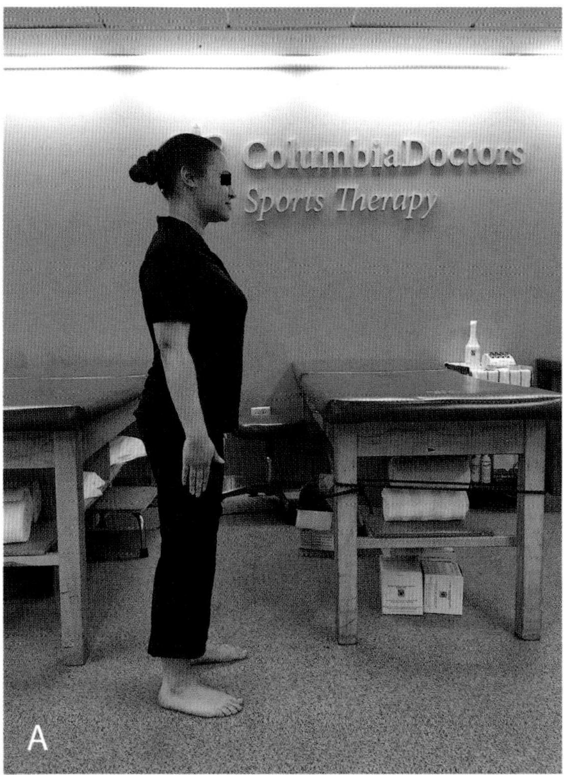

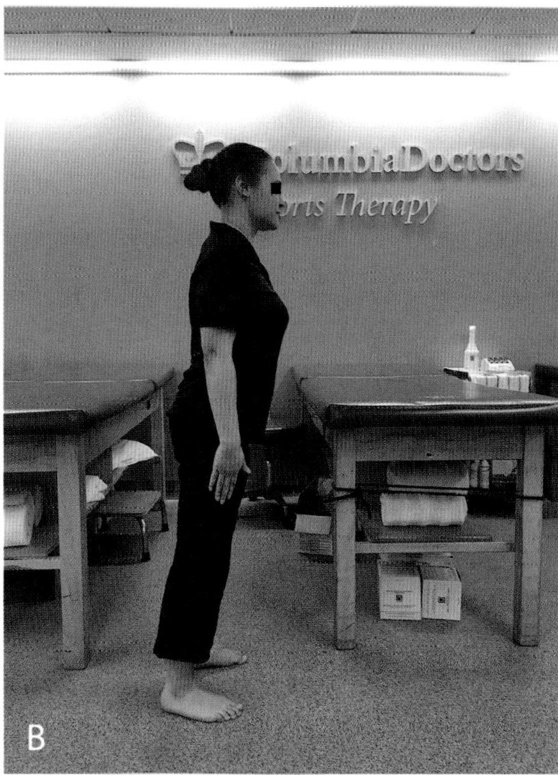

Figure 53.1 **A**, **B**, Photographs of sways: The patient stands with feet shoulder width apart and shifts weight forward as far as possible just prior to the point of the heel coming up, then returns to the start position. The patient engages foot intrinsic muscles and the peroneus longus. Advancement comes by having the patient hold the end position for longer periods of time.

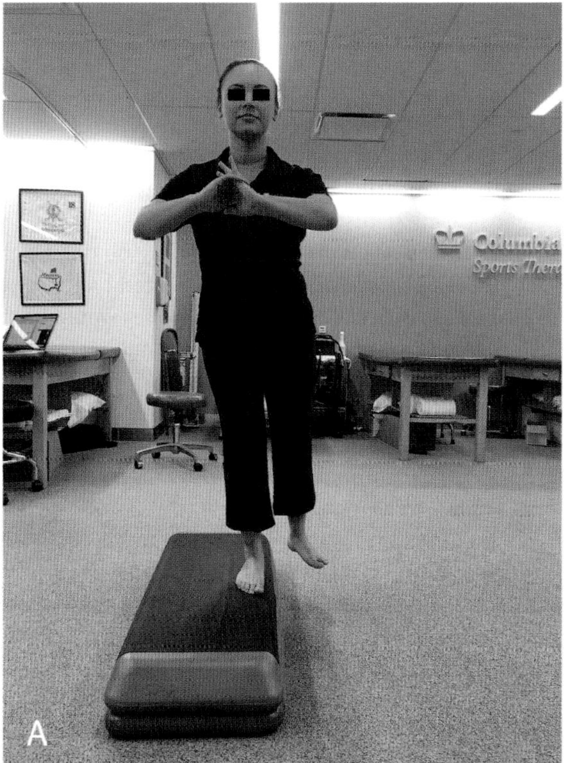

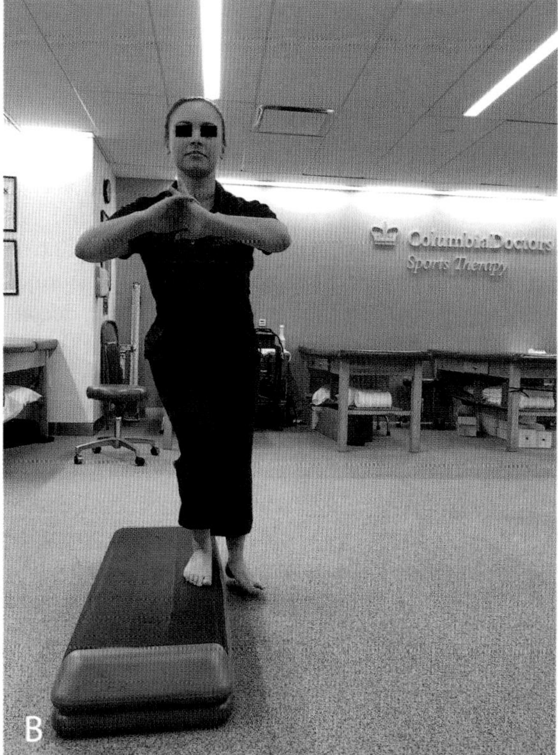

Figure 53.2 **A**, **B**, Photographs of medial step-down: The patient stands off the edge of a step and lowers the body, maintaining level hips and knee aligned over the foot until the nonworking leg taps the ground, at which point the patient returns to the starting position. Advancement comes by having the patient stand on an unstable surface.

© 2018 American Academy of Orthopaedic Surgeons

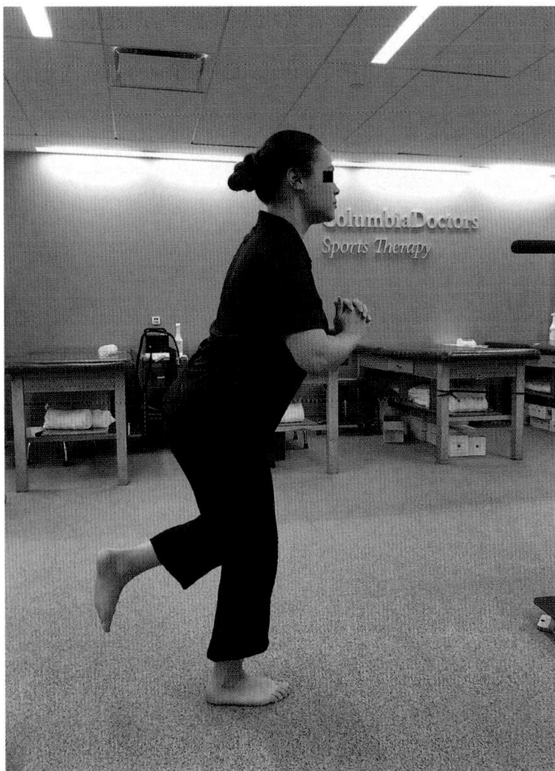

Figure 53.3 Photograph of single-limb stance. The patient stands on one leg, maintaining balance to engage foot and ankle stabilizers as well as hip musculature. Advancement comes by having the patient perform dynamic movements with the upper body and maintaining balance.

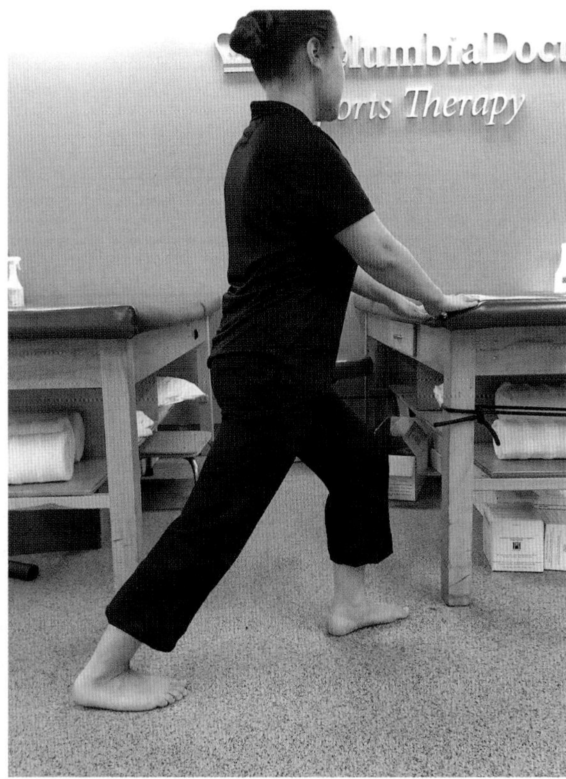

Figure 53.4 Photograph of gastrocnemius stretch: The patient places the involved foot back with toes pointed directly forward and heel on the ground. The back knee must remain straight. With the front leg, the patient leans forward until a moderate stretch is felt. Maintain for 30 seconds to 1 minute.

the foot, knee, and even the hip. In addition, the quality of the scar mobility is assessed and manually addressed to minimize restriction.

Initially, the goal is to achieve appropriate weight acceptance in the foot to allow the patient to restore normal gait patterns. To accomplish this goal, the neuromuscular control, balance, mobility, and ROM is addressed to allow smooth transition into a normalized gait. As discussed earlier, deconditioning is often a big issue. The foot and the rest of the leg need to be conditioned but not overloaded to allow the lower extremity to accommodate the stresses of walking.

Physical therapy will start with first allowing the patient to get comfortable placing weight through the surgical leg. Weight acceptance, gait training, and mobility are addressed on the first few visits of therapy to coincide with general strengthening and conditioning of the lower extremity. In addition to light weight-bearing activities, patients can also perform light nonimpact activities such as a stationary bicycle to improve circulation and endurance, and to enhance quality of motion after being immobilized.

It is important to get the patient performing exercises that will lead into normal movement patterns. Starting with frontal and sagittal sways and progressing to marches and step-throughs is a successful way to start training an individual for normalized gait patterns. ROM exercises—such as gastrocnemius/soleus stretching (Figures 53.4 and 53.5), ankle pumps, ankle alphabets, and balance board (Figure 53.6)—certainly improve the mobility throughout the foot and ankle. Hip musculature exercises are also incorporated, and can be advanced depending on weight-bearing status and strength level.

Once the patient can tolerate standing on one leg, bilateral strengthening—such as squats and bilateral leg presses—can be progressed to unilateral. These exercises would be activities such as step-ups, anterior step-downs, standing hip abduction, and balance exercises to incorporate the whole leg and challenge the neuromuscular and proprioceptive systems. Isolated ankle strengthening, including standing dorsiflexion and plantarflexion, are incorporated when patients' pain levels allow for these specific movements.

As a patient starts progressing to higher-level activities, it is important to discuss what activities the patient typically participates in to cater the exercises toward these movements. This higher-level training can begin once strength is 80% of the uninvolved side.

Exercise Description

- *Sways (Frontal Plane):* The patient starts in the standing position with weight mostly on the uninvolved side. The patient then slowly shifts weight onto surgical side. Once more comfortable with this, the patient can increase the

 © 2018 American Academy of Orthopaedic Surgeons

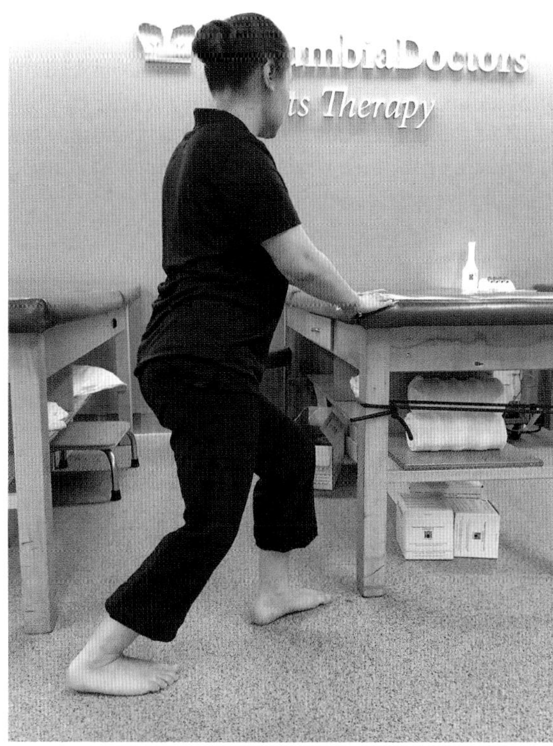

Figure 53.5 Soleus stretch: The patient places the involved foot back, with toes pointed directly forward and heel on the ground. The back leg must be bent. With the front leg, the patient leans forward until a moderate stretch is felt. Maintain for 30 seconds to 1 minute.

amount of weight being accepted onto the surgical side until almost all of it is accommodated.

- *Sways (Sagittal Plane):* The patient starts in the standing position with weight even between both feet. The patient sways forward, with the pivot point being talocrural just prior to the heels coming off the ground, then pushes back with the feet to neutral position.
- *Marches:* The patient stands and alternates picking up one leg into the air. The patient initially starts with using a stable point to hold onto and gradually works into not needing any assistance. In addition, the amount of time the patient spends on the surgical side is gradually increased.
- *Step-throughs:* The patient starts with the nonsurgical leg behind the surgical leg. Then, have the patient step forward with the nonsurgical leg in a normal step length and accept the weight through that leg. Then, have the patient take that same leg and step backward, back to the starting position. This allows the pivot point foot to get conditioned for movement in a normal gait pattern. This process is then mirrored, performing the same exercise, but now the other leg is the pivot point.
- *Single Leg Stance:* The patient stands on the involved side using a stable surface for assistance and progresses to not needing any assistance.
- *Overexaggerated Gait:* Set up cones in a straight line 1.5 feet apart. Have the patient lift the leg in a marching position and step forward, striking with the heel and locking the

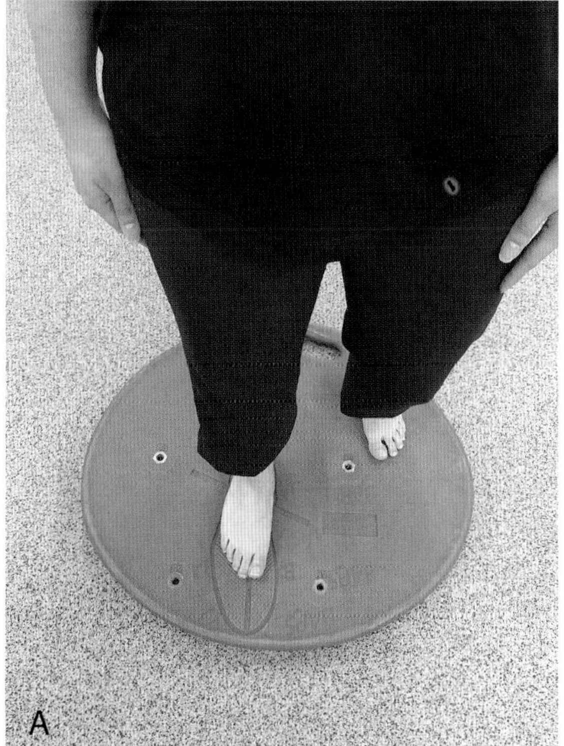

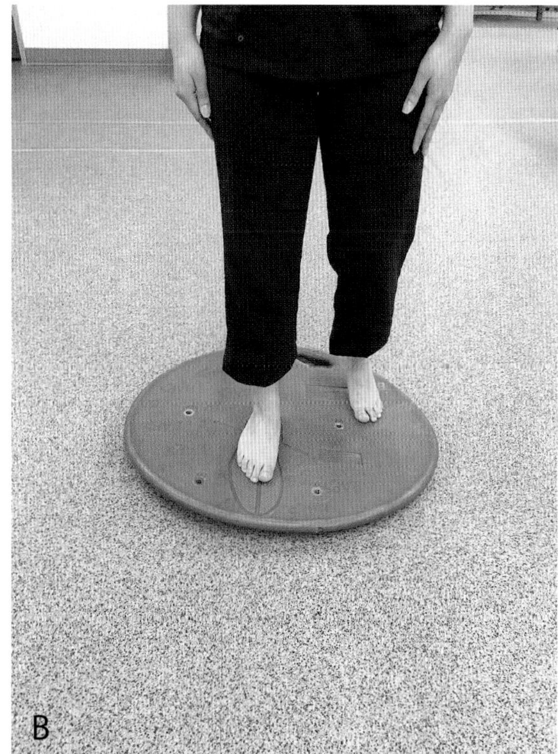

Figure 53.6 **A**, **B**, Photographs of balance board: The patient stands on BAPS board with involved foot and rolls board on its edge in clockwise and counterclockwise movements to engage foot intrinsic and ankle musculature.

© 2018 American Academy of Orthopaedic Surgeons

knee (contracting quadriceps), and then step through with the other leg, performing the same sequence.

Evidence Review

The literature for physical therapy following bunion operations is currently limited. Schuh et al. looked at rehabilitation following osteotomy surgery, specifically assessing plantar pressure parameters. After a 4-week course of physical therapy and gait training, there was improved weight bearing of the first ray and great toe following treatment. In addition, the same group found improved loading of the hallux following a multimodal course of physical therapy after osteotomy. They concluded that Chevron osteotomy alone did not restore physiologic forefoot loading, but if combined with physical therapy, may lead to restoration of proper foot loading.

PEARLS

- 65° of hallux dorsiflexion is necessary for level walking.
- 80° of hallux dorsiflexion is necessary for stair climbing.
    - 10° of talocrural joint dorsiflexion is necessary for gait evaluate with knee flexed and extended to dinstiguish achilles vs gastrocnemius tightness.

BIBLIOGRAPHY

Schuh R, Hofstaetter SG, Adams SB Jr, Pichler F, Kristen KH, and Trnka HJ. Rehabilitation after hallux valgus surgery: importance of physical therapy to restore weight-bearing of the first ray during the stance phase. *Phys Ther* 2009 Sep; 89(9):934–945.

© 2018 American Academy of Orthopaedic Surgeons

54 Flatfoot Surgery

Margaret J. Lobo, MD, and Samantha Francucci, PT, DPT

INTRODUCTION

The degenerative breakdown of the medial longitudinal arch is commonly referred to as adult acquired flatfoot and is a separate entity from a congenital arch deformity. It is a common biomechanical problem with a complex etiology. The medial longitudinal arch is comprised of both static and dynamic stabilizers. The bony longitudinal arch and the supporting ligaments—the spring and deltoid ligaments—are the static components, while the posterior tibial tendon, flexor digitorum longus, flexor hallucis longus, and the gastrocnemius/soleus complex are the main dynamic arch stabilizers. A breakdown of the medial longitudinal arch occurs when the dynamic stabilizers of the arch weaken, placing increased stresses and ultimately failure of the ligaments that support the bony arch (Table 54.1). The characteristic acquired flatfoot deformity consists of hindfoot valgus, subtalar eversion and forefoot abduction as the foot rotates dorsally and laterally relative to the talus (Figure 54.1).

Although some cases of acquired flatfoot may be managed with orthotics and shoe modifications, surgery is indicated in cases of pain, progressive deformity, and difficulty with ambulation. The goals of the surgical procedure are to preserve the mechanics of the foot, providing push off while walking. Flatfoot surgery usually includes osseus and soft-tissue procedures to correct the static and dynamic imbalances. The common soft-tissue procedures done for flatfoot reconstruction include a gastrocnemius recession (lengthening) and a flexor digitorum longus transfer (to augment the posterior tibial tendon). The bone procedures may include a medial slide calcaneal osteotomy, an anterior lengthening calcaneal osteotomy, and fusions or osteotomies of medial column joints, such as a first metatarsal medial cuneiform fusion (the Lapidus procedure) and the navicular cuneiform fusion. When the talonavicular joint, subtalar joint, and calcaneocuboid joint have significant degeneration, a triple arthrodesis is performed. A rigid adult acquired flatfoot deformity is also best treated with a deformity correcting hindfoot fusion (see Chapter 55). A preoperative assessment, including clinical examination and radiographs, is used to determine the combination of procedures required to correct the flatfoot deformity, particularly assessing the stiffness and degree of the deformity.

Postoperative rehabilitation is a critical component in the recovery of these patients. The flatfoot deformity occurs slowly over several years and results in weakening of the foot intrinsic musculature as well as contractures and imbalance of the calf. The deformity and altered gait pattern associated with flatfoot affects the knee, hip, and back. All of these areas need rehabilitation postoperatively.

Surgical Indications

- Dysfunction of the posterior tibial tendon
- Progressive planovalgus deformity
- Pain refractory to orthotics and shoe modifications

Contraindications

- Limited ambulator
- Neuropathy or peripheral vascular disease posing high risk for wound healing problems and infection
- Medical conditions precluding safe surgery

SURGICAL PROCEDURES

Flexor Tendon Transfer

In the flatfoot deformity, the posterior tibial tendon (PTT) is compromised. The PTT may have significant tendinopathy, an interstitial tear, or be completely ruptured at the time of surgery. The flexor digitorum longus (FDL) tendon is used to either augment or replace the injured PTT. The FDL is transferred to the medial aspect of the navicular, the primary insertion site for the posterior tibial tendon. This muscle is directly posterior to the PTT and acts at the same phase of the gait cycle, making it a good candidate for transfer (Figure 54.2). The FDL tendon may be transferred to the navicular bone without significant loss of lesser toe flexion.

This procedure is performed through a longitudinal skin incision along the PTT from the tip of the medial malleolus to

Neither of the following authors nor any immediate family member has received anything of value from or has stock or stock options held in a commercial company or institution related directly or indirectly to the subject of this article: Dr. Francucci and Dr. Lobo.

© 2018 American Academy of Orthopaedic Surgeons

Table 54.1 FLATFOOT DEFORMITY INSTIGATING FACTORS

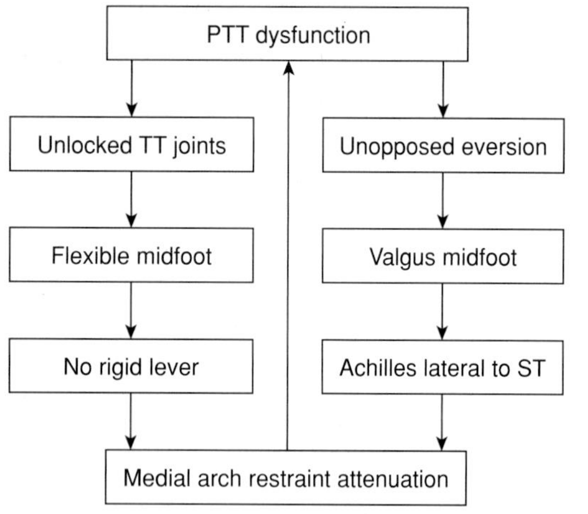

PTT = posterior tibial tendon, ST = subtalar joint, TT = transverse tarsal joints.

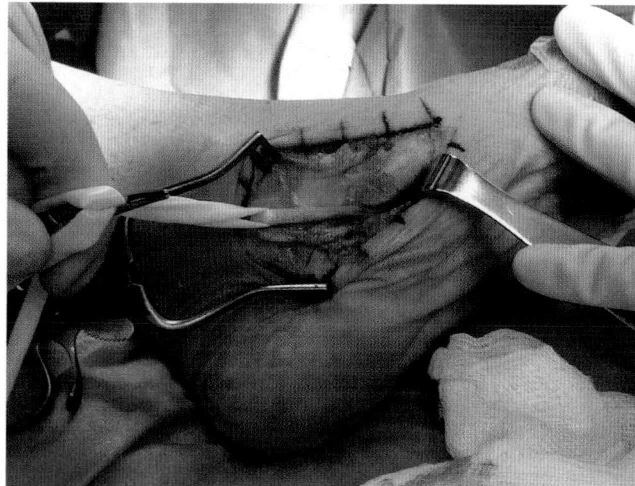

Figure 54.2 Clinical photograph demonstrating flexor digitorum longus tendon just posterior to the posterior tibial tendon. The posterior tibial tendon has been removed and the remaining 1 cm of the tendon is visualized at the navicular.

the navicular cuneiform joint. The sheath is opened and the PTT is exposed and assessed. A section of the PTT is resected 1 cm proximal to the navicular insertion and at the level of the medial malleolus. The FDL tendon is located by making a small incision in the posterior aspect of the PTT sheath. It is sharply dissected to the level of the knot of Henry, then sectioned at this level. A bone tunnel is made from the plantar to dorsal aspect of the medial navicular for passage of the FDL tendon. Once the other bone and soft-tissue procedures are completed, the FDL tendon is sutured to the remaining PTT and itself. The tendon is tensioned with the ankle in dorsiflexion and slight inversion when securing the tendon transfer. Approximately

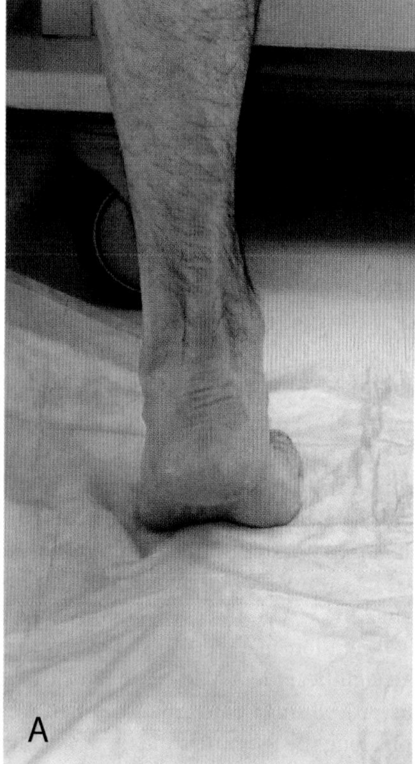

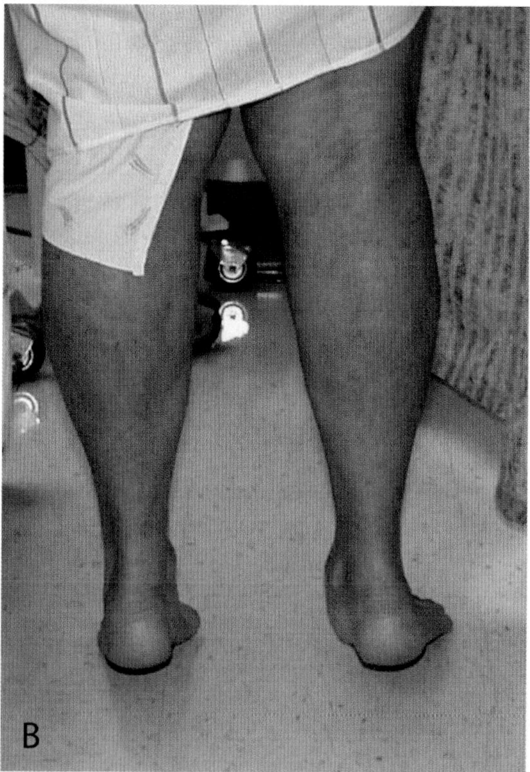

Figure 54.1 Photographs of a single-limb heel rise demonstrating normal heel height and inversion (**A**) in comparison to hindfoot valgus with double-limb heel rise (**B**). Note that the Achilles and calcaneal tuberosity are lateral to the midline in the flatfoot deformity.

© 2018 American Academy of Orthopaedic Surgeons

8 to 12 weeks is required for the tendon to become strongly incorporated into the bony tunnel. Thus, passive range of motion (PROM) and active strengthening exercises should be limited and gentle until weeks 8 to 10.

Gastrocnemius Recession

The gastrocnemius muscle originates on the distal femur and joins the soleus muscle in the lower leg coalescing to the Achilles tendon, which inserts on the calcaneal tuberosity. With a contracture of the Achilles tendon, or isolated to the gastrocnemius muscle, a plantigrade heel can only be achieved with abduction through the transverse tarsal joints. Consequently, a valgus hindfoot results. This contracture can be the primary cause of the adult acquired flatfoot deformity or a secondary cause occurring after the arch collapse. An integral part of flatfoot reconstruction is releasing the contracture of the gastrocnemius muscle. An isolated contracture of the gastrocnemius can be determined by the Silfverskiöld test, which tests passive ankle dorsiflexion with the knee extended and then flexed. Insufficient dorsiflexion with the knee extended, and increased ankle dorsiflexion with the knee bent confirms a gastrocnemius contracture.

The gastrocnemius recession can be done via a posterior or medial approach, but is typically approached medially in combination with flatfoot reconstruction. An incision is made at the musculotendinous junction of the gastrocnemius and soleus, approximately two fingerbreadths posterior to the tibia. Blunt dissection is then performed to locate the superficial posterior fascia. Care must be taken to identify and protect the saphenous nerve and vein. The gastrocnemius muscle is then bluntly separated from the fascia posteriorly and the soleus muscle anteriorly. The foot is brought into dorsiflexion and the tendinous portion of the gastrocnemius tendon is cut sharply. The gastrocnemius lengthens until the soleus is tense (the soleus is still intact); thus, overlengthening is usually not possible. The incision is then closed in layers, including the fascia, subcutaneous tissue, and skin.

During the rehabilitation process, it is important to maintain gastrocnemius flexibility. Emphasis should be placed on maintaining the foot in a dorsiflexed position while immobilized and daily stretching of the gastrocnemius/soleus complex once out of a cast. Strengthening of the gastrocnemius will be important after the third month.

Posterior Calcaneal Osteotomy (Medial Slide)

The flatfoot deformity includes hindfoot valgus, a condition in which the heel tuber is lateral to the midline. The medial calcaneal slide (Figure 54.3) repositions the heel to be centered under the midline axis. This allows the Achilles vector to pull the hindfoot in varus in the toe-off phase of gait and thereby assists in locking the transverse tarsal joints.

The procedure is performed via a lateral approach. An oblique incision is made from the superior to the inferior calcaneal recess. Once the skin is incised, blunt dissection is used to reach the periosteum. An osteotomy in line with the skin incision is made anterior to the Achilles tendon and exiting

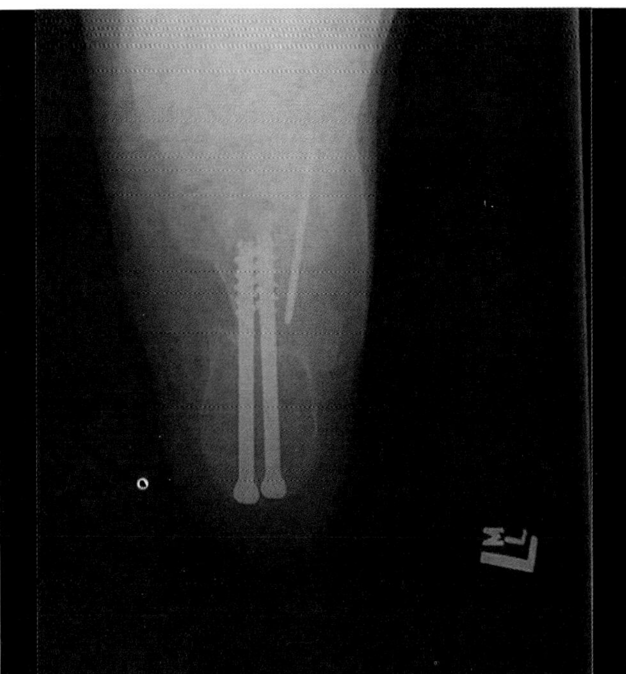

Figure 54.3 A tangential radiograph of the calcaneus demonstrating a medial slide osteotomy.

in the inferior recess of the calcaneus. The plantar calcaneal tuberosity is then translated medially up to 1 cm. It is secured by large screws placed percutaneously from the point of the heel. Bone healing occurs rapidly in this osteotomy, but occasionally pain may be experienced from the screw heads during the initial transition to full weight bearing (FWB).

Anterior Calcaneal Osteotomy (Lateral Column Lengthening)

A "lateral column lengthening" (Figure 54.4) is performed to bring the forefoot back medially around the talus, correcting forefoot abduction, hindfoot valgus, and medial arch sag. By extending the length of the calcaneus at the location of the talonavicular joint, the talonavicular joint can be rotated from an abducted to neutral alignment. There are minor variations to this procedure.

The Evans osteotomy (common variety of lateral column lengthening) is a transverse osteotomy made in line with the calcaneocuboid joint. A longitudinal skin incision is made along the anterior aspect of the calcaneus from the sinus tarsi to the calcaneocuboid joint. The periosteum and tendon is then elevated off the calcaneocuboid joint and the calcaneus. The osteotomy is made parallel to the calcaneocuboid joint and approximately 1 cm proximal to the joint surface. An opening wedge is made ranging from 4 to 12 mm and filled with structural graft secured with either a plate or screws. Care must be taken to prevent superior migration of the distal portion of the osteotomy as well as to avoid overlengthening the lateral column, as this will lead to stiffness with eversion and pain. Closure is performed in layers of the fascia, subcutaneous tissue, and the skin.

© 2018 American Academy of Orthopaedic Surgeons

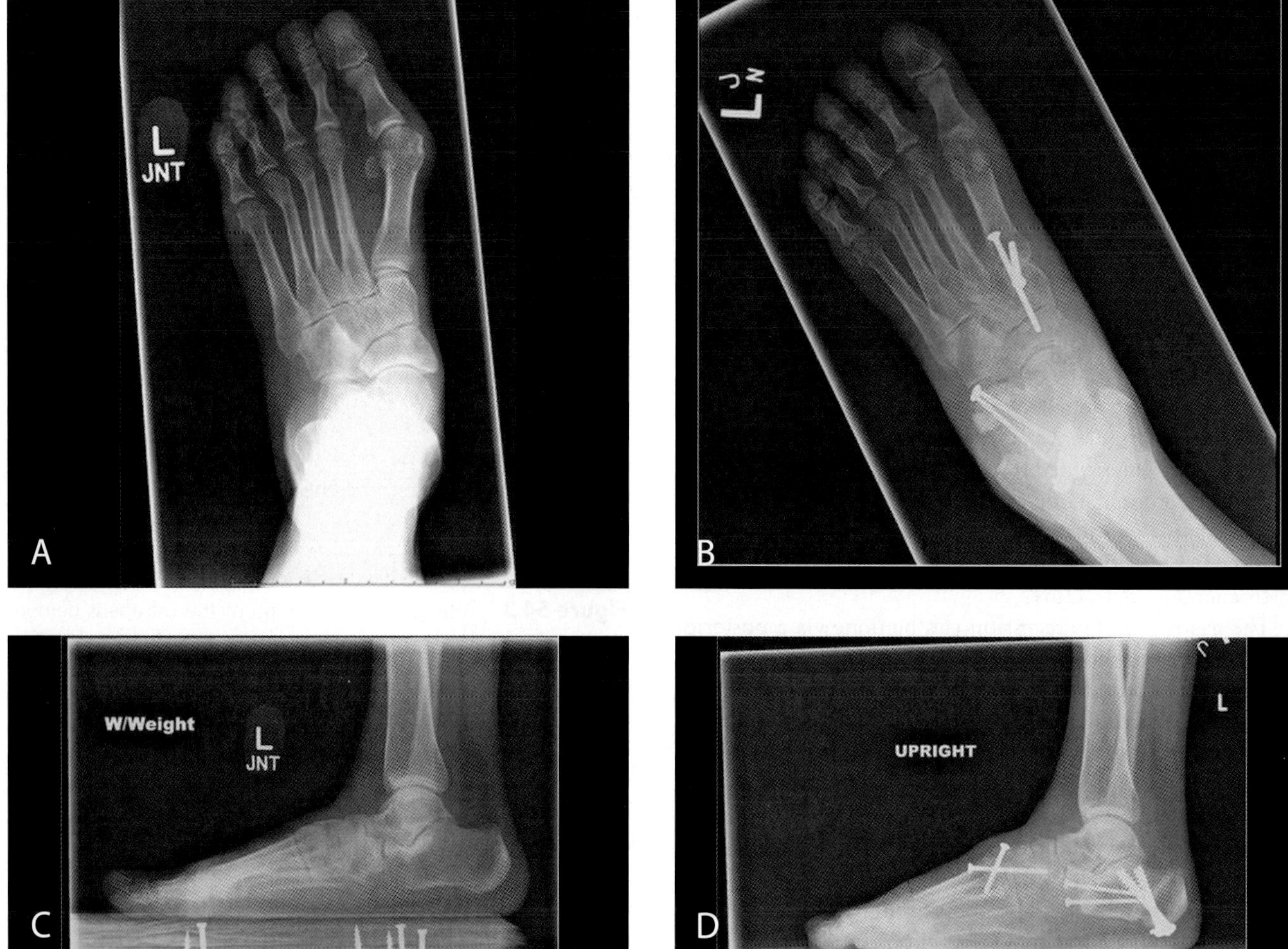

Figure 54.4 Anteroposterior and lateral radiographs demonstrating a lateral column lengthening, first tarsometatarsal fusion, and medial slide osteotomy and flexor digitorum longus transfer preoperatively and postoperatively. **A**, **C**, Preoperative planovalgus foot; note in **C** the plantar gapping demonstrating medial arch instability. **B**, **D**, Correction with medial and lateral bone and soft-tissue work.

This osteotomy is performed in close proximity to the calcaneocuboid joint. Stiffness in eversion may result; active range of motion (AROM) exercises allowing for inversion and eversion help decrease loss of eversion.

First Tarsometatarsal Fusion and Navicular Cuneiform Fusion

Fusions of the medial column may be required to address the flatfoot deformity. Sagging of the medial column is common for an acquired flatfoot. Instability of these joints will present as a hallux valgus deformity as well as plantar gapping of the first tarsometatarsal and/or navicular cuneiform joints. In this situation, fusion of the involved joints is required to stabilize the medial column to restore the medial longitudinal arch (see Figure 54.4).

Fusion of these joints requires an exposure of the joint by either a medial longitudinal approach or a dorsal approach centered on the involved joint. Once the soft tissue has been dissected and the joint is exposed, the cartilage is removed from both surfaces and prepared to create a healthy bleeding cancellous surface for fusion. The joint is reduced and secured with either a plate or screws. The soft tissues are then closed in a layered fashion.

Complications

Perioperative complications are primarily related to the incisions in the form of delayed wound healing, infection, and bleeding. Swelling also limits range of motion (ROM) in the postoperative period and needs to be aggressively managed with frequent, daily elevation. Stiffness in the forefoot, midfoot, and transverse tarsal joints is also common, and ROM must be practiced frequently. Other possible complications include nonunion, hardware failure, nerve damage, deep vein thrombosis, pulmonary embolism, persistent pain, and recurrent flatfoot deformity.

© 2018 American Academy of Orthopaedic Surgeons

POSTOPERATIVE REHABILITATION

Introduction

While a variety of surgical procedures are utilized to correct the flatfoot deformity, the recovery for these procedures is similar. The recovery is lengthy, requiring a period of immobilization prior to functional rehabilitation (Table 54.2). Immobilization is required for both bone healing and tendon-to-bone healing. While immobilization is required, it is important to recommend ROM and strengthening exercises for uninvolved joints (hip, knee, and especially toes) to prevent stiffness, minimize atrophy, and allow for a successful return to function.

Additionally, the deformity is insidious over years, creating adaptations that require correction during recovery. The leg may also show extensive deconditioning prior to surgery, worsened by months of rest after the procedure. As a result, rehabilitation is a long, grueling process.

Postoperative rehabilitation should focus on creating dynamic stability of the medial foot, ankle, and arch. Preoperative muscle and mechanical impairments must be

Table 54.2 THE SIX PHASES OF REHABILITATION, REHABILITATION GUIDELINES, AND GOALS

Phase of Rehabilitation	Rehabilitation Guidelines	Goals
Preoperative	Strengthen core and upper extremities Maintain flexible lower extremities NWB training with assistive device	Safe NWB gait Independence with ADLs while NWB
Perioperative (week 2)	NWB in splint Strict elevation "toes to nose" Hip and knee ROM Focus on proper NWB mechanics Selfmonitoring	Edema management Pain control Learn ADLs while maintaining safe NWB practices Ensure healing process
Immobilization Phase I (casting) First Month	NWB in cast Frequent elevation Hip and knee ROM and strength Pelvic and core strengthening Toe ROM Isometrics of calf musculature	Edema management Pain control Minimize atrophy Maintain forefoot ROM
Immobilization Phase II (CAM walker boot) Second Month	Progressive weight bearing in boot Gait training AROM to ankle, hindfoot, and forefoot Gentle gastrocnemius stretching Closed-chain exercises Double-limb proprioceptive exercises Scar mobilization Stationary bike in boot Core/upper and lower extremity strengthening Elevation	FWB with supportive shoe and no assistive device Normal gait Increase ROM Edema management
Functional Rehabilitation (Months 36)	Balance/proprioceptive training Maintain gastrocnemius/soleus flexibility Resistive ankle exercises AROM/PROM to extremity Joint mobilizations Strength training Elevation	Single-limb heel rise Reciprocal stair negotiation Edema management
Return to Daily Life (Months 6 plus)	Plyometrics/agility drills Elevation	Return to recreational activities Edema management

ADLs = activities of daily living, AROM = active range of motion, CAM = controlled ankle motion, NWB = non-weight bearing, PROM = passive range of motion, ROM = range of motion.

© 2018 American Academy of Orthopaedic Surgeons

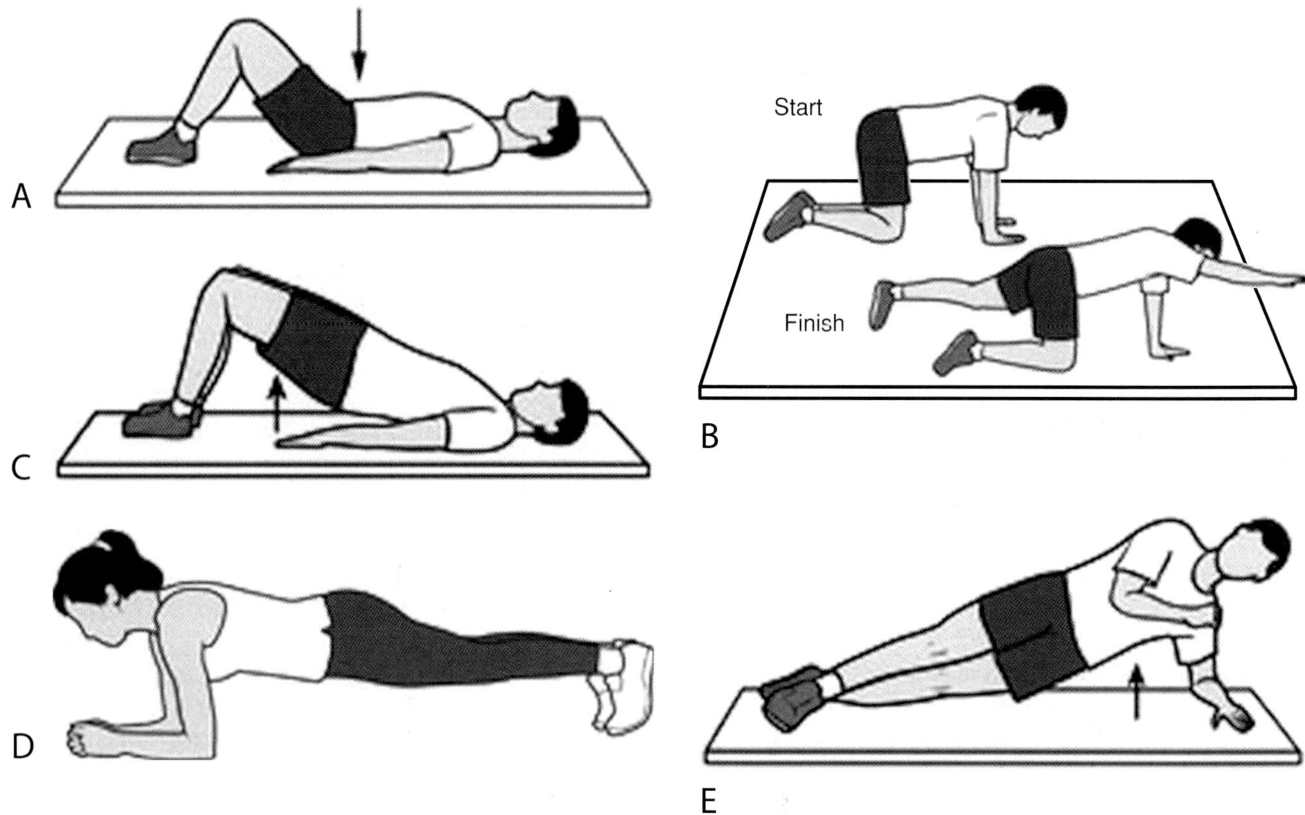

Figure 54.5 **A–E**, Illustrations of preoperative exercises focusing on pelvic and core strengthening. **A** and **B** can be performed postoperatively as long as the patient is able to maintain weight-bearing precautions.

addressed in order to support the surgical procedures and ensure a successful outcome.

Authors' Preferred Protocol

Preoperative Period

Strengthening of pelvic and core stabilizers, including the hip abductors, will be required as well as stretching of hip flexors, hamstrings, and the remainder of the posterior column. Patients should perform upper body exercises with focus on triceps strength to prepare for assistive device use.

Goals

Maximize strength and endurance of core stabilizers (Figure 54.5) as well as upper and lower extremities.

Perioperative Period

The patient is placed in a short-leg splint covering the posterior, medial, and lateral aspects of the lower leg. Care is taken to make sure that the ankle is in neutral dorsiflexion and occasionally slight inversion to take the tension off the tendon transfer. Most patients are admitted to the hospital overnight for strict elevation and physical therapy for instruction on non–weight bearing (NWB) of the affected extremity to ensure independence with transfers, mobility, and stair negotiation. The patient is discharged from the hospital by postoperative day one or two with orders of strict elevation (Figure 54.6). The importance of deep breathing for pulmonary health, frequent weight shifts to prevent skin breakdown, and keeping the foot elevated for 50 minutes of every hour is stressed. Elevation is the key to prevent restrictive swelling that increases the risk of wound complications, impairs joint mobilization, and causes pain. Continued hip and knee ROM exercises will also help with pain control. Patients should be taught how to self-monitor for sensation, color, and temperature changes.

Goals

Edema and pain management are the goals of this phase, as well as patient independence with self-monitoring techniques and maintaining NWB for optimal function in the household.

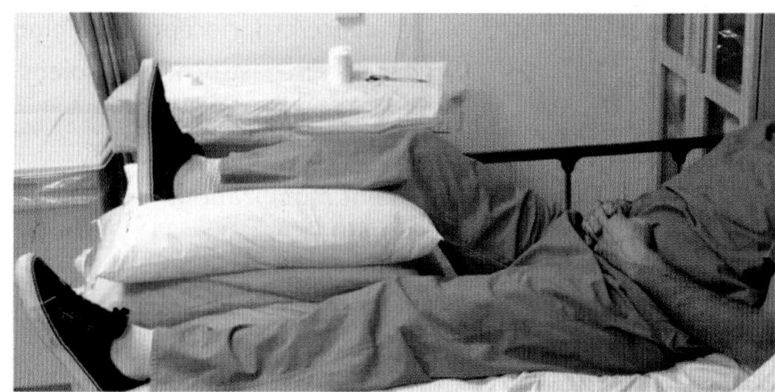

Figure 54.6 Photograph of proper elevation following reconstructive foot surgery.

© 2018 American Academy of Orthopaedic Surgeons

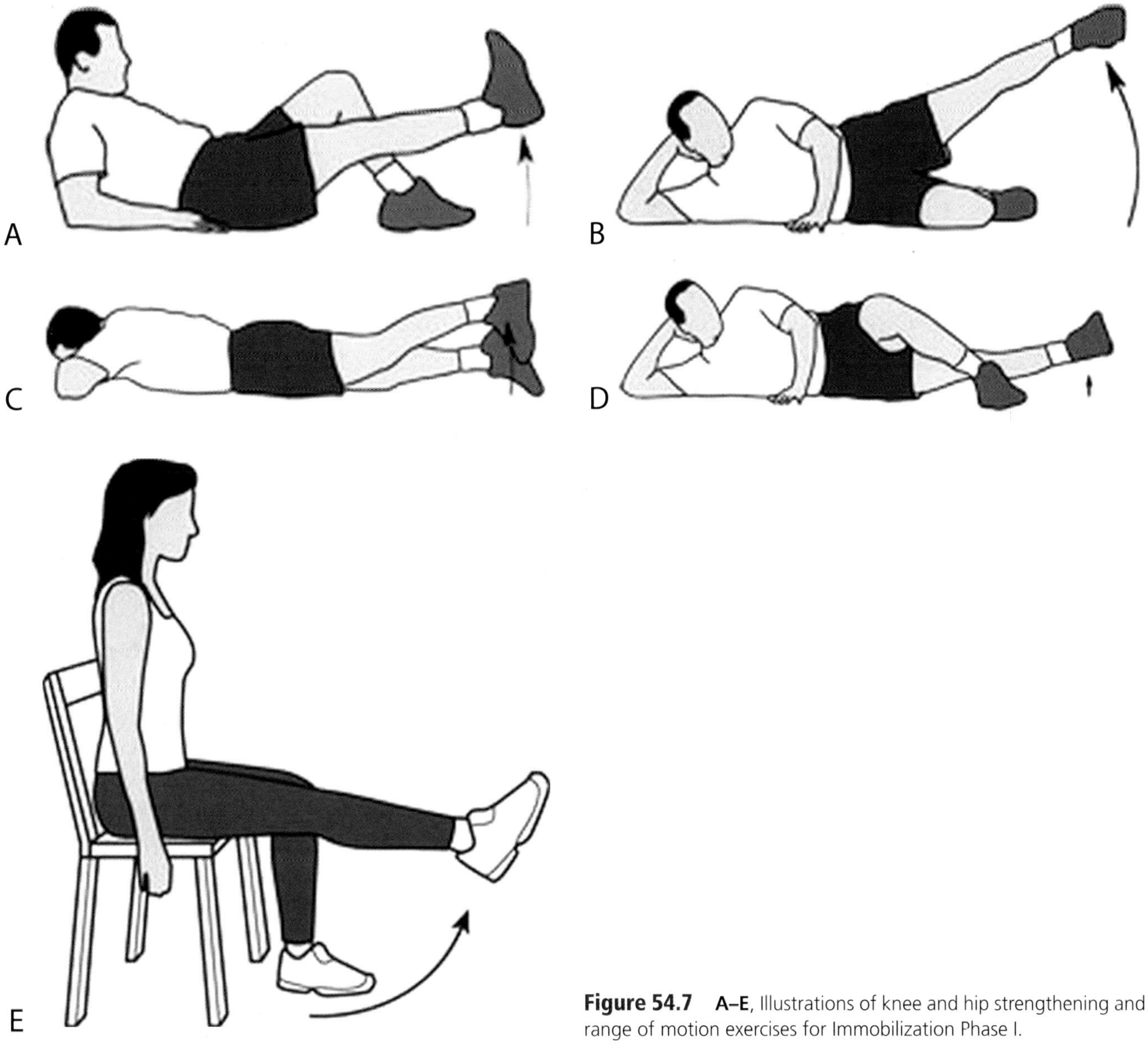

Figure 54.7 **A–E**, Illustrations of knee and hip strengthening and range of motion exercises for Immobilization Phase I.

Restrictions

No weight bearing during this phase. The affected extremity should not be left in a dependent position for more than 10 minutes at a time.

Immobilization Phase I (Rigid)

The stitches are typically removed around day 14 and the patient is placed in a short-leg cast or cast boot. Stress is placed on the importance of knee and hip strength and flexibility. Examples of strengthening exercises while maintaining NWB precautions include straight-leg raises in all four directions and long arc quads (Figure 54.7). Care must be taken while doing these exercises, as they are weighted by the cast on the operative leg. Hamstring stretches (Figure 54.8) should also be performed. Pelvic and core stabilizer strengthening exercises should continue as tolerated. ROM is encouraged to the

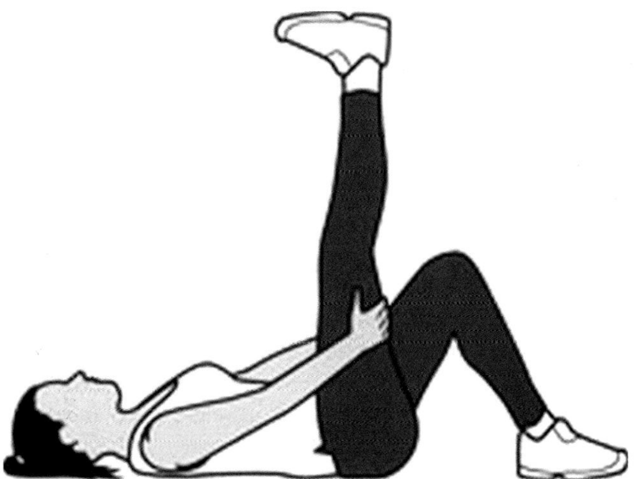

Figure 54.8 Illustration of hamstring stretch for Immobilization Phase I.

© 2018 American Academy of Orthopaedic Surgeons

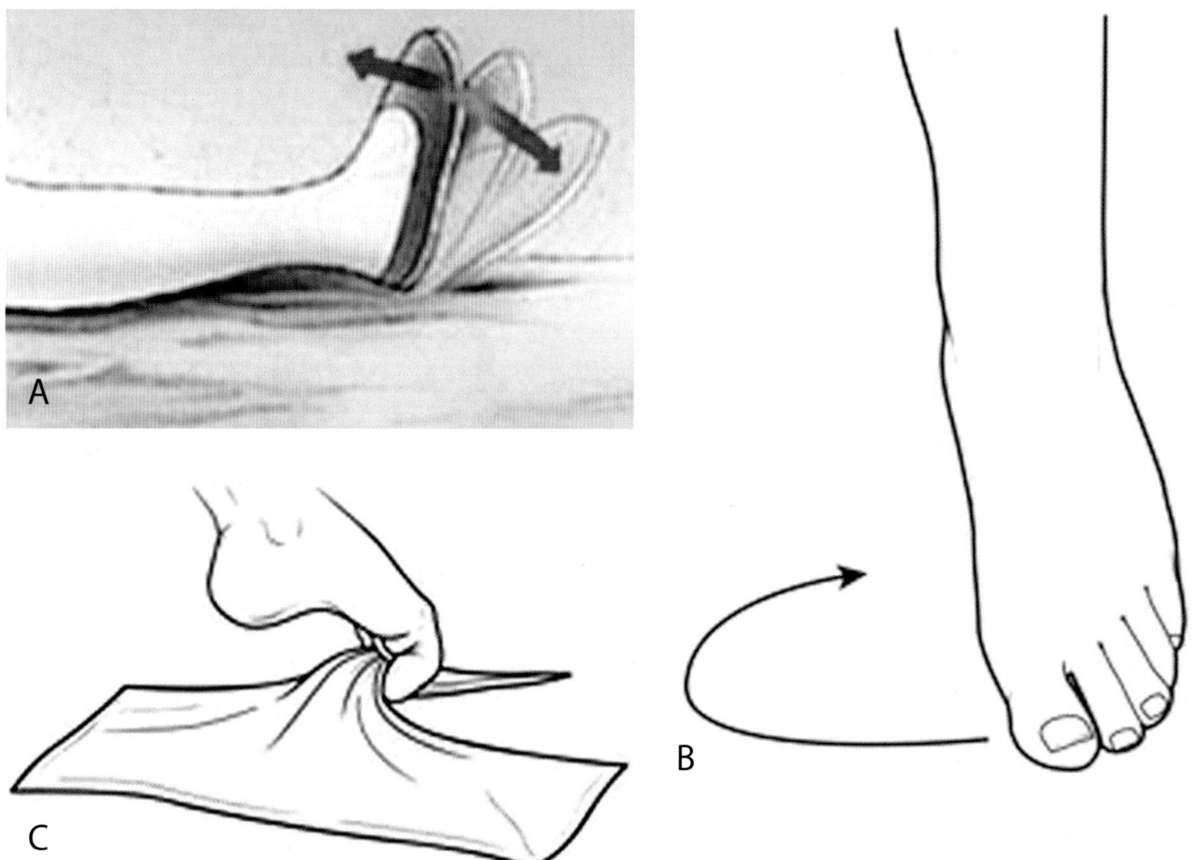

Figure 54.9 Illustrations of ankle and hindfoot range of motion exercises for Immobilization Phase II. **A**. Ankle pump. **B**. Ankle rotation in both directions. **C**. Known as the towel scrunch, this forefoot exercise aids in toe range of motion and intrinsic strengthening.

toes and the patient is instructed on isometric ankle exercises in four directions to perform while in the cast.

Goals

Goals of this phase of rehabilitation include pain and edema management, maintenance of nonimmobilized joints, minimizing atrophy, and strengthening of proximal and distal muscle groups. Continued focus of safe NWB gait is also stressed.

Restrictions

No weight bearing during this phase.

Immobilization Phase II (Protective Brace)

In weeks 6 to 12, rehabilitation focus is on gait reeducation and progressive weight bearing with appropriate assistive device. Recommendations are made to begin weight bearing at 20 pounds on the operative extremity and advance approximately 20 pounds every 4 days until full weight bearing in a controlled ankle motion (CAM) boot has been achieved. This process will be gradual, starting with weight shifts and small periods of walking. Stress is placed on moving deliberately forward but slowly with proper foot and ankle mechanics. Rehabilitation should address any gait deviations, including the patient's ability to control pronation and supination. Typically, a patient will take 3 to 4 weeks to obtain full weight bearing in a boot. Then, the boot can be slowly discontinued over 2 weeks in favor of a supportive tie shoe. Patients should make progressions to the least restrictive assistive device and discharge its use once gait is normalized.

Every effort should be made to build medial stability through muscle activity; however, orthotics to reduce pronation can act as a complement to rehabilitation. Education should be provided on appropriate shoewear to prevent hyperpronation.

Ankle and hindfoot AROM exercises in all directions are prescribed and should be performed three times a day for 10 minutes a session. Forefoot exercises, such as towel scrunches, are also introduced in this phase. Foot and ankle exercises are performed in this phase of rehabilitation (Figure 54.9). Emphasis is placed on performing the exercises slowly and holding the terminal limit of motion for at least 10 seconds. Performing the exercises bilaterally is recommended so that the patient can visualize normal motion and work toward that goal.

The patient should perform gentle gastrocnemius and soleus stretches at this time (Figure 54.10), and maintain flexibility of other tight structures as appropriate. As weight bearing increases, the patient may begin double-limb proprioceptive

© 2018 American Academy of Orthopaedic Surgeons

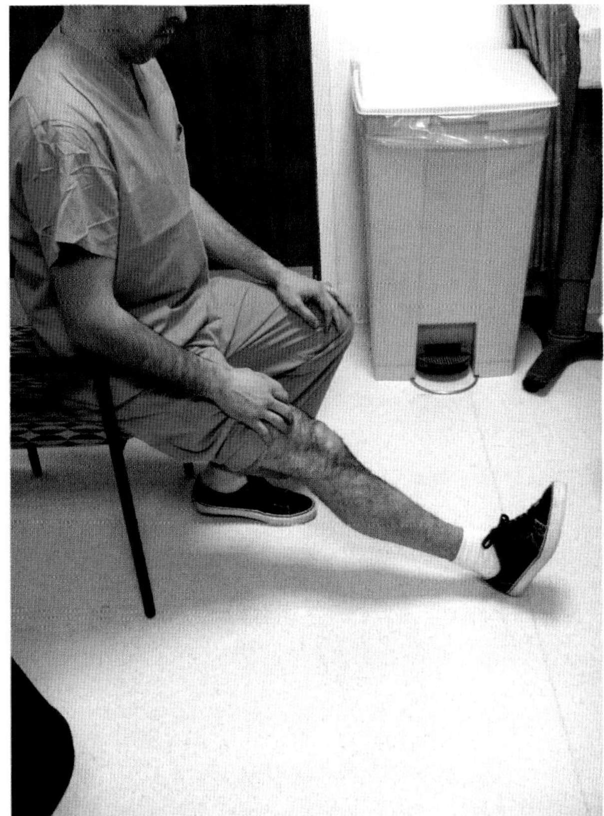

Figure 54.10 Photograph of gastrocnemius stretching with ankle actively dorsiflexed.

and balance exercises (Figure 54.11). The exercises should recruit the flexor hallucis longus and intrinsic muscles to provide stability to the arch and allow the patient to actively reduce excessive pronation force. One technique that therapists use to recruit the medial musculature and build dynamic arch support is instructing patients to shift their body weight over the lateral aspect of the foot while performing weight-bearing exercises, essentially forcing the foot and ankle out of the abducted, everted, and hyperpronated position.

Scar mobilization is also indicated in this phase of recovery. In order to maintain cardiovascular health, stationary biking while wearing the boot is recommended.

Goals

In Immobilization Phase II, progressive weight bearing is utilized until FWB has been achieved. Continued strengthening and ROM is utilized to achieve independence from the CAM walker boot by the end of this phase. Continued proximal strengthening and edema management is necessary to enter the functional rehabilitation phase of recovery.

Restrictions

The tendon transfer and midfoot fusions (if applicable) are still healing. Passive stretching should not be attempted until month 3. AROM in eversion should be carefully monitored to avoid placing significant stress on healing bone and transferred tendons.

Functional Rehabilitation

Once motion and FWB out of the boot have been achieved, attention and effort is placed on balance and strengthening. Balance and proprioception can be improved performing tandem and single-limb stance activities starting at a counter or stable surface and gradually adding challenges, such as balancing on foam or a pillow or a narrow double-limb stance on a balance device (Figure 54.12).

ROM exercises may progress to active assisted and passive. A wall lunge stretch is a powerful exercise to achieve terminal dorsiflexion and stretch the gastrocnemius and soleus muscles (Figure 54.13). In order to achieve sufficient ROM for proper gait and stair negotiation, manual therapy techniques can be progressed to include soft-tissue and joint mobilizations as appropriate while being mindful of which joints are fused.

Resisted exercises (Figure 54.14) may be initiated, using caution with combined plantarflexion and inversion. Single-limb heel rises may also be initiated. This strengthening test marks the end of functional rehabilitation and will often not be achieved until the postoperative month 6. The exercise may be broken down into easier submovements. We recommend beginning with a double-limb heel rise. Compare bilaterally for height of heel rise and demonstration of hindfoot inversion. Look for symmetry in both measurements (Figure 54.15). Once this is achieved with minimal upper extremity support, then single-limb descents of the operative side over 5 seconds may be performed. Once single-limb descents are achieved, single-limb heel rises can be started. Healthy patients should be able to lift their heel the same height as during the single-leg heel rise as they can during the double-leg heel rise. Recommendations are made for slow, progressive advancement and moderation in these activities. Ten-minute sessions, two to three times a day, are sufficient. Symmetry in heel rise with proper mechanics is crucial.

Continued advancement in ROM and strengthening allows normal gait and stair negotiation to be achieved by the end of this phase. Exercise programs, such as cycling with resistance and rowing, may begin as soon as FWB in a shoe has been achieved. Treadmill walking may take longer to achieve, but may begin when normal stair descent has occurred.

Goals

In functional rehabilitation, all patients must achieve single-limb heel rises and a reciprocal stair pattern as they demonstrate full ROM, strength, and proprioception. A long-term home exercise program should be established.

Restrictions

No formal restrictions exist in this phase of rehabilitation. However, moderation and slow increases in activity are required.

Return to Daily Living and Outcomes

This program continues until the patient's goals are achieved. This may not occur until 1 year after surgery. There is continual,

© 2018 American Academy of Orthopaedic Surgeons

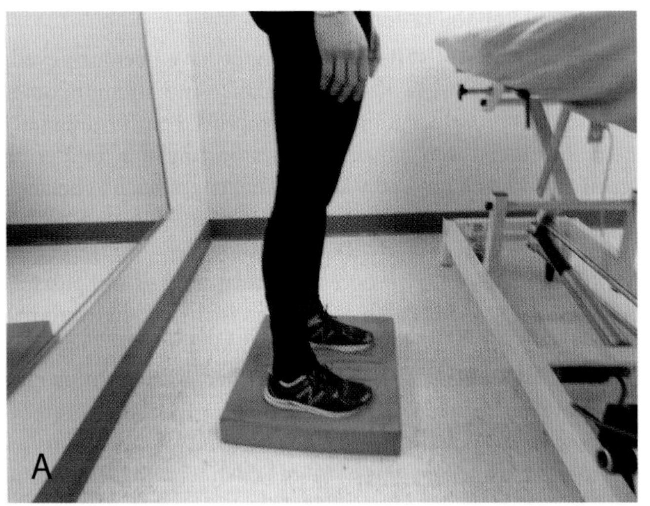

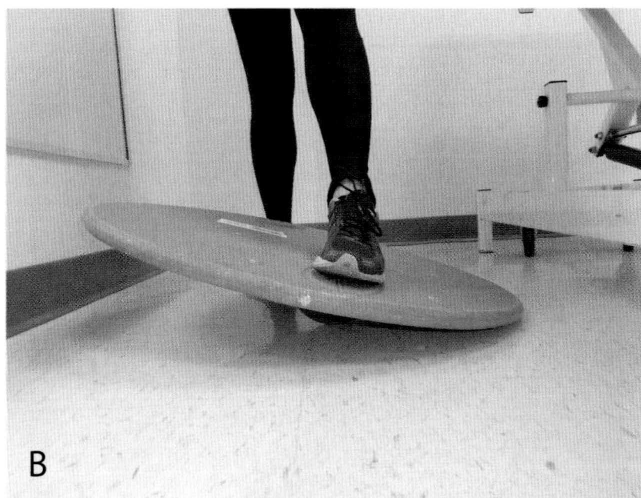

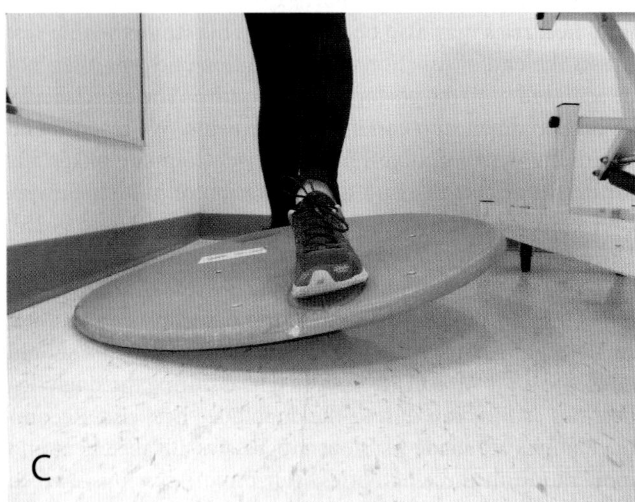

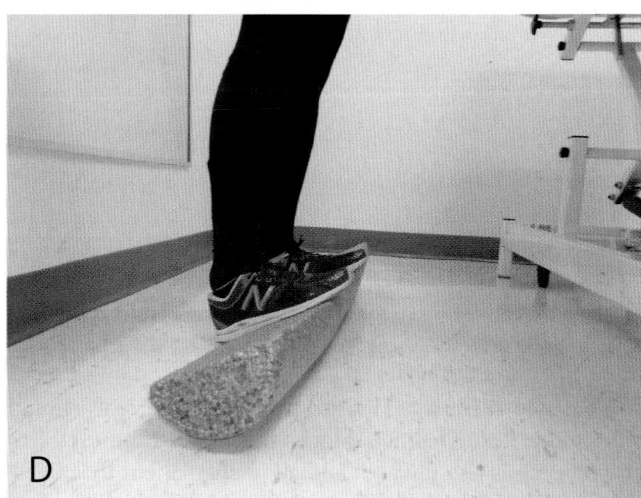

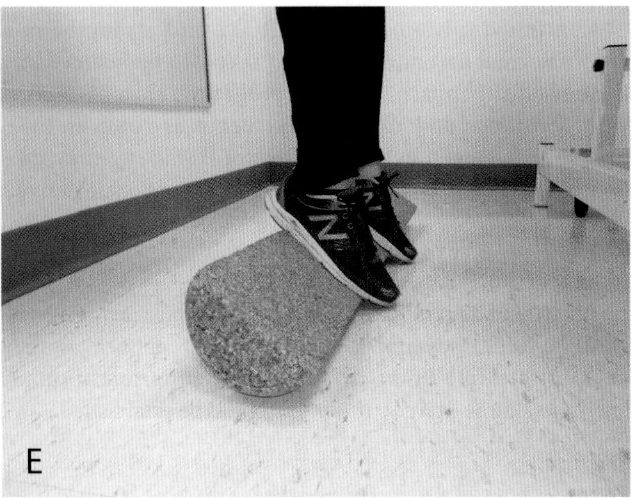

Figure 54.11 Double and single limb balance and proprioception exercises with **A**, foam; **B**, **C**, balance board; **D**, **E**, half round cylinder.

 © 2018 American Academy of Orthopaedic Surgeons

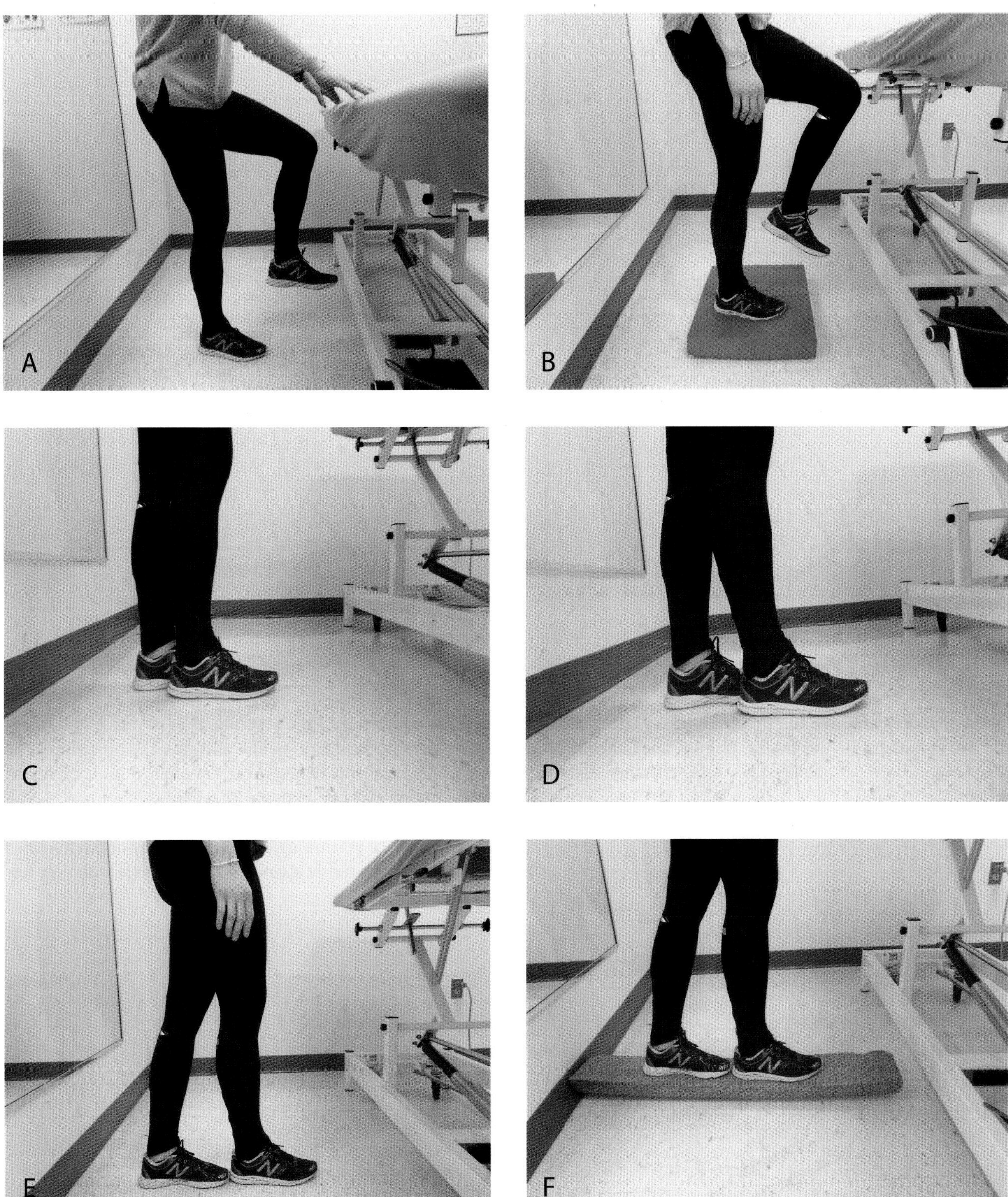

Figure 54.12 Photographs of stance progression; **A**, **B**, Single-limb stance progressions for Functional Rehabilitation phase. **C–F**, Tandem stance progressions for Functional Rehabilitation phase.

© 2018 American Academy of Orthopaedic Surgeons

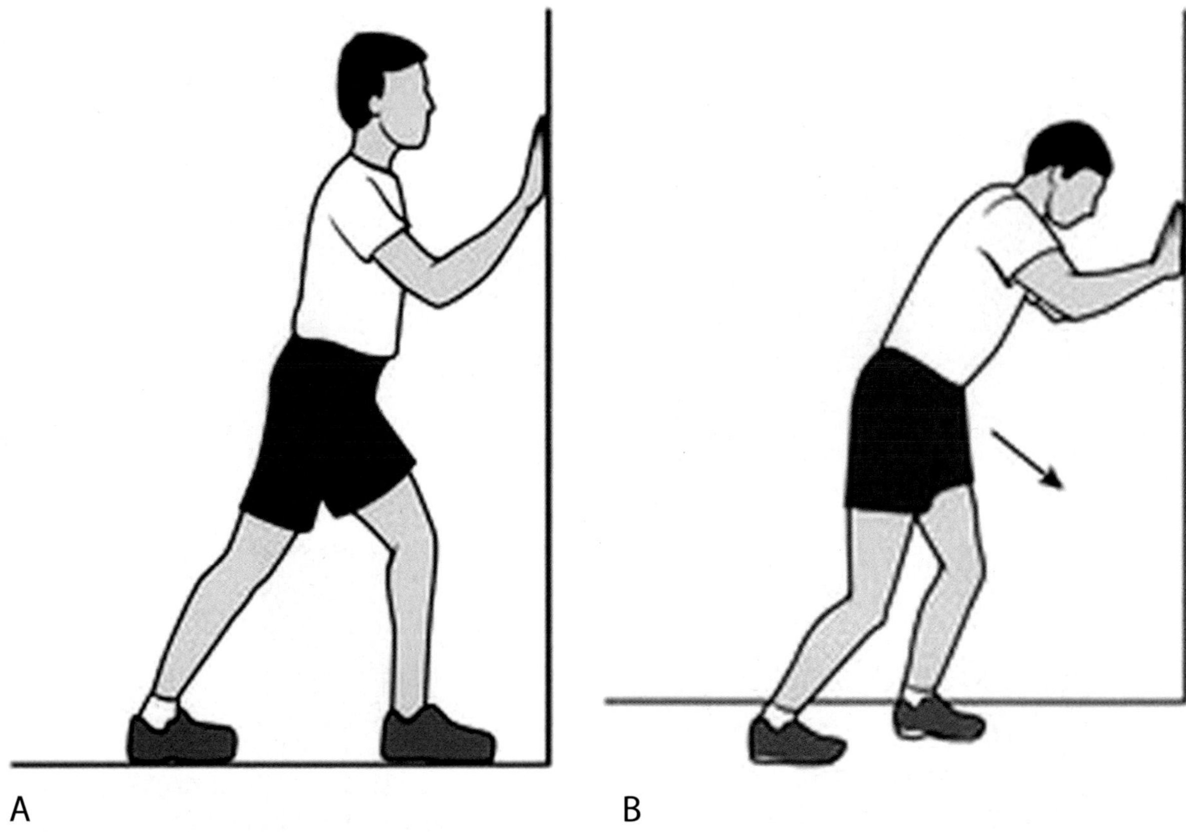

Figure 54.13 Illustrations of calf stretches. **A**, Gastrocnemius stretch. **B**, Soleus stretch.

subtle improvement over the first year, as the edema abates and strength returns to the lower extremity. The final outcome of flatfoot reconstruction depends on many factors including patient age, weight, health status, and activity level prior to surgery, adherence to the rehabilitation protocol, and integrity of the foot structures before and after the procedure. The expectation is that patients will achieve full AROM and return to their prior level of function with regard to low-impact activities, such as walking, biking, and swimming. High-impact recreation, such as running and jumping, may not be tolerated postsurgery. The newly aligned joint is durable with very low failure rates.

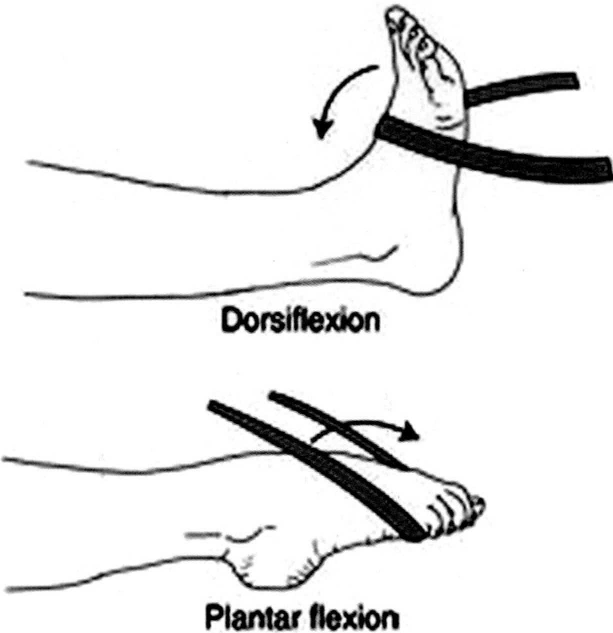

Figure 54.14 Illustraiton of resisted ankle exercises for Functional Rehabilitation phase.

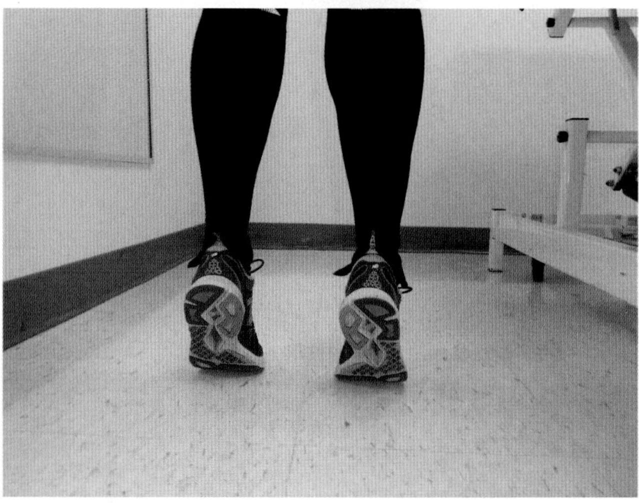

Figure 54.15 Photograph of symmetrical double-limb heel rise.

© 2018 American Academy of Orthopaedic Surgeons

PEARLS

- The rehabilitation of this procedure is long and exhaustive to the surgeon, therapist, and patient.
- Recovery continues well into the second postoperative year.
- Continued patience and focus on edema management, ROM and gentle strengthening will be required to achieve a full recovery.

BIBLIOGRAPHY

Guyton GP, Jeng C, Kreiger LE, Mann RA: Flexor digitorum longus transfer and medial displacement calcaneal osteotomy for posterior tibial tendon dysfunction: a middleterm clinical followup. *Foot Ankle Int* 2001;22(8):627 632.

Haddad SL, Mann R: Flatfoot deformity in adults, in Coughlin MJ, Mann RA, Saltzman CL, eds: *Surgery of the Foot and Ankle,* ed 8. Philadelphia, PA, Mosby Elsevier, 2007, pp 1007–1082.

Hiller L, Pinney SJ: Surgical treatment of acquired flatfoot deformity. what is the state of practice among academic foot and ankle surgeons in 2002? *Foot Ankle Int* 2003;24(9):701–705.

Johnson KA, Strom DE: Tibialis posterior tendon dysfunction. *Clin Orthop Relat Res* 1989;(239):196–206.

Orthopaedic Specialists of North Carolina: Galland/Kirby Posterior Tibial Tendon Reconstruction (FDL Transfer and Calcaneal Osteotomy) Postsurgical Rehabilitation Protocol. Available at: http://www.orthonc.com/sites/default/files/forms/kirby/Posterior_Tibial_Tendon_Reconstruction.pdf Accessed February 1, 2014.

Peninsula Orthopaedic Associates: PostOp Flexible Flatfoot Reconstruction. Available at: http://www.peninsulaortho.com/downloads/Flexible%20Flatfoot%20Reconstruction.pdf Accessed January 27, 2014.

Royal National Orthopaedic Hospital: Rehabilitation Guidelines for Patients Undergoing Surgery for Tibialis Posterior Reconstruction. Available at: https://www.rnoh.nhs.uk/sites/default/files/downloads/physiotherapy_rehabilitation_gudelines_ti bialis_posterior_reconstruction.pdf. Accessed February 1, 2014.

© 2018 American Academy of Orthopaedic Surgeons

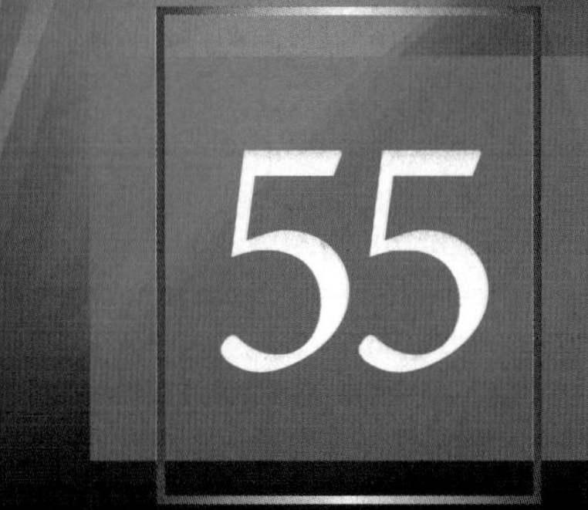

55 Ankle and Hindfoot Fusions

Craig S. Radnay, MD, MPH

INTRODUCTION

Arthritis is second only to cardiovascular disease in producing chronic disability that directly impacts the quality of life. Arthritis is also the leading cause for decreased work performance in the United States. The ankle and hindfoot joints are exposed to enormous joint reactive forces during gait and activity, 3 to 4 times more than that experienced in the hip and knee, with a smaller contact area and higher peak contact stresses. Fortunately, activity-limiting ankle arthritis is less common than degenerative disease of other major weight-bearing joints.

Ankle arthritis is most commonly posttraumatic, following a fracture of the ankle. For this reason, ankle and hindfoot arthritis patients tend to be younger than their hip/knee counterparts. Other causes for ankle and hindfoot arthritis include chronic joint instability, rheumatoid or inflammatory arthritis, neuropathy, postsepsis, and osteonecrosis with talar collapse.

While there have been numerous recent design advances in screw and plate technology, a successful outcome for an ankle or hindfoot fusion procedure still relies on the same concepts: appropriate preparation of the joint surfaces and rigid multiplanar internal fixation. Once the joint is successfully fused, after 3 to 4 months, functional rehabilitation will continue to help patients adjust to lack of motion at the fused joint. Most patients will be satisfied with their pain relief and surrounding joints may accommodate to allow resumption of most regular activities.

While a hip or knee fusion is poorly tolerated, patients with an ankle fusion generally do well. This is largely because adjacent joints (subtalar and talonavicular) provide compensatory motion in plantarflexion (PF) and dorsiflexion (DF). Conversely, patients with stiff hindfoot joints may be not as good candidates for fusion.

When considering surgery for someone with ankle arthritis, the patient should have failed nonoperative management, including shoewear and activity modification, physical therapy, exercise, weight loss, pain medications, and bracing. Total ankle replacement may be an alternative surgical option for some patients. Risks of complications are higher for ankle replacement, although some patients may see better function. Certainly, patients who are not as good candidates for ankle fusion (those with hindfoot stiffness) may be the best candidates for ankle replacement. Patients with advanced arthritis of the hindfoot (subtalar or calcaneocuboid joints) may benefit from arthrodesis/fusion of these joints. Most hindfoot arthritis is posttraumatic as well, although some fusions are performed for deformity, as in an advanced flatfoot deformity. Rare patients will have arthritis of both ankle and hindfoot, in which case combined fusions of multiple joints may be necessary. Patients with such "pantalar" fusions tend to have not as good results, with much more stiffness and less ability to compensate.

Selective arthrodesis is employed to achieve as much pain relief and stability with deformity correction as possible while preserving as many joints as possible. Pantalar arthrodesis is now limited as a salvage procedure for extreme posttraumatic pathology across multiple joints or for advanced Charcot reconstruction. The pain relief, restoration of alignment, improved soft-tissue status, and return to ambulation achieved in these cases, however, still justifies the use of this technique.

Contraindications to ankle or hindfoot fusions include active infection, especially with an open or arthroscopic approach. Relative contraindications include history of infection in the joint, advanced arthritis, and/or fusions at surrounding joints.

SURGICAL APPROACH

Ankle Arthrodesis

Ankle arthrodesis is often performed in a supine position through a direct anterior approach, utilizing the interval between the tibialis anterior and extensor hallucis longus tendons. Alternately, a lateral approach can be made, with an incision over the fibula. The fibula is cut and rotated externally, and the ankle joint is entered from the lateral side. With either approach, the tibiotalar joint is exposed, and any loose bodies and prominent osteophytes are carefully removed. The joint

Dr. Radnay or an immediate family member is a member of a speakers' bureau or has made paid presentations on behalf of OrthoDevelopment and Wright Medical Technology; serves as a paid consultant to OrthoDevelopment and Wright Medical Technology; and serves as a board member, owner, officer, or committee member of the American Orthopaedic Foot and Ankle Society.

© 2018 American Academy of Orthopaedic Surgeons

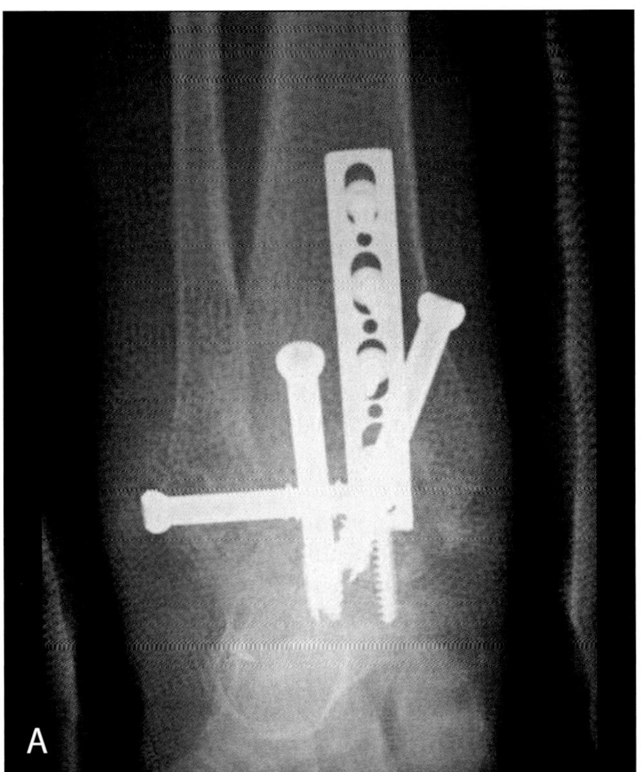

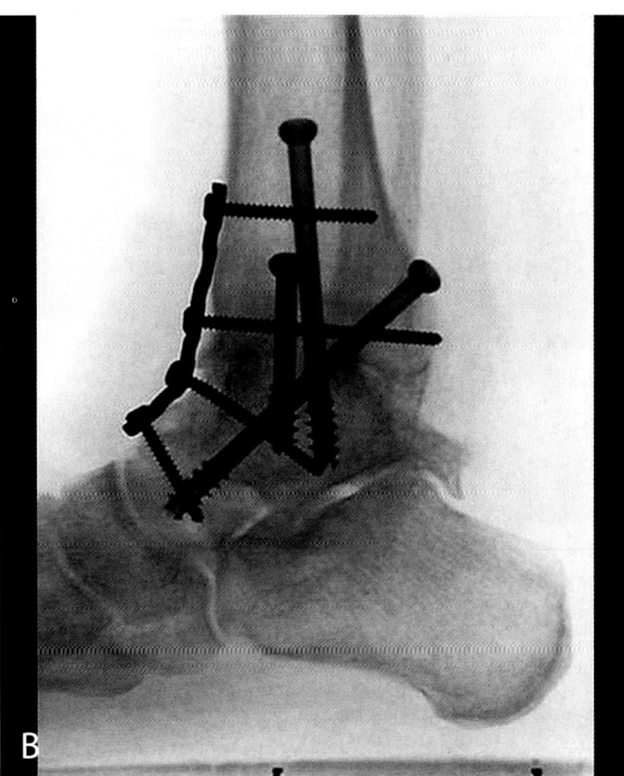

Figure 55.1 **A**, **B**, Anteroposterior and lateral radiographs of ankle fusion with anterior neutralization plate.

is distracted with the use of laminar spreaders or pin distraction clamps, and the remaining articular cartilage is sharply débrided with the use of sharp periosteal elevators. Setting the ankle in the correct position for fusion is essential. This should also be planned out preoperatively, considering the entire lower leg, ankle, and foot. The tibiotalar joint should be in neutral DF/PF, 5° of external rotation and 5° of valgus. The anterior aspect of the talar dome should be positioned at the anterior border of the tibial plafond. Any deformity is corrected at this time; supplemental bone graft is utilized as needed for defects, although not routinely. With a rigid foot, a few degrees of ankle DF may be preferred. The position of the knee and the bow of the tibia should also be examined prior to surgical stabilization. For example, with quadriceps weakness, the arthrodesis should be positioned with the foot in 10° of equinus, which can help stabilize the knee joint. An equinus foot will force the knee into hyperextension, which is helpful if the quadriceps is weak.

In rare cases, persistent equinus deformity may be corrected with a percutaneous Achilles lengthening or gastrocnemius recession. In general, both equinus and calcaneus positioning should be minimized to prevent a back-knee thrust or excessive heel strike, respectively. In addition, rigid-foot deformity might necessitate slight overcorrection at the ankle or additional selective osteotomy or arthrodesis to create a plantigrade foot.

As an alternative to lag screws, a plate can be placed anteriorly or laterally. (Figure 55.1, A and B). An anterior plate neutralizes the PF, DF, and torsion moments across the joint, increasing rigidity and decreasing micromotion at the ankle fusion interface in the sagittal, coronal, and axial planes. Alternative approaches may be considered in special situations, such as ankles with soft-tissue concerns or a revision procedure. A lateral transfibular approach can be utilized, with the fibula preserved with internal fixation at the conclusion to provide greater stability and options for potential future surgical procedures. A posterior midline approach could also be utilized in a complex posttraumatic or revision situation from the prone position.

Arthroscopic Ankle Arthrodesis

Arthroscopic ankle arthrodesis has gained increasing popularity, with reports of shorter hospital stays, shorter time to solid fusion, equivalent to improved union rates, and earlier functional improvement when compared with open arthrodesis. Arthritic ankles with minimal deformity are excellent candidates for this procedure. With increasing experience with ankle arthroscopy and improved instrumentation, this technique can also be utilized for more complex deformities. The minimal soft-tissue disruption via an arthroscopic approach may also reduce the degree of permanent functional impairment of the joints and soft tissues adjacent to the fusion site. Arthroscopic fusion can extend surgical indications to patients with a compromised soft-tissue envelope or vasculopathy, which might otherwise be a relative contraindication to an open procedure. Patients with global inflammatory, postseptic, or hemophilic arthritis are also good candidates. Contraindications to the arthroscopic technique include the same as those for an open approach, as well as significant focal bone loss and deformity, and extremely stiff, immobile ankles, which preclude arthroscopy.

© 2018 American Academy of Orthopaedic Surgeons

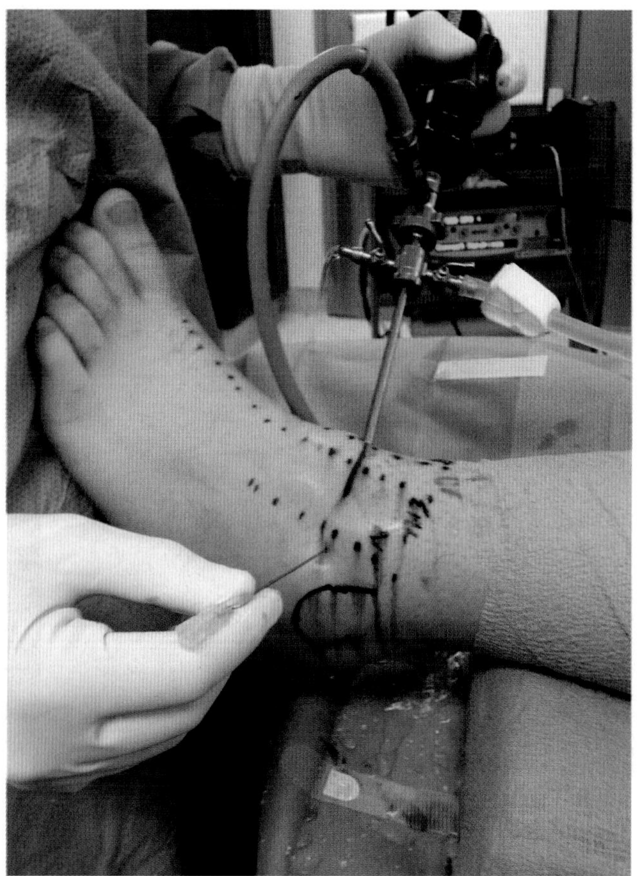

Figure 55.2 Photograph of set-up for arthroscopic ankle arthrodesis.

The arthroscopic procedure is performed utilizing standard anteromedial and anterolateral portals (Figure 55.2). Removal of the articular cartilage is achieved with the use of an aggressive soft-tissue resector and the hard chondral bone is cleared down to softer, bleeding subchondral bone with the use of a high-speed burr. The fusion is stabilized, in appropriate alignment, with 2 or 3 large fragment compression screws, as described for the open technique. Pin and screw placement is verified utilizing multiplanar fluoroscopy.

Hindfoot Fusions

Hindfoot fusion approaches are specific to the pathology. The subtalar and calcaneocuboid joints can be easily accessed through either a lateral Ollier incision or via a longitudinal incision extending from distal to the fibular tip in line with the fourth metatarsal. The talonavicular joint can be approached through a medial incision utilizing the plane between the anterior and posterior tibial tendons.

Rigid internal fixation utilizing large fragment screws and/or plates is confirmed with multiplanar fluoroscopy (Figure 55.3). For an isolated subtalar joint fusion, the prepared joint should be positioned in slight valgus (5°) alignment, with the calcaneus positioned underneath the talus. Residual forefoot varus should be eliminated. Bone graft is utilized in revision procedures, and as needed in primary cases.

Extended ankle and hindfoot fusion cases are approached from either a direct anterior or extensile lateral exposure. The anterior approach usually requires an additional small lateral subtalar incision. The extended fusions via the extensile

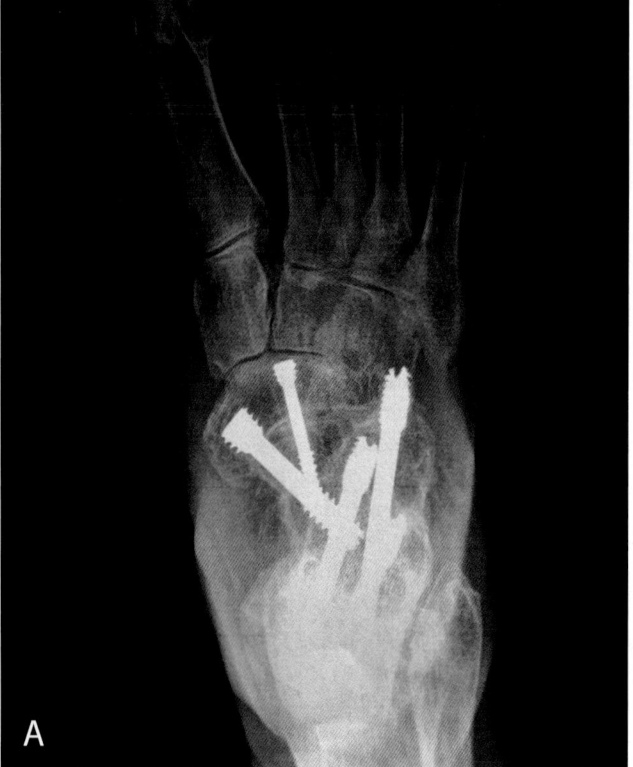

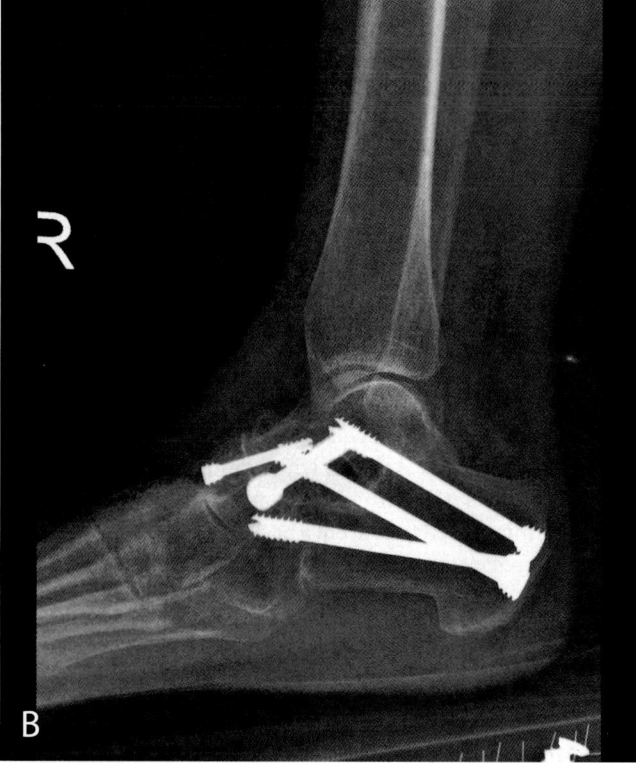

Figure 55.3 **A**, **B**, Multiplanar radiographs following triple hindfoot (subtalar, talonavicular, calcaneocuboid) arthrodesis.

© 2018 American Academy of Orthopaedic Surgeons

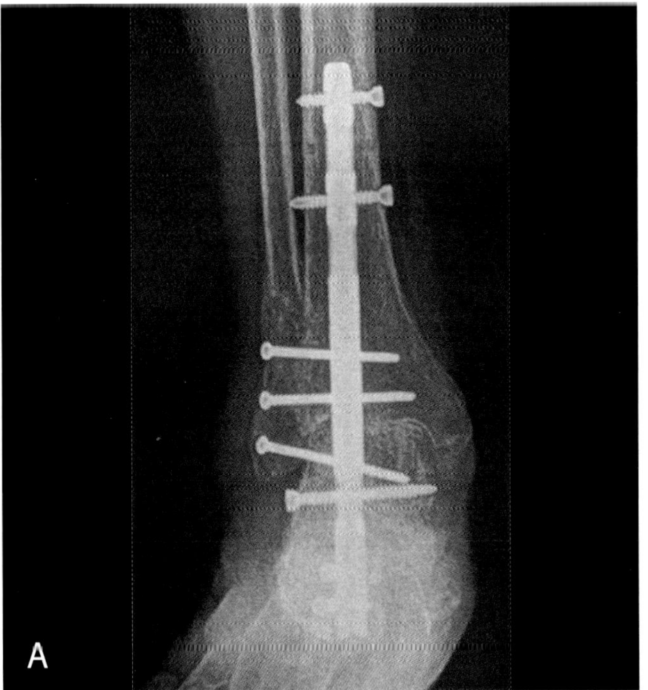

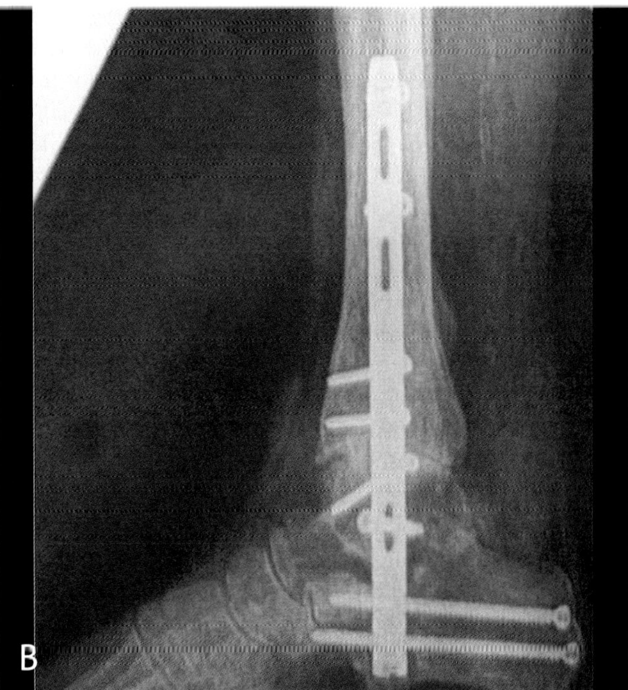

Figure 55.4 **A**, **B**, Anteroposterior and lateral radiographs following tibiotalocalcaneal fusion with intramedullary nail, tibiofibular fusion, and supplemental stabilization.

lateral approach is performed with an incision along the fibula curving anteriorly in line with the fourth metatarsal, with an additional medial window at the tibiotalar joint. The fibula is osteotomized above the level of the ankle joint to expose the ankle and subtalar joints; the fibula is débrided of soft tissue, decorticated, and fused to the lateral tibia at the end of the case. Alternatively, the fibula can be removed, morselized, and used as autograft across the articular surfaces. The tibiotalocalcaneal joint is then stabilized with either an intramedullary nail placed in compression in retrograde fashion, or with anterior and/or posterior plating (Figure 55.4, A and B).

Postoperatively, patients are followed closely for the first 6 to 12 weeks to ensure proper wound healing and compliance with non–weight bearing, to maximize bony consolidation and fusion. Follow-up with the surgeon is typically scheduled at 2 weeks, 6 weeks, 3 months, 6 months, and 1 year. Multiplanar radiographs are warranted at each visit to help assess bony healing, hardware, and alignment. If patients do not seem to be improving clinically or radiographically, CT scan is recommended by the 6-month visit for additional assessment.

Complications of Ankle and Hindfoot Fusions

- Infection
- Delayed wound healing
- Nerve disruption or entrapment
- Nonunion (5%–40%)
- Malunion
- Painful, prominent hardware
  - Penetration of surrounding joints
- Stiffness, decreased ROM
  - Transfer stresses to surrounding joints
- Gait changes, increased energy expense
  - Decreased stride length, cadence
  - Abnormal motion at the subtalar joint
- Persistent pain despite union
- Compensatory painful arthritis
  - Develops in 50% at 8 years, nearly 100% at 20 years

POSTOPERATIVE REHABILITATION

In this section are some general guidelines for initial stage recovery and relative progression of rehabilitation. Patients are placed in a well-padded bulky plaster splint in the operating room. They remain non–weight bearing, with the leg elevated as much as possible for the first 2 weeks, until wounds are inspected and stitches removed. Most patients will be placed back into a well-padded non–weight bearing cast for the next 4 weeks. Many surgeons prefer a cast to a removable CAM boot. Weight bearing is restricted until there are radiographic signs of healing since weight bearing generates torque on the ankle, which is detrimental to fusion. In general, removable casts/boots may not provide adequate immobilization because of the lever arm created by the foot and the tibia. Soft-tissue related issues and pain tolerance may require specific changes in the program. These changes will be made by the surgeon and physical therapist as deemed appropriate for the individual patient.

Patients are informed preoperatively and reminded peri- and postoperatively that full functional recovery can take up to 1 year—including pain relief, swelling, range of motion (ROM), gait, and function. It is normal to have some pain and discomfort during recovery, especially as the activity level

© 2018 American Academy of Orthopaedic Surgeons

increases. It is paramount when discussing surgery with these patients to be honest about the length and limitations of their recovery period, and to remind patients to be patient in the postoperative period. The more the patient is informed, the more improved will be the patient's pain control, anxiety level, hospital length of stay (LOS), and satisfaction. The patient and family should be engaged in and understand the postoperative plan, which will instill confidence and help motivate them in the patient's recovery.

Multimodal pain management is utilized in the pre-, peri-, and postoperative periods. Multiple studies have shown that postoperative pain and rapid rehabilitation protocols correlate with the quality of recovery. Effective analgesia should be provided, minimizing the use of opioids and their side effects. For ankle and hindfoot fusion surgery, a combination of regional anesthetic or peripheral nerve blocks is combined with oral and intravenous medication pre-, intra-, and postoperatively to attempt to block pain generation at several different stages in the pain pathway. Improved postoperative pain scores will leave patients more alert and oriented, and allow them to be more engaged with their physical therapy, which is important to improve ROM in the short and long term.

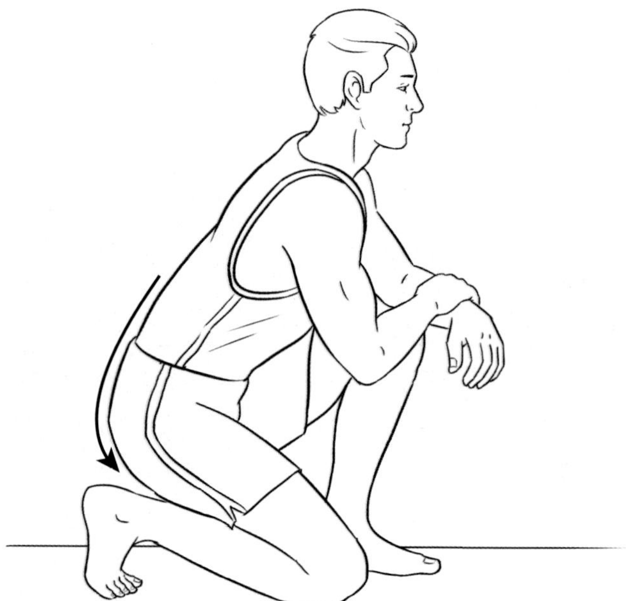

Figure 55.6 Illustration of toe extension/ankle dorsiflexion with kneeling.

Phase I: Date of Surgery to 6 Weeks

- Objective: Healing, protection of fusion, elevation/edema control, pain management.
- Immobilization: Cast splint. After 2-week follow-up: cast versus CAM boot.
- Weight-Bearing Status: Non–weight bearing.

Phase II: Weeks 6 to 8

- Objective: Continued promotion of healing, edema management.
- Immobilization: Use of removable walker boot.
- Weight-Bearing Status: Begin progression to full weight bearing.
- Therapy: 2 to 3 times per week with a focus on swelling reduction, pain control, home care/exercise instructions for motion, pain/swelling control.
- Sagittal motion after ankle fusion is predominantly in PF through the transverse tarsal joints (Figures 55.5, 55.6, 55.7); focus on subtalar inversion/eversion following ankle fusion (Figure 55.8).
- Subtalar fusions: Ankle ROM starting 6 weeks postoperatively (Figure 55.9).

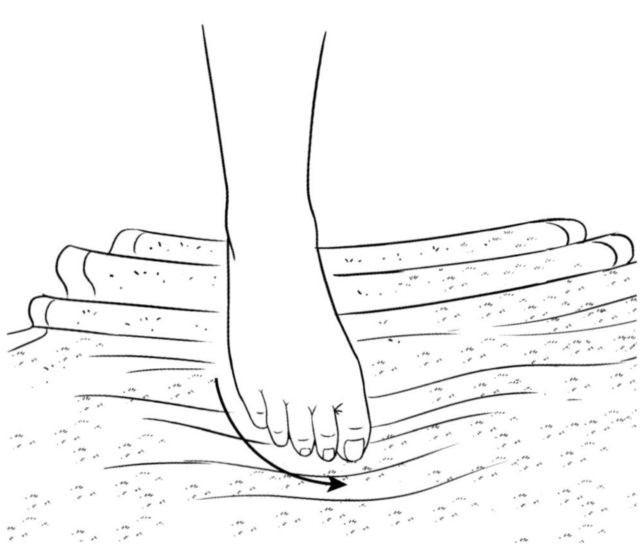

Figure 55.5 Illustration of unilateral toe curl and tarsometatarsal flexion. Rest foot on towel and bunch up towel by curling toes.

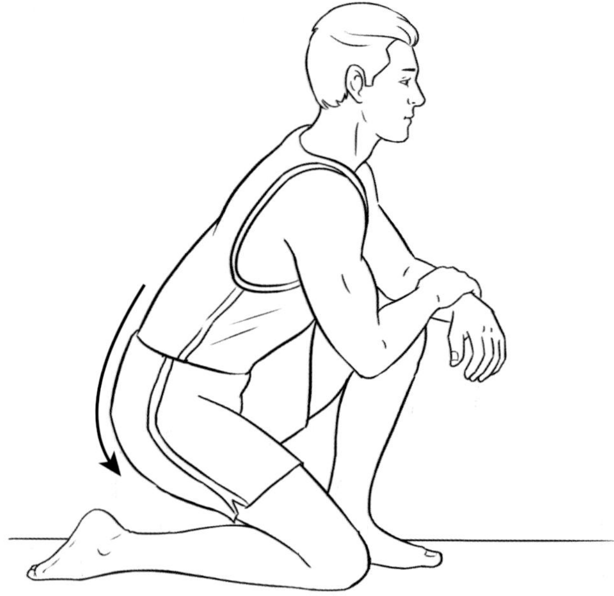

Figure 55.7 Illustration of ankle plantarflexion from kneeling.

© 2018 American Academy of Orthopaedic Surgeons

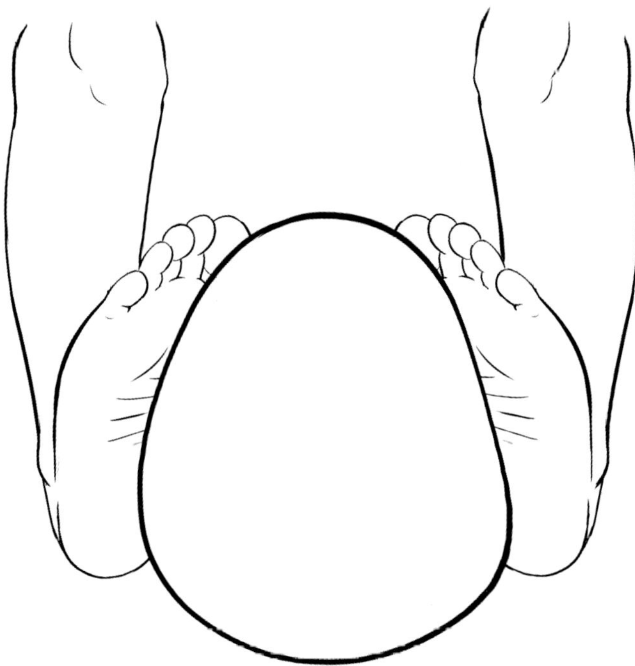

Figure 55.8 Illustration of ankle/foot inversion (isometric). Press inner border of feet into ball or rolled pillow.

Phase III: Weeks 8 to 16

- Objective: Swelling reduction, increase in ROM, neuromuscular re-education, develop baseline of ankle control/strength.

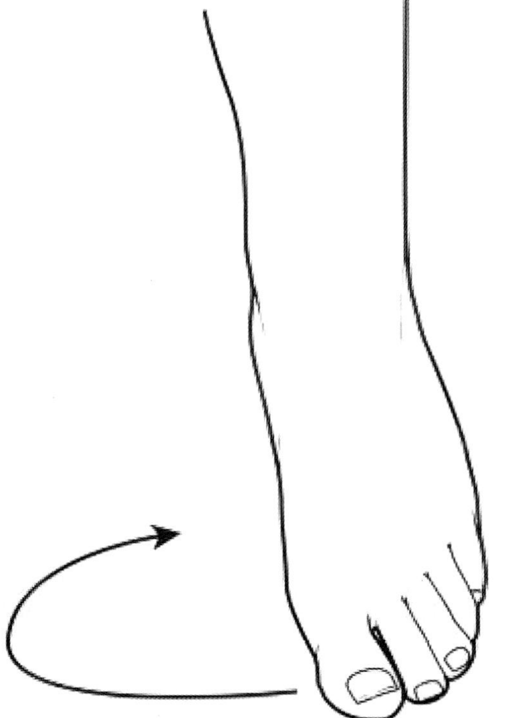

Figure 55.9 Illustration of trace and spell alphabet with ankle. (Reproduced with permission from OrthoInfo. © American Academy of Orthopaedic Surgeons. Available at: http://orthoinfo.aaos.org.)

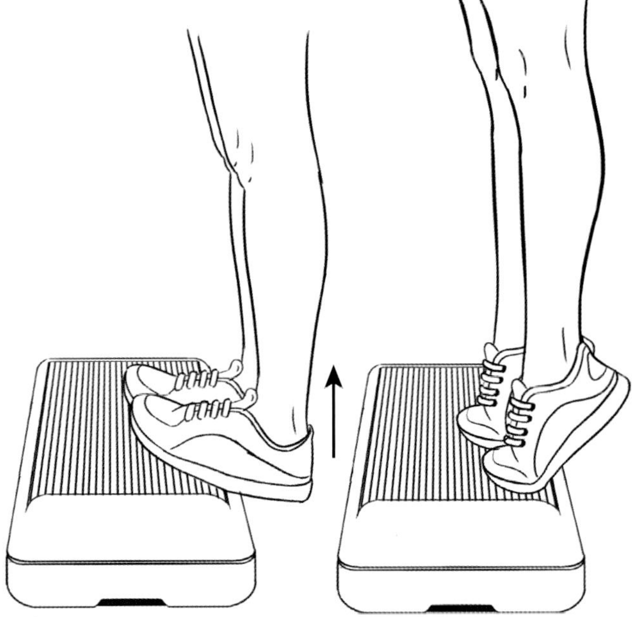

Figure 55.10 Illustration of heel raise with toes on board.

- Immobilization: Wean boot to brace, orthotics, or regular shoes.
- Weight-Bearing Status: Progression to full weight bearing, progressive reduction in crutch or other assistive device.
- Therapy: 2 to 3 times per week based on patient's initial presentation. Frequency may be reduced as the patient exhibits good recovery and progress toward goals, instructions in home care, and exercise program to complement clinical treatment.
- Rehabilitation Program
  - Strength: Techniques should begin with isometrics in four directions with progression to resistance band/isotonic strengthening for DF and PF (Figures 55.10 and 55.11). Hindfoot eversion and inversion isometric strengthening should continue with introduction of resistance bands (Figures 55.12 and 55.13). Resistance bands should progress from mild to heavier resistance, as tolerated. Aquatic therapy and stationary biking allowed, as tolerated.
  - Proprioception: May begin with seated balance board and progress to standing balance exercises as tolerated (Figures 55.14–55.16).

Phase IV: Weeks 16 to 24

- Objective: Functional ROM, strength within functional limits, adequate proprioception for stability and balance, normalized gait, tolerance for a full day of ADLs/work, return to reasonable recreational activities.
- Weight-Bearing Status: Full, patient should exhibit normalized gait. Extended fusions/neuropathic (Charcot) fusion transition to double upright calf brace for 1 year.
- Therapy: Once every 2 to 4 weeks based on patient status and progression, to be discharged to an independent

© 2018 American Academy of Orthopaedic Surgeons

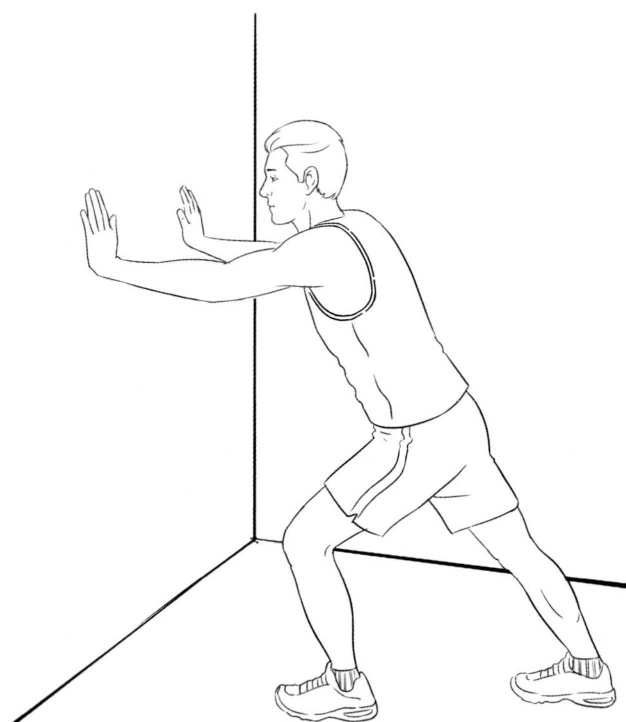

Figure 55.11 Illustration of gastrocnemius stretch with back leg straight, heel on floor.

exercise program once goals are achieved. Patient to be instructed in appropriate home/gym exercise program.

- Rehabilitation Program
  - Strength: Progression to full body weight resistance exercises with goal of ability to perform a single-leg heel raise (raise height may be limited by location and extent of fusion).

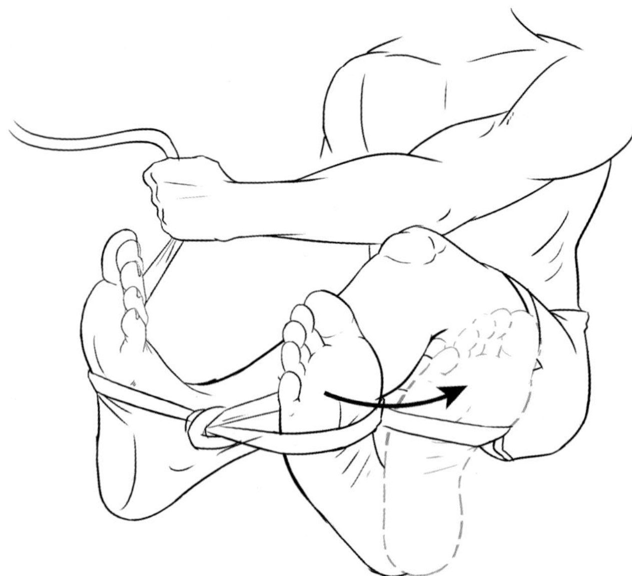

Figure 55.12 Illustration of resisted ankle inversion with crossed legs using resistance bands.

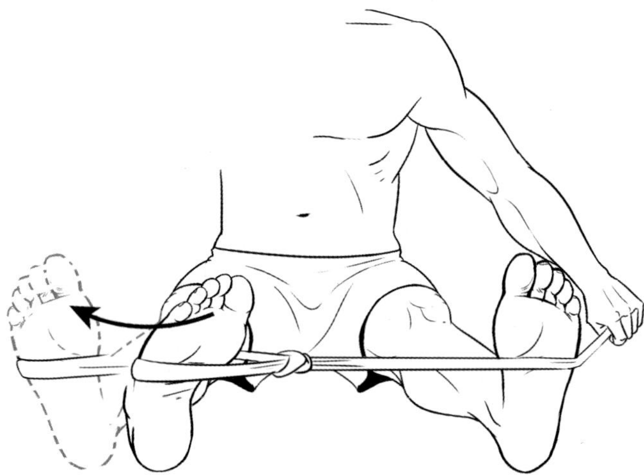

Figure 55.13 Illustration of resisted ankle eversion using resistance bands.

  - Proprioception: The patient should be instructed in proprioceptive drills that provide both visual and surface challenges to balance.
  - Agility: Cone/stick drills, leg press, plyometric exercises, soft landing drills (Figures 55.17 and 55.18).
  - Sports: Prior to return to any running or jumping activity, the patient must display a normalized gait and have strength to perform repetitive single-leg heel raises. Note

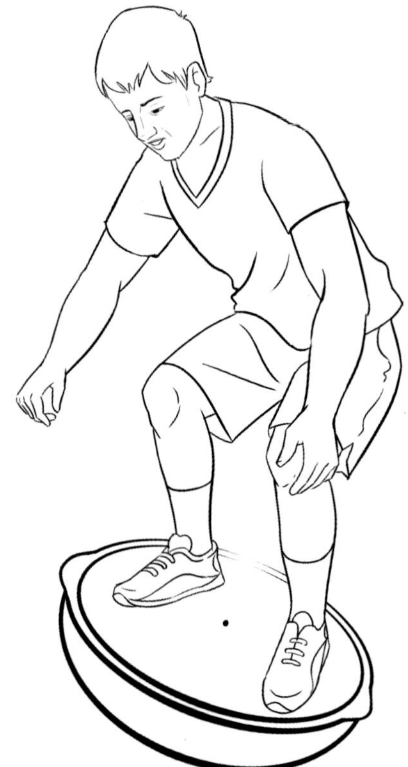

Figure 55.14 Illustration of balance and proprioception with seated balance board; rotate foot clockwise and counterclockwise.

© 2018 American Academy of Orthopaedic Surgeons

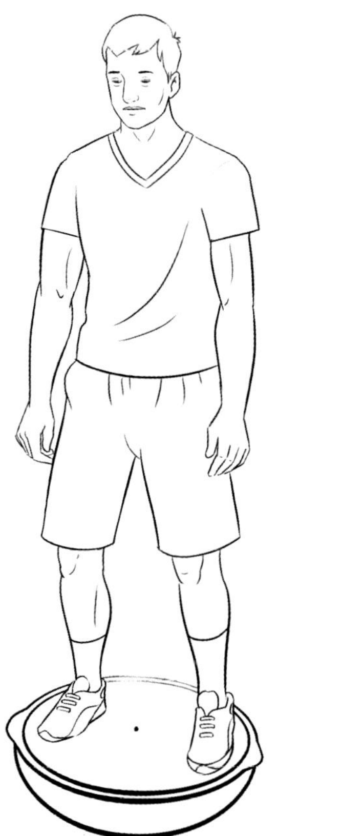

Figure 55.15 Illustration of balance board with 2 feet standing and rotating.

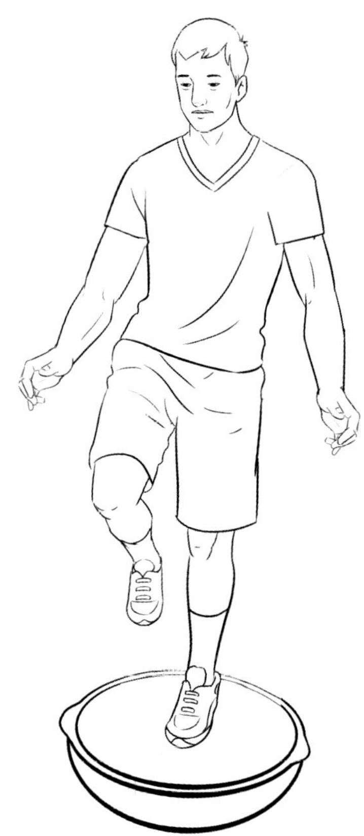

Figure 55.16 Illustration of balance board, standing and rotating, with one foot.

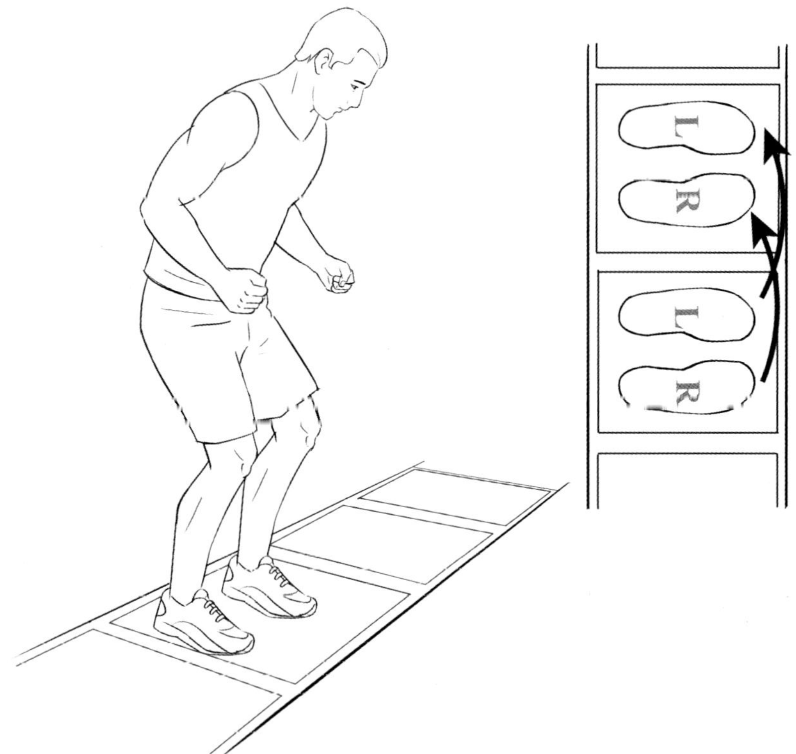

Figure 55.17 Illustration of lateral shuffle with floor ladder.

© 2018 American Academy of Orthopaedic Surgeons

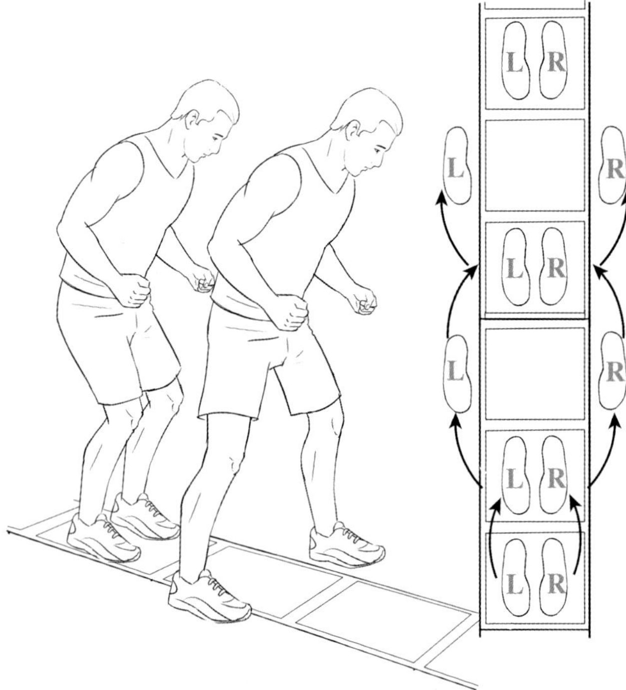

Figure 55.18 Illustration of hopscotch through floor ladder.

that nonimpact activities (bicycle, elliptical, swimming) are, in general, better tolerated by patients following ankle or hindfoot fusion. Some patients with an isolated hindfoot fusion (i.e., isolated subtalar fusion) might be able to tolerate some type of activity with running/jumping, if adequate gait and strength are achieved postoperatively.

PEARLS

- Dissect soft tissue carefully.
- Consider arthroscopic fusion with compromised soft-tissue envelope.
- Joint reduction and provisional alignment confirmed with multiplanar fluoroscopy.
- Avoid varus malalignment.
- Multimodal pain management.

- Rehabilitation focused on strength, proprioception, agility and periarticular ROM.
  - Postoperative non–weight wearing until bony consolidation demonstrated.
  - Progressive weight bearing in CAM walker boot.
  - Initial focus on wound healing, swelling control, edema management.
  - Work on ROM after fusion compensatory through adjacent joints.
  - Strength training progression from isometric to isotonic.
  - Progression toward increased resistance training, aquatic therapy, stationary biking.
  - Proprioception and balance board exercises for balance training.
  - Work on agility and plyometric exercises.
  - Increase tolerance for return to ADLs and recreational activities.
  - Discharge with instructions for independent home exercise program.

BIBLIOGRAPHY

Cooke PH, Jones IT: Arthroscopic ankle arthrodesis. *Techniques in Foot & Ankle Surgery* 2007;6:210–217.

Coughlin MJ, Mann RA, Saltzmann CL: Arthrodesis of the foot and ankle. *Surgery of the Foot and Ankle,* ed 8. Mosby, 2007, pp 923–952, 1087–1112.

Muir DC, Amendola A, Saltzman CL: Long term outcome of ankle arthrodesis. *Foot Ankle Clin* 2002;7:703–708.

Saltzman CL, Blanchard GM, Huff T, Hayes A, Buckwalter JA, Amendola A: Epidemiology of ankle arthritis: report of a consecutive series of 639 patients from a tertiary orthopaedic center. *Iowa Orthop J* 2005;25:44–46.

Stauffer RN, Chao EY, Brewster RC: Force and motion analysis of the normal, diseased, and prosthetic ankle joint. *Clin Orthop Related Res* 1977;127:189–196.

Tarkin IS, Mormino MA, Clare MP, Haider H, Walling AK, Sanders RW: Anterior plate supplementation increases ankle arthrodesis construct rigidity. *Foot & Ankle International* 2007;28:219–223.

Townshend D, DiSilvestro M, Krause F, Penner M, Younger A, Glazebrook M, Wing K: Arthroscopic versus open ankle arthrodesis: A multicenter comparative case series. *J Bone Joint Surg Am* 2013;95:98–102.

© 2018 American Academy of Orthopaedic Surgeons

Ankle Arthroplasty

May Fong Mak, FRCSEd (Ortho), Xavier Crevoisier, MD, and Mathieu Assal, MD, PD Dr.

INTRODUCTION

Ankle arthroplasty was developed in the 1970s as an alternative to ankle arthrodesis for the treatment of end-stage ankle osteoarthritis (OA). Conservation of a functional range of motion (ROM) of the ankle remains a primary advantage of total ankle arthroplasty (TAA) over arthrodesis. Forty years of progress, through three generations of prosthesis designs and improvements in surgical technique, have seen a rise in TAA survivorship in ranges of 70% to 98% at 3 to 6 years, and 80% to 95% at 8 to 12 years, as well as patient return to light recreation and sports, in terms of overall function.

This chapter focuses on postoperative rehabilitation following TAA. Optimal rehabilitation starts with identification of relevant preoperative factors, is dependent on good surgical technique, and relies heavily on a team-based approach to postoperative care. Rehabilitation should not be viewed only as a postoperative activity. Elderly patients with decreased muscle strength and coordination may benefit from therapy preoperatively. In addition, the value of patient education in the consultation room cannot be overlooked, as an informed patient is better equipped to understand and anticipate the process that is to come.

Surgical Procedure

Surgical success is a synthesis of systematic preoperative assessment, meticulous surgical planning, and methodical performance of the operative procedure.

A prerequisite for success is correct patient selection. The ideal candidate is an elderly individual with limited physical demands, low body mass index, a well-aligned and stable hindfoot, normal bone stock, good preservation of peripheral vascularity, and healthy periarticular soft tissues. TAA is indicated to preserve remaining motion in special circumstances in which end-stage OA affects both ankles, or is present in a foot stiffened by adjacent joint degeneration or previous subtalar or midfoot arthrodesis. TAA should be avoided in young patients with high functional demands, severe hindfoot malalignment, neuroarthropathy, active infection, talar avascular necrosis, and poor soft-tissue envelope.

Modern TAA designs are cementless three-component systems comprised of two metallic components and an interposed ultra-high-molecular-weight polyethylene (UHMWPE) insert. Irrespective of manufacturer, the surgical approach and general operative principles are similar.

Most surgeons favor an anterior approach to the ankle. A 15-cm longitudinal incision is made over the anterior aspect of the ankle. The extensor retinaculum is incised, the interval between the tendons of the tibialis anterior and extensor hallucis longus (EHL) is entered, and the joint capsule is incised longitudinally to expose the ankle joint. The most distal part of the anterior tibial margin and its osteophytes are removed with an osteotome to expose the tibial plafond and talar dome. The tibial resection parameters that must be considered for correct component placement are varus/valgus alignment, slope, height, rotation, and translation. The tibial and talar cuts are made with the specific instrumentation provided. The medial and lateral gutters must routinely be cleared of osteophytes and impinging soft tissue. Trial implants are sized and inserted, and their position and ankle alignment verified by fluoroscopy and on-table clinical assessment of ankle ROM. The final prosthesis is subsequently implanted, and once again final position and alignment are confirmed clinically and radiologically. Meticulous hemostasis is ensured to avoid a postoperative hematoma that can exert pressure on the surrounding soft tissues, leading to skin necrosis, or can act as a source of infection. Careful closure is performed, beginning with the joint capsule. Careful attention is given to the extensor retinacular repair, as it forms an important barrier between the ankle joint and the more superficial incision. The subcutaneous layer and skin are closed in layers. Staples are not recommended for closure, particularly in the tenuous central portion of the incision directly overlying the ankle joint. A soft dressing and postoperative splint are carefully applied.

The TAA procedure can be fraught with technical errors, as demonstrated by the literature validating the existence of

Dr. Crevoisier or an immediate family member serves as a board member, owner, officer, or committee member of the Swiss Foot and Ankle Society. Neither of the following authors nor any immediate family member has received anything of value from or has stock or stock options held in a commercial company or institution related directly or indirectly to the subject of this article: Dr. Assal and Dr. Mak.

© 2018 American Academy of Orthopaedic Surgeons

a "learning curve" during which surgeons acquire skills and experience before they become proficient at performing TAA. Keeping in mind several technical pearls will contribute to a better surgical outcome. Careful soft-tissue dissection, the avoidance of unnecessary retraction, and methodical wound closure cannot be overemphasized since good soft-tissue handling is paramount to successful wound healing. Repair of the extensor retinaculum is crucial, as it prevents bowstringing of the tibialis anterior tendon exerting direct pressure on the undersurface of the surgical wound, which can rapidly culminate in disastrous wound necrosis or dehiscence. Long-standing soft-tissue contractures must be recognized and released in order to balance the ankle joint. Clearance of the gutters must be a routine part of each surgery to avoid postoperative impingement pain. Preexisting ankle instability may predispose to prosthesis subluxation or dislocation, and must therefore be recognized and corrected through ligamentous reconstructive procedures during TAA surgery. Tendon pathology—such as fissures, ruptures, or dislocations—should be addressed. Achilles tendon lengthening is indicated in patients with heel equinus contracture, but should be used sparingly and cautiously due to the risk of chronic heel cord pain postoperatively. Symptomatic peritalar joint arthritis should be considered for fusion in the same setting. Hindfoot and first ray osteotomies and tendon transfers may be required in some cases to balance the foot.

POSTOPERATIVE REHABILITATION

The final outcome following ankle arthroplasty is subject to a multitude of factors, including (1) preoperative ROM, strength, functional level, and related comorbid conditions; (2) intraoperative restoration of the anatomic ankle joint line, the accuracy of tibial and talar cuts, prosthesis design, instrumentation, positioning, and fixation; and (3) postoperative complications and rehabilitation.

Postoperative rehabilitation is integral in influencing the final outcomes pertaining to ROM, strength, proprioception, balance, and gait. The ideal rehabilitation protocol should be supervised, well defined, structured, goal oriented, and can be adjusted with consideration for tissue healing, joint mobility, muscle strength, and capability of the individual patient.

In TAA, the goals of rehabilitation are:

- Decrease pain and edema, and protect through immobilization.
- Achieve full ROM.
- Achieve full power and endurance.
- Achieve full proprioception and coordination, and adoption of normal gait.

A multidisciplinary team comprising foot and ankle surgeons, anesthesiologists, rehabilitation physicians, physical therapists, occupational therapists, and social workers must work closely together to support the patient through the rehabilitative process. Advancement from one phase to the next is determined by the patient's progress in achieving rehabilitation milestones, and should not be based solely on a generic time frame. A rehabilitation protocol is represented in Table 56.1.

Pain Relief

- Early pain relief is a basic principle of acute rehabilitation, as unresolved pain will delay progress toward the next phase of therapy.

Table 56.1 A PROTOCOL FOR POSTOPERATIVE REHABILITATION AFTER STANDARD TOTAL ANKLE ARTHROPLASTY

Rehabilitation Phase	Estimated Time Frame	Emphasis	Components
Acute	First 2 weeks	Protection	• Pain relief • Wound care • Immobilization • Basic rehabilitation
Early	Next 10 weeks	Weight bearing Motion Strength	• Static weight bearing • Unsupported weight bearing • Early ROM exercises • Strength training
Late	Beyond 12 weeks	Neuromuscular	• Proprioception • Balance • Coordination • Gait retraining • Terminal ROM exercises • Intensified strength training

ROM = range of motion.

 © 2018 American Academy of Orthopaedic Surgeons

- Regional anesthetic infusions are increasingly used with other analgesics following orthopaedic surgery. Postoperative continuous popliteal sciatic nerve blockade effectively decreases pain and the need for rescue opioids after surgery, improving patient satisfaction and recovery.
- Patient-controlled analgesia in the form of intermittent intravenous boluses of opioids is another commonly used modality.
- Oral medications are generally introduced early and continued after analgesic infusions have been discontinued.
- There is ongoing controversy over the use of traditional nonsteroidal anti-inflammatory drugs (NSAIDs) as laboratory data suggest that its inhibition of prostaglandins impairs bone formation and bony in-growth. Although its clinical significance remains uncertain, some surgeons limit the use of NSAIDs for postoperative pain, especially in patients who have other risk factors for delayed bone healing.
- The effectiveness of pain relief can be monitored using the visual analog scale (VAS).

Wound Care

- On the first postoperative day, the operated ankle is inspected under aseptic conditions for undetected bleeding, excessive soft-tissue tension, compartment syndrome, and neurovascular deficit.
- The suction drain is removed 48 to 72 hours postoperatively.

Immobilization

- Ankle immobilization after TAA is critical to protect the soft tissues for complete undisrupted healing, and the prosthesis–bone interface for sufficient osteointegration before unsupported ambulation is resumed.
- The ankle is immobilized in slight dorsiflexion (DF) to avoid the common problem of postoperative ankle equinus contracture (Figure 56.1), and to encourage future motion within the DF arc.
- Immobilization is achieved with a well-padded below-knee univalve cast (Figure 56.2).

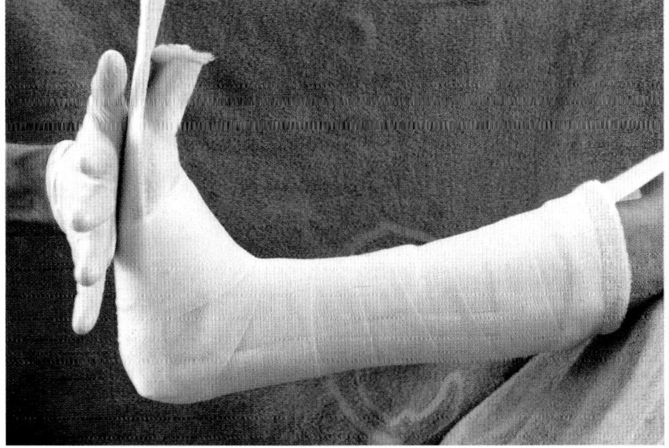

Figure 56.1 Photograph of ankle immobilization in 5° of dorsiflexion from the first postoperative day lasting for 6 weeks.

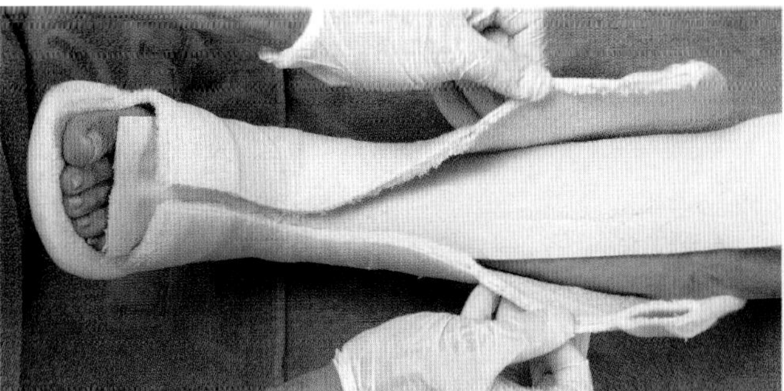

Figure 56.2 Photograph of univalved cast for protection of the soft-tissue envelope and total ankle arthroplasty.

- Patients after routine TAA are typically immobilized for 6 weeks.
- The operated limb is not allowed to bear weight or to be in a dependent position, to minimize swelling for the first 2 weeks.
- Patient compliance is paramount. Each patient is given clear instructions about cast care, related complications, and weight-bearing restrictions.

Phase I: Acute Rehabilitation Swelling and Pain Control (Weeks 0–2)

- Physical and occupational therapy commence after acute postoperative medical and surgical issues have resolved, and is enhanced with a good relationship between the patient and therapist.
- Patients are taught basic skills for their safe return home, focusing on independent transfers, safe ambulation with walking aids, and self-care with adaptive equipment.

Elevation, immobilization, and nonweight bearing are emphasized to ensure wound healing. Control of swelling also limits pain exacerbation.

Phase II: Early Weight Bearing and Motion (Weeks 2–12)

Weight Bearing (Static)

- Static weight bearing with increasing graduations of 15 kg per week will commence from the third postoperative week for 4 weeks. In this concept, the patient progressively bears weight with crutches, while the ankle remains immobilized within the cast.
- The cast is fitted with a removable cast shoe to enable walking (Figure 56.3).
- Weight bearing may be delayed in the presence of adjunctive bony or soft-tissue procedures.
- At least 6 weeks of immobilization postoperatively is typical. Though seemingly lengthy, in our experience, it has reduced the incidence of complications associated with soft-tissue healing with no detrimental effect on the final ROM.

Weight Bearing (Unsupported)

- After the sixth postoperative week, the cast is removed and, for the first time since surgery, the ankle is unsupported.

© 2018 American Academy of Orthopaedic Surgeons

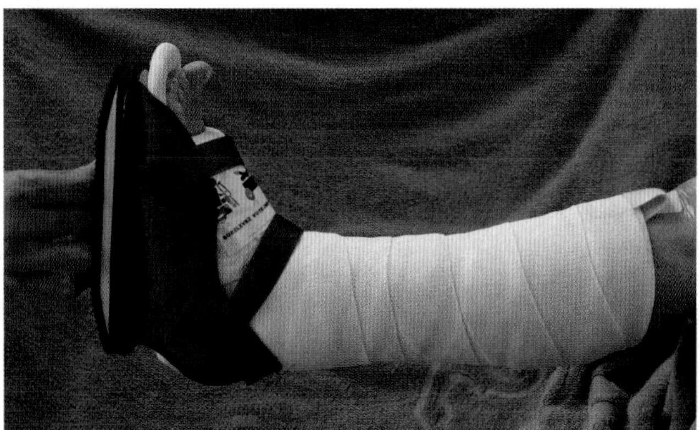

Figure 56.3 Photograph of shoe fitted to the cast for static weight bearing.

- Appropriate shoewear can make a substantial difference to recovery. Shoes that are large enough to accommodate postoperative swelling—such as running shoes with a thick rocker sole to reduce mechanical stresses in the ankle—are recommended for a minimum of 6 weeks.
- Compressive stockings are used concurrently to control postoperative edema.
- At the end of 10 weeks, most patients will achieve aid-free full weight bearing.

Early Range of Motion Exercises

- Motion exercises are initiated once the cast has been removed. Patients undergo an average of two supervised physiotherapy sessions a week.
- Therapy generally involves active and passive flexion/extension exercises, as tolerated by the patient.
- Forced inversion and eversion are generally not encouraged at this stage, but gentle active motion is allowed.

Strength Training

- Most patients progress to gentle active resistance exercises for strength training 2 weeks after commencement of motion exercises.
- An effective modality used in strength training is aquatic therapy. Walking in deep pool water exerts a compressive effect to reduce swelling, provides resistance for strength training while minimizing excessive movement, and enables virtually impact-free weight bearing.

Radiographic Assessment

- Standard anteroposterior (AP) and lateral ankle weight bearing radiographs are reviewed at postoperative weeks 2, 6, and 12.
- At postoperative months 6, 12, and 24, in addition to the AP view (Figure 56.4), flexion-extension lateral views may be performed to radiographically assess ROM (Figure 56.5).
- Radiographs are also evaluated for development of stress fracture, osteolysis, implant loosening, thinning of the polyethylene component, component subsidence or migration, formation of bone cysts, bony impingement, heterotopic ossification, and adjacent joint arthritis.

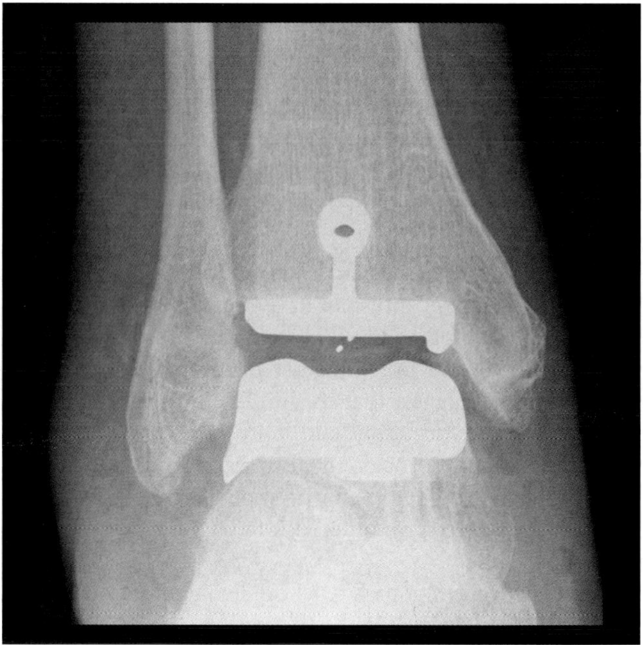

Figure 56.4 Anteroposterior radiograph of weight-bearing ankle showing a well-aligned three-component total ankle arthroplasty.

Phase III: Advanced Functional Rehabilitation (Week 12+)

Usually, at 3 months, adequate bony healing has occurred to permit the limits of rehabilitation to be pushed to achieve advanced functional goals.

Neuromuscular Retraining

- Neuromuscular rehabilitation forms the final step of rehabilitation that is integral to the functional success of the TAA. It encompasses proprioception, balance, coordination, and gait retraining.
- Patients learn tasks requiring interaction of neuromuscular skills with increasing complexity that are relevant to their future activity.
- Balance boards, treadmills, and stepping drills are useful in this phase, while endurance can be built with an exercise bicycle or other machines.

Terminal Range of Motion Exercises

- The extremes of the motion range may be achieved through supervised stretching exercises performed using a resistance band.
- It is widely accepted that the postoperative ROM after TAA is dependent on its preoperative range; however, the sagittal arc of motion can improved through surgery to encompass more DF, desirable for gait mechanics. DF is necessary for initial heel contact and clearance during the swing phase.
- The objective of motion rehabilitation should be to achieve the intraoperative arc of motion.
- Patients typically achieve an average final range of 25° to 30° of motion, with 5° to 10° of dorsiflexion and 15° to 20° of plantarflexion (PF).

© 2018 American Academy of Orthopaedic Surgeons

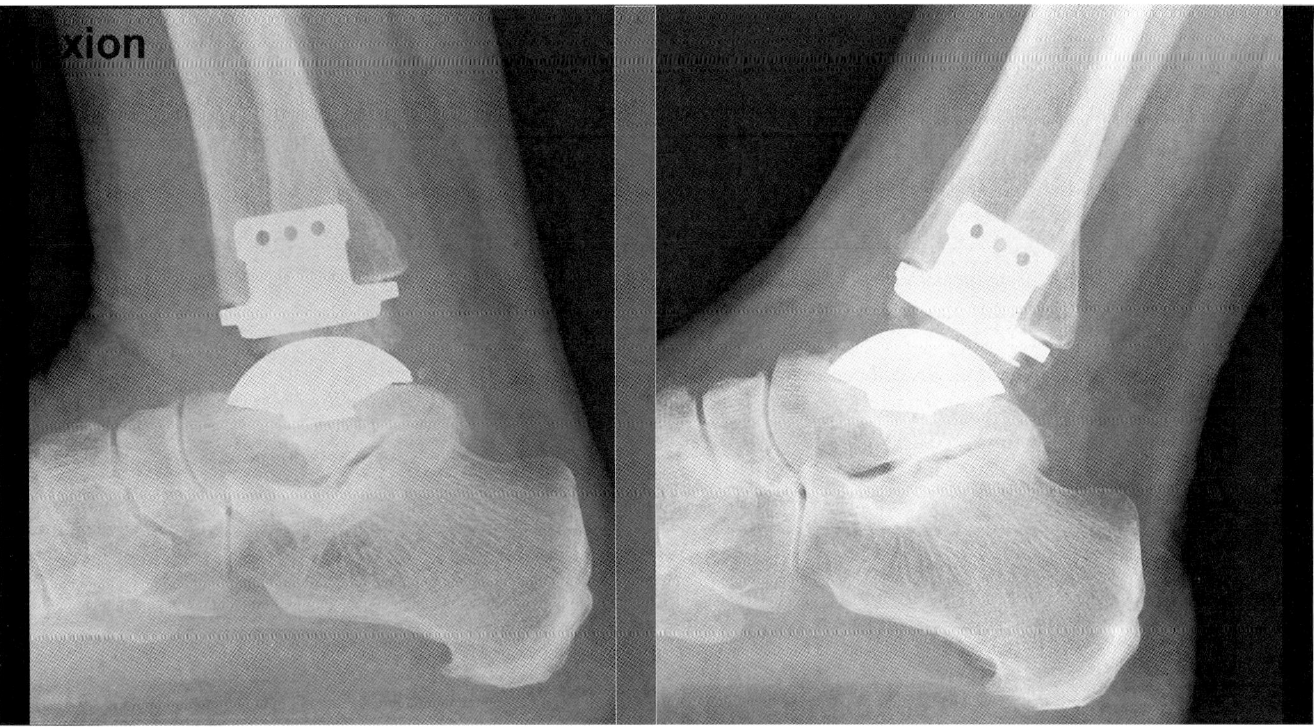

Figure 56.5 Flexion-extension radiographic views showing 15° of ankle dorsiflexion and 30° of plantarflexion.

- It should be stressed that the primary cause of arthritis has bearing on the final ROM. For example, TAA for posttraumatic OA in equinus with posterior soft-tissue scarring is more likely to produce a stiffer ankle postoperatively compared to TAA for inflammatory arthritis.

Intensified Strength Training

- Power training is intensified through isometric and isotonic exercises, and can take the form of closed- or open-chain exercises.
- It must be remembered that an ankle that is still painful, swollen, and stiff will hinder progress in power training, mandating decreasing the intensity and volume of rehabilitation.

The therapist-led program ends upon recovery of full function, including return to low-demand recreational and sporting activities such as walking, cycling, boating, golf, and swimming. The patient is encouraged to persevere with maintenance exercises that may be performed independently and safely in the home setting.

Precautions

In the course of rehabilitation, the therapist should not hesitate to discuss with the surgeon any issues they may encounter pertaining to the progress of the patient. These include, but are not limited to, patient-reported symptoms or therapist-observed signs, such as subjective (functional) or objective (mechanical) instability, dislocation, acute swelling, acute pain, inability to weight bear, regression in function, or wound complications. Early intervention is required for any suggestion of infection or fracture to limit the risk of failure of the procedure.

OUTCOMES

Several conclusions have been made with regard to postoperative gait, ROM, proprioception, muscle function, and return to sports:

- Successful TAA can restore near-normal gait patterns, as demonstrated in a study that found no differences in spatiotemporal variables of gait analysis in patients after TAA compared with normal controls 1 year postoperatively.
- A recent review comparing ankle ROM before and after TAA suggested only marginal improvements, with a mean increase in the flexion-extension arc ranging from 3° to 14°.
- No difference in proprioception was found between arthritic ankles after TAA and contralateral healthy ankles.
- Muscle function in arthritic ankles improved after TAA compared with their preoperative level, but did not achieve the level of the contralateral unaffected leg.
- Patients who have undergone TAA can expect to resume light sports and recreation, but rarely strenuous sporting activities.

The outcomes of TAA reported in the literature cannot be directly attributed to rehabilitation. While it is difficult to isolate the influence that rehabilitation has on TAA outcomes, it is widely accepted that even a technically superior operation must be complemented by good rehabilitation for optimal restoration of function.

© 2018 American Academy of Orthopaedic Surgeons

BIBLIOGRAPHY

Ajis A, Henriquez H, Myerson M: Postoperative range of motion trends following total ankle arthroplasty. *Foot Ankle Int* 2013;34(5):645–656.

Bonnin MP, Laurent JR, Casillas M: Ankle function and sports activity after total ankle arthroplasty. *Foot Ankle Int* 2009; 30:933–944.

Coetzee JC, Castro MD: Accurate measurement of ankle range of motion after total ankle arthroplasty. *Clin Orthop Relat Res* 2004;424:27–31.

Conti SF, Dazen D, Stewart G, et al: Proprioception after total ankle arthroplasty. *Foot Ankle Int* 2008;29:1069–1073.

Easley ME, Adams SB Jr, Hembree WC, DeOrio JK: Results of total ankle arthroplasty. *J Bone Joint Surg Am* 2011;93(15): 1455–1468.

Fukui A, Tanaka Y, Inada Y, Samato N, Ito K, Oshima M, Takakura Y: Turndown retinacular flap for closure of skin fistula after total ankle replacement. *Foot Ankle Int* 2008; 29:624–626.

Valderrabano V, Nigg BM, von Tscharner V, Stefanyshyn DJ, Goepfert B, Hintermann B: Gait analysis in ankle osteoarthritis and total ankle replacement. *Clin Biomech (Bristol, Avon)* 2007;22:894–904.

Valderrabano V, Nigg BM, von Tscharner V, Frank CB, Hintermann B: Total ankle replacement in ankle osteoarthritis: an analysis of muscle rehabilitation. *Foot Ankle Int* 2007;28:281–291.

Vuolteenaho K, Moilanen T, Moilanen E: Non-steroidal anti-inflammatory drugs, cyclooxygenase-2 and the bone healing process. *Basic Clin Pharmacol Toxicol* 2007;102: 10–14.

White PF, Issioui T, Skrivanek, GD, Early JS, Wakefield C: The use of a continuous popliteal sciatic nerve block after surgery involving the foot and ankle: does it improve the quality of recovery? *Anesth Analg* 2003;97:1303–1309.

 © 2018 American Academy of Orthopaedic Surgeons

57 Osteochondral Lesions of the Talus: Rehabilitation

Daniel C. Farber, MD, Erik Freeland, PT, DO, and Sarah Tyndall, MPT, OCS

INTRODUCTION

Historically, terms including osteochondritis dessicans, transchondral talus fracture, and osteochondral talus fracture have been used to describe what are now referred to as osteochondral lesions of the talus (OLTs). OLTs form a subset of osteochondral lesions that occur in various typical areas of the skeleton. While most lesions are unilateral, patients do have bilateral lesions. The lesions usually occur in two areas of the dome of the talus. Medial osteochondral lesions are more common than lateral osteochondral lesions. Medial lesions have been described as deeper, extending into subchondral bone and often developing into cystic lesions. Lateral lesions are more commonly associated with a traumatic injury and are described as shallow, with a greater tendency to become displaced.

The etiology of an OLT can be divided into nontraumatic and traumatic defects. Most authors believe that a traumatic etiology has an integral role in the pathogenesis of a vast majority of OLTs. It is hypothesized that they represent the chronic phase of a talar dome compression fracture. A single event of macrotrauma or repetitive microtrauma may initiate the lesion in an individual already predisposed to talar dome ischemia. The development of a symptomatic OLT depends on various factors. The primary mechanism is damage and insufficient repair of the subchondral bone plate.

CLINICAL PRESENTATION

The diagnosis of an OLT is rarely made immediately after an acute ankle injury. In most cases, it is associated with chronic ankle pain that develops after a traumatic incident, commonly an inversion injury to the lateral ligamentous complex. Patients presenting with an OLT often describe prolonged pain, recurrent ankle swelling, weakness, and subjective instability. The pain is commonly described as deep in the ankle. Patients may also report mechanical symptoms, including catching, clicking, and locking. The physical examination often reveals tenderness at the level of the ankle mortise anteriorly or posteriorly. Ligamentous insufficiency or laxity may be present and should always be evaluated, as it will help guide potential treatment. The examination, however, may be benign; thus, the history is usually the best way to assess for the possibility of an OLT. A high index of suspicion for an OLT must be maintained when evaluating patients with chronic ankle pain.

IMAGING/CLASSIFICATION

Advanced imaging modalities have significantly increased our ability to accurately diagnose OLTs. CT is predominantly utilized as an adjunct for a more comprehensive evaluation and preoperative planning of known lesions. MRI is the preferred imaging study for detection of a suspected OLT that is not seen on initial plain radiographs (Figure 57.1). It is also extremely useful for further evaluation and staging of a known OLT. MRI provides improved three-dimensional localization and sizing of the lesion. It also aids in the assessment of stability and determination of the presence of a cystic component.

NONSURGICAL TREATMENT

A trial of nonoperative management for OLTs is appropriate for nondisplaced lesions. While several authors recommend a 3-month period of conservative treatment, there remains no clear consensus on the ideal regimen. Nonoperative treatment ranges from non–weight bearing in a cast to protected weight bearing in a boot.

Nonoperative treatment should include a course of physical therapy following immobilization. The active treatment progression may follow a very similar course as the postoperative regimen, although the speed of progression will be

Dr. Farber or an immediate family member has stock or stock options held in JMEA Corporation; has received research or institutional support from Innocoll; and serves as a board member, owner, officer, or committee member of the American Academy of Orthopaedic Surgeons. Neither of the following authors nor any immediate family member has received anything of value from or has stock or stock options held in a commercial company or institution related directly or indirectly to the subject of this article: Dr. Freeland and Dr. Tyndall.

© 2018 American Academy of Orthopaedic Surgeons

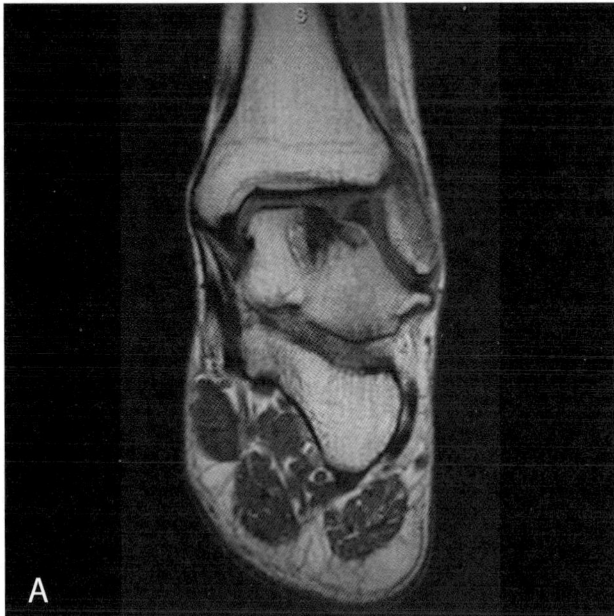

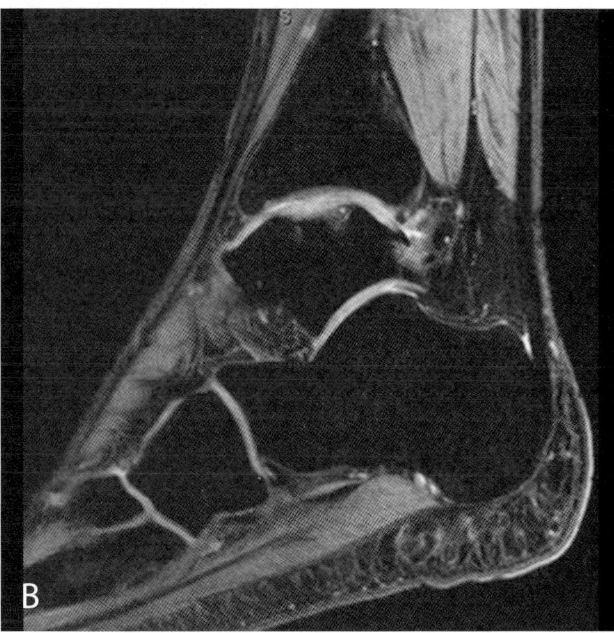

Figure 57.1 **A**, Coronal T1-weighted MRI depicting a large lateral uncontained OCLT. **B**, Sagittal T2-weighted MRI of the same patient. (Adapted from Mintz DN, Tashjian GS, Connell DA, Deland JT, O'Malley M, Potter HG: Osteochondral lesions of the talus: A new magnetic resonance grading system with arthroscopic correlation. *Arthroscopy* 2003;9:353–359.)

based primarily on patient symptoms and response rather than time. Most patients will also benefit from manual therapy. Components of manual therapy include joint mobilizations to distract the talus, which allows for better anterior-posterior or medial-lateral alignment. Soft-tissue release to the peroneals, gastrocnemius-soleus complex, and anterior compartment may allow for decompression of the joint that occurs due to compensatory overuse of the lower leg musculature.

SURGICAL TREATMENT

Surgical intervention is indicated for acute displaced osteochondral lesions and for those lesions refractory to conservative care. The surgical approach and objectives of surgery are variable and dictated by the type of lesion. Furthermore, patient-specific goals must be strongly considered prior to proceeding with surgical management. Goals may include removal of a loose fragment or securing a larger fragment anatomically. However, the primary objective is to create an environment for functional fibrocartilaginous proliferation or resurfacing with hyaline cartilage to restore more normal joint function.

The primary traditional approach includes open-ankle arthrotomy. Numerous exposure methods have been described, including several variations of medial malleolar osteotomies, distal tibial osteotomies, along with combined anterior and posterior arthrotomies. Open approaches involve significant tissue trauma and, as a result, may be associated with postoperative stiffness, prolonged rehabilitation time, and poor cosmetic appearance.

Ankle arthroscopy has established itself as a useful tool in both the diagnosis and treatment of osteochondral lesions of the talus. Compared to an extensive open approach, arthroscopy has proven to provide superior visualization of the talar dome along with improved access to the lesion. As a result of recent advances, arthroscopic management of osteochondral lesions of the talus is now the preferred technique whenever possible.

A wide variety of procedures that vary in complexity have been described for the treatment of OLTs. Treatment strategies generally are categorized as primary repair, reparative techniques, or restorative techniques. Primary repair techniques involve stabilizing large, acute, displaced fragments with commercially available metal or bioabsorbable implants. Reparative treatments are marrow-stimulation techniques, which include abrasion arthroplasty, microfracture, and drilling techniques. On occasion, these techniques may require bone grafting of the defect, then marrow stimulations techniques later. The goal of these various techniques is to stimulate fibrocartilaginous proliferation to resurface the talus. Restorative techniques primarily include autologous chondrocyte implantation (ACI), osteochondral autologous transfer system (OATS and mosaicplasty) and fresh osteochondral allograft. The primary goal of these techniques is resurfacing with hyaline cartilage. ACI is a two-stage operation. The first step involves harvesting of the patient's own chrondrocytes, which are then cultured and grown in a laboratory and followed by a surgical procedure for implantation of the chondrocyte suspension beneath a sutured periosteal flap. The OATS is a single stage procedure that involves harvesting an osteoarticular plug, typically from the ipsilateral knee, and implanting it into the talus in a press-fit technique. Mosaicplasty is a term that describes harvesting and transfer of multiple smaller osteoarticular plugs to fill a single large void. Osteochondral allograft involves harvesting a sized matched portion of a fresh cadaveric talus that is often secured to the native talus via screws but may also

© 2018 American Academy of Orthopaedic Surgeons

be implanted in an OATS-type fashion. Future directions in restorative techniques for OLTs include matrix/membrane ACI (MACI), collagen-covered autologous chondrocyte implantation (CACI), arthroscopic allograft/autograft (AAP) with platelet-rich plasma (PRP) implantation, stem cell–mediated cartilage implants, and other scaffolds.

When selecting the appropriate treatment option, there are several important variables to consider. It is imperative to delineate—primarily from advanced imaging (MRI and/or CT)—the type, stability, and displacement of the lesion. Chronicity, size, location, and containment are other important factors to consider. Reparative treatments generally are indicated for lesions that do not involve the extreme medial or lateral margins of the talus and are less than 1.5 cm^2 in size. These techniques are relatively inexpensive, with low morbidity and a high success rate. Restorative techniques are considered for larger and deeper lesions that are not amenable to the reparative techniques previously described.

POSTOPERATIVE REHABILITATION

Due largely to insufficient research, no true consensus exists regarding a formal rehabilitation program and return to sport times after surgical treatment of OLTs. Furthermore, a vast array of literature with high variability in surgical techniques and postoperative treatment protocols limits any definitive conclusions.

Since arthroscopic treatment is the most common surgical intervention, our postoperative rehabilitation protocol is primarily aimed at treatment after excision, curettage of the OLT, and subsequent bone marrow stimulation. Variations of this protocol exist and are dependent primarily on the type, size, and location of the lesion. Often, a more conservative approach is deemed necessary if restorative techniques are utilized to allow time for bone healing.

The general trend of postoperative rehabilitation in recent years has been to move away from "time-based" protocols to more functional or "criteria-based" protocols. This allows each program to be tailored to the deficits and weaknesses of each patient, as well as to their sport-specific goals. Our protocol consists primarily of time-based phases early, with the primary goal of ensuring bone and cartilage healing and patient symptom control. As the patient progresses and healing has taken place, we transition to functional criteria for progression.

Rehabilitation begins at week 2 following an initial period of postoperative immobilization and non–weight bearing (Table 57.1). The protocol initiates with active ankle range of motion (ROM) and proximal strengthening at 2 weeks postoperatively. The patient remains non–weight bearing, and efforts are focused on edema control and pain management.

Once weight bearing is initiated in a CAM boot at 6 weeks postoperatively, progressive resistance exercises are introduced along with gentle stretching maneuvers. Around week 10, the patient is weaned from CAM boot immobilization for weight-bearing rehabilitation activities. At approximately 12 weeks, the patient may start weaning from the boot for daily activities, although a lace up ankle brace may be used to supplement ankle strength for prolonged standing or walking, if needed. At this point, proprioceptive, cardiovascular, and closed kinetic chain training are introduced while progressive resistance exercises are advanced. Manual treatments to aid in ROM improvements and activity advancement are also included.

At 3 months after surgery, strengthening continues; proprioceptive training intensifies through the sixth month. Once the patient is approximately 6 months postoperative and given adequate clinical improvement and without radiographic or surgical concerns, the patient can be advanced to impact and sport-specific training, and back to actual sport activity as soon as adequate strength and stability are demonstrated.

Throughout this prolonged period of recovery, it is important to consider the patient's insurance benefits for therapy. Treatment quality should never be compromised, but understanding of potential treatment limitations—such as allowed number of visits, copay amounts, and other confounding variables—can help to determine the optimal rehabilitation schedule. It may be beneficial for patients to be seen for 1 to 2 visits during the early phases and to initiate proximal strengthening and resistance band ankle strengthening as a home program. This allows the patient to maximize visits for functional recovery.

Monitoring of patient progress is critical for a successful rehabilitation program. One element of this is standardizing assessments of ROM and strengthening. Dorsiflexion range can be measured in many ways. A reproducible method of measurement has the patient in long-sitting position, while instructing the patient to keep the forefoot inverted and actively dorsiflexing. This allows the therapist to palpate Achilles and hindfoot alignment while visualizing subtalar and talar neutral positions. In this position, both the talar surface is protected and chronic midfoot deviations can be minimized while gastrocnemius-soleus flexibility loss can be assessed. Most patients will be able achieve up to 8° to 10° of dorsiflexion with this measurement technique at full recovery.

Inversion and eversion ROM and strength assessments can also vary. By performing ROM and manual strength testing in a plantar-flexed position, the posterior tibialis and peroneals can be isolated from the extensor compartment, resulting in more accurate grading of medial-lateral muscular stability and excursion. This also allows the patient to perform medial-lateral motion of the talus without compressing the repaired talar surface. Full 5/5 strength is assessed over 5 seconds of progressive resistance without failure or dorsiflexion compensation.

Gastrocnemius-soleus strength testing should initially be performed in non–weight bearing to determine the patient's ability to activate or sustain a muscle contraction. However, as the patient progresses through rehabilitation, this should be advanced to a weight-bearing heel raise assessment. A patient should be able to perform a full double-leg heel raise, then achieve repetitive single-leg eccentric control prior to completing single-leg heel raises. The strength assessment should include observation for loss of height, knee flexion compensation, or even inversion/eversion off the midline second ray. Full

© 2018 American Academy of Orthopaedic Surgeons

Table 57.1 POSTOPERATIVE PROTOCOL FOR OSTEOCHONDRAL LESIONS OF THE TALUS

Phase	Therapy

Phase 1: Protective NWB (weeks 0–6)	• Cast × 2 weeks
	• Weeks 2–6 CAM boot with AROM of ankle
	• Initiate proximal strengthening program
	  • Straight Leg Raises (SLR) × 4 planes
	  • Clamshells
	  • Upper Body Ergometer (UBE) and upper body strengthening
	  • Mat core stabilization program
	• Instruct patient in edema control (modalities, elevation)

Phase 2: Protective WB (weeks 6–9)	• Progressive PWB in CAM boot, as tolerated
	• Initiate 4-way resistance bands
	• Inversion/eversion strengthening performed in plantarflexed position (Figures 57.2 and 57.3)
	  • Performed twice daily
	  • Build from 30–90 reps before progressing resistance level
	• Initiate light gastrocnemius towel stretching with the forefoot inverted (Figure 57.4)
	• Continue edema control

Phase 3: Normalize Gait (weeks 10–12)	• Initiate weight-bearing out of boot during therapy activities
	• Continue resistance band strengthening at home
	• Progress to WB lunge or slantboard gastrocnemius stretches in subtalar neutral
	• Initiate soleus stretching within pain-free capacity
	• Start proprioceptive training within pain-free capacity
	  • Singe Limb Stance (SLS) progression
	• Start WB cardio
	  • Bike first, progress to elliptical, as tolerated
	• Start light closed kinetic chain (CKC) stabilization
	  • Bridges, mini-squats, forward step-up, light shuttle or leg press
	• Progress ankle strength weight-bearing double-leg heel raises
	• Manual treatment, as needed
	  • Soft tissue work to release lower leg muscles, scar tissue around incision (Figure 57.5)
	  • Posterior talar glides in midrange (pain-free) (Figure 57.6)
	• Modalities for edema/effusion, if needed (ice, electrical stimulation, elevation)

Phase 4: Progressive strengthening (week 12 to 6 months)	• Wean out of boot for daily activities • Advance proprioceptive training once gait is normalized • Initiate step-down, eccentric drills, advanced CKC stabilization • Progress heel rises from double-leg to eccentrics to single leg, as tolerated; add directional resistance with bands
Phase 5: Impact training (6–9 months)	Criteria: • Surgeon clearance • Full proximal chain strength • Minimal 8° of active dorsiflexion* • Minimal repetition 15 single-leg heel raises and 5/5 inversion/eversion strength** • No more than 1 cm difference edema on figure-8 girth assessment • If available, begin with deweighted jumps on shuttle leg press or pilates reformer • Progress to light jog on treadmill • Must use a graded running program • Advance into agility and sport-specific noncontact training when running gait is symmetrical without pain, residual effusion

AROM = active range of motion, NWB = non–weight bearing, PWB = partial weight bearing, WB = weight bearing.
*Measured in long-sit position, forefoot adducted to approximate subtalar neutral.
**Heel raise assessed in single-leg stance to full height in straight leg without knee flexion (quadriceps compensation) or weight bearing on upper extremities. Patient may use light "fingertip" touch for balance. Inversion/eversion strength assessed in plantarflexion position to isolate peroneals and posterior tibialis.

 © 2018 American Academy of Orthopaedic Surgeons

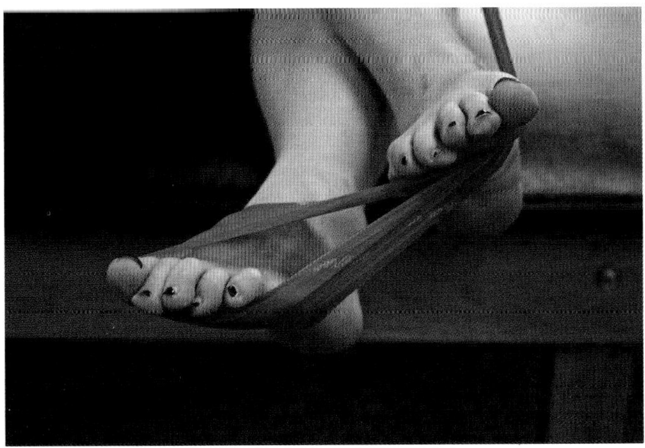

Figure 57.2 Photograph of resisted inversion exercise of the left ankle performed in plantarflexion to isolate the posterior tibialis and off-load the talar surface.

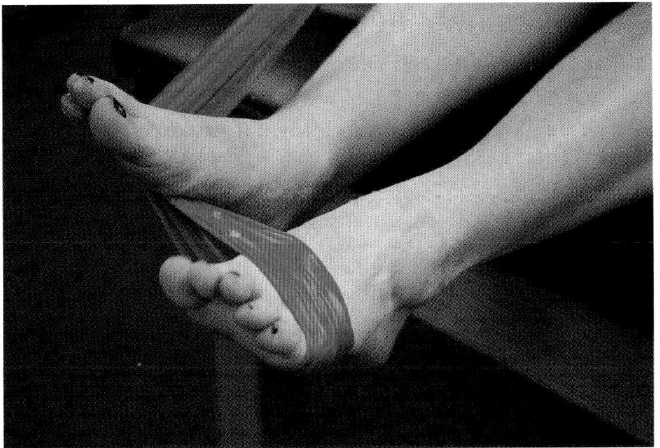

Figure 57.3 Photograph of resisted eversion exercise of the left ankle also performed in plantarflexed position to isolate the peroneals to improve lateral ankle stability.

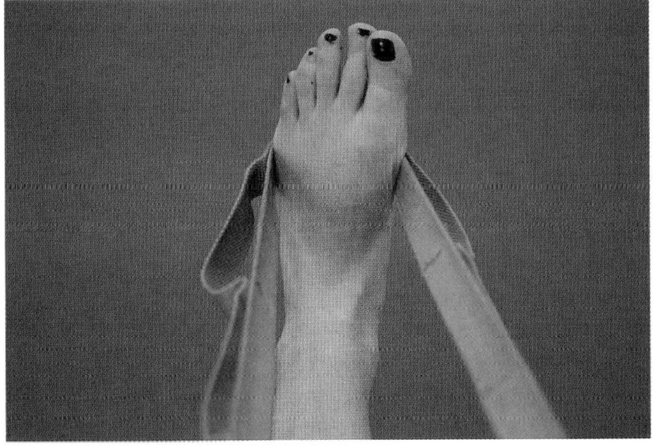

Figure 57.4 Photograph of gastrocnemius towel stretch performed with forefoot adduction, as seen from the patient view. It is important to instruct the patient how to visually find a position not only as close to subtalar neutral as possible, but also within pain-free range.

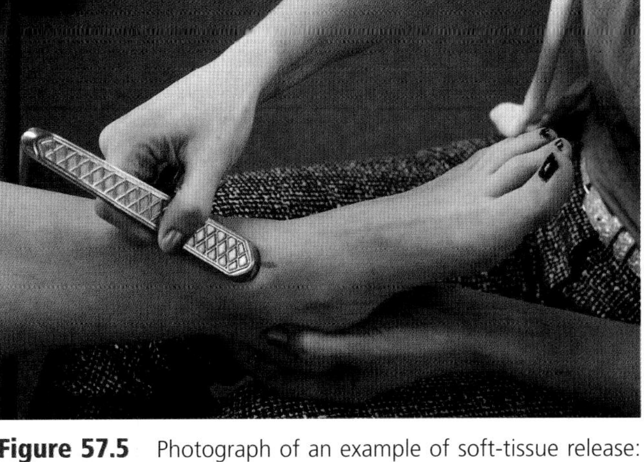

Figure 57.5 Photograph of an example of soft-tissue release: instrument-assisted soft-tissue mobilization (IASTM) performed to medial scar incision to reduce scar-tissue formation and improve anterior capsule mobility.

strength is considered to be at least 20 single-leg heel raises without compensation. Talar or surgical site pain should be considered an important factor in both assessments and activity should be limited to within pain tolerance during the early phases.

Restoring normal gait can be a daunting task for any patient postoperatively, but especially following chronic ankle pain with an OLT. Common compensatory changes to reduce the load on the affected extremity in weight-bearing include proximal chain or hip external rotation and contralateral

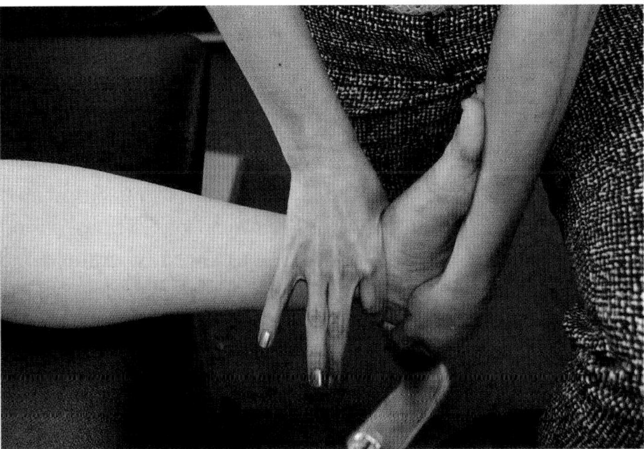

Figure 57.6 Photograph of manual posterior talar glide to the left ankle performed by a therapist. Central dome of talus is placed in the webspace of the right hand while the left hand places the calcaneus in the subtalar neutral position. Manual pressure is applied in an anterior-posterior direction to improve posterior capsule mobility and simulate necessary mechanics to restore the weight-bearing dorsiflexion range needed for gait, stairs, and higher-level impact activities. Other variations can include simple joint distraction through a long axis, or applying a posterior-inferior glide with the mobilizing hand to decrease shear forces over the talar surface.

© 2018 American Academy of Orthopaedic Surgeons

trunk shift, as well as forefoot abduction and hindfoot pronation or supination. Prolonged compensatory strategies can lead to secondary weaknesses of the hip stabilizers, lower abdominal and lower back core musculature, tightness in the gastrocnemius-soleus complex and shortened or lengthened medial-lateral ankle stabilizers. A comprehensive therapy program should focus on eliminating all of these deleterious compensatory measures when present. Computerized gait assessment tools can help, although it is the authors' opinion that this is not required unless gait deviations persist and limit progression of care.

Access to advanced equipment—such as an underwater treadmill or other devices that limit forces of weight bearing—may be limited, but can aide in attaining functional goals at any point in the rehabilitation process. Progressive weight bearing can be initiated without a CAM boot between 6 to 10 weeks postoperatively in a deweighted situation (i.e., 25%–50% body weight, increasing gradually) to allow for neuromuscular re-education of proper gait mechanics. Off-weighted jump training and running can also be performed to advance strength and cardiovascular endurance once a patient is 6 months postoperative. This may be especially helpful for those who may not have achieved all the strength benchmarks for advancement to full body weight impact activities listed in the protocol in Table 57.1.

OUTCOMES

Minimally symptomatic lesions appear to do well over time, with only minor progression. However, Elias et al revealed in a review of serial MRIs of 29 patients who had OLTs that were treated nonsurgically that 45% showed progression, 24% improved, and 31% remained unchanged. Furthermore, a systematic review in 2010 demonstrated that nonsurgical treatment in more symptomatic patients demonstrated only a 53% success rate. This same systematic review of 52 published reports describing the results of 65 treatment groups indicated that most recent publications on treatment of OLTs involving arthroscopic excision and curettage—followed by either bone marrow stimulation, ACI, or OATS—had success rates of 85%, 76%, and 87%, respectively. Success in this review is variably defined by several subjective and objective measures, including resolution of pain and return to preinjury level of function, including sports. In 2013, van Bergen confirmed maintenance of short-term results at 8 to 20 years following surgically treatment with 78% excellent or good results. Polat et al looked at 5-year follow-up of their surgically treated OLTs and found that 42.6% of patients were asymptomatic and 23.1% had minimal symptoms after high-level activity. Almost one-third of their patients had 1 stage of progression of arthrosis (Takakura classification).

There is vast diversity in the literature regarding treatment methods and postoperative protocols, making the results overall quite variable and difficult to compare. While the precise natural history of surgically treated OLTs is unclear, most good results appear to persist over time but with nearly a quarter of patients experiencing lesser outcomes. Overall, however, progression to end-stage osteoarthritis of the ankle has been shown to be an uncommon final outcome.

SUMMARY

The goal of treatment for OLTs is relief of pain and restoration of function. Following surgical intervention, whether reparative or restorative, proper rehabilitation is crucial to returning patients to function and maximally improving their quality of life. Further research and collaboration may help to fine-tune and improve protocols to achieve these goals. Most important, however, focusing on each individual's unique objectives and customizing a comprehensive rehabilitation program to fit the patient provides the greatest chance for success.

BIBLIOGRAPHY

Alexander AH, Lichtman DM: Surgical treatment of transchondral talar-dome fractures (osteochondritis dissecans): Long-term follow-up. *J Bone Joint Surg Am* 1980;62:646–652.

Bauer M, Jonsson K, Lindén B: Osteochondritis dissecans of the ankle. A 20-year follow-up study. *J Bone Joint Surg Br* 1987;69(1):93–96.

Elias I, Jung JW, Raikin SM, Schweitzer MW, Carrino JA, Morrison WB: Osteochondral lesions of the talus: Change in MRI findings over time in talar lesions without operative intervention and implications for staging systems. *Foot Ankle Int* 2006;27(3):157–166.

Elias I, Zoga AC, Morrison WB, Besser MP, Schweitzer ME, Raikin SM: Osteochondral lesions of the talus: localization and morphologic data from 424 patients using a novel anatomical grid scheme. *Foot Ankle Int* 2007;28:154–161.

Ferkel RD, Dierckman BD, Phisitkul P: Arthroscopy of the Foot and Ankle, in Coughlin MJ, Saltzman CL, Anderson RB, eds: *Surgery of the Foot and Ankle,* ed 9. Philadelphia, PA, Elsevier, 2014:1748–1758.

Giannini S, Vannini F: Operative treatment of osteochondral lesions of the talar dome: current concepts review. *Foot Ankle Int* 2004;25:168–175.

Hermanson E, Ferkel RD: Bilateral osteochondral lesions of the talus. *Foot Ankle Int* 2009;30(8):723–727.

Kim HN, Kim GL, Park JY, Woo KJ, Park YW: Fixation of a posteromedial osteochondral lesion of the talus using a three-portal posterior arthroscopic technique. *J Foot Ankle Surg* 2013;52(3):402–405.

Klammer G, Maquieira GJ, Spahn S, Vigfusson V, Zanetti M, Espinosa N: Natural history of nonoperatively treated osteochondral lesions of the talus. *Foot Ankle Int* 2015;36: 24–31.

Polat G, Erşen A, Erdil ME, Kızılkurt T, Kılıçoğlu Ö, Aşık M: Long-term results of microfracture in the treatment of talus osteochondral lesions. *Knee Surg Sports Traumatol Arthrosc* 2016;24(4):1299–1303.

© 2018 American Academy of Orthopaedic Surgeons

van Bergen CJ, Kox LS, Maas M, Sierevelt IN, Kerkhoffs GM, van Dijk CN: Arthroscopic treatment of osteochondral defects of the talus: outcomes at eight to twenty years of follow-up. *J Bone Joint Surg Am* 2013;20;95(6):519–525.

van Dijk CN, Reilingh ML, Zengerink M, van Bergen CJ: Osteochondral defects in the ankle: why painful? Knee Surg Sports. *Traumatol Arthrosc* 2010;18(5):570–580.

Verhagen RA, Struijs PA, Bossuyt PM, van Dijk CN: Systematic review of treatment strategies for osteochondral defects of the talar dome. *Foot Ankle Clin* 2003;8:233–242, viii–ix.

Zengerink M, Struijs PA, Tol JL, van Dijk CN: Treatment of osteochondral lesions of the talus: a systematic review. *Knee Surg Sports Traumatol Arthrosc* 2010;18:238–246.

Zinman C, Wolfson N, Reis ND: Osteochondritis dissecans of the dome of the talus. Computed tomography scanning in diagnosis and follow-up. *J Bone Joint Surg Am* 1988;70: 1017–1019.

© 2018 American Academy of Orthopaedic Surgeons

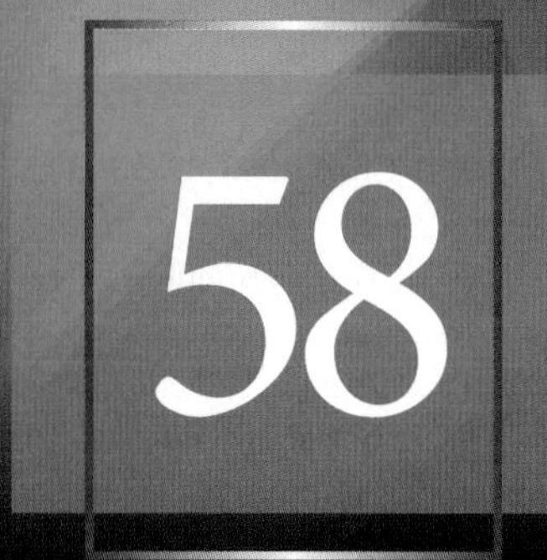

Ankle Instability Surgery

Lan Chen, MD, CarolLynn Meyers, PT, and Oliver Schipper, MD

INTRODUCTION

Lateral ankle ligament complex injuries are a common sport-associated injury. The most common mechanism of injury is inversion and internal rotation of the foot. Nonoperative management, including functional rehabilitation, is the mainstay of treatment for acute injuries. Up to 20% of acute injuries may not respond to conservative management and progress to chronic lateral ankle pain and instability.

The lateral ankle is supported by both static and dynamic restraints. Static structures include the bony congruity of the tibiotalar joint and the lateral ankle ligaments: the anterior talofibular ligament (ATFL), calcaneofibular ligament (CFL), and the posterior talofibular ligament (PTFL). The ATFL is the most commonly injured, and may be the first or only ligament injured with ankle inversion injuries. It acts to limit anterior displacement of the talus when the ankle is in neutral. The ATFL is most commonly composed of two bands (varies from one to three bands) separated by perforating arterial branches. The inferior band is taut in ankle dorsiflexion while the superior band is taut in ankle plantarflexion. The ATFL originates at the anterior edge of the lateral malleolus and runs anteromedially to insert on the lateral talar neck. The ligament is near horizontal with the ankle in neutral position.

The CFL originates from the distal tip of the lateral malleolus just inferior to the ATFL and runs posterior, inferior, and medial to insert on the posterolateral calcaneus. It lies just deep to the peroneal tendons. Laxity in the CFL leads to increased talar tilt when the ankle is stressed to inversion at 90° of neutral position.

The PTFL is the strongest of the three lateral ankle ligaments, and is rarely injured. It originates from the medial surface of the lateral malleolus, deep to the peroneal tendons, and inserts on the lateral tubercle of the talus, just lateral to the flexor hallucis longus. In plantarflexion and neutral, the PTFL is relaxed; in dorsiflexion, the ligament is taut.

The lateral ankle is further supported by the peroneus brevis and peroneus longus tendons, which serve as dynamic stabilizers of the lateral ankle. The tendons run posterior to the fibula in the peroneal groove, held in place by the superior peroneal retinaculum. The tendons then course superficial to the PTFL and CFL to run along the lateral calcaneus under the inferior peroneal retinaculum.

EVALUATION AND TREATMENT OPTIONS

Conservative management is the primary treatment choice for the majority of acute lateral ankle ligament complex injuries, and consists of a short period of immobilization in a walking boot (less then 3 weeks), activity modification, and functional rehabilitation. Physical therapy should emphasize peroneal tendon strengthening, decreasing edema, stretching, gait training, and proprioception. Surgery is reserved for high-level athletes and patients with continued ankle instability despite a course of supervised aggressive physical therapy.

Chronic lateral ankle instability may be defined as mechanical instability of the lateral ankle with or without persistent pain after 3 to 6 months of conservative management. Surgery is contraindicated in patients with lateral ankle pain in the absence of lateral ankle instability. Relative contraindications include connective tissue disorders (e.g., Ehlers-Danlos syndrome), peripheral vascular disease, and patients that cannot follow postoperative protocols. An MRI without contrast is obtained preoperatively to evaluate the ankle for other pathologies, including concomitant osteochondral lesions, peroneal tendon pathology, bone bruising, or impingement. An MRI can also show lax or wavy ligaments or nonvisualization of the lateral ankle ligaments. Another important preoperative consideration is the presence of hindfoot deformity. A varus hindfoot increases the risk of lateral ankle ligament complex injuries, and increases stress on the lateral ligament complex repair. All pathologies that are associated with chronic ankle stability should be addressed at the time of surgery. The presence of these concomitant findings may alter final rehabilitation protocol based on severity of pathology and clinician preference.

None of the following authors or any immediate family member has received anything of value from or has stock or stock options held in a commercial company or institution related directly or indirectly to the subject of this article: Dr. Chen, Dr. Meyers, and Dr. Schipper.

© 2018 American Academy of Orthopaedic Surgeons

SURGICAL PROCEDURE

Modified Bröstrom Procedure

Anatomic lateral ankle complex reconstruction is favored over nonanatomic reconstruction. The modified Bröstrom procedure is an anatomic repair of the lateral ankle ligaments indicated for chronic ankle instability despite conservative treatment. Ankle baseline motion and stability are evaluated under anesthesia.

Ankle arthroscopy is frequently indicated for patients with any intra-articular pathology as determined by preoperative imaging. The patient is positioned supine with a small bump under the ipsilateral hip to internally rotate the ankle. If arthroscopy is indicated, a noninvasive ankle distractor is applied, and the joint is insufflated. A standard anteromedial portal is created using a blunt trocar for a 2.7-mm arthroscope. An anterolateral portal is created via transillumination to avoid superficial peroneal nerve branches and dorsal veins of the ankle. Intra-articular pathology is addressed, followed by lateral ligament repair or reconstruction.

A posterior curved incision that starts posterior to the fibula is used. This incision allows repair of the peroneal tendons along with the lateral ankle ligaments. The proximal edge of the inferior extensor retinaculum is dissected first and mobilized. The superficial peroneal and sural nerves are avoided. The peroneal tendons just inferior to the fibula tip are retracted distally to allow visualization of the CFL.

A U-shaped incision of the deeper tissues along the anterior inferior border of the distal fibula is performed, being careful to resect the soft tissue close to the bone of the distal fibula. The anterior talofibular ligament/capsular confluence is examined, and often found to be attenuated. The CFL is visualized as well.

The origin of the ATFL and CFL is débrided to create a healing bed. Two suture anchors or bone tunnels are then placed at the origin of the ATFL and CFL. Prior to tightening the repair, the foot is placed in neutral and slight eversion with a posterior force placed on the foot. The lax ATFL and CFL are then reapproximated and secured to their respective origins.

The repair is reinforced by repairing the inferior extensor retinaculum to the periosteum of the distal fibula with interrupted sutures (Gould modification). The peroneal tendons are now also examined for synovitis or tearing. The ankle is ranged prior to closure of the skin. A final check of the anterior drawer and talar tilt is performed to confirm stability. The patient is placed in a well-padded splint in the neutral position.

Graft Reconstruction

Graft reconstruction or augmentation is indicated for patients with attenuated, irreparable ligament tissue, obese patients, or high-demand athletes who place more stress on their ankles. Graft options include the peroneus brevis, gracilis, plantaris, or allograft tendon. The gracilis or plantaris tendon is preferred over use of the peroneus brevis because the peroneus brevis is an important dynamic stabilizer of the lateral ankle. Allograft tendon can be used in patients who wish to avoid donor site morbidity.

An extensile lateral ankle incision is used starting along the peroneal tendons and extending it over the lateral malleolus. This is a larger exposure than that used in the modified Bröstrom technique. Again, the proximal edge of the inferior peroneal retinaculum is visualized and mobilized. The ATFL/anterolateral ankle joint capsule is incised, as is the CFL. If the ligaments are not repairable, a gracilis autograft is used.

Multiple techniques have been described for fixation of the tendon autograft, including drill tunnels in the fibula, talus, and calcaneus. Many surgeons prefer using interference screw fixation at the insertion of the ATFL and CFL. First, the graft size is measured. With an appropriately sized drill for the graft size, a fibula tunnel is started at the origin of the CFL, exiting posteriorly on the fibula. The peroneal tendons are retracted posteriorly for visualization of the tunnel exit on the fibula. Another drill hole is started at the origin of the ATFL and also exists posterior to the fibula, about 1 cm proximally, giving a 1-cm posterior fibula bone bridge. The gracilis graft is passed through the ATFL and CFL bone tunnels. Fixation at the respective insertions of the ATFL and CFL on the lateral talar neck and lateral calcaneus is performed with interference screw fixation. Stress testing is performed with anterior drawer and inversion stress of the ankle.

It is important to avoid anterior translation of the talus when tensioning the graft by placing a bump under the distal tibia and avoiding placing a bump under the heel.

Complications of Surgery

The most common postoperative complications of lateral ankle ligament repair and reconstruction are nerve-related. Other complications include wound problems, infection, loss of motion of the ankle, recurrent instability, and deep vein thrombosis. Nerve injury is often treated with desensitization. In the case of recurrent instability, revision surgery may be offered in select cases depending on the index surgery and causes of failure.

POSTOPERATIVE REHABILITATION

Rehabilitation after lateral ankle ligament repair or reconstruction is started after a short period of immobilization and the skin incision has healed. It is focused on restoration of ankle motion, strength, proprioception, balance, and muscle endurance. Improvements in neuromuscular control lead to decreased risk of reinjury following rehabilitation and, ultimately, improved global function and return to sport.

Protocol

0 to 5 Weeks

- Cast immobilization, non–weight bearing for 2 weeks, progressive weight bearing in cast from week 3 to 5.

5 to 12 Weeks

- Cast removal, weight bearing as tolerated in walking boot, initiate formal physical therapy
  - Functional goals for this stage of rehabilitation: achieve double-limb balance on solid surface, then unstable surface, initiate single limb balance
    1. Active range of motion (AROM)/passive range of motion (PROM) for plantarflexion, dorsiflexion,

© 2018 American Academy of Orthopaedic Surgeons

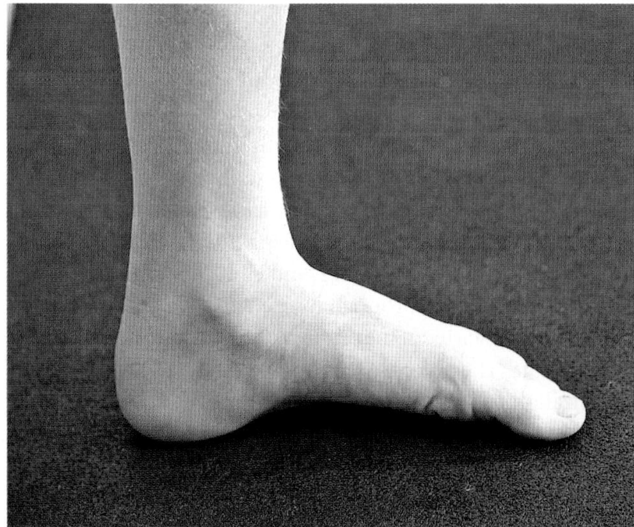

Figure 58.1 Photograph of patient in sitting position with foot on floor, actively lifting arch for intrinsic strengthening.

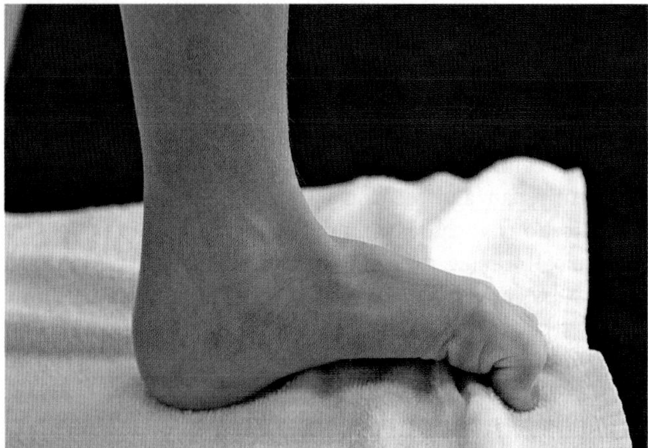

Figure 58.2 Photograph of seated towel curl strengthening exercise.

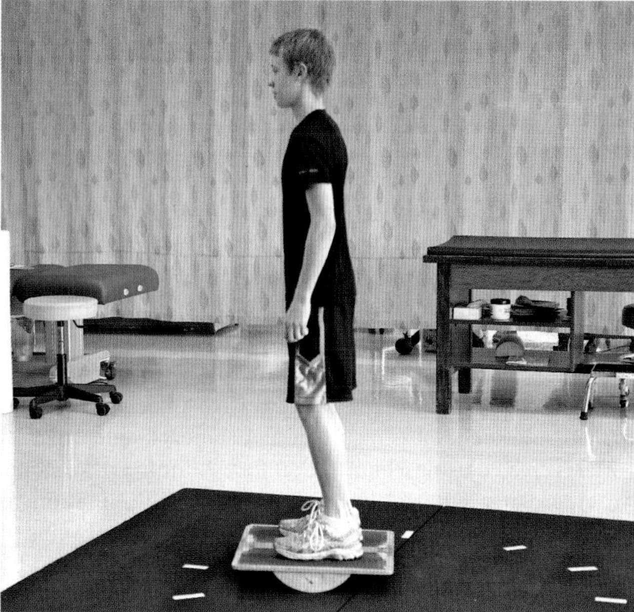

Figure 58.4 Photograph of basic static balance exercise with bilateral support on unstable surface.

and eversion of the ankle, AROM/PROM digits, foot intrinsic muscle strengthening (Figures 58.1 and 58.2).

2. No active or passive inversion of the ankle (until 12 weeks).
3. Gastrocnemius and soleus stretches in non–weight bearing and weight-bearing positions (i.e., setting and standing).
4. Edema control: cryotherapy, compression stockings, compression bandaging techniques.
5. Ice for pain and swelling control.
6. Scar and soft tissue mobilization.
7. Initiate and progress through balance and functional exercises (Figures 58.3–58.8), including star excursion balance exercises (Figures 58.9 and 58.10).

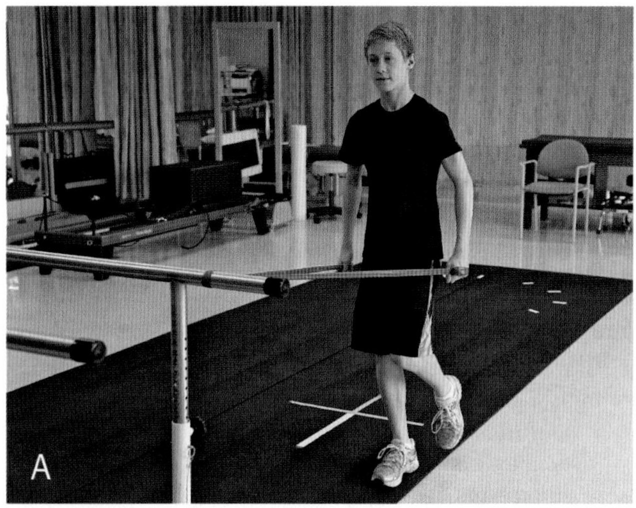

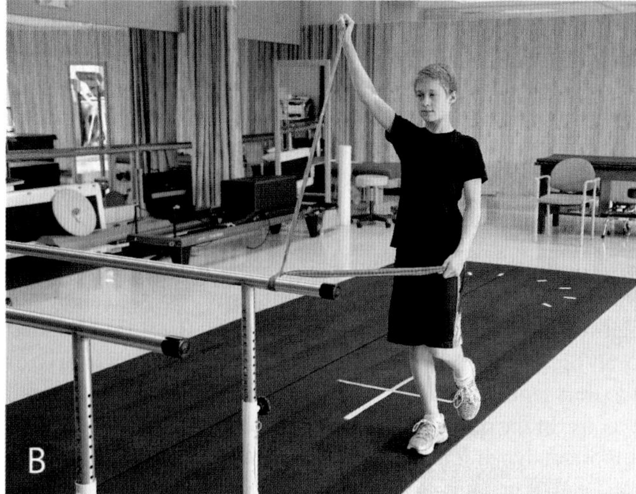

Figure 58.3 **A**, **B**, Photograph of unilateral balance activity on stable surface with upper extremity resistance. Movement patterns can be simulated to be sport- or activity-specific.

 © 2018 American Academy of Orthopaedic Surgeons

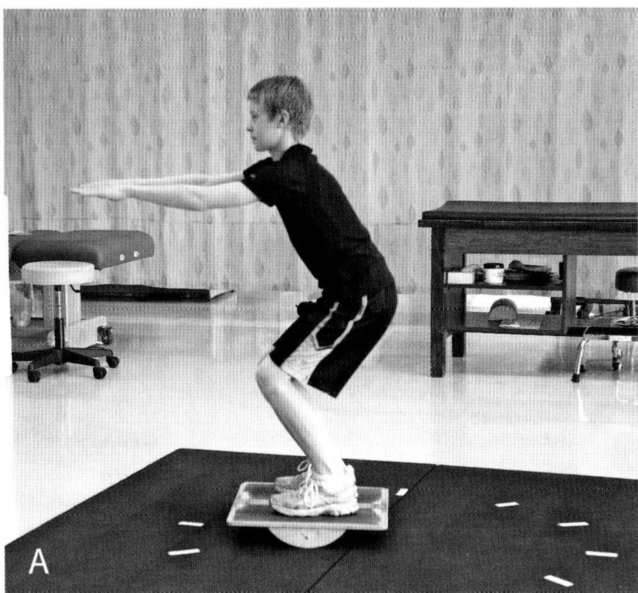

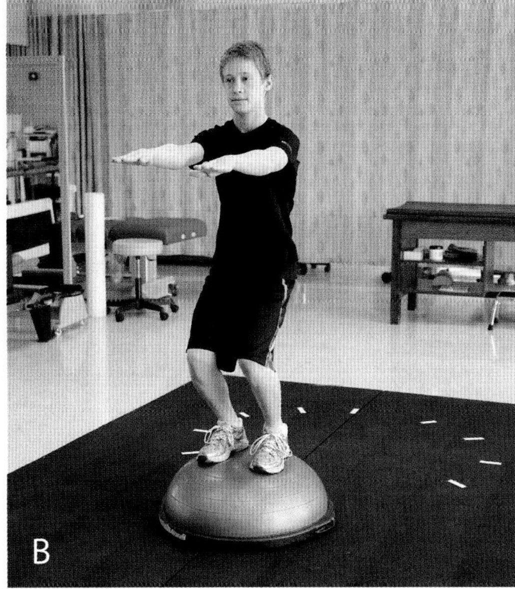

Figure 58.5 **A**, **B**, Photograph of dynamic balance exercises combining unstable surface with functional movement.

12 to 16 Weeks

- Progress to supportive, athletic shoe with lace-up ankle brace.
    - Functional goals for this stage of rehabilitation: achieve single-limb balance on solid surface, then unstable surface with supportive brace or taping.
        1. Continue above PT progression, initiate plyometrics and agility drills.

16 Weeks

- Progress to shoes only, no ankle supportive device.
    - Functional goals for this stage of rehabilitation: achieve and improve performance agility drills, start running, back to sport and sport-specific drills are started, perform functional outcome testing with star excursion balance testing and hop testing (Figure 58.11)

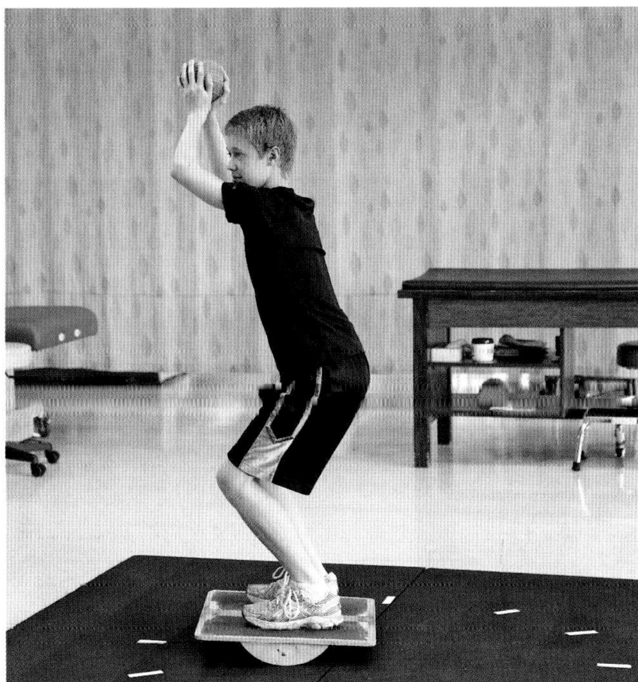

Figure 58.6 Photograph of advanced dynamic balance exercise with use of unstable surface and resisted upper extremity motion with weight (ball weight).

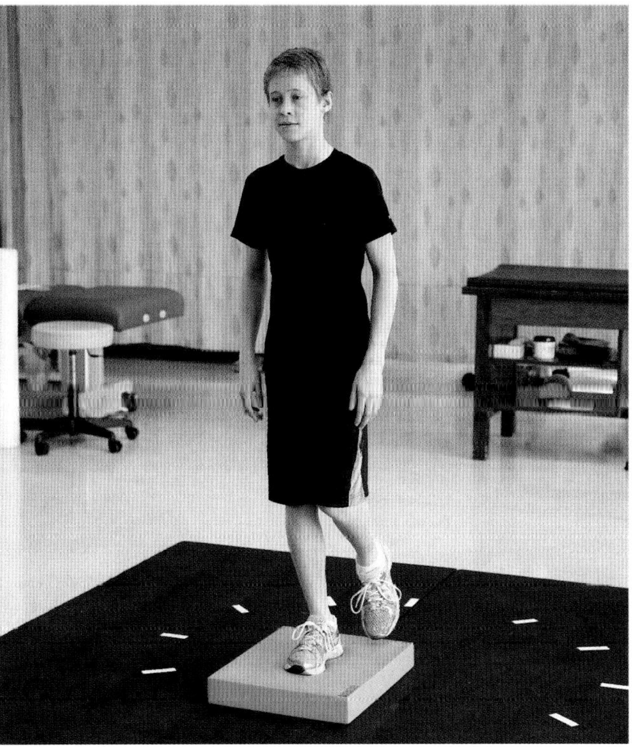

Figure 58.7 Photograph of single-leg balance on unstable surface.

© 2018 American Academy of Orthopaedic Surgeons

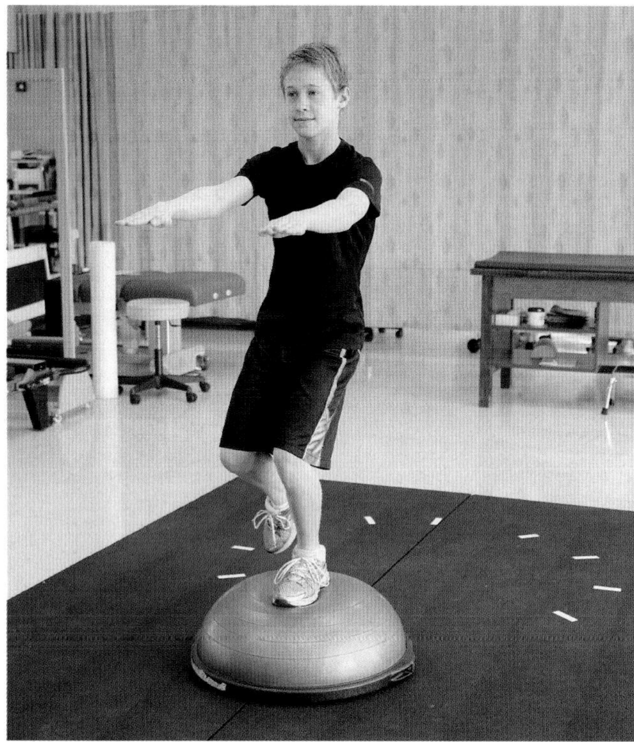

Figure 58.8 Photograph of single-leg balance on unstable surface with functional upper extremity reaches.

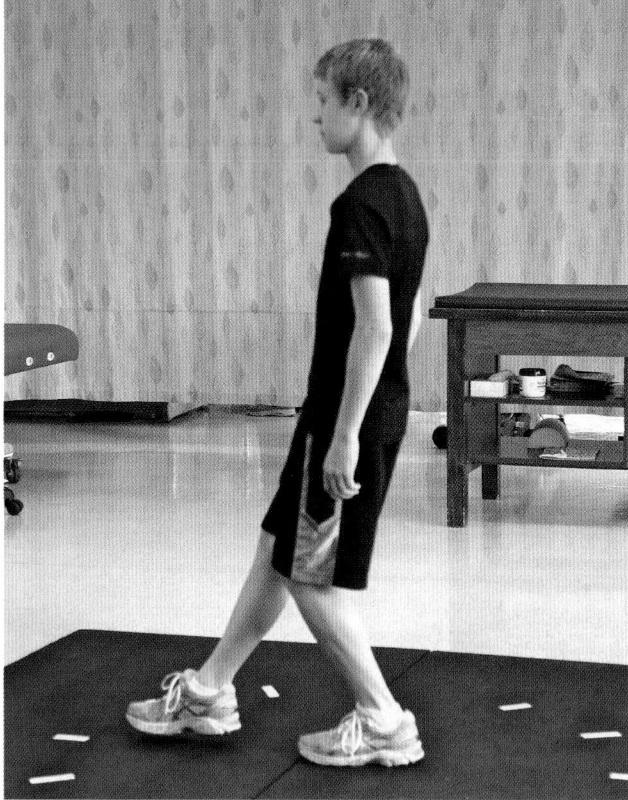

Figure 58.9 Photograph of anterior lower extremity reach exercise.

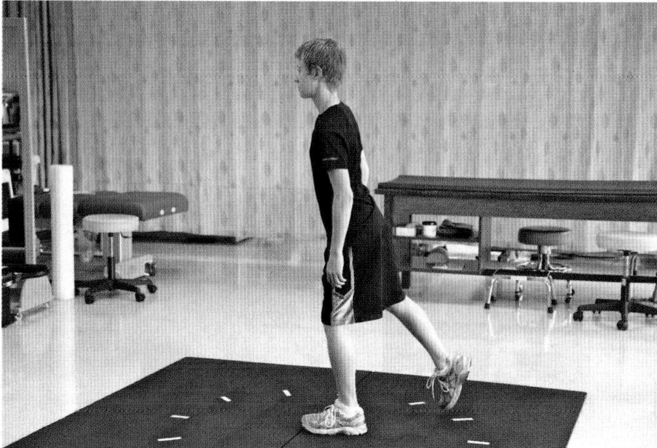

Figure 58.10 Photograph of posterior lower extremity reach exercise.

1. Progress plyometrics, agility exercises for return to sport practice and competition when functional targets are met.

Physical Therapy Specifics

- Active and passive motion of the digits, foot intrinsic muscle strengthening
- Balance and functional exercises:
  Static balance activities should be a precursor to more dynamic activities. Static activities can be initiated as soon as able to weight bear on the lower extremity. General progression of static balance activities is from bilateral to unilateral and from stable to unstable surfaces (foam mat,

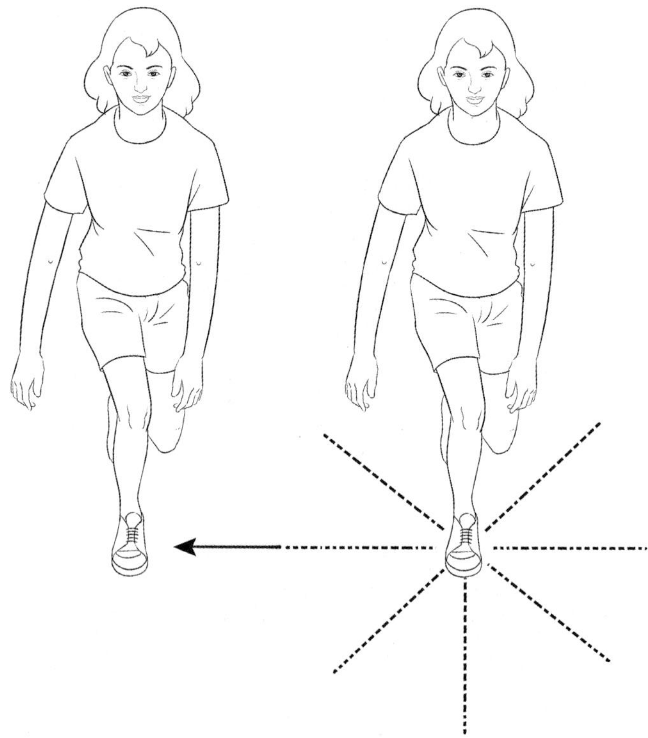

Figure 58.11 Illustration of the hop test.

© 2018 American Academy of Orthopaedic Surgeons

balance boards, balance ball). As the activity becomes easier to perform, activities to distract concentration can be added, such as throwing or catching a ball). Forces added by throwing and catching a ball simulate balance reactions needed for the progression to plyometric activities.

Star Excursion Balance Exercises

These functional exercises include reaches, lunges, and jumping progressions. Initial work is in the frontal plane, with progression to the sagittal and then transverse planes of motion. Progress is determined by tolerance of repetitions and excursion of the exercises. These can also be progressed from performance on a stable surface to an unstable surface, such as a foam mat.

Plyometrics/Agility Drills

Double-leg jump rope is a good tool for early plyometric activity. Progression can be to alternate leg jumping. Initiate a straightforward running program, with a progression of distance first and then speed. Initiate progression to cutting activities, direction changes, and tempo changes. Multidirectional drills or more advanced agility work is important, especially in the athletic population. Include jumping with 2-foot take-off and 2-foot landing, hopping with one-foot take-off and same-foot landing. Also include bounding with-one foot take-off and opposite-foot landing. Add obstacles and direction changes for further challenges.

OUTCOMES

Ankle instability surgery is most commonly performed to return patients to high functional demand activity, such as sport or dance. In general, these goals are attained in the motivated patient with good rehabilitation and well-performed surgery. The time frame is variable but may take 6 or more months depending on the specific needs and the injury. Minor symptoms may persist but do not preclude high-level activity. A graded return to activity is critical. Functional testing may be useful in this regard.

Functional Outcome Tests

A patient's performance on these two tests is used starting at week 16 to assess improvement of the operated extremity compared to the contralateral extremity. These objective measurements help guide a patient's return to sport.

Star Excursion Balance Tests

The patient stands on one foot and reaches as far as possible in each of 8 directions with the other foot, touching down on the return and completing the task upon returning to the starting position. The 8 directions extend out into a circle, and each target line is 45° from the adjacent lines (anterior reach, anteromedial reach, medial reach, posterior medial reach, posterior, posterolateral reach, lateral reach, anterior lateral reach). The quality and control of movement is assessed, as well as comparison of distance of reach right and left.

Hop Testing

There are a variety of hop test options for assessing performance with lateral movements and direction changes. The lateral hop for distance and the side hop tests are appropriate for the lateral ankle instability and postoperative modified Bröstom patient. The lateral hop for distance measures the distance that an individual travels laterally in 3 continuous hops on a single limb. The goal is 80% or greater when compared to the uninjured side. Another hop test is the side hop, in which the amount of time needed to hop lateral back and forth over a 30-cm distance for 10 repetitions is measured.

BIBLIOGRAPHY

Bell SJ, Mologne TS, Sitler DF, Cox JS: Twenty-six-year results after Bröstrom procedure for chronic lateral ankle instability. *Am J Sports Med* 2006;34:975–978.

Boyer DS, Younger AS: Anatomic reconstruction of the lateral ankle ligament complex of the ankle using a gracilis autograft. *Foot Ankle Clin* 2006;11:585–595.

Coughlin MJ, Schenck RC Jr, Grebing BR, Treme G: Comprehensive reconstruction of the lateral ankle for chronic instability using a free gracilis graft. *Foot Ankle Int* 2004;25:231–241.

Gólano P, Vega J, de Leeuw PAJ, Malagelada F, Manzanares MC, Götzens V, van Dijk CN: Anatomy of the ankle ligaments: a pictorial essay. *Knee Surg Sports Traumatol Arthrosc* 2010;18:557–569.

Jakubietz MG, Jakubietz DF, Gruenert JG, Zahn R, Meffert RH, Jakubietz RG: Adequacy of palmaris longus and plantaris tendons for tendon grafting. *J Hand Surg Am* 2011;36(4):695–698.

Maffulli N, Ferran N: Management of acute and chronic ankle instability. *J Am Acad Orthop Surg* 2008;16:608–615.

Vienne P, Schöniger R, Helmy N, Espinosa N: Hindfoot instability in cavovarus deformity: static and dynamic balancing. *Foot Ankle Int* 2007;28(1):96–102.

Wiesel SW, ed. *Operative Techniques in Orthopaedic Surgery*. Philadelphia, Wolters Kluwer/Lippincott Williams & Wilkins, 2011, vol 2, pp 4301–4346.

© 2018 American Academy of Orthopaedic Surgeons

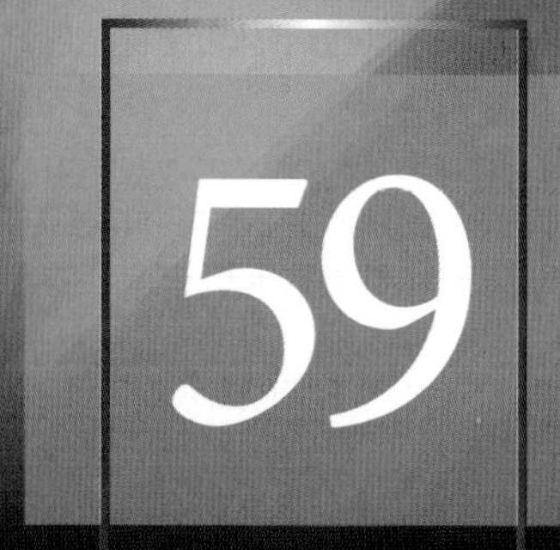

Achilles Tendon Reconstruction

Heather E. Hensl, PA-C, MPH, Anthony D'Angelo, MS, PT, ACT, CSCS, and Andrew K. Sands, MD

INTRODUCTION

The Achilles tendon is the conjoined tendon of the gastrocnemius, soleus, and plantaris, which inserts into a 2 cm × 2 cm area on the posterosuperior aspect of the calcaneus. It is the longest and strongest tendon in the human body, withstanding forces up to 10 times body weight during running and jumping activities. The Achilles derives its blood supply from the muscle tissue proximally and the calcaneal insertion distally, leaving the midsection to rely on the paratenon encasing it. A hypovascular watershed area is often described from 2 to 6 cm above the insertion. Given the strength demands on the Achilles and the vascularity surrounding it, proper postoperative rehabilitation is crucial in promoting the dynamic nature of the tendon, capable of responding to progressive stresses, while still protecting the tendon repair from tensile forces during the healing process.

Surgical repairs of the Achilles fall into the following categories: (1) direct repair for acute Achilles rupture, (2) reconstruction of the Achilles with flexor hallucis longus (FHL) transfer for chronic ruptures or tendinopathy unresponsive to nonoperative treatment, or (3) débridement of degenerative tissue with partial calcanectomy and proximal calf lengthening for chronic insertional Achilles tendinosis.

Diagnosis is usually made by physical examination. Imaging studies, such as MRI and ultrasound, might be helpful in assessing the quality of the tendon, the size of the gap and possible approximation of the tendon if nonoperative closed treatment is considered. These factors are important in deciding on the type of reconstruction chosen.

SURGICAL PROCEDURES

Primary Repair of Acute Achilles Tendon Rupture

Diagnosis is made by history and physical examination. Patients will report hearing a pop or feeling a snap in the posterior leg, followed by acute pain and difficulty walking. They will not be able to rise on their toes. There will be a palpable gap within the tendon itself, most typically in that watershed region 2 to 6 cm proximal to the calcaneal insertion. The Thompson test will be abnormal, demonstrating no ankle plantar flexion with the patient prone.

Open repair of the Achilles may facilitate an earlier return to normal activities and return to work than nonoperative treatment. Many surgeons feel that an accurate repair of the tendon gives the patient the best chance at restoration of functional strength, with to a faster return to sports, and a potentially lower incidence of re-rupture in younger patients and explosive sporting activities. In patients with histories significant for diabetes, morbid obesity, renal failure, chronic corticosteroid use, or chronic peripheral edema, nonoperative treatment should be considered. Vascular insufficiency is considered a relative contraindication to operative treatment. Recently, nonoperative functional treatment has shown increasing success, however, with re-rupture rates approaching the low rates seen in surgically treated ruptures without the surgical complications of tendon adhesion, wound dehiscence, and infection. Functional treatment is therefore an option in a compliant patient not participating in elite-level sport. Ultimately, the decision for the form of treatment is made by the surgeon and patient.

Dr. Sands or an immediate family member is a member of a speakers' bureau or has made paid presentations on behalf of Synthes; serves as a paid consultant to Synthes; has stock or stock options held in Amgen and Pfizer; has received research or institutional support from Synthes; has received nonincome support (such as equipment or services), commercially derived honoraria, or other non-research–related funding (such as paid travel) from Saunders/Mosby-Elsevier; and serves as a board member, owner, officer, or committee member of the AO Foundation. Neither of the following authors nor any immediate family member has received anything of value from or has stock or stock options held in a commercial company or institution related directly or indirectly to the subject of this article: Dr. D'Angelo and Dr. Hensl.

© 2018 American Academy of Orthopaedic Surgeons

The goal of the procedure is to restore the integrity of the tendon at the appropriate length to allow for rehabilitation. Theoretically, delaying surgery by approximately 1 week after rupture allows for the consolidation of tendon ends and decreased soft-tissue swelling, making the repair technically easier. Straight posterior or posteromedial approaches are the two most commonly used incisions. Supine positioning with a large contralateral bump through the posteromedial approach offers a decreased chance of skin problems and easy access should FHL transfer be needed unexpectedly. Some surgeons prefer the prone position.

The surgical incision is made just posteromedial over the medial tendon. This approach also prevents injury to the sural nerve. To minimize wound complications, careful soft-tissue techniques must be performed, taking care not to traumatize skin edges or make any flaps. The dissection should be performed sharply directly down to the paratenon. To minimize subsequent adhesions between the tendon repair and the skin, the paratenon should be opened with care to allow its closure after the repair. The tendon repair should be made with the ankle in neutral position, not in maximum plantar flexion. If the repair cannot be achieved in neutral position, an FHL transfer may be used to bridge any gap. A strong, braided, nonabsorbable suture is used in performing the repair, typically following a Bunnell or Krachow-Hungerford pattern. Alternately, or additionally, a suture anchor may be employed to further secure the repair, and is inserted into the calcaneus. Care should be taken to bury knots under or within the tendon whenever possible, as prominent suture knots are irritating to the patient and can lead to complications in skin healing. Meticulous wound closure in layers is performed to include the paratenon, followed by a bulky compressive dressing and plaster splint application, with the ankle placed in a neutral position. This splint remains on for 10 to 12 days postoperatively.

Complications of Achilles repair can include sural nerve injury, infection, wound healing problems, and scar sensitivity.

Repair of Achilles with Excision/Débridement of Nonviable Tissue and FHL Transfer

This technique is used for acute-on-chronic ruptures or chronic Achilles tendinopathy unresponsive to nonoperative treatment. Acute-on-chronic ruptures should be suspected in patients who report a previous history of calf tightness, Achilles tendonitis, plantar fasciitis or history of playing sports with ankle sprains and Achilles strains, with concomitant equinus contracture on physical examination. A gastrocnemius contracture plays a definitive role in Achilles pathology, and isolated tightness of the gastrocnemius can place excess tension on the Achilles, leading to Achilles and plantar fascia disorders. Be sure to examine the patient's contralateral leg for equinus contracture (Silfverskiöld test), and to evaluate lateral radiographs for evidence of calcifications within the Achilles tendon or posterosuperior calcaneal spurs, all suggestive of a more longstanding tendinopathy. In the presence of such findings, especially in older patients or sports participants, surgical repair should include primary repair of the Achilles, with débridement of any diseased tissue, and augmentation with a FHL transfer.

Delayed diagnosis or missed injury may also result in the need for reconstruction with tendon transfer because of tendon retraction and a gap present on attempted direct repair.

The surgery is similar to a direct repair. In addition to the medial incision made for the Achilles repair, a second incision is performed along the medial aspect of the foot (the medial utility incision), in order to retrieve the FHL tendon more distally, with sufficient length for the transfer. The muscle belly of the FHL runs more distally in the leg, right to the back of the ankle joint. Transferring the FHL into the Achilles brings this vascular muscle belly into the relatively avascular, diseased Achilles tendon. In addition to bringing vascularity, a transfer of the FHL makes a stronger repair (more tissue) and potentially more strength to the patient (additional muscle to plantarflex the ankle). Layered closure and plaster splint application is identical to that performed in primary repairs.

The downside to performing the FHL transfer is the need for a second incision, resulting in occasional mild complaints related to a decrease in push-off strength in the hallux. It is possible to harvest the FHL for transfer without a second incision, although the tendon will be shorter and the repair to the calcaneus may be weaker.

Potential complications are the same as those in a primary rupture repair.

Surgical Treatment for Chronic Insertional Achilles Tendinosis

Chronic insertional Achilles tendinosis is treated with débridement of degenerative tissue with partial calcanectomy and proximal calf lengthening.

In insertional Achilles tendinosis, patients develop focal tenderness and prominence of the distal tendon above or over the posterior tuber. Lateral radiographs may show ossification/calcification of the Achilles insertion on the calcaneus or a Haglund's deformity (a bony prominence of the calcaneal tuberosity). When nonoperative measures fail to relieve the discomfort, surgical treatment should be sought. If a gastrocnemius contracture is identified in a patient undergoing surgical treatment of Achilles tendinopathy, simultaneous gastrocnemius lengthening should be performed.

The mainstay of surgical treatment involves débridement of the diseased tendon. The patient is placed in the prone position. Two incisions are used. The proximal incision is at the gastrocnemius musculotendinous interface to perform a Strayer procedure or gastrocnemius recession. It is placed medial to the midline to decrease the possibility of sural nerve injury. The subcutaneous tissues can be retracted, which allows direct visualization of the gastrocnemius tendon. The space between the gastrocnemius tendon and the soleus tendon can be opened; the gastrocnemius tendon is released and allowed to retract. The distal incision is a midline incision over the tuber and distal Achilles tendon. The incision is carried straight down through the paratenon and periosteum without raising flaps. The tendon can then be dissected subperiosteally

© 2018 American Academy of Orthopaedic Surgeons

medially and laterally, taking care to not completely detach it from the tuber. If present, a Haglund's deformity is resected, along with any inflammatory tissue between the calcaneus and the Achilles tendon just above the insertion (retrocalcaneal bursitis). A suture anchor inserted into the tuber, tangential to the line of pull, can secure the Achilles to the tuber, yielding a more secure repair of the tendon. Closure and immobilization mirrors that of the previously described repairs.

Complications

Complications of surgical management of Achilles tendinosis are related to the two wounds, with potential sural nerve injury possible not only at the level of the distal Achilles, but also at the level of the gastrocnemius lengthening. Particular care should be taken in closing the fascia and subcutaneous layers of the calf incision to avoid muscle herniation and puckering, and ultimately a poorer cosmetic result.

POSTOPERATIVE REHABILITATION

Introduction

While postoperative rehabilitation is best tailored to the individual patient, there are general guidelines for rehabilitating an Achilles repair. The initial postoperative stages involve only the patients themselves, and as healing progresses, formal physical therapy is incorporated. Progression is best individualized based on a given patient's specific needs, pain level, physical examination, functional progress, and the development of any complications during the postoperative course. Precautions and contraindications to rehabilitation progression can include signs of infection, delayed wound healing, neurovascular complications (i.e., deep vein thrombosis [DVT]), increased laxity of the Achilles/possible re-rupture, and increased swelling, redness, or pain.

Authors' Preferred Protocol

Immediately following Achilles repair, the patient is kept immobilized in a well-padded short-leg plaster splint in neutral position. Additionally, the patient must be non–weight bearing (NWB), utilizing crutches, a walker, or a rolling knee walker. Patients may perform activities of daily living (ADLs) as tolerated, provided they rest/elevate the operative leg appropriately. They may also do active range of motion (AROM) of the hip, knee, and especially toes in lying and standing positions. The goal during this time is to control swelling and pain after surgery. This short course of immobilization for wound healing continues for 10 to 12 days postoperatively, at which point they are transferred into a removable controlled ankle motion (CAM) boot, and the postoperative rehabilitation portion of recovery commences.

Phase 1: Maximum Protection Phase (1–8 Weeks Postoperatively)

Gait

- *Goals:* Initially, maintain ipsilateral hip and knee ROM, improve core, hip, and knee strengths, and ambulate safely on an assistive device. Next, progress from NWB with crutches to weight bearing as tolerated (WBAT) with crutches/cane (progression of WB is based on the individual patient's ability to ambulate with proper biomechanics).
- Typical progression from NWB to partial weight bearing (PWB) in CAM boot begins at approximately 6 weeks, using two crutches and removing one wedge every 2 weeks staring at 6 weeks (if wedges are utilized).
- WBAT may begin in a CAM boot as early as 6 weeks, with the patient beginning with two crutches and progressing to a cane by 8 weeks.

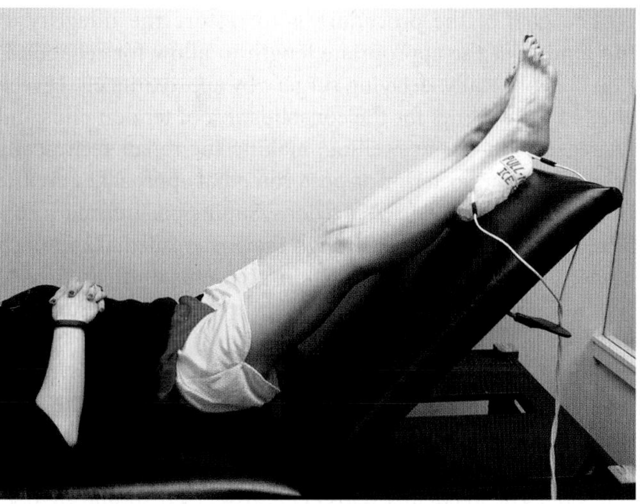

Figure 59.1 Photograph of cryotherapy and electrical stimulation in elevation.

Modalities

In this phase, several modalities may be used after the wound has closed.

- *2–6 weeks:* Early cryotherapy maybe used in elevation for pain and edema control (Figure 59.1)
- *4–6 weeks:* Ultrasound only if wound is completely closed and healing well to promote circulation and remodeling of tissue.
- *6 weeks:* Moist heat can begin with light ROM stretch to *neutral* to promote remodeling of tissue, and must comply with surgeon restrictions (Figure 59.2).

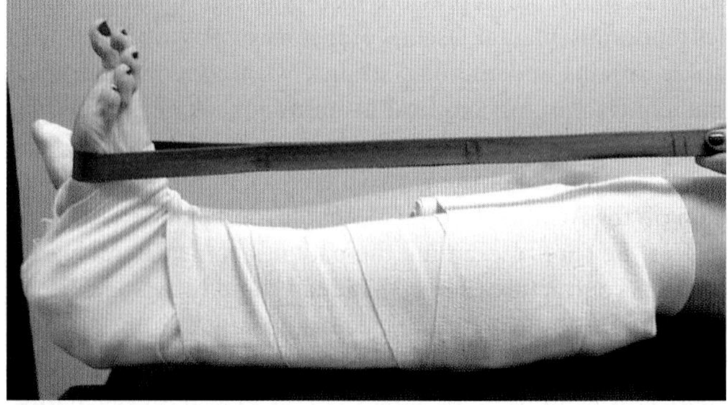

Figure 59.2 Photograph of cryotherapy gastrocnemius/soleus on stretch to neutral.

© 2018 American Academy of Orthopaedic Surgeons

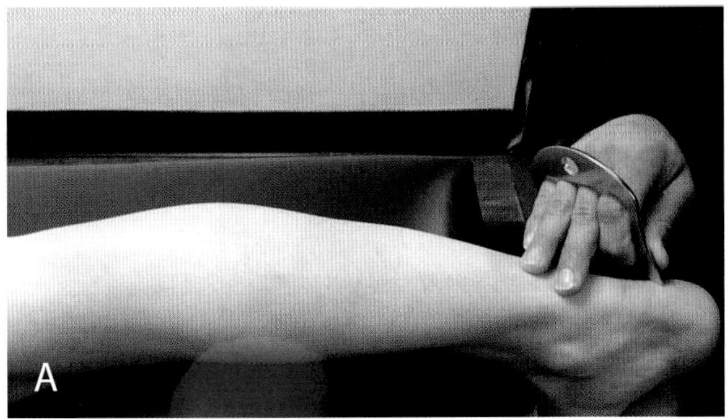

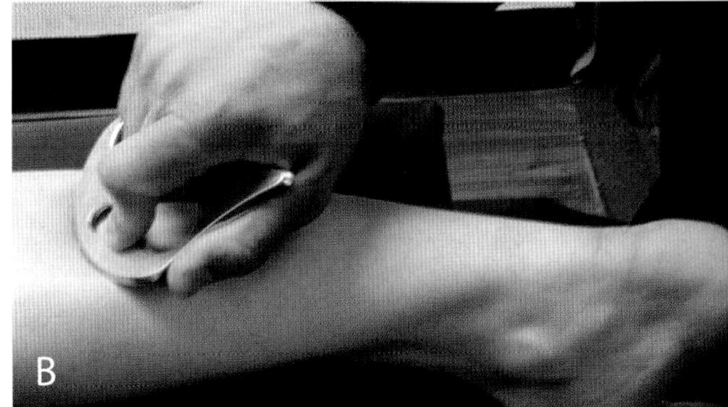

Figure 59.3 Photographs of myofascial massage. **A**, Myofascial massage to scar site. **B**, Myofascial massage to gastrocnemius/soleus complete.

Therapy

- Limit active dorsiflexion ROM to neutral with knee flexed at 90° for 6 weeks
- *No* passive heel cord stretching
- Inversion/eversion ROM
- Bicycle with brace on; no resistance
- Proximal hip and knee strengthening (progressive resistance exercise [PREs]; open kinetic chain)
- Core strengthen on table in CAM boot: bridges, clams, straight-leg raising (SLR) all planes with focus on lateral abductors
- Stretching (gluteus maximus, gluteus medius, piriformis, rectus femoris)
- Upper extremity exercises: arm pulleys/resistance band diagonals, as tolerated
- Joint and soft-tissue mobilization

Myofascial and Scar Mobilization

- *3–6 weeks*
  - Dependent on healing of surgical site
  - Electrical stimulation to gastrocnemius/soleus complex may begin first to reduce spasm, pain and promote circulation until the superficial surgical site is completely healed.
  - Once the site has healed, soft-tissue massage, which may incorporate appropriate tools, can be used to promote fibroblastic production, enhancing the remodeling of myofascial tissue and collagen fibers (Figure 59.3).

Phase 2 Intermediate Protection Phase (8–12 Weeks Postoperatively)

Gait: Weight Bearing as Tolerated

- A CAM boot is designed to promote early knee flexion to unload the surgical site; thus, correction of improper biomechanics should be stressed when beginning transition to weight bearing without a CAM boot and into a cushioned running sneaker.
- Patients are instructed in WBAT without a CAM boot using two crutches at 8 weeks. Patient education focuses initially on proper mechanics, beginning with heel strike, progressing to full knee extension during the stance phase. Patients are instructed on how to sufficiently unload the repair, allowing for proper mechanics during ambulation.
- Early motion and proper mechanics during the loading phase has been shown to improve remodeling of the tissue and promote improved alignment of the surgical site's collagen.
- Patients are instructed to perform a full home exercise program (HEP) and practice ambulation without the CAM boot daily to help with transition to FWB out of CAM by weeks 10 to 12.
- For simple repairs of acute ruptures, some surgeons progress weight bearing more quickly, so that the patient is full weight bearing in the CAM boot at 4 to 5 weeks and out of the boot at 8 weeks.

Modalities: Cryotherapy, Ultrasound, and Electrical Stimulation, as Needed

As described earlier; Premodulated electrical stimulation may be continued for pain control along with cryotherapy on stretch for tissue lengthening and reorganization (12 weeks) (Figure 59.4).

Therapy

- The goal is to restore normal gait, discontinue crutches when gait is not antalgic, and discontinue the CAM boot by the end of week 12.

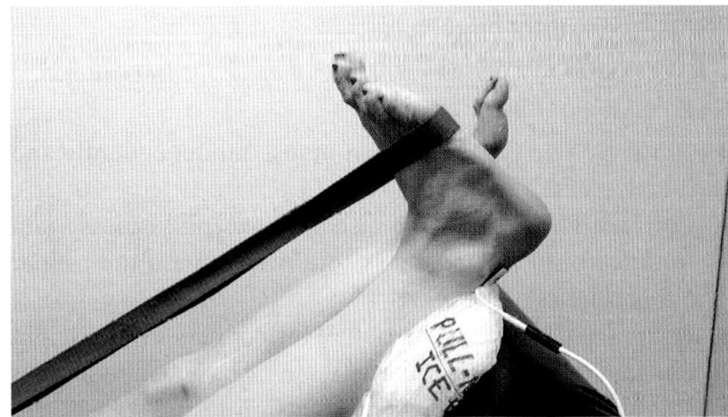

Figure 59.4 Photograph of cryotherapy in elevation on full stretch to gastrocnemius/soleus.

© 2018 American Academy of Orthopaedic Surgeons

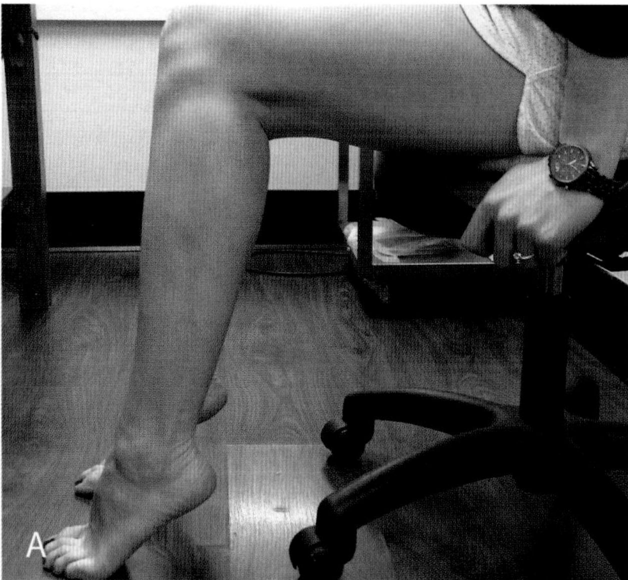

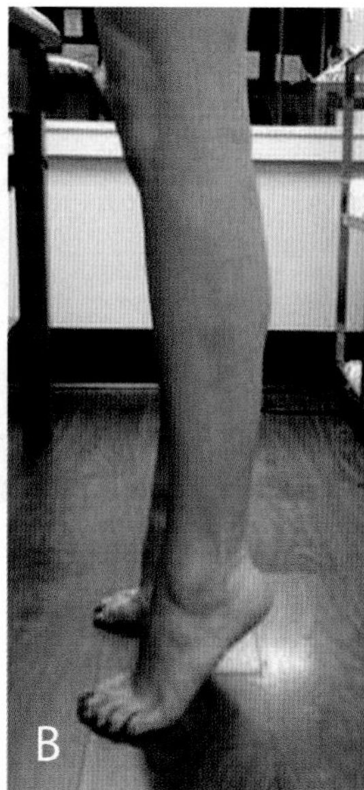

Figure 59.5 Photographs of heel raises. **A**, Seated soleus heel raises. **B**, Bilateral standing gastrocnemius/soleus heel raise.

- At week 8, begin gentle plantarflexion (PF) and dorsiflexion (DF) PREs. Begin with the knee flexed and gradually progress to the knee extended position. The goal is to increase DF to allow the boot to come off (Figure 59.5).
- Inversion and eversion isometrics; progress to isotonics.
- Static single-leg balance and standing bilateral heel raise at 10 to 12 weeks
- Closed kinetic chain leg strengthening (leg press/squats/step-ups)
- Continue bicycle; can start to add tension

Myofascial and Scar Mobilization

- Deep tissue and trigger point work to gastrocnemius/soleus region
- Myofascial and deep scar mobilization techniques may continue throughout this phase with focus to the scar; soft-tissue mobilization of the plantar fascia and FHL.
- Medial and lateral mobilization to the tendons should also be performed to minimize adhesion formation.

Phase 3: Strengthening Phase (12–16 Weeks Postoperatively)

Gait: Full Weight Bearing (FWB)

- *10 weeks:* The CAM boot can be used independently and cane weaned.
- *12 weeks:* The CAM boot is discontinued and a cane is again resumed until the patient is comfortable with the proper biomechanics of gait.
- Focus again should be placed on proper heel strike, weight transfer to the stance phase, with focus on the patient's ability to maintain full knee extension in the stance, and follow through phases of gait.
- Goal is normal gait pattern at FWB.
- Cushioned running sneakers are often recommended in transitioning to back-to-normal shoe wear.

Modalities

- Cryotherapy, ultrasound, and e-stimulation, PRN

Therapy

- Restore normal ankle ROM.
- Normalize gastrocnemius/soleus muscle flexibility; progress to standing calf stretch.
- Normalize Achilles tendon flexibility.
- Aggressive plantarflexion and dorsiflexion strengthening (emphasize eccentrics; Figure 59.6).
- Heel and toe walks in FWB; progress to standing single-leg heel raises.
  - Begin with a cane, as needed, during the toe walk phase to assist isotonic PF.
  - The patient will have difficulty maintaining FWB in PF and will eccentrically drop the heel to the floor. This is a normal progression which will improve with time.
- Aggressive inversion and eversion strengthening
- Begin proprioception/balance activities.
- Begin retro treadmill program (start with 10% grade and progress to 0% grade)
- Continue closed kinetic chain lower extremity strengthening
- Stairmaster or Versaclimber, as tolerated

Phase 4: Functional Strengthening and Agility Phase (16–24 Weeks Post-op)

Modalities

- Ice, as needed, post-exercise

Therapy

- Continue ankle and leg strengthening.
- Maintain calf and Achilles flexibility equal to uninvolved limb.

© 2018 American Academy of Orthopaedic Surgeons

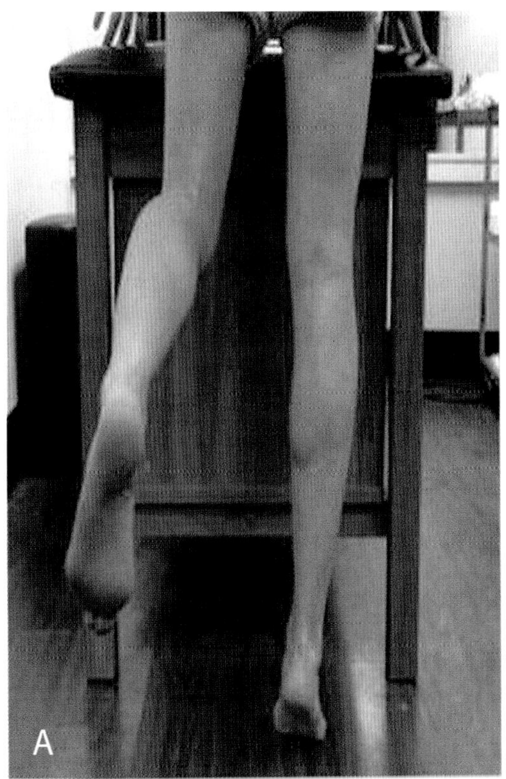
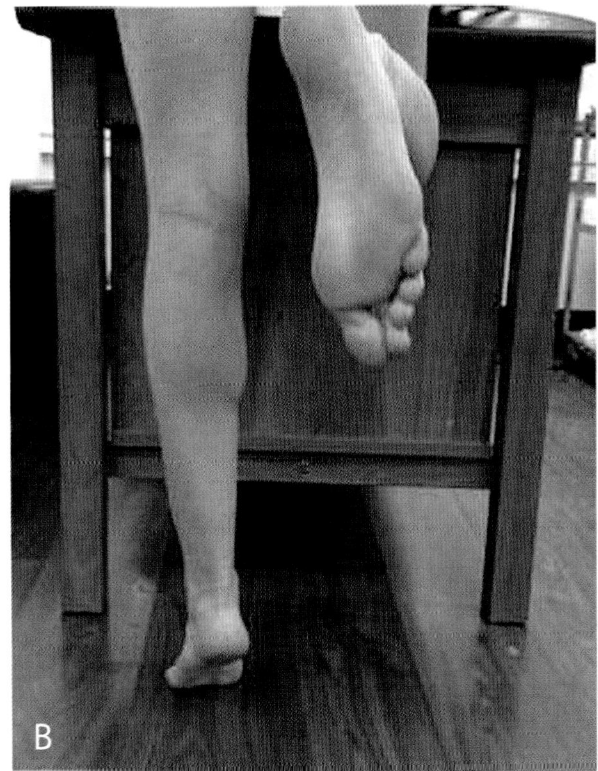

Figure 59.6 Photographs of heel raises. **A**, Unilateral standing gastrocnemius/soleus heel raise. **B**, Eccentric unilateral gastrocnemius/soleus heel raise.

- Continue muscle endurance training.
- Begin stretch shortening cycle (SSC) drills, low-level plyometric program.
- Progress to agility and higher-level plyometric program (symptom-free).
- Begin interval running program.
- Limited return to sporting activities.
- Progress to full home program.

Goals

- Normal ankle ROM
- Ankle strength to manual muscle testing: 5/5
- No swelling in foot and ankle
- Maximum function

Return to Sport Criteria

Patients are assessed for return to sports through several functional tests. They must do the following:

- Repeatedly perform a lateral step-down for 2 sets at 15 repetitions.
- Concentrically perform eccentric heal raise on the effected side, 2 sets at 15 repetitions
- Perform bilateral toe walks with fully contracted gastrocnemius/soleus complex with no heel drops during weight bearing weight shifts to contralateral lower extremity.
- *Triple hop test:* 3 consecutive jumps on the affected side for distance. It must be 90% of the unaffected lower extremity.
- Perform plyometric hops on 6-inch box, 3 sets for 30 seconds. Two planes anterior-posterior and lateral.
- Run for 5 minutes with no deviations or misalignment at heel strike.

Sports-specific activities related to individual sports—that is, cutting drills, high-jump drills, and sprints—are gradually incorporated into exercise routines as symptoms and performance allow. Return to competitive activity requires stepwise progression, with care not to exacerbate symptoms.

OUTCOMES

Outcomes of surgical repair of the Achilles are generally favorable. However, the patient must be prepared for a lengthy recovery period that may extend to 6 or even 12 months, particularly if interested in return to high-level sport activity. Residual soreness and incomplete but mild deficit in muscle strength are common. Wound healing problems and contracture exert a major negative influence on outcome, thus must be avoided.

PEARLS

- The surgeon must maintain meticulous technique to minimize soft-tissue complications. In many cases, the benefits of surgical repair depend on the ability to achieve soft-tissue healing without complications. If any concerns develop

© 2018 American Academy of Orthopaedic Surgeons

regarding the wound, the surgeon should be notified for timely management.

- As with most other ankle reconstructive procedures, a brief period of immobilization is important postoperatively to minimize chance for infection. Mobilization can begin once the soft tissues have begun recovering from the acute inflammation.
- Total recovery time will be long, typically more than 6 months. Many patients and therapists use the single-leg heel raise as a test of success. This test will not be normal for more than 6 months. It is better to focus on double-leg heel raises, and other strengthening exercises, to put the focus on good technique in strength and endurance.

BIBLIOGRAPHY

Erickson BJ, Mascarenhas R, Saltzman BM, Walton D, Lee S, Cole BJ, Bach BR Jr: Is operative treatment of Achilles tendon ruptures superior to nonoperative treatment? a systematic review of overlapping meta-analyses. *Orthop J Sports Med* 2015;3:2325967115579188.

Gulati V, Jaggard M, Al-Nammari SS, et al: Management of Achilles tendon injury: A current concepts systematic review. *World J Orthop* 2015;6(4):380–386.

Holm M, Kjaer M, Eliasson P: Achilles tendon rupture–treatment and complications: A systematic review C. *Scand J Med Sci Sports* 2015;25(1):e1–e10.

Hunt KJ, Cohen BE, Davis WH, Anderson RB, Jones CP: Surgical treatment of insertional Achilles tendinopathy with or without flexor hallucis longus tendon transfer: a prospective, randomized study. *Foot Ankle Int* 2015;36: 998–1005.

Maffulli N, Tallon C, Wong J, Lim KP, Bleakney R: Early weight-bearing and ankle mobilization after open repair of acute midsubstance tears of the Achilles tendon, http://ajs.sagepub.com/content/31/5/692.short

Martin RL, Manning CM, Carcia CR, Conti SF: An outcome study of chronic Achilles tendinosis after excision of the Achilles tendon and flexor hallucis longus tendon transfer. *Foot Ankle Int* 2005;26(9):691–697.

Ng CO, Ng GY, See EK, Leung MC: Therapeutic ultrasound improves strength of Achilles tendon repair in rats. *Ultrasound Med Biol* 2003;29:1501–1506.

Ozkaya U, Parmaksizoglu AS, Kabukcuoglu Y, Sokucu S, Basilgan S: Open minimally invasive Achilles tendon repair with early rehabilitation: Functional results of 25 consecutive patients. Available at: http://www.sciencedirect.com/science/article/pii/S002013830800483X

Speck M, Klaue K: Early full weightbearing and functional treatment after surgical repair of acute Achilles tendon rupture. Available at: http://ajs.sagepub.com/content/26/6/789.short

Suchak AA, Spooner C, Reid DC, Jomha NM: Postoperative rehabilitation protocols for Achilles tendon ruptures: a meta-analysis. *Clin Orthop Relat Res* 2006;445:216–221.

Wegrzyn J, Luciani JF, Philippot R, Brunet-Guedj E, Moyen B, Besse JL: Chronic Achilles tendon rupture reconstruction using a modified flexor hallucis longus transfer. *Int Orthop* 2010;34(8):1187–1192.

© 2018 American Academy of Orthopaedic Surgeons

Calcaneus, Talus, Midfoot, and Lisfranc Fractures

Thomas C. Dowd, MD, and Eric M. Bluman, MD, PhD

INTRODUCTION

Fractures of the tarsal bones have long been associated with significant pain, dysfunction, and deformity. Advances in surgical management have allowed for rigid fixation, permitting more rapid return to motion and weight bearing. Isolated injuries can occur; however, these fractures are often encountered in patients who have sustained multiple injuries (polytrauma). Well-timed fracture reduction and fixation allows for minimized morbidity and complications, improved deformity correction, and optimal restoration of anatomic relationships. While foot fracture fixation allows for earlier return to motion about the ankle and foot, premature weight bearing can be associated with failure of fixation. Rehabilitation has to achieve a balance between early mobilization and protection of the fixation. Common surgical interventions for fractures about the tarsal bones are described in this chapter, along with an explanation of the typical postoperative physical therapy regimen.

CALCANEUS FRACTURES

There are several varieties of fractures that occur about the calcaneus. Commonly encountered patterns include joint depression, tongue-type calcaneus fractures, and anterior process fractures. Joint depression fractures are often treated with open reduction and internal fixation (ORIF). Comminution of the posterior facet is of central importance in determining the severity of the fracture. The system described by Sanders is used for classification of these fractures (Table 60.1). Surgical treatment varies depending on the patient, fracture pattern, and surgeon preference. The goals of surgical intervention are the restoration of calcaneal height, elimination of varus deformity, and optimization of the subtalar joint articulations. Subsequent rehabilitation should be aimed at preservation and restoration of motion without compromising fracture union.

Operative Treatment of Calcaneal Fractures

Indications

Nonoperative management of calcaneus fractures is frequently utilized, in part because of the difficulty of fracture repair surgery in restoring normal joint function. Calcaneus fractures with intra-articular fragment displacement, significant loss of height (Figure 60.1), and avulsion type fractures, especially those with posterior distal leg skin compromise (Figure 60.2). are appropriately treated with surgical intervention. Certain patient characteristics—such as smoking history, impaired vascular supply, poorly controlled diabetes, and inability to follow postoperative instructions—may be contraindications to surgical intervention. Additionally, severe intra-articular comminution frequently portends poor outcome; nonoperative intervention or acute subtalar arthrodesis may be performed in specific cases.

Procedure

ORIF of the calcaneus has traditionally been performed through an extensile approach to the hindfoot. This L-shaped approach includes a vertical limb centered between the Achilles and the peroneal tendons, overlying the sural nerve at its proximal extent. The horizontal limb is extended parallel and just dorsal to the glabrous skin (Figure 60.3). The soft-tissue flap is elevated in a full-thickness fashion and includes the peroneal tendons. The peroneal tendons must be evaluated at the completion of fracture reduction and fixation to assess for potential dislocation from within the sheath at their retrofibular location. The primary at-risk structures are lateral and superficial

Dr. Bluman or an immediate family member serves as a paid consultant to Stryker; has stock or stock options held in EDC and Neutin; has received nonincome support (such as equipment or services), commercially derived honoraria, or other non-research–related funding (such as paid travel) from Rogerson Orthopaedics and Wolters Kluwer Health–Lippincott Williams & Wilkins; and serves as a board member, owner, officer, or committee member of the American Academy of Orthopaedic Surgeons, Advanced Reconstruction of the Foot & Ankle 2, *the American Orthopaedic Foot and Ankle Society, FootCareMD, and* Techniques in Foot & Ankle Surgery. *Dr. Dowd or an immediate family member has received research or institutional support from Zimmer; and serves as a board member, owner, officer, or committee member of the American Orthopaedic Association, the American Orthopaedic Foot and Ankle Society, and the AAOS.*

© 2018 American Academy of Orthopaedic Surgeons

Table 60.1 SANDERS CLASSIFICATION OF CALCANEUS FRACTURES

Classification	Description
Type I	Nondisplaced posterior facet fractures (any number of fragments)
Type II	Two fragments at posterior facet (one fracture lines with displacement)
Type III	Three fragments at posterior facet (two fracture lines with displacement)
Type IV	Four or more fragments at posterior facet (at least three fracture lines with displacement)

This classification is based on the coronal CT scan images at the widest point through the sustentaculum tali.
Fracture lines may be subclassified according to their medial to lateral location: A = lateral fracture, B = central fracture, C = medial fracture.
(Data from Buckley RE, Tough S. Displaced Intra-articular Calcaneal Fractures. *Journal of the American Academy of Orthopaedic Surgeons* 2004;12:172–178. Adapted with permission from Sanders R: Intra-articular fractures of the calcaneus: Present state of the art. *J Orthop Trauma* 1992;6:252–265.)

to the bone. However, fixation screws may impinge on structures medial to the calcaneus, especially if they are excessively long or malpositioned relative to the sustentaculum tali (Figure 60.4). Wound closure is performed in layers and great care is taken to minimize any damage to the soft tissue, which could potentially lead to healing delay, necrosis, or infection.

Alternate approaches to the calcaneus for ORIF have gained popularity. One of these is the sinus tarsi approach. This approach is of variable length, oriented along a line from the tip of the distal fibula to the fourth metatarsal base (Figure 60.5). The extensor digitorum brevis muscle is encountered and elevated dorsally. The peroneal tendons are again encountered in the flap of tissue overlying the calcaneus, but should be elevated with the skin and subcutaneous tissue, minimizing dissection of the full-thickness tissue bed. Care must be taken to preserve the tendons and the superior peroneal retinaculum with proximal extension of this incision.

In certain cases, the posterior facet has sustained such damage that subtalar arthrodesis is performed in conjunction with ORIF of the displaced fracture. This may be performed via either approach and entails removal of the remaining articular cartilage, preparation of subchondral bone, and compressive fixation between the calcaneus and talus.

Tongue-type or posterior avulsion patterns involve fracture with displacement between the proximal Achilles insertion site and the remainder of the calcaneus, and may involve part of the posterior facet. Displaced fractures may place posterior skin under pressure, requiring urgent reduction and fixation. These are often addressed with a percutaneous technique or a posterior approach. Anterior process avulsion fractures occur at the dorsal anterior aspect of this portion of the calcaneus. They usually are produced with an inversion injury of the foot. The superior portion of the calcaneocuboid joint may be involved with large fragments. Treatment for small fragments is usually non-operative, but may occasionally involve resection if persistent pain can be attributed to nonunion. Larger fragments may be best treated with ORIF. All these fractures should be considered distinct from the displaced, intra-articular calcaneus fracture, especially with respect to the focus of rehabilitation efforts.

Complications

- Wound healing delay
  - Related to thin soft-tissue envelope
  - Requires careful tissue handling
- Infection
  - Most problematic of complications and related to wound healing problems
  - Requires early detection and treatment
- Subtalar arthrofibrosis, stiffness
- Posttraumatic subtalar arthritis
- Peroneal tendon instability/impingement
- Anterior ankle impingement, especially with loss of calcaneal height

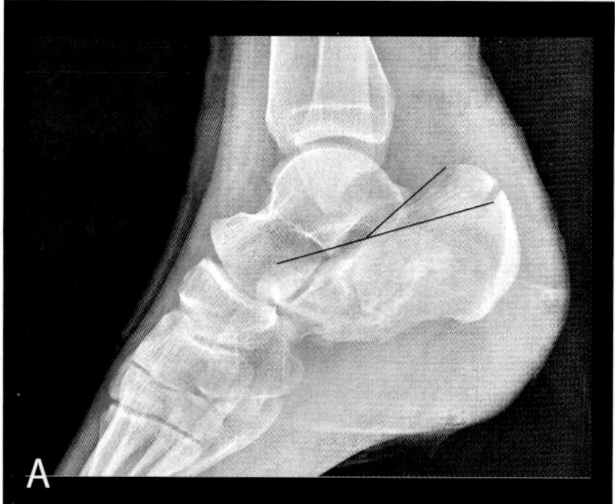

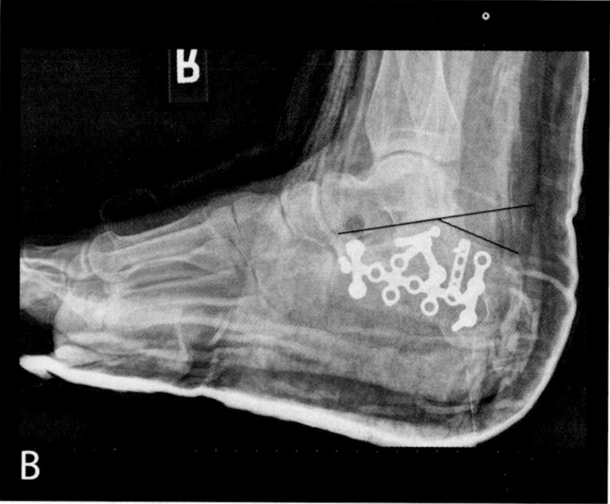

Figure 60.1 **A**, Radiograph showing a Bohler angle, measured to assess the degree of depression of the calcaneus fracture. In this case, the angle between the lines is flattened considerably. **B**, Radiograph showing restored Bohler angle after open reduction and internal fixation of the calcaneus.

© 2018 American Academy of Orthopaedic Surgeons

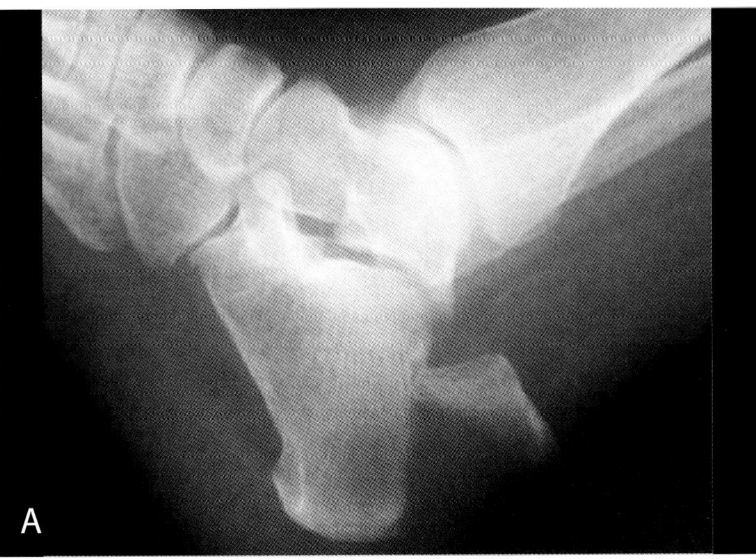

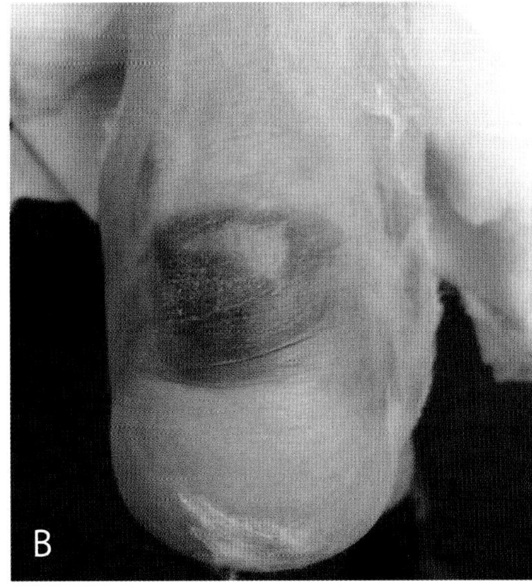

Figure 60.2 **A**, Radiograph demonstrating avulsion of the tuberosity of the calcaneus. **B**, Clinical photograph demonstrating skin compromise associated with fracture. (From Banerjee R, Chao JC, Taylor R, Siddiqui A. Management of calcaneal tuberosity fractures. *J Am Acad Orthop Surg* 2012;20(4):253–8. doi: 10.5435/JAAOS-20-04-253.)

- Gastrocnemius/Achilles contracture
- Sural nerve Injury
- Compartment syndrome
  - Claw toes

Postoperative Rehabilitation for Calcaneus Fractures

General rehabilitation principles are discussed at end of chapter.

- Subtalar stiffness, with loss of inversion/eversion motion, is a common challenge following calcaneus surgery.
- Subtalar arthrodesis will require modification of protocol to eliminate subtalar mobilization efforts.
- For a variety of reasons, it is unusual to have any limitation of dorsiflexion following calcaneus fracture. In fact, some patients have increased dorsiflexion of the ankle compared to the opposite leg. Limited ankle dorsiflexion may be a product of Achilles/gastrocnemius contracture or from

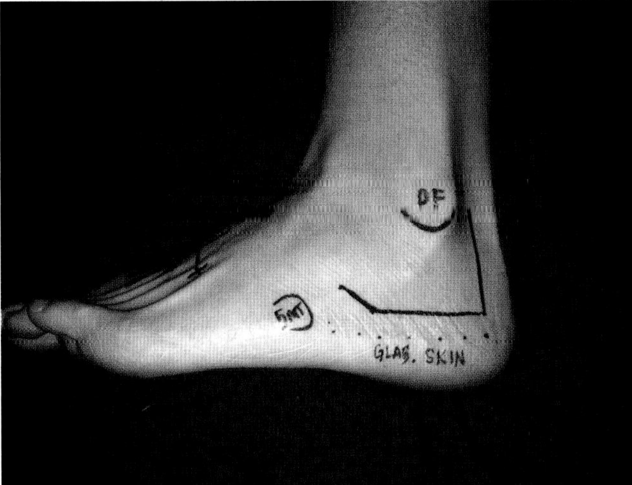

Figure 60.3 Schematic of extensile lateral approach to the calcaneus. DF = distal fibula, 5MT = fifth metatarsal base, GLAB. SKIN = glabrous skin (plantar to dotted line).

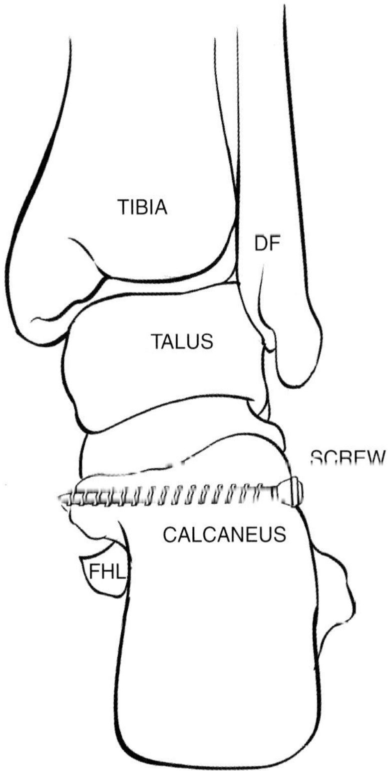

Figure 60.4 Illustration of the coronal section of the hindfoot demonstrating the relationship between the interfragmentary lag screw, sustentaculum tali and flexor halluces longus tendon.

© 2018 American Academy of Orthopaedic Surgeons

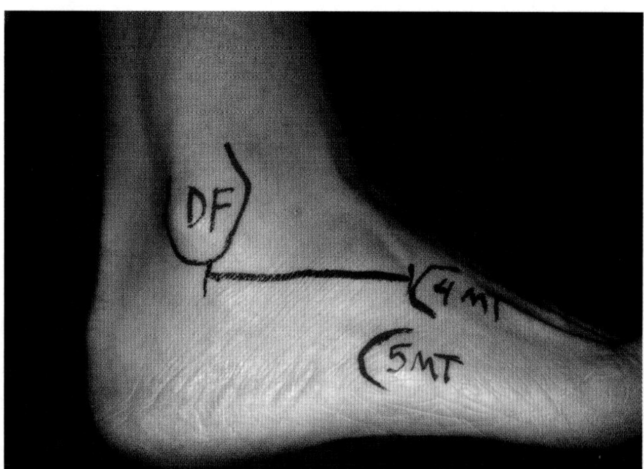

Figure 60.5 Photograph demonstrating the sinus tarsi approach for treatment of a fractured calcaneus. Sinus tarsi approach to the calcaneus (*solid black line*). DF = distal fibula, 5MT = fifth metatarsal base, 4MT = fourth metatarsal base.

anterior ankle impingement secondary to diminished restoration of calcaneal height. It is important to distinguish one from the other and address both.

- In the rare instance of concomitant peroneal tendon stabilization, efforts to mobilize the subtalar joint should be delayed. The joint may require more extensive physiotherapy to counteract arthrofibrosis, but the trade-off is successful healing of the superior peroneal retinaculum, peroneal tendon, and/or sheath repair.

TALUS FRACTURES

The talus is a bone with a complex shape, in which fractures occur at specific locations (body, neck, head, lateral/posterior processes). As with calcaneal fractures, talus fracture may be associated with polytrauma. A unique aspect of the talus is its limited blood supply and lack of tendon attachments. There are no tendon insertions on the talus. The stability of the talus is governed by bony constraints and ligaments.

Talar neck and body fractures are frequently associated with subluxation or dislocation about the surrounding joints (subtalar, ankle, talonavicular). Talar neck fractures are classified according to the Hawkins system, as modified by Canale (Table 60.2). Fracture of the body of the talus may necessitate osteotomy about the ankle (medial or lateral malleolus) in order to perform articular reduction, adding another "injury" to the healing. Recent advances include arthroscopic assisted reduction and fixation. These injuries are difficult to treat and often result in stiffness, deformity, pain, arthritis, avascular necrosis, and dysfunction even after satisfactory ORIF.

Surgical Procedure

Indications

Owing to the association with four distinct bones and their articular surfaces, talar neck fractures with displacement are typically treated operatively to prevent joint malalignment (Figure 60.6). Talar neck fractures without displacement may also be treated operatively in order to optimize progression to early range of motion (ROM) and activities. Talar body fractures with displacement are treated with surgical intervention in order to restore articular congruity of the tibiotalar and subtalar joints. Symptomatic lateral process fractures may be treated operatively if they are of significant size, associated with instability about the ankle, or persistently painful after trial of nonoperative management. Relative contraindications include smoking, impaired vascular supply, poorly controlled diabetes, or limited potential for restoration of function.

Table 60.2 MODIFIED HAWKINS CLASSIFICATION OF TALAR NECK FRACTURE

Classification	Description
Type I	Nondisplaced fracture
Type II	Displaced fracture with subtalar subluxation/dislocation
Type III	Displaced fracture with subtalar and ankle dislocation
Type IV	Displaced fracture with subtalar, ankle, and talonavicular dislocation

Based on Canale ST, Kelly FB. Fractures of the neck of the talus. Long-term evaluation of seventy-one cases. *J Bone Joint Surg Am* 1978;60(3):143–56.

Procedure

Open Reduction and Internal Fixation of the Neck of the Talus

Talar neck ORIF is often performed through a lateral approach. However, a combined lateral and medial approach is often recommended for those fractures with medial comminution and risk for developing a varus deformity. It is essential to prevent varus deformity in order to maintain appropriate transverse tarsal joint function. In addition, an osteotomy of the distal

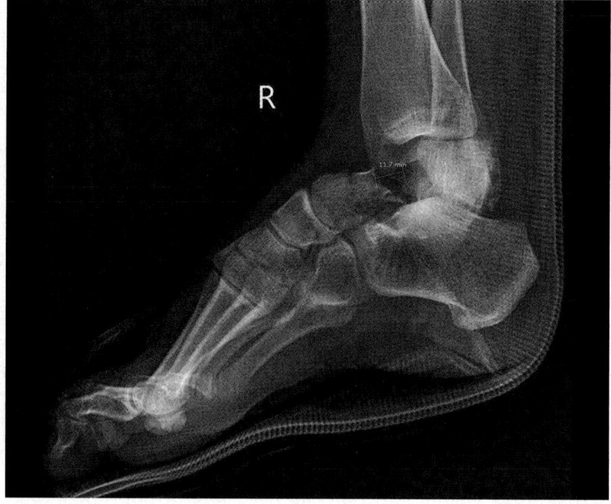

Figure 60.6 Radiograph of talus neck fracture with rotation and displacement of the talar body fragment.

© 2018 American Academy of Orthopaedic Surgeons

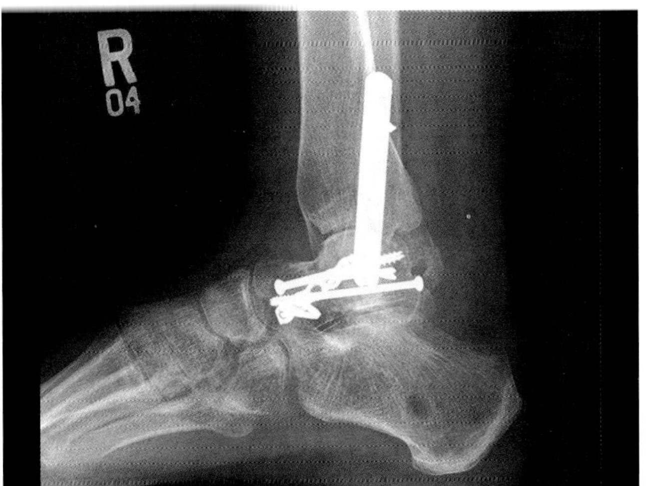

Figure 60.7 Postoperative radiograph demonstrating reduction and fixation of talus neck fracture using anterior to posterior and posterior to anterior screws with a medial plate. Osteotomy was not necessary due to ipsilateral distal fibula fracture.

fibula or medial malleolus is occasionally employed to assist in visualizing the fracture site prior to reduction and fixation (Figure 60.7).

The lateral approach to the talus is performed in a linear fashion, dorsal to the line formed by the tip of the distal fibula and the fourth metatarsal base. This puts branches of the superficial peroneal nerve at risk for traction or transection injury. The medial approach to the talar neck is performed in line with and plantar to the anterior tibialis tendon (Figure 60.8). Branches of the saphenous nerve and vein must be protected.

Depending on fracture pattern, associated injuries and surgeon preference, screws will be placed from posterior to anterior or anterior to posterior. Posterior to anterior screws are placed through the posterolateral interval, exploiting the internervous plane between the flexor hallucis longus and the peroneal tendons. The sural nerve remains superficial at the entry site for these screws and is at risk. Placement of the screws requires great caution to ensure appropriate depth and orientation to avoid irritation of the surrounding tendons and articular surfaces (posterior ankle and posterior facet of the subtalar joint). Anterior to posterior screws are placed near the talar head, placing at risk those medial and dorsal structures near the entry site (anterior tibialis tendon, posterior tibialis tendon, extensor hallucis longus tendon, and saphenous and deep peroneal nerve branches). For fractures with comminution, small bridging plates may be used to stabilize the bone.

Open Reduction and Internal Fixation of the Body of the Talus

Talar body fractures are posterior to the lateral process of the talus. These fractures often involve a significant portion of the articular surface of the tibiotalar joint and/or the posterior facet of the subtalar joint. These fractures regularly require a distal fibular or distal tibial (commonly medial malleolus) osteotomy to aid in visualization, reduction, and fixation.

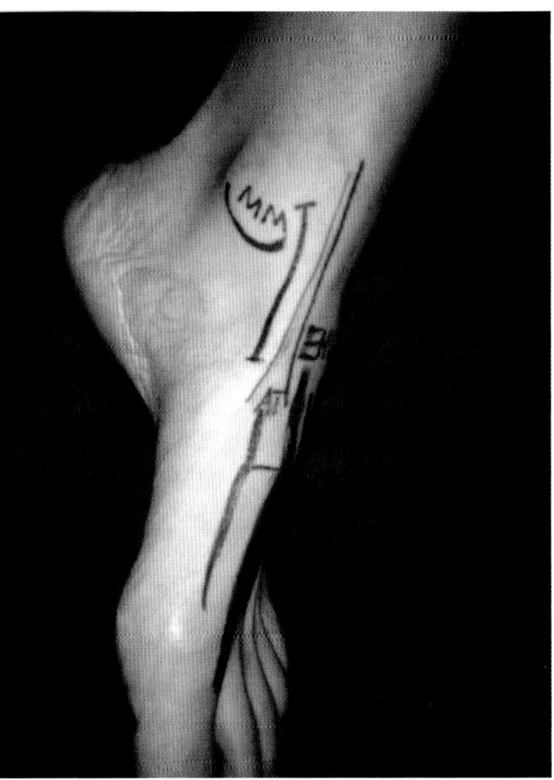

Figure 60.8 Photograph demonstrating the medial approach to the neck of the talus (*solid line*). This is often referred to as an extension of the anteromedial ankle arthroscopy portal. MM = medial malleolus, AT = anterior tibial tendon. Dotted line: saphenous vein and nerve.

Open Reduction and Internal Fixation/Excision of the Lateral Process of the Talus

Lateral process of the talus fractures are commonly treated with immobilization and rest. However, some fractures will remain symptomatic and require excision. Some fractures of the lateral process of the talus are large enough to prompt reduction and fixation when associated with displacement. Associated injuries should be considered; these include syndesmosis injury as well as peroneal tendon dislocation/tear.

Complications

- Wound healing
  - Infection
- Varus malunion
- Non-union
- Arthrofibrosis of ankle and/or subtalar joint
- Posttraumatic arthritis of the ankle, subtalar, or talonavicular joints
- Nerve Injury (saphenous, sural, superficial and deep peroneal nerves)
- Osteonecrosis
  - Common sequelae but does not always lead to collapse and arthritis
  - Hawkin's sign seen on ankle radiographs 1–3 months post injury is predictive of revascularization of the body of the talus

© 2018 American Academy of Orthopaedic Surgeons

Specific Rehabilitation Considerations

- In the setting of varus malunion, efforts to restore motion will be unsuccessful (the foot is fixed in varus/inversion) and corrective osteotomy may be necessary.
- If osteonecrosis develops, coordination between the orthopaedic surgeon and physical therapist is essential to set treatment goals. Often osteonecrosis is asymptomatic requiring no intervention.

MIDFOOT/LISFRANC FRACTURES

Introduction

Fractures about the midfoot, specifically Lisfranc and cuboid injuries, are often missed and difficult to treat. Patients presenting with midfoot tenderness, edema, and plantar midfoot ecchymosis should be regarded with a high index of suspicion for these injuries. The Lisfranc complex includes the first through fifth tarsometatarsal joints. The Lisfranc ligament is a complex ligamentous structure that serves to stabilize the second metatarsal base in its position as the keystone of the "Roman arch" of the foot. The cuboid articulates with the fourth and fifth metatarsals distally and the calcaneus proximally. Injuries to these structures may occur together or in isolation. Serial radiographs (especially weight-bearing radiographs if tolerated), stress radiographs, MRI and CT scanning should be employed to make a definitive diagnosis and guide treatment (Figure 60.9). Efforts should be aimed at maintaining the functional architecture of the foot and avoiding shortening, in particular, valgus and lateral column shortening (with cuboid fracture). In general, cuboid fractures and Lisfranc injuries are treated with surgical intervention, if displaced at all.

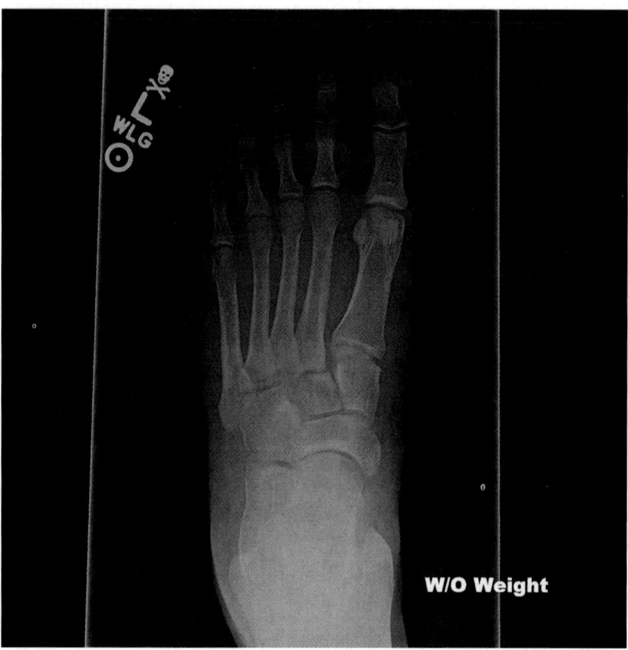

Figure 60.9 Radiograph of the foot demonstrating Lisfranc injury with associated "fleck" sign.

Lisfranc Injury

Indications

Surgical indications include dislocation of the joints about the Lisfranc complex and displaced fracture(s) in the region of the first through third tarsometatarsal joints. These injuries often involve extension into the naviculo-cuneiform articulation(s). It is essential to perform anatomic reduction and stabilize these joints with rigid fixation. Relative contraindications include history of smoking, impaired vascular supply, poorly controlled diabetes, and inadequate soft-tissue coverage. However, if soft-tissue coverage can be performed in order to perform limb salvage, then ORIF is performed.

Procedure

Lisfranc Open Reduction and Internal Fixation

ORIF of Lisfranc joint may be performed through a variety of approaches to the dorsal and medial midfoot region. These incisions are created in a longitudinal fashion. The incisions are determined by a variety of factors, including fracture orientation, specific joint involvement, associated open injuries and surgeon preference.

The medial approach is centered over the first tarsometatarsal joint (TMTJ). This incision overlies terminal branches of the saphenous nerve and vein, and the medial branches of the superficial peroneal nerve. As dissection progresses deep to the subcutaneous fat, the anterior tibialis tendon is encountered. Care should be taken to preserve the insertion of this tendon. If release is necessary, the tendon should be repaired and/or anchored near its native insertion.

Dorsal incisions may be made over the first TMTJ or between adjacent, involved TMTJs. Proper planning will allow optimal exposure of injured structures with preservation of a wide, full-thickness skin bridge between incisions. The typical incision exploits the interval between the extensor hallucis longus and brevis. Dorsal structures encountered include the anterior tibialis and extensor digitorum longus tendons, terminal branches of the superficial peroneal nerve, deep peroneal nerve, and dorsalis pedis artery (as well as the perforating artery that passes plantarly between the first and second metatarsal bases; Figure 60.10).

Fixation of these fractures depends on fracture orientation, extent of comminution, soft-tissue integrity, and surgeon preference. After reduction, stability may be conferred by simple screw placement. However, plate and screw constructs may be necessary (Figure 60.11). The surgical aim is to create a stable construct that will support proper healing while allowing for early ROM to preserve flexibility at nearby joints, particularly the ankle, and subtalar and talonavicular joints. Later removal may be necessary for transarticular and/or prominent, symptomatic hardware.

At times, the injury progresses laterally. Fractures and/or dislocations may result in fourth and fifth TMTJ instability. In these situations, open or closed reduction is performed with pin fixation of the affected joints. Pins are maintained for approximately 6 weeks before removal. Permanent rigid fixation and

 © 2018 American Academy of Orthopaedic Surgeons

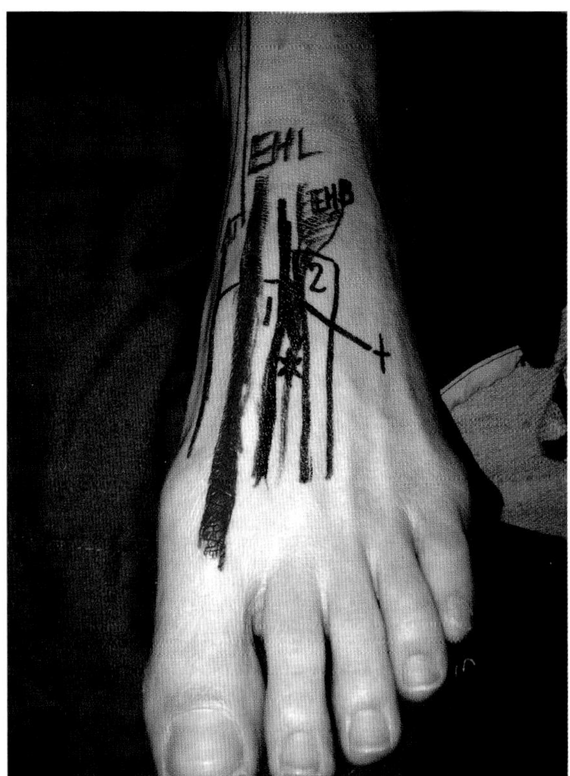

Figure 60.10 Photograph demonstrating plantar perforating branch of the dorsalis pedis artery (*), arcuate branch (+), and relationship with Lisfranc joint, EHL, EHB.

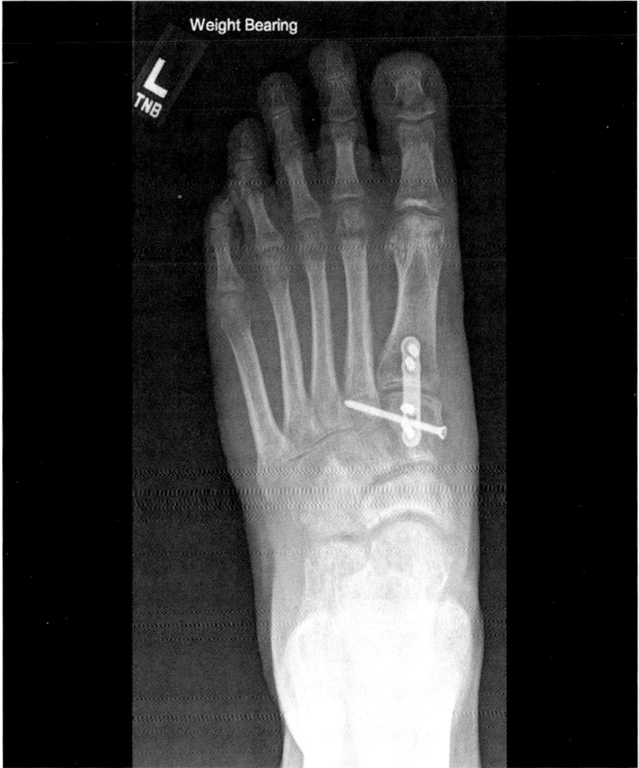

Figure 60.11 Radiograph of the foot demonstrating fixation of Lisfranc injury with a plate spanning the first tarsometatarsal joint. (Note disuse osteopenia.)

arthrodesis is not recommended at the fourth and fifth TMTJs owing to subsequent stiffness and inability to accommodate to uneven ground.

Lisfranc Arthrodesis

Arthrodesis of the Lisfranc joint is often performed for purely ligamentous injuries at the Lisfranc complex or in articular fractures with extensive comminution as definitive initial treatment. These injuries are addressed in a manner similar to that described for ORIF. Additionally, the articular sites selected for arthrodesis are denuded of cartilage and rigidly fixed. On occasion, an autograft or allograft will be interposed prior to placement of fixation. If the autograft is harvested from the proximal tibia or the iliac crest, this will have additional rehabilitation implications, particularly if there is extensive dissection through the iliotibial band for proximal tibial bone graft harvest.

Open Reduction Internal Fixation of the Cuboid

Indications

Indications for ORIF of cuboid fractures include dislocation, significant displacement, intra-articular extension and lateral column shortening. Relative contraindications include smoking, impaired vascular supply, and poorly controlled diabetes.

Surgical Procedure

ORIF of the cuboid is performed for those cuboid fractures associated with lateral column shortening or significant intra-articular involvement and displacement. The cuboid is crushed between the adjacent bones when an abduction force or axial load is placed. The injury rarely occurs in isolation; thus, medial midfoot structures must be assessed. The cuboid has extensive articulations engaging the calcaneus, lateral cuneiform, navicular, and lateral metatarsal bases. The goals of surgical intervention include restoration of length and minimizing posttraumatic arthritis. Typically, an open approach to the cuboid is performed with a laterally based longitudinal incision exploiting the interval between the peroneus brevis and extensor digitorum brevis (Figure 60.12). The incision is carried from the anterior process of the calcaneus to the fourth metatarsal base, and the extensor digitorum brevis muscle is elevated dorsally. Bone graft may be used to fill any void associated with the collapse of the underlying cancellous bone.

Often, a small external fixator is used to maintain length of the cuboid during surgery. Occasionally, the device is kept in place for 6 weeks after surgery (Figure 60.13). Alternatively, internal fixation may span the joints to hold the lateral column out to length. If there is intra-articular comminution and the calcaneocuboid joint cannot be reasonably preserved, an arthrodesis may be performed. However, every effort should be made to preserve the articulation between the cuboid and the metatarsal bases. Further, the plantar surface of the cuboid should be assessed at the peroneal sulcus to ensure reduction of the tendon as it passes medially. The goals are to maintain length and joint function. Arthrodesis across the calcaneocuboid joint is well tolerated, but it is worth reiterating that arthrodesis across the fourth and fifth TMTJs is poorly tolerated.

© 2018 American Academy of Orthopaedic Surgeons

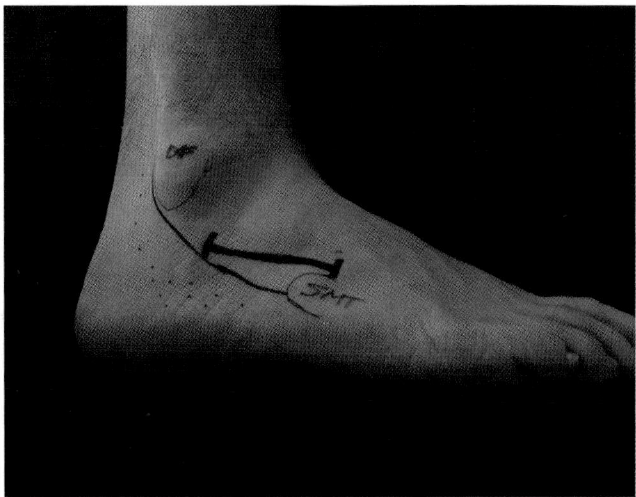

Figure 60.12 Photograph demonstrating the lateral approach to cuboid. Incision (*purple line with vertical border lines*) is plantar to the extensor digitorum brevis muscle belly, dorsal to peroneal tendon(s) (*straight black line*) and fifth metatarsal base (5MT), centered over the cuboid and distal to distal fibula (DF).

Complications

- Wound healing issue
  - Infection
- Equinus contracture
- Deformity:
  - Flatfoot
  - Forefoot abduction
- Midfoot (Lisfranc/Chopart joint) arthrosis
- Peroneus longus tendinopathy
- Toe stiffness
- Nerve injury

Specific Rehabilitation Consideration for Midfoot Injuries

- Sagittal plane motion is limited to less than 10° at the medial and middle column of the midfoot. There is limited role for attempts to restore motion at these joints. The lateral column is far more mobile; efforts should be made to optimize motion and avoid rigidity at these joints (cubometatarsal).
- Owing to significant soft-tissue damage about the midfoot and ensuing surgical dissection, there is significant risk for contracture and scarring about the flexors and extensors of the toes. Mobilization efforts should be focused about these tendons to minimize contracture (usually in extension) and loss of function about the toes.

GENERALIZED REHABILITATION PROTOCOL FOR FOOT INJURIES

Early Wound Healing Phase

Early efforts are focused on immobilization in a well-fitting, appropriately padded posterior short-leg splint with side gussets, applied in neutral positioning at the ankle and foot. This should be removed after the wound is healed (typically at least 2 weeks postoperatively). Active toe flexion exercises (intrinsic contractions) can keep blood flowing in the plantar venous plexus.

Range of Motion Advancement/Edema Diminishment Phase

After the wound has healed, patients who are compliant with non–weight bearing instructions may be placed in a removable immobilization device such as a controlled-ankle-motion (CAM) boot. Efforts at this stage are focused on the return of ROM at the subtalar joint and ankle. Therapeutic activities may include active and gentle active assist/passive efforts. The limb

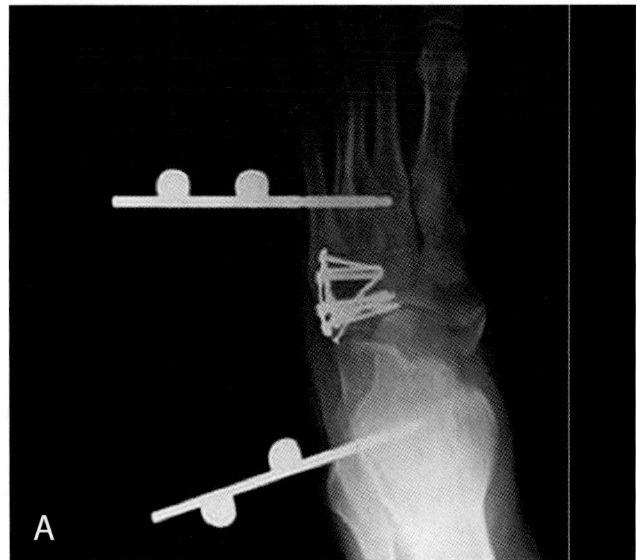

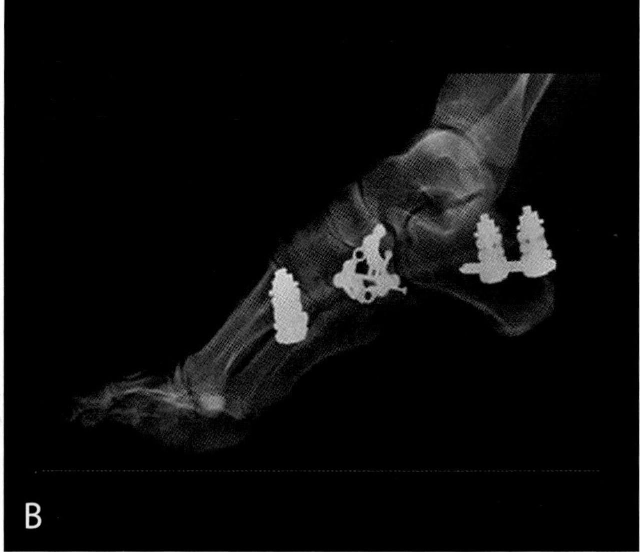

Figure 60.13 **A**, Radiograph demonstrating anteroposterior view of cuboid fracture external and internal fixation. **B**, Radiograph demonstrating lateral view of cuboid fracture external and internal fixation. (From Borrelli J Jr, De S, VanPelt M. Fracture of the cuboid. *J Am Acad Orthop Surg* 2012;20(7):472–7. doi: 10.5435/JAAOS-20-07-472.)

 © 2018 American Academy of Orthopaedic Surgeons

may be suspended off the treatment table in multiple planes in order to employ gravity to initiate plantarflexion, dorsiflexion, inversion, and eversion. Persistent edema may restrict rehabilitation efforts and should be addressed. ROM and return of calf function will assist greatly and can be augmented with application of ice packs and/or compression devices (foot pumps, cold therapy, cold compression units). Desensitization may be employed, especially if sural nerve injury has occurred. The patient should maintain strict non–weight bearing status until clinical and potentially radiographic evidence of fracture healing has occurred.

Strengthening and Restoration of Function Phase

After the fracture has progressed to clinical and radiographic healing, the orthopaedic surgeon may initiate progression to weight bearing and return to footwear (typically 8–12 weeks postoperatively). If necessary, accommodative/offloading orthotics can be used to alleviate pain from heel fat pad injury/atrophy and any residual plantar prominences. It is often critical to provide support for the medial arch following Lisfranc injury. Further, ankle–foot orthoses (including spring-leaf devices) may be employed to stabilize the weakened ankle as rehabilitation progresses. After injury and prolonged immobilization, weakness and atrophy often manifest, particularly about the musculature of the leg. Strengthening efforts progress with advancement of weight bearing but may be augmented with use of focused resisted ankle/hindfoot plantarflexion, dorsiflexion, inversion, and eversion with resistance band(s). Attention is also placed to optimizing active toe motion and strength, with activities such as towel grabs. As pain subsides and the fracture remodels and strengthens, advanced strengthening efforts should progress with use of weighted equipment for focused strengthening of the musculature about the leg.

Proprioception

After injury, and subsequent immobilization, proprioception declines. Appropriate treatment of the ensuing deficits should be employed to optimize function and minimize the risk of recurrent injury to the affected limb. Once fracture healing has progressed to allow prolonged stance phase on the injured limb, balance activities should progress. Initial efforts begin with bilateral stance on even ground with eyes open. As progress allows, uneven ground or use of a balance board should be introduced with eyes open and closed (Figure 60.14). Once these activities are successfully performed on both feet, therapy should advance to include unilateral stance.

Agility and Return to Activity

Once healing has progressed to allow strengthening and proprioception therapies, a focused effort should be made to optimize the function and return the patient to preinjury activity levels. Final stages of therapy include education regarding optimization of mechanics and gait to minimize overload on the injured extremity and limit advancement of arthritis at the adjacent joints. Focused monitoring, education, and instruction should be provided for daily activities, lateral and cutting

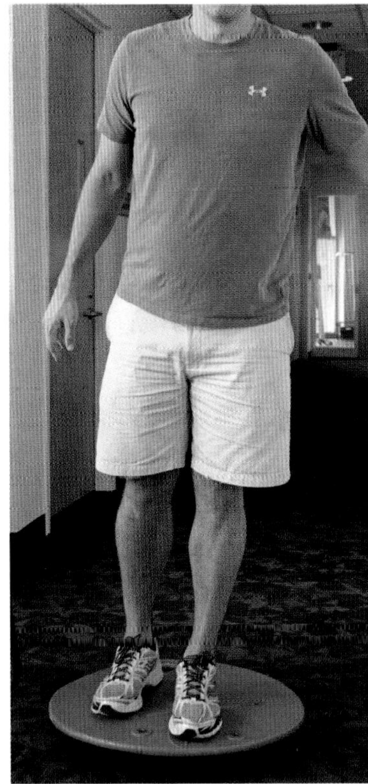

Figure 60.14 Representative photograph of BAPS use. (Image courtesy of Robert D'Angelo, PA-C)

activities, jumping, and sports/vocation-specific activities. These are tailored to the patient's specific needs.

Certain patients will not be able to return to full activity. It is particularly difficult for laborers to return to their prior functional level following Lisfranc injuries and calcaneus fractures. If limitations are noted and rehabilitation efforts plateau, a multidisciplinary plan should be made to minimize pain and optimize function. This plan may include activity modifications, anti-inflammatory medications, diagnostic injections, advanced custom orthoses, selective arthrodesis, or even amputation. Recent advances have been made with the development of the Intrepid Dynamic Exoskeletal Orthosis (IDEO™) and similar devices that may allow for limb salvage efforts to be associated with satisfactory return to function (Figure 60.15).

PEARLS

Surgical

- Restore height, eliminate varus, restore the articular surface of the posterior facet and morphology of the tuber in calcaneus fractures.
- Restore articular relationships and avoid varus malunion in talus fractures.
- Achieve stability and articular congruity with Lisfranc injuries. Consider arthrodesis with severe comminution.
- Avoid permanent rigid fixation of the lateral column of the midfoot.

© 2018 American Academy of Orthopaedic Surgeons

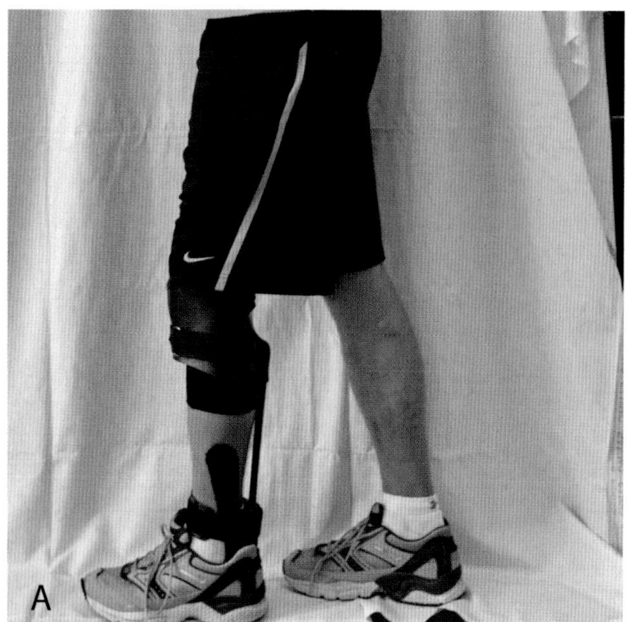

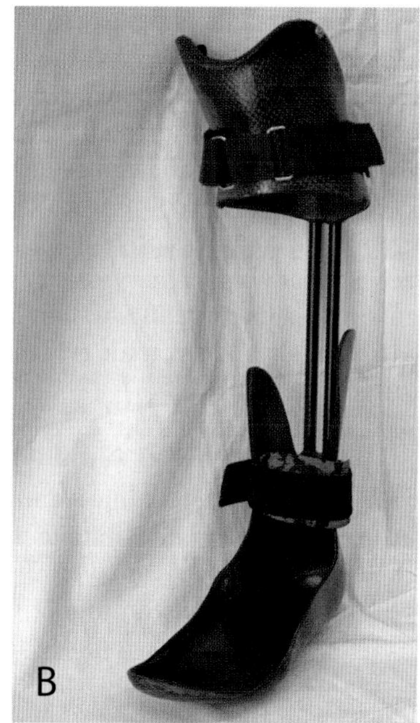

Figure 60.15 **A**, Photograph of IDEO on patient. **B**, Photograph of IDEO. (Images courtesy of Robert D'Angelo, PA-C)

Rehabilitation

- Early efforts should focus on edema control.
- ROM is typically limited, at least until wound healing has occurred. Mobilization of soft tissues and joints then progresses consistently.
- Full weight bearing is typically limited until consolidation of fractures is demonstrated (around 8–12 weeks).
- The goal is restore the foot to one that functions on uneven ground in all preinjury activities. This may be difficult to achieve. Bracing, arthrodesis, and amputation may be considered if the injury and its subsequent healing and rehabilitation fail to allow for achievement of patient-specific functional goals.

BIBLIOGRAPHY

Borrelli J Jr, De S, VanPelt M: Fracture of the cuboid. *J Am Acad Orthop Surg* 2012;20(7):472–477.

Desmond EA, Chou LB: Current concepts review: Lisfranc injuries. *Foot Ankle Int* 2006;27(8):653–660.

Fortin PT, Balazsy JE: Talus Fractures: evaluation and treatment. *J Am Acad Orthop Surg* 2001;9(2):114–127.

Hsu JR, Bosse MJ: Challenges in severe lower limb injury rehabilitation. *J Am Acad Orthop Surg* 2012;20(suppl 1): S39–S41.

Ly TV, Coetzee JC: Treatment of primarily ligamentous Lisfranc joint injuries: primary arthrodesis compared with open reduction and internal fixation. A prospective, randomized study. *J Bone Joint Surg Am* 2006;88(3):514–520.

Patzkowski JC, Blanck RV, Owens JG, Wilken JM, Kirk KL, Wenke JC, Hsu JR; STReC: Comparative effect of orthosis design on functional performance. *J Bone Joint Surg Am* 2012; 94(6):507–515.

Sanders R: Displaced intra-articular fractures of the calcaneus. *J Bone Joint Surg Am* 2000;82(2):225–250.

 © 2018 American Academy of Orthopaedic Surgeons

SECTION 7

Spine

61 Rehabilitation After Spine Surgery—Relevant Anatomy

David Alex Stroh, MD, Bradley Moatz, MD, and P. Justin Tortolani, MD

INTRODUCTION

A thorough understanding of the anatomy of the spine, spinal cord, and surrounding structures forms the basis for sound surgical treatment, as well as successful postoperative rehabilitation. A stable axial skeleton is the cornerstone of ambulation and the support for the major organ spaces (head, thorax, abdomen, and pelvis). The particular structure and biomechanics of the vertebral column and musculature dictate what techniques and exercises will help patients achieve balance, correct posture, functionality, or accommodate postoperative difficulties in mobilization. While an extensive review is beyond the scope of this chapter, the reader is referred to classic works for further learning; the basic principles presented here will provide a framework for spine kinesiology as well as a rationale for what constitutes *safe* postoperative physical therapy.

ANATOMY OF THE ADULT SPINE

Topical Anatomy

Pertinent topical anatomy starts with the occiput at the posterior base of the skull, from which a ridge of bone (the superior nuchal line) extends laterally. As one works inferiorly, the spinous processes increase in size, with the most easily palpable at C7 (the vertebral prominens). The thoracic spinous processes gradually angulate inferiorly from cranial to caudal, so that the vertebral body may be located at times superior to the palpable spinous process. Examination of the topical landmarks provides useful information. First, there should be no step-off between spinous processes, which otherwise may indicate spondylolisthesis. The posterior superior iliac spine (PSIS) may be palpated with the thumbs, and the fingers curled anteriorly to define the "version" (inclination in the sagittal plane) of the pelvis. On the Adams forward bending test, the spinous processes and ribs serve as landmarks in the evaluation of scoliosis. Various topical landmarks are useful in estimating the level of spinal vertebrae (Table 61.1).

Vertebral Elements

The spine is organized into cervical (C1–C7), thoracic (T1–T12), lumbar (L1–L5), fused sacral (S1–S5), and fused coccygeal (4 total) segments, as shown in Figure 61.1, with additional lumbar and cervical vertebrae or sacralized terminal lumbar vertebrae being common variations. Four transition zones are notable. The region from the occiput to the first and second cervical vertebrae is highly specialized, with C1 forming a flattened ring to both cradle the skull and rotate about the dens (or axis) of C2. Two junctions within the vertebral column itself accompany the transition from the lordotic cervical and lumbar regions to the kyphotic thoracic region. Finally, the lumbosacral junction provides a connection to the bony pelvis via the relatively immobile sacroiliac (SI) joints. These junctions are unique in that they are areas of transition from a relatively immobile spinal segment (thoracic and sacral) to a more mobile one (cervical and lumbar). As a result, these areas are under relatively higher stress and are particularly vulnerable to injury.

Dr. Moatz or an immediate family member has received nonincome support (such as equipment or services), commercially derived honoraria, or other non-research–related funding (such as paid travel) from Globus Medical and Vertebral Technologies Incorporated. Dr. Tortolani or an immediate family member has received royalties from Globus Medical; serves as a paid consultant to Globus Medical, Innovasis, and Spineology; has received research or institutional support from Spineology; and serves as a board member, owner, officer, or committee member of the Journal of Spinal Deformity, *Medstar Union Memorial Hospital, and Surgical Neurology International. Neither Dr. Stroh nor any immediate family member has received anything of value from or has stock or stock options held in a commercial company or institution related directly or indirectly to the subject of this article.*

© 2018 American Academy of Orthopaedic Surgeons

Table 61.1	TOPICAL LANDMARKS AND SPINAL LEVELS
Mandible	C2–C3
Hyoid cartilage	C3
Thyroid cartilage	C4–C5
Cricoid cartilage	C6
Vertebral prominens	C7
Scapular spine	T3
Sternal angle	T4–T5
Inferior scapular angle	T7
Umbilicus	T10
Iliac crests	L4
Posterior superior iliac spine	S2

All typical vertebrae share certain features (Figure 61.2): ventrally a cylindrical body, dorsally a vertebral arch, and paired pedicles connecting the two and completing the ring of the vertebral foramen. The body is composed of mostly cancellous bone with a thin cortical rim. On each side, three processes emanate from the region where the pedicle meets the remainder of the vertebral arch (the posterior elements). The transverse process lies between the superior and inferior processes, and serves as a bony lever arm for the attachment of ligaments and muscles. The bony isthmus between the superior and inferior processes is the pars interarticularis, an area prone to stress fracture with repetitive translational motion of adjacent vertebrae. Two flattened laminae spread dorsally from the isthmus, completing the vertebral arch and coalescing into an elongated posterior spinous process.

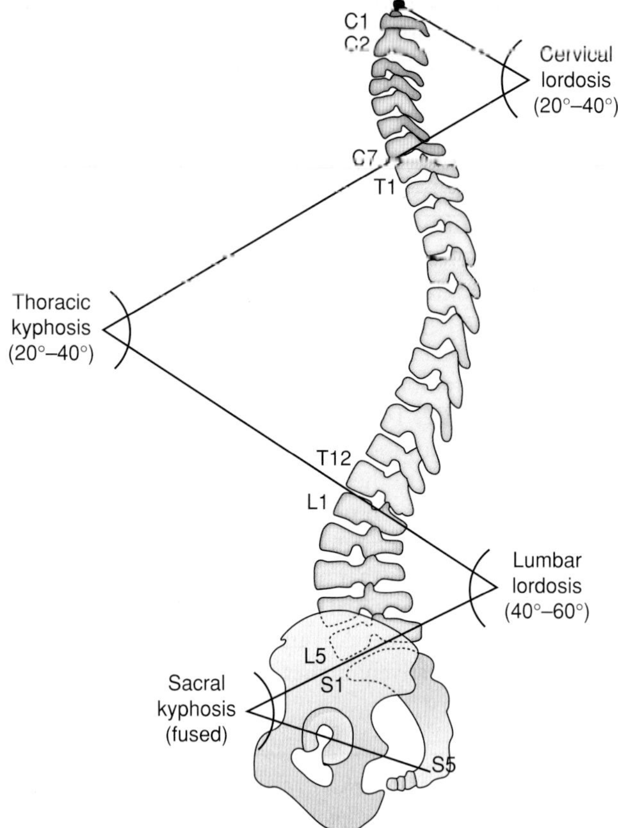

Figure 61.1 Sagittal view of the vertebral column and pelvis demonstrating cervical and lumbar lordosis, thoracic and sacral kyphosis, and the fused coccyx. (Adapted from Roussouly P, Pinheiro-Franco JL: Sagittal parameters of the spine: biomechanical approach. *Eur Spine J* 2011;20(Suppl 5):609–618.)

Regional variations in vertebral morphology balance the need for both stability and range of motion (ROM). From cephalad to caudad, body size increases to support the increased weight borne by the lumbar spine. The orientation of facet joints slowly shifts from roughly 45° from the sagittal plane (semicoronal) to nearly parallel. This restricts the amount of permissible rotation in the lumbar spine. Pedicle diameter increases almost linearly from C3 to T1, decreases linearly from T1 to T4–T6, then increases almost exponentially from T6 to S1 (with the notable exception that the L1 pedicles are often smaller than T12). In the axial plane, their orientation also becomes more medially angulated in the inferior segments. These variations make pedicle screw placement more difficult in the cranial regions of the thoracic and cervical spine, to the point at which screws placed in the lateral mass are commonly used for posterior cervical fixation. Finally, the anterior lip of a cervical vertebra slightly overlaps the disc inferiorly, and from C3 to C7 there are superiorly directed uncinate processes on the lateral peripheries of the superior endplates that articulate with a groove (the uncus) on the inferior endplate of the body above.

Anterior to the transverse process exists some form of costal element. In the cervical spine, this fuses anteriorly to the body to form the transverse foramen for the vertebral artery. The anterior portions of the C7 transverse processes inconsistently form anomalous cervical ribs, a risk factor in the development of thoracic outlet syndrome. The costal element of the thoracic spine is a facet and its corresponding rib, which in some cases spans two vertebrae and serves to stiffen the thoracic segments. The costal element in the lumbar vertebrae is split to form the mammillary, accessory, and part of the transverse processes. In the sacrum, the costal elements fuse to the transverse processes above and below to present the contiguous articulating surface of the SI joint.

The vertebrae of the upper cervical and sacral regions are highly specialized. The atlas (C1) and axis (C2) lack formal vertebral bodies; instead, they comprise anterior and posterior arches. C1 has concave facets both superiorly and inferiorly on C1 to accept the curved occiput and the lateral mass (a fusion of the pedicle and the articular facets) of C2. The dens of C2 is held anteriorly against C1 primarily by the transverse, alar, and apical ligaments, as well as the tectorial membrane (a continuation of the posterior longitudinal ligament). The fused sacrum presents a continuous lateral articulation for the SI joint, a middle sacral crest representing the fused spinous processes, lateral crests which create a groove for the multifidus, and sacral foramina to transmit the sacral nerve roots.

© 2018 American Academy of Orthopaedic Surgeons

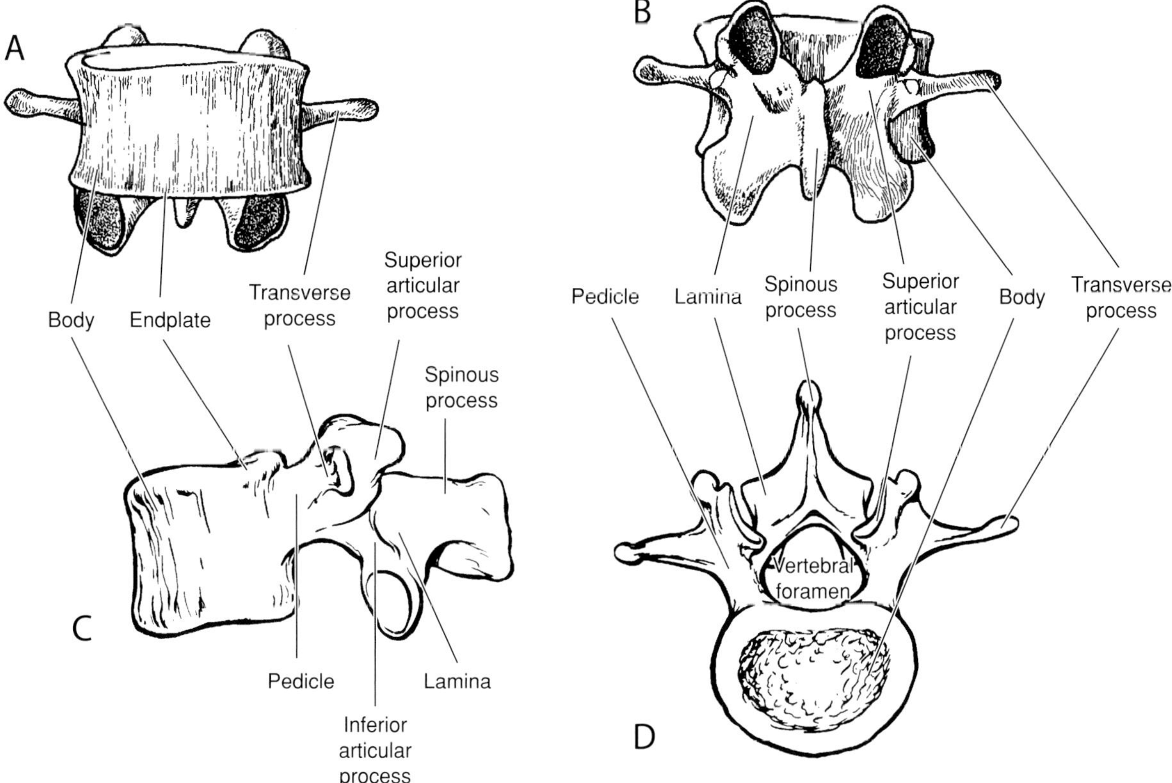

Figure 61.2 Features of a typical vertebra, demonstrated from anterior (**A**), posterior (**B**), lateral (**C**), and superior (**D**) views. (Reproduced with permission from MediClip, copyright (c) 2003, Philadelphia, PA, Lippincott Williams & Wilkins. All rights reserved.)

Joints and Ligaments of the Vertebral Column

A variety of joints are found throughout the vertebral column. All typical vertebrae contribute superior and inferior articular processes to the facet or zygapophyseal joints, so named because they "yoke" together two adjacent vertebrae. Facet joints are relatively mobile and permit gliding motion to accommodate flexion–extension and some degree of rotation. From C3 to C7, the inferior vertebral body contacts the superior body at the lateral periphery via the uncovertebral joints, which permits flexion–extension but limits lateral flexion. In the thoracic spine, costal facets articulate with same-leveled ribs both on the vertebral bodies and on certain transverse processes to permit rib motion.

The intervertebral disc is an arthrodial joint that separates adjacent vertebrae and cushions axial load. It comprises an outer annulus (primarily type 1 collagen) and an inner nucleus pulposus (relatively high proteoglycan content). The hydrophilic proteoglycans draw in water and hydrate the nucleus, which allows it to resist compression. Injuries to the disc may include incomplete annular tears, full-thickness tears, and herniations of the nucleus pulposus. These are categorized into disc bulges (intact, but weakened, annulus expands broadly under pressure), protrusions (disc material breaks through the annulus), or extrusions (nuclear material breaks off into the vertebral foramen). The disc does not receive any blood vessels, and most of the nutrients necessary to the cells within the disc are delivered via diffusion from vessels in the endplate.

Ligamentous restraints in the spinal column (Figure 61.3) include the anterior longitudinal ligaments (ALL) and posterior longitudinal ligaments (PLL), facet joint capsule, ligamentum flavum, interspinous ligament, and supraspinous ligament (and its cervical continuation, the ligamentum nuchae). These ligaments restrict safe vertebral motion and stabilize the spine. Ligaments contacting the intervertebral or spinal foramina

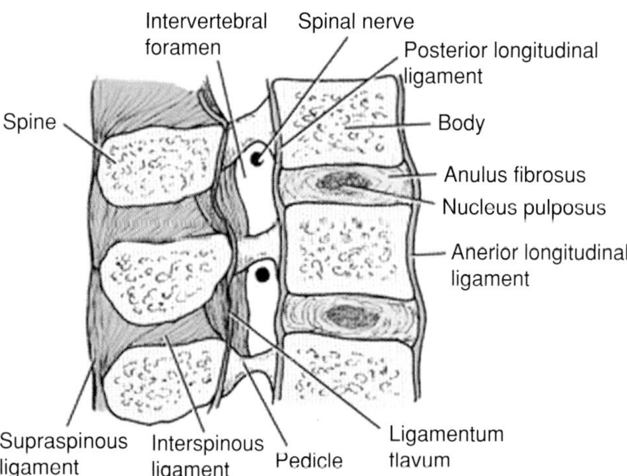

Figure 61.3 Ligamentous structures of the spinal column in oblique and sagittal cross-section. (Reproduced with permission from Snell RS: *Clinical Neuroanatomy.* Philadelphia, PA, Lippincott Williams & Wilkins, 2009.)

© 2018 American Academy of Orthopaedic Surgeons

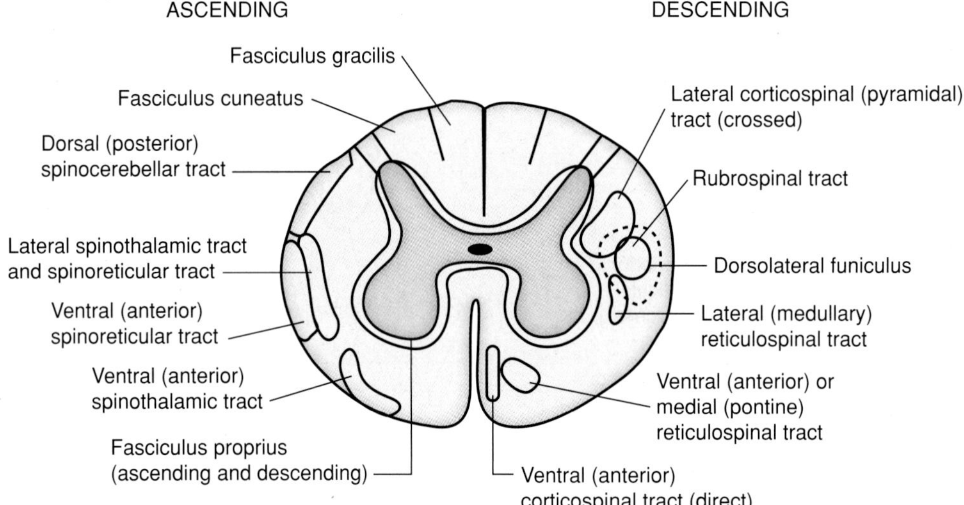

Figure 61.4 Cross-section of the spinal cord with outlines of longitudinal motor and sensory tracts. (Reproduced with permission from Ballantyne JC: *Massachusetts General Hospital Handbook of Pain Management*. Philadelphia, PA, Lippincott Williams & Wilkins, 2005.)

(PLL, facet capsule, ligamentum flavum) may cause nerve compression if they become hypertrophic.

Nervous System Anatomy and Pathoanatomy

The spinal cord is divided into longitudinal tracts (Figure 61.4) well organized by function (ascending sensory vs. descending motor/inhibitory), region (cervical, thoracic, lumbar, and sacral), and cell type (gray matter vs. white matter). The white matter tracts of the spinal cord are located peripherally, compared to the central gray matter of motor neuron bodies. Paired dorsal (ascending axons of sensory neurons in the dorsal root ganglion) and ventral roots (descending axons of motor neurons) emanate from the spinal cord, coalescing into the proper spinal nerve before exiting the vertebral foramen and splitting into dorsal and ventral rami. Various motor, sensory, and reflex physical examination findings are attributed to specific nerve roots, as shown in Table 61.2.

In considering disc herniations, two facts help the investigator correlate imaging findings with expected radicular symptoms to determine the spinal nerve affected. First, from C3 to C7, the nerve roots are located above the pedicle bearing their name (e.g., C7 exits above the C7 pedicle), a pattern that changes at T1 since no C8 vertebra exists for the C8 nerve root (T1 exits below the T1 pedicle). Second, the exit angle of the nerve roots is shallow in the cervical spine (nearly horizontal) and becomes steeper caudally. Because of this, cervical disc herniations will almost always affect one nerve root (usually the higher-numbered nerve), while lumbar herniations may affect either the exiting/lower-numbered nerve root (if sufficiently lateral to the foramen) or the traversing/higher-numbered nerve root (more central). The spinal cord ends in most at the L1 to L2 level, terminating in a swelling known as the conus medullaris. Stenosis of the vertebral foramen from any cause in levels above this carries a risk of spinal cord compression, which can lead to myelopathy. Below L2, only nerve roots can be compressed, leading to radiculopathy. In cases of complete occlusion of the vertebral foramen beneath L2, cauda equina syndrome may develop.

Vascular Anatomy

The blood supply to the spinal cord is derived from two anterior and one posterior spinal arteries. These receive other vessels throughout the length of the cord (segmental medullary and intercostal arteries) from the subclavian/vertebral arteries, or directly from the aorta. The largest of these segmental medullary arteries, the artery of Adamkiewicz, enters in the midthoracic spine and can be interrupted by endovascular grafts, retroperitoneal dissection, or thrombosis leading to spinal cord ischemia. Traveling within the vertebral foramina are anterior and posterior radicular branches from the dorsal branches of the intercostal arteries, which may be a source of bleeding with aggressive dissection in this area. Venous drainage is achieved through a convoluted internal vertebral plexus that spans the length of the spinal cord. These vessels also receive venous drainage from the pelvis and thorax via the Batson venous plexus, a valveless system that has been implicated in the spread of metastatic tumors and infections to the vertebral column.

The course of the vertebral artery is especially important in dissection and instrumentation of the cervical spine. The vessel travels through the transverse foramen at all cervical levels except C7. It then makes a sharp curve after exiting the foramen of C1 and travels medially, before turning superiorly to enter the foramen magnum. Surgical dissection any more than 2 cm lateral to the vertebral body risks damage to the vertebral artery.

Spinal Musculature

The muscles of the neck are arranged into anterior groups (superficial, suprahyoid, infrahyoid, and deep) and posterior

 © 2018 American Academy of Orthopaedic Surgeons

Table 61.2 PHYSICAL EXAMINATION OF SPINAL NERVE ROOTS

Spinal Level	Sensory (Light Touch or Pinprick) (0, Absent; 1, Altered; 2, Normal)	Motor (0, Paralysis; 1, Twitch only; 2, Moves without gravity; 3, Resists gravity; 4, Resists external force; 5, Normal)	Reflex (0+, None; 1+, Diminished; 2+, Normal; 3+, Hyperactive; 4+, Hyperactive with clonus)
Upper Extremity			
C5	Shoulder (axillary)	Abduct shoulder (axillary)	Biceps
C6	Base of thumb (radial)	Flex arm (C5 < C6/musculocutaneous) Resisted wrist extension for C6 (radial side weak) and C7 (ulnar side weak)	Brachioradialis
C7	Middle finger (median)	Extend arm (radial) Resisted wrist flexion for C7 (radial side weak) and C8 (ulnar side weak)	Triceps
C8	Small finger (ulnar)	Resisted finger flexion and thumb extension	
T1	Medial arm (medial brachial cutaneous)	Resisted finger abduction	
Lower Extremity			
L1	Inguinal region		
L2	Medial thigh (obturator)	Hip flexion (L2 > L3/femoral)	
L3	Medial knee	Quadriceps extension (L3 + L4/ femoral)	
L4	Medial foot (saphenous) and anterior knee	Ankle dorsiflexion (L4 > L5/deep peroneal)	Quad tendon
L5	Dorsum foot (superficial peroneal)	Great toe dorsiflexion (deep peroneal)	
S1	Lateral foot (sural)	Ankle plantarflexion (posterior tibial)	Achilles tendon
S2	Popliteal fossa	Knee flexion (L5–S2/sciatic)	Anal wink (S2–S5)
S3–S4	Anus (S3–S4)	Lesser toe flexion (S2–S4), voluntary sphincter contraction (S2–S4)	

groups (superficial, suboccipital triangle), as seen in Table 61.3. These muscle groups are separated by the superficial, pretracheal, and prevertebral fascias. The typical anterior approach to the spine utilizes a transverse, left-sided incision (to avoid the more vulnerable recurrent laryngeal nerve on the right) that splits the platysma and longus colli, leaving all other muscles intact. The midline posterior cervical approach, like all midline spine incisions, passes through the fasciotendinous junction of the paraspinal muscles, then continues beneath the periosteum once bone is reached. As in the posterior lumbar approach, dissection laterally from the spinous process potentially disrupts the dorsal rami, innervating the paraspinal musculature. Since these muscle tracts are segmentally innervated, no significant paresis or deficit occurs.

All remaining back muscles are organized into extrinsic, intrinsic (superficial, intermediate), and abdominal (anterior and posterior) groups. The three layers of the thoracolumbar and lumbodorsal fascias separate these muscles further. Anterior approaches to the spine traverse the layers of the abdominal wall (midline or paramedian), and retract the intra-abdominal contents either as a whole within the peritoneum or through the peritoneum. The retroperitoneal fascia is then incised and the great vessels avoided, allowing direct access to the anterior spine. Alternatively, a retroperitoneal approach through the muscle bellies of the transverse and oblique abdominal muscles allows direct access to the plane between the peritoneum and retroperitoneum. An incision off midline may represent a posterolateral/Wiltse approach to the spine, which takes a plane between the multifidus and longissimus muscles. Although more invasive of the muscle than a midline approach, this approach typically does not lead to significant muscle transection that would compromise movement. Finally, an extremely far lateral incision is used in the lateral transpsoas approach. This approach transects the psoas fibers to reach the anterolateral aspect of the vertebral body. At-risk structures include the lumbar nerve roots, which pass through the psoas muscle before exiting and converging into the lumbar plexus (Table 61.4).

© 2018 American Academy of Orthopaedic Surgeons

Table 61.3 MUSCULATURE OF THE NECK

Muscle	Origin	Insertion	Function	Nerve
Anterior Neck: Superficial				
Platysma	Superior border of clavicle	Anterior surface of mandible and skin overlying lower face and neck	Tightens skin for facial expression; depresses jaw	Cervical branch of facial nerve
Sternocleidomastoid	Manubrium and clavicle	Mastoid process and superior nuchal line	Flexes and rotates head toward opposite side. *Antagonist: Trapezius*	Spinal accessory nerve
Anterior Cervical Triangle: Suprahyoid				
Diagastric	Mandible and mastoid	Hyoid	Opens jaw. *Antagonist: Masseter*	Mylohyoid and facial nerve
Mylohyoid	Mandible		Elevates hyoid, depresses mandible, elevates the floor of the oral cavity. *Antagonist: Infrahyoid group*	Mylohyoid nerve
Stylohyoid	Styloid process of temporal bone			Facial nerve
Geniohyoid				Hypoglossal nerve
Anterior Cervical Triangle: Infrahyoid				
Sternohyoid	Manubrium	Hyoid	Depresses hyoid and larynx. *Antagonist: Suprahyoid group*	Ansa cervicalis
Omohyoid	Scapula			
Thyrohyoid	Thyroid cartilage			Ventral rami of C1
Sternothyroid	Manubrium	Thyroid cartilage	Depresses hyoid and elevates larynx. *Antagonist: Suprahyoid group*	Ansa cervicalis
Anterior Neck: Deep				
Longus capitis	Transverse processes of C3–C6	Inferior occiput	Flexes vertebral column. *Antagonist: Trapezius*	Ventral rami of C2–C6
Longus colli		Basilar surface of occiput		Ventral rami of C1–C4
Posterior Neck: Superficial				
Scalene	Transverse processes of C2–C7	Posterior border of ribs 1 and 2	Laterally flexes neck, elevates ribs	Ventral rami of C5–C8
Posterior Neck: Suboccipital Triangle				
Rectus capitis posterior major/minor	Posterior spine or tubercle of atlas and axis	Inferior nuchal line	Extends, rotates, and laterally flexes head *Antagonist: Sternocleidomastoid*	Suboccipital nerve
Obliquus capitis superior/inferior	Spine of axis and transverse process of atlas	Occiput and transverse process of atlas	Extends and rotates head. *Antagonist: Sternocleidomastoid*	

 © 2018 American Academy of Orthopaedic Surgeons

Table 61.4 MUSCULATURE OF THE BACK

Muscle	Origin	Insertion	Function	Nerve
Extrinsic				
Trapezius	Medial aspect of superior nuchal line, external occipital protruberance, ligamentum nuchae C7–T12	Clavicle, acromion and scapular spine	Elevates, adducts, medially rotates scapula. Extends neck. *Antagonist: Serratus anterior, sternocleidomastoid*	Spinal accessory nerve
Rhomboid minor	Spinous processes C7–T1	Medial border of scapula	Adducts and medially rotates scapula. *Antagonist: Serratus anterior*	Dorsal scapular nerve (C5)
Rhomboid major	Spinous processes T2–T5			
Levator scapulae	Transverse processes of atlas, axis, C3, C4		Elevates scapula	Dorsal scapular nerve and dorsal rami of C3–C4
Latissimus dorsi	Thoracolumbar fascia (spinous processes of T7 through ilium)	Floor of intertubercular sulcus of humerus	Extends, adducts, and internally rotates humerus *Antagonist: Deltoid, subscapularis*	Thoracodorsal nerve
Serratus posterior superior	Spinous processes of C7–T3	Superior border ribs 2–5	Elevates ribs	Ventral rami of T1–T4 (intercostal nerves)
Serratus posterior inferior	Spinous processes of T11–L3	Inferior border ribs 9–12	Depresses ribs	Ventral rami of T9–T12 (intercostal nerves)
Intrinsic: Superficial Layer/Spinotransverse Group				
Splenius capitis	Inferior aspect of ligamentum nuchae, C3–T4	Superior nuchal line and mastoid process	Extend, or rotate and laterally flex, neck. *Antagonist: Sternocleidomastoid, longus colli*	Dorsal rami of spinal nerves
Splenius cervicus	Spinous processes of T1–T6	Transverse process of C1–C4		
Intrinsic: Intermediate Layer/Sacrospinalis Group (Erector Spinae)				
Spinalis	Sacrum, iliac crest, lumbar spinous processes	Spinous processes of C2–T8	Extends, rotates, and laterally flexes vertebral column. *Antagonist: Sternocleidomastoid, longus colli, abdominals*	Dorsal rami of spinal nerves
Longissimus		Mastoid process, spinous processes of cervical and thoracic spine		
Iliocostalis		Inferior border of ribs and transverse processes of C4–C7		

Continued on following page

© 2018 American Academy of Orthopaedic Surgeons

Table 61.4 MUSCULATURE OF THE BACK *(Continued)*

Muscle	Origin	Insertion	Function	Nerve
Intrinsic: Deep Layer/Transversospinalis Group				
Semispinalis capitis	Transverse processes of C7–T7	Nuchal ridge of occiput	Extends and rotates head to opposite side	Dorsal rami of spinal nerves
Semispinalis thoracis	Transverse processes of T1–T10	Spinous processes of C2–T4		
Multifidus	Transverse processes of C3–S4	Spinous processes of superior vertebrae (C2–S4)	Laterally flex and rotate vertebral column to opposite side	
Rotatores		Spinous process of adjacent superior vertebra	Rotate adjacent superior vertebra to opposite side	
Levator costarum		Superior border of adjacent inferior ribs	Elevate inferior rib	
Intertransversarii		Transverse processes of C3–S4	Laterally flex superior vertebra	
Interspinales	Spinous processes of C3–S4	Spinous process of adjacent superior vertebra	Extend superior vertebra	
Anterior Abdominal Wall				
Rectus abdominis	Pubis	Xiphoid and inferior border of costal cartilage for ribs 5–7	Main flexor of vertebral column. *Antagonist: Erector spinae, multifidus, interspinales*	Thoracoabdominal nerves (T7–T12)
Transversus abdominis	Iliac crest and inguinal ligament, thoracic surface of ribs 6–12	Pubic crest, pectineal line	Reduces intra-abdominal volume, increases intra-abdominal pressure	Dorsal rami of T7–T12; iliohypogastric, ilioinguinal, and genitofemoral nerves
External oblique	Anterior and inferior borders of ribs 4–12	Iliac crest and inguinal ligament	Rotates vertebral column to same side, reduces intra-abdominal volume, increases intra-abdominal pressure	Dorsal rami of spinal nerves T5–T12
Internal oblique	Iliac crest and inguinal ligament	Anterior and inferior borders of ribs 4–12, xiphoid, linea alba		Dorsal rami of spinal nerves T8–T12; iliohypogastric and ilioinguinal nerves
Posterior Abdominal Wall				
Diaphragm	Thoracic surface of the xiphoid and ribs 6–12	Central tendon	Ascent and descent alter intrathoracic and intra-abdominal volume and pressure	Phrenic nerve and dorsal rami of lumbar spinal nerves
Psoas major/ minor	Transverse processes and lateral body surfaces of L1–L4	Lesser trochanter of femur	Flex and externally rotate hip. *Antagonist: Gluteus maximus*	Lumbar plexus (L1–L3)
Iliacus	Iliac fossa		Flex hip, rotate spine towards	Femoral nerve
Quadratus lumborum	Iliolumbar ligament and iliac crest	Inferior border of last rib and transverse processes of L1–L4	Lateral flexion of vertebral column; depression of ribs	Ventral rami of T12–L4

© 2018 American Academy of Orthopaedic Surgeons

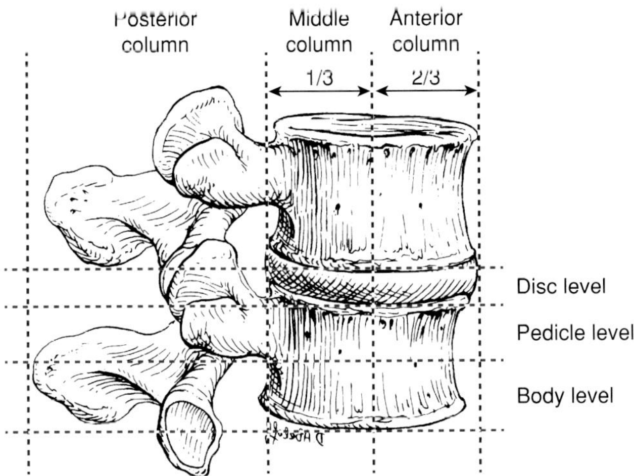

Figure 61.5 Spinal motion segment (functional spinal unit), divided into three columns (blue) and three levels (red). (Reproduced with permission from MediClip, copyright (c) 2003, Philadelphia, PA, Lippincott Williams & Wilkins. All rights reserved.)

OVERVIEW OF BIOMECHANICS

A spinal motion segment (or functional spinal unit, Figure 61.5) is the smallest collection of spinal elements that replicates the kinematics/dynamics of the entire vertebral column. It comprises two adjacent vertebrae, their interposed disc, and all ligamentous connections in between. This segment can be separated conceptually into three columns and three rows on a lateral view. In the coronal plane, the anterior column spans from the ALL to two-thirds through the vertebral body. The middle column follows from the posterior two-thirds of the body to the PLL. Finally, the posterior column runs from the posterior to the PLL to the posteriormost portion of the spinal process. Spinal stability is compromised when two of the three columns are disrupted (either by bony or ligamentous injury). Across the disc, pressure in each "column" will vary based on posture, with supine, standing, and seated postures having increasing degrees of intradiscal pressure. Pain that is greater in the seated position is more likely due to pressure on the disc rather than nerve compression, since neural foramina open wider in flexion and relieve pressure on nerve roots. The observation that a greater percentage of body weight is borne by the anterior and middle columns has led to the successful use of interbody devices (designed to restore the integrity of the anterior spine).

In the axial plane, the level of the intervertebral disc, the pedicle, and the body can be separated. In the balanced spinal segment, structures in any two of these levels will never be coplanar. This helps describe imaging findings, localize structures intraoperatively, and provide information about what the source of any nerve compression/irritation might be (e.g., disc material at the disc level, facet cyst at the pedicle level, osteophyte at the body level, and so on).

The S-shaped curve of the adult vertebral column is due in part to genetics and to human upright posture. Infants are born with a C-shaped vertebral column, lacking the cervical lordosis that later develops in response to holding the head up against gravity. Excessive lordosis or kyphosis leads to altered distribution of tensile and compressive forces across the tripod of the segment (one leg is the disc, two are the facet joints), leading to degeneration of either the disc or facet joints. As this spinal motion segment loses mobility, adjacent motion segments must bear greater load and experience accelerated degeneration.

The vertebral column is mobile in sagittal (flexion–extension), coronal (lateral flexion), and axial (rotation) planes. These motions are initiated by the surrounding musculature and continue to the extent permitted by bony and ligamentous restraints. ROM in each direction varies throughout the spine. In general, most of the total flexion–extension of the spine is accomplished from motion in the cervical and lumbar regions, with only minor thoracic contribution. Most rotation is achieved from the C1 to C2 articulation, followed by the upper thoracic spine. The contribution to lateral flexion is relatively equal in each region. The specialized C1 to C2 relationship permits a large amount of both rotation and flexion–extension, creating a region that is highly mobile but also relatively unstable. Relative motion of one vertebra around another rarely occurs in one plane. Coupled motion describes the tendency of one vertebra to rotate with respect to an adjacent vertebra with lateral flexion. In order to distribute soft-tissue tension and keep the facet joints located, rotation must follow the bending of any curved rod such as the spine (as is frequently seen in scoliosis).

In the isolated spine (without accounting for muscle actions), imbalance may occur in the sagittal or coronal planes. The spine naturally attempts to correct an unbalanced curve with curvature in another part of the vertebral column. Common measurements describing spinal stability, balance, and curvature are shown in Figure 61.6. Spinal muscles permit the vertebrae to flex and extend variably to accommodate the center of gravity in each region. When a load borne by the vertebral column acts over a larger distance (i.e., holding an object at arm's length instead of close to the torso), tensile and compressive forces across the loaded vertebrae increase and lead to muscle overuse. A large protuberant abdomen is commonly one such force with an increased lever arm. Long-term, imbalance of "agonist–antagonist" muscle groups contributes to instability, as muscle tonicity changes with injury or inflammation. Tonically active stabilizers, such as the multifidus, may be inactive after surgery, with no obvious deficits until synergistic muscles are fatigued. The multifidi and longus colli/capiti become relatively inactive, whereas the trapezius, sternocleidomastoid, and erector spinae become hyperactive in response to inflammation. Focused rehabilitation of these inactive groups may improve patient balance and help control postoperative pain.

Anteriorly, the three regions spanned by the vertebral column (thorax, abdomen, and pelvis) operate under different biomechanical principles. The bony thorax is relatively stiff and limits its motion. The abdomen may be conceptualized as an airbag anterior to the spinal column. Increasing the intra-abdominal pressure provides a rigid anterior strut for support. This is accomplished with strengthening of the muscles that surround the abdomen (diaphragm above, pelvic floor below, rectus

© 2018 American Academy of Orthopaedic Surgeons

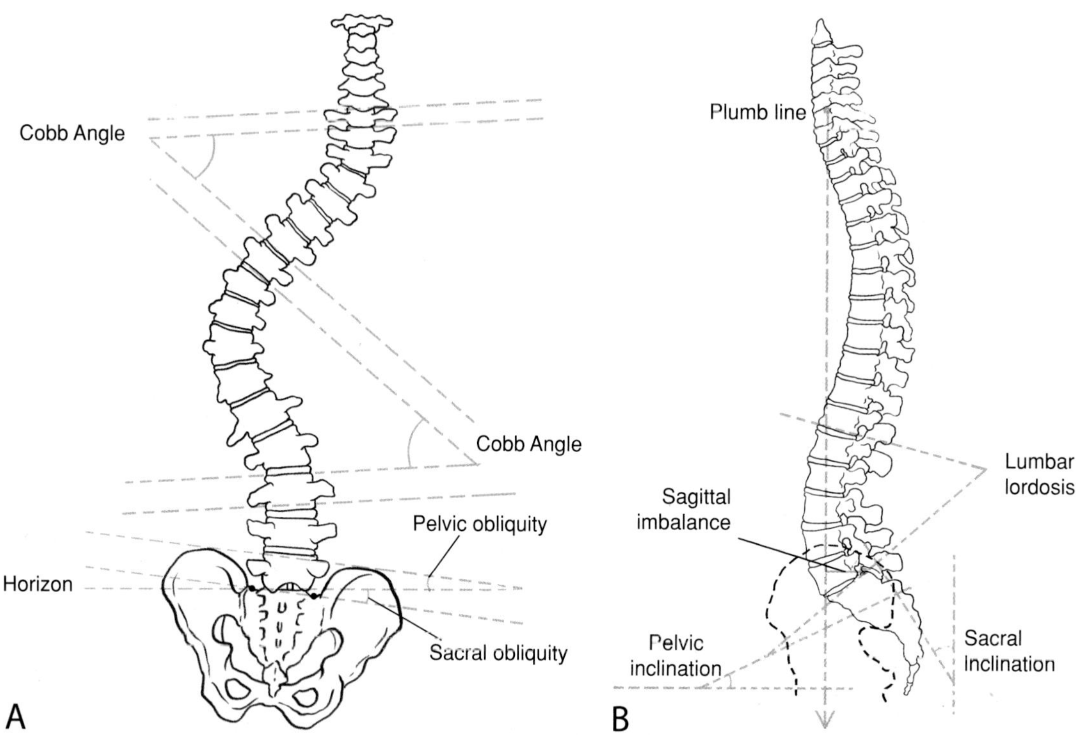

Figure 61.6 Biomechanical angles and lines of the spine. **A**, Coronal view depicting scoliosis and the measurement of Cobb angles, and pelvic and sacral obliquity. **B**, Sagittal view depicting measurement of lordosis angle, C7 plumb line for sagittal imbalance, and pelvic and sacral inclination (related to pelvic incidence). (Adapted from Lenke L [Terminology Committee of the Scoliosis Research Society]. SRS Terminology Committee and Working Group on Spinal Classification Revised Glossary of Terms. Available at http://www.srs.org/professionals/glossary/SRS_revised_glossary_of_terms.htm. Accessed on January 29, 2014.)

abdominis, and obliques). The pelvis is the terminal bony attachment for the spine; as such, its orientation is often crucial when considering spinal balance. In the coronal plane, the degree of deviation is called obliquity. Pelvic obliquity follows when the line connecting the iliac crests is not parallel to the horizontal of ground level. The obliquity of the sacrum usually follows the pelvis, but may rarely be different. In the sagittal plane, the degree of deviation is known as inclination or version, with the sacrum and pelvis inclined separately. The relative degree of sacral and pelvic inclination, as well as the location of the femoral head within the hip joint, determine pelvic *incidence,* which can be correlated with the propensity of L5 to "slip" on S1, leading to spondylolisthesis.

With procedures that destabilize the spine by removing load-bearing structures, care must be taken with postoperative activity. The safety of postoperative rehabilitation is determined by whether three-column support is restored to the spine. If bony fusion has yet to occur, excessive segmental motion may compromise instrumentation and bracing may be useful. The counterpoint to this is that a back brace does the work of spinal musculature, leading to paraspinal atrophy with prolonged use.

BIBLIOGRAPHY

Alderink GJ: The sacroiliac joint: review of anatomy, mechanics, and function. *J Orthop Sports Phys Ther* 1991;13(2):71–84.

Choi G, Raiturker PP, Kim MJ, Chung DJ, Chae YS, Lee SH: The effect of early isolated lumbar extension exercise program for patients with herniated disc undergoing lumbar discectomy. *Neurosurgery* 2005;57(4):764–772; discussion 764–772.

Cresswell AG, Grundström H, Thorstensson A: Observations on intra-abdominal pressure and patterns of abdominal intra-muscular activity in man. *Acta Physiol Scand* 1992; 144(4):409–418.

Danielsen JM, Johnsen R, Kibsgaard SK, Hellevik E: Early aggressive exercise for postoperative rehabilitation after discectomy. *Spine (Phila Pa 1976)* 2000;25(8):1015–1020.

Dolan P, Greenfield K, Nelson RJ, Nelson IW: Can exercise therapy improve the outcome of microdiscectomy? *Spine (Phila Pa 1976)* 2000;25(12):1523–1532.

Erdogmus CB, Resch KL, Sabitzer R, et al: Physiotherapy-based rehabilitation following disc herniation operation: results of a randomized clinical trial. *Spine* 2007;32:19.

Foley BS, Buschbacher RM: Sacroiliac joint pain: anatomy, biomechanics, diagnosis, and treatment. *Am J Phys Med Rehabil* 2006;85(12):997–1006.

Gejo R, Matsui H, Kawaguchi Y, Ishihara H, Tsuji H: Serial changes in trunk muscle performance after posterior lumbar surgery. *Spine (Phila Pa 1976)* 1999;24:(10):1023–1028.

Gray S: *Gray's Anatomy,* Random House Digital, Inc., 2011.

Hakkinen A, Ylinen J, Kautiainen H, Tarvainen U, Kiviranta I: Effects of home strength training and stretching versus stretching

© 2018 American Academy of Orthopaedic Surgeons

alone after lumbar disk surgery: a randomized study with a 1-year follow-up. *Arch Phys Med Rehabil* 2005;86(5):865–870.

Hebert JJ, Marcus RL, Koppenhaver SL, Fritz JM: Postoperative rehabilitation following lumbar discectomy with quantification of trunk muscle morphology and function: a case report and review of the literature. *J Orthop Sports Phys Ther* 2010;40(7):402–412.

Hides J, Gilmore C, Stanton W, Bohlscheid E: Multifidus size and symmetry among chronic LBP and healthy asymptomatic subjects. *Man Ther* 2008;13(1):43–49.

Hides J, Wilson S, Stanton W: An MRI investigation into the function of the transversus abdominis muscle during "drawing-in" of the abdominal wall. *Spine (Phila Pa 1976)* 2006;31(6):E175–E178.

Hides JA, Stokes MJ, Saide M, Jull GA, Cooper DH: Evidence of lumbar multifidus muscle wasting ipsilateral to symptoms in patients with acute/subacute low back pain. *Spine (Phila Pa 1976)* 1994;19(2):165–172.

Hodges P: Is there a role for transversus abdominis in lumbo-pelvic stability? *Man Ther* 1999;4(2):74–86.

Hodges P, van den Hoorn W, Dawson A, Cholewicki J: Changes in the mechanical properties of the trunk in low back pain may be associated with recurrence. *J Biomech* 2009;42(1):61–66.

Hyun SJ, Kim YB, Kim YS, Park SW, Nam TK, Hong HJ, Kwon JT: Postoperative changes in paraspinal muscle volume: comparison between paramedian interfascial and midline approaches for lumbar fusion. *J Korean Med Sci* 2007;22(4):646–651.

Kjellby-Wendt G, Carlsson SG, Styf J: Results of early active rehabilitation 5–7 years after surgical treatment for lumbar disc herniation. *J Spinal Disord Tech* 2002;15(5):404–409.

Kjellby-Wendt G, Styf J: Early active training after lumbar discectomy. A prospective, randomized, and controlled study. *Spine (Phila Pa 1976)* 1998;23(21):2345–2351.

Lenke L (Terminology Committee of the Scoliosis Research Society): *SRS Terminology Committee and Working Group on Spinal Classification Revised Glossary of Terms.* Available at http://www.srs.org/professionals/glossary/SRS_revised_glossary_of_terms.htm. Accessed on January 29, 2014.

Magnusson ML, Pope MH, Wilder DG, Szpalski M, Spratt K: Is there a rational basis for post-surgical lifting restrictions? 1. Current understanding. *Eur Spine J* 1999;8(3):170–178.

Mannion AF, Denzler R, Dvorak J, Müntener M, Grob D: A randomised controlled trial of post-operative rehabilitation after surgical decompression of the lumbar spine. *Eur Spine J* 2007;16:(8):1101–1117.

Mayer TG, Mooney V, Gatchel RJ, Barnes D, Terry A, Smith S, Mayer H: Quantifying postoperative deficits of physical function following spinal surgery. *Clin Orthop Relat Res* 1989; 244:147–157.

McGregor AH, Dore CJ, Morris TP, Morris S, Jamrozik K: Function after spinal treatment, exercise and rehabilitation (FASTER): improving the functional outcome of spinal surgery. *BMC Musculoskelet Disord* 2010;11(1):1.

Mercer SR, Bogduk N: Joints of the cervical vertebral column. *J Orthop Sports Phys Ther* 2001;31(4):174–182; discussion 183.

Millisdotter M Strömqvist B: Early neuromuscular customized training after surgery for lumbar disc herniation: a prospective controlled study. *Eur Spine J* 2007;16:19–26.

Newsome RJ, May S, Chiverton N, Cole AA: A prospective, randomised trial of immediate exercise following lumbar microdiscectomy: a preliminary study. *Physiotherapy* 2009;95(4):273–279.

Ostelo RW: Rehabilitation following first-time lumbar disc surgery: a systematic review within the framework of the Cochrane collaboration. *Spine (Phila Pa 1976)* 2003;28(3):209–218.

Ostelo RW, de Vet HC, Berfelo MW, Kerckhoffs MR, Vlaeyen JW, Wolters PM, van den Brandt PA: Effectiveness of behavioral graded activity after first-time lumbar disc surgery: short term results of a randomized controlled trial. *Eur Spine J* 2003;12(6):637–644.

Pope MH, Magnusson ML, Wilder DG, Goel VK, Spratt K: Is there a rational basis for post-surgical lifting restrictions? 2. Possible scientific approach. *Eur Spine J* 1999;8(3):179–186.

Rantanen J, Hurme M, Falck B, et al: The lumbar multifidus muscle five years after surgery for a lumbar intervertebral disc herniation. *Spine (Phila Pa 1976)* 1993;18(5):568–574.

Rothman RH: *The Spine,* ed 6. Philadelphia, PA, WB Saunders Company, 2011.

Roussouly P, Pinheiro-Franco JL: Sagittal parameters of the spine: biomechanical approach. *Eur Spine J* 2011;20(Suppl 5):609–618.

Solomonow M, Zhou BH, Harris M, Lu Y, Baratta RV: The ligamento-muscular stabilizing system of the spine. *Spine (Phila Pa 1976)* 1998;23(23):2552–2562.

Taylor H, McGregor AH, Medhi Zadeh S, Richards S, Kahn N, Zadeh JA, Hughes SP: The impact of self-retaining retractors on the paraspinal muscles during posterior spinal surgery. *Spine (Phila Pa 1976)* 2002;27(24):2758–2762.

Tesh KM, Dunn JS, Evans JH: The abdominal muscles and vertebral stability. *Spine (Phila Pa 1976)* 1987;12:501–508.

Thompson JC: *Netter's Concise atlas of Orthopaedic Anatomy.* ICON Learning Systems 2002.

Vora AJ, Doerr KD, Wolfer LR: Functional anatomy and pathophysiology of axial low back pain: disc, posterior elements, sacroiliac joint, and associated pain generators. *Phys Med Rehabil Clin N Am* 2010;21(4):679–709.

Wagner H, Anders C, Puta C, et al: Musculoskeletal support of lumbar spine stability. *Pathophysiology* 2005;12(4):257–265.

Ward SR, Kim CW, Eng CM, Gottschalk LJ, Tomiya A, Garfin SR, Lieber RL: Architectural analysis and intraoperative measurements demonstrate the unique design of the multifidus muscle for lumbar spine stability. *J Bone Joint Surg Am* 2009;91(1):176–185.

Wegley RS, Kumore AI: Posterior cervical paraspinal musculature morphology: a cadaveric and CT scan study. *J Orthop Sports Phys Ther* 1986;8(1):15–26.

White AA: *Clinical biomechanics of the spine,* Philadelphia, PA, J. B. Lippincott, 1990.

Wilke HJ, Wolf S, Claes LE, Arand M, Wiesend A: Stability increase of the lumbar spine with different muscle groups. A biomechanical in vitro study. *Spine (Phila Pa 1976)* 1995;20(2):192–198.

Wood PM: Applied anatomy and physiology of the vertebral column. *Physiotherapy* 1979;65(8):248–249.

Zoidl G: Molecular evidence for local denervation of paraspinal muscles in failed-back surgery/postdiscotomy syndrome. *Clin Neuropathol* 2003;22(2):71–77.

© 2018 American Academy of Orthopaedic Surgeons

62 Lumbar Laminectomy and Microdiscectomy

Samuel C. Overley, MD, and Sheeraz Qureshi, MD

INTRODUCTION

Lumbar disc herniation is one of the most common degenerative pathologies that the orthopaedic spine surgeon encounters in practice. A herniated disc or herniated nucleus pulposus is a seemingly simple problem with an equivalently simple definitive surgical treatment. However, there is much controversy regarding how long a herniated disc should be observed and treated conservatively prior to addressing the pathology surgically. Much of the consideration of operative versus nonoperative treatment of herniated discs lies in individual patient factors. Global considerations that must be taken into account when considering any spinal procedure—such as patient age, associated comorbidities, and subjective patient evaluation by the surgeon—are integral to appropriate patient selection, which is paramount.

Once a disc herniation is identified with correlative physical examination findings, a discussion of the natural history of the disease should ensue. This is an area of much controversy and conflicting opinions among experts, though most can agree that a course of nonoperative treatment is a reasonable and necessary step for the first-time presenter, the cornerstone of which is physical therapy and rehabilitation. A commonly quoted study by Saal and Saal found a 90% good or excellent outcome in patients with a symptomatic herniated disc treated nonoperatively. Subsequent studies have not been able to reproduce as high of a success rate; however, more recent highly powered, long-term prospective trials such as the Maine Lumbar Spine Study and the Spine Patient Outcomes Research Trial (SPORT) show good results in over 50% of patients treated nonoperatively. The authors' preferred time frame for nonoperative treatment of radicular pain without motor impairment, cauda equina syndrome, or progressive neurologic symptoms is 3 months.

After failure of nonoperative treatment in a patient with a single-level symptomatic herniated disc with correlative physical examination and imaging findings, the treating surgeon may offer the patient a microdiscectomy or laminectomy. There are two basic ways to perform such a procedure: through a mini-open approach or through a minimally invasive surgical technique. Each procedure accomplishes the same goal of removing the offending disc bulge/herniation with minimal osseous disruption and neural tissue manipulation. The mini-open approach does, however, involve a subperiosteal muscle dissection, whereas the minimally invasive technique employs a muscle-sparing approach. The salient points of each surgical procedure, primarily as they relate to postoperative rehabilitation implications, will be discussed further in the surgical procedure section.

Lumbar spinal stenosis is another common disease process in the adult spine. We will primarily reference the congenital form of stenosis, though there are acquired etiologies that are beyond the scope of this chapter. The presentation, patient population, and etiology of spinal stenosis differs from that of a single level herniated disc, thus necessitating a different approach by the surgeon. Congenital spinal stenosis is an anatomic diagnosis by definition, primarily affecting the elderly population. It is the result of degenerative changes in the lumbar spine that ultimately lead to a stenotic canal. It is postulated that varying degrees of spinal stenosis take place in everyone as they age by virtue of its degenerative nature. However, it is uncertain why certain individuals have accelerated rates of stenosis compared to others, though it has been shown that genetics play a large role in the disease process. Additionally, not all patients with spinal stenosis are symptomatic, and there is no direct objective correlation to degree of stenosis and symptomatology. Those who are symptomatic typically present with vague, ill-defined lower back pain that radiates to

Dr. Qureshi or an immediate family member has received royalties from Zimmer; is a member of a speakers' bureau or has made paid presentations on behalf of Globus Medical, Medtronic Sofamor Danek, and Stryker; serves as a paid consultant to Medtronic, Orthofix, Stryker, and Zimmer; and serves as a board member, owner, officer, or committee member of the American Academy of Orthopaedic Surgeons, the Cervical Spine Research Society, Clinical Orthopaedics and Related Research, Contemporary Spine Surgery, Global Spine Journal, *the Musculoskeletal Transplant Foundation, the North American Spine Society, the journal* Spine, *and* The Spine Journal. *Neither Dr. Overley nor any immediate family member has received anything of value from or has stock or stock options held in a commercial company or institution related directly or indirectly to the subject of this article.*

© 2018 American Academy of Orthopaedic Surgeons

the gluteal region and, in some cases, to the lower extremities. This phenomenon, referred to as neurogenic claudication, is typically exacerbated by standing and activities such as walking uphill or up stairs, causing hyperextension of the lumbar spine. Symptoms are relieved by flexion of the lumbar spine, which translates into a patient's description of relief when sitting or leaning forward onto an object, such as a walker or shopping cart.

Similar to that of herniated discs, there is a wealth of literature that aims to determine the optimal treatment for patients with spinal stenosis. Many recent long-term prospective studies, including the two previously mentioned (Maine Lumbar Spine Study and SPORT) have looked at both operative and nonoperative treatment of spinal stenosis. The results are not conclusive but are tangible and powered sufficiently to permit the North American Spine Society to conclude in their evidence-based guidelines that in one-third to one-half of patients with mild to moderate lumbar spinal stenosis, nonoperative treatment may be favorable.

In patients who fail nonoperative treatment, the primary surgical goal is to increase the space of the stenotic canal. Lumbar spinal stenosis is the most common reason for spinal surgery in the elderly population (age >65 years). In the absence of instability, laminectomy remains the gold standard for definitive treatment of adult spinal stenosis. As with microdiscectomy, a laminectomy may be accomplished via both a mini-open exposure and a minimally invasive approach.

SURGICAL PROCEDURE

Microdiscectomy

Indications

The most commonly encountered absolute indication for a lumbar microdiscectomy is a progressive neurologic deficit. Contrary to most patients' perception, radicular pain is the least worrisome symptom relevant to patient safety and potential long-term irreversible nerve damage. Such pain is the most common indication for a trial of nonoperative treatment. However, a progressive deficit that affects motor function, commonly a footdrop (L4–L5 nerve root), is a serious matter that deserves urgent attention. In this scenario, operative treatment is indicated in lieu of conservative treatment to prevent potential permanent nerve damage or progression to cauda equina syndrome.

Other relative indications are typically unique to each patient but universally revolve around a case of severe radicular pain that has not responded adequately to nonoperative treatment. One absolute prerequisite for discectomy is radiologic identification (usually in the form of MRI or CT myelogram) of a compressive disc pathology that is concordant with patient symptomatology and physical examination findings. It is on the onus of the surgeon and patient to develop a strategy for treatment of such conditions that takes into account the risks and benefits of surgery with the expectations of the patient. Generally speaking, a radicular pain pattern and physical examination findings that correlate with imaging have the highest predictability of success when treated surgically.

Contraindications

While there are not true absolute contraindications to lumbar microdiscectomy, the central theme of both peer-reviewed literature and anecdotal evidence is to avoid microdiscectomy in patients with primarily mechanical low back pain. Other factors that are by no means absolute contraindications—but that have been shown to be associated with worse outcomes after microdiscectomy—are work-related injury, absence of correlative findings on physical examination, lack of radicular pain distribution, and central disc bulges.

Laminectomy

Indications

As is true of microdiscectomy for lumbar disc herniations, the one absolute indication for laminectomy is the presence of a progressive neurologic deficit or, more commonly seen with spinal stenosis, cauda equina syndrome. In the absence of these alarming and potentially permanent disease states, a combination of patient desire for surgery and a failed course of nonoperative treatment will be the driving forces for ultimate surgical treatment of lumbar spinal stenosis. Attempts to demonstrate objective outcomes measures have been helpful to aid in the decision-making process for both patient and surgeon; however, definitive prognostic indicators have still not been determined. Deen et al showed that the most common causes of early failed laminectomy was the absence of classical symptoms of neurogenic claudication in combination with lack of objective radiographic evidence of stenosis.

Contraindications

Instability must be assessed and considered when contemplating a laminectomy for spinal stenosis. Instability is a dynamic process that may not always be overtly present on static imaging studies. A thorough and dynamic radiographic examination is often required to diagnose instability. The diagnosis of instability is paramount in any patient with spinal stenosis because, if present, a laminectomy will likely require augmentation with a stabilizing procedure such as a fusion. For this reason, it is generally accepted that patients with spinal stenosis and evidence of lumbar instability should not be treated with an isolated laminectomy, as their failure rates are significantly higher than those without objective instability.

Procedure

Microdiscectomy

Anatomy

The functional components of the lumbar intervertebral disc are the outer fibrous layer known as the annulus fibrosus, the inner gelatin-like layer of the nucleus pulposus, and the hyaline cartilage endplates of the vertebral bodies abutting the cranial and caudal ends of the disc. The annulus fibrosus acts a barrier to the inner nucleus pulposus, converting axial loads through

© 2010 American Academy of Orthopaedic Surgeons

the spine into hoop stresses. The hyaline cartilage endplates allow for diffusion of nutrients into the inner nucleus pulposus while also serving to absorb metabolic waste products. In early disc degeneration, the endplates lose diffusion capacity, metabolic waste products accumulate in the nucleus pulposus, and annular support weakens, allowing herniation of the nucleus pulposus. Integrity of the pars interarticularis is critical to stability of the posterior elements. This is important to keep in mind when removing os to create adequate exposure in the interlaminar window. The ligamentum flavum is the final layer encountered before the epidural space. This ligament may have adhesions to the dura; therefore, extreme caution must be used when resecting the ligament. The dural sac contains the spinal nerve roots that collectively comprise the cauda equina after termination of the spinal cord at or around L1. Understanding the anatomic relation of the exiting and traversing nerve roots is critical during any spinal procedure. The exiting nerve root of a level exits out of the infrapedicular foramen of that level, while the traversing nerve root of the level below passes the disc space just lateral to the dural sac. Close attention must be paid to the traversing nerve while performing a microdiscectomy to avoid damaging it.

Technique

When performing a mini-open microdiscectomy, a midline incision is made over the spinous processes of the desired intervertebral disc. Subcutaneous dissection is carried down to the spinous processes and interspinous ligament with care to not disrupt the ligament, as it contributes stability to the posterior elements. The paravertebral musculature, comprised of the multifidus and erector spinae, are dissected subperiosteally unilaterally on the side of the disc herniation. The lamina, pars, and facets of the vertebrae on the side of the pathology are exposed without disrupting the facet joint capsules. The interlaminar space is identified and limited bony resection of the laminae with a Kerrison rongeur will provide adequate exposure of the compressed nerve root. The ligamentum flavum is resected carefully, revealing the traversing nerve root and the intervertebral disc below. The nerve root is retracted medially and protected with a nerve root retractor, while the remaining annulus surrounding the disc bulge is incised with an 11-blade scalpel. The pathologic nucleus pulposus is resected with a micropituitary. After the diseased nucleus pulposus is removed, hemostasis is achieved. Closure of the fascia overlying the spine is critical to prevent dehiscence and deep wound infection. The subcutaneous tissue is closed with an absorbable suture and the skin is closed with either a running subcuticular absorbable suture or interrupted nylon sutures.

The minimally invasive technique is similar to the mini-open except for its muscle-sparing approach. A slightly lateral incision is made in a predetermined location to allow for an obliquely placed tube to dock on the interlaminar space. Sequential dilator tubes are placed in a "Russian doll" fashion, which displaces the spinal musculature rather than traumatically dissecting it from its osseous insertions.

Laminectomy

Anatomy

The pertinent anatomy is similar to the anatomy listed earlier for microdiscectomy. Some more relevant anatomy pertains to the bony structure of the lamina, specifically at the pars–laminar interface. As mentioned previously, extreme care must be taken not to destabilize the pars intra-articularis. This is accomplished by not extending the laminectomy too far lateral and into the pars. A minimum distance of 5 mm from the lateral edge of the pars must be maintained in order to prevent iatrogenic pars fracture.

Technique

The approach for a laminectomy is identical to that for the mini-open microdiscectomy. However, with a true laminectomy, a bilateral dissection of the paravertebral muscles is necessary in order to expose the entire lamina. In some instances, a hemilaminectomy may be performed in which the same unilateral exposure described earlier for microdiscectomy will be sufficient. Once the bilateral lamina and facet joints have been exposed, it is necessary to identify the far lateral borders of the pars inter-articularis. As mentioned earlier, in order to prevent iatrogenic pars fracture, a minimum distance of 5 mm from the lateral pars must be maintained throughout the laminectomy. A midline laminotomy is performed of the undersurface of the cephalad vertebra and carried cephalad to the insertion of the ligamentum flavum. The laminectomy is continued to the subarticular zone laterally to include no more than 50% of the medial facet (superior articulating process of the caudal lamina) and into the medial lamina of the caudal vertebra. After this is accomplished bilaterally, the entire spinous process can be removed, allowing direct visualization of the underlying ligamentum flavum, which often is removed with the spinous process. Care must be taken to avoid a durotomy while removing the ligament, as it may have attachments to the dura. At this point, the dural sac and traversing nerve roots are visible and any further decompression via osteophyte resection or foraminotomy may be accomplished.

Complications

Microdiscectomy

There are a range of complications, though at an acceptably low occurrence rate, that may occur following a lumbar microdiscectomy. The most pertinent to a postoperative rehabilitation protocol is recurrence. Recurrence rates vary in the literature and range from 0% to 18%, depending on the definition of recurrence. Many surgeons have sought to find risk factors associated with recurrence, and while some patient and surgeon factors—such as obesity and open approach, respectively—have shown to be correlated with significant rates of recurrence, there is little evidence linking recurrence to postoperative activity or rehabilitation. Though there is a paucity of literature supporting it, many surgeons still limit activity and refer for physical therapy postoperatively. Quite to the contrary, a prospective trial in *Physiotherapy* concluded that

© 2018 American Academy of Orthopaedic Surgeons

patients who underwent immediate exercise following a single-level microdiscectomy became independently mobile and returned to work sooner. True recurrence, defined as a recurrent herniation at the same level and same side, has an incidence of only 2% to 3%.

Incidental durotomy has been cited to occur in up to 4% of microdiscectomy cases. These patients were shown to have a lower rate of symptom resolution as well as an increased incidence of chronic pain and headaches.

Other complications that pertain less to the scope of this book include wound infections, reported in 0% to 3% of cases, pyogenic discitis, noted to occur in only 0.2% of cases, and rare intraoperative vascular injury.

Laminectomy

Complications of lumbar laminectomy are similar to microdiscectomy, including durotomy, infection, vascular injury, and recurrence of symptoms. However, due to the increased dissection typically performed for adequate exposure as well as the amount of bony resection and unroofing of the spinal canal, a significant risk of epidural hematoma exists. An epidural hematoma typically presents within the first 24 to 48 hours postoperatively with new-onset lower extremity sensorimotor deficits, and usually results in an urgent take-back for hematoma removal and canal decompression. Patients are also at an increased risk of deep venous thrombosis (DVT) and pulmonary embolism secondary to their limited activity and lack of pharmacologic DVT prophylaxis (for risk of epidural hematoma) following a lumbar laminectomy.

Instability following lumbar laminectomy is a real concern as well. The rate of clinical instability following decompression without arthrodesis is around 5%. Many factors have been shown to be associated with a higher rate of postlaminectomy instability, including presence of preoperative spondylolisthesis, abnormal motion on dynamic films preoperatively, decompression at degenerative L3 or L4 levels, and multilevel wide decompression. Attention should be paid during postoperative rehabilitation to patients satisfying one or more of these risk factors, as they are more likely to develop postlaminectomy instability.

POSTOPERATIVE REHABILITATION

Introduction

Minimally invasive surgery (MIS) techniques can be used in a wide variety of spinal pathologies, certainly including, but not limited, to microdiscectomy and laminectomy as previously described. The idea of MIS was conceived with the idea of accomplishing intended goals of surgery—decompression, fusion, and/or realignment—while causing minimal insult to the soft-tissue envelope about the spine. Specifically, MIS aims to decrease muscular crush injuries due to excessive retraction; avoid muscular dissection and resection of tendonous insertions of the multifidus and erector spinae on to the posterior bony elements, as well as eliminate massive denervation of these muscle groups; and decrease disruption of the dorsolumbar fascia, which serves as a conduit for inferred spinal stability from the abdominal musculature. Preserving the stabilizing spinal musculature via an MIS technique has been shown to result in an increase of over 50% postoperative extension strength when compared to a traditional midline open approach. This increased extension strength also correlates to the cross-sectional area of the multifidus as measured on MRI, a finding that has been reproduced by other similar prospective studies.

A study by Shivonen aimed to establish a clinical significance in patient outcomes based on denervation of the multifidus. The results showed a significant correlation between failed back syndrome and denervation of the multifidus with histologic changes in the muscle consistent with muscle atrophy, marked fibrosis, and fatty infiltration. The importance of maintaining this muscular integrity is paramount when considering postoperative rehabilitation planning. A neurovascularly intact paraspinal muscle unit with minimally disrupted dorsolumbar fascia enables the physiatrist or physical therapist to pursue an aggressive strengthening rehabilitation regimen during the minimum protection phase early in the postoperative period. The goals of rehabilitation focus primarily on strengthening the stabilizing musculature of the spine through a series of exercises, stretches, and joint mobilization procedures that will be outlined in detail later.

Another key advantage of MIS as a result of decreased soft tissue destruction is decreased postoperative pain. This is beneficial to the patient not only in the obvious sense of a more comfortable postoperative period and faster return to activity and work, but also allows for tolerance of a more aggressive, higher-intensity rehabilitation program that has been shown to result in less short-term pain and disability than low-intensity programs.

Though both post microdiscectomy and laminectomy patients generally have little activity restrictions from their operating surgeon, there are a few activities that should be avoided in the 3- to 4-week postoperative period. For patients who have undergone microdiscectomy, avoidance of activities that overload axial compression—such as jumping, running, and other gravity-dependent impact activities—should be avoided. Increased axial impact across the disc carries the theoretical risk of increasing the rate of reherniation through the small annulotomy created at the time of surgery.

Additionally, extreme rotational activities should be avoided for the same time period in those that have undergone either a microdiscectomy or laminectomy. These types of motion are most commonly associated with golf, tennis, and baseball.

Authors' Preferred Protocol

Start exercises at 3 to 4 weeks postoperatively.

- Patients will be seen in clinic approximately 2 weeks postoperatively and instructed exactly when to begin exercises as well as given a requisition form for therapy.
- Number of repetitions should be tailored to the patient's pain tolerance and specific surgeon recommendations.

© 2018 American Academy of Orthopaedic Surgeons

Table 62.1 POST-OPERATIVE REHABILITATION PROTOCOL

Exercise Type	Muscle Group	Number of Reps/Sets	Number of Days per Week	Number of Weeks
Posterior pelvic tilt (draw-in)	Spinal stabilizers	1 minute reps, 10 sets	7	10–12
Draw-in double leg lift	Spinal stabilizers + abdominal	10 reps, 10 sets	5–7	6–8
Draw-in single leg lift	Spinal stabilizers + trunk extensors	30 second reps, 10 sets	5–7	6–8
Lumbar spine stretch (like a cat)	Spinal stabilizers	30 seconds, in between every exercise set	7	10–12
Quadruped limb load	Multifidus + erector spinae	10 reps, 10 sets	3–4	6–8
Prone Superman	Multifidus + erector spinae	10 second reps, 10 sets	3–4	6–8

- These exercises should not cause pain. If at any point the patient begins to experience pain, cease the exercise. If the patient continues to experience pain, consult with the surgeon.
- Exercises should be carried out under a high-intensity model.
- Muscular soreness similar to the feeling after a high-intensity weight training or aerobic workout is to be expected following these exercises. If the patient complains of pain, especially that of a radicular nature, consult with the surgeon (Table 62.1).

Posterior Pelvic Tilt (Draw-In)

- This is the most important maneuver to perform correctly, as it is the starting position for all supine exercises.
- Begin supine in a relaxed position, with knees slightly flexed and heels on the ground,
- Draw in the abdomen with a slow, deep breath, bringing the belly button as close to the spine as possible,
- Keeping that position, activate the abdominal muscles as though bracing for a punch to the abdomen,
- Actively tilt the pelvis posteriorly, attempting to straighten the lumbar spine, and bring the small of the back down to the ground,
- Hold this position for 1 minute, rest for 30 seconds, and repeat for a total of 10 sets,

Draw-In Limb Loading

- Begin in the supine position.
- Obtain the posterior pelvic tilt starting position.
- Slowly flex both legs to 90° of knee flexion.
- Lift both legs off the mat to achieve 90° of hip flexion. Hold for 10 seconds.
- Slowly lower legs until heels hit the ground.
- Extend legs straight by sliding heels on the ground.
- Slowly lift straight legs together to 45° and hold for 10 seconds.
- Repeat 10 times. Do a total of 10 sets with lumbar stretch (arch spine toward the ceiling, like a cat) between each set.

Draw-In Single-Leg Lift

- Begin in the supine position
- Obtain the Posterior pelvic tilt starting position
- Slowly flex both legs to 90° of *knee flexion*
- Slowly flex the Right leg to 90° of *hip flexion*
- Extend the Left leg, and slowly raise it 4 to 5 inches off of the ground
- Hold this position for 30 seconds, then perform the same exercise using opposite legs—this is one complete set
- Assume lumbar stretch (cat) position for 30 seconds, and repeat to accomplish 10 sets

Lumbar Spine Stretch (Like a Cat)

- Begin in quadruped position
- Slowly arch the spine toward the ceiling, like a cat.
- After maximum arch of the back is obtained, slowly begin to sit, bottom back toward the heels.
- While sitting back on the heels, extend arms forward, trying to stretch arms as far away from the body as possible while letting the head relax in a forward flexed position.
- Hold this pose for 30 seconds.

Quadruped Limb Load

- Begin in the quadruped position.
- Attempt to create the posterior pelvic tilt position while on all fours.
- Slowly lift the right arm until parallel with the ground.
- Lift the left leg by extending at the hip until the leg is parallel with the ground.
- Hold this position for 30 seconds, then slowly return to starting position and repeat with the opposite arm/leg for a total of 10 sets.

Prone Superman

- Start in the prone position with arms extended overhead, lying flat on the ground.
- Contract abdominal muscles.

© 2018 American Academy of Orthopaedic Surgeons

- Slowly lift legs, arms, and head off the ground simultaneously.
- Continue to lift extremities until you are at the point of maximum spinal arch.
- Hold position for 10 seconds, return to starting position for 30 seconds, and repeat for a total of 10 sets.

Functional Goals and Restrictions

The functional goals for a microdiscectomy and laminectomy are simple: return to normal activity, work, and a pain-free state with the help of an intense rehabilitation protocol. Patients should permanently refrain only from heavy weight-bearing squats. All other activity is permitted as tolerated.

The ultimate goals of the outlined rehabilitation protocol is to maximally stabilize the spine by strengthening muscle groups of the paraspinal and abdominal muscles, as well as the iliopsoas, hip extensors, and upper back musculature. It takes a coordination of effort on the part of the surgeon, physiatrist, physical therapist, and, most important, the patient, adhering to a dynamic postoperative stretching, stabilizing, and strengthening regimen to achieve maximum benefit after a microdiscectomy or laminectomy.

PEARLS

Microdiscectomy

- Most lumbar disc herniations respond well to conservative treatment, and approximately 80% to 90% will not require surgery after a 3-month course of treatment with activity modification, nonsteroidal anti-inflammatory drugs (NSAIDs), physical therapy, and/or corticosteroid injections.
- However, in those who fail 3 months of conservative therapy, surgery has shown statistically significant outcomes compared to continued nonoperative therapy.
- Progressive neurologic signs and symptoms, especially footdrop, should alert the surgeon to potential permanent nerve damage, and may be an indication to pursue surgery irrespective of the time frame of symptoms.
- Careful patient selection with rigorous scrutiny of correlation of symptoms and physical examination with imaging is crucial to good outcomes for surgical treatment.
- MIS techniques decrease muscle destruction and denervation as well as postoperative pain, and may lead to quicker return to work and normal activity, along with a lower rate of failed back syndrome.
- Patients should be cautioned that lumbar microdiscectomy is a procedure that is most reliable at alleviating leg pain, and is less predictable for back pain, numbness, and weakness.

Laminectomy

- MIS surgical technique is not an excuse for an inadequate exposure. It is vital to clearly identify the midlateral pars and facet capsule to avoid too far lateral bony resection that may lead to iatrogenic pars fracture.
- It is imperative to remain >5 mm from the lateral edge of the pars intra-articularis to avoid iatrogenic pars fracture.
- Decompression should begin centrally from the caudal portion of the superior lamina, which has the ligamentum flavum protecting the dura, advancing cranially and laterally to the medial pedicle.
- Patients with radiographic evidence of instability may benefit from a fusion along with decompression, rather than an isolated laminectomy.
- The SPORT has demonstrated significant efficacy of operative over nonoperative treatment of symptomatic spinal stenosis at 2-year follow-up.

BIBLIOGRAPHY

Abramovitz JN, Neff SR: Lumbar disc surgery: results of the Prospective Lumbar Discectomy Study of the Joint Section on Disorders of the Spine and Peripheral Nerves of the American Association of Neurological Surgeons and the Congress of Neurological Surgeons. *Neurosurgery* 1991;29(2):301–307, discussion 307–308.

Atlas SJ, Keller RB, Wu YA, Deyo RA, Singer DE: Long-term outcomes of surgical and nonsurgical management of sciatica secondary to a lumbar disc herniation: 10 year results from the Maine Lumbar Spine Study. *Spine (Phila Pa 1976)* 2005;30(8):927–935.

Atlas SJ, Keller RB, Wu YA, Deyo RA, Singer DE: Long-term outcomes of surgical and nonsurgical management of lumbar spinal stenosis: 8 to 10 year results from the Maine Lumbar Spine Study. *Spine (Phila Pa 1976)* 2005;30(8):936–943.

Deen HG Jr, Zimmerman RS, Lyons MK, Wharen RE Jr, Reimer R: Analysis of early failures after lumbar decompressive laminectomy for spinal stenosis. *Mayo Clin Proc* 1995;70(1):33–36.

Fox MW, Onofrio BM, Hanssen AD: Clinical outcomes and radiological instability following decompressive lumbar laminectomy for degenerative spinal stenosis: a comparison of patients undergoing concomitant arthrodesis versus decompression alone. *J Neurosurg* 1996;85(5):793–802.

Kim DY, Lee SH, Chung SK, Lee HY: Comparison of multifidus muscle atrophy and trunk extension muscle strength: percutaneous versus open pedicle screw fixation. *Spine (Phila Pa 1976)* 2005;30(1):123–129.

Moliterno JA, Knopman J, Parikh K, et al: Results and risk factors for recurrence following single-level tubular lumbar microdiscectomy. *J Neurosurg Spine* 2010;12(6):680–686.

Nasca RJ: Rationale for spinal fusion in lumbar spinal stenosis. *Spine (Phila Pa 1976)* 1989;14(4):451–454.

Newsome RJ, May S, Chiverton N, Cole AA: A prospective, randomised trial of immediate exercise following lumbar microdiscectomy: a preliminary study. *Physiotherapy* 2009; 95(4):273–279.

Ostelo RW, Costa LO, Maher CG, de Vet HC, van Tulder MW: Rehabilitation after lumbar disc surgery. *Cochrane Database Syst Rev* 2008;(4):CD003007.

Saal JA, Saal JS: Nonoperative treatment of herniated lumbar intervertebral disc with radiculopathy. *An outcome study. Spine (Phila Pa 1976)* 1989;14(4):431–437.

© 2018 American Academy of Orthopaedic Surgeons

Saxler G, Krämer J, Barden B, Kurt A, Pförtner J, Bernsmann K: The long-term clinical sequelae of incidental durotomy in lumbar disc surgery. *Spine (Phila Pa 1976)* 2005;30(20):2298–2302.

Sihvonen T, Herno A, Paljärvi L, Airaksinen O, Partanen J, Tapaninaho A: Local denervation atrophy of paraspinal muscles in postoperative failed back syndrome. *Spine (Phila Pa 1976)* 1993;18(5):575–581.

Stevens KJ, Spenciner DB, Griffiths KL, Kim KD, Zwienenberg-Lee M, Alamin T, Bammer R: Comparison of minimally invasive and conventional open posterolateral lumbar fusion using magnetic resonance imaging and retraction pressure studies. *J Spinal Disord Tech* 2006;19(2):77–86.

Tronnier V, Schneider R, Kunz U, Albert F, Oldenkott P: Postoperative spondylodiscitis: results of a prospective study about the aetiology of spondylodiscitis after operation for lumbar disc herniation. *Acta Neurochir (Wien)* 1992;117(3–4):149–152.

Valdes AM, Hassett G, Hart DJ, Spector TD: Radiographic progression of lumbar spine disc degeneration is influenced by variation at inflammatory genes: a candidate SNP association study in the Chingford cohort. *Spine (Phila Pa 1976)* 2005;30(21):2445–2451.

Watters WC 3rd, Baisden J, Gilbert TJ, et al: Degenerative lumbar spinal stenosis: an evidence-based clinical guideline for the diagnosis and treatment of degenerative lumbar spinal stenosis. *Spine J* 2008;8(2):305–310.

Weinstein JN, Tosteson TD, Lurie JD, et al: Surgical versus nonsurgical therapy for lumbar spinal stenosis. *N Engl J Med* 2008;358(8):794–810.

 © 2018 American Academy of Orthopaedic Surgeons

Lumbar Spine Fusion

Adam E.M. Eltorai, MD, and Alan H. Daniels, MD

INTRODUCTION

The goal of lumbar spine fusion surgery is to alleviate pain, numbness, paresthesias, and/or weakness due to vertebral segment pathology or instability. Each of the various surgical approaches includes adding a bone graft or bone graft substitute to elicit physiologic bony union of adjacent vertebrae to reduce motion.

LUMBAR SPINE FUSION

Indications

Indications for lumbar spine fusion include select cases of degenerative disc disease, spondylolisthesis (isthmic, degenerative, or postlaminectomy); spinal stenosis; instability (as measured by anterior/posterior translation or endplate angulation); fractures; tumors; infections; and deformity (such as scoliosis, lordosis, or kyphosis).

Contraindications

There are several factors that may negatively impact the outcome of spinal fusion surgery. These relative contraindications include current smoking status; multilevel degenerative lumbar disease; disability >1 year prior to consideration of fusion; failure to return to work for ≥6 months after previous spine surgery; being severely deconditioned; and psychiatric comorbidities, including factitious disorder, somatization, or history of substance abuse.

Procedure

Relevant Anatomy

Figures 63.1 and 63.2 show the anatomy that is relevant to lumbar spine fusion.

Techniques

There are numerous lumbar fusion surgery techniques available. The most common operations include posterolateral gutter fusion, posterior lumbar interbody fusion (PLIF), transforaminal lumbar interbody fusion (TLIF), far-lateral lumbar interbody fusion (XLIF), anterior lumbar interbody fusion (ALIF), and anterior/posterior (AP) lumbar fusion.

Posterolateral gutter fusion surgery involves the placement of bone graft in the posterolateral portion of the spine. In PLIF, bone graft and/or an interbody cage is placed into the disc space in the front of the spine. TLIF involves the removal of an entire facet joint, enabling greater disc space access and less neural retraction than PLIF. During ALIF surgery, bone graft is placed with a plate or interbody cage within the cleared disc space through an incision in the abdomen. XLIF surgery is performed through a lateral incision and allows access to the upper lumbar vertebral levels (L1–L4). AP lumbar fusion can achieve the greatest stability, but requires anterior and posterior incisions combining XLIF or ALIF and posterolateral gutter fusion procedures.

Complications

As with any type of surgery, there is a risk of infection, bleeding, and anesthetic complications. Specific postoperative complications of lumbar spine fusion include failure to alleviate lower back pain; pseudoarthrosis (when the vertebrae do not fuse together properly); pedicle screws may break or loosen; migration of anterior grafts or cages; and nerve damage that may result in loss of leg strength or sensation, loss of bowel or bladder control, or ejaculation difficulty (especially in anterior L4–S1 fusion surgeries).

POSTOPERATIVE REHABILITATION

Introduction

Early physical therapy consultation makes postoperative rehabilitation more successful. Although surgical technique and unique patient characteristics will dictate certain aspects of rehabilitation (such as the use of brace or bone growth

Dr. Daniels or an immediate family member serves as a paid consultant to DePuy, A Johnson & Johnson Company, Globus Medical, Orthofix, and Stryker; serves as an unpaid consultant to Osseus; and has received research or institutional support from Orthofix. Neither Mr. Eltorai nor any immediate family member has received anything of value from or has stock or stock options held in a commercial company or institution related directly or indirectly to the subject of this article.

© 2018 American Academy of Orthopaedic Surgeons

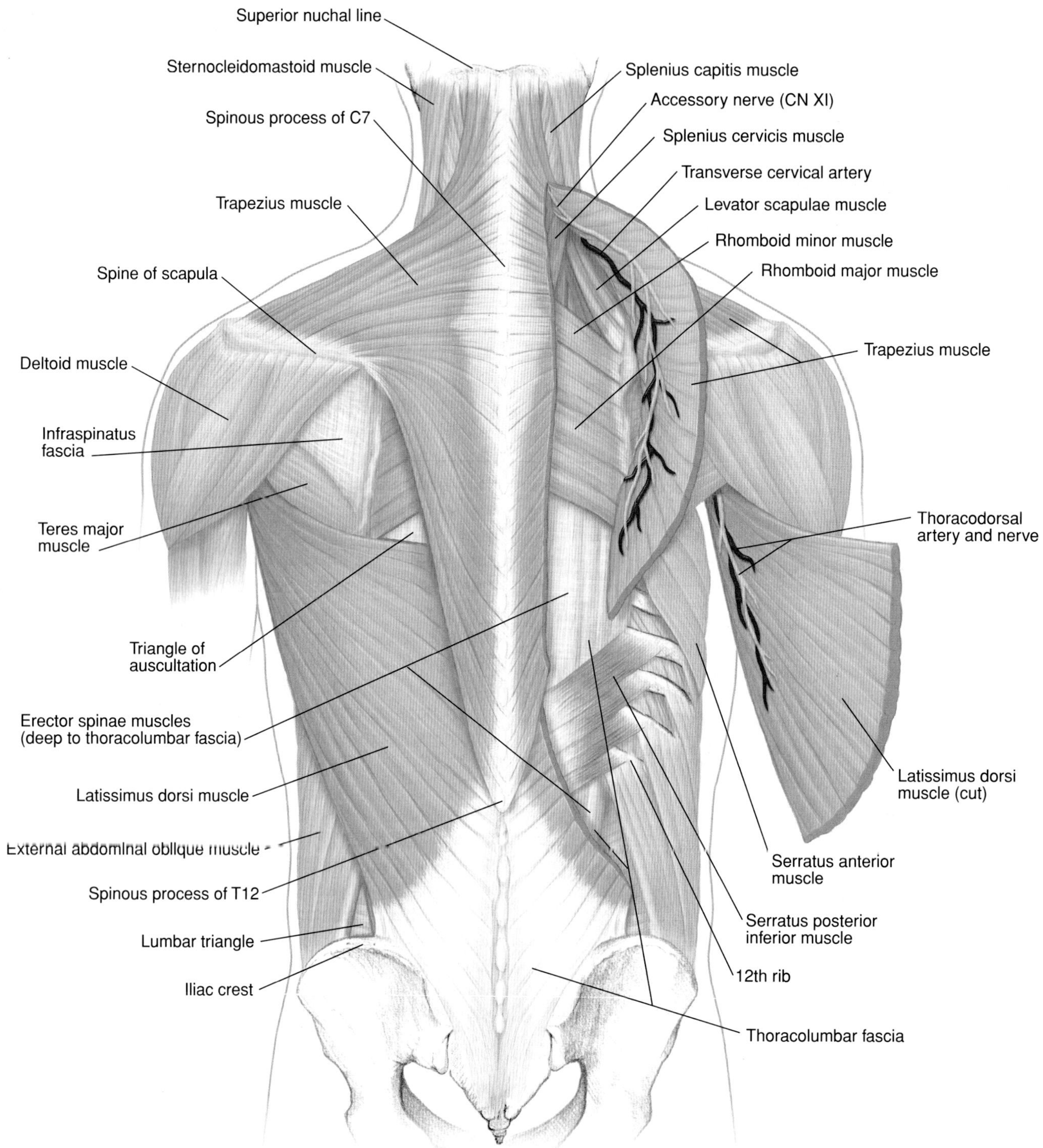

Figure 63.1 Illustration of muscles of the back. (Reproduced with permission from Tank PW, Gest TR: *Lippincott Williams & Wilkins Atlas of Anatomy*. Baltimore, Wolters Kluwer Health, 2009.)

stimulation), there are general rehabilitation principles that all lumbar fusion surgery patients should keep in mind. First and foremost, rehabilitation requires time and energy commitment. Preoperatively, patients should understand that the surgery is just the beginning of the healing process. Although the traditional teaching following lumbar fusion was to avoid all twisting and bending postoperatively, it is now believed that some torso movement may be beneficial; modern fixation techniques allow for safe mobility postoperatively following lumbar spinal fusion. While twisting, bending, and lifting

© 2018 American Academy of Orthopaedic Surgeons

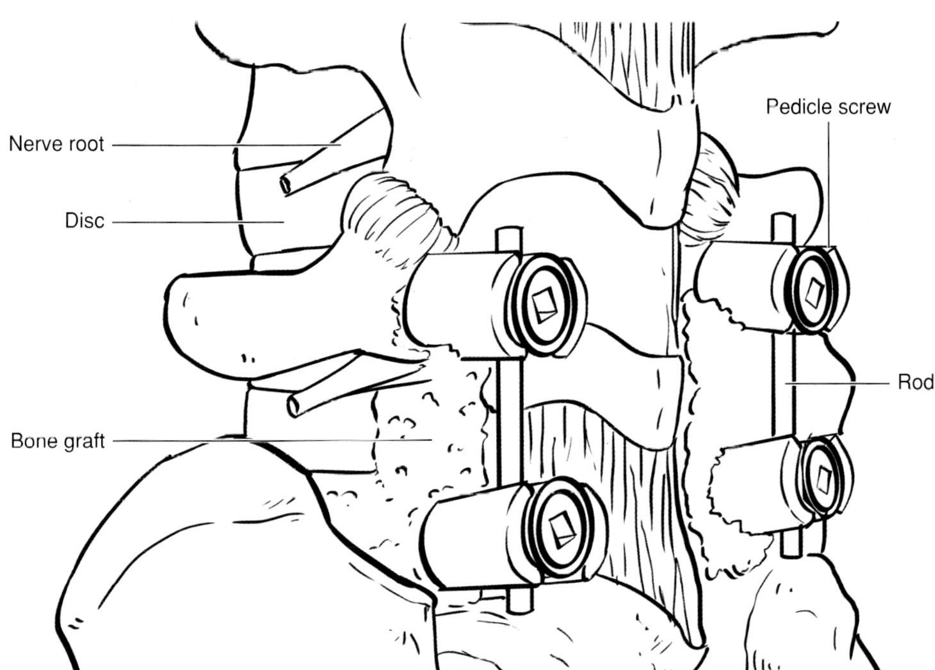

Figure 63.2 Illustration of surgical anatomy and technique.

should be avoided initially, gentle stretching, strengthening, and conditioning are beneficial as they promote restorative blood flow, activation of stabilizing support muscles, and continued flexibility in addition to prevention of venous thromboembolism. Bone fusion achieves initial maturity by 3 to 6 months, although it may take years for the fusion to completely mature. Gentle stress on the graft actually promotes bone growth; therefore, activity and mobility are beneficial.

Authors' Preferred Protocol

- Immediately postoperatively, the patient can begin stretching, stabilization exercises that do not involve trunk movement, and walking, as tolerated.
- By postoperative week 6, stabilization exercises that involve trunk movement should be incorporated. Goals progress toward improving lumbar and core strength.
- By postoperative week 9, aerobic conditioning should be incorporated to improve overall fitness and help burn excess body weight that may strain the lumbar spine (Table 63.1).

Stretches: Low Back, Hamstrings, and Quadriceps

Low Back

- Stretching the low middle back may help prevent adhesions of the nerve roots.
- Lie on the back with legs on the ground, slowly lift one leg until stretch is felt in the lower back.
- Use a hand to support the raised leg and extend your ankle in a "pumping the gas" motion for 5 to 10 seconds.
- Switch legs.
- Repeat every two hours (Figure 63.3).

Hamstrings: Lying or Seated Options

Lying Option

- Lie on the back, bend both knees.
- Straighten one leg and use a hand to support the raised leg.
- Push heel toward the ceiling until a stretch is felt in the back of the thigh.
- Hold for 30 seconds.
- Switch legs.
- Repeat 3 times, twice a day (Figure 63.4).

Seated Option

- Sit on the edge of the chair.
- Straighten one leg with toes up and heel on the ground.
- Hold the sides of the chair and move your bottom off the chair.
- Keep the chest up while feeling a stretch in back of the extended thigh.
- Hold for 30 seconds.
- Switch legs.
- Repeat 3 times, twice a day (Figure 63.5).

Quadriceps

- Lie on the stomach.
- Bring the heel as close to your bottom as you can.
- Hold for 30 seconds.
- Switch legs.
- Repeat 3 times, twice a day (Figure 63.6).

Pelvic Tilt

- Lie on the back with bent knees.
- Push the back to the floor, straightening the back and tilting the pelvis.

© 2018 American Academy of Orthopaedic Surgeons

Table 63.1 REHABILITATION PROGRAM FOR LUMBAR SPINE FUSION SURGERY

Exercise Type	Main Muscle Groups	Number of Repetitions/Sets	Number of Days per Week	Number of Weeks
Low back stretch	Erector spinae (iliocostalis, longissimus, spinalis), latissimus dorsi	2 repetitions/8 sets	7	Postop day 1 and onward
Hamstring stretch	Hamstrings (semitendinosus, semimembranosus, biceps femoris)	3 repetitions (30-s holds)/2 sets	7	Postop day 1 and onward
Quadriceps stretch	Quadriceps (vastus lateralis, vastus intermedius, vastus medialis, rectus femoris)	3 repetitions (30-s holds)/2 sets	7	Postop day 1 and onward
Pelvic tilt	Erector spinae, latissimus dorsi	2 repetitions (15-s holds)/2 sets	7	Postop day 1 and onward
Lying march	Quadriceps	"March" for 30 s/ 4 sets	7	Postop day 1 and onward
Bridge	Gluteus maximus/medius, hamstrings, abdominals (rectus abdominis, internal/ external obliques)	5–10 repetitions/ 2 sets	7	Postop day 1 and onward
Back extension	Trapezius, latissimus dorsi, erector spinae	3 repetitions/2 sets	7	Postop day 1 and onward
Prone hip extension	Hamstrings	3 repetitions/2 sets	7	Postop day 1 and onward
Seated row	Trapezius, latissimus dorsi, erector spinae, teres major/minor	5 repetitions/2 sets	5	Postop day 1 and onward
Diagonal abdominal curls	Erector spinae, abdominals (+ transverse abdominis), quadratus lumborum	5–10 repetitions/ 2 sets	5	Postop week 6 and onward
Opposite limb raise	Trapezius, erector spinae, deltoid, gluteus maximus/minimus, quadriceps, hamstrings	3–5 repetitions/ 2 sets	5	Postop week 6 and onward
Lean back	Trapezius, latissimus dorsi, erector spinae	Hold for 30 s/3 sets	5	Postop week 6 and onward
Oblique pull	Abdominals, deltoid, latissimus dorsi	5–10 repetitions/ 2 sets	5	Postop week 6 and onward
Exercise ball opposite limb lift	Triceps brachii, transverse abdominis, serratus posterior, psoas, iliacus	10–20 repetitions/ 1 set	5	Postop week 6 and onward
Exercise ball leg extension	Hamstrings	5–10 repetitions/ 1 set	5	Postop week 6 and onward
Hip raise	Gluteus maximus/medius, hamstrings, abdominal	5–10 repetitions/ 1 set	5	Postop week 6 and onward
Aerobic conditioning	All organ systems	≥30 min	5	Postop week 9 and onward

- Hold for 20 seconds.
- Repeat 3 times, twice a day (Figure 63.7).

Lying March

- Lie on the back with bent knees,
- Lift alternating legs off the ground several inches in a marching motion.
- Keep the pelvis stationary.
- "March" for 30 seconds three times a day (Figure 63.8).

Bridge

- Lie on the back.
- Raise the hips off the floor while keeping the back straight.
- Repeat 5 to 10 times, twice daily (Figure 63.9).

Back Extension

- Lie on the stomach with a pillow under the abdomen.
- Lift the head and shoulders 1 to 2 inches off the ground.

© 2018 American Academy of Orthopaedic Surgeons

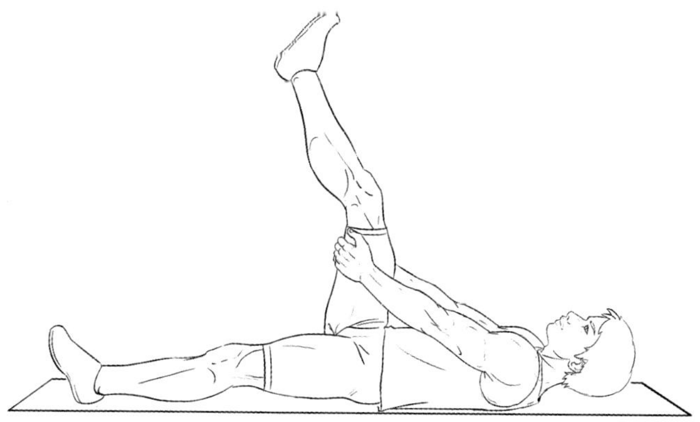

Figure 63.3 Illustration of low back stretch.

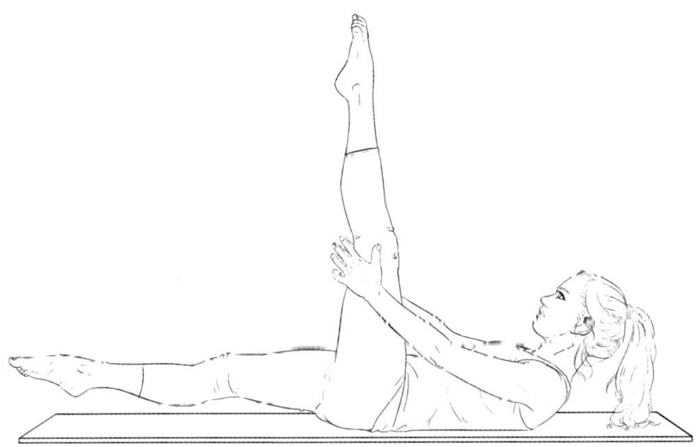

Figure 63.4 Illustration of hamstring lying stretch.

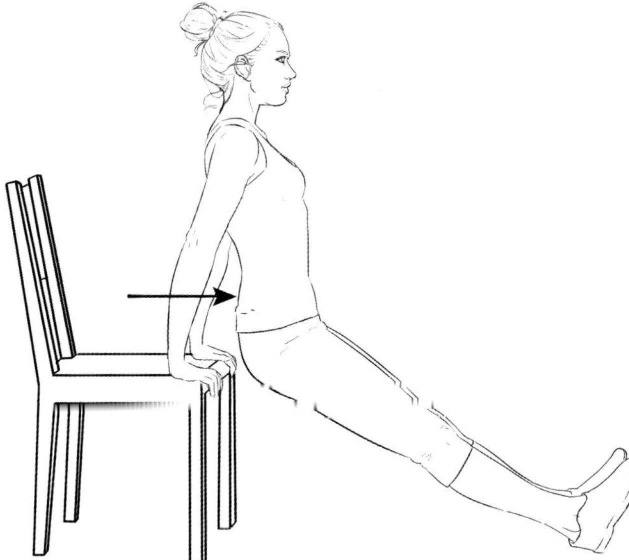

Figure 63.5 Illustration of hamstring seated stretch.

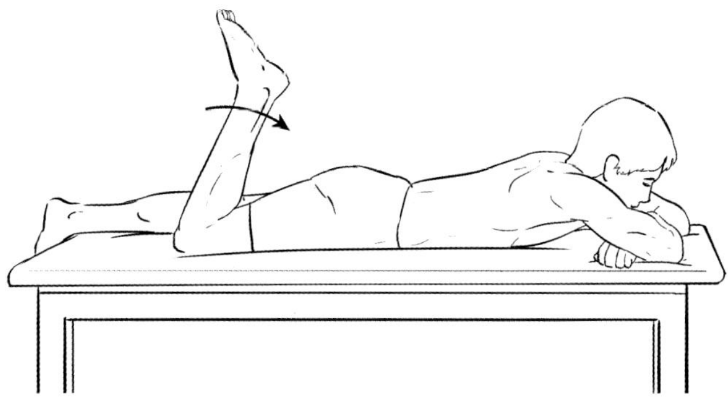

Figure 63.6 Illustration of quadriceps stretch.

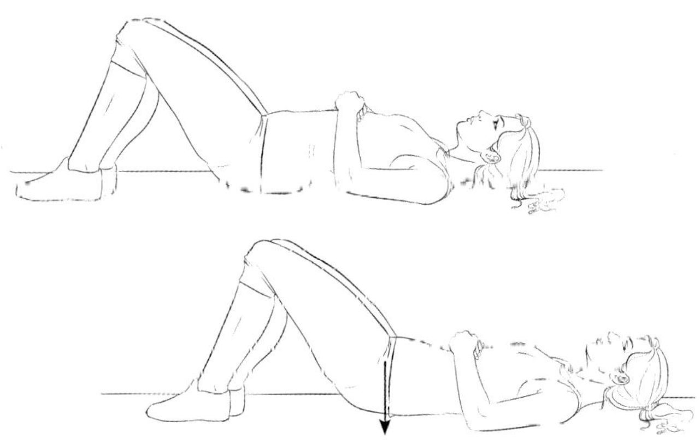

Figure 63.7 Illustration of pelvic tilt.

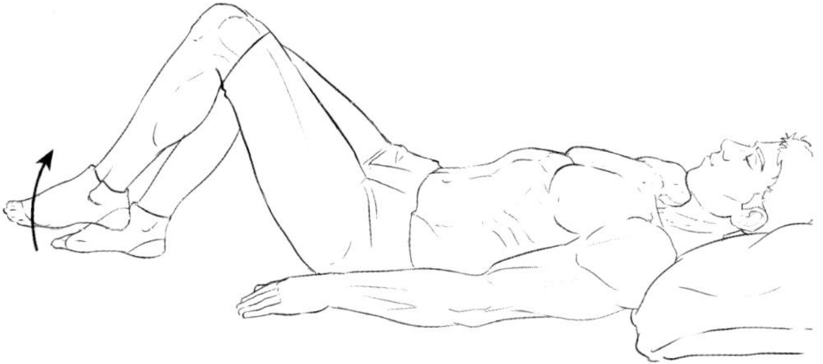

Figure 63.8 Illustration of lying march.

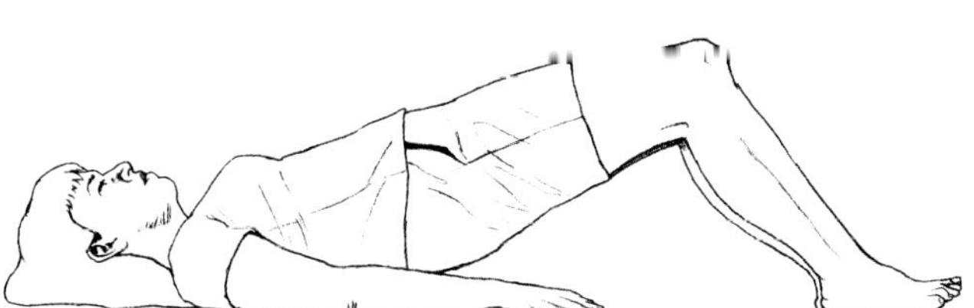

Figure 63.9 Illustration of bridge stretching exercise. (Anatomical Chart Company, *Trigger Points FlipBook: Understanding Myofascial Pain and Discomfort.* ed 2. Philadelphia, Wolters Kluwer, 2007.)

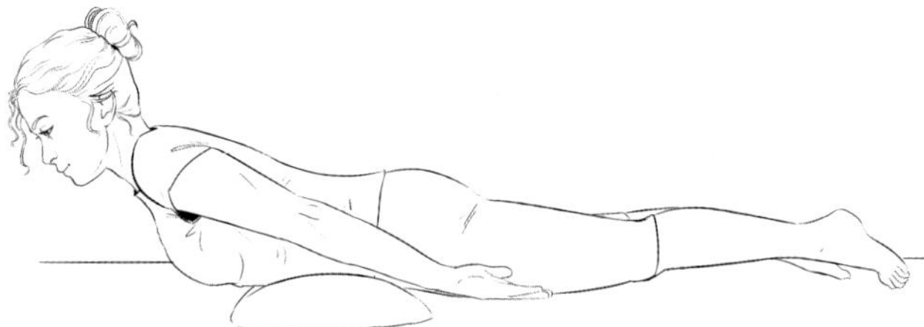

Figure 63.10 Illustration of back extension.

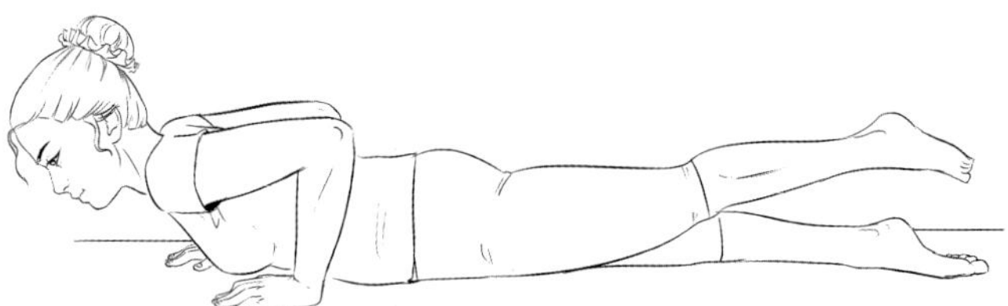

Figure 63.11 Illustration of prone hip extension.

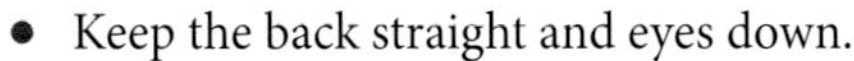

- Keep the back straight and eyes down.
- Repeat three times, twice daily (Figure 63.10).

Prone Hip Extension

- Lie on the stomach.
- Raise one heel toward the ceiling while keeping your pelvis squarely on the ground.
- Keep the other leg on the ground.
- Alternate legs three times, twice daily (Figure 63.11).

Seated Row

- Secure an elastic band to a fixed, stationary object (e.g., closed door).
- Sit upright on a chair.
- Pull the elastic band horizontally, squeezing the shoulder blades together.
- Repeat 3 times, twice daily (Figure 63.12).

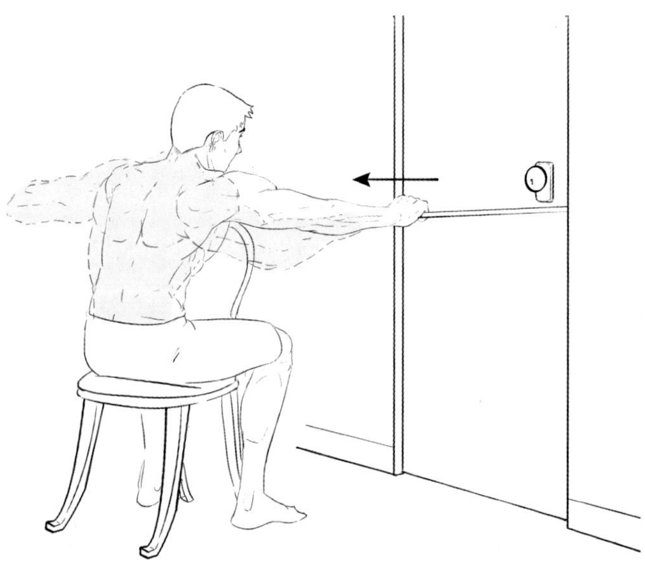

Figure 63.12 Illustration of seated row exercise.

Diagonal Abdominal Curls

- Lie on your back with bent knees.
- Raise right shoulder 4 inches off the ground toward the left hip.
- Set the shoulder down.
- Raise the left shoulder 4 inches off the ground toward the right hip.
- Set the left shoulder down.
- Repeat 5 to 10 times, twice daily (Figure 63.13).

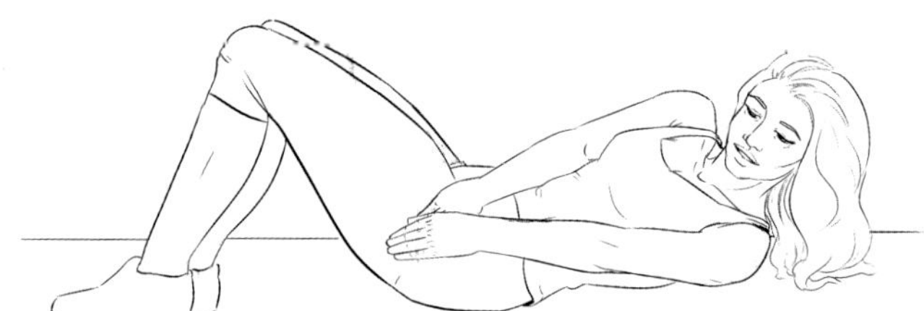

Figure 63.13 Illustration of diagonal abdominal curls.

Opposite Limb Raise

- Position on your hands and knees.
- Raise one arm and the opposite leg toward a horizontal plane.
- Perform with the alternate limbs.
- Repeat 3 to 5 times, twice daily (Figure 63.14).

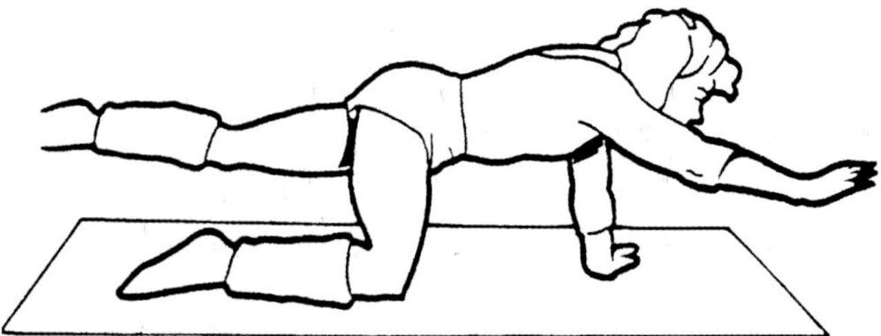

Figure 63.14 Illustration of opposite limb raise. (MediClip image (c) 2003, Philadelphia, Lippincott Williams & Wilkins. All rights reserved.)

Lean Back

- Secure an elastic band to a fixed, stationary object (e.g., closed door).
- With straight arms, lean backward to stretch the back (Figure 63.15).

Oblique Pull

- Secure an elastic band to a fixed, stationary object that is close to the ground (e.g., couch leg).

© 2018 American Academy of Orthopaedic Surgeons

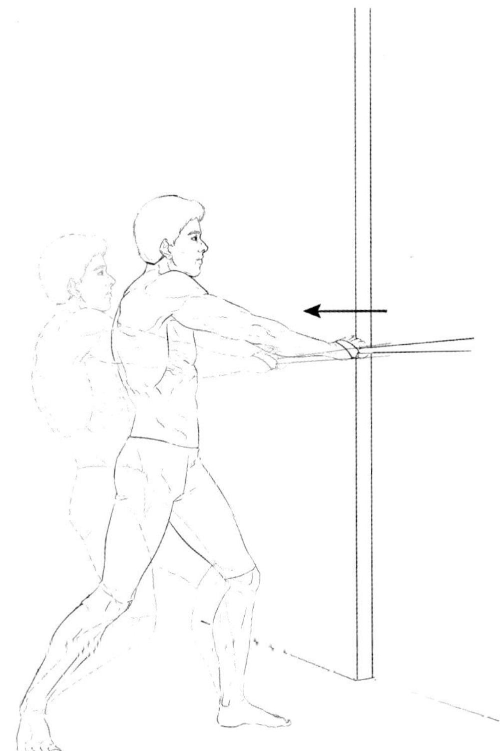

Figure 63.15 Illustration of lean back exercise.

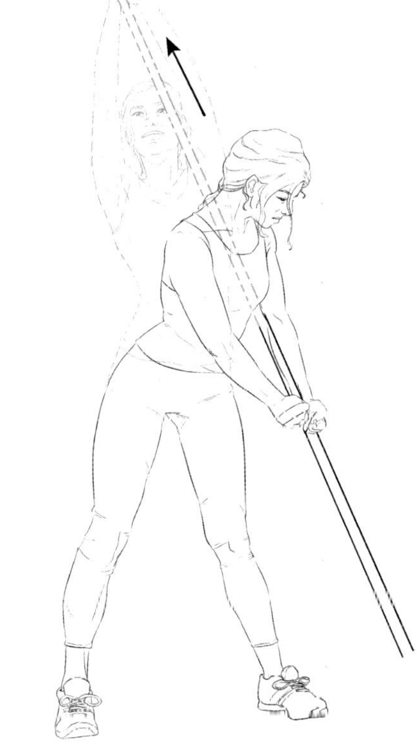

Figure 63.16 Illustration of oblique pull exercise.

- Stand with feet below the shoulders with the band down beside the torso.
- With two hands, pull the band over the opposite shoulder 5 to 10 times.
- Perform with the opposite side.
- Repeat twice daily (Figure 63.16).

Exercise Ball Opposite Limb Lift

- Sit on an exercise ball.
- Raise one leg and the opposite arm toward the ceiling while maintaining balance.
- Perform with alternate limbs.
- Repeat 10 to 20 times (Figure 63.17).

Exercise Ball Leg Extension

- Lie on the exercise ball with your stomach.
- Slide forward until the ball is under the thighs and hands are securely on the ground.
- Raise one heel toward the ceiling while keeping the opposite thigh on the ball.
- Alternate legs 5 to 10 times (Figure 63.18).

Hip Raise

- Lie on the back.
- Position the exercise ball under the calves.
- Raise your hips toward the ceiling, straightening the back and tightening the abdominal muscles.
- Repeat 5 to 10 times (Figure 63.19).

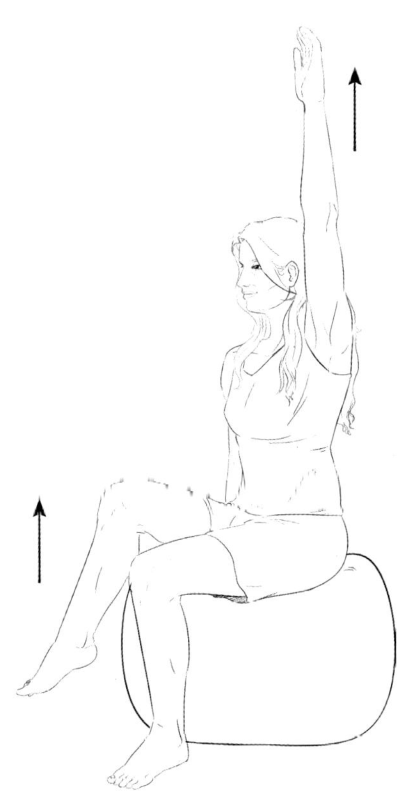

Figure 63.17 Illustration of exercise ball opposite limb lift exercise.

© 2010 American Academy of Orthopaedic Surgeons

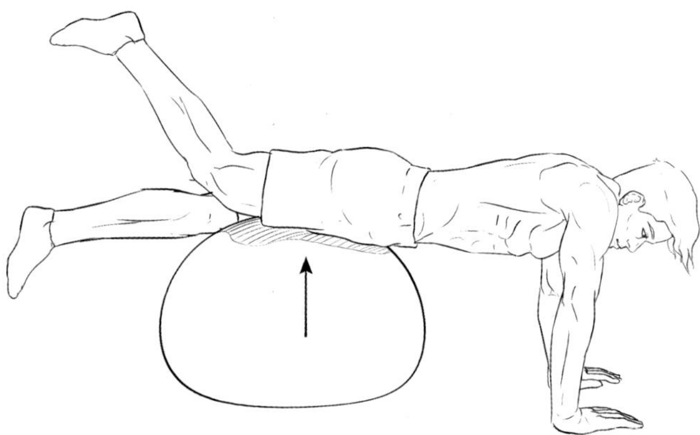

Figure 63.18 Illustration of exercise ball leg extension exercise.

Aerobic Conditioning

- Before starting, obtain physician approval to ensure that the back and heart will tolerate such activities.
- Start slow as strength and fitness are regained.
- Gradually increase intensity and duration with eventual goal of ≥30 minutes of aerobic exercise 5 times per week.
- Focus on low-impact exercises, such as swimming, speed walking, stationary bicycles, or elliptical trainers.
- Avoid high-impact exercises with abrupt start–stop and direction changes, such as running, jumping, or contact sports.

Functional Goals and Restrictions

See Table 63.2 for details.

Evidence Review

Several prospective randomized trials have been performed to assess the efficacy of specific rehabilitation protocols following lumbar spinal fusion, although these trials provide low-level evidence for efficacy. Based on the available low-quality data, it appears that physical therapy may improve pain and function when provided after lumbar spinal fusion. Several systematic reviews have concluded that due to the lack of high-quality studies and the variation in the physical therapy techniques assessed in the available literature, the current evidence provides only limited guidance for physical therapy following lumbar fusion.

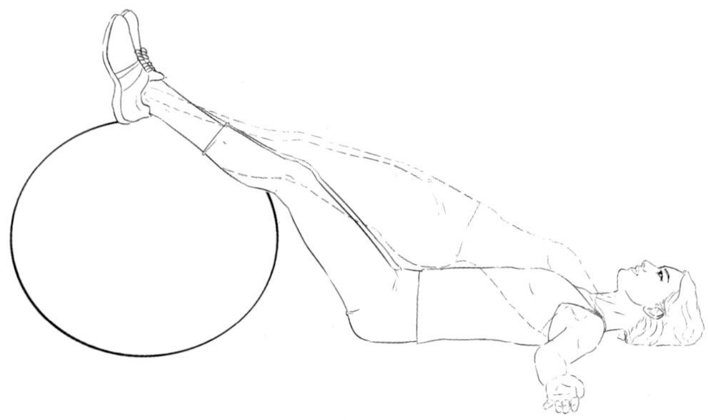

Figure 63.19 Illustration of hip raise exercise.

Table 63.2 FUNCTIONAL GOALS AND RESTRICTIONS BY POSTOPERATIVE WEEK

Postoperative Week	Functional Goals
1	Walking and stretching
1	Stabilization exercises with stationary trunk
6	Stabilization exercises involving mild trunk movement
9	Aerobic conditioning
12	Activity as tolerated

PEARLS

Immediately after lumbar spine fusion surgery, patients will experience pain and most experience some limitations in mobility. There are several things that patients can do preoperatively to make the postoperative recovery go more smoothly, such as organizing their home, arranging assistance, and quitting smoking. Preparing the home may involve placing commonly used household items in easy-to-reach places. Initially, a second set of hands around the house will make (independent) ADLs easier. Finally, smoking cessation is critical. There is substantial evidence demonstrating that nicotine impairs bone growth and smokers have worse surgical outcomes. Furthermore, determining where physical therapy will be performed postoperatively, and considering initiation of physical therapy preoperatively to learn the exercises may be beneficial.

BIBLIOGRAPHY

Abbott AD, Tyni-Lenne R, Hedlund R: Early rehabilitation targeting cognition, behavior, and motor function after lumbar fusion: a randomized controlled trial. *Spine* 2010;35:848–857.

Abbott AD, Tyni-Lenne R, Hedlund R: The influence of psychological factors on pre-operative levels of pain intensity, disability and health-related quality of life in lumbar spinal fusion surgery patients. *Physiotherapy* 2010;96:213–221.

Archer KR, Coronado RA, Haug CM, et al: A comparative effectiveness trial of postoperative management for lumbar spine surgery: changing behavior through physical therapy (CBPT) study protocol. *BMC Musculoskelet Disord* 2014;15:325.

Christensen FB, Laurberg I, Bunger CE: Importance of the backcafe concept to rehabilitation after lumbar spinal fusion: a randomized clinical study with a 2-year follow-up. *Spine* 2003;28:2561–2569.

© 2018 American Academy of Orthopaedic Surgeons

Gilmore SJ, McClelland JA, Davidson M: Physiotherapeutic interventions before and after surgery for degenerative lumbar conditions: a systematic review. *Physiotherapy* 2015; 101(2):111–118.

McGregor AH, Probyn K, Cro S, et al: Rehabilitation following surgery for lumbar spinal stenosis. *Cochrane Database Syst Rev* 2013;(12):CD009644.

Oestergaard LG, Nielsen CV, Bünger CE, et al: The effect of early initiation of rehabilitation after lumbar spinal fusion. *Spine* 2012;37:1803–1809.

Rushton A, Eveleigh G, Petherick EJ, et al: Physiotherapy rehabilitation following lumbar spinal fusion: a systematic review and meta-analysis of randomised controlled trials. *BMJ Open* 2012;2:e000829.

© 2018 American Academy of Orthopaedic Surgeons

64 Adult and Adolescent Scoliosis

Abigail K. Allen, MD, Elizabeth Zhu, MD, and Samuel K. Cho, MD

INTRODUCTION

Adolescent Scoliosis

Adolescent scoliosis is a spinal deformity in the coronal and sagittal planes that is broadly categorized into neuromuscular, congenital, and idiopathic etiologies. Of these, adolescent idiopathic scoliosis (AIS) accounts for 80% to 85% of cases and is most common. Congenital scoliosis results from the failure of formation or segmentation of vertebral precursors that allow asymmetric vertebral growth and curvature. Neuromuscular scoliosis has many etiologies, such as cerebral palsy, muscular dystrophy, spinal muscular atrophy, and myelomeningocele. AIS will be the focus of discussion in this chapter.

Scoliosis is radiographically defined by the curvature of the spine in the coronal plane greater than 10° using the Cobb method (Figure 64.1). Anatomically, scoliosis is a 3-dimensional deformity that includes vertebral rotation as well. Although present in 2% to 4% of children between ages 10 and 16 years, only about 10% of patients with AIS progress and require medical intervention. Without treatment, severe curves may cause chronic back pain, respiratory dysfunction, and degenerative arthritis. Risk factors for progression include large curve magnitude, skeletal immaturity, and female gender. In general, surgery is performed for curves greater than 45° to 50°. Spinal fusion is the current gold standard; its aim is to correct the deformity and prevent further progression.

Adult Scoliosis

When scoliosis occurs in a skeletally mature patient, it is called adult scoliosis. Reported rates of scoliosis in adults vary widely. As in adolescents, curvature greater than 10° as measured by the Cobb method is defined as scoliosis. However, most adults that seek treatment have curves that exceed 30°. Adult scoliosis may simply be progression of untreated adolescent scoliosis, or it may be caused by other spinal conditions such as degeneration, osteoporosis, or osteomalacia. In addition, adult scoliosis occurs frequently with spinal stenosis, rotatory subluxation, and nerve compression. Adults with scoliosis may also have loss of height, shortness of breath, and early satiety. Unlike in AIS, patients usually present with axial back and radicular leg pain, sometimes along with progressive truncal imbalance. The pain may be related to the curve or to the compression of the spinal nerves. There is considerable variability in management of adult scoliosis, including nonoperative care, decompression, limited stabilization, and long fusions. Surgical intervention is indicated for patients with pain and functional limitations unresponsive to nonoperative care, progression of deformity, neural impairment, and lung function impairment.

SURGERY

The goal of surgery is to achieve a solid, well-balanced spinal fusion to prevent long-term dysfunction and disability. Posterior spinal fusion is the mainstay of treatment in scoliosis. Other surgical approaches include anterior and combined anterior–posterior spinal fusions. The surgical approach used depends on a number of factors, including curve magnitude, flexibility, location, as well as surgeon preference and experience. Currently, segmental pedicle screws, hooks, and wires provide better correction and less frequent implant failures. The pedicle, the hardest part of the vertebral body, serves as an excellent anchor point for fixation devices.

The posterior spinal musculature consists of deep and superficial layers (Figure 64.2). The superficial erector spinae includes the iliocostalis, longissimis, and sacrospinal muscles. The deep layer includes the short rotators (multifidus and rotators), intertransversarii, and interspinous muscles. The spinal musculature is innervated segmentally by the dorsal rami of the thoracolumbar nerve roots. The blood supply is

Dr. Cho or an immediate family member serves as a paid consultant to DePuy, A Johnson & Johnson Company, Medtronic, Stryker, and Zimmer; has received research or institutional support from Zimmer; and serves as a board member, owner, officer, or committee member of the AOSpine North America, the Cervical Spine Research Society, the North American Spine Society, and the Scoliosis Research Society. Neither of the following authors nor any immediate family member has received anything of value from or has stock or stock options held in a commercial company or institution related directly or indirectly to the subject of this article: Dr. Allen and Dr. Zhu.

© 2018 American Academy of Orthopaedic Surgeons

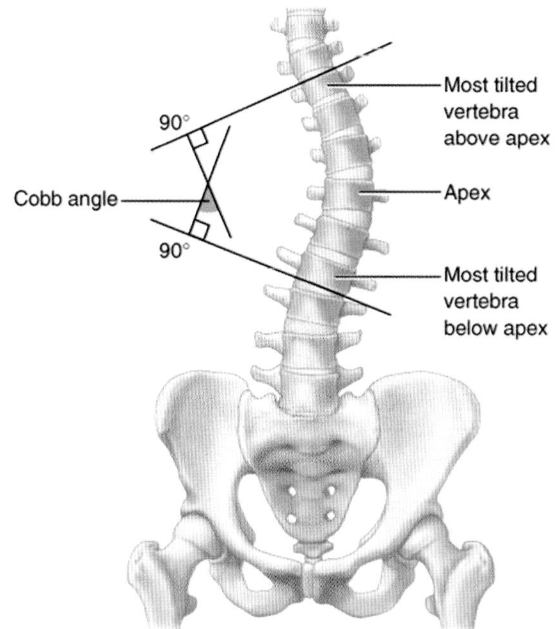

Figure 64.1 Cobb method. (Reproduced with permission from Flynn JM, ed: *Operative Techniques in Pediatric Orthopaedics*. Philadelphia, PA, Wolters Kluwer Health, 2010.)

segmentally distributed from the dorsal branches of the posterior intercostal arteries.

Typically, a straight midline back incision is used for the posterior surgical approach. The skin and subcutaneous fat are transected until the thoracolumbar fascia is reached. The thoracolumbar fascia is dissected between the tips of the spinous processes and dissection is carried out to the transverse processes. Surgery exposes and traumatizes paravertebral muscles, which serve as important stabilizers, especially in the lumbar spine. Posterior dissection of the spine also carries risk of denervation of the paraspinal musculature and decrease in trunk strength. Prolonged retraction during surgery can cause ischemic damage to the paraspinal muscles as well. Postoperative complications are rarer in adolescents than adults, and may include neural injury, neural compression, infection, nonunion, instability, and medical complications such as myocardial infarction, stroke, deep vein thrombosis, and pulmonary embolism. Last, spinal fusion leads to loss of range of motion (ROM) to varying degrees dependent on the site and length of the fusion (Figures 64.3–64.6).

POSTOPERATIVE REHABILITATION

The main goal of postoperative rehabilitation for scoliosis patients is to optimize function following surgery. Primarily, rehabilitation interventions aim to decrease pain and restore function in activities of daily living (ADLs). Rehabilitation protocols following spinal fusion have not been well established, and differ from surgeon to surgeon. There are not any comprehensive guidelines that are agreed upon. Therefore, the rehabilitation protocols described are the authors' based on our clinical experience.

Postoperative care as currently practiced can be divided into three phases: immediate postoperative care and mobilization, back-specific rehabilitation, and return to functional activity level. In the immediate postoperative care phase, the therapist evaluates the patient's physical capacity and addresses any special needs. Therapy centers on transfer, gait, and basic back care after surgery. In the back-specific rehabilitation phase, the patient gradually increases muscular coordination, strength, and endurance through a home or subacute rehabilitation exercise program under the guidance of the physician. Therapy centers on maximizing functional status. When patients enter the final phase to help them return to their baseline functional activity level, the patients progress further in exercise tolerance and aerobic conditioning, while continuing to focus on back stretching and strengthening.

The health care team—consisting of the orthopaedic surgeon, pain service, physical therapist, and ancillary staff—should encourage patients to mobilize soon after surgery. Pain is a poor indicator of determining exercise program duration and intensity. Kool et al. found that patients who were trained to stop exercising because of pain fared worse in all measures, including strength, ROM, disability, limping, guarding, pain killer dosage, and health care seeking. In contrast, patients who were trained to continue with therapy despite pain had decreased disability overall. Therefore, psychological support to overcome fear about pain, injury, and function should be given in addition to active physical treatment.

Immediate Postoperative Care and Mobilization

The goal of rehabilitation between surgery and discharge from the hospital is independent ambulation and regaining some of ADLs. ADLs refers to the basic tasks of life, such as eating, bathing, dressing, toileting, and transferring. In addition to postoperative wound and medical care, patients require physical, and occasionally occupational, therapy. Prior to initiating physical therapy, a comprehensive medical evaluation—including pain control, postoperative hemoglobin levels, and cardiovascular and neurologic status—should be performed. For pain, we use patient-controlled anesthesia (PCA) immediately after surgery (given to the patient in the recovery room) with transition to oral medications as soon as the patient can tolerate oral intake. Adequate pain control is essential to the rehabilitation process.

External bracing is typically not necessary. Early mobilization avoids deconditioning following surgery. Therefore, patients are encouraged to sit up in bed on the day of surgery, and to stand and walk on postoperative day one with support from the physical therapist. For patients who had spinal fusion that spans the lumbosacral junction, it is paramount to have their body positioned close to the head of the bed such that elevation of the head to sit up the patient does not break the bed through the lumbosacral region, but rather the hip joint. Physical therapists should also teach deep diaphragmatic breathing

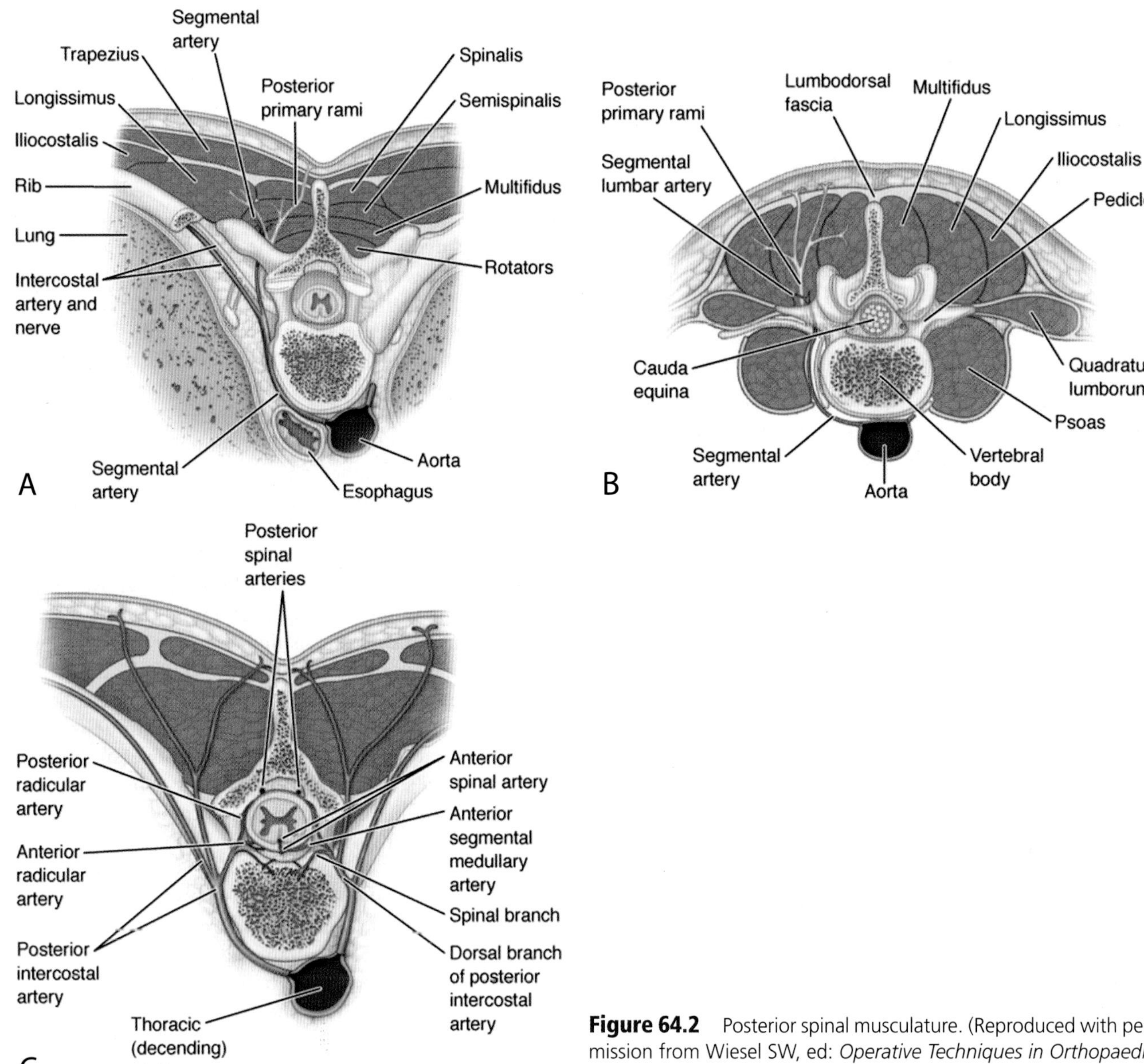

Figure 64.2 Posterior spinal musculature. (Reproduced with permission from Wiesel SW, ed: *Operative Techniques in Orthopaedic Surgery,* ed 2. Philadelphia, PA, Wolters Kluwer Health, 2016.)

to promote full chest expansion, and ankle ROM to promote circulation and avoid blood clot development from inactivity. Bending, lifting, and twisting maneuvers are avoided and discouraged. Before discharge, the patient should demonstrate ability to ambulate, including being able to walk up a flight of stairs (Table 64.1).

Postdischarge Home or Subacute Exercise Program

Immediately after discharge, the focus is on recuperation with or without some basic and gentle back conditioning. The home exercise program depends on a number of factors, including age, medical comorbidities, and length of fusion. Since spinal arthrodesis takes place gradually over several months after surgery, spinal fusion precaution should be taken. This includes avoiding any twisting, bending forward, heavy lifting, driving, abdominal straining, prolonged sitting, and excessive physical activity. Patients should walk, take stairs, lie down with proper back alignment, and have living areas arranged to prevent bending, stooping, and reaching. While changing body positions, patients should continue to use the logrolling and transferring techniques learned in the inpatient setting.

After discharge from the hospital, AIS and adult scoliosis patients differ in their postoperative rehabilitation, since younger, healthier patients tend to recover from surgery more quickly. AIS patients may return to school 4 to 6 weeks after surgery. Adolescents must be aware of their limitations immediately following surgery and should not begin athletic activities until cleared by the surgeon. Return to sports depends

© 2018 American Academy of Orthopaedic Surgeons

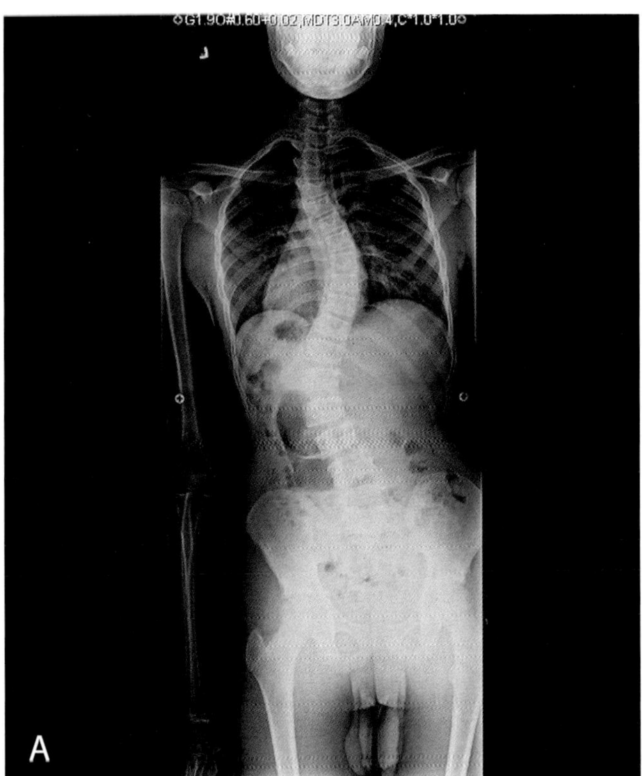

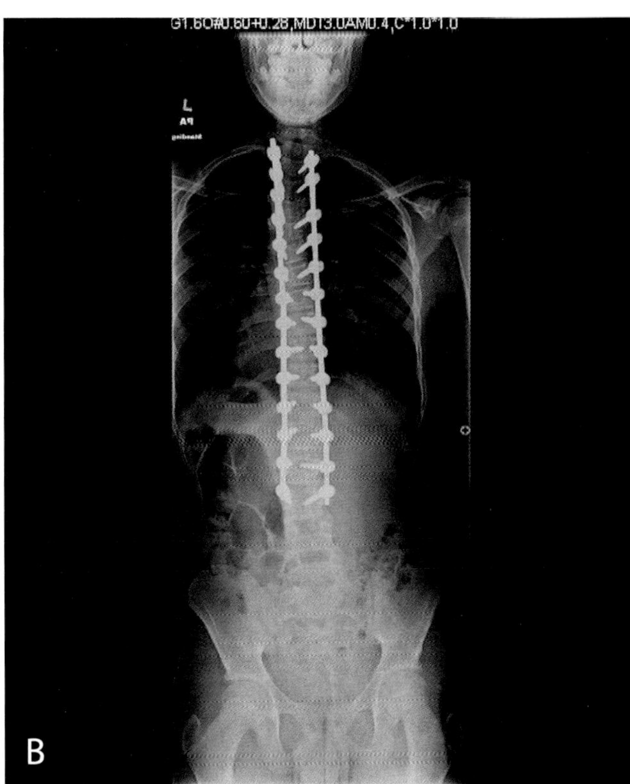

Figure 64.3 Posteroanterior radiographs demonstrating preoperative and postoperative images of posterior spinal fusion in adolescent idiopathic scoliosis.

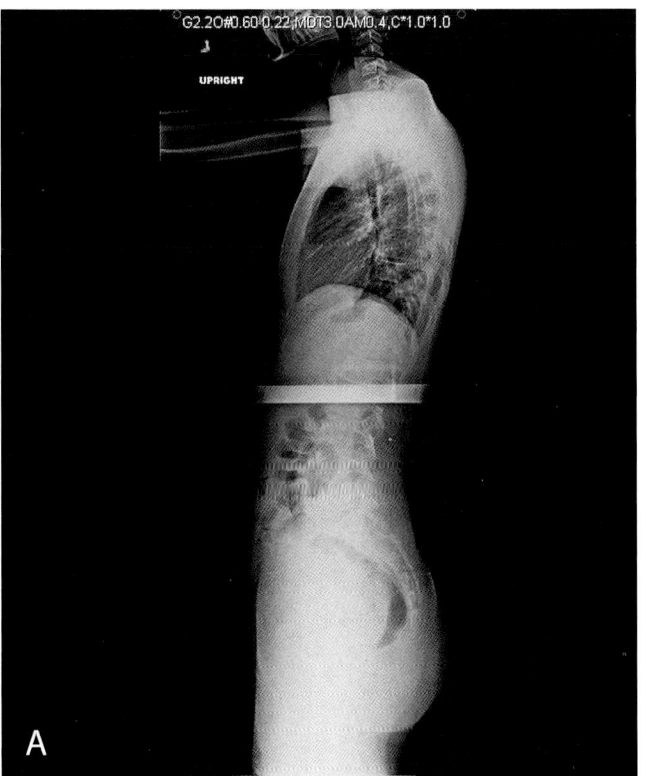

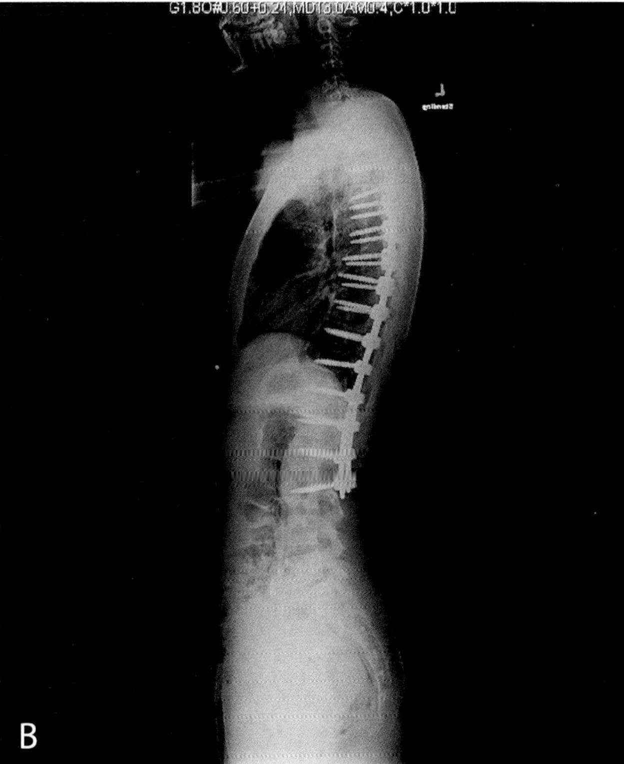

Figure 64.4 Lateral radiographs of the same patient in Figure 64.3 demonstrating preoperative and postoperative images of posterior spinal fusion in adolescent idiopathic scoliosis.

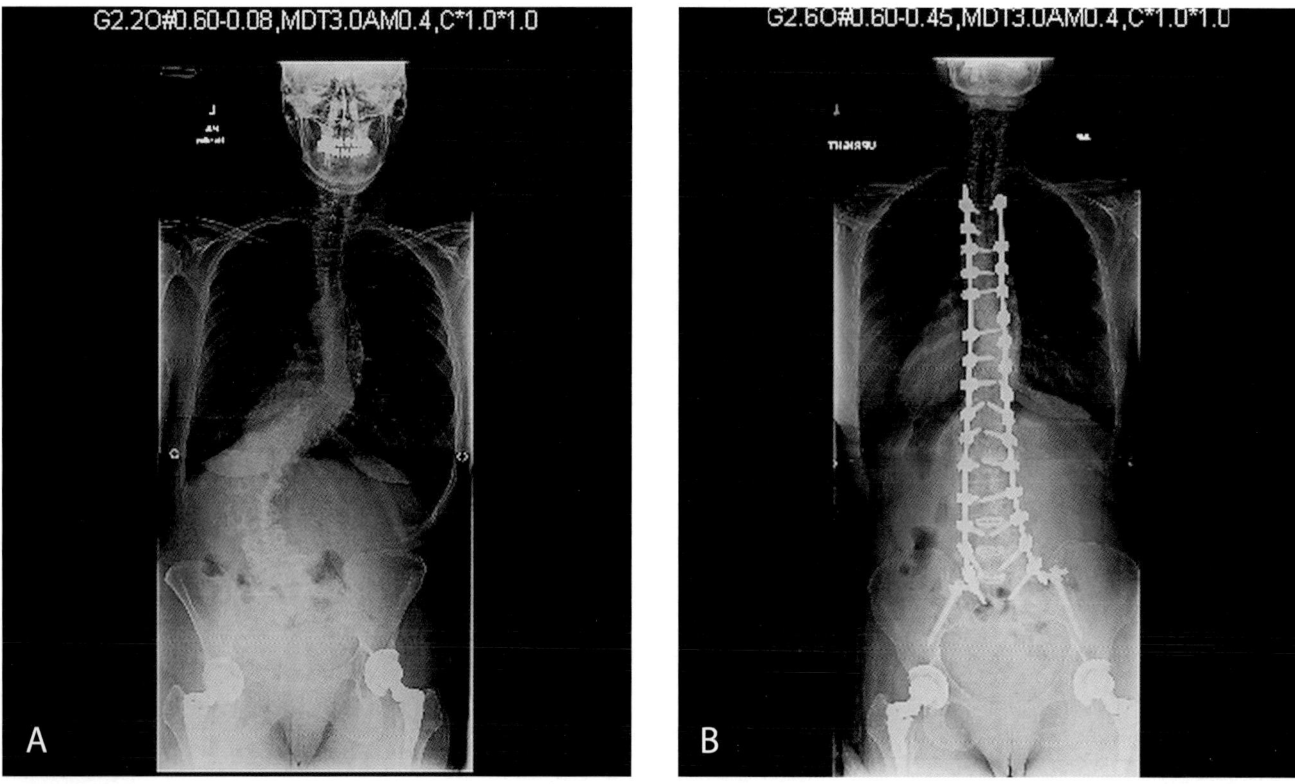

Figure 64.5 Posteroanterior radiographs demonstrating preoperative and postoperative images of posterior spinal fusion in adult scoliosis.

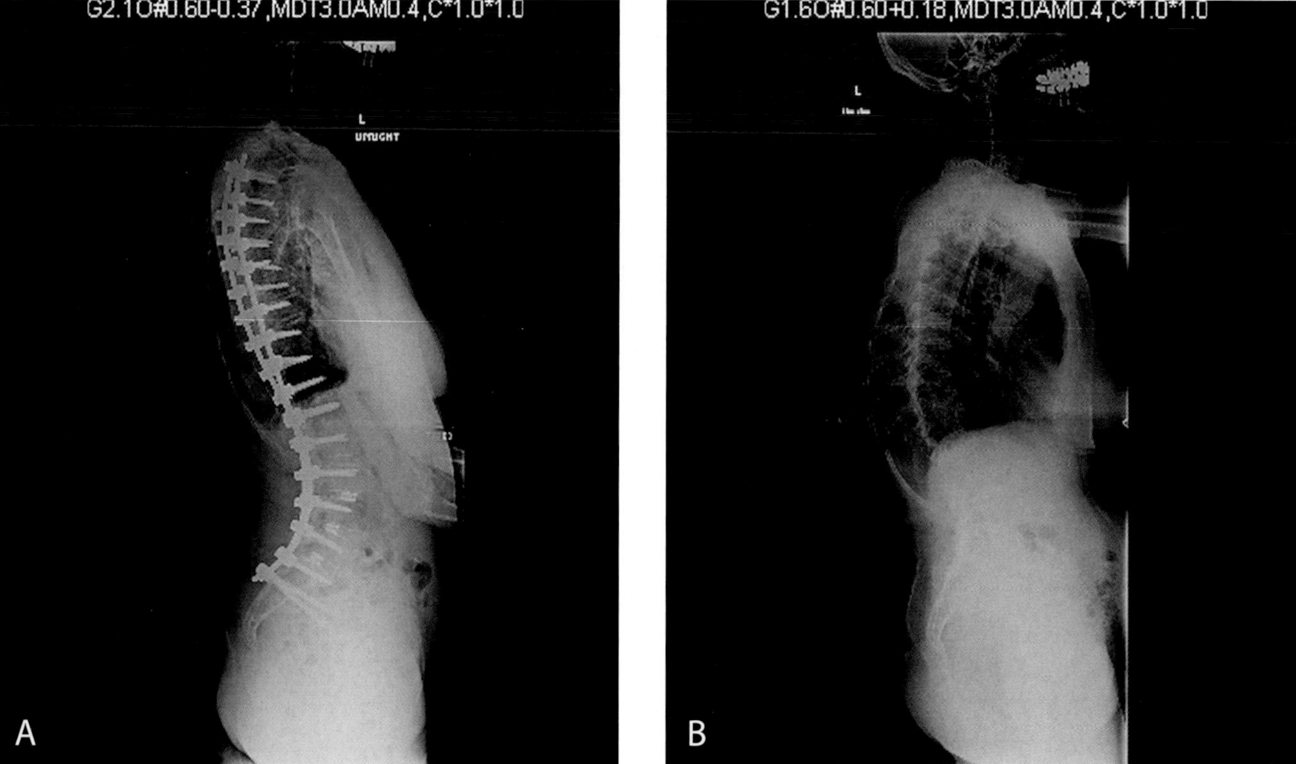

Figure 64.6 Lateral radiographs of the same patient in Figure 64.5 demonstrating preoperative and postoperative images of posterior spinal fusion in adult scoliosis.

 © 2018 American Academy of Orthopaedic Surgeons

Table 64.1 MOBILITY AFTER SURGERY

Task	Goal
Log rolling 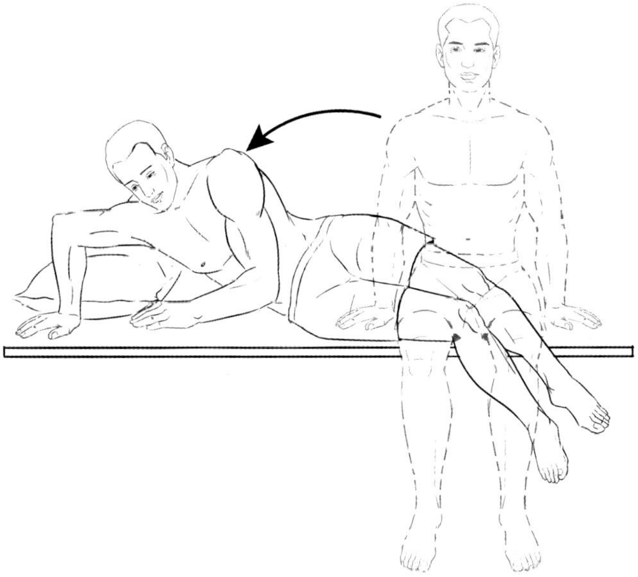	Limit rotation and enable the patient to use the arms as support for independent transfer from supine to sitting. May require side grab bar to be added to bed.
Transferring 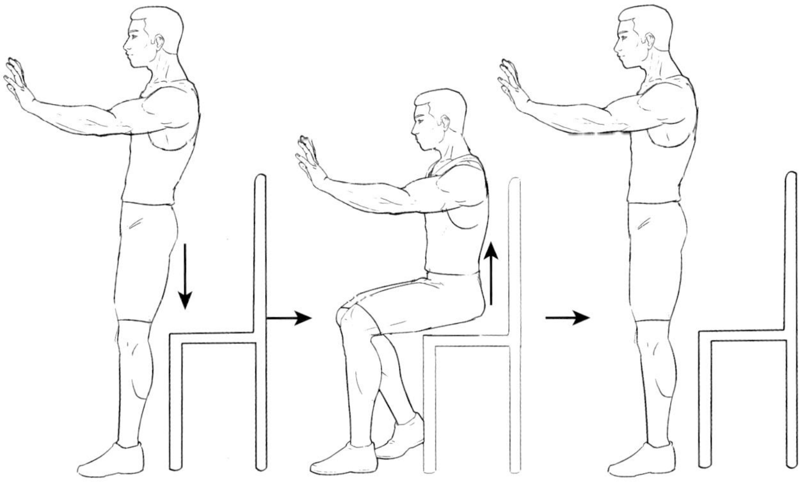	Promote independence in sit-to-stand transfer. May require grab bar or elevated commode in presence of weak arms or quadriceps.
Ambulation	Promote independence in ambulation from level surface to stairs to inclines. May require rolling walker or cane.

on surgeon preference, typically ranging from 6 to 12 months postoperatively. In one study, patients self-progressed their activity starting 4 months postoperatively if they were pain free and had no radiographic signs of implant migration or curve progression. One report stated that if there are less than three free lumbar segments, sports with axial and rotatory burdens, such as football and gymnastics, should be discouraged. However, most patients studied returned to full clearance, including contact sports, by 7 months. Though postoperative return to sports depends on several factors, many patients return to athletic competition at or above their preoperative level.

For adult scoliosis patients, therapy is more involved since it may take longer to achieve full functional recovery compared to adolescents. The extent of fusion has important

© 2018 American Academy of Orthopaedic Surgeons

implications for the kinds of therapy prescribed. For example, patients who had fusion to the sacrum are taught to minimize pelvic motion to optimize chances of fusion at L5–S1. In the first 4 to 6 weeks postoperatively, patients are encouraged to ambulate. During this time period, patients develop muscle coordination and should be able to perform exercises without fatigue in the target muscles of the back and legs. Daily stretching and stabilization exercises may be performed up to every 2 hours for those patients without lumbosacral fusion. This program promotes body awareness and patient self-confidence in independent care. Adults with desk jobs may return to work and resume normal activities at home by 2 to 3 months after surgery. Patients should avoid bending, twisting and heavy lifting (Table 64.2).

- *Note:* Exercises that utilize pelvic motion are not suitable for patients who had fusion that extends down to the sacrum.

Adult Scoliosis Back-Specific Exercise Program

After gaining muscle coordination in the immediate postdischarge period, the back-specific exercise stage of the rehabilitation program helps the patient without lumbosacral fusion to improve control of the neutral lumbar spine as well as increase trunk and hip muscle coordination and strength. In addition

Table 64.2 STATIC STABILIZATION EXERCISES FOR MOBILITY

Stretch	Description
Supine hamstring 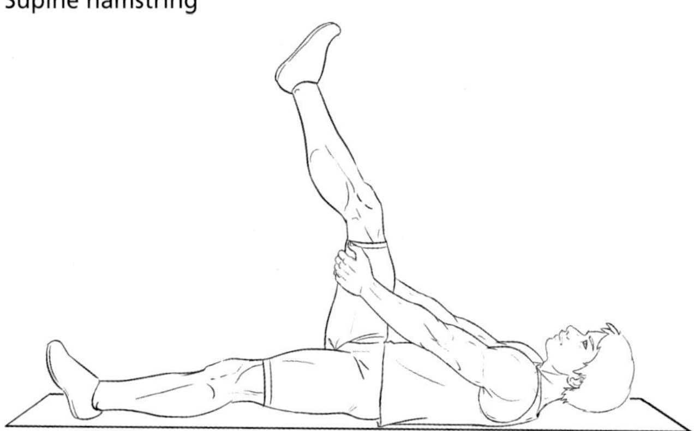	Lying on the back, bend both knees. Slowly straighten one leg and push the heel toward the ceiling until the stretch is felt. Alternate legs. Not suitable for lumbosacral fusion.
Quadriceps flexion 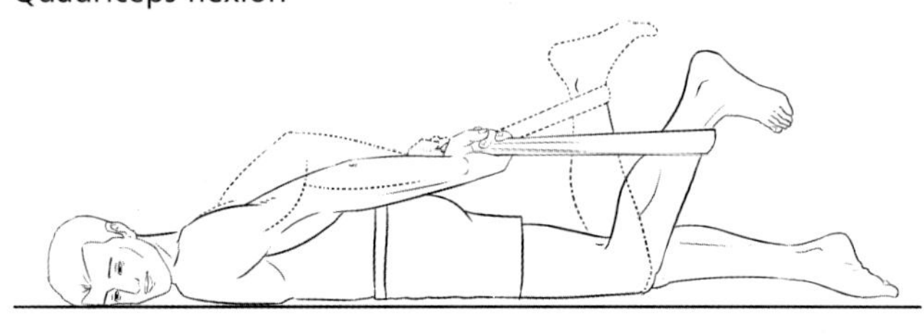	Lying on the stomach, bring the heel toward the buttocks as far as possible. Not suitable for lumbosacral fusion.
Pelvic tilt 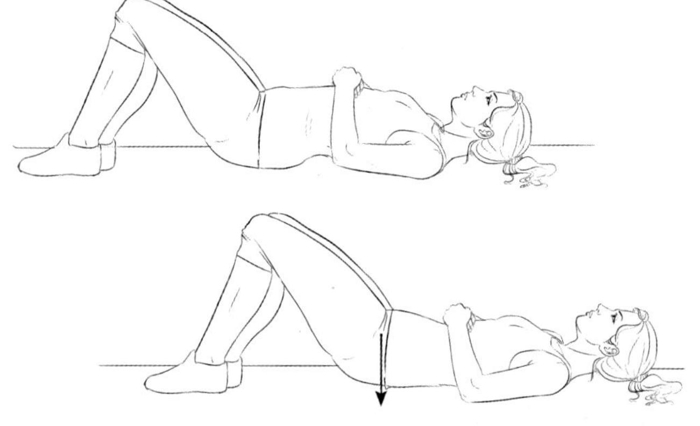	Lying on the back, bend both knees. Pull the belly downward and inward toward the spine. Not suitable for lumbosacral fusion.

© 2018 American Academy of Orthopaedic Surgeons

Table 64.2 STATIC STABILIZATION EXERCISES FOR MOBILITY *(Continued)*

Stretch	Description
Hip extension	Lying on the stomach, raise one leg at the time while holding the knee straight. Do not rock the pelvis. Alternate legs.
Upper body extension 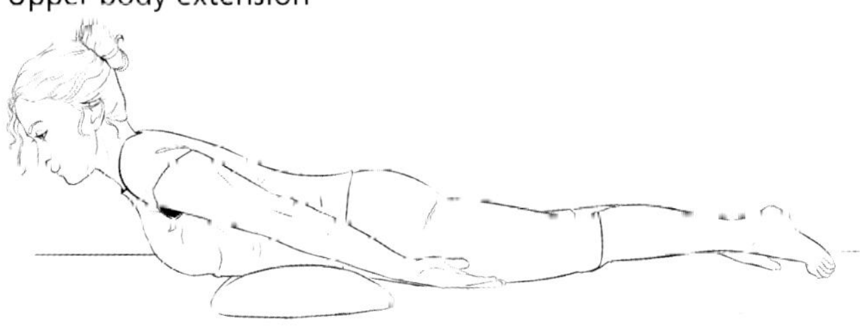	Lying on the stomach, squeeze the shoulder blades together while raising the head and shoulders off the floor. Not suitable for lumbosacral fusion.
Pelvic bridge 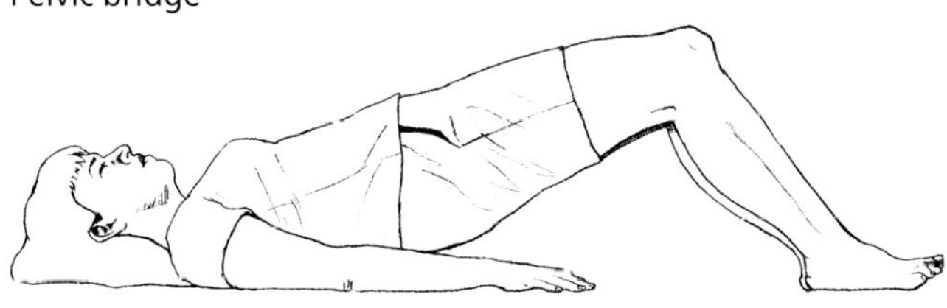 (Reproduced with permission from *ACC Trigger Points FlipBook*. Philadelphia, PA, Wolters Kluwer Health, 2007.)	Lying on the back, bend both knees. Raise the hips from the floor and keep a straight line from shoulders to hips. Not suitable for lumbosacral fusion.

to increasing muscle strength and endurance, these exercises teach patients how to properly lift objects to avoid injury. By the end of this period, patients should be able to perform 8 to 14 repetitions of each exercise with a 5-kg maximum load. Patients perform these home exercises at least two to three times per week in addition to walking for 20 to 30 minutes a day. For patients who had their lumbosacral spine fused, these exercises are discouraged, as they place undue stress on the instrumentation and may lead to implant failure or nonunion (Table 64.3).

- *Note:* Exercises that utilize pelvic motion are not suitable for patients who had fusion that extends down to the sacrum.

Return to Function

After clinical and radiographic evidence of fusion, exercises can be progressed as tolerated by the patient with a goal of returning to desired function and athletic activity. Physical activity is encouraged for long-term outcome. Patients can intensify stretching and strengthening exercises in addition to increasing aerobic conditioning. Aerobic exercise is beneficial, though there is no evidence regarding whether one specific type of exercise is more effective than the other. Additionally, long-term pain disability after spinal surgery is negatively correlated with psychological aspects such as mental stress and job satisfaction. Addressing psychosocial factors in addition to continued physical activity is important to the restoration of optimal patient function. All patients should be aware that full functional recovery may take a year or longer.

PEARLS

- Rehabilitation following scoliosis surgery requires a multidisciplinary approach involving the patient, surgeon,

Table 64.3 BACK-SPECIFIC EXERCISES

Exercise	Description
Squat	From a standing position, move the hips back and flex the knees and hips to lower the torso so that the crease of the hip falls below the top of the knee. Return to an upright position.
Deadlift	From a standing position with feet under hips, hinge the hips, driving the hips backward while keeping the torso tight and straight. Grab a light weight (under 5 kg) and brace the core and latissimi. Pull up on the weight by driving the knees outward with a leg press. As the weight passes the knees, drive the hips forward and lock the body in a straight position. Reverse the movement.
Abdominal crunch 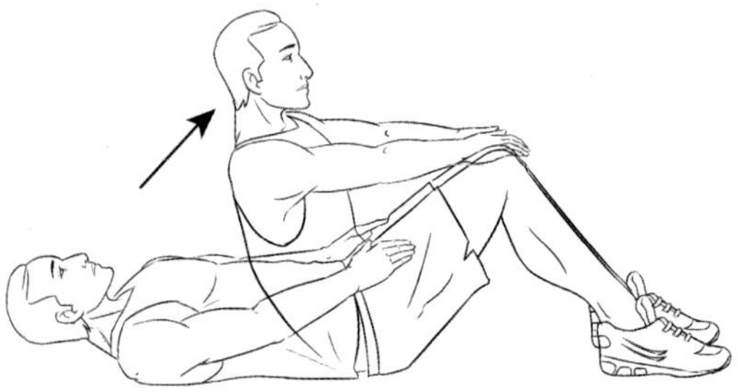	Lying on the back with knees bent, curl the shoulders toward the pelvis with hands crossed over the chest.
Hip abduction 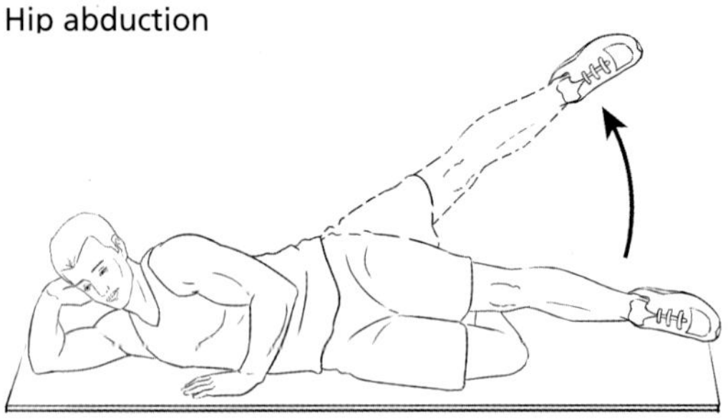	Lying on one side, abduct the leg upward with knee extended. Lower leg back down. Alternate sides.
Hip extension 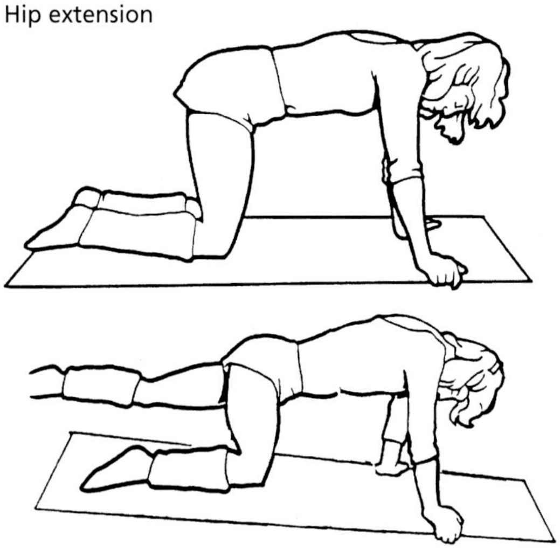 (Reproduced with permission from MediClip, copyright (c) 2003, Philadelphia, PA, Lippincott Williams & Wilkins. All rights reserved.)	On hands and knees with shoulders above hands and hips above knees, lift one leg into the air until sole of the foot is upward and the thigh is parallel to the floor. Lower the knee. Alternate legs.

© 2018 American Academy of Orthopaedic Surgeons

Table 64.3 BACK-SPECIFIC EXERCISES *(Continued)*

Exercise	Description
Shoulder extension and flexion 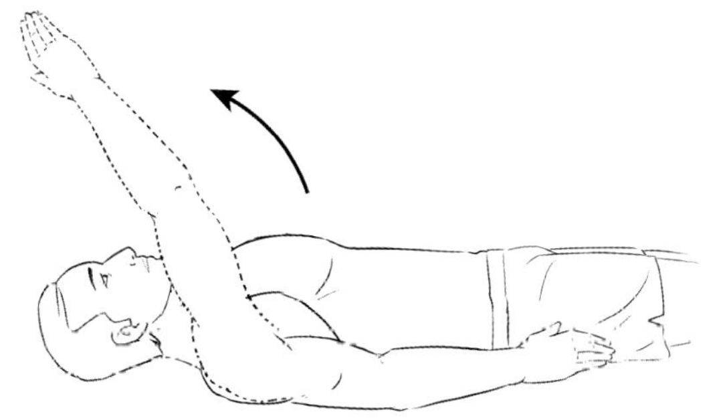	Lying on back, lift arm upward to the ceiling with elbow straight as possible. Repeat with other arm.
Shoulder adduction and abduction 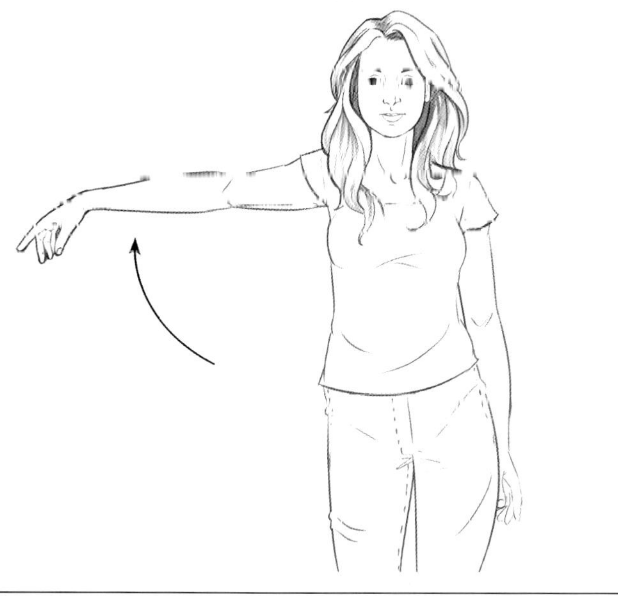	Standing, raise arm out to side with elbow straight and palm downward. Hold and release arms back to sides.
Forward lunge 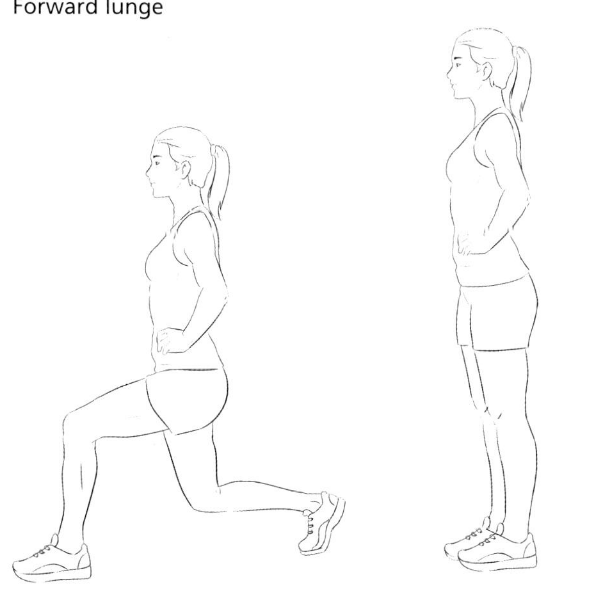	Standing with feet together, step forward with one leg and lower the body so that both knees are flexed to 90°. Keep the knees above the plane of the toes. Push back up to the starting position. Alternate legs.

© 2018 American Academy of Orthopaedic Surgeons

anesthesiologist and pain service, physical therapist, ancillary staff, as well as the parent or caretaker.

- The physician must establish the patient's understanding and expectations of the surgery and postoperative rehabilitation.
- The immediate goal following surgery is for the patient to return to ADLs as soon as possible. The treatment team works together to decrease risk factors for delayed recovery, including attention to psychosocial factors.
- Recognize that each patient is different. Some patients may need formal physical therapy during the rehabilitation phase after surgery, while others may need encouragement to return to physical movement and activity. Some patients, especially adolescents, may need to be dissuaded in the early postoperative phase from returning too quickly to athletic activity.

BIBLIOGRAPHY

Alaranta H, Hurme M, Einola S, Kallio V, Knuts LR,Törmä T: Rehabilitation after surgery for lumbar disc herniation: results of a randomized clinical trial. *Int J Rehabil Res* 1986;9:247–257.

Bas P, Romagnoli M, Gomez-Cabrera MC, Bas JL, Aura JV, Franco N, Bas T: Beneficial effects of aerobic training in adolescent patients with moderate idiopathic scoliosis. *Eur Spine J* 2011;20:415–419.

Bradford DS, Tay BK, Hu SS: Adult scoliosis: surgical indications, operative management, complications, and outcomes. *Spine (Phila Pa 1976)* 1999;24:2617–2629.

Bridwell KH: Surgical treatment of idiopathic adolescent scoliosis. *Spine (Phila Pa 1976)* 1999;24:2607–2616.

Carter OD, Haynes SG: Prevalence rates for scoliosis in the US adults: results from the first National Health and Nutrition Examination Survey. *Int J Epidemiol* 1987;16:537–544.

Dolan P, Greenfield K, Nelson RJ, Nelson IW: Can exercise therapy improve the outcome of microdiscectomy? *Spine (Phila Pa 1976)* 2000;25:1015–1020.

Fabricant PD, Admoni S, Green DW, et al: Return to athletic activity after posterior spinal fusion for adolescent idiopathic scoliosis: analysis of independent predictors. *J Pediatr Orthop* 2012;32:259–265.

Gejo R, Matsui H, Kawaguchi Y, Ishihara H, Tsuji H: Serial changes in trunk muscle performance after posterior lumbar surgery. *Spine (Phila Pa 1976)* 1999;24:1023–1028.

Howard A, Donaldson S, Hedden D: Improvement in quality of life following surgery of adolescent idiopathic scoliosis. *Spine (Phila Pa 1976)* 2007;32:2715–2718.

Kjellby-Wendt G, Styf J: Early active training after lumbar discectomy: a prospective, randomized and controlled study. *Spine (Phila Pa 1976)* 1998;23:2345–2351.

Kool JP, Oesch PR, Bachmann S, et al: Increasing days at work using function-centered rehabilitation in nonacute nonspecific low back pain: a randomized controlled trial. *Arch Phys Med Rehabil* 2005;86:857–864.

Lonstein JE: Scoliosis: surgical versus nonsurgical treatment. *Clin Orthop* 2006;443:248–259.

Mahomed N, Liang M, Cook E, et al: The importance of patient expectations in predicting functional outcomes after total joint arthroplasty. *J Rheumatology* 2002;29:1273–1279.

Maruyama T, Takeshita K: Surgical treatment of scoliosis: a review of techniques currently applied. *Scoliosis* 2008;3:6.

Medicine ACoS: *Guidelines for Exercise Testing and Prescription.* Lea & Febiger, Philadelphia, PA, 1991.

Parsch D, Gärtner V, Brocai DR, Carstens C, Schmitt H: Sports activity of patients with idiopathic scoliosis at long-term follow-up. *Clin J Sport Med* 2002;12:95–98.

Reamy BV, Slakey JB: Adolescent idiopathic scoliosis: review and current concepts. *Am Fam Physician* 2001;64:111–116.

Rubery PT, Bradford DS: Athletic activity after spine surgery in children and adolescents: results of a survey. *Spine (Phila Pa 1976)* 2002;27:423–427.

Sarwahi V, Wollowick AL, Sugarman EP, Horn JJ, Gambassi M, Amaral TD: Minimally invasive scoliosis surgery: an innovative technique in patients with adolescent idiopathic scoliosis. *Scoliosis* 2011;6:16.

Simmons ED Jr, Kowalski JM, Simmons EH: The results of surgical treatment for adult scoliosis. *Spine (Phila Pa 1976)* 1993;18:718–724.

Stambough JL: Matching patient and physician expectations in spine surgery leads to improved outcomes. *Spine J* 2001;1:234.

Suk SI, Lee SM, Chung ER, Kim JH, Kim SS: Selective thoracic fusion with segmental pedicle screw fixation in the treatment of thoracic idiopathic scoliosis: more than 5-year follow-up. *Spine* 2005;30:1602–1609.

Von Strempel A, Scholz M, Daentzer M: Sports capacity of patients with scoliosis. *Sportverletzung Sportschaden* 1993;7: 58–62.

Weber BR, Grob D, Dvorak J, Muntener M: Posterior surgical approach to the lumbar spine and its effect on the multifidus muscle. *Spine (Phila Pa 1976)* 1997;22:1765–1772.

Wright A, Ferree B, Tromanhauser S: Spinal fusion in the athlete. *Clin Sports Med* 1993;12:599–602.

© 2018 American Academy of Orthopaedic Surgeons

65 Anterior Cervical Diskectomy and Fusion: Technique, Complications, and Rehabilitation

Sreeharsha V. Nandyala, BA, Alejandro Marquez-Lara, MD, David S. Cheng, MD, and Kern Singh, MD

INTRODUCTION

Degenerative disease of the cervical spine is a frequent finding that may result in symptomatic cervical radiculopathy. Radiographic evidence demonstrates at least one degenerative finding in the cervical spine on radiographs by age 65 years in nearly 95% of men and 70% of women. Cervical total disc replacement (TDR) and anterior cervical discectomy and fusion (ACDF) are both indicated surgical interventions for this condition.

ACDF was first described in the 1930s. Significant ensuing modifications have improved patient safety and clinical outcomes. This procedure involves the decompression of neural elements from a herniated disc or degenerative disc disease causing spinal stenosis along with concurrent bony fusion of the affected spinal levels.

Prospective randomized studies demonstrate that a structured regimen of postoperative physical therapy is associated with improved functional outcomes, less opioid utilization, and faster recovery. The goal of postoperative rehabilitation is to improve neck range of motion (ROM); improve muscle endurance; and address procedural complications, including dysphagia and dysphonia. This chapter provides a discussion of ACDF and highlights the postoperative complications, restrictions, recovery, and rehabilitation goals.

SURGICAL PROCEDURE: ANTERIOR CERVICAL DISKECTOMY AND FUSION

Indications

- Persistent neck pain and/or arm pain, numbness, or tingling despite 6 weeks of conservative management with rest, physical therapy, and nonsteroidal anti-inflammatory drugs (NSAIDs)
- Diagnostic studies (MRI, CT ± myelogram) that demonstrate degenerative disc disease or herniated disc disease with corresponding symptoms
- Myelopathy (balance disturbances, slow-wide based gait)
- Tumor/trauma

Contraindications

- Superficial infection
- Tracheostomy
- History of anterior neck radiation

Surgical Technique

- Superficial anatomic landmarks include
  - Hyoid at C3
  - Thyroid cartilage at C4–C5
  - Cricoid cartilage at C6
- Step 1
  - A horizontal incision is made medial to the sternocleidomastoid (SCM) muscle.
  - The side of approach should be determined based on the surgeon's comfort and experience.
- Step 2
  - The platysma is divided in line with the skin incision.
  - The external jugular vein helps to identify the tracheosophageal groove.
- Step 3
  - The SCM and carotid sheath are retracted laterally while the tracheoesophageal complex is retracted medially.
  - The recurrent laryngeal nerve lies in the tracheoesophageal groove and is susceptible to injury.

Dr. Singh or an immediate family member has received royalties from Pioneer, Stryker, and Zimmer; serves as a paid consultant to DePuy, A Johnson & Johnson Company, Stryker, and Zimmer; has stock or stock options held in Avaz Surgical and Vital 5; has received nonincome support (such as equipment or services), commercially derived honoraria, or other non-research-related funding (such as paid travel) from SLACK Incorporated, Thieme, and Wolters Kluwer Health–Lippincott Williams & Wilkins; and serves as a board member, owner, officer, or committee member of the American Academy of Orthopaedic Surgeons, the Cervical Spine Research Society, ISASS—the International Society for the Advancement of Spine Surgery, the Scoliosis Research Society, SMISS—the Society for Minimally Invasive Spine Surgery, Spine Surgery Today, *the Vertebral Columns–ISASS, and Wolters Kluwer Health–Lippincott Williams & Wilkins. None of the following authors or any immediate family member has received anything of value from or has stock or stock options held in a commercial company or institution related directly or indirectly to the subject of this article: Dr. Cheng, Dr. Marquez-Lara, and Dr. Nandyala.*

© 2018 American Academy of Orthopaedic Surgeons

- Step 4
  - The longus coli are swept laterally to expose the superficial disc space.
  - The sympathetic chain lies superficial to the longus coli; thus, care must be taken to position the retractors deep to this muscle.
- Step 5
  - A knife or electrocautery is utilized to perform the annulotomy.
  - Straight and curved curettes are utilized to remove the disc material.
- Step 6
  - A microcurette or nerve hook with a 1-mm Kerrison rongeur is utilized to remove the posterior longitudinal ligament.
- Step 7
  - A high-speed burr is utilized to decorticate the endplates to improve bone graft contact.
- Step 8
  - A trial sizer is placed to approximate the intervertebral space and an appropriately sized bone graft is gently impacted into place.
- Step 9
  - An anterior cervical plate is applied and cervical screws are placed through the plate typically measuring 12 mm to 16 mm.
  - The choice between fixed versus variable screws depends on the surgeon's preference.
- Step 10
  - The retractors are removed, and the muscle and skin incisions are closed primarily.
  - The utilization of a drain (e.g., Penrose) depends on the surgeon's preference.

Complications

Pseudarthrosis

Patients may present with recurrent pain that gradually worsens over a period of months. Proper patient selection is paramount in reducing the risk of pseudarthrosis. Risk factors include smoking, osteoporosis, chronic steroid use, obesity, and malnutrition. Pseudarthrosis can also be associated with implant failure and fracture, thus requiring reinstrumentation. Patients with worsening pain in the postoperative period must be evaluated clinically and radiographically for evidence of pseudarthrosis.

Adjacent Segment Degeneration

Although an ACDF is widely accepted and considered the classic interventional management for cervical degenerative pathology, the reduction in adjacent level kinematics, progression of adjacent level degeneration, and an increased intradiscal pressure and facet forces eventually cause wear and tear of the adjacent spinal levels and produces pain. As such, postoperative physical therapy and home exercise should focus on maintaining adequate neck ROM to strengthen the neck musculature as well as endurance in an effort to reduce pain and improve postoperative kinematics.

Dysphagia

Postoperative dysphagia is a well-published complication of ACDF, with a rate of 1.7% to 50.3%. The pathophysiology of postoperative dysphagia is not fully understood and is subject to further study. Video-fluoroscopic swallow studies in patients who underwent anterior cervical spine surgery reported a range of etiologies that spanned all stages of swallowing. Notably, prevertebral soft-tissue swelling, posterior pharyngeal wall residue, and impaired upper esophageal sphincter opening are possible etiologies. Hypoglossal, glossopharyngeal, and recurrent laryngeal nerve injuries are also proposed explanations for postoperative dysphagia. Postoperative dysphagia has been reported to improve with time, with a mean incidence of 19.8% at 6 months, 16.8% at 12 months, and 12.9% at 24 months after ACDF. Some radiographic studies have reported an incidence of 50% in the early postoperative period in cervical surgery with anterior instrumentation.

Dysphonia

Postoperative hoarseness and dysphonia are also well-known complications of anterior cervical spine surgery. The published rates range from 0.1% to 21%. A wide range of etiologies have been suggested; the most common is believed to be pharyngeal and laryngeal edema by virtue of retraction devices and the natural postoperative healing process. Other causes include injury to the recurrent laryngeal nerve (RLN) from stretching, direct lesion, or retraction. In addition, laryngeal injury from endotracheal intubation is also a suspected cause of postoperative hoarseness and dysphonia. Some authors have implemented protocols to monitor the intraoperative endotracheal cuff pressure to limit the extent of laryngeal injury. Postoperative hoarseness and dysphonia can be long-standing, with up to 12% of patients having persistent symptoms for more than 6 months.

Postoperative Rehabilitation

Physical therapy should focus on improving the patient's functional status and neck stability. Patients should be encouraged to maintain adequate activity within the pain-free range under the guidance and discretion of the therapist. The goals of physical therapy include improving neck muscle strength, endurance, and facilitating stabilization. In general, until fusion is achieved, patients should avoid neck extension since an anterior fusion was utilized.

The recommendations and goals in Table 65.1 should be utilized as the basis for an individualized treatment regimen for the patient. It must be noted that, currently, there is no optimal evidenced-based physical therapy regimen. The proposed time frame should be utilized as a rough timeline only. Early mobilization after surgery is of paramount importance.

Dysphagia

- Patients can expect to have dysphagia in the early postoperative period. The majority of cases will resolve as the swelling improves and with laryngeal recovery.

© 2018 American Academy of Orthopaedic Surgeons

Table 65.1 PHASES OF REHABILITATION AFTER ACDF PROCEDURES

Rehabilitation Phase	Recommendations	Goals
Acute/Postoperative Phase (Weeks 0–4)	• Walking • Exercise bike • Stair stepper • Cervical collar and traction (Figure 65.1) • Therapeutic ultrasound is a deep-heating modality that is contraindicated during acute inflammation. • Begin with active-assisted ROM with stretching short and tight muscles: cervical paraspinals, scalenes, levator scapulae, upper trapezius	• Reduce pain and inflammation (Ice compression, TENS unit, medications PRN) • Restoration of ADLs • Sitting in chair with back support (20-min intervals)
Recovery Phase (Weeks 5–10)	• Cervical isometric strengthening exercises (Figures 65.2–65.5) • Shoulder and scapular strengthening exercises (Figures 65.6, 65.7) • No lifting greater than 20 lbs • Posture education • Active neck ROM without extension • Upper extremity strength and endurance with resistance training (Figure 65.8)	• Pain-free neck ROM • Neck and shoulder stability without support • Improve neuromuscular control • Cardiovascular and resistance training for at least 30 min
Functional Recovery (Weeks 10+)	• Individualized home exercise per therapist and physician • Review problems with ADLs	• Improved power and endurance of neck, shoulder, and arm muscles • Functional ADLs • Aerobic cardiovascular activity for more than 60 min

ADLs = activities of daily living, PRN = when necessary, ROM = range of motion, TENS = transcutaneous electrical nerve stimulation.

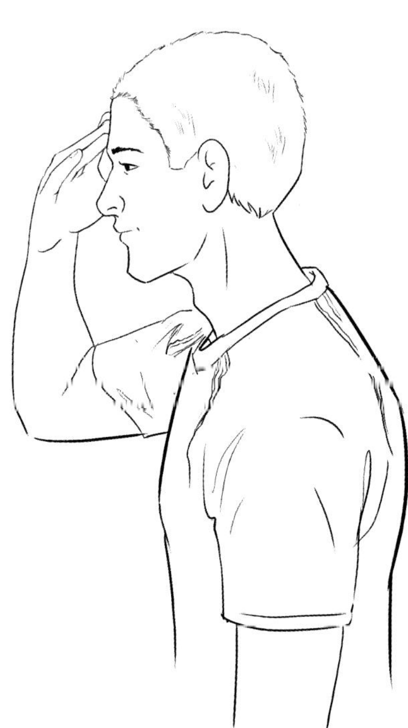

Figure 65.1 Flexion isometric strengthening.

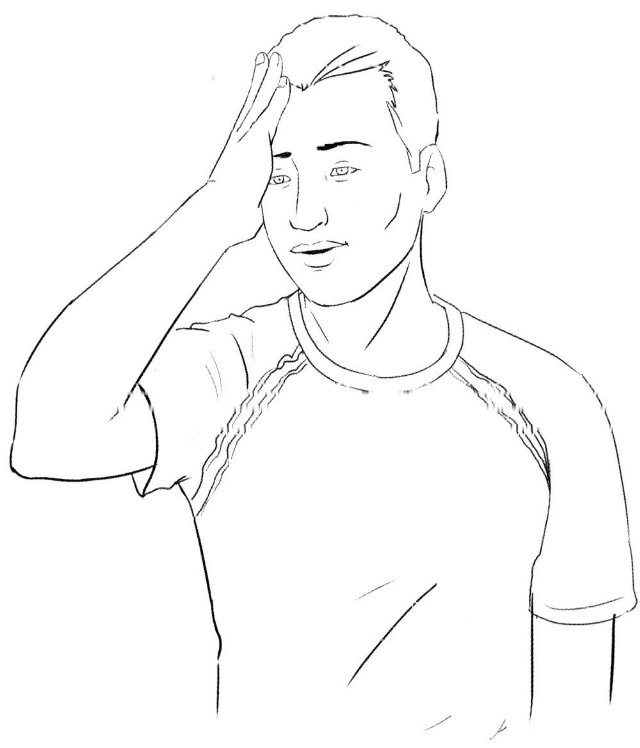

Figure 65.2 Lateral cervical isometric rotation.

© 2010 American Academy of Orthopaedic Surgeons

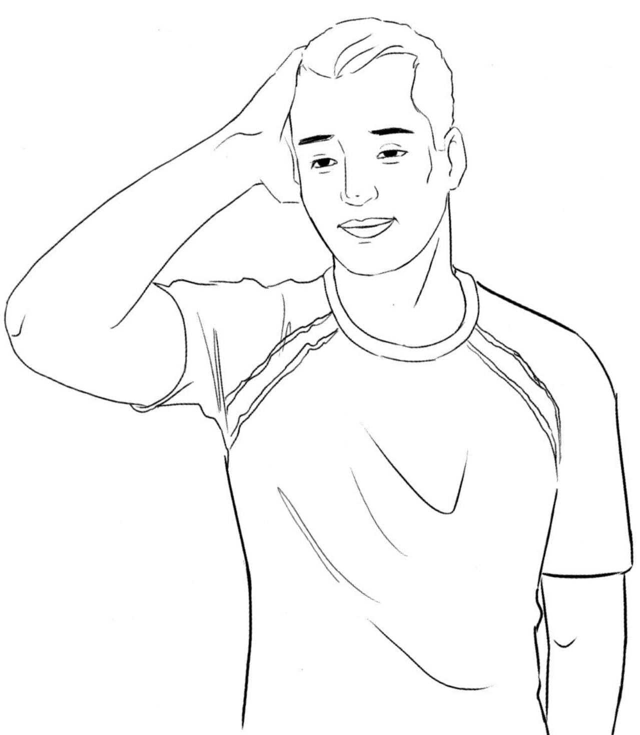

Figure 65.3 Lateral cervical isometric side bending.

- Dysphagia that persists greater than 48 hours must be investigated in a multidisciplinary approach.
- Video-fluoroscopic studies should be utilized to assess the anatomy and physiology of the muscles. Speech pathologists should evaluate the patient with solids and liquids and propose a treatment regimen and swallowing exercises/maneuvers.

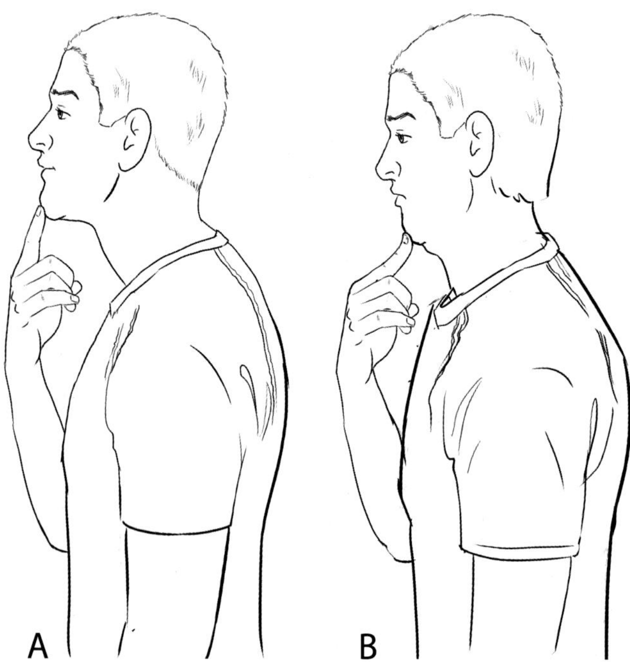

Figure 65.4 A, Starting position chin tuck. B, Final position chin tuck.

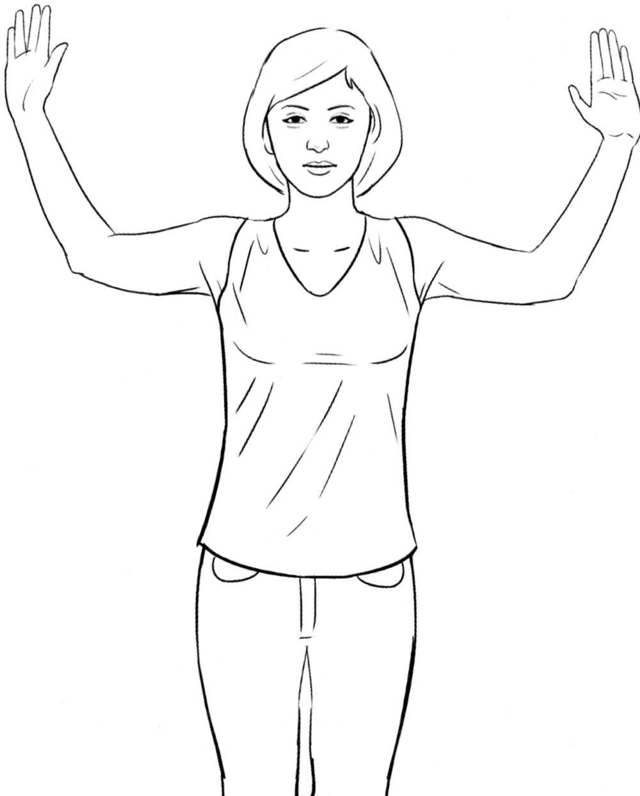

Figure 65.5 Scapular retraction.

- A gastroenterologist may assess for esophageal dysmotility and/or stricture with esophagogastroduodenoscopy.
- A neurologist may utilize electromyography to assess for potential nerve injury.
- If the root cause is identified, an individualized treatment protocol should be implemented.

Dysphonia

- This majority of patients with dysphonia will likely recovery spontaneously as the swelling resolves and scar tissue is mobilized with physical therapy.

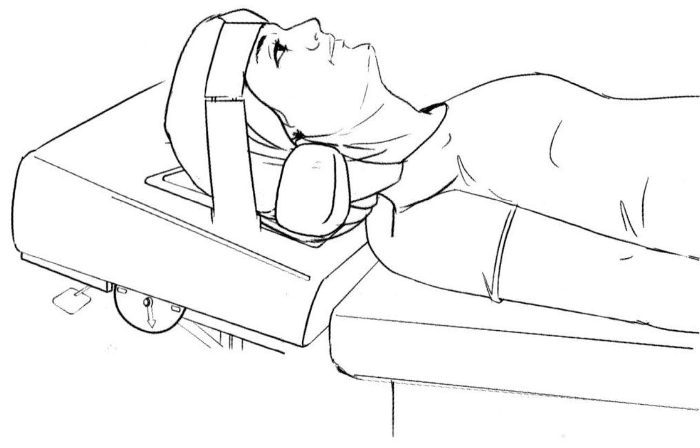

Figure 65.6 Cervical traction.

© 2018 American Academy of Orthopaedic Surgeons

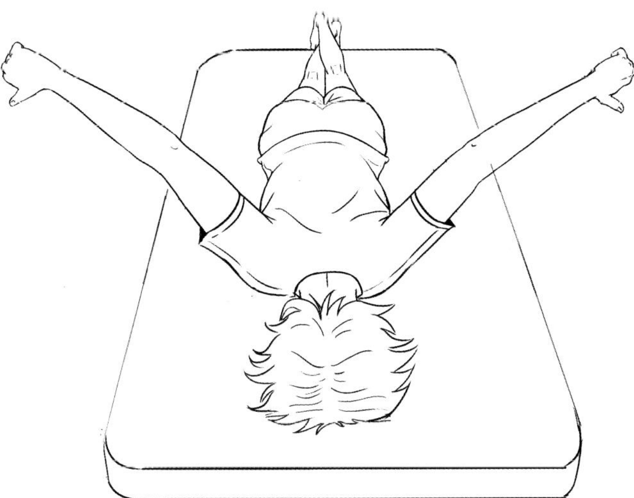

Figure 65.7 Supine abduction pullout.

- Around 12% of patients may demonstrate evidence of hoarseness and dysphonia that lasts greater than 6 months. Patients who develop RLN injury will demonstrate symptoms of dysphagia, hoarseness, shortness of breath, or aspiration.
- Speech therapy may enable patients to compensate for vocal cord paralysis until the RLN has time to recover.
- Consultation with an otolaryngologist is warranted if symptoms persist for greater than 3 months.
- True vocal cord medialization involves temporary vocal fold injection into the paralyzed vocal cord with short-term biodegradable substances. These biomaterials "push" the paralyzed cord to the midline.
- Surgical options include true vocal cord medialization laryngoplasty. This procedure involves the placement of an implant into the paralyzed vocal cord, which "pushes" the vocal cord to the midline.

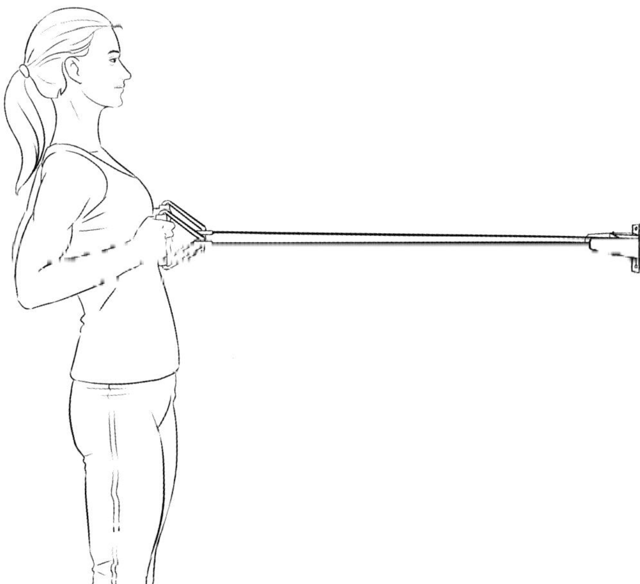

Figure 65.8 Standing row with resistance band.

PEARLS

- During the surgical approach, the recurrent laryngeal nerve should be identified (when possible) and care should be taken to limit retraction.
- Retractors should not abut the sympathetic nerve plexus.
- A strict rehabilitation regimen to improve stability, neck muscle strength, and endurance should be utilized.
- The care team must be cognizant of the procedural complications, including dysphagia and dysphonia.

BIBLIOGRAPHY

Bazaz R, Lee MJ, Yoo JU: Incidence of dysphagia after anterior cervical spine surgery: a prospective study. *Spine (Phila Pa 1976)* 2002;27(22):2453–2458.

Boden SD, McCowin PR, Davis DO, Dina TS, Mark AS, Wiesel S: Abnormal magnetic-resonance scans of the cervical spine in asymptomatic subjects. A prospective investigation. *J Bone Joint Surg Am* 1990;72(8):1178–1184.

Caspar W, Barbier DD, Klara PM: Anterior cervical fusion and Caspar plate stabilization for cervical trauma. *Neurosurgery* 1989;25(4):491–502.

Frempong-Boadu A, Houten JK, Osborn B, Opulencia J, Kells L, Guida DD, Le Roux PD: Swallowing and speech dysfunction in patients undergoing anterior cervical discectomy and fusion: a prospective, objective preoperative and postoperative assessment. *J Spinal Disord Tech* 2002;15(5):362–368.

Gao Y, Liu M, Li T, Huang F, Tang T, Xiang Z: A meta-analysis comparing the results of cervical disc arthroplasty with anterior cervical discectomy and fusion (ACDF) for the treatment of symptomatic cervical disc disease. *J Bone Joint Surg Am* 2013;95(6):555–561.

Gore DR, Sepic SB, Gardner GM, Murray MP: Neck pain: a long-term follow-up of 205 patients. *Spine* 1987;12(1):1–5.

Kishen TJ, Diwan AD: Fusion versus disk replacement for degenerative conditions of the lumbar and cervical spine: quid est testimonium? *Orthop Clin North Am* 2010;41(2):167–181.

Lee MJ, Bazaz R, Furey CG, Yoo J: Risk factors for dysphagia after anterior cervical spine surgery: a two-year prospective cohort study. *Spine J* 2007;7(2):141–147.

Lee MJ, Bazaz R, Furey CG, Yoo J: Influence of anterior cervical plate design on dysphagia: a 2-year prospective longitudinal follow-up study. *J Spinal Disord Tech* 2005;18(5):406–409.

Lee YJ, Lim MR, Albert TJ: *Dysphagia after anterior cervical spine surgery: Pathophysiology, incidence, and prevention.* Cervical Spine Research Society, 2007.

Lehto IJ, Tertti MO, Komu ME, Paajanen HE, Tuominen J, Kormano MJ: Age-related MRI changes at 0.1 T in cervical discs in asymptomatic subjects. *Neuroradiology* 1994;36(1):49–53.

Leonard R, Belafsky P: Dysphagia following cervical spine surgery with anterior instrumentation: evidence from fluoroscopic swallow studies. *Spine (Phila Pa 1976)* 2011;36(25):2217–2223.

© 2018 American Academy of Orthopaedic Surgeons

Martin RE, Neary MA, Diamant NE: Dysphagia following anterior cervical spine surgery. *Dysphagia* 1997;12(1):2–8; discussion 9–10.

Peolsson A, Kjellman G: Neck muscle endurance in nonspecific patients with neck pain and in patients after anterior cervical decompression and fusion. *J Manipulative Physiol Ther* 2007;30(5):343–350.

Razfar A, Sadr-Hoisseini SM, Rosen CA, Snyderman CH, Gooding W, Abla AA, Ferris RL: Prevention and management of dysphonia during anterior cervical spine surgery. *Laryngoscope* 2012;122(10):2179–2183.

Riley LH, 3rd, Skolasky RL, Albert TJ, Vaccaro AR, Heller JG: Dysphagia after anterior cervical decompression and fusion: prevalence and risk factors from a longitudinal cohort study. *Spine (Phila Pa 1976)* 2005;30(22):2564–2569.

Saunders RL, Bernini PM, Shirreffs TG Jr., Reeves AG. Central corpectomy for cervical spondylotic myelopathy: a consecutive series with long-term follow-up evaluation. *J Neurosurg* 1991;74(2):163–170.

Schneeberger AG, Boos N, Schwarzenbach O, Aebi M: Anterior cervical interbody fusion with plate fixation for chronic spondylotic radiculopathy: a 2- to 8-year follow-up. *J Spinal Disord* 1999;12(3):215–220; discussion 21.

Singh K, Marquez-Lara A, Nandyala SV, Patel AA, Fineberg SJ: Incidence and risk factors for dysphagia after anterior cervical fusion. *Spine (Phila Pa 1976)* 2013;38(21):1820–1825.

Smith-Hammond CA, New KC, Pietrobon R, Curtis DJ, Scharver CH, Turner DA: Prospective analysis of incidence and risk factors of dysphagia in spine surgery patients: comparison of anterior cervical, posterior cervical, and lumbar procedures. *Spine (Phila Pa 1976)* 2004;29(13):1441–1446.

Stewart M, Johnston RA, Stewart I, Wilson JA: Swallowing performance following anterior cervical spine surgery. *Br J Neurosurg* 1995;9(5):605–609.

Vaidya R, Carp J, Sethi A, Bartol S, Craig J, Les CM: Complications of anterior cervical discectomy and fusion using recombinant human bone morphogenetic protein-2. *Eur Spine J* 2007;16(8):1257–1265.

Vanderveldt HS, Young MF: The evaluation of dysphagia after anterior cervical spine surgery: a case report. *Dysphagia* 2003 Fall;18(4):301–304.

Winslow CP, Winslow TJ, Wax MK: Dysphonia and dysphagia following the anterior approach to the cervical spine. *Arch Otolaryngol Head Neck Surg* 2001;127(1):51–55.

Wyss J, Patel A. Therapeutic programs for musculoskeletal disorders. New York, NY, Demos Medical Publishing, 2013.

Yue WM, Brodner W, Highland TR. Persistent swallowing and voice problems after anterior cervical discectomy and fusion with allograft and plating: a 5- to 11-year follow-up study. *Eur Spine J* 2005;14(7):677–682.

© 2018 American Academy of Orthopaedic Surgeons

66 Posterior Cervical Laminectomy Fusion and Laminoplasty

Brett A. Braly, MD, and John M. Rhee, MD

INTRODUCTION

Cervical myelopathy, which results from compression of the cervical spinal cord, is a challenging condition for all health care professionals. Early signs and symptoms of subtle cervical myelopathy are difficult to appreciate and often underdiagnosed, leading to potential delayed treatment and further complicating the rehabilitation process.

The natural history of cervical myelopathy is generally thought to be a gradual stepwise decline in function. Although proper strengthening and functional training are important to optimize independence, these and other nonoperative modalities do not halt disease progression. As such, cervical myelopathy is generally considered to be a surgical disorder unless the patient is unwilling or unable to have surgery.

Cervical myelopathy can be caused by single- or multiple-level spinal cord compression. Compression is generally degenerative in nature and can result from disc pathology, spondylosis, structural instability, kyphosis, congenital narrowing of the spinal canal, or any combination of these. Less common causes of myelopathy include tumors or infections.

Surgical management of cervical myelopathy typically involves decompression of the spinal cord, with or without adjunctive stabilization. Anterior and/or posterior approaches can be used, depending on the clinical circumstances. In general, posterior surgery is favored for multilevel (≥3-level) compression and is most commonly performed by one of two methods: laminoplasty or laminectomy with fusion. Though the treatment goals and indications are similar, the postoperative course and rehabilitation goals for each are very different.

SURGICAL PROCEDURE

Presentation

Practitioners participating in patient rehabilitation should be aware of the signs and symptoms of myelopathy in order to help identify early signs of newly diagnosed or (in the case of a surgical complication) recurrent myelopathy. The difficulty in recognizing myelopathy lies within its breadth of clinical complaints, with no single pathognomonic finding. Often, patients will complain of balance or coordination problems, difficulties with fine motor control of the hands, progressive weakness, numbness or tingling of the hands, issues with dropping items, or problems controlling bowel or bladder function. Pain, either in the neck or arms, may or may not be present. Patients may display a wide-based unstable gait, weakness (particularly of the hands), numbness, hyperreflexia or other provocative signs (Hoffman, Babinski, clonus, inverted radial reflex). However, because approximately 20% of patients with cervical myelopathy may not demonstrate any focal findings on physical examination, it is important to understand that the absence of physical findings does not rule out the diagnosis. Imaging studies such as MRI or CT-myelograms should demonstrate correlative compression of the spinal cord. The primary indication for surgery is symptomatic myelopathy.

Decision Making

In appropriate circumstances, the spinal cord can be decompressed either anteriorly or posteriorly. In patients with anterior compressive lesions—such as disc herniations, spondylotic bone spurs, or OPLL—performing a posterior decompression requires a neutral or lordotic alignment such that the cord can drift posteriorly away from the anterior lesions following

Dr. Rhee or an immediate family member has received royalties from Biomet; is a member of a speakers' bureau or has made paid presentations on behalf of BiometDepuy and Zimmer; serves as a paid consultant to Biomet Synthes; has stock or stock options held in Alphatec Spine and Phygen; has received research or institutional support from DePuy, A Johnson & Johnson Company and KineflexMedtronic; has received nonincome support (such as equipment or services), commercially derived honoraria, or other non-research–related funding (such as paid travel) from Wolters Kluwer Health–Lippincott Williams & Wilkins; and serves as a board member, owner, officer, or committee member of the Cervical Spine Research Society. Neither Dr. Braly nor any immediate family member has received anything of value from or has stock or stock options held in a commercial company or institution related directly or indirectly to the subject of this article.

© 2018 American Academy of Orthopaedic Surgeons

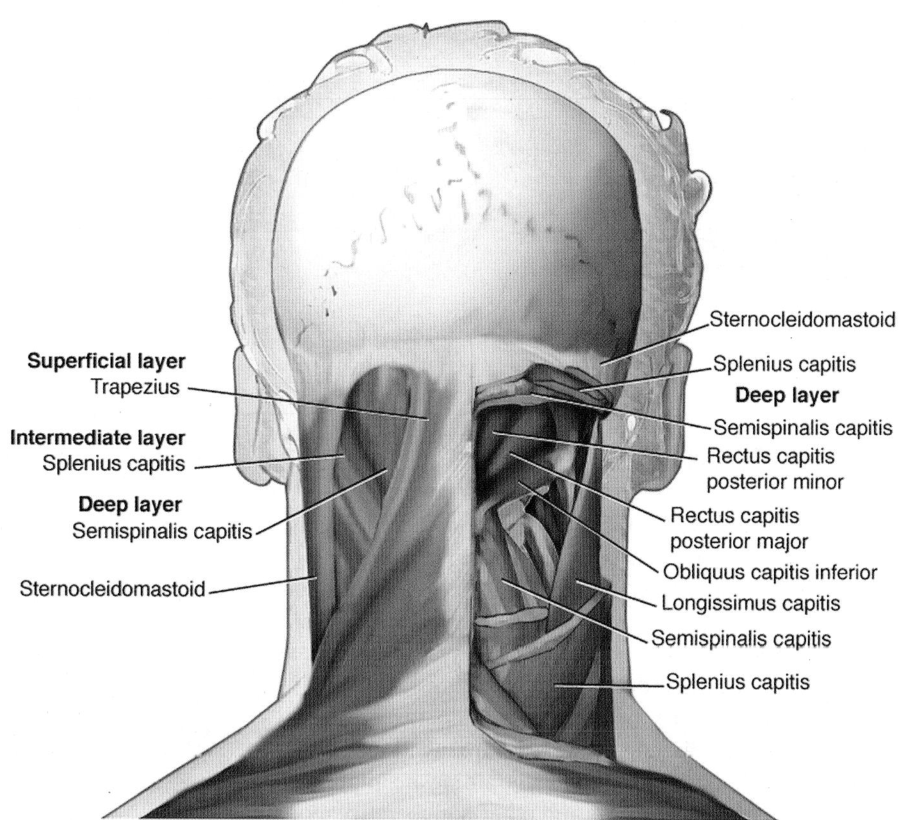

Figure 66.1 Superficial, intermediate, and deep layers of the posterior cervical musculature are shown. The suboccipital muscles lie deep to these muscles and are shown on the right. (Reproduced with permission from Rao R, Marawar SV: Posterior cervical approach. In: Wiesel SW, ed. *Operative Techniques in Orthopaedic Surgery* (Section editor: Rhee JM). Volume 4. Philadelphia, PA: Wolters Kluwer; 2011:4517.)

removal or opening of the lamina. If the alignment is kyphotic and the impinging structures are anterior, a posterior approach may not afford a satisfactory decompressive effect. Relative contraindications that are procedure specific are debatable. Smoking may hinder a patient's ability to heal a fusion mass and thus favor a nonfusion approach. Axial neck pain arising from spondylosis may be better treated by a stabilizing procedure such as fusion rather than a motion-preserving operation such as laminoplasty, although there is no conclusive data to substantiate this notion, and proponents of either method would argue that both are equally viable treatment options for cervical myelopathy.

In all cases of cervical myelopathy, the primary goal of surgical treatment is to prevent progression. Although, as a general rule, approximately 50% improvement in myelopathic symptoms may be anticipated postoperatively, improvement in myelopathic symptoms or pain may not occur in any given patient depending on a number of factors, including the severity of underlying spinal cord damage. As such, patients must be extensively counseled that arrest of progression constitutes surgical success even in the absence of any symptomatic improvement.

Procedure

Anatomy

The cervical spine is composed of seven cervical vertebrae, which, along with an extensive ligamentous complex, connect the occiput to the thoracic spine. These vertebrae are designed to provide stability to the head, allow for motion of the head in all planes, and provide protected passage of the spinal cord, allowing nerve roots to exit and supply the muscles of the neck and arms (Figures 66.1 and 66.2).

The upper two vertebrae have unique functions in movement of the head and are much less commonly involved in the development of cervical myelopathy. The lower cervical spinal vertebrae (C3–C7) are more uniform in appearance and progress through similar degenerative changes, leading to the development of myelopathy.

Posterior decompressive surgery focuses on eliminating the compressive force of the lamina and ligamentum flavum. This can be accomplished through laminectomy, completely removing the lamina and usually requiring fusion to maintain alignment, or through laminoplasty, hinging open the lamina to provide space for the cord. Opening the canal posteriorly provides three mechanisms of decompression: (1) a direct decompressive effect from structures causing dorsal compression (such as posterior osteophytes and ligamentum flavum); (2) general enlargement of the canal (such as in those with a congenitally narrowed canal); and (3) an indirect decompressive effect away from anterior structures (such as disc herniations, annular bulges, spondylotic bars, ossification of the posterior longitudinal ligament [OPLL]) if the overall alignment of the spine is sufficiently lordotic to allow the cord to drift posteriorly.

Laminectomy and Fusion

Laminectomy is the complete removal of the lamina from the cervical canal. Historically, multilevel laminectomy was

 © 2018 American Academy of Orthopaedic Surgeons

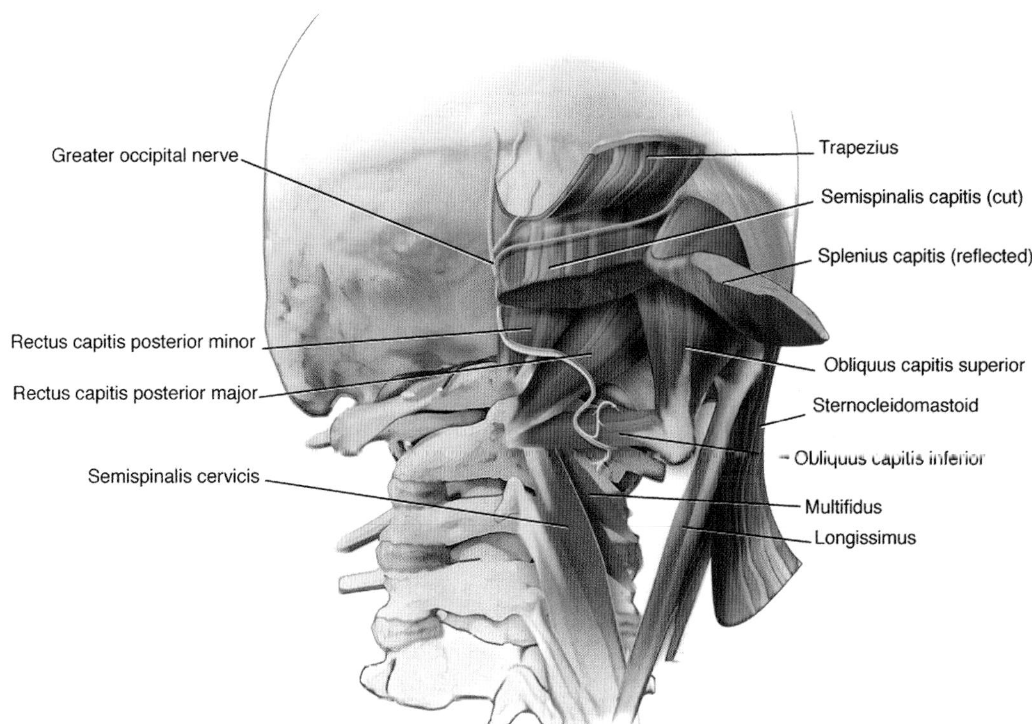

Figure 66.2 Anatomy of the suboccipital triangle. The suboccipital triangle lies between the rectus capitus posterior major, the obliquus superior, and the obliquus inferior. The greater occipital nerve is seen crossing the suboccipital triangle along its medial angle. The posterior arch of the atlas with the vertebral artery is seen in the floor of the suboccipital triangle. (Reproduced with permission from Rao R, Marawar SV: Posterior cervical approach. In: Wiesel SW, ed. *Operative Techniques in Orthopaedic Surgery* (Section editor: Rhee JM). Volume 4. Philadelphia, PA: Wolters Kluwer; 2011:4517.)

commonly used as a stand-alone decompressive procedure. However, due to substantial limitations associated with multilevel laminectomy alone—namely, postlaminectomy kyphosis and spondylolisthesis, both of which can lead to pain and/or recurrent spinal cord compression—instrumentation and fusion are currently performed in conjunction with laminectomy. Fusion procedures require bony healing for a successful outcome, whether in the cervical spine or anywhere in the body. Similar to casting a broken arm, immobilization is critical to providing the environment amendable to fusion healing. This is the rationale behind instrumentation with screws and rods to provide structural stability to the cervical spine, allowing the bone graft to heal into a solid fusion mass (Figure 66.3).

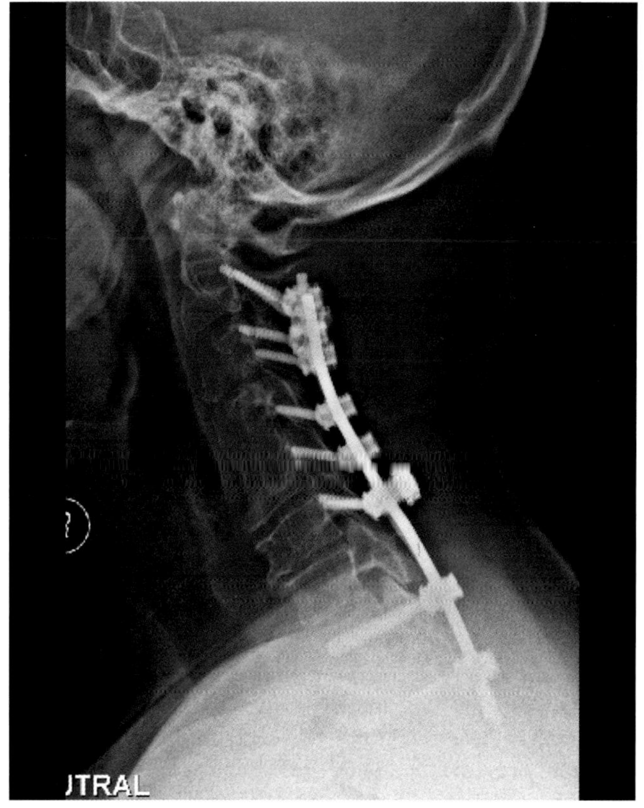

Figure 66.3 Laminectomy and fusion.

Laminoplasty

The goals of laminoplasty are threefold: (1) to decompress the spinal cord, (2) preserve stability and alignment better than that achievable with laminectomy alone, (3) and maintain range of motion (ROM). By hinging open the lamina without completely removing it, there is maintenance of inherent stability as well as surface area for the reattachment of the posterior cervical musculature. The hinged lamina can be held open by a variety of methods, ranging from suture to bone grafts to plate fixation (Figure 66.4). While there is expected bony healing of the hinge site, no fusion is performed across motion segments. Therefore, a postoperative period of rigid immobilization is generally not recommended when the

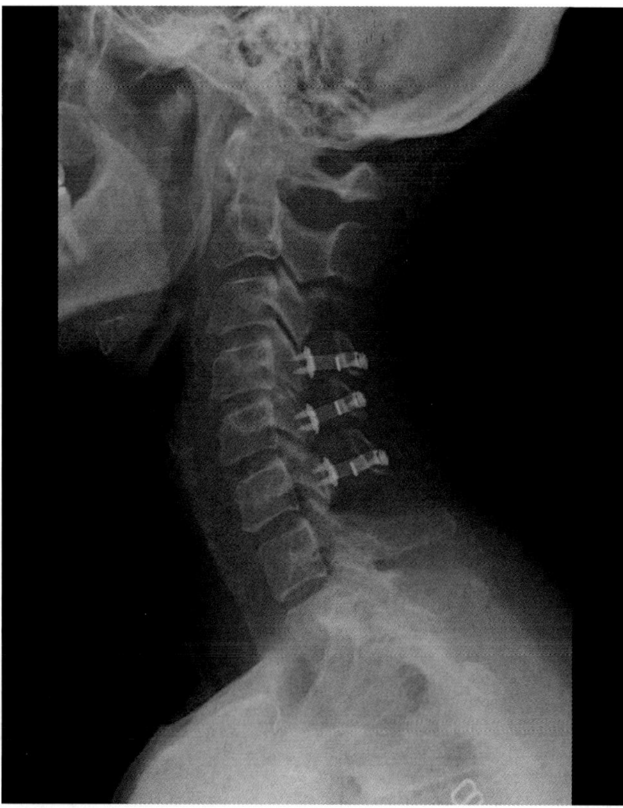

Figure 66.4 Laminoplasty.

laminoplasty is stabilized rigidly with plates, which is one of the reasons why we favor plate fixation. Immobilization has historically been recommended when less rigid forms of fixation, such as sutures or bone grafts, are used to prop open the laminoplasty.

The literature demonstrates that both laminoplasty and laminectomy with fusion are similarly effective methods of treating myelopathy in the appropriately chosen patient, keeping in mind again that the primary determinant of success is arrest of progressive neurologic worsening. No clear evidence shows a superiority of one procedure over the other in all cases. As such, the choice of procedure should be tailored to each patient's particular case.

Complications

As mentioned earllier, it is important to recognize the signs and symptoms of myelopathy because one major complication of surgery, though rare, is recurrence. Postoperative worsening or recurrence may arise from epidural hematoma, infection, hinge collapse, malpositioned instrumentation, instability, or acute adjacent segment involvement. Not infrequently, those with severe preoperative cord compression may develop postoperative worsening of weakness or numbness in the absence of any discernable mechanical complication, presumably due to cord edema, stretch, or reperfusion-type injury as a result of decompression. C5 palsies occur in approximately 5% to 10% of cases. They typically occur several (2–4) days postoperatively but may occur immediately or, less commonly, several weeks after surgery. The etiology is likely multifactorial but, again, may be related to root and/or cord edema along with stretch on the nerve root as the cord drifts posteriorly after decompression. Pain is often absent. The literature conflicts as to whether C5 palsies occur more commonly with laminoplasty versus laminectomy and fusion. Our anecdotal impression is that it occurs more commonly in our practice with the latter. If a C5 palsy occurs, we recommend physical therapy to maintain shoulder ROM and prevent frozen shoulder as well as strengthening exercises as motor recovery progresses.

A common complication of fusion procedures is nonunion of the fusion mass. Multiple factors have been shown to affect a patient's healing potential, many of which are outside of a practitioner's control. Careful protection of the fusion bed by immobilization cannot be understated in attempting to heal successfully.

Aggressive therapy, poor host factors, surgical technique, or a combination of these can result in the diastasis of the posterior spinal fascia and musculature. The result is the anterior migration of the extensor muscles to the extent that they may exert a flexor mechanism on the cervical spine. In nonfusion operations, this can contribute to postoperative kyphosis.

POSTOPERATIVE REHABILITATION

Introduction

Postoperative rehabilitation of a myelopathic patient has two major goals in mind: restoration of functional loss from the compressive myelopathy itself and successful recovery from the surgery. As mentioned earlier, not all postoperative courses are created equally. Though the primary goal of decompressing the cervical spine is similar in both the laminectomy/fusion and laminoplasty groups, the postoperative course and rehabilitation recommendations can be quite different. It is critically important to be able to differentiate between these procedures and not simply lump them together as posterior cervical spine surgery.

Functional recovery from myelopathy is patient dependent. Multiple factors—such as the nature, severity, and timeline of compression—affect the expected rehabilitation potential. Patients with long-standing, severe myelopathy may not be expected to show as much clinical improvement as a patient with early-onset mild compressive symptoms. Rehabilitation in this arena is patient specific but often involves gait and stability training, coordination control, and strengthening of those muscular groups affected.

Rehabilitation specific to postoperative recovery depends on the surgical technique. Laminoplasty patients may begin to focus on early ROM in an effort to avoid stiffness and compensatory loss of motion, whereas laminectomy patients are generally immobilized in a cervical orthosis and educated to limit neck motion during the initial phases of fusion healing.

Laminectomy and fusion patients may be immobilized in a collar for a period of 6 weeks or longer, depending on

 © 2018 American Academy of Orthopaedic Surgeons

Table 66.1 CERVICAL REHABILITATION PROTOCOL

Postoperative Stage	Laminoplasty	Laminectomy and Fusion
Immediate postop (Days 1–4)	Patient-directed ROM focusing on extension and avoiding flexion	Rigid collar immobilization
Weeks 1–6	Patient-directed ROM focusing on extension and avoiding flexion	Rigid collar immobilization
Weeks 7–12	AROM and gentle AAROM, gentle strengthening	Rigid/soft collar, depending on the length of the construct and patient healing potential
Months 3–6	AROM and PROM, progressive strengthening	Isometric strengthening with gentle ROM
Months 6+	Activities as tolerated	Activities as tolerated; aggressive ROM if fusion is healed appropriately.

AAROM = active assisted range of motion, AROM = active range of motion, PROM = passive range of motion.

the patient and the length of the construct. During this time, strengthening the posterior neck musculature may be difficult to accomplish. Isometric strengthening exercises may show benefit but should be held until the posterior fascia and musculature have had a chance to heal. Some loss of ROM is expected in a fusion procedure depending on the number and location of the levels fused. Because the adjacent motion levels above and below the fusion cannot be manipulated independently from the fusion mass, they must also be immobilized throughout the course of the fusion healing period.

Laminoplasty patients are instructed to move their necks early and often. Collar use, either rigid or soft, is surgeon dependent and varies widely. In general, when plate fixation is used, immediate ROM can be performed. If less rigid forms of fixation are utilized, such as bone struts or sutures, a period of postoperative immobilization is generally recommended even after laminoplasty to prevent early laminoplasty closure. Strengthening of the posterior spinal musculature can be more aggressive in laminoplasty patients compared to the fusion cohort but should be employed judiciously in the early phase while the muscles heal in order to avoid diastasis.

Authors' Preferred Protocol

Laminectomy and Fusion (Table 66.1)

- Isometric muscular strengthening may be instituted after initial muscle and wound healing. This consists of resisted extension of the cervical spine in a neutral position. The patient can put both hands at the posterior apex of the skull and then provide isometric neck extension force against hand resistance for a count of ten. Ten repetitions are performed at a time. Patients are encouraged to do this as much as possible throughout the day, but should do a minimum of three times per day.
- Early immobilization is critical to prevent implant loosening and allow the fusion mass to heal.
- Once the fusion has healed to an appropriate extent, ROM can be instituted.

Laminoplasty

- Overall rehabilitation goals are extensor muscle strengthening and preserving ROM. Early extension exercise within a short ROM can be instituted immediately postoperatively. The exercise is similar to that described for the laminectomy and fusion patient, with the exception that the neck is allowed to extend as tolerated during the exercise. Ideally, the neck and the occiput should extend posteriorly, such that the patient is looking up during application of maximal hand resistance.
- Rehabilitation is time dependent to allow for wound healing.
- Early patient-directed ROM is appropriate.
- Guided ROM can begin at 6 weeks.
- Extreme muscular strengthening should be delayed until the deep closure has had a chance to progress appropriately (3–6 weeks).
- The secondary goal of surgery is to avoid loss of motion.

Functional Goals and Restrictions

Recovery from spinal cord compression can be a lengthy and slow process. Rehabilitation should be aggressive in promoting patient independence for as long as improvement is noted. Functional recovery from the surgical procedure is a shorter time requirement and, again, patient dependent. Fusion healing takes, on average, 6 to 9 months to mature, though many surgeons will agree to isometric strengthening and removal of the collar at 6 to 12 weeks. Recovery from laminoplasty can take 3 to 6 months before the posterior musculature has settled and the initial stiffness that the patient experiences subsides.

Evidence Review

Worsening axial neck pain after posterior cervical surgery is not common in our experience but may occur. Postoperative kyphosis, nonunion of fusion surgery, and infection can be potential sources. Increasingly recognized is the importance of properly maintaining the function of the posterior extensor muscles when performing laminoplasty. Suggested techniques

© 2018 American Academy of Orthopaedic Surgeons

include muscle-sparing dissections and avoiding detachment of the C2 extensor insertions whenever possible. Maintenance of the posterior musculature appears important for preserving cervical alignment, which, in turn, may limit recurrent cord compression as well as fatigue-related neck pain.

Iizuda et al were the first to publish data showing that the duration of postoperative immobilization had an effect on ROM after laminoplasty. Patients who wore a collar for 4 weeks had better overall ROM than those who wore a collar for 8 weeks. Since that time, surgeons have become more aggressive in limiting collar wear. No clear protocol is universal and collar wear can vary surgeon to surgeon from 2 weeks or more to no collar or a soft orthosis postoperatively. We recommend use of a collar as needed for up to no more than 2 to 3 weeks postoperatively from laminoplasty.

PEARLS

Laminoplasty

- Limit surgical dissection to the lamina–lateral mass junction.
- Maintain extensor attachments to C2 and every other level not decompressed.
- Remove spinous processes to limit stress on fascial repair and facilitate closure.
- Patient education on goal of maintaining motion is important.
- Cervical rehabilitation is balanced with functional rehabilitation from spinal cord compression, which should begin immediately postoperatively.

Laminectomy and Fusion

- Careful fusion bed preparation and bone grafting techniques impact fusion rates.
- Cervical immobilization is critical during the healing process of the fusion mass.
- Isometric muscle strengthening is appropriate once fascial repair has healed.
- Some decrease in motion is expected. Improving ROM should await appropriate healing of the fusion mass.
- Cervical rehabilitation is balanced with functional rehabilitation from spinal cord compression, which should begin immediately postoperatively.

BIBLIOGRAPHY

Iizuda H, Nakagawa Y, Shimegi A, Tsutsumi S, Toda N, Takagishi K, Shimizu T: Clinical results after cervical laminoplasty: differences due to the duration of wearing a cervical collar. *J Spinal Disord Tech* 2005;18(6):489–491.

Kato Y, Iwasaki M, Fuji T, Yonenobu K, Ochi T: Long-term follow-up results of laminectomy for cervical myelopathy caused by ossification of the posterior longitudinal ligament. *J Neurosurg* 1998;89:217–223.

Mikawa Y, Shikata J, Yamamuro T: Spinal deformity and instability after multilevel cervical laminectomy. *Spine (Phila Pa 1976)* 1987;12:6–11.

Rhee J, Heflin JA, Hamasaki T, Freedman B: Prevalence of physical signs in cervical myelopathy: a prospective, controlled study. *Spine (Phila Pa 1976)* 2009;34(9):890–895.

© 2018 American Academy of Orthopaedic Surgeons

67 Rehabilitation After the Compression Fracture

Soo Yeon Kim, MD, Jeffrey Algra, MD, MS, and Alok D. Sharan, MD, MHCDS

INTRODUCTION

The health care expenditures attributable to osteoporotic vertebral compression fractures (VCF) in the United States exceed a billion dollars a year, with most costs related to inpatient and nursing home services. The incidence of VCF rises significantly with age especially for Asian and Caucasian postmenopausal women with low bone mass density (BMD); the risk for vertebral fracture increases twofold for each single standard deviation (SD) decrease in lumbar spine BMD.

Only a third of all VCFs diagnosed on imaging mandate medical care and 10% will mandate a hospital admission. Consequences of VCFs are increased mortality and morbidity such as chronic back pain, loss of function, difficulties in activities of daily living (ADLs), and increased risk for subsequent fractures. Although not all fractures are symptomatic, back pain, kyphosis, and loss of height are common signs. In the acute phase, pain can last from weeks to months and most fractures will have significant pain reduction at 3 months, even though some fractures do show a protracted course. Conservative treatment consists of pharmacotherapy, a short period of bed rest, physical therapy, and back bracing. Vertebral augmentation is an acceptable option after conservative treatment has failed for VCFs as well as for painful benign and malignant spinal tumors (hemangiomas, multiple myeloma).

Vertebroplasty and balloon kyphoplasty are both minimally invasive vertebral augmentation options performed by injecting bone cement into the vertebral body (VB). Both augmentation methods have end goals of relief of fracture-related pain and stabilization of the deformed spine, but kyphoplasty will additionally attempt to restore VB height.

The optimal timing and indication for the procedure is debatable, but it seems that both percutaneous vertebroplasty (PVP) and percutaneous kyphoplasty (PKP) are safe and adequate treatments for acute fracture-related pain when conservative treatment has failed. PVP seems to be indicated for persistent pain after 6 weeks to 3 months of conservative treatment and PKP is best indicated in the window of 3 weeks to 6 weeks after diagnosis, especially for more complex spinal deformity.

Physical therapy is one of the major treatments for VCF. There are only a handful of studies on what constitutes appropriate postoperative rehabilitation treatment. There are studies showing improvement in pain, posture, physical function, and quality of life after comprehensive physical therapy especially targeting the back extensor muscles in hyperkyphotic elderly with or without compression fractures. Also, physical therapy after vertebroplasty has been shown to decrease subsequent fracture recurrence.

The correlation of the severity of hyperkyphosis to the degree of weakness of the back extensor muscles would make back extensor muscle exercises a primary focus for postoperative vertebral augmentation rehabilitation.

SURGICAL PROCEDURE

Vertebral Cementoplasty (VC): Vertebroplasty and Balloon Kyphoplasty (Table 67.1)

Indications

- VCFs of the thoracolumbar spine due to osteoporosis with kyphotic VB deformity with a loss of VB height causing pain are the main indication for performing VC.
- VCFs due to metastasis or hematopoietic and lymphoid neoplasms (e.g., multiple myeloma)
- Vertebral body neoplasm or vascular tumors without fracture (e.g., hemangioma) with pain as primary symptom

Patient Selection and Vertebral Level

The best clinical outcome will be obtained when patients are selected based on diagnosis of acute compression fracture as the main pain generator and the level of augmentation is selected precisely. Multilevel augmentation can be indicated in cases of severe instability but should be performed in a multistep process (one to two levels/day). Correlation of symptoms (acute, focal,

Dr. Sharan or an immediate family member serves as a paid consultant to Paradigm Spine; and serves as a board member, owner, officer, or committee member of Wolters Kluwer Health–Lippincott Williams & Wilkins. Neither of the following authors nor any immediate family member has received anything of value from or has stock or stock options held in a commercial company or institution related directly or indirectly to the subject of this article: Dr. Algra and Dr. Kim.

Table 67.1 INDICATIONS AND CONTRAINDICATIONS FOR KYPHOPLASTY AND VERTEBROPLASTY

	Indications	Contraindications	
		Absolute	**Relative**
Kyphoplasty	• VCF of TL spine with pain and kyphotic deformity and loss of VB height • VCF due to metastasis or neoplasm • VB neoplasm or vascular tumor with pain and without fracture	• Spinal infection • Coagulation disorder • Allergy to PMMA, contrast • Defined sensory deficits • Bowel or bladder involvement • Pregnancy	• Pulmonary comorbidity limiting prone-lying position • Marked obscured anatomic landmarks due to morbid obesity or prior instrumentation • Mild posterior cortex instability • Spinal canal stenosis due to posterior displaced bone fragments
Vertebroplasty	• VCF of TL spine with pain • VCF due to metastasis or neoplasm • VB neoplasm or vascular tumor with pain and without fracture	Same as kyphoplasty *with the addition of:* • spinal canal stenosis due to posterior displaced bone fragments	Same as kyphoplasty *with the addition of:* Vertebra plana *and excluded:* • Spinal canal stenosis due to posterior displaced bone fragments

PMMA = polymethyl methacrylate, TL = thoracolumbar, VB = vertebral bodies, VCF = vertebral compression fractures.

or referred axial back pain) per history and on examination with radiologic findings—magnetic resonance imaging (MRI) with short tau inversion recovery (STIR) images showing bone edema, bone scan showing increased uptake or computed tomography (CT) scan—is essential for precise identification of the acute fracture.

Contraindications

Absolute contraindications include recent spinal infection, uncorrected coagulation disorder, allergy to polymethyl methacrylate (PMMA) or contrast, pregnancy and neurologic compromise with defined sensory deficits, or bowel and bladder involvement.

Relative contraindications include, but are not limited, to pulmonary comorbidity limiting the patient's ability to adequately ventilate while prone during the procedure, marked obesity, or prior spinal instrumentation obscuring adequate fluoroscopically guided anatomic landmarks, and mild posterior displaced bone fragment.

Procedure

Relevant Anatomy

The VB is the target of this procedure and is augmented by filling with cement. For osteoporotic compression fractures, the most involved levels are lower thoracic and upper lumbar vertebrae, especially T12 and L1.

For the transpedicular approach, which is the most performed and preferred, the pedicles form the target direction. The orientation of the thoracic pedicles is more anterior and medially angled while the lumbar pedicle axis is more parallel to the sagittal plane. This leads to an alternative and sometimes necessary parapedicular approach for thoracic levels (above T10) to ensure cement filling in the center (both in a sagittal and axial plane) of the VB (Figure 67.1).

Compression fractures mostly involve the superior endplate with a collapsed anterior vertebral cortex in a typical wedge pattern, although lateral cortex collapse is very common. Imaging should clarify the precise VB deformation/destruction and, most important, posterior cortex integrity should be assessed prior to augmentation (Figure 67.2).

Technique

A single or biplanar fluoroscope is used and preferred for most typical approaches, with every step being confirmed through anteroposterior (AP) as well as lateral views. CT-assisted guidance augmentation can be performed for adequately trained and qualified professionals for complex cases involving complete destruction of the posterior vertebral cortex or severe vertebra plana.

The target zone for VC is the anterior third of the VB, which is reached through either a parapedicular (along the lateral cortex of the pedicle) or more commonly performed transpedicular approach. The parapedicular approach is used for the following:

- high thoracic levels (above T10)
- small, fractured or tumor-invaded pedicles
- inadequate pedicle visualization

With the parapedicular approach, the needle will enter the VB at the pedicle–VB junction and will allow for a more medially, centrally placed needle tip position. When placed correctly, a single-needle method could cover the entire target zone, but VC usually involves bilateral placement (Figure 67.3). In

 © 2018 American Academy of Orthopaedic Surgeons

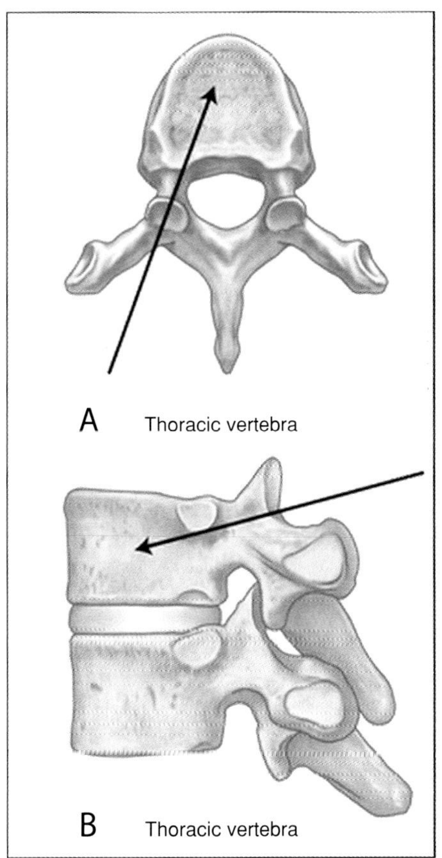

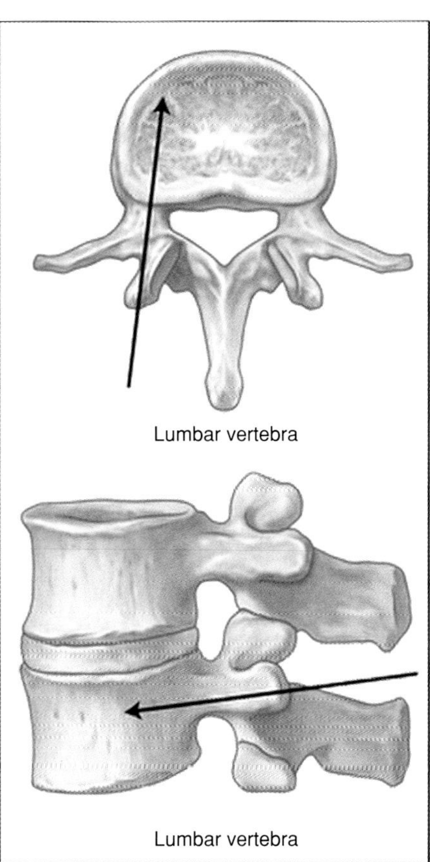

Figure 67.1 Illustration of the orientation of the pedicles on the (**A**) axial cross-section and (**B**) sagittal view for both the thoracic and lumbar vertebrae.

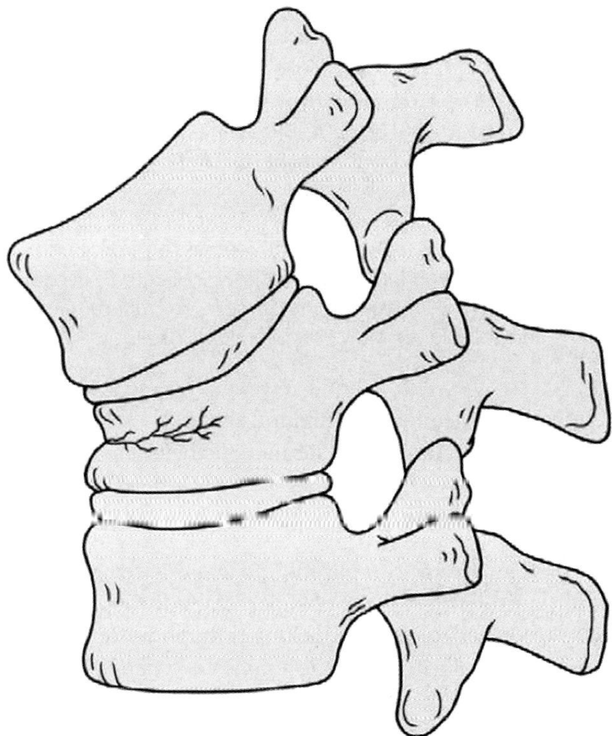

Figure 67.2 This illustration shows the typical anterior wedging pattern seen with a compression fracture. (Reproduced with permission from Raj PP: *Interventional Pain Management. Image-guided Procedures*, ed 2. Philadelphia, PA, Elsevier, 2008.)

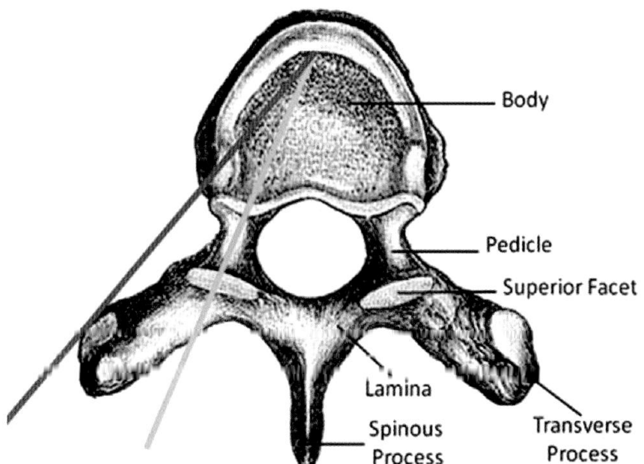

Figure 67.3 The *green arrow* in this illustration depicts the typical transpedicular approach to the vertebroplasty. When this approach is difficult, a parapedicular approach (*red arrow*) may be used. (Reproduced with permission from Molina G, Campero A, Feito R, Pombo: Kyphoplasty in the treatment of osteoporotic vertebral compression fractures (VCF), in Alexandrea A, ed: *Advances in Minimally Invasive Surgery and Therapy for Spine and Nerves*. Wien: Springer, 2011.)

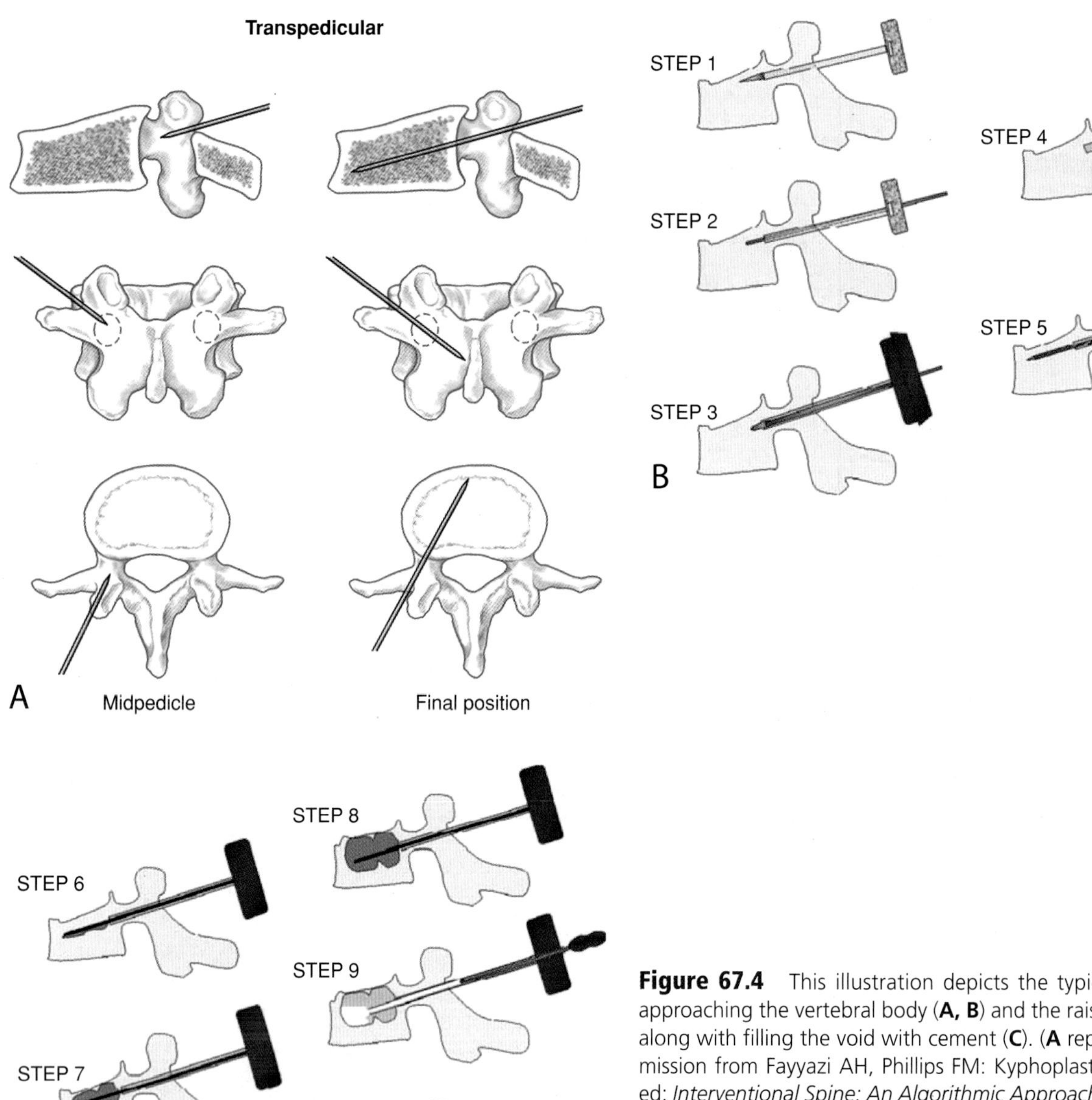

Figure 67.4 This illustration depicts the typical steps taken in approaching the vertebral body (**A, B**) and the raising of the balloon along with filling the void with cement (**C**). (**A** reproduced with permission from Fayyazi AH, Phillips FM: Kyphoplasty, in Slipman CW, ed: *Interventional Spine: An Algorithmic Approach.* Philadelphia, PA, Elsevier, 2008. **B** and **C** reproduced with permission from Bono CM, Garfin SR: Thoracic and lumbar kyphoplasty, in Ozgur B, Benzel EC, Garfin SR: *Minimally Invasive Spine Surgery: A Practical Guide to Anatomy and Techniques.* New York, Springer, 2009.)

kyphoplasty, the balloon tamp is used to create a cavity in the VB and correct the kyphotic deformity prior to cement filling (Figure 67.4).

The endpoint of cement fill is reached when reaching close to the posterior cortical margin or endplate. Relative low cement fill is especially recommended for osteoporotic patients with low BMD.

When the patient has fully recovered from the anesthesia, many surgeons will keep the patient in a supine position for at least 15 to 30 minutes to ensure complete cement hardening.

Complications

- Cement extravasation
- Venous uptake causing pulmonary emboli
- Hematoma (epidural, paraspinal)
- Infection (osteomyelitis, epidural abscess)
- Iatrogenic fractures (ribs, sternum, pedicle)
- Pneumothorax
- Postprocedure pain

The most important complication to avoid is cement extravasation outside the VB either superficially through endplate cracks or posterior cement tracking through posterior cortex damage, especially in metastatic lesions. In kyphoplasty, due to the created void, the pressure of cement filling is much lower compared to vertebroplasty, which is the main reason for the lower incidence of cement extravasation.

When leakage into the spinal canal with neurologic deficits does occur, immediate spinal surgery consult should be obtained.

 © 2018 American Academy of Orthopaedic Surgeons

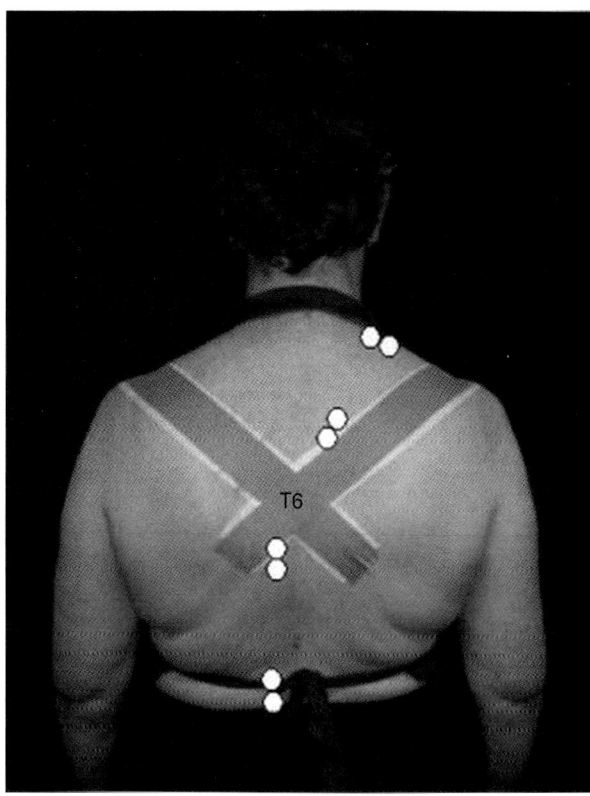

Figure 67.5 Photograph of taping after a compression fracture aims to maintain thoracic hyperextension. (Reproduced with permission from Greig AM, Bennell KL, Briggs AM, Hodges PW: Postural taping decreases thoracic kyphosis but does not influence trunk muscle electromyographic activity or balance in women with osteoporosis. *Man Ther* 2014;13:249–257.)

Be mindful of progressive pain postprocedure even without neurologic deficits; there should be a low threshold for obtaining a CT scan.

Although not an immediate complication but debatably considered iatrogenic are adjacent-level compression fractures. Significantly increased strain, especially on the superior level VB and intervertebral disc, may cause up to fourfold more compression in osteoporotic spines with low BMD and with high cement fill.

POSTOPERATIVE REHABILITATION

Introduction

Pharmacotherapy and cementoplasty aimed at pain control are the primary treatment for individuals with VCF. However, they do not directly address patients' physical and functional impairment that accompanies VCF, especially in the geriatric population. A multimodal physical therapy program for VCF includes a wide range of interventions, including orthosis, manual therapies, or various therapeutic exercises. The key to a successful outcome is a highly individualized program, for both exercise selection and intensity, based on patients' physical abilities and impairment and progress based on patient tolerance to avoid new injury. The therapy program should consider the patient's previous functional level, current deconditioned level, degree of kyphosis, level of injury, and severity of osteoporosis.

Physical Therapy

In the early stage, utilize modalities to decrease pain and facilitate mobilization as quickly as possible.

i. Postural taping: aims to encourage a retracted scapular and pectoral girdle posture and promote thoracic spine extension (Figure 67.5)
   1. Apply a protective skin barrier.
   2. Instruct patients to elongate the crown of the head toward the ceiling and gently draw shoulder blades down and together and maintain the position during the application of the tape.
   3. Apply nonrigid, hypoallergenic tape to provide skin protection.
   4. Apply the rigid therapeutic tape firmly from the anterior aspect of the acromioclavicular joint, coursed over the muscle bulk of upper trapezius, and then diagonally toward the spinous process of T6. Bilateral tapes intersect at T6.

ii. Orthosis (Figure 67.6): Orthoses are used in the acute phase up to 6 months after the fracture to decrease pain by stabilizing the spine and facilitating early mobilization. For thoracic and high lumbar factures, traditional sagittal three-point hyperextension braces (Jewett and cruciform anterior spinal hyperextension [CASH]) to limit flexion only, or a thoracic lumbar orthosis (TLO; Knight-Taylor brace, clam shell) that limits flexion and side bending, can be used. For severe VCF, a custom-molded TLO fitted in hyperextension to limit overall restriction in all planes is

© 2018 American Academy of Orthopaedic Surgeons

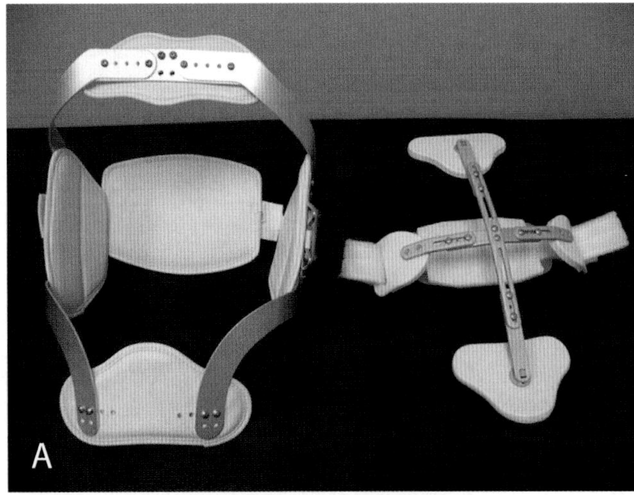

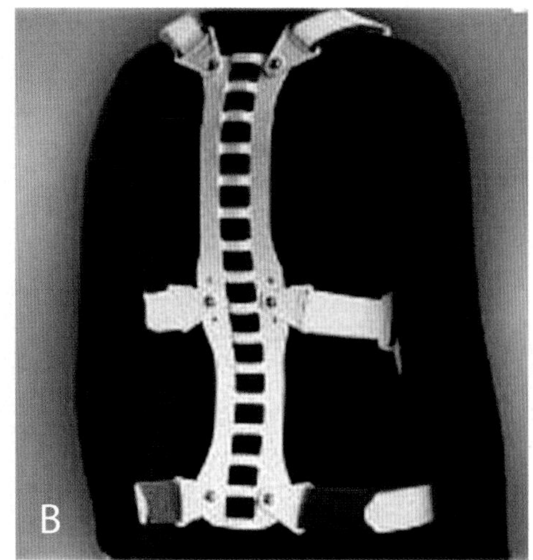

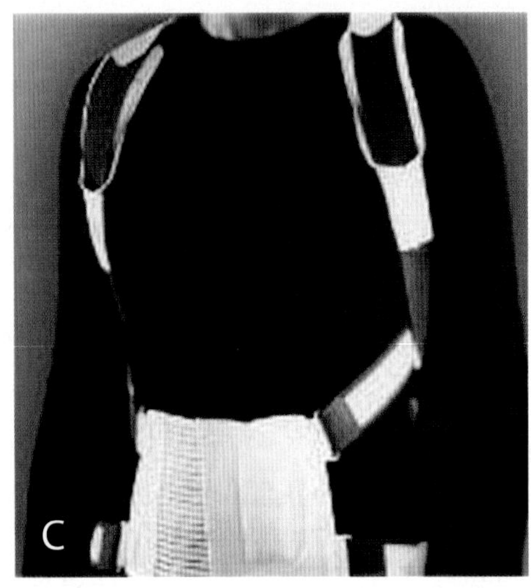

Figure 67.6 **A**, **B**, **C**, Photographs of types of orthoses. The goal of bracing after a compression fracture is to limit flexion. Typical braces used include Jewitt, CASH, or TLO braces.

needed. However, due to its rigidity and weight, there has been an issue with compliance with traditional orthoses. Newly developed orthoses (Spinomed, posture-training support brace) are lighter, easier to wear, and are shown to perform their desired function.

iii. Soft-tissue massage and passive mobilization technique on the thoracic spine can be performed at each treatment session by a therapist.

Subacute Stage

Acute pain following a VCF often improves within a few weeks. There is no guideline that suggests when to start strengthening exercises. However, it is generally accepted to start once acute resting pain is controlled. There are two main purposes of exercise in the treatment of VCF: the first is to improve axial stability through safe strengthening of axial musculature, especially spinal extensors; the second is to enhance proprioception to improve posture and locomotion and decrease risk of future fracture and fall.

iv. Exercises in the sitting position: Sitting forward on a chair with chin retraction, scapular retraction, and transverse abdominus contraction

1. Elbow back in the sitting position (Figure 67.7)
   a. Place hands behind the head with elbows pointing out to the side, press elbows back by performing scapular retraction.
   b. 5 seconds, hold for 5 repetitions

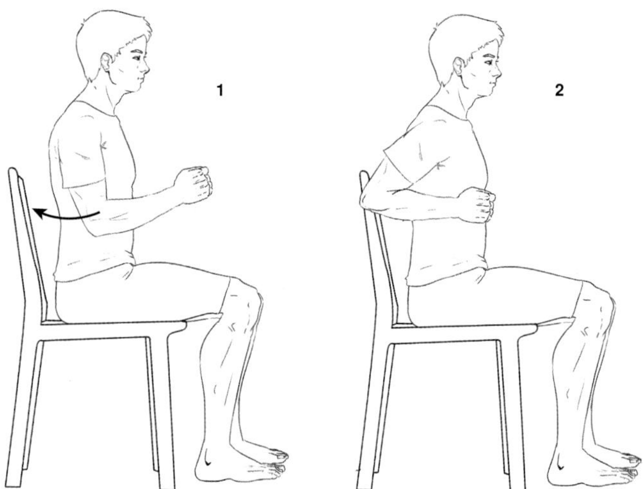

Figure 67.7 Illustration of elbow back in the sitting position.

© 2018 American Academy of Orthopaedic Surgeons

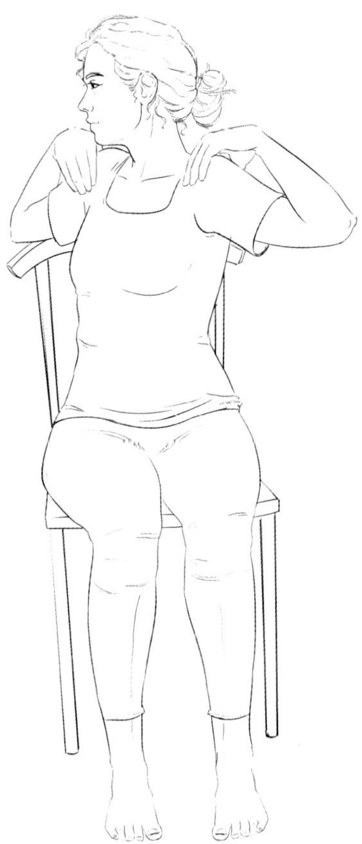

Figure 67.8 Illustration of trunk mobility in the sitting position.

2. Trunk mobility in the sitting position (Figure 67.8)
    a. Place hands on the shoulders, rotate the trunk gently in both directions, and flex laterally to each side.
    b. 5 repetitions in each direction
3. Scapular retraction in the sitting position (with or without resistance band) (Figure 67.9)
    a. Holding resistance band in both hands with elbows at the sides and flexed to 90°, pull the band back to retract the scapula.
    b. 8 to 10 repetitions for 2 sets

v. Exercises in the supine position
1. Transversus abdominis muscle contraction in the supine position (Figure 67.10)
    a. Lying supine with the knees at 30° of flexion, place the fingertips on the lower abdomen, then activate the transversus abdominis and the pelvic floor at the same time.

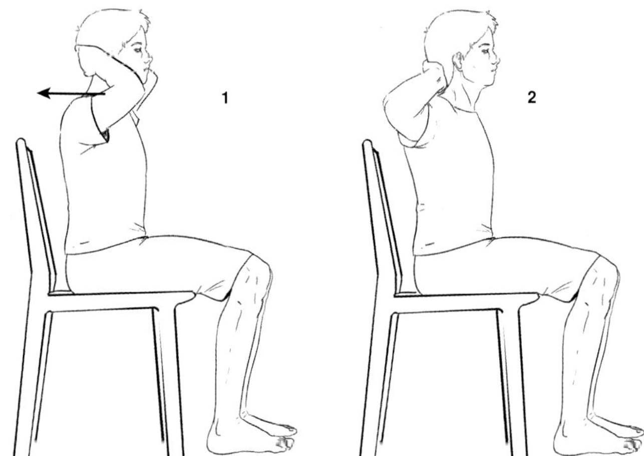

Figure 67.9 Illustration of scapular retraction in the sitting position.

    b. Progress to lifting the neck off the ground as tolerated without flexing the back.
    c. Hold for 5 to 10 seconds for 8 to 10 repetitions.
2. Bridging in the supine position (Figure 67.11)
    a. Lying supine with the knees flexed 90° with feet flat and both arms on the ground, push through the feet and arms to lift the back and pelvis off the ground.
    b. Hold for 5 to 10 seconds for 5 repetitions.

vi. Exercises in the prone position
1. Progressive resistive back extension exercise (Figure 67.12)
    a. Lying prone with 2 standard pillows under the lower half of the abdomen (approximately 30° of flexion of the spine), extend the back up to the neutral position.
    b. Progress to the same exercise with a weighted backpack starting with 30% of the maximum strength of back extensor strength. Increase the weight of the backpack as back extensor strength improves.
    c. Lift 5 seconds followed by 5 seconds rest for 10 repetitions.
2. Four-point kneeling with one-arm lift (Figure 67.13)
    a. Start in a 4-point kneeling position with hands underneath the shoulders and the knees under the hips, then lift one arm slowly off the ground.
    b. 8 to 10 repetitions for each leg
    c. Progress to one arm and leg lift.

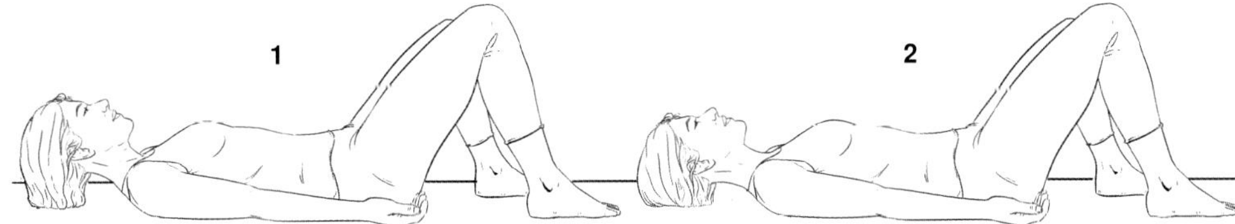

Figure 67.10 Illustration of transversus abdominis muscle contraction in the supine position. (Reproduced with permission from *ACC Trigger Points FlipBook*, Philadelphia, PA, Wolters Kluwer, 2007.)

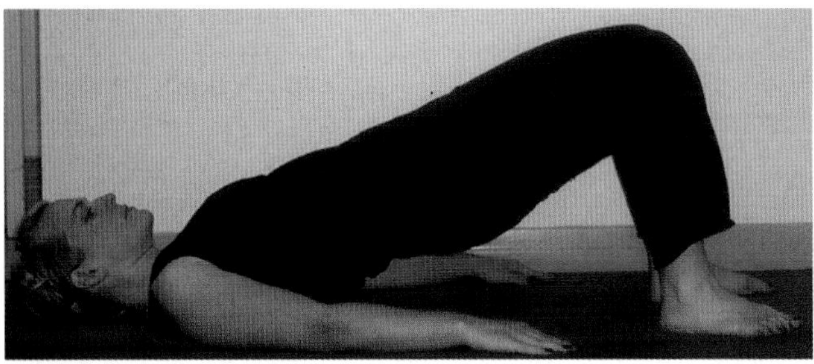

Figure 67.11 Photograph of bridging in the supine position.

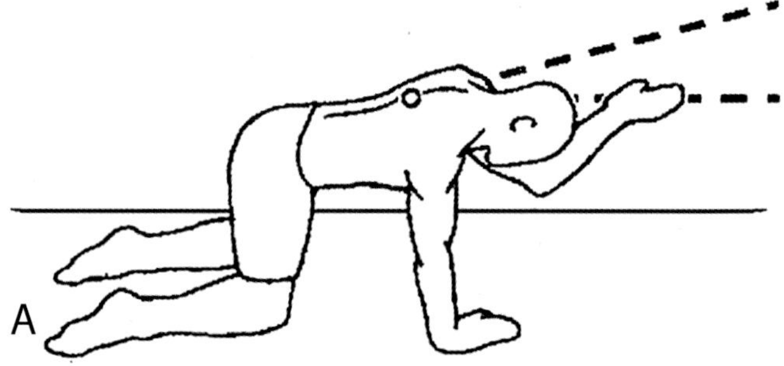

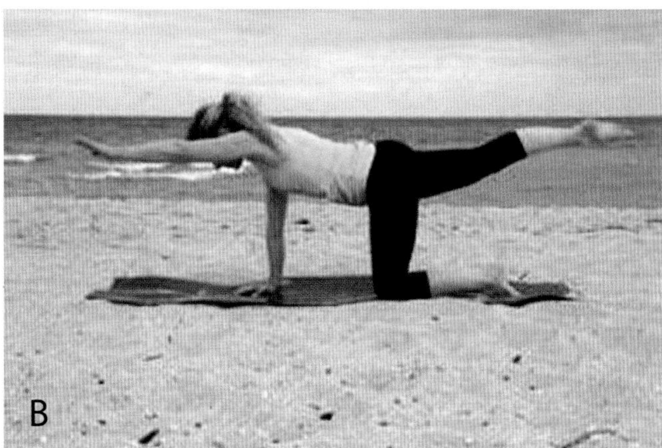

Figure 67.13 **A**, Illustration of four-point kneeling with one-arm lift. **B**, Photograph of four-point kneeling with one-arm lift.

vii. Balance exercise
   1. Sit-to-stand exercise (Figure 67.14)
      a. Sitting forward in the chair, shift weight forward and slowly lift up off the chair using leg the muscles. The patient may hold onto the chair for support only.
      b. Standing straight with a chair immediately behind with the knees just in front of the seat, lean forward slightly and return to a sitting position.
      c. 10 repetitions
   2. Knee raise (Figure 67.15)
      a. Hold the bar or the back of the chair to stabilize the body and lift one leg at a time.
      b. 10 seconds for 10 repetitions.
      c. Progress to one-leg support with eyes open without support.

Functional Goals and Restrictions

Goals of Treatment of VCF

- Alleviate pain and promote early mobilization.
- Promote healing of injured tissue.
- Relieve muscle spasm.
- Restore normal range of motion (ROM) and decrease kyphosis and proprioceptive afferents for the spine and lower limbs.
- Increase strength and balance and improve aerobic capacity.
- Educate the patient about healthy lifestyle and risk factors of falls to prevent further episodes.
- Return the patient to ADLs.

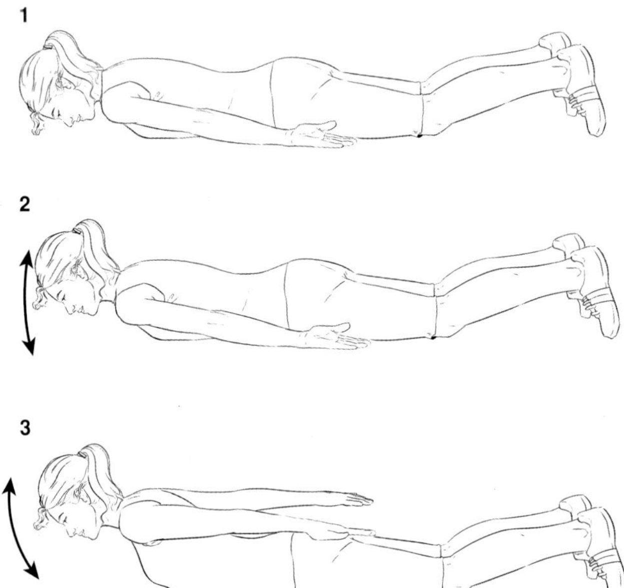

Figure 67.12 Illustration of progressive resistive back extension exercise. (Reproduced with permission from MediClip Images (c) 2003, Philadelphia, PA, Lippincott Williams & Wilkins. All rights reserved.)

General Considerations

Osteoporotic VCFs frequently occurs in the geriatric population. Elderly patients usually present with multiple problems, which may include motor, sensory, and cognitive dysfunction. Therefore, the initial assessment should include not only the patient's current level of function, motor control, balance, and sensorium, but also motivation, support system, and environment for home exercises. The physical therapy program has to be designed based on the patient's initial assessment by a specialist. Elderly patients tend to be rather cautious; thus, overactivity is rarely a problem. However, a safe environment with proper safeguards and supervision, as well as close monitoring and follow up, are essential.

Special Considerations for VCF Patients

The major concern for exercises after VCF is refracture. There is a report that showed no significant elevated risk of new-onset

© 2018 American Academy of Orthopaedic Surgeons

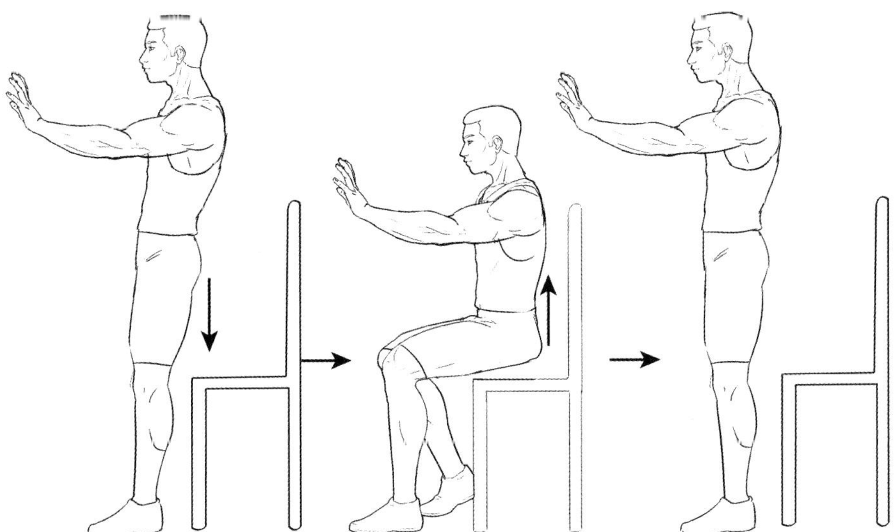

Figure 67.14 Illustration of sit-to-stand exercise.

fracture after vertebroplasty with increased physical activity. However, patients should be carefully counseled after vertebroplasty to optimize medical therapy for osteoporosis and to use extreme care when engaging in even moderate physical activity. Strenuous spinal flexion exercise may increase risk of VCF. The therapeutic exercise program has to avoid excessive flexion exercises and has to focus on spinal extension, which has shown positive effects on physical impairments, function, and quality of life after VCF.

PEARLS

Difference Between Kyphoplasty and Vertebroplasty

- Kyphoplasty is better for posterior cortex wall involvement as it shows lower cement extravasation
- Kyphoplasty is better for kyphotic deformity and will restore VB height with better realignment.

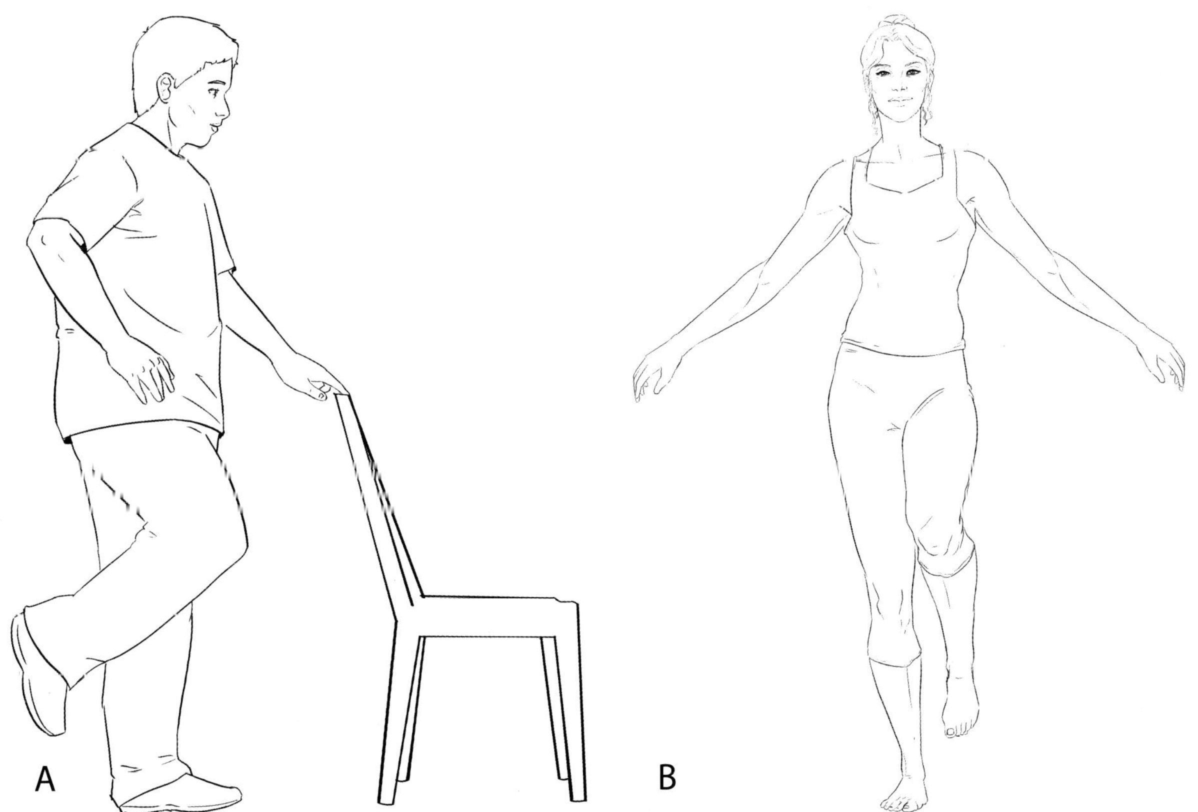

Figure 67.15 **A**, **B**, Illustrations of knee raise.

© 2018 American Academy of Orthopaedic Surgeons

- Kyphoplasty is mostly bilateral placement, while VP can achieve adequate cement coverage by single-needle placement.

Surgical

- Do not breach the medial wall of the pedicle while traversing the pedicle.
- The endpoint for needle placement is in the anterior third of the VB.
- Slow cement injection to observe cement extravasation.
- Low cement fill in low BMD VCF is better for prevention of adjacent-level VCF.
- In the case of neurologic deficit with spinal canal compromise, posterior and/or posterior decompression and fusion is indicated.

Rehabilitation

- Early immobilization with TLSP upon diagnosis
- Prompt physical therapy will yield the best results.
- An individualized physical therapy program is of utmost importance.
- Avoid strenuous flexion exercises.
- A structured home exercise program must be maintained to prevent further refracture.

BIBLIOGRAPHY

Anselmetti GC, Bernard J, Blattert T, et al: Criteria for the appropriate treatment of osteoporotic vertebral compression fractures. *Pain Physician* 2013;16(5):E519–E530.

Bansal S, Katzman WB, Giangregorio LM: Exercise for improving age-related hyperkyphotic posture: a systematic review. *Arch Phys Med Rehabil* 2014,95(1).129–140.

Bautmans I, Van Arken J, Van Mackelenberg M, Mets T: Rehabilitation using manual mobilization for thoracic kyphosis in elderly postmenopausal patients with osteoporosis. *J Rehabil Med* 2010;42:129–135.

Bennell KL, Matthews B, Greig A, et al: Effects of an exercise and manual therapy program on physical impairments, function and quality-of-life in people with osteoporotic vertebral fracture: a randomised, single-blind controlled pilot trial. *BMC Musculoskelet Disord* 2010;11:36.

Cumming SR, Melton JL: Epidemiology and outcomes osteoporotic fractures. *Lancet* 2002;359(9319):1761–1767.

DVO Guideline 2009 for Prevention, Diagnosis and Therapy of Osteoporosis in Adults. *Osteologie* 2011;20:55–74.

Granito RN, Aveiro MC, Renno AC, Oishi J, Driusso P: Comparison of thoracic kyphosis degree, trunk muscle strength and joint position sense among healthy and osteoporotic elderly women: a cross-sectional preliminary study. *Arch Gerontol Geriatr* 2012;54:e199–e202.

Greig AM, Bennell KL, Briggs AM, Hodges PW: Postural taping decreases thoracic kyphosis but does not influence trunk muscle electromyographic activity or balance in women with osteoporosis. *Man Ther* 2008;13(3):249–257.

Huntoon EA, Schmidt CK, Sinaki M: Significantly fewer refractures after vertebroplasty in patients who engage in back-extensor-strengthening exercises. *Mayo Clin Proc* 2008;83(1):54–57.

Longo UG, Loppini M, Denaro L, Maffulli N, Denaro V: Conservative management of patients with an osteoporotic vertebral fracture: a review of the literature. *J Bone Joint Surg Br* 2012;94(2):152–157.

Mika A, Fernhall B, Mika P: Association between moderate physical activity, spinal motion and back muscle strength in postmenopausal women with and without osteoporosis. *Disabil Rehabil* 2009;31:734–740.

Nagaraja S, Awada HK, Dreher ML, Gupta S, Miller SW: Vertebroplasty increases compression of adjacent IVDs and vertebrae in osteoporotic spines. *Spine J* 2013;13(12):1872–1880.

Papaioannou A, Watts NB, Kendler DL, Yuen CK, Adachi JD, Ferko N: Diagnosis and management of vertebral fractures in elderly adults. *Am J Med* 2002;113:220–228.

Pneumaticos SG, Triantafyllopoulos GK, Giannoudis PV: Advances made in the treatment of thoracolumbar fractures: Current trends and future directions. *Injury* 2013;44(6):703–712.

Radcliff K: Surgical planning for the treatment of thoracolumbar fractures: Anterior, posterior, or combined approach? *Seminars in Spine Surgery* 2012;24:244–251.

Sinaki M, Itoi E, Wahner HW, et al: Stronger back muscles reduce the incidence of vertebral fractures: a prospective 10 year follow-up of postmenopausal women. *Bone* 2002;30(6):836–841.

Sinaki M: Critical appraisal of physical rehabilitation measures after osteoporotic vertebral fracture. *Osteoporos Int* 2003; 14(9).773–779.

Sinaki M: The role of physical activity in bone health: a new hypothesis to reduce risk of vertebral fracture. *Phys Med Rehabil Clin N Am* 2007;18(3):593–608, xi–xii.

Sinaki M: Exercise for patients with osteoporosis: management of vertebral compression fractures and trunk strengthening for fall prevention. *PM R* 2012;4(11):882–888.

Sinaki M: Yoga spinal flexion positions and vertebral compression fracture in osteopenia or osteoporosis of spine: case series. *Pain Pract* 2013;13(1):68–75.

Venmans A, Lohle PN, van Rooij WJ: Pain course in conservatively treated patients with back pain and a VCF on the spine radiograph (VERTOS III). *Skeletal Radiol* 2013.

Wong CC, McGirt MJ: Vertebral compression fractures: a review of current management and multimodal therapy. *J Multidiscip Healthc* 2013;6:205–214.

Xu GJ, Li ZJ, Ma JX, Zhang T, Fu X, Ma XL: Anterior versus posterior approach for treatment of thoracolumbar burst fractures: a meta-analysis. *Eur Spine J* 2013;22(10):2176–2183.

© 2018 American Academy of Orthopaedic Surgeons

SECTION 8

Trauma

68 General Principles of Fracture Treatment and Rehabilitation

Roman Hayda, MD, COL (ret)

INTRODUCTION

Fracture treatment aims to restore function to the maximal extent possible. Fundamentally, fractures require immobilization not only for comfort and pain control, but also for healing. However, immobilization leads to joint stiffness, muscle atrophy, and even generalized patient deconditioning. Current fracture care has evolved to balance the immobilization and support required to achieve fracture healing with motion to limit joint contracture and muscle atrophy. Fixation of fractures with intramedullary devices, plates and screws, or external fixation provides fracture stabilization with appropriate alignment while allowing joint and, more important, patient mobilization. The goal is to restore normal function as early as possible. Optimizing the physical and psychological factors that affect fracture healing and functional recovery is critical in the recovery process. Exercise, performed with or without a therapist, is vital in this process. However, understanding all of the factors that affect therapy—including, but not limited to, weight-bearing status and joint motion parameters and their progression—is critical in the return of the patient to preinjury state of function.

In the past, lacking the surgical implants and techniques to effectively fix fractures, most fractures were treated with casts, braces, or traction. These methods led to "cast disease": bone and muscle atrophy, joint contracture, and pressure sores. When bed rest was required with traction, systemic sequelae such as pneumonia, ileus, thromboembolic disease, and urinary tract infection were common complications. Nonetheless, today, using a cast is still an effective form of treatment, especially in pediatric patients, most of whom are treated with casts or braces for fractures. Rapid healing and high remodeling capacity in the pediatric patient result in typically excellent outcomes. In adults, cast treatment is effective in minimally displaced and stable injuries, particularly in the upper extremity, where some deformity is well tolerated. Otherwise, surgical management may be the preferred treatment.

CONSIDERATIONS FOR SURGICAL FRACTURE MANAGEMENT

Subsequent chapters will discuss considerations for surgical treatment of fractures in particular anatomic areas, with the techniques employed and their implications for therapy. In general, fracture surgery is performed when adequate alignment cannot otherwise be achieved and maintained during the healing process. Fracture displacement, healing capacity, tolerance of deformity, patient functional needs, and ability or willingness to undergo surgery all factor in the decision for surgery. Aside from a single fracture in a limb, which is described in subsequent chapters, it is useful to consider three scenarios: multiple fractures in a single limb, fractures in multiple limbs, and fracture treatment in a patient with multiple system injury.

Multiple Fractures in a Single Limb

An important consideration in choosing surgical treatment of fractures is whether the fracture is isolated or whether the limb or patient has multiple fractures. A limb with multiple fractures is difficult to adequately stabilize nonsurgically even if an individual fracture can be treated in this manner. In this circumstance, all fractures in the limb are surgically stabilized,

Dr. Hayda or an immediate family member is a member of a speakers' bureau or has made paid presentations on behalf of AONA and Synthes; serves as an unpaid consultant to BioIntraface; has received research or institutional support from Stryker; and serves as a board member, owner, officer, or committee member of the American Academy of Orthopaedic Surgeons, Clinical Orthopaedics and Related Research, *the* Journal of Bone and Joint Surgery–American, *the* Journal of Orthopaedic Trauma, *METRC, and the Orthopaedic Trauma Association.*

© 2018 American Academy of Orthopaedic Surgeons

allowing for mobilization. For instance, a "floating elbow" consisting of a humerus fracture and forearm fracture will usually have both surgically fixed. Even though many isolated humerus fractures can be treated with bracing, in a combined fracture, surgery is done so that the shoulder, elbow, and wrist can be mobilized, reducing stiffness of those joints and disability. The same holds true in the floating-knee situation regardless of whether the tibia fracture is amenable to cast treatment.

Fractures in Multiple Limbs

The multiply fractured patient presents a different challenge to the team of surgeons and therapists. Multiple limbs with fractures can impair the patient's ability to perform even the most basic ADLs. In such cases, surgery is performed to allow for patient participation in self-care. Even a fracture as simple as bilateral wrist fractures may benefit from surgical fixation to allow such basic activities as feeding, toileting, and grooming since casts are not required.

In patients with fractures of the upper and lower extremities, the upper extremity fracture may require fixation to assist with patient mobilization. A humeral shaft fracture may be treated with a rod or plate to allow the use of crutches or walker in a patient with a combined lower extremity injury when otherwise it may be adequately treated with a brace to provide mobility and support. The method and extent to which weight bearing is allowed in the upper extremity is dependent on the location and complexity of the fracture, which determines the degree of stability that can be achieved with fixation. An intra-articular fracture of the distal humerus will not allow weight bearing until the fracture is adequately healed. A complex fracture of the wrist or forearm might not allow immediate weight bearing through traditional crutches or walker, but may allow for weight bearing through a platform. In such cases, the method of weight bearing and timing of progression should be made through communication between the surgeon and therapist.

Fracture Treatment in a Patient with Multiple System Injury

The multiply injured patient with a number of organ systems affected presents yet another challenge to the surgical and rehabilitation teams. Head injury, chest or abdominal injury, and spine fracture or dislocation with or without neurologic injury, combined with fractures of the extremities all require evaluation and treatment. Often, there are competing priorities that require careful coordination of the teams to achieve the optimal result. Data have shown that fixation of femur fractures within 24 hours of injury in the multiply injured patient leads to shorter intensive care unit (ICU) stays and fewer systemic complications, such as pulmonary failure. Fixation lessens systemic stress and allows for more optimal patient positioning and mobilization, reducing morbidity and length of stay in the ICU. However, in the most severely injured patient, even this degree of surgery may be too much, leading to complications. Surgery may induce a second hit on overtaxed systems, leading to organ failure. In such a case, "damage control" surgery may be undertaken to allow for further stabilization and resuscitation of the patient. An external fixator may be applied and converted to a rod when the patient is deemed stable and not susceptible to secondary inflammatory insults of surgery, typically after 5 to 7 days. Current protocols emphasize early resuscitation with fixation of most fractures within 48 hours, reducing complications and length of stay. A patient with head injury may be delayed even if adequately resuscitated since hypotension associated with extensive surgery in the first 4 to 5 days of injury will adversely affect neurologic recovery.

INITIATION OF THERAPY IN THE INJURED PATIENT

In the hospitalized fracture patient, rehabilitation can be started as soon as the extent of injuries and treatment plan is established. Uninjured limbs are exercised to maintain their strength and flexibility. Instruction in using these limbs for mobilization and transfers reestablishes the patient's sense of independence and control. Physiologic benefits of maintenance of strength and circulation also assist in the recovery of the patient. Active ankle pumping exercise may also reduce swelling and diminish the risk of thromboembolism.

As fractured limbs are repaired, they should also be incorporated into the therapeutic regimen. Doing so will reestablish the belief by the patient that even a severely injured limb may be restored to a functional status. Conversely, waiting until the fracture is healed or pain free will lead to atrophy of surrounding musculature and the development of scar, restricting motion. Therefore, mobilization is advanced as the nature of the injury and the quality of repair allows.

Even in the obtunded, intubated, or neurologically impaired patient, some form of therapy should be instituted early. The goals may obviously be different than in patients able to participate in their own therapy, but equally important. Therapy in these cases is directed toward avoiding complications related to disuse, namely, contracture and decubitus ulcers. Early institution of such measures is important, as the duration of intubation or impaired neurologic status may be hard to determine. Passive stretching of major joints—along with protective splinting of the hand, wrist, and ankle—are important. The hand is splinted in the "safe position" or intrinsic plus, with the wrist slightly extended and the metacarpophalangeal (MCP) joints in flexion with the interphalangeal (IP) joints extended. It is also important to keep the thumb abducted to avoid a contracture of the first web space. The ankle is splinted or braced in neutral position to keep the foot plantigrade. Equinus contracture is an all too common complication of the lower extremity that is not allowed to bear weight. The bed- or chair-bound patient is also subject to knee flexion contracture, which must be avoided. All providers must be reminded that contracture can occur in both injured and uninjured limbs. Obtunded, head-injured, paralyzed, or otherwise impaired patients are particularly prone to contracture. Frequent position changes and protective padding and mattresses reduce the

© 2018 American Academy of Orthopaedic Surgeons

risk of decubitus ulcer formation. In many cases, the nursing team can be instructed in measures to limit contracture and pressure ulcer formation.

In all fracture cases, therapy should focus on regaining control of the limb as the extremity injury and the overall patient condition allows. This includes active contraction of major muscle groups, gross movement of the limb, passive and active motion of the joint, and ultimately coordinated functional use of a limb. In the acute setting, the patient may not even be able to fire major motor groups in the fractured limb even when neurologically intact due to pain inhibition. Activities geared to muscle reeducation are critical to recovery.

Occult Injury

The entire treatment team, including therapists, should be vigilant in detecting occult injuries in the multiply injured patient. In the acute period, certain injuries may not be apparent to the physicians evaluating and treating the patient. There are a number of reasons for delayed diagnosis. The limb may not have had any external signs of injury, while the patient may not be able to verbalize or may be distracted by other injuries. Injuries may also be radiographically occult due to suboptimal radiographs or simply by virtue of being nondisplaced. The femoral neck is one such injury prone to delays in diagnosis, with the potential for severe consequences such as displacement, nonunion, and avascular necrosis. Fractures in the foot and hand may also suffer delays in diagnosis. Finally, neurologic injuries may be diagnosed late because of the inability to assess their status in the obtunded, intubated, or head-injured patient. Cooperative evaluation among surgeons and therapists helps limit long-term sequelae associated with delayed diagnosis. Therefore, it is important to communicate new or unexpected findings of pain, block to motion, or neural deficits.

BIOMECHANICAL PRINCIPLES OF FRACTURE IMPLANTS

Subsequent chapters will discuss the various options for fracture fixation in specific anatomic locations and the rehabilitation implications. However, understanding the biomechanical principles behind the fixation techniques will be useful, as they influence not only fracture fixation, but also rehabilitation of the extremity.

Intramedullary rods or nails are used to stabilize long bones, especially in the lower extremity. They come in a variety of lengths and diameters to accommodate anatomic variations. Interlocking screws at both ends of the nail allow for maintenance of axial length and rotation (Figure 68.1). To a degree, angular control is also allowed. Rods can be inserted through small incisions, although at times opening the fracture site is required to allow for reduction or avoid injury to critical structures. These devices are considered load sharing, potentially allowing full weight bearing with the exception of when the fracture extends into the joint or involves the metaphyseal area. In the metaphysis, intimate contact is lacking between the cortex and the nail, allowing for potential loss of reduction with weight-bearing forces. Most diaphyseal fractures of the femur and tibia are treated with nails, as well as select fractures of the humerus.

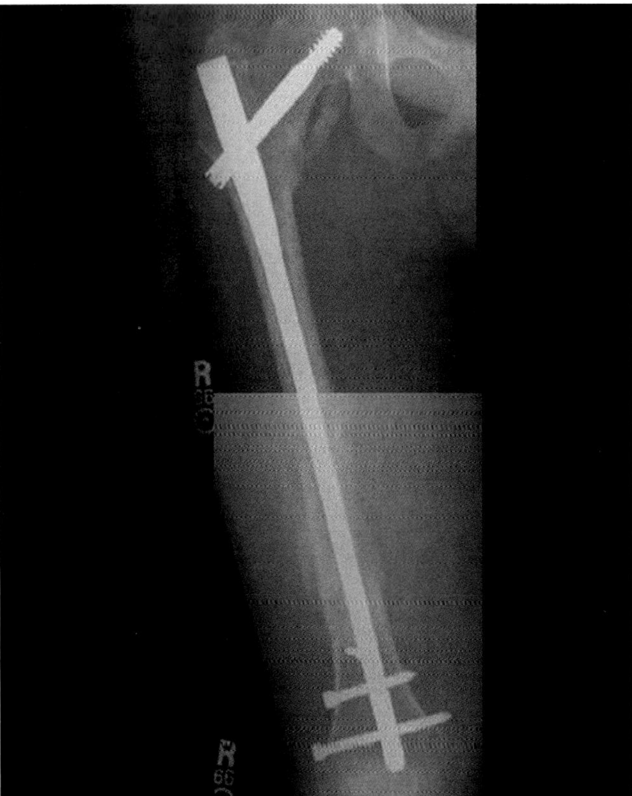

Figure 68.1 Radiograph of an intramedullary rod for a femur fracture.

Plates and screws are also used to maintain fracture reduction while the fracture heals. Such devices allow for precise control of fracture fragments at the potential expense of requiring greater surgical exposure (Figure 68.2, A and B). Plates and screws are most commonly used in fractures around joints in the lower extremity, and in the upper extremity for periarticular and diaphyseal fractures. In certain applications, they may be implanted through small incisions, affording the advantages of limited dissection and preservation of blood supply. Plates may be used in diaphyseal fractures as well, but are load bearing, limiting initial weight bearing if used in the lower extremity. However, studies have supported allowing weight bearing in plated humeral shaft fractures.

External fixation is a minimally invasive technique that stabilizes fractures by means of pins inserted through the soft tissues into bone, with an external frame providing stability. Two general types exist: planar and circular. Planar frames are often used a temporary fixation during damage-control surgery, open fractures, or temporary reduction and stabilization of unstable fractures of the ankle or around the knee pending internal fixation. They may also be used as definitive fixation through minimally invasive techniques for the wrist or ankle. It may also be used as definitive fixation when soft-tissue

© 2018 American Academy of Orthopaedic Surgeons

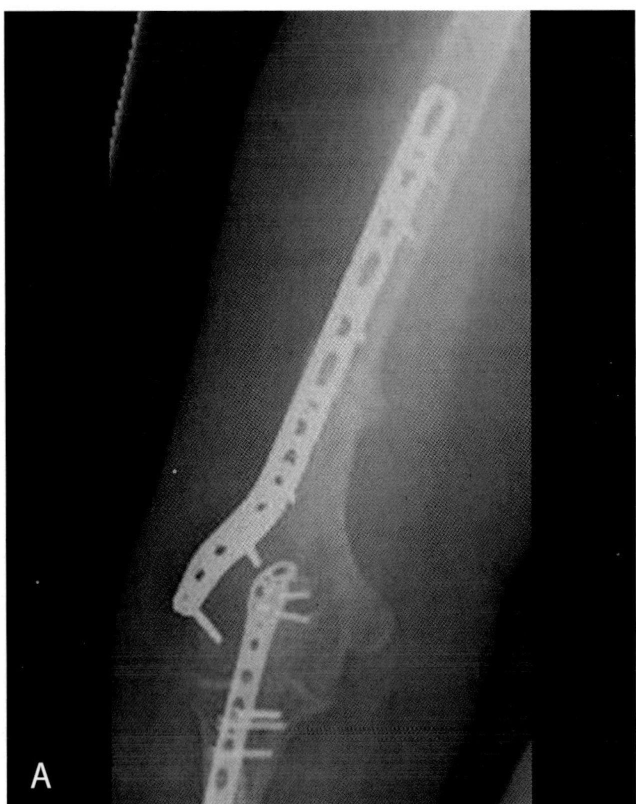

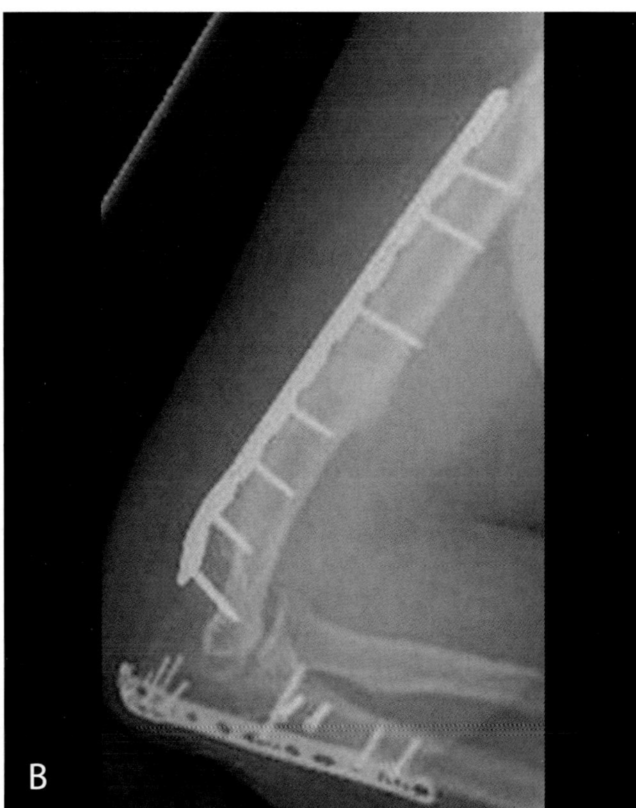

Figure 68.2 Radiographs of plating of a humerus and proximal ulna fracture. **A**, Anteroposterior view. **B**, Lateral view.

considerations do not allow the use of nails or plates. A circular frame is bulkier but allows for multiplanar control of the fracture (Figure 68.3). Pins or tensioned wires fixed to rings provide stability in multiple planes. Some devices allow for gradual correction of complex deformities. Biomechanically, since the frame is more distant from the fracture compared to rods or plates, less precise control is achieved, but still may be adequate for fracture healing. Although external fixation may be used in any extremity, external fixators are most often used for definitive fixation in the tibia and wrist, where pin insertion locations are least likely to injure nerves or vessels or transfix muscle. Since the pins are inserted through the skin, there is risk of infection and pin loosening. When pins become infected, they may require antibiotic treatment or pin removal and replacement.

Splints, braces, and even casts may be used in conjunction with surgical fixation of fractures for a number of reasons. In the immediate postoperative period, splints limit motion and maintain a desired position while wounds heal. They may also assist in swelling control. Perhaps most important, the immobilization may limit initial postoperative pain. These may be maintained for several days or weeks until therapy is initiated. Longer-term external supports may be utilized if there remain concerns regarding fixation quality due to bone quality or limitations of fixation. Other potential reasons for casting are to limit effects of patient noncompliance at the cost of joint stiffness or to limit joint motion in the case of joint instability.

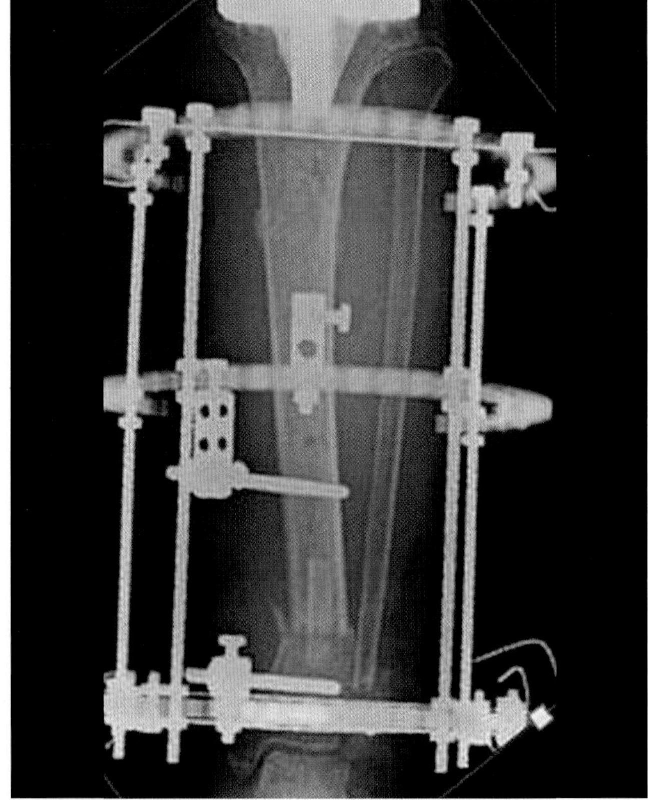

Figure 68.3 Radiograph of a circular frame treatment of an open distal tibia fracture.

© 2018 American Academy of Orthopaedic Surgeons

PITFALLS TO SUCCESSFUL REHABILITATION OF FRACTURE SURGERY

Potential pitfalls to successful rehabilitation of surgically treated fractures must be recognized in order to mitigate their effects. These may be related to patient physical, mental, or psychological factors, or extrinsic factors. Some of these factors may be modified and controlled while others cannot be modified.

Injury severity and patient comorbidities are examples of unmodifiable factors that influence outcome. These must be taken into account when performing surgery and during the rehabilitation period. They may also be useful in setting patient expectations regarding outcome. An intra-articular fracture with a high degree of comminution is likely to develop stiffness and posttraumatic arthritis in spite of accurate reduction and stable fixation. However, early appropriate therapy can limit severe motion limits and enhance function. Severe osteoporosis is associated with fracture comminution and limited fixation stability. In such situations, it may be impossible to restore preinjury anatomy. A surgeon may even consider joint replacement. Among fixation implants, intramedullary devices and locking plate screw constructs offer enhanced stabilization in osteoporotic bone. Regardless, it may be inappropriate to allow weight bearing or early motion delaying progression of rehabilitation. Other systemic conditions—such as rheumatoid arthritis, lupus, and other connective tissue disorders—are associated with osteoporosis and challenges fracture fixation. Similarly corticosteroids used in these disorders as well as others contribute not only to osteoporosis, but affect wound healing in the short term and should be taken into account.

Diabetes also has a profound effect on fracture treatment that is only partially modifiable. Patients with diabetes have delays in bone healing while also having a higher risk of poor wound healing and infection. Neuropathy associated with diabetes may also limit normal feedback due to loss of pain receptors that protect patients from overcoming the limits of fracture fixation. Nonunion is a distinct risk in these patients. For these reasons, immobilization and weight-bearing limitations may be prolonged in diabetics, especially those with neuropathy. Good control of blood sugar level has been shown to limit the risk of infection, which is beneficial in surgically treated fractures. However, direct effects on fracture healing are unknown.

Nutrition and Smoking

Modifiable factors influencing fracture healing and recovery are smoking and nutrition. Smoking and use of tobacco products is clearly related to delayed union and nonunion of fractures. Reversal of the ill effects of smoking on bone and soft-tissue healing can happen in a matter of weeks, making tobacco cessation efforts worthwhile in fracture patients, although notoriously difficult to achieve. Provider counseling is an important factor in cessation efforts.

Adequate nutrition is also vital in healing fractures. Patients may be malnourished prior to injury. Geriatric fracture patients and indigents are often chronically malnourished. Injury may induce or magnify malnourishment by increasing metabolic demands while appetite may be depressed following injury. In other cases, diet may be restricted due to abdominal injury or oral intake limited by multiple trips to the operating room. Therefore, multiply injured patients and others at risk for malnutrition benefit from early nutrition intervention. Nutritional supplementation with balanced protein shakes, in addition to standard meals, are effective strategies. Oral alimentation is preferred; if not possible, gastric tube feeding is acceptable. If either is not possible, parenteral intravenous nutrition should be considered.

Pain Control

Pain control in fracture patients is a complex topic about which volumes can be written, but is equally important in instituting effective therapeutic regimens. Simply stated, all pain cannot be eliminated during rehabilitation, especially during the initial phases of recovery, but reasonable pain control is required for effective rehabilitation. In fact, pain is an important modulating factor during initial treatment to limit activity, which allows healing. At some point, pain response may become counterproductive, inhibiting functional restoration. Narcotics have been the traditional mainstays of pain control, but tolerance, dependence, and hyperalgesia have become increasingly recognized side effects. Multimodal strategies that involve various pharmacologic agents are being increasingly recognized as more effective strategies. Agents include acetaminophen, nonsteroidal anti-inflammatory drugs (NSAIDs), gabalin and pregabalin, and tricyclics, among others, which can be used synergistically with narcotics. Although NSAIDs may affect fracture healing if used long term, they are not associated with nonunion when used in the immediate postoperative period. Nerve blocks are useful acutely. Biofeedback, massage, acupuncture, and desensitization can also be useful, and have been used in posttraumatic complex regional pain syndrome.

Neurologic and Psychological Factors

Neurologic and psychological factors are known to be powerful modifiers to effective rehabilitation. Traumatic brain injury and its effects on cognition limit the patient's ability to actively participate or understand the rehabilitation process. Meanwhile, the timing and extent of recovery are unpredictable. Comatose patients with severe injury felt to be unrecoverable initially do at times recover with a decreased, although functional, capacity. Therefore, in such patients, early rehabilitation should focus on establishing conditions that allow functional return by avoiding contractures. As the condition improves, therapeutic exercises of increasing complexity are instituted to return to functions of daily living. Sitting, feeding, grooming, and walking are reestablished as neural function allows.

Depression and posttraumatic stress disorder (PTSD), which are common in the trauma patient, may impair the patient's ability to participate in rehabilitation as well. Sleep disorders associated with these conditions, as well as other issues, affect engagement in rehabilitation. Furthermore, recovery

© 2018 American Academy of Orthopaedic Surgeons

from complex injury is marked by setbacks that further place doubt in the patient's sense of ability to recover. Therefore, depression and PTSD should be screened for and treatment instituted to allow for optimal rehabilitation of patients. A supportive and proactive program instituting realistic goals, not only in rehabilitation but also in vocational and avocational pursuits, is critical in optimal patient recovery.

SUMMARY

The successful rehabilitation of the surgically treated fracture patient requires a close cooperation between the patient, surgeon, and therapist. Effective communication between all three parties limits complications and enhances results. Understanding the fracture and its fixation in the context of the whole patient can establish realistic goals in the progression of therapy. The following chapters will provide principles of therapy of fractures in particular anatomic locations.

BIBLIOGRAPHY

Bhandari M, Busse JW, Hanson BP, Leece P, Ayeni OR, Schemitsch EH: Psychological distress and quality of life after orthopedic trauma: an observational study. *Can J Surg* 2008;51(1):15–22.

Bone LB, Johnson KD, Weigelt J, Scheinberg R: Early versus delayed stabilization of femoral fractures. A prospective randomized study. *J Bone Joint Surg Am* 1989;71:336–340.

Borrelli J Jr, Pape C, Hak D, Hsu J, Lin S, Giannoudis P, Lane J: Physiological challenges of bone repair. *J Orthop Trauma* 2012;26(12):708–711.

D'Alleyrand JC, O'Toole RV: The evolution of damage control orthopedics: current evidence and practical applications of early appropriate care. *Orthop Clin North Am* 2013;44(4):499–507.

Enderson BL, Reath DB, Meadors J, Dallas W, DeBoo JM, Maull KI: The tertiary trauma survey: a prospective study of missed injury. *J Trauma* 1990;30(6):666–669; discussion 669–670.

Friedemann-Sánchez G, Sayer NA, Pickett T: Provider perspectives on rehabilitation of patients with polytrauma. *Arch Phys Med Rehabil* 2008;89(1):171–178.

Griffiths RD: Specialized nutrition support in critically ill patients. *Curr Opin Crit Care* 2003;9(4):249–259.

Harwood PJ, Giannoudis PV, van Griensven M, Krettek C, Pape HC: Alterations in the systemic inflammatory response after early total care and damage control procedures for femoral shaft fracture in severely injured patients. *J Trauma* 2005;58(3):446–454.

Herkowitz HN, Dirschl DR, Sohn DH: Pain management: the orthopaedic surgeon's perspective. *J Bone Joint Surg Am* 2007;89(11):2532–2535.

Kang H, Ha YC, Kim JJ, Woo YC, Lee JS, Jang EJ: Effectiveness of multimodal pain management after bipolar hemiarthroplasty for hip fracture: a randomized, controlled study. *J Bone Joint Surg Am* 2013;95(4):291–296.

Keene DD, Rea WE, Aldington D: Acute pain management in trauma. *Trauma* 2011;13:167–179.

Kempen GI, Sanderman R, Scaf-Klomp W, Ormel J: The role of depressive symptoms in recovery from injuries to the extremities in older persons. A prospective study. *Int J Geriatr Psychiatry* 2003;18(1):14–22.

Koval KJ, Maurer SG, Su ET, Aharonoff GB, Zuckerman J: The effects of nutritional status on outcome after hip fracture *J Orthop Trauma* 1999;13(3):164–169.

Lee JJ, Patel R, Biermann JS, Dougherty PJ: The musculoskeletal effects of cigarette smoking. *J Bone Joint Surg Am* 2013;95(9):850–859.

Liu J, Ludwig T, Ebraheim NA: Effect of the blood HbA1c level on surgical treatment outcomes of diabetics with ankle fractures. *Orthop Surg* 2013;5(3):203–208.

Miller AG, Margules A, Raikin SM: Risk factors for wound complications after ankle fracture surgery. *J Bone Joint Surg Am* 2012;94(22):2047–2052.

Nåsell H, Adami J, Samnegård E, Tønnesen H, Ponzer S: Effect of smoking cessation intervention on results of acute fracture surgery: a randomized controlled trial. *J Bone Joint Surg Am* 2010;92(6):1335–1342.

Ozkalkanli MY, Ozkalkanli DT, Katircioglu K, Savaci S: Comparison of tools for nutrition assessment and screening for predicting the development of complications in orthopedic surgery. *Nutr Clin Pract* 2009;24(2):274–280.

Ricci WM, Streubel PN, Morshed S, Collinge CA, Nork SE, Gardner MJ: Risk factors for failure of locked plate fixation of distal femur fractures: an analysis of 335 cases. *J Orthop Trauma* 2014;28(2):83–89.

Reuben SS, Buvanendran A: Preventing the development of chronic pain after orthopaedic surgery with preventive multimodal analgesic techniques. *J Bone Joint Surg Am* 2007;89(6):1343–1358.

Tingstad EM, Wolinsky PR, Shyr Y, Johnson KD: Effect of immediate weightbearing on plated fractures of the humeral shaft. *J Trauma* 2000;49(2):278–280.

© 2018 American Academy of Orthopaedic Surgeons

Acetabulum

Kerellos Nasr, MD, Stephanie Dickason, PT, and Rahul Banerjee, MD

INTRODUCTION

Fractures of the acetabulum, or hip socket, account for 10% of injuries to the pelvis. These fractures have a bimodal distribution. Young patients sustain these fractures through high-energy mechanisms, such as motor vehicle collisions or falls from a height. Elderly patients sustain lower energy injuries, such ground-level falls.

The treatment of acetabular fractures is determined by the characteristics of the patient and the specific nature of the fracture. Most nondisplaced acetabular fractures may be treated without surgery. Displaced acetabular fractures in younger patients require surgical treatment to restore a stable, congruent articular surface. Anatomic restoration of the articular surface helps to prevent the development of future hip arthritis in this patient population. Elderly patients with displaced acetabular fractures often still require surgery in order to have a stable functional hip. However, in many cases, surgical treatment will include total hip arthroplasty in this patient population.

Due to the varied nature of acetabular fractures, the surgical approach and subsequent rehabilitation is unique depending on the specific characteristics of the fracture, the type of treatment, and, in cases of operative treatment, the surgical approach.

CLASSIFICATION

Letournel and Judet classified acetabular fractures into two groups; elementary fracture patterns and associated fracture patterns (Figure 69.1). Elementary fracture patterns (with the exception of the transverse fracture) involve a fracture of a single column of the acetabulum and include:

- Anterior wall fractures
- Anterior column fractures
- Posterior wall fractures
- Posterior column fractures
- Transverse fractures (a single fracture line that spans both columns)

The associated fracture patterns include fractures that have at least two elementary forms and are more complex in nature. These include:

- Posterior wall posterior column fractures
- Anterior column (or wall) posterior hemitransverse fractures
- Transverse posterior wall fractures
- T-type fractures
- Both column fractures

The classification is useful in describing the fracture pattern and helps to determine the surgical approach, as discussed later.

MANAGEMENT OF ACETABULAR FRACTURES

Many acetabular fractures will require surgical treatment in order to restore a stable congruent joint. In select cases, nonoperative treatment may be preferred. Indications for nonoperative treatment include:

- Nondisplaced fractures (<2 mm)
- Displaced fractures not involving weight-bearing dome
- Hip joint stability is maintained
- Both column fractures that retain secondary congruency of the hip joint
- Medical conditions that make the risks of surgery outweigh its benefits

Most acetabular fractures will require surgical treatment to achieve anatomic reduction of the articular surface, create a stable congruent joint, and provide stable fixation to allow

Dr. Banerjee or an immediate family member is a member of a speakers' bureau or has made paid presentations on behalf of AO North America and Smith & Nephew; serves as a paid consultant to Smith & Nephew; and serves as a board member, owner, officer, or committee member of the American Academy of Orthopaedic Surgeons. Neither of the following authors nor any immediate family member has received anything of value from or has stock or stock options held in a commercial company or institution related directly or indirectly to the subject of this article: Mr. Dickson and Dr. Nasr.

© 2018 American Academy of Orthopaedic Surgeons

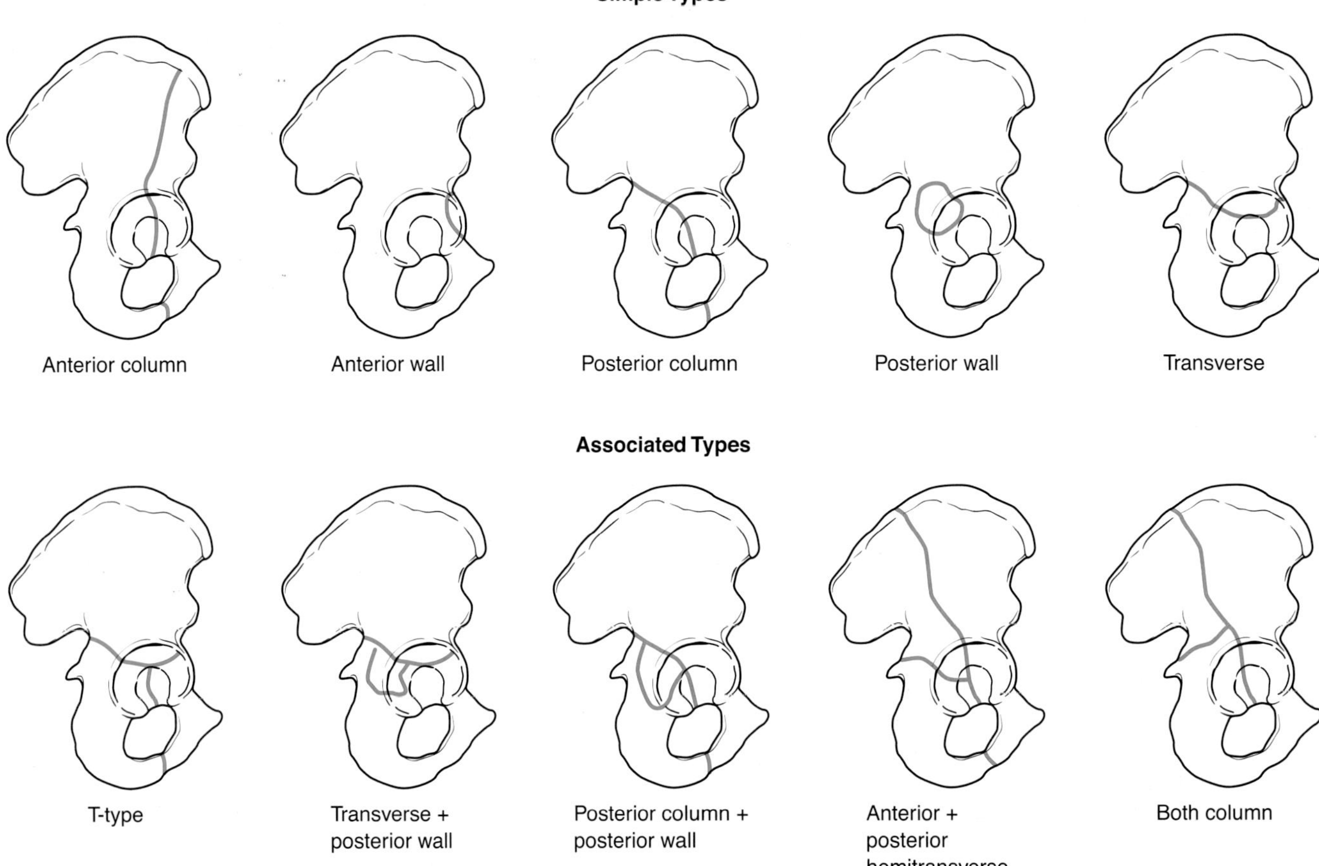

Figure 69.1 Illustration of the Letournel Acetabular Fracture Classification. (Reproduced with permission from Bucholz RW, Heckman JD: *Rockwood & Green's Fractures in Adults*, ed 5. Philadelphia, PA, Lippincott Williams & Wilkins, 2001.)

early range of motion (ROM). Indications for surgical treatment include:

- Fractures involving the weight-bearing dome with 2-mm displacement
- Hip joint instability or incongruity
- Intra-articular incarcerated fragments
- Irreducible fracture dislocations

In elderly patients, surgical treatment will often include total hip arthroplasty in conjunction with or instead of internal fixation. The indications for total hip arthroplasty include:

- Osteoporotic bone that prevents stable fixation
- Extensive comminution that would not allow adequate joint reduction
- Extensive injury to the articular cartilage of the acetabulum or femoral head
- Previous history of degenerative joint disease

SURGICAL APPROACH

Surgical treatment of acetabular fractures is performed through one of several commonly used approaches. The surgical approach is chosen based on the fracture pattern. Three of the main surgical approaches include the Kocher-Langenbeck approach, the ilioinguinal approach, and the extensile iliofemoral approach. The choice of surgical approach is determined by fracture pattern and surgeon preference, and impacts the postoperative rehabilitation.

Kocher-Langenbeck Approach

The Kocher-Langenbeck approach allows access to the posterior and superior surface of the acetabulum, thus is well suited for treatment of fractures of the posterior column or posterior wall and certain types of transverse fractures (Figure 69.2). It is similar to the posterior approach for hip replacement but exposes more of the ischium and outer table of the ilium.

The skin is incised a few centimeters lateral and distal to the posterior superior iliac spine and carried to the greater trochanter, then curved distally following the lateral aspect of the femoral shaft, ending distal to the gluteus maximus insertion. Sharp dissection is taken down to the fascia over the gluteus maximus proximally and the iliotibial (IT) band distally in line with skin incision. The IT band is sharply incised inline with the skin incision and the gluteus maximus is bluntly split, making sure to not injure the superior gluteal neurovascular bundle.

The trochanteric bursa is dissected posteriorly to allow exposure of the short external rotators: the piriformis, gemelli, and obturator internus. Care should be taken to achieve hemostasis during this exposure. The gluteus maximus insertion may

 © 2018 American Academy of Orthopaedic Surgeons

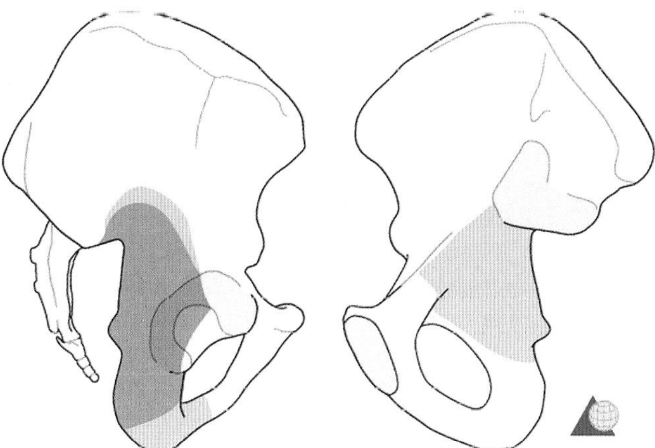

Figure 69.2 Illustration of the Kocher-Langenbeck approach. (Copyright AO Foundation, Switzerland. Available at: www.aosurgery.org.)

be partially or totally incised in order to increase exposure, if needed. The sciatic nerve can now be carefully visualized; it typically runs anterior (or deep) to the piriformis and posterior (or superficial) to the rest of the external rotators. It is at risk from the injury and during surgery, particularly the peroneal division. The short external rotators are then incised 1 cm lateral to their femoral insertions to avoid damaging the medial circumflex artery, which carries the majority of the femoral head blood supply. Injury to the quadratus femoris should be avoided for the same reason. Injury to the blood supply from the trauma or surgery may lead to avascular necrosis in the postoperative period. The short external rotators are reflected posteriorly, protecting the sciatic nerve. With the placement of retractors, the greater and lesser sciatic notches and ischial spine are exposed, thus the posterior column is now visible. The hip joint can be inspected with the use of a capsulotomy and distraction of the joint, utilizing traction through the femur.

Performing a trochanteric osteotomy may extend the Kocher-Langenbeck approach. The osteotomy allows for greater exposure superior and anterior to the acetabulum, and is useful with certain posterior fracture patterns and some transverse fractures. The osteotomy is carried from the tip of the trochanter to the vastus tubercle. The osteotomized fragment, which has the insertions of the gluteus medius and minimus (depending on the technique, it may also have the insertion of the vastus lateralis) is reflected anteriorly. By reflecting the fragment, cephalad exposure is increased, which also allows for surgical hip dislocation for direct visualization of the articular surface. After surgical fixation, the osteotomized fragment is reduced and stabilized with lag screws.

After completion of fixation, thorough débridement of any necrotic muscle, especially the gluteus medius and minimus, and loose bony fragments should be removed to decrease the incidence of heterotopic ossification. The short external rotators are reattached to the femur and the gluteus maximus and IT band are repaired.

The Kocher-Langenbeck approach requires release of the short external rotators of the hip and retraction of the abductor muscles. As a result of this and in combination with the injury, these muscle groups are often weak after surgery and should be addressed during rehabilitation.

Ilioinguinal Approach

The ilioinguinal approach, as developed by Letournel, is an anterior approach to the acetabulum that allows for access of the anterior column (Figure 69.3). This approach is predominantly used for anterior wall or anterior column fractures, anterior column posterior hemitransverse fractures, T-type fractures, transverse fractures, and associated both-column fractures. This approach does not allow direct exposure of the articular surface of the acetabulum; therefore, the joint is reduced indirectly by careful reduction of extra-articular anatomy.

The skin is incised 1 to 2 cm proximal to the pubic symphysis and curved to the iliac crest; the external oblique is released, leaving tissue to repair, allowing the surgeon to subperiosteally elevate the iliacus, exposing the internal iliac fossa. The external oblique aponeurosis is cut from the anterior superior iliac spine (ASIS) moving superior to the external inguinal ring, ending at the lateral border of the rectus sheath. In the medial aspect of the wound, the spermatic cord (in males) or the round ligament (in females) is mobilized; the transversus abdominis is released starting from the ASIS to the conjoint tendon and the pubic tubercle from the inguinal ligament. The ilioinguinal and lateral femoral cutaneous nerves must be protected as they are encountered. The external iliac artery and vein cross the surgical field, and are scrupulously protected as the surgeon works around them.

With deep dissection through the ilioinguinal approach, three windows are created through which reduction of fracture fragments is performed and fixation can be implanted. The lateral window is lateral to the iliopsoas and provides access from the sacroiliac (SI) joint to iliopectineal eminence, thus the internal iliac fossa. The middle window lies between the iliopsoas and the external iliac vessels. Through this window, the surgeon can work on the pelvic brim, quadrilateral plate,

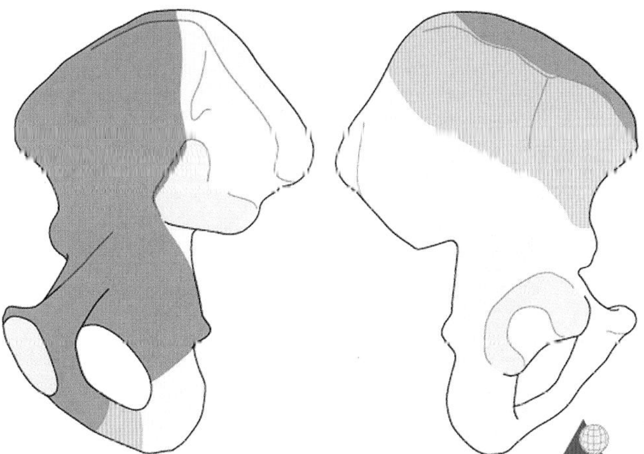

Figure 69.3 Illustration of the ilioinguinal approach. (Copyright AO Foundation, Switzerland. Available at: www.aosurgery.org.)

and the lateral third of the superior pubic ramus. The medial window is medial to the external iliac vessels. During the deep dissection, the surgeon must investigate any retropubic anastomoses between the obturator and external iliac (or inferior epigastric) vessels, known as the corona mortis. If present, the anastomoses should be ligated.

Direct exposure of the quadrilateral lamina and the interior aspect of the pelvic brim is possible through the anterior intrapelvic approach, which is often used in conjunction with the ilioinguinal approach. In these cases, the medial and middle window of the ilioinguinal approach may be replaced by the anterior intrapelvic approach.

To perform the anterior intrapelvic approach, a transverse incision Pfannenstiel-type incision is made approximately 1 to 2 cm proximal to the pubic symphysis. Dissection is taken down to the musculature. The rectus abdominus fascia is incised through the linea alba, giving entrance to the space of Retzius between the bladder and the bony pubis. The distal insertion of the rectus should be maintained as the more proximal posterior insertion is elevated from the posterior surface of the pubic rami. The surgeon stands on the contralateral side from the fracture and must release the iliopectineal fascia to enter the true pelvis. The corona mortis must be identified and ligated. With subperiosteal elevation of the iliopsoas and retraction of the external iliac vessels, the pelvic brim is now seen. Direct exposure of the medial aspect of the quadrilateral lamina is possible through this approach. The obturator neurovascular bundle is encountered and should be protected.

Closure of the ilioinguinal approach includes careful repair of the inguinal ligament and the fascia of the external oblique aponeurosis. The abdominal wall muscles are repaired to their insertion along the iliac crest, just proximal to the origin of the abductor muscles.

Extended Iliofemoral Approach

The extended iliofemoral approach allows complete visualization of the lateral innominate bone (Figure 69.4); it is indicated with certain transverse fractures, T-type fractures, or both-column fractures. It is typically used when there is a delay in fixation (usually >3 weeks) or in corrective surgeries for malunions or nonunions since it offers the widest direct exposure of the acetabulum. This approach should be done in patients who can handle an extended recovery period, and is avoided in the elderly and obese.

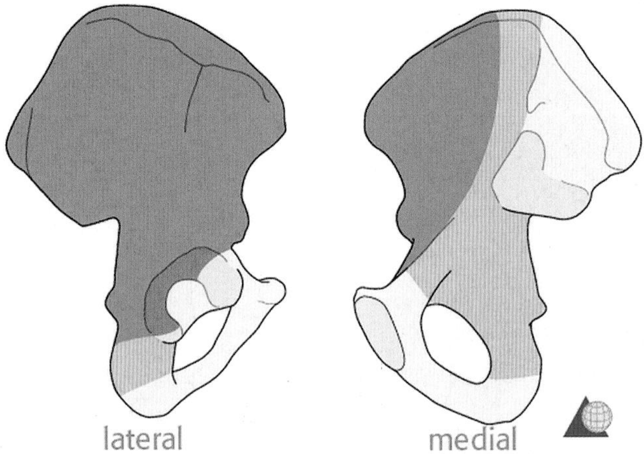

Figure 69.4 Illustration of the extended iliofemoral approach. (Copyright AO Foundation, Switzerland. Available at: www.aosurgery.org.)

Although it provides excellent exposure, the extended iliofemoral approach has drawbacks in that it has the highest complication rate of all the approaches and is technically demanding. Since the abductors are elevated from their origin and insertion, they are considerably weaker; the approach also has a problem with heterotopic ossification. In addition, the superior gluteal artery and vessels can be damaged during this approach, leading to significant bleeding, necessitating embolization or more extensive surgery to control hemorrhage. As the superior gluteal vessels are at risk, so is the accompanying nerve (further increasing abductor weakness); the sciatic nerve may be injured with this procedure as well. Furthermore, branches from the lateral femoral cutaneous nerve are always transected, leading to paresthesias of the lateral thigh.

The incision is from the posterior superior iliac spine (PSIS) taken along the iliac crest to the ASIS; it is then carried distally in a slight posterior direction along the femur. The intervals between the abdominal and gluteal muscles at the iliac crest and between the tensor fasciae latae (TFL) and sartorius are developed. The TFL is elevated from the ASIS and taken laterally; the fascia lata is longitudinally dissected distally.

The gluteal muscles are lifted off from their insertion on the iliac crest in an anterior superior to posterior inferior direction until the PSIS and greater sciatic notch are reached. The lateral branches of the anterior femoral circumflex vessels are ligated, allowing more lateral retraction of the TFL and fascia lata. The direct head of the rectus femoris is elevated from the anterior inferior iliac spine. The insertions the gluteus medius and minimus are tagged for later repair and then released. This is also done for the short external rotators, taking care not to damage the medial circumflex artery. Care must be taken to guard the superior gluteal neurovascular bundle and sciatic nerve. The hip capsule is then released if not already opened from the injury, to allow intra-articular visualization. If access is needed in the internal iliac fossa, the abdominal musculature can be incised and the iliacus can be elevated.

Modifications to the extended iliofemoral approach have also been described. The T-extensile approach (or Big T) utilizes osteotomies of the iliac crest, ASIS, and greater trochanter in order to mobilize the abductors. In contrast to the conventional extended iliofemoral approach, these osteotomies allow for bony healing.

During closure, the hip capsule and external rotators are repaired. The gluteus medius must be anatomically reinserted and with robust sutures while the leg is abducted. If osteotomies are performed instead, these are repaired with lag screws. The rectus femoris is reapproximated to its insertion through bone tunnels while the knee is extended. The remaining muscles are repaired, and the fascia and skin are closed.

© 2018 American Academy of Orthopaedic Surgeons

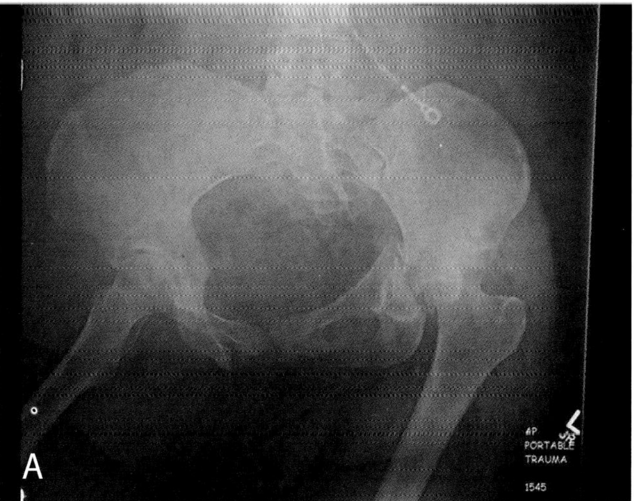

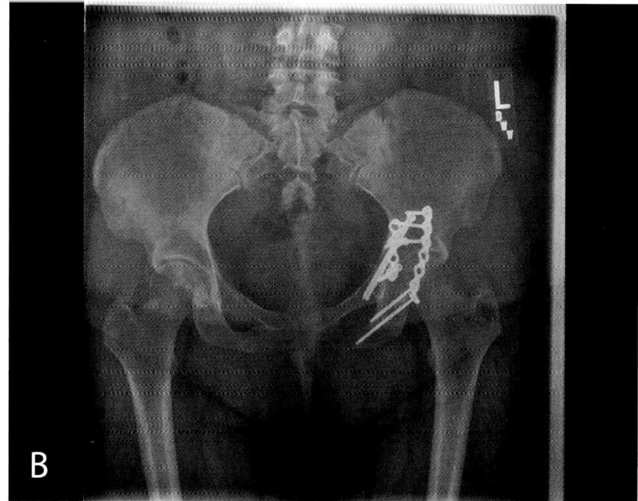

Figure 69.5 **A**, Radiograph of a 20-year-old female's posterior hip dislocation and transverse posterior wall acetabular fracture, sustained in a motor vehicle accident. **B**, Radiograph of the same patient in **A**, treated with open reduction and internal fixation using a Kocher-Langenbeck approach. After reduction, the anterior column is stabilized with a 6.5-mm lag screw. The posterior wall and posterior column are stabilized with lag screws and small fragment buttress plates.

The extended iliofemoral approach requires release of both the origin and insertion of the abductor muscles. Therefore, these muscles are significantly weakened and require special attention during rehabilitation.

Internal Fixation of Acetabular Fractures

After surgical exposure, the fractured acetabulum is anatomically reduced and stabilized with small fragment screws and plates. The goal of internal fixation is to provide a stable, congruent hip that allows for early ROM. Lag screws may be utilized for larger fragments with simple fracture patterns. Buttress plates are often required for posterior wall fractures. Larger screws may be utilized to stabilize fractures of the anterior or posterior column (Figure 69.5).

Minimally Invasive Reduction and Fixation of Acetabular Fractures

In certain cases, reduction of the acetabular fracture may be achieved by minimally invasive techniques. These methods are technically challenging, but have the benefit of avoiding large surgical approaches, which decreases pain and may facilitate recovery.

COMPLICATIONS

Complications after operative treatment of acetabular fractures that impact rehabilitation include posttraumatic arthritis, avascular necrosis, heterotopic ossification, peroneal nerve injury, deep vein thrombosis, pulmonary embolism, and abductor weakness. Posttraumatic arthritis is the most common complication. These patients may present with gradually increasing hip pain over time. Avascular necrosis of the femoral head occurs with injury to the femoral head blood supply, which may occur at the time of surgery, with associated hip dislocation, or by iatrogenic injury during surgery. Heterotopic ossification occurs with use of the extended iliofemoral approach and the Kocher-Langenbeck approach. Prophylactic treatment is necessary to decrease the risk of hip ankylosis; this includes either low-dose external radiation therapy or the use of indomethacin. Peroneal nerve injury may occur at the time of injury or secondary to manipulation of the sciatic nerve during exposure. This may result in an inability of the patient to actively dorsiflex the foot. Abductor weakness is common, particularly with any approach that involves a posterior approach or manipulation to the gluteus musculature.

POSTOPERATIVE REHABILITATION

Rehabilitation after acetabular fracture can be divided into the acute injury/postoperative phase and the posthealing phase. Initially, the focus of therapy interventions centers on mobility training and patient-specific education, including home exercise instruction and weight-bearing limitations. The emphasis is on encouraging maximal activity while waiting for soft-tissue and bony healing. The principle of "active waiting" is to prepare each patient for the posthealing phase so that return to functional independence and preinjury activities can occur as quickly as possible.

Acute Phase (0–12 Weeks)

The physical therapy evaluation consists of the following elements:

1. Obtaining a preinjury functional history, including any previous functional or gait limitations, use of assistive devices or braces, level of mobility (household, community), job or recreational activities, need for assistance for mobility and activities of daily living (ADLs).

2. Pain assessment and visual inspection of extremities to check for edema, joint effusions, or ecchymosis not otherwise noted by other providers. As patients with acetabular fracture often also have concomitant injuries, including posterior cruciate ligament (PCL) injuries and sciatic nerve injuries, it is important for the physical therapist to be vigilant in observation of patients. It is not unusual for additional injuries to be discovered after the patient begins to become more mobile.
3. Lower quarter strength and sensation screening should be done to assess for concomitant nerve injury. The peroneal portion of the sciatic nerve is often injured, particularly during posterior hip dislocations with posterior wall fractures.
4. Mobility assessment, including bed mobility, transfers, and gait training with assistive device of choice.

Based on the evaluation findings, the physical therapist can develop goals and a plan of care specific to each patient's needs and limitations.

The physical therapy treatment should include the following elements:

1. *Instruction in weight-bearing limitations.* Typically, foot-flat weight bearing is prescribed to minimize contact pressures across the femoral head and acetabulum. This allows for relaxation of the hip musculature, resulting in only ground reaction force from the weight of the limb to cross the joint. Toe-touch weight-bearing is also occasionally prescribed for the same reason, but is generally avoided due to the risk of developing contractures of the hip flexors, hamstrings, and ankle plantarflexors over the 12 weeks typically required to heal these fractures. Non–weight bearing is to be avoided due to the increase in loading across the joint when the hip musculature is contracted.
2. *Hip precautions.* Depending on the type of surgical approach used and injury pattern, certain precautions or limitations of hip ROM may be required to protect the surgical repair and allow for recovery of the muscles. In cases associated with posterior hip dislocations and posterior wall fractures, posterior hip precautions should be maintained during the initial 12-week postoperative recovery period. Posterior hip precautions include limiting hip flexion to less than 90°, avoiding active hip flexion, and limiting active internal rotation of the hip. If an osteotomy of the greater trochanter has been performed or, in the case of the extended iliofemoral approach, if the abductor muscle insertion or origin has been surgically disrupted, active abduction should be avoided during the initial 12-week recovery period.
3. *Home exercise program.* The focus of exercise prescription in the initial healing phase should be on gentle active ROM to decrease edema, facilitate movement of synovial fluid in the joint, and to prevent and/or minimize muscle atrophy and contracture. Patients should be instructed in the amount of exercise that will prepare their limb for the posthealing phase without interfering with fracture healing.

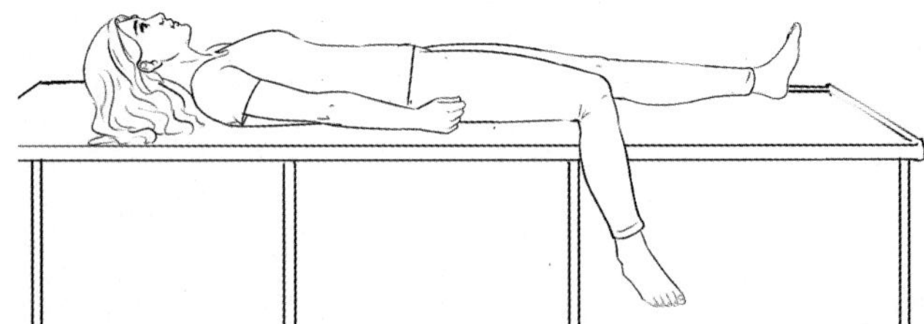

Figure 69.6 Illustration of the supine hip flexor stretch.

Home Exercise Program for Acute Acetabular Fracture With or Without Repair

- All exercises should be performed through the full arc of active ROM without overpressure.
- Performing the exercise multiple times/day for a smaller number of repetitions is preferable to longer sessions 2 to 3 times/day.

Supine Hip Flexor Stretch (Figure 69.6)

- Lie on your back at the edge of your bed.
- Let your leg lower over the edge, allowing your knee to bend, until you feel a stretch in the front of your hip.
- Hold for 30 seconds, then slowly lift your leg back onto the bed.
- Perform 1 repetition 5 times/day.

Heel Slides (Figure 69.7)

- Lie on a firm, flat surface.
- Starting with your knee straight and toes toward the ceiling, slide your heel toward your buttocks. Bend as far as you can comfortably.
- Slowly lower your leg back to a straight position.
- Perform 5 to 10 repetitions 5 times/day.

Supine Hip Abduction (Figure 69.8)

- Lie on your back with legs together.
- Slide your leg out to the side, keeping your toes toward the ceiling.
- Go as far as you are able, keeping in mind that you might not be able to go very far initially.
- Slide your leg back toward the starting position.
- Perform 5 to 10 repetitions 5 times/day.

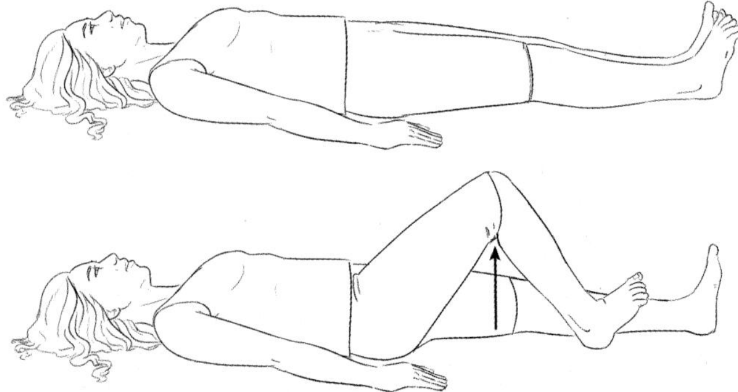

Figure 69.7 Illustration of heel slides.

© 2018 American Academy of Orthopaedic Surgeons

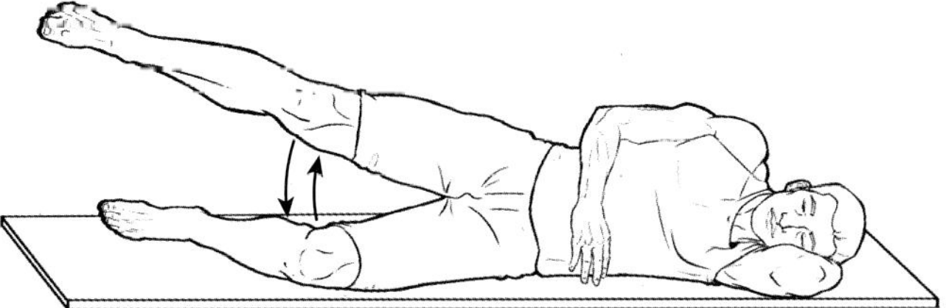

Figure 69.8 Illustration of supine hip abduction.

Post-Healing Phase (>8–12 Weeks)

Generally, patients are cleared at 12 weeks postoperatively or postinjury to advance weight bearing. The goals of rehabilita tion in this phase are restoration of ROM and strength of the limb, restoring normal gait patterns, and preparing the patients to return to the demands of their daily activities. In this phase, the patients' exercise program will progress to include progressive resistance exercises and closed-chain exercises. Advancement of gait from more supportive to less supportive assistive devices is often used as patients show strength gains. Continued abductor strengthening is important during this phase. Adjuncts such as pool therapy and/or use of a stationary bike are also useful during this phase.

Exercises for Healed Acetabular Fractures

- Muscle soreness and small, transient joint effusions are not uncommon as weight-bearing status is advanced. Patients should be advised that this is normal and resolves quickly.
- Apply ice for 15 to 20 minutes to any area of soreness or effusion to decrease inflammation.
- Notify your physical therapist immediately if any exercise results in severe pain.
- The following exercises are a progression from easiest to most difficult.

Standing Weight Shift (Figure 69.9)

- With arms relaxed at your side, stand with even weight on both feet.

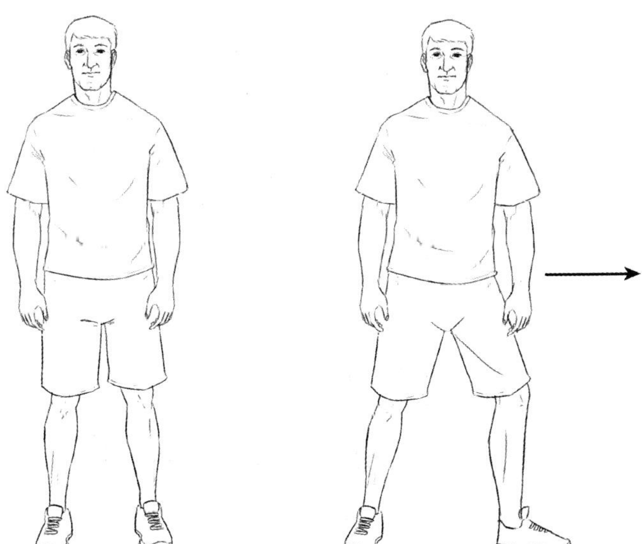

Figure 69.9 Illustration of standing weight shift.

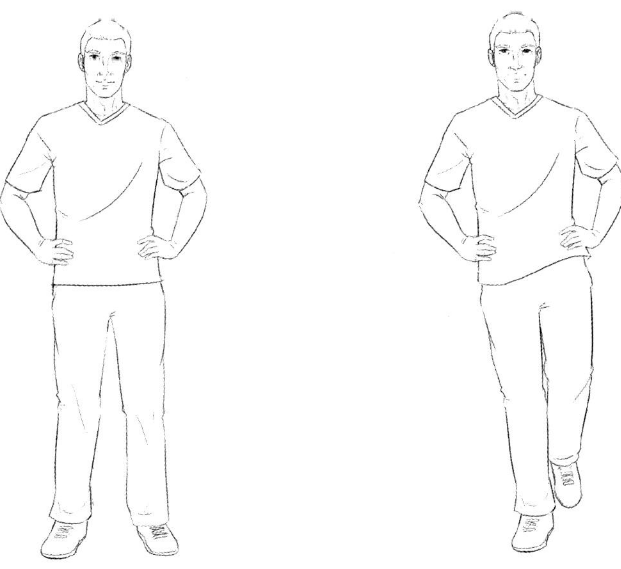

Figure 69.10 Illustration of single-limb stance.

- Slowly shift weight over your involved leg, keeping your foot flat.
- Shift as far as you are able, hold that position for 1 to 2 seconds, then slowly push back to the starting position with your involved leg.
- Perform 10 repetitions 3 times/day.

Single-Limb Stance (Figure 69.10)

- Holding on to a solid object, such as the kitchen counter with one hand, place the other on your hip.
- Slowly bend the knee of your uninvolved leg, putting all your weight on your involved leg.
- Be sure to keep your pelvis level.
- Hold for 5 seconds, then slowly lower your foot back to the floor.
- Perform 10 repetitions, 3 times/day.

Single-Limb Stance with Pelvic Lift (Figure 69.11)

- Holding on to a solid object with one hand, place the other hand on your hip. It is best to have your hand on the hip of your uninvolved leg.
- Hike your pelvis bone up toward your ribs, keeping your balance on your involved leg.
- Slowly lower your pelvis to the level position. Do not let your pelvis sag down.
- Perform 10 repetitions, 3 times/day.

Single-Leg Mini-Squats (Figure 69.12)

- Standing with your hands on your hips, stand on your involved leg. You may hold on to a sturdy surface, such as the kitchen counter, with one hand for balance as needed for safety.
- Bend your knee slowly, keeping your hips level and knee in line with your toes.
- Straighten your knee slowly, but do not let your knee pop into hyperextension.
- Perform 10 repetitions, 3 times/day.

© 2019 American Academy of Orthopaedic Surgeons

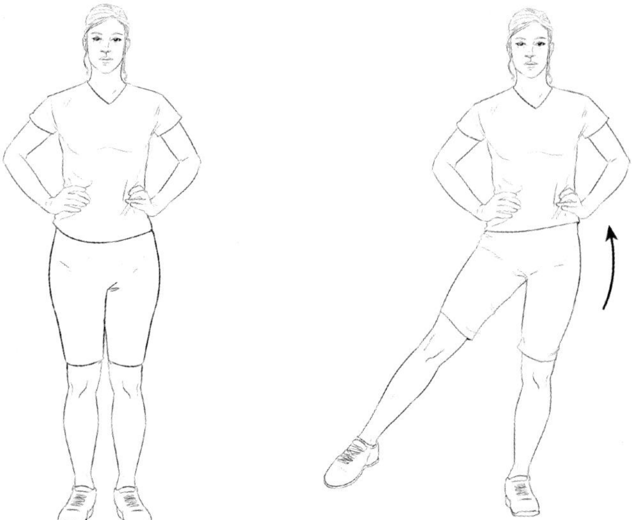

Figure 69.11 Illustration of single-limb stance with pelvic lift.

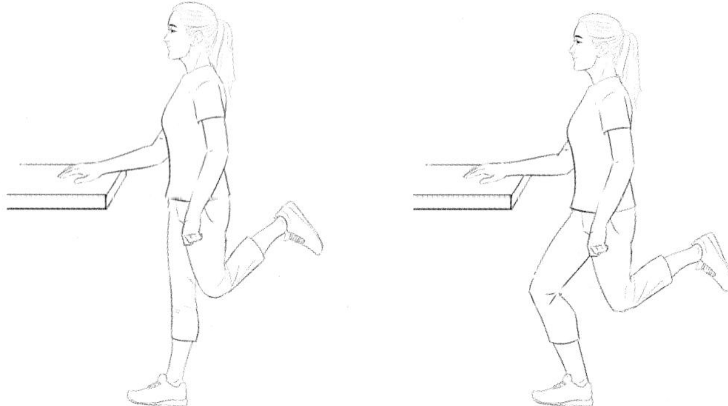

Figure 69.12 Illustration of single-leg mini-squats.

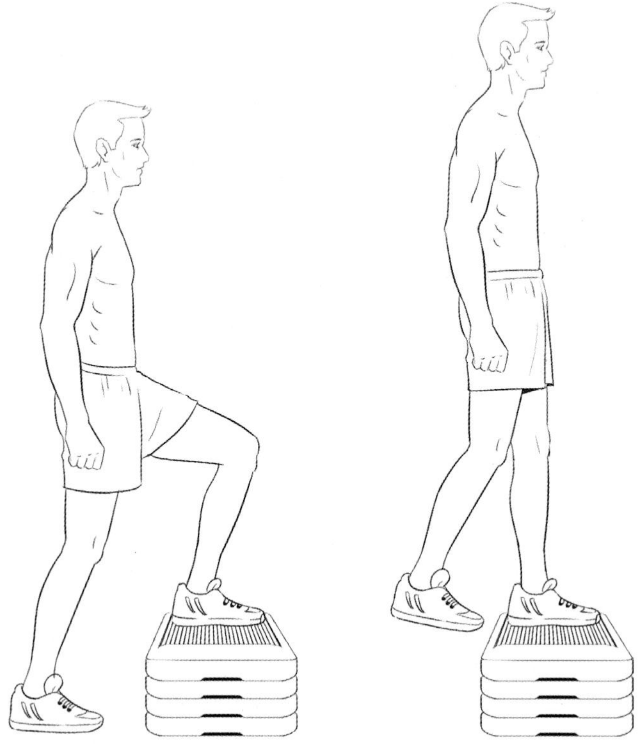

Figure 69.13 Illustration of step-ups.

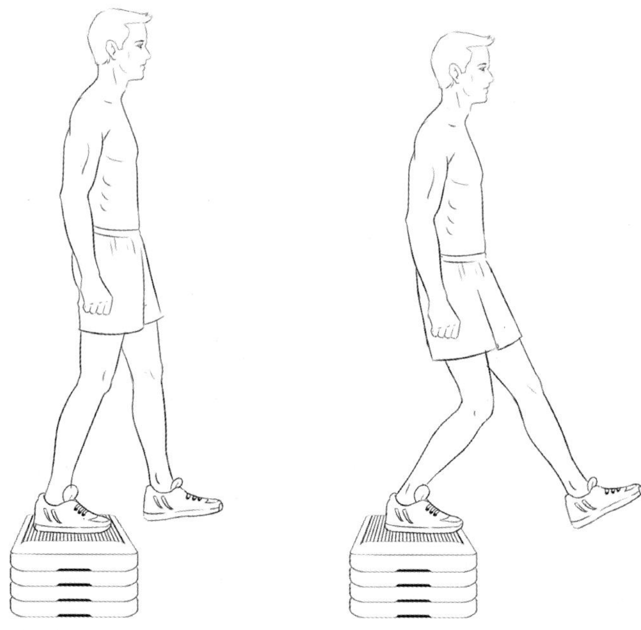

Figure 69.14 Illustration of step-downs.

Step-Ups (Figure 69.13)

- Place your involved leg on a step.
- Step up slowly, keeping your pelvis level until your knee is straight.
- Slowly bend your knee, returning your foot to the starting position.
- Start with this exercise by holding on with 2 hands, then progress to 1-hand support on the uninvolved side, then finally, to no-hand support.
- Perform 10 repetitions, 3 times/day.

Step-Downs (Figure 69.14)

- Stand on a step. Keep your involved foot on the step.
- Slowly step down with the uninvolved leg. Keep the pelvis level and knee in line with your toes.
- Push back up with your involved leg and bring your foot back up to the step.
- As with step-ups, this exercise can be progressed from 2-hand support, to 1, then no-hand support.
- Perform 10 repetitions, 3 times/day.

All exercises start with 10 repetitions but should be progressed in 3 to 5 repetition increments until reaching 20 repetitions.

CLINICAL PEARLS

- Both the obturator nerve and femoral nerve are at risk during anterior surgical approaches. Excessive retraction during an ilioinguinal approach or anterior intrapelvic approach may result in injury to these nerves. Even a transient femoral nerve palsy makes it difficult for the patient to extend the knee and can significantly increase recovery

 © 2018 American Academy of Orthopaedic Surgeons

time after surgery. Similarly, obturator nerve injury may result in abductor weakness.

- Acetabular fractures result in weakness of the hip abductors due to injury. This is often worsened by retraction or release of the abductor muscles during posterior or extensile approaches. The surgeon should attempt to minimize injury to the abductor muscles, as this may result in prolonged recovery.
- Heterotopic ossification occurs frequently in the gluteus minimus, as it is adjacent to the acetabulum and often injured with posterior wall and column fractures and posterior hip dislocations. Excision of injured muscle at the time of surgery helps to reduce the risk of heterotopic ossification.
- Patients may find performing their exercises in front of a mirror easier at first. Exercising with visual feedback can help patients know that their limbs and pelvis are in the desired position.
- Patients who are diligent in performing their home exercise program while healing are generally able to return to ambulation without an assistive device with a normal or near normal gait pattern in approximately 12 to 14 weeks after surgery. This time frame may be longer in older patients or those with concomitant injuries. Beyond 12 weeks, patients are no longer restricted and may pursue more advanced activities (e.g., swimming and biking) based on their confidence and comfort. Patients should be counseled that full recovery often requires 9 to 12 months.

BIBLIOGRAPHY

Borrelli J Jr, Ricci WM, Anglen JO, Gregush R, Engsberg J: Muscle strength recovery and its effects on outcome after open reduction and internal fixation of acetabular fractures. *J Orthop Trauma* 2006;20(6):388–951.

Kubota M, Uchida K, Kokubo Y, et al: Changes in gait pattern and hip muscle strength after open reduction and internal fixation of acetabular fracture. *Arch Phys Med Rehabil* 2012;93(11):2015–2021.

Letournel, E, Judet, R: *Fractures of the Acetabulum,* Springer Berlin Heidelberg, 1993.

Norkin C, Levangie P: *Joint Structure and Function: A Comprehensive Analysis,* ed 4. Philadelphia, PA, F. A. Davis, 2005.

© [illegible] American Academy of Orthopaedic Surgeons

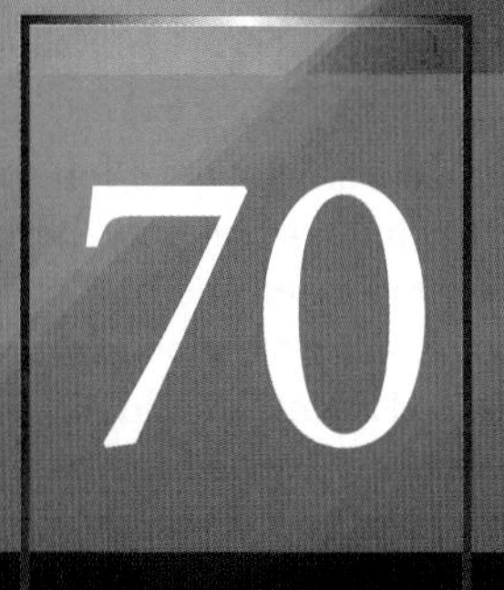

70 Rehabilitation After Pelvic Ring Injury

Richard D. Wilson, MD, MS, Michelle Kenny, MS, PT, and Heather A. Vallier, MD

INTRODUCTION

Pelvic ring injuries are a common occurrence. Low-energy injuries, frequent after falls from a standing height, are seen in older patients. However, injuries from a high-energy mechanism affect patients of all ages and can result in various fracture patterns, depending on the magnitude and direction of the injury forces. Treatment is based on fracture location and associated displacement and instability. It follows that activity limitations and other aspects of the rehabilitative process would be determined by these features as well.

CLASSIFICATION

The Young-Burgess classification, based on force vectors, is used to describe pelvic ring injuries and to determine associated injuries, transfusion requirements, and type of treatment. Most fractures fall into one of three types: lateral compression, anteroposterior compression, and vertical shear patterns. Lateral compression injuries are most common. These result from force applied to the lateral aspect of the pelvis and greater trochanter. A fall directly onto the lateral aspect of the hip and a motor vehicle collision with side impact are two frequent mechanisms of injury. One or more pubic ramus fracture may occur, and the sacrum is fractured and compressed on the side of the force. Unless the posterior pelvis ring is completely fractured and displaced, these injuries are treated nonoperatively. However, with high-energy injuries, the posterior pelvis on the side of impact can be unstable with sacral and/or iliac fractures. Less commonly, the contralateral hemipelvis can be affected, resulting in anterior sacroiliac disruption. Surgery would be indicated for such injuries in order to reduce the fracture, restoring rotational alignment of the pelvis (Figure 70.1). Fixation also reduces pain and maintains alignment until the fractures are healed.

Anteroposterior compression injuries occur when a force is directed through the anterior and/or posterior aspects of the pelvis. These result in symphyseal disruption, and can cause complete sacroiliac dislocations unilaterally or bilaterally when the force is very large. Injuries with wide displacement of the posterior pelvic ring may be associated with life-threatening hemorrhage from the sacral venous plexus and rarely from adjacent arteries. Initial treatment includes expeditious pelvic reduction with a sheet or binder, which promotes blood clot formation in most cases. Surgical treatment is indicated for wide symphyseal disruptions in association with partial or complete sacroiliac injuries (Figure 70.2). If the posterior ring is not injured, surgery is not indicated.

Vertical shear pelvic ring fractures occur when an axial force is directed through one side of the pelvis, for example, when a patient falls from a height and lands on one leg, or when a motorcycle crash occurs and force is directed through one leg. The anterior ring is disrupted through the pubic rami or symphysis, and the posterior ring is disrupted with sacroiliac dislocation or fracture dislocation, resulting in cephalad displacement of the injured hemipelvis. Surgery is indicated to restore pelvic ring alignment, to provide stability and pain relief, and to promote mobility from bed.

SURGICAL TREATMENT

Indications and Contraindications

Most high-energy lateral compression, anteroposterior compression, and vertical shear injuries are treated surgically. Surgery is generally indicated to restore pelvic ring alignment and to provide stability, relieve pain, and promote mobility from

Dr. Vallier or an immediate family member serves as a board member, owner, officer, or committee member of the American Academy of Orthopaedic Surgeons, the Center for Orthopaedic Trauma Advancement, the Journal of Orthopaedic Trauma, *and the Orthopaedic Trauma Association. Dr. Wilson or an immediate family member serves as a paid consultant to SPR Therapeutics; has received research or institutional support from SPR Therapeutics, and serves as a board member, owner, officer, or committee member of the Association of Academic Psychiatrists. Neither Dr. Kenny nor any immediate family member has received anything of value from or has stock or stock options held in a commercial company or institution related directly or indirectly to the subject of this article.*

© 2018 American Academy of Orthopaedic Surgeons

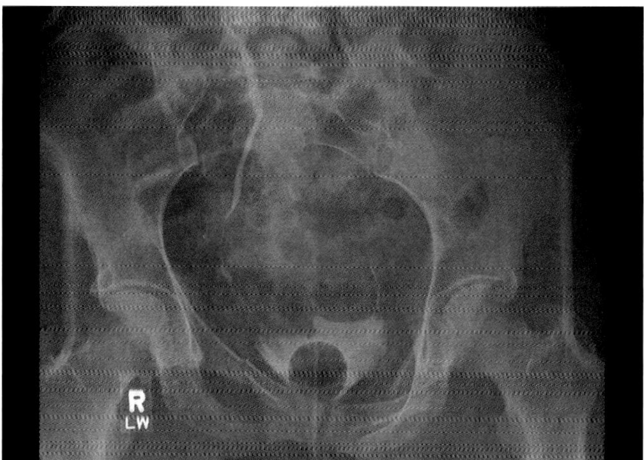

Figure 70.1 Radiograph of a lateral compression pelvic ring injury. Force directed through the right hemipelvis in a T bone motor vehicle collision generates bilateral ramus fractures and a right sacrum fracture, with internal rotation deformity of the right side and external rotation deformity of the left side. Surgery is indicated to improve alignment and to provide stability.

bed. Various procedures may be indicated based on the location and displacement of the fractures; the age, habitus, and functionality of the patient; the quality of the bone; and the presence of open fractures and/or degloving wounds. Pelvic ring injuries may be treated with open reduction and internal fixation (ORIF) anteriorly, laterally, or posteriorly. Percutaneous techniques are also commonly employed for both anterior and posterior ring fractures. Contraindications to surgery would include severe underlying medical illness or life-threatening head injury that precludes general anesthesia.

Open Reduction and Internal Fixation of the Anterior Pelvic Ring

ORIF for the anterior ring is recommended for anteroposterior compression or vertical shear injuries that have displacement of

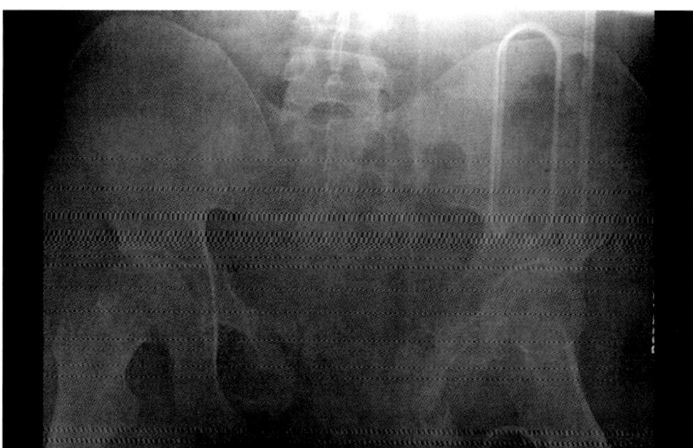

Figure 70.2 Radiograph of an anteroposterior compression pelvic ring injury. Symphysis disruption and left sacroiliac dislocation can be associated with massive bleeding. This injury is treated surgically to control bleeding and to improve pelvic alignment and stability.

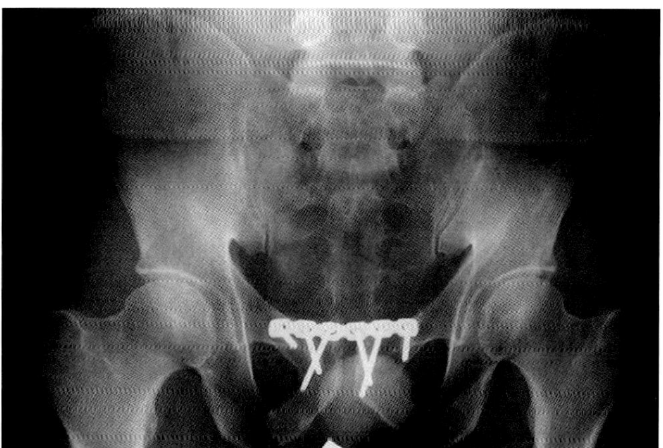

Figure 70.3 Radiograph showing plate fixation of a symphysis disruption. Ambulation is limited for 8 to 12 weeks. Lifting or abdominal exercises are avoided for approximately 8 weeks to permit soft-tissue healing and muscle recovery.

the pubic symphysis (Figure 70.3). A Pfannenstiel exposure is performed. The rectus raphe is divided in the midline, and the rectus tendons are elevated from the rami, but not detached. The pubic symphysis is reduced, and plate fixation is placed. Often, tears in the rectus muscle or insertions are present; care should be taken to repair these after the fracture is reduced and stabilized. Bladder ruptures may also be present, which should be addressed with bladder repair by urologists or general trauma surgeons once the fracture has been reduced and stabilized. Layered repair of the rectus raphe, along with the dermal and epidermal tissues, is then performed. Lifting and abdominal exercises that would strain the injured and healing rectus should be avoided for approximately 8 weeks.

Anterior External Fixation

Another way to reduce and stabilize the anterior pelvic ring is with external fixation. Anterior pelvic external fixation may be indicated as a supplement for posterior ring fixation in patients who have lateral compression injuries and multiple pubic rami fractures. External fixation could also be used as an alternative to symphyseal plating in patients with open pelvis fractures in order to minimize the risk of infection. Pins are placed in the ileum using radiographic guidance. Most often, one pin is placed on each side, and reduction maneuvers can be performed by manipulating these pins to improve pelvis alignment. Anterior bars are placed to connect the pins. The external fixator may be left in place for 6 to 12 weeks depending on the severity of the injury and the need for added stability. Pins placed in the anterior inferior ileum prevent upright sitting, while pins placed in the lateral ileum permit sitting upright (Figure 70.4).

Percutaneous Fixation of the Posterior Pelvic Ring

Percutaneous reduction and fixation of the posterior pelvic ring with iliosacral screws is the most common surgical treatment for unstable posterior fractures. This technique is performed in the supine position, as are symphyseal plating and external fixation.

© 2010 American Academy of Orthopaedic Surgeons

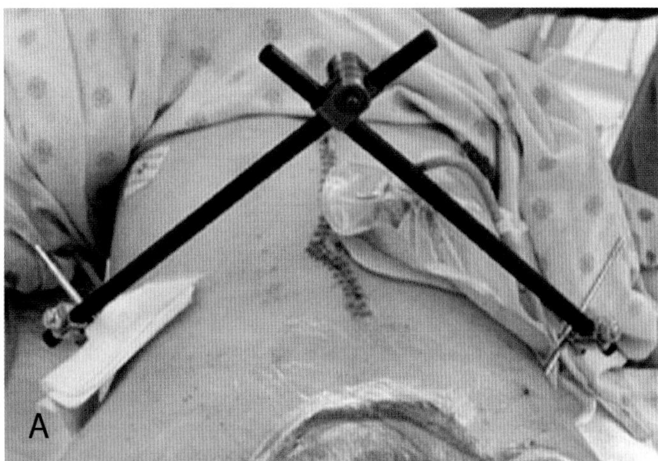

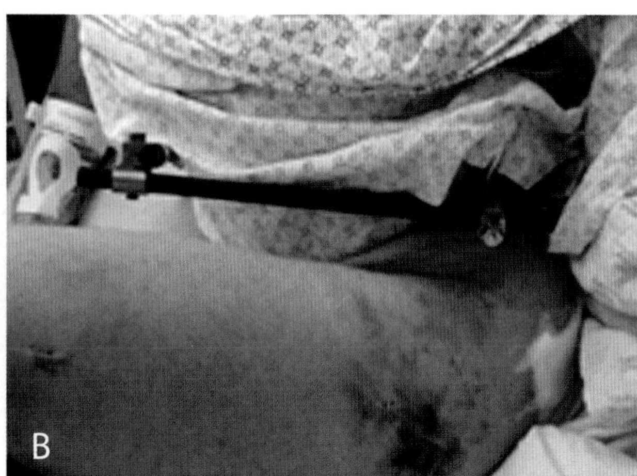

Figure 70.4 Photographs of external fixation for treatment of pelvic ring fracture. **A**, Pins are placed in the lateral ileum with bars over the abdomen. **B**, Patient is able to sit upright with lateral ileum pins.

Multiplanar radiography is used to insert a guidewire into the first and or second sacral segment to facilitate cannulated screw placement. Such screws are used to treat the posterior injuries associated with lateral compression, anteroposterior compression, and vertical shear fractures (Figure 70.5). Care must be taken to scrutinize bone and implant position to avoid iatrogenic injury to nerves from the lumbosacral plexus. Displaced posterior ring injuries, especially vertical shear patterns, often are associated with lumbosacral plexus injuries, generating deficits on the side of fracture displacement.

Open Reduction and Internal Fixation of the Posterior Pelvic Ring

Open reduction of the posterior pelvic ring is recommended infrequently. Indications would include unusual anatomic variants that preclude placement of percutaneous iliosacral screws. Some complex pelvis ring fractures may also have adjacent lower lumbar fractures of dislocations. These patients may be best served with lumbopelvic fixation. This technique is generally undertaken by spine surgeons and orthopaedic trauma surgeons working together, with the patient in the prone position. Implants may include lumbar and/or sacral pedicle screws, iliac bolts, and iliosacral screws. A mechanically robust construct is achieved; however, surgical times and associated hemorrhage are increased, and the risk of wound complication or soft-tissue irritation is moderately high (Figure 70.6).

COMPLICATIONS

Many complications may occur in the post-acute care phase for those with pelvic ring fractures. The high-energy injury that causes many pelvic ring fractures typically results in comorbid injuries, often in multiple organ systems. The risks for complications and mortality are most associated with the severity of injury and associated injuries rather than the stability of the pelvic ring fracture. Not only is it necessary to be vigilant for typical postoperative complications for those who undergo

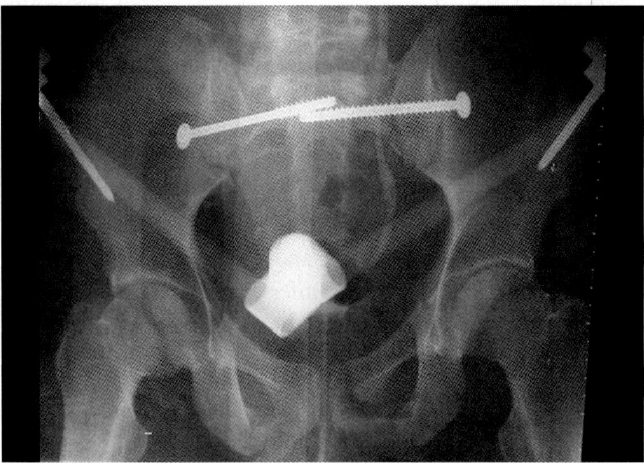

Figure 70.5 Radiograph showing iliosacral screw fixation of bilateral sacral fractures used in conjunction with anterior external fixation to stabilize this pelvic ring injury.

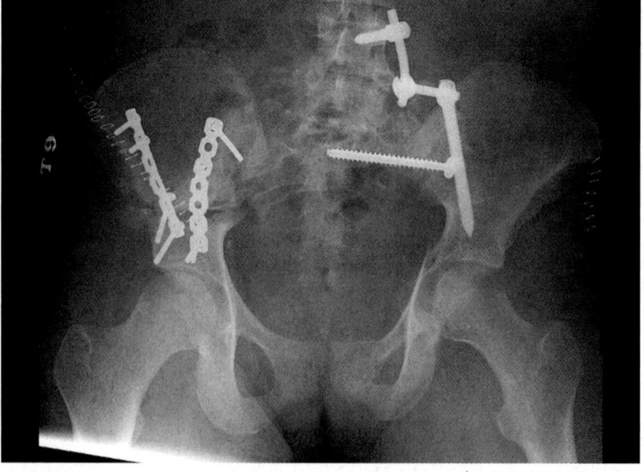

Figure 70.6 Radiograph showing lumbopelvic fixation securing lumbosacral disruption, on the left side of this example. Open reduction and plate fixation of the right ileum was also performed.

© 2018 American Academy of Orthopaedic Surgeons

surgical repair, there are additional complications associated with pelvic ring fractures, in particular. The complications relevant to the postacute phase of care will be focused on here.

Skin

Many risks to the skin exist after pelvic ring fracture. The immobility associated with recovery increases the possibility of pressure sores at the sacrum and heels due to the time spent supine, at the ischia from time sitting, and for sores related to orthoses, casts, or splints required for treatment or mobility. The ability to avoid pressure sores is dependent on frequently turning the patient, positioning properly, managing bowel and bladder incontinence, optimizing nutrition, and performing suitable inspection. Surgical wounds and pin sites from external fixators also need appropriate care and frequent inspection to reduce occurrence of infection. In spite of these efforts, many surgical wounds may require repeated débridement and vacuum closure devices to achieve healing.

Genitourinary

Bladder and urethral trauma are commonly sustained from injuries that involve pelvic ring disruption; thus, management of acute injuries, such as bladder or urethral disruption, will be guided by urologists. Urinary retention is a frequently encountered complication in the postacute phase due to pain, trauma from the injury or catheterization, bladder overdistension, neurologic injury, and pharmaceuticals (particularly opioid analgesics). The initial management is bladder decompression by catheterization, with urologic consultation when the catheter is unable to be advanced due to the high risk of urethral and bladder injury associated with pelvic ring disruption. A urinalysis should be obtained to evaluate for bladder infection, as risk will be high in those who underwent catheterization during acute hospitalization and had infection treated. Following bladder decompression, serial postvoid residuals should be obtained to ensure adequate bladder emptying. The value indicating persistent retention is controversial, but should be less than 150 mL on multiple occasions to indicate adequate voiding. If a spontaneous void has not occurred within 6 to 8 hours or if bladder fullness is perceived, the bladder should be emptied via clean intermittent catheterization (CIC). For most, urinary retention will be temporary, and can be treated with CIC until resolution. Those with slow recovery of adequate voiding will need to undergo training for self-catheterization, particularly those with prostatic hypertrophy or injury to the sacral or peripheral nerves. If function or preference prevents intermittent catheterization, then indwelling catheterization and follow-up with urologic specialists should be planned. Special consideration should be paid to men who are at risk for concurrent prostatic hypertrophy that may require co-treatment with α-adrenergic antagonists.

Deep Venous Thrombosis and Pulmonary Embolism

There is a high risk for deep venous thrombosis (DVT) following pelvic ring disruption due to immobility, potential for vascular injury, and coagulopathy. While the greatest risk is at the time of injury and immediately following, risk remains elevated for days and weeks following the injury. Without a contraindication, all patients who have mobility impairment should receive chemoprophylaxis with aspirin, low-dose heparin, or low-molecular-weight heparin. Mechanical prophylaxis by graduated compression stockings or intermittent pneumatic compression should be used in conjunction with chemoprophylaxis, or as sole prophylaxis in those whom chemoprophylaxis is contraindicated. It is not recommended to place vena caval filters for primary prevention, even in those who have a contraindication to chemoprophylaxis. There is not a consensus on duration of treatment, although those who undergo nonoperative care should be treated until mobilizing adequately (e.g., ambulating 50 feet with or without a device). Those who are treated surgically may receive prophylaxis for a longer duration. Screening for DVT by Doppler ultrasound is not recommended, although those with symptoms of increased leg edema, leg discoloration, or increased leg pain should undergo evaluation. For those with dyspnea, chest pain, or acute hypoxia, an urgent evaluation for pulmonary embolism should be considered.

Neurologic Injury

Nerve injury is common with pelvic ring disruption (10%–15%), particularly those with sacral or sacroiliac disruption or with vertical shear injury (near 50%). Nerve injuries may occur by transection, compression, avulsion, or traction. The injuries are often multiple and can affect the lumbosacral plexus, cauda equina, or peripheral nerves. It is imperative that all patients with a pelvic ring disruption undergo a full neurologic examination, including perineal sensory testing, to evaluate for sacral level lesions that carry risk for genitourinary dysfunction. When a neurologic injury is suspected, an electrodiagnostic study can aid in diagnosing and prognosticating the extent of neurologic injury and the likelihood of recovery. Many will have gait abnormalities associated with neurologic injury that may require an orthotic prescription, such as an ankle-foot orthosis to treat weakness of ankle dorsiflexors. Some patients will experience recovery of nerve injuries, while others will have a permanent disability.

Pain

Pain is nearly universal in this patient group. Adequate pain control is necessary for patients to mobilize early and to reap the greatest benefit during rehabilitation. The extensive nature of injuries associated with high-energy trauma, frequently including nerve damage, can be associated with a greater severity of pain that will require higher doses and a larger variety of analgesics. Balance must be sought between pain control and medication side effects, particularly side effects of opiate analgesics that can complicate recovery. Multimodal analgesia (MMA) is a comprehensive approach that reflects the numerous neurophysiologic pain pathways and neurochemical pain mediators involved in the perception of pain. The strategy combines analgesics with differing mechanisms of

© 2018 American Academy of Orthopaedic Surgeons

action to effectively control pain, and may also allow a reduction in the dose of each individual analgesic. Regimens often include acetaminophen and nonsteroidal anti-inflammatory drugs (NSAIDs), which may have greater efficacy when used together versus separate, adjunctive medications such as gabapentinoids, and opiate analgesics as needed. For those with pain that is inadequately controlled with MMA, it might be necessary to prescribe long-acting opiate analgesics. The use of long-acting opiate analgesics may achieve a lower overall narcotic dose for those in severe pain. Many examples of MMA protocols have been described in the literature, although protocols are best implemented with input from the multidisciplinary health care team of providers. Careful evaluation of the risk and benefit of each analgesic for each individual is also necessary to reduce morbidity related to treatment.

Closed Head Injury

It is estimated that 20% to 45% of those with pelvic ring disruption will also sustain a closed head injury. Closed head injuries, with resultant injury to the brain, can be a cause of disability with poor long-term outcomes if left untreated. For some, the brain injury will cause greater disability and will take higher priority during the recovery period than the pelvic ring disruption. For others, the brain injury will be less severe; however, even mild brain injuries can cause long-term sequelae that may prevent return to prior levels of functioning. It is important for all patients with pelvic ring disruption to have a careful cognitive examination to evaluate for injury to the brain. If a brain injury is suspected, appropriate treatment with a speech and language pathologist and a brain injury specialist should be initiated.

Mood

Physical injury is associated with psychological distress that can affect recovery and long-term outcomes. The prevalence of mood disorders after physical injury is high, affecting more than 40% of trauma survivors. Development of a mood disorder after a physical injury may not be associated with severity of injury, and all survivors of physical injury are at risk. Mood disorders that are common in trauma survivors include depression, anxiety, acute stress disorder, and adjustment disorder. As recovery continues to later phases, survivors may be diagnosed with posttraumatic stress disorder (PTSD). The treatment team should be vigilant for symptoms such as insomnia, anorexia, anxiety, poor participation, poor concentration, hypervigilance, and sadness. Identification of symptoms is imperative to diagnosis, implementing proper treatment, and offering appropriate care by mental health professionals.

POSTOPERATIVE REHABILITATION

Introduction

It is important that all who sustain a pelvic ring fracture undergo some form of rehabilitation therapy, with the goals of reducing disability and hastening return to the level of prior functioning. The severity of comorbid injuries, functional limitations, and amount of social support will determine the level at which rehabilitation is delivered. It is preferable that rehabilitation start as soon as possible, often postoperative or posttrauma day 1. Those with less severe injuries, greater function, and adequate social support will be able to undergo rehabilitation in the community. Many who experience pelvic ring disruptions will require rehabilitation in an inpatient setting prior to discharge to the community.

Table 70.1 WEIGHT-BEARING RESTRICTIONS AFTER PELVIC RING FRACTURE

Injury and Treatment	Weight Bearing
Stable, nonoperative lateral compression or anteroposterior compression injury	Progressive weight bearing as tolerated
Unilateral posterior injury with fixation for lateral compression, anteroposterior compression, or vertical shear injury	Touch down weight bearing for 8–12 weeks. Twelve weeks for pure dislocations (vs. fracture–dislocations) and medically compromised patients or fractures with severe initial displacement.
Bilateral posterior injury, unilateral posterior fixation	Pivot transfer on the nonoperative side, touch down weight bearing on the stabilized side for 12 weeks.
Bilateral posterior injury, bilateral posterior fixation	Bed-to-chair transfers for 10–12 weeks

Note: Avoid straight leg raises for 8 weeks on the injured side(s).

Rehabilitation Protocol

All patients who sustain a pelvic ring disruption will have impairments in mobility. The degree to which mobility is affected is based on three factors (Table 70.1):

1. Severity and type of injury (lateral compression, anteroposterior compression, vertical, or posterior)
2. Nonoperative injury versus injury requiring fixation
3. Restrictions in weight bearing, as dictated by the orthopaedist (weight bearing as tolerated, non–weight bearing unilaterally or bilaterally, or partial weight bearing [touch down weight bearing])

Acute Hospital Stay (Hospital Admission Until Medically Able to Tolerate Rehabilitation Therapies)

- Goal: To promote range of motion (ROM) within pain tolerance, early mobility out of bed
- Maintain ROM within pain tolerance: hip/knee flexion in supine position
- Mobilization: Out of bed to chair day 1 while maintaining weight-bearing restrictions using a walker or transfer board. Progress to ambulation as tolerated, based on weight-bearing restrictions.

© 2018 American Academy of Orthopaedic Surgeons

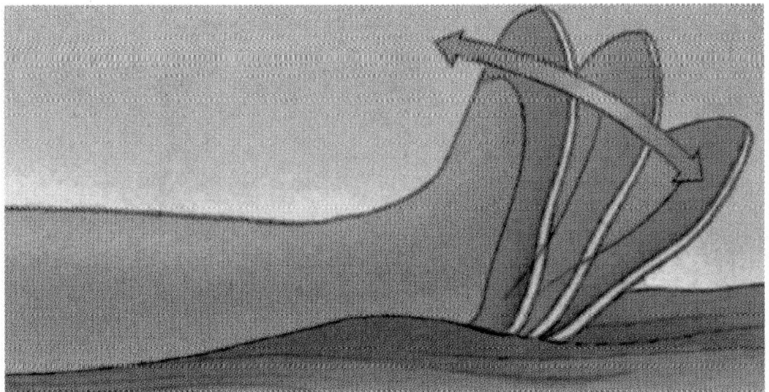

Figure 70.7 Illustration of ankle pump exercise.

- Therapeutic Exercises
  - Ankle pumps (Figure 70.7; 3 sets of 10 repetitions, 1 time per day)
  - Gluteal sets (Figure 70.8; 3 sets of 10 repetitions, 1 time per day)
  - Quad sets (Figure 70.9; 3 sets of 10 repetitions, 1 time per day)
  - Long arc quads (Figure 70.10; 3 sets of 10 repetitions, 1 time per day)

Acute/Subacute Rehabilitation (from Admission Until Able to Discharge to Home)

- *Goal:* To prepare for discharge to the community within weight-bearing restrictions with adequate pain control to allow for strengthening and mobility. To encourage a high level of overall body conditioning; general deconditioning at baseline will slow functional recovery.
- Avoid flat supine and side lying if these make the patient uncomfortable. Initially, when lying supine, a wedge should be used to elevate the head and shoulders along with a bolster to keep the hips and knees flexed. Several times each day, remove the bolster from the lower limbs to encourage full knee extension to neutral as well as hip extension to neutral.
- *Ambulation:* 3-point gait with walker or axillary crutches. Using a device with bilateral upper limbs promotes decreased pressure through lower limbs and pelvis.
- *Lower extremity orthosis:* Assess patient for lower-limb orthosis if nerve injury is present. Foot drop should be corrected prior to gait training.
- *Stair climbing:* Nonalternating steps using bilateral upper limbs on rails or 1 rail or crutch
- Therapeutic exercises
- Continue those listed for the acute hospital stay and add the following:
  - Heel slides (Figure 70.11; 3 sets of 10 repetitions, 1 time per day)
  - Short arc quads (Figure 70.12; 3 sets of 10 repetitions, 1 time per day)
  - Gentle hip abduction/adduction with gravity eliminated (Figure 70.13, 3 sets of 10 repetitions, 1 time per day)

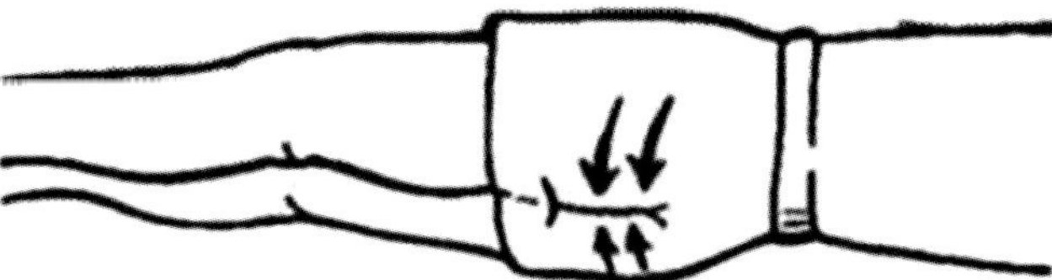

Figure 70.8 Illustration of gluteal sets.

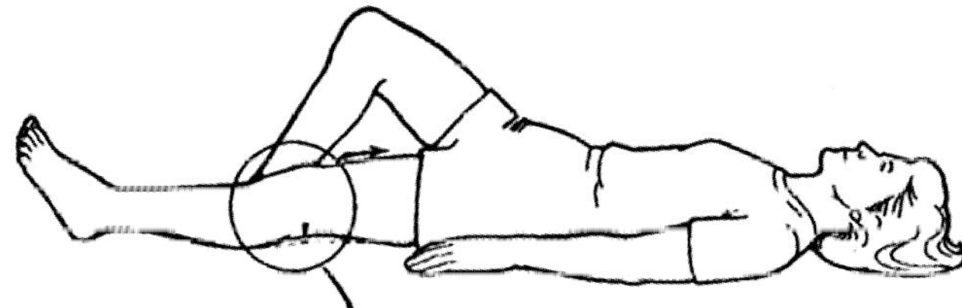

Figure 70.9 Illustration of quad sets.

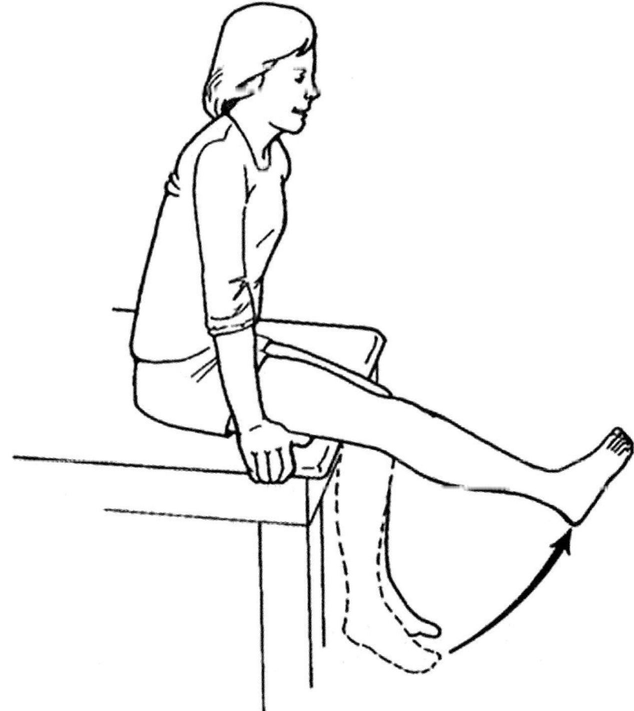

Figure 70.10 Illustration of long arc quad sets.

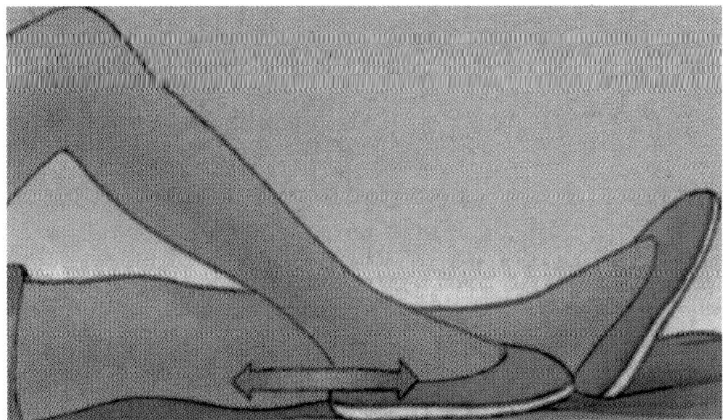

Figure 70.11 Illustration of heel slide exercise.

© 2018 American Academy of Orthopaedic Surgeons

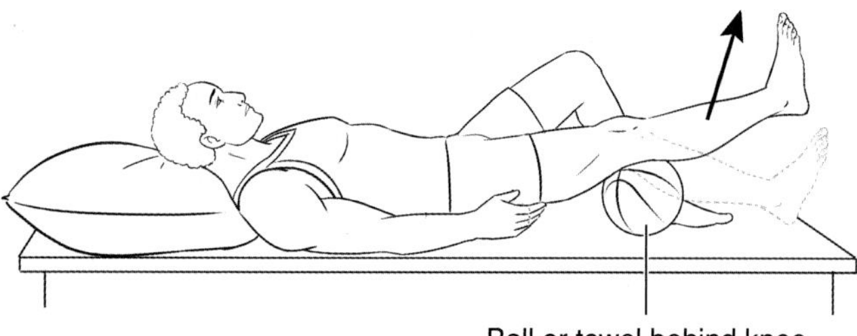

Figure 70.12 Illustration of short arc quads.

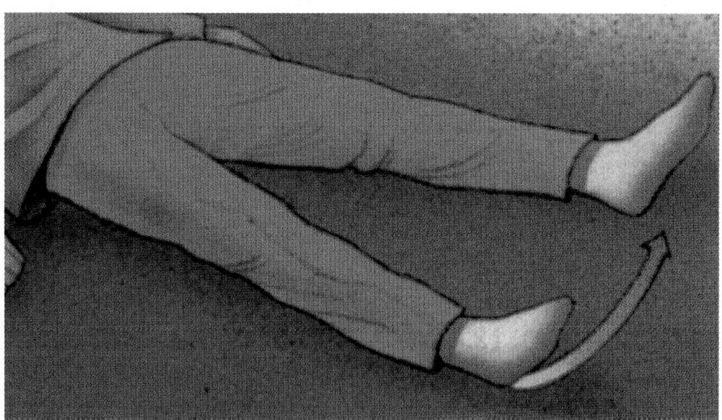

Figure 70.13 Illustration of gentle hip abduction/adduction with gravity eliminated.

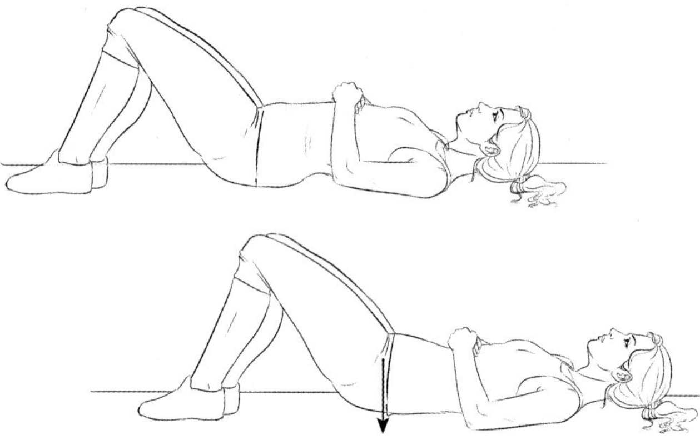

Figure 70.14 Illustration of pelvic tilt.

- Mobility-Related Activities of Daily Living (MRADLs): Pelvic fractures affect MRADLs to the extent that the patient has weight-bearing restrictions and concomitant limitations in overall mobility. An occupational therapist should be consulted to address impairments.

Outpatient Rehabilitation (Community Discharge Until Achievement of Full Weight Bearing and Progression to Prior Functional State)

- *Goal:* To return to previous level of mobility as the pelvic injury heals while concurrently stabilizing the muscles surrounding the injury to reestablish pelvic rhythm and lumbar stability during gait. Depending on severity of injury, full functional recovery can exceed 12 months.

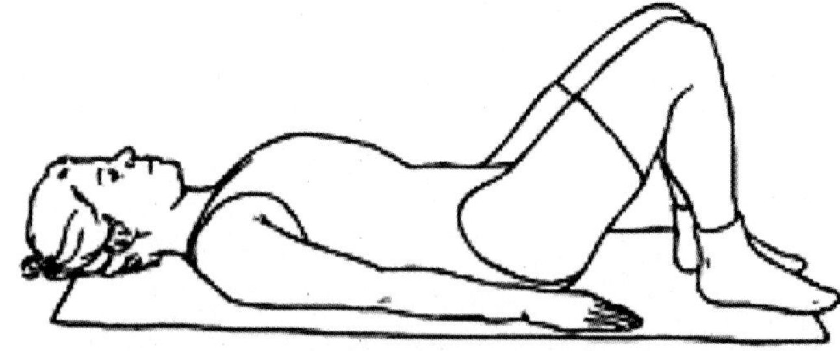

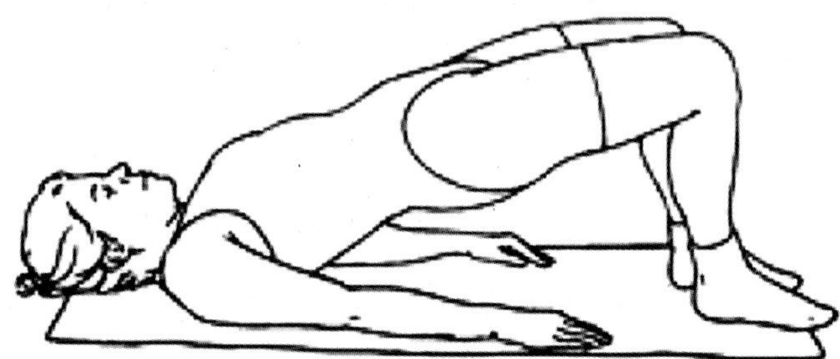

Figure 70.15 Illustration of bridge.

- Progression from bilateral device for ambulation to unilateral device (straight cane or axillary crutch on uninjured side) and stair climbing using alternating steps. Weight bearing is typically without restrictions at 12 weeks.
- The determinants of gait describe pelvic rotation in the transverse plane during swing, pelvic rotation in the frontal plane (slight lateral pelvic drop during swing), and lateral displacement of the pelvis over the support leg during stance.
- Therapeutic Exercises
  - Lumbar stabilization (Figures 70.14–70.17; pelvic tilt, bridge, prone-opposite arm/leg lifts, quadruped leg left with neutral spine)
  - Standing progression (Figures 70.18–70.21; balance, side stepping, step-ups, single leg stance, mini knee bends)
  - Adjuncts to strengthening and conditioning may include aquatic therapy

OUTCOMES

Following surgical treatment of pelvic ring injury, patients generally recover function and ambulatory capacity. Given the magnitude of these high-energy injuries, full recovery is generally lengthy and may take up to a year. Residual deficits are often related to associated injuries to other extremities and nerves of the lumbosacral plexus, which are in the zone of injury. Some level of pain, especially in the posterior pelvis, is common but does not preclude normal daily functions. However, work involving manual labor and high-level sports are often difficult. Given the proximity of the genitourinary organs, sexual activity may be compromised to a degree.

 © 2018 American Academy of Orthopaedic Surgeons

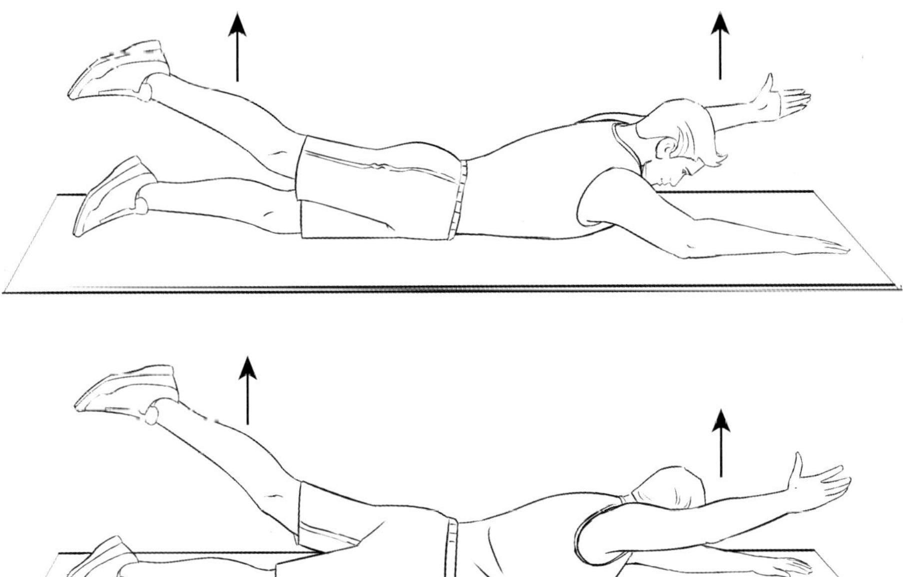

Figure 70.16 Illustration of prone-opposite arm/leg lifts.

Appropriate therapy restoring strength and flexibility emphasizing posture and mechanics can mitigate sequelae of these major injuries.

PEARLS

- Identification of mechanism of injury in conjunction with radiography will determine locations of mechanical instability of a pelvic fracture. This will guide treatment decision making (operative vs. nonoperative) and weight-bearing restrictions.
- Multidisciplinary care is essential in acute management of pelvic ring injury to address associated soft-tissue, urologic, gastrointestinal, and other system injuries. Multidisciplinary care expands to include the rehabilitation team as the fracture treatment plan is determined.
- Bladder dysfunction is common after pelvic ring disruption. Patients should be screened for bladder retention by serial postvoid residual measurements and appropriate management initiated for those with high volumes.
- Lumbosacral plexus injuries and other nerve injuries are common in association with sacral fractures and/or

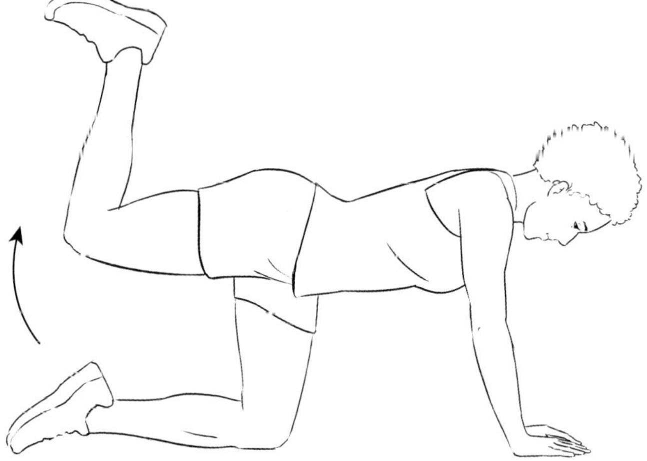

Figure 70.17 Illustration of quadruped leg lift with neutral spine.

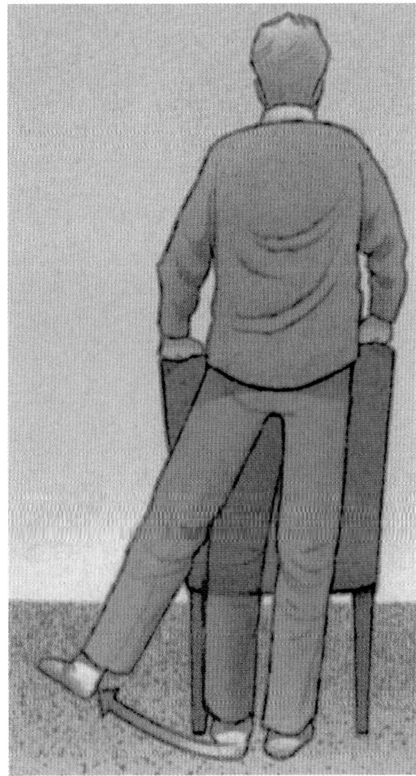

Figure 70.18 Illustration of side stepping. (Reproduced from OrthoInfo. © American Academy of Orthopaedic Surgeons. http://orthoinfo.aaos.org.)

© 2018 American Academy of Orthopaedic Surgeons

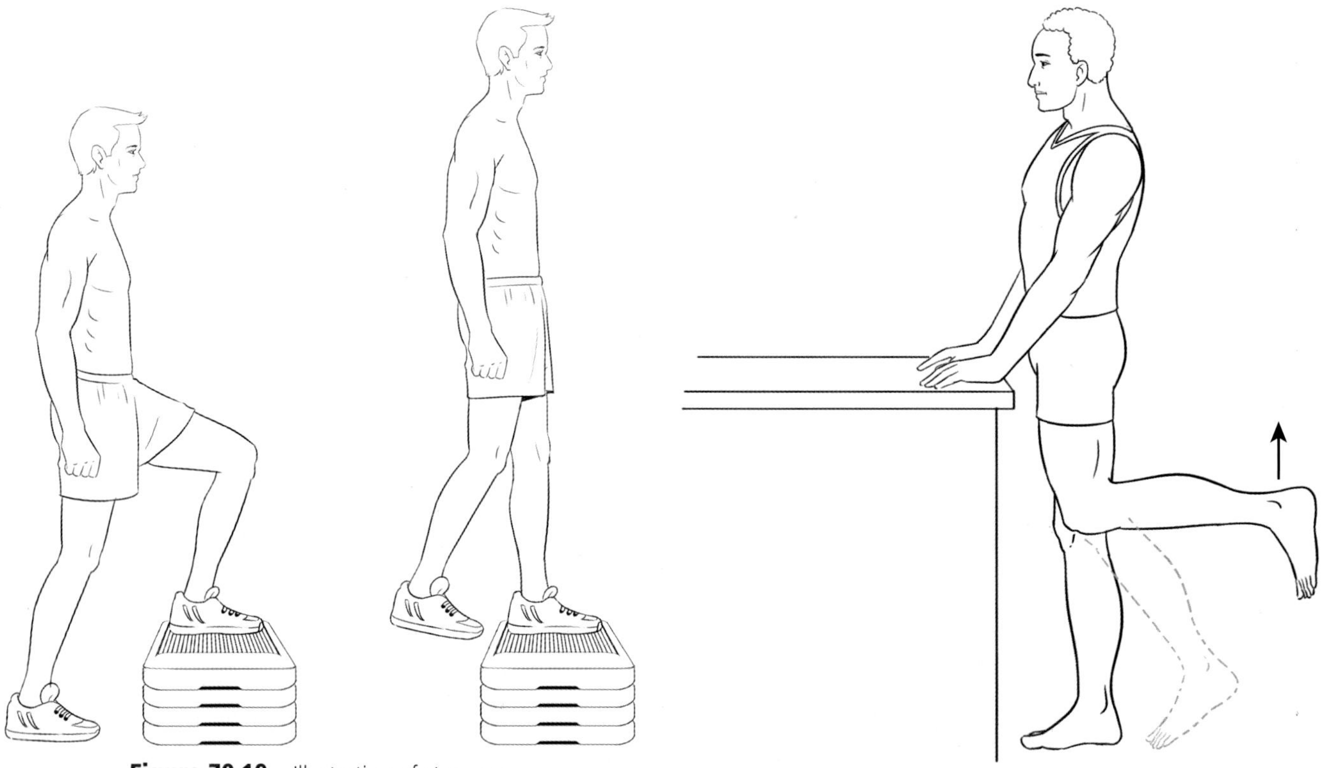

Figure 70.19 Illustration of step-ups.

Figure 70.20 Illustration of single-limb stance.

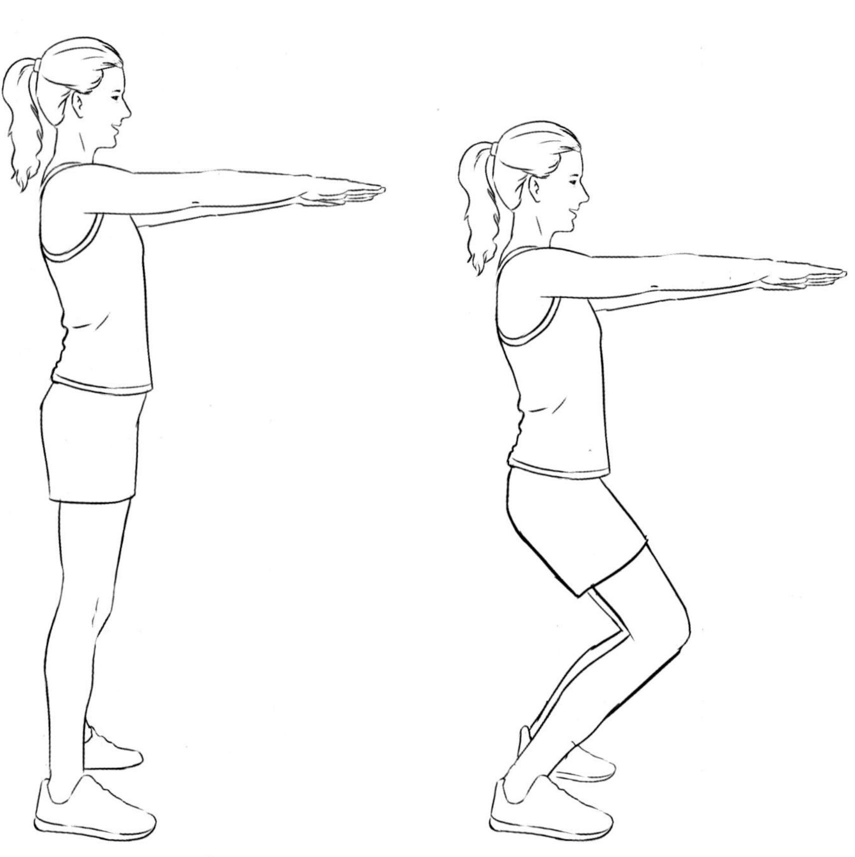

Figure 70.21 Illustration of mini knee bends.

© 2018 American Academy of Orthopaedic Surgeons

posterior pelvic displacement. Diagnosis and treatment, especially pain medications, should be expedited.

- Pain may be severe after pelvic ring disruption and can interfere with rehabilitation if not adequately controlled. Multiple classes of analgesics may be required to control pain while limiting side effects.
- Mood disorders often accompany injuries and can slow recovery. The health care team should be observant for symptoms of psychosocial distress such as insomnia, anorexia, anxiety, poor participation, poor concentration, hypervigilance, and sadness.
- Promote early mobility while maintaining weight bearing restrictions. Avoid flat supine positioning during rehabilitation.
- Restore normal gait during the outpatient phase of rehabilitation.

BIBLIOGRAPHY

Crichlow RJ, Andres PL, Morrison SM, Haley SM, Vrahas MS: Depression in orthopaedic trauma patients: prevalence and severity. *J Bone Joint Surg Am* 2006;88:1927–1933.

Dalal SA, Burgess AR, Siegel JH, Young JW, Brumback RJ, Poka A, Dunham CM, Gens D, Bathon H: Pelvic fracture in multiple trauma: classification by mechanism is key to pattern of organ injury, resuscitative requirements, and outcome. *J Trauma* 1989;29(7):981–1000; discussion 1000–1002.

Falck-Ytter Y, Francis CW, Johanson NA, et al: Prevention of VTE in orthopedic surgery patients: Antithrombotic Therapy and Prevention of Thrombosis, 9th ed: American College of Chest Physicians Evidence-Based Clinical Practice Guidelines. *Chest* 2012;141(2_suppl):e278S–e325S.

Gustavo Parreira J, Coimbra R, Rasslan S, Oliviera A, Fregoneze M, Mercadante M: The role of associated injuries on outcome of blunt trauma patients sustaining pelvic fractures. *Injury* 2000;31:677–682.

Huittinen VM, Slatis P: Fractures of the pelvis, trauma mechanism, types of injury and principles of treatment. *Acta Chir Scand* 1972;138:563–569.

Kurmis AP, Kurmis TP, O'Brien JX, Dalen T: The effect of nonsteroidal anti-inflammatory drug administration on acute phase fracture-healing: A review. *J Bone Joint Surg Am* 2012;94:815–823.

O'Donnell ML, Creamer M, Bryant RA, Schnyder U, Shalev A: Posttraumatic disorders following injury: an empirical and methodological review. *Clin Psy Rev* 2003;23:587–603.

Saunders JS, Inman VT, Eberhart HD: The major determinants in normal and pathological gait. *J Bone Joint Surg Am* 1953; 35A:543–558.

Sembler Soles GL, Lien J, Tornetta P 3rd: Nonoperative immediate weightbearing of minimally displaced lateral compression sacral fractures does not result in displacement. *J Orthop Trauma* 2012;26(10):563–567.

Tini PG, Wieser C, Zinn WM: The transitional vertebra of the lumbosacral spine: Its radiological classification, incidence, prevalence, and clinical significance. *Rheumatol Rehabil* 1977; 16:180–185.

Toker S, Hak DJ, Morgan SJ: Deep vein thrombosis prophylaxis in trauma patients. *Thrombosis* 2011;50:53–73.

© 2018 American Academy of Orthopaedic Surgeons

71 Proximal Femur Fractures: Neck, Intertrochanteric, and Subtrochanteric

Mark K. Solarz, MD, John J. Walker, PT, DPT, MBA, and Saqib Rehman, MD

INTRODUCTION

Hip fractures, to which the various fractures of the proximal femur are commonly referred, occur most commonly from low-energy mechanisms in the elderly population due to decreased bone mineral density. They also occur in younger populations from high-energy mechanisms such as motor vehicle accidents and falls from height. Management of such injuries depends on the fracture pattern as well as the baseline function of the individual. Equally if not more important as fracture management is the rehabilitation process, followed by aims to regain function in the injured limb and restore baseline ambulatory ability. It is commonly said that the elderly patient with a fractured hip will lose one level of mobility even after recovery. While there may be some truth in this, the goals of rehabilitation after a hip fracture, regardless of patient age, are early mobilization to prevent complications of recumbency, such as pressure ulcers, pneumonia, and deconditioning.

Hip fractures and their related comorbidities continue to be a significant burden on health care expenditures, and are predicted to continue increasing as our population ages. These fractures accounted for 20% of Medicare claims from 1986 to 2005, with 77% of those patients being female. Women, especially those of Caucasian race, account for a higher percentage of proximal femur fractures as a result of their increased risk of low bone mineral density.

Rehabilitation of patients with proximal femur fractures is frequently complicated by multiple medical comorbidities and/or malnutrition in the elderly, or associated traumatic injuries in the young patient. These clearly impact the course of rehabilitation, both early after management and later after discharge from the hospital. Mobilization of patients out of bed as soon as possible is paramount in both the elderly and the young patient, as decubiti, pneumonia, and related sequelae from recumbency can have both immediate and long-lasting effects. For instance, a patient with a successfully repaired hip may not be able to comfortably ambulate for months due to a heel decubitus.

The team caring for the elderly with proximal femur fracture should also evaluate reasons for the patient falling. Risk factors such as vestibular issues, blood pressure, cardiac issues, or osteoporosis prior to initiating the rehabilitation phase after surgery should be identified. Previous falls are accurate indicators of future falls. In the first year after initial fracture, there is a 6 to 20 times higher incidence of a new fracture; therefore, institution of fall prevention strategies is important in the overall management of these patients.

Challenges with the rehabilitation of patients with hip fractures are severalfold. In addition to the issues with treating elderly and polytrauma patients, hip fracture patients are at high risk for falls due to potential problems with balance, fatigue from anemia, abductor weakness, and syncope. Falls can lead to additional injuries, including intracranial bleeding in an anticoagulated patient. While most postoperative patients are allowed to weight bear as tolerated, in certain cases, there are restrictions to motion aimed at preventing postoperative dislocation or weight-bearing limitations to optimize fracture healing. Many patients either live alone or with elderly companions, and must learn how to perform basic activities of daily living (ADLs). The physical therapist and rehabilitation specialist are therefore in a position to make a difference not only with helping the patient regain hip strength, coordination, gait, and balance, but also to gain independence, safety, and overall well-being.

ANATOMY OF THE PROXIMAL FEMUR

The proximal femur can be divided into three anatomically distinct regions: the femoral neck, intertrochanteric, and

Dr. Rehman or an immediate family member is a member of a speakers' bureau or has made paid presentations on behalf of Synthes; has received nonincome support (such as equipment or services), commercially derived honoraria, or other non-research–related funding (such as paid travel) from Jaypee Medical Publishing; and serves as a board member, owner, officer, or committee member of the Orthopaedic Trauma Association and Orthopedic Clinics of North America. Neither of the following authors nor any immediate family member has received anything of value from or has stock or stock options held in a commercial company or institution related directly or indirectly to the subject of this article: Dr. Solarz and Dr. Walker.

© 2018 American Academy of Orthopaedic Surgeons

subtrochanteric regions. The femoral neck is located just distal to the femoral head and proximal to a line between the greater and lesser trochanters. Fractures of this region can be further divided into subcapital, transcervical, and basicervical, depending on the location of the fracture within the femoral neck. These fractures are intracapsular, making them particularly prone to nonunion in comparison to other proximal femur fractures. The major blood supply to the femoral head is the medial femoral circumflex artery and its tributary, the lateral epiphyseal artery, which travel retrograde along the femoral neck, making the femoral head prone to osteonecrosis with displaced fractures in this area.

The intertrochanteric region of the femoral metaphysis lies between the greater and lesser trochanters. There is a rich blood supply, unlike the femoral neck, leading to a lower rate of nonunion. There are typically four main parts, consisting of the greater and lesser trochanters, the femoral neck, and the femoral shaft. Intertrochanteric fractures range from a simple nondisplaced fracture through the intertrochanteric region to separation of all four parts. These fractures are either stable or unstable depending on the condition of the femoral calcar (posteromedial cortex) and the orientation of the fracture line. Those that exhibit reverse obliquity and subtrochanteric extension below the lesser trochanter are particularly unstable and require specific types of fixation during definitive treatment.

Subtrochanteric fractures occur in the region of the femur from the lesser trochanter to within 5 cm distal to this landmark. These display a typical displacement pattern with the proximal fragment in flexion, external rotation, and abduction due to the influence of the iliopsoas, short external rotators, and gluteus medius and minimus, respectively.

Treatment of proximal femur fractures is surgical in almost all cases, other than in patients who are too medically unstable to undergo an operation or nonambulators in minimal discomfort. There are several surgical options for the treatment of proximal femur fractures, though the type and pattern of the specific fracture typically orients the surgeon toward a particular type of fixation.

SURGICAL PROCEDURES

Femoral Neck Fractures

Closed or Open Reduction with Cannulated Screw or Sliding Hip Screw Fixation

Indications

Indications for using cannulated screw fixation with open or closed reduction are impacted or minimally displaced femoral neck fractures in any patient or displaced femoral neck fractures in the younger patient (<60–65 years old; Figure 71.1). The sliding hip screw is another construct providing stable fixation useful in fixation of the femoral neck fracture in a younger patient. It may be necessary to perform an open reduction if a satisfactory reduction of the fracture cannot be achieved by closed means. Surgical treatment of the displaced femoral neck fracture in the younger patient is considered a

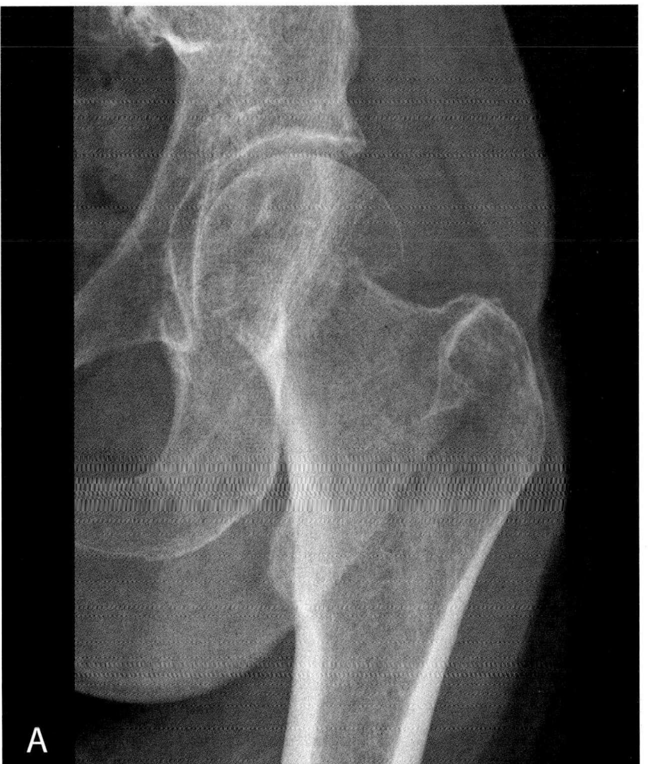

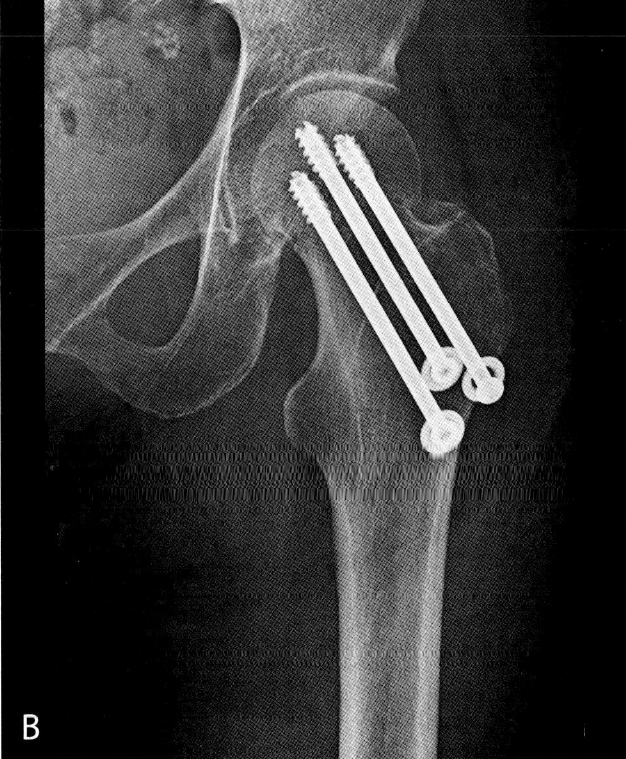

Figure 71.1 Preoperative (**A**) and postoperative (**B**) radiographs of a femoral neck fracture treated with closed reduction and cannulated screw fixation.

© 2018 American Academy of Orthopaedic Surgeons

surgical emergency due to the increased risk of osteonecrosis and nonunion with these injuries that are believed to be increased with surgical delay.

Contraindications

Contraindications for cannulated screw fixation of a femoral neck fracture include any active infection in the affected hip or in those patients who are not stable enough to tolerate a surgical procedure for medical reasons.

Procedure

Cannulated screw fixation is accomplished using three large (7.3-mm or 6.5-mm) cannulated screws that are placed over guidewires once adequate reduction is accomplished. If three independent cannulated screws are used, they are typically placed in an inverted triangle position across the fracture site to engage the femoral head. The most inferior screw is placed along the inferior cortex of the femoral neck to support the calcar; the other two screws are placed in the anterosuperior and posterosuperior positions. The starting point for the inferior screw is at or above the level of the lesser trochanter to prevent a stress riser in the subtrochanteric region, which can increase the risk of subtrochanteric fractures. Maximal spread of the screws within the femoral neck provides the most stable construct. If placed percutaneously, there is minimal soft-tissue disruption. However, open reduction is commonly performed in the younger patient with displaced femoral neck fractures in order to anatomically reduce the fragments and lessen the insult on the vascular supply to the femoral head. Weight-bearing restrictions after this treatment varies considerably, with bone quality, surgeon preference, and patient age each playing a role. Toe-touch or touch-down weight bearing on the surgical extremity is usually preferred to protect the reduction until fracture healing is confirmed clinically and radiographically. However, many elderly patients are unable to tolerate this due to loss of strength and balance. Therefore, they may weight bear as tolerated with an assistive device in order to preserve and promote as much mobility as possible.

Sliding hip screw fixation is preferred by some surgeons for fixation of midcervical and basicervical femoral neck fractures. It may offer biomechanical advantages while requiring more exposure. This technique is described in the intertrochanteric section to follow. When used in the femoral neck, a separate cannulated screw may be placed more proximally for rotational control.

Complications

Complications include osteonecrosis of the femoral head, nonunion or malunion, and screw penetration into the hip joint. These would present with acutely increased and persistent pain in the hip or groin region, which can limit rehabilitation. The abductors are rarely violated during this procedure; thus, postoperative Trendelenberg gait is not frequently seen. The occurrence of dislocation is generally very low; therefore, postoperative hip precautions are typically not necessary. As with all proximal femur fractures, there is a high risk of deep venous thrombosis (DVT) and/or pulmonary embolus (PE); thus, mechanical and chemical (when appropriate) prophylactic measures are essential to avoid this complication.

Hemiarthroplasty and Total Hip Arthroplasty

Indications

Indications for hemiarthroplasty include displaced femoral neck fractures in low-functioning, elderly patients (Figure 71.2). Those elderly patients who are higher functioning or those with preexisting hip osteoarthritis are candidates for the more costly total hip arthroplasty. The osteoporotic bone precludes reliable fixation, while the expected increased activity level may induce wear on the acetabular cartilage and pain.

Contraindications

Contraindications include any active infection within the hip or those who are not medically stable to undergo the operation.

Procedure

Hemiarthroplasty involves removal of the femoral neck and head, and replacement with a prosthetic device. A bipolar hemiarthroplasty also contains an outer bearing over the prosthetic head that serves to theoretically decrease wear on the native articular surface of the acetabulum, while a unipolar hemiarthroplasty does not contain this outer bearing. A total hip arthroplasty replaces the femoral neck and head with a prosthetic component while replacing the acetabular surface with a prosthetic cup as well.

Anterolateral, direct anterior, and posterior surgical approaches are commonly used for hemiarthroplasty and total hip arthroplasty. Anterolateral approaches either utilize the intermuscular plane between the tensor fasciae latae and the gluteus medius, thereby sparing the abductors (Watson-Jones approach), or can split the gluteus medius anteriorly and detach a portion of the abductors from the greater trochanter. The direct anterior approach (Smith-Peterson, and its variants) utilizes an internervous plane between the sartorius (femoral nerve) and the tensor fascia lata (superior gluteal nerve), often detaching a portion of the reflected head of the rectus femoris. In both the anterolateral and direct anterior approaches, an anterior capsulotomy is performed to gain access to the hip joint. The posterior approach splits the gluteus maximus muscle and detaches the short external rotators prior to a posterior capsulotomy, leaving the abductors unviolated aside from intraoperative retraction. In each case, the proximal fracture fragment, including the femoral head, is removed and the neck is prepared with a cut perpendicular to the longitudinal orientation of the neck. The femoral canal is prepared with a series of broaches in order to accept the final implant. Femoral stems can either be cemented or uncemented depending on surgeon preference and the quality of the bone. In a total hip arthroplasty, the acetabular cup is then prepared with a series of reamers to medialize and position the replacement cup with appropriate anteversion and inclination. Once the components are implanted and reduced, care is taken to repair the capsulotomy. The abductors are then repaired in the case

© 2018 American Academy of Orthopaedic Surgeons

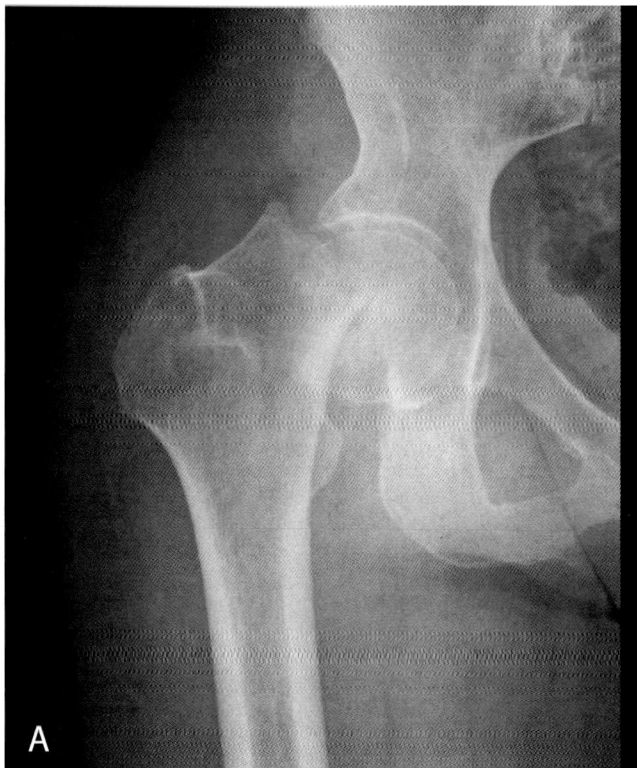

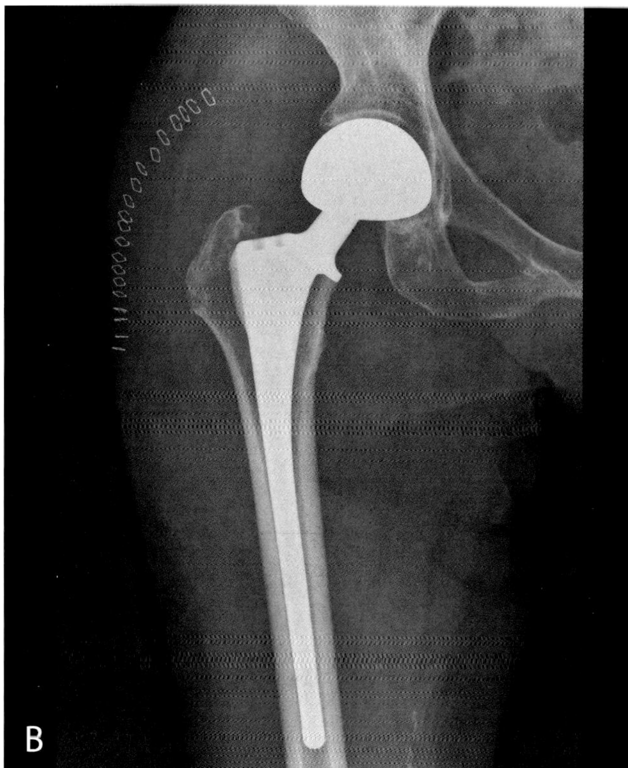

Figure 71.2 Preoperative (**A**) and postoperative (**B**) radiographs of a displaced transcervical femoral neck fracture treated with bipolar uncemented hemiarthroplasty.

of the anterolateral approach and the short external rotators are repaired in the case of the posterior approach. The subcutaneous tissues and skin are closed according to surgeon preference. Patients can weight bear as tolerated following hemiarthroplasty or total hip arthroplasty, though they often must maintain hip precautions during the initial postoperative period to decrease the risk of dislocation. For a posterior surgical approach to the hip and posterior capsulotomy, the hip is most unstable in flexion, adduction, and internal rotation. Thus, typical posterior hip precautions include no hip flexion past 70°, no adduction past the midline of the body, and no internal rotation of the hip past neutral. Typically, the patient is placed in a wedge-shaped abduction pillow postoperatively to prevent adduction while in bed. Also, low chairs and toilets are avoided to prevent excessive hip flexion. For anterior approaches to the hip with anterior capsulotomies, most instability occurs with abduction and external rotation. Patients are cautioned against such positioning, though specific devices are not as commonly needed to prevent these unwanted positions.

Complications

Complications include deep infection, periprosthetic fracture, dislocation, and wear of the acetabulum. Buttock or groin pain following hemiarthroplasty may be a sign of acetabular cartilage erosion or acetabular protrusion. Total hip arthroplasty has a higher rate of postoperative dislocation than hemiarthroplasty, and the posterior approach has a higher rate of dislocation when compared to the direct anterior or anterolateral approach. Specific hip precautions, depending on the surgical approach, are recommended to decrease the risk of dislocation. In the case of the anterolateral approach, there is increased risk of postoperative Trendelenberg gait or limp due to intraoperative violation of the abductor complex. As both hemiarthroplasty and total hip arthroplasty do not rely on bony union across a fracture site, there is no risk for nonunion or malunion. Mechanical and chemical (when appropriate) DVT/PE prophylaxis should be employed, as these are a common complication following hip arthroplasties.

Intertrochanteric Fractures

Open Reduction and Internal Fixation with a Sliding Hip Screw Construct or Fixed-Angle Plate

Indications

Indications for open reduction internal fixation (ORIF) with a sliding hip screw (SHS) are basicervical femoral neck fractures and stable or unstable intertrochanteric fractures (Figure 71.3).

Contraindications

Active hip infection or medically unstable patient would be general contraindications for this procedure. Specific surgical contraindications for a standard SHS construct include significant lateral wall comminution, a reverse obliquity component, or subtrochanteric extension. Subtrochanteric fractures can be treated with a fixed-angle plate construct, though this is usually reserved for when the femoral canal is unable to accept an intramedullary construct.

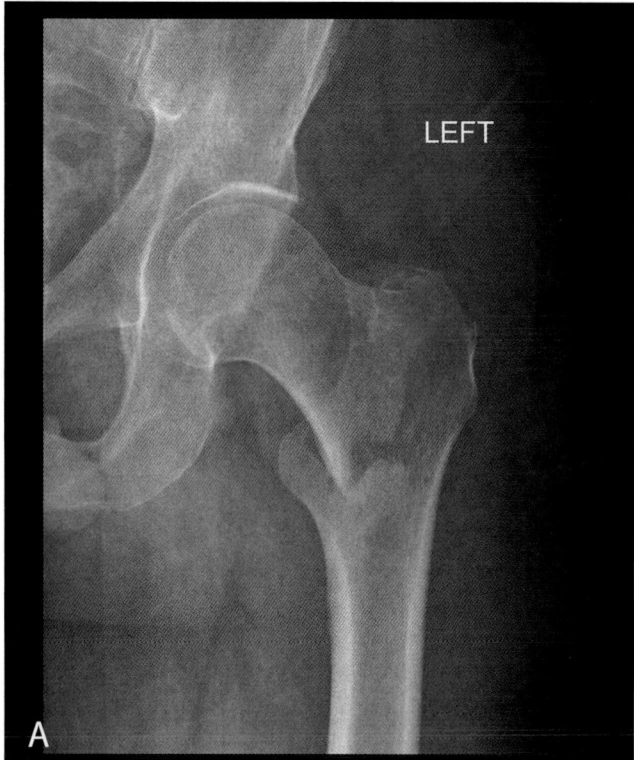

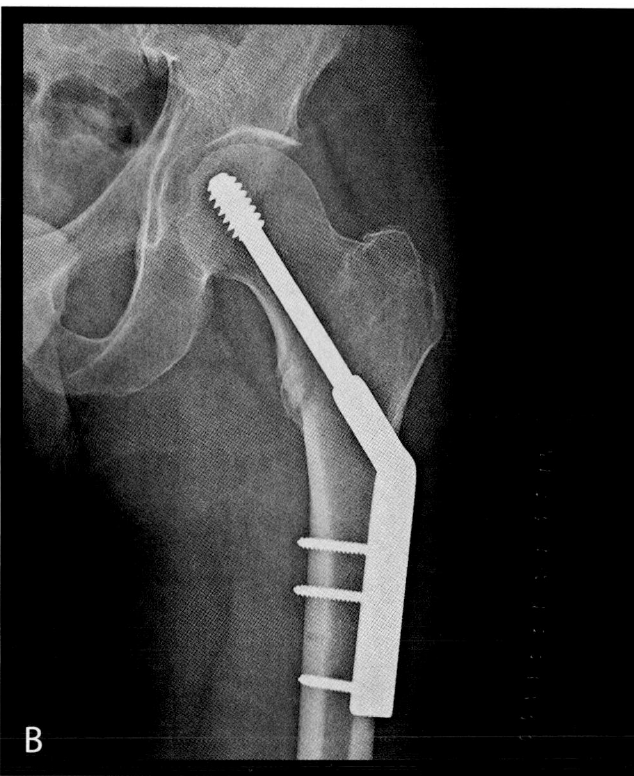

Figure 71.3 Preoperative (**A**) and postoperative (**B**) radiographs of an intertrochanteric femur fracture treated with open reduction and a standard sliding hip screw construct.

Procedure

The surgical approach is directly lateral through the fascia lata and vastus lateralis muscle. The vastus lateralis is either split or retracted anteriorly to expose the lateral aspect of the proximal femur. The fracture is reduced and a guidewire is inserted for the lag screw across the fracture site and into the femoral head. Correct positioning of the lag screw in the head reduces the risk of construct failure. The lag screw is inserted across the fracture site and secured into a laterally placed compression plate. The barrel in the plate allows for the lag screw to slide, providing controlled compression. Care is taken to repair the fascia lata along with the surgeon's preferred subcutaneous and skin closure. Patients are encouraged to weight bear on this construct, providing compression at the fracture site.

With a fixed-angle plate, the same approach as for the SHS is used to the lateral aspect of the proximal femur once the fracture is reduced. Typically, an angled blade or locking plate is chosen to obtain proximal fixation into the proximal femur fragment while distal fixation is obtained with cortical screws through the plate. Again, care is taken to close the fascia lata followed by subcutaneous and skin closure according to surgeon preference. In many cases, the patients are toe-touch weight bearing according to surgeon preference and the amount of comminution present in the fracture. However, as stated previously, elderly patients are often unable to restrict their weight bearing due to loss of strength and balance, thus are allowed to weight bear as tolerated with an assistive device.

Complications

Complications include deep infection, screw cutout or penetration, and component collapse (especially in the case of an SHS used for a fracture with lateral wall comminution or reverse obliquity). A trochanteric stabilizing plate can be added to decrease the risk of component collapse and femoral shaft medialization. Painful hardware can result from the sliding screw irritating the soft tissues lateral to the construct, though this typically occurs. As with all fractures, there is a risk of nonunion or malunion. Due to the rich blood supply of the intertrochanteric region, nonunion is less of a risk than in the femoral neck, but malunion from a poor surgical reduction or failure of reduction postoperatively. As with the treatment of all hip fractures, mechanical and chemical (when appropriate) DVT/PE prophylaxis should be employed according to surgeon preference.

An increasing number of intertrochanteric fractures are being treated with cephalomedullary nails. These are preferred when treating unstable patterns, such as 4-part fractures, reverse obliquity patterns, and those with extension into the subtrochanteric region. The technique is described in the next section.

Subtrochanteric Femur Fractures

Cephalomedullary Nailing

A cephalomedullary nail (CMN) is a construct that includes an intramedullary nail into the femoral canal with a lag screw through the proximal portion of the nail into the femoral

© 2018 American Academy of Orthopaedic Surgeons

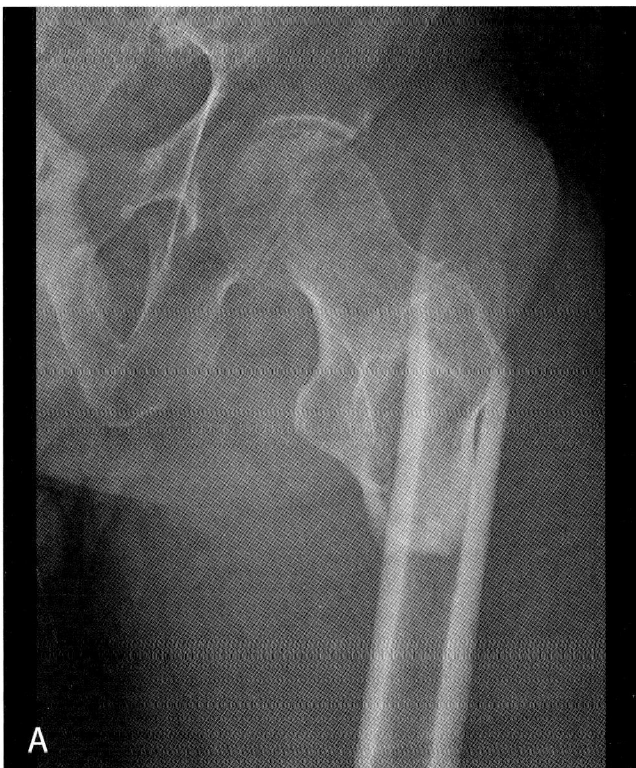

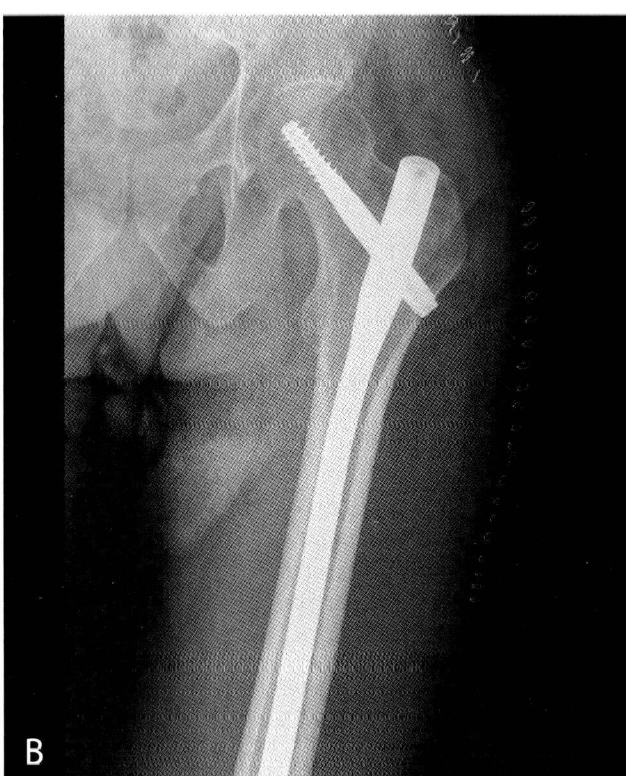

Figure 71.4 Preoperative (**A**) and postoperative (**B**) radiographs of a subtrochanteric femur fracture treated with cephalomedullary nailing.

head. Indications for a CMN include stable or unstable intertrochanteric fractures and subtrochanteric fractures (Figure 71.4).

The patient is positioned in a supine or lateral position on a traction or flat radiolucent table, respectively, and the fracture is reduced with a combination of traction and lower extremity manipulation. A short incision is made proximal to the greater trochanter and carried down through the fascia lata. The abductors can be injured during the surgical approach as well as with instrumentation for nail preparation and insertion. Trochanteric entry nails use the superiormost tip of the greater trochanter for a starting point while piriformis entry nails utilize the piriformis fossa. A guidewire is inserted from the appropriate starting position into the medullary canal and an opening reamer creates the cortical window for passage of the nail. A ball-tipped wire is then passed through the entry site across the fracture and down the medullary canal. Short nails do not require any further reaming, while long nails require that the medullary canal is reamed in preparation for the implant. Once the nail is positioned down the canal, an aiming guide is used to place the lag screw from the lateral cortex into the femoral head. The nail can then be locked distally if the surgeon prefers. The fascia lata is repaired upon closure along with subcutaneous and skin closure.

Complications

Complications include deep infection, fracture at the distal tip of the nail due to the resultant stress riser (especially with short CMNs), malrotation and/or shortening. A postoperative Trendelenberg gait can be due to intraoperative injury to the abductors or varus malreduction of the fracture. Like intertrochanteric fractures, nonunion of subtrochanteric fractures is less commonly seen than in femoral neck fractures, though delayed union among bisphosphonate-related subtrochanteric fractures is well documented. When using a long CMN, anterior cortex perforation of the femoral shaft can occur if there is mismatch between the curvature of radius of the nail and the bone, especially in weaker osteoporotic bone. Mechanical and chemical (when appropriate) DVT/PE prophylaxis should be employed according to surgeon preference.

POSTOPERATIVE REHABILITATION

Postoperative rehabilitation following surgical fixation of a hip fracture typically begins either the day of surgery or the first postoperative day. In the elderly, rehabilitation is crucial to decreasing the high mortality rates seen after hip fractures. These patients are mobilized to sitting and even standing with weight bearing as tolerated within the first several days of surgery to reduce complications. The young patient is similiarly mobilized, although weight bearing may be restricted in certain fracture patterns and constructs.

Phase I: Postoperative Safety (0–1 Weeks)

The time period immediately following proximal femur fracture repair, typically the first week, is characterized by pain

© 2018 American Academy of Orthopaedic Surgeons

management and prevention of complications associated with recumbency. These complications include:

- Wound infection
- DVT/PE
- Pressure ulcers
- Respiratory and urinary tract infection

By monitoring patient signs and symptoms, these complications can be avoided and the rehabilitative process can begin. The most important treatment is the mobilization out of bed. Appropriate pain control and support with therapy and nursing teaches the patient to sit up, transfer to a chair, and stand and walk with appropriate ambulatory aids and precautions. Important in this effort is instruction in ADLs to include safe bathing, dressing, and toileting. Regaining a sense of independence also assists the patient in regaining a feeling of control.

Modalities are often used in the outpatient setting to both stimulate the hip girdle musculature and reduce edema that often slows healing at the surgical site. Common modalities and reasoning for their use include the following.

- Ultrasound: Tissue healing, increasing tissue flexibility/heating effect
- Neuromuscular stimulation (NMES): Muscle strengthening, muscular reeducation, edema reduction
- Transcutaneous electrical nerve stimulation (TENS): Pain control
- Vasopneumatic compression: Pain control, swelling reduction

Phase II: Restoration of Motion and Progression to Ambulation (1–4 Weeks)

Once a physical therapist (PT), physician, nurse (RN), or athletic trainer (ATC) educates the patient on precautions and compensated ADL training, a structured rehabilitation program can begin. The first 4 weeks of the recovery after fracture surgery includes protection of the healing structures, reduction of inflammation, restoration of range of motion (ROM) and progression toward ambulatory independence. Outpatient rehabilitation, in comparison to home therapy, has displayed better outcomes in terms of muscular strength, gait speed, balance and ADLs. In the initial rehabilitation sessions, hip ROM and strength will become the rehabilitation focus with the goal to regain active muscular control of the limb. Because the hip is a "ball and socket" joint, it is vulnerable to ROM loss through muscular contractures and capsular adhesions. To ensure that ROM and flexibility are maintained, the clinician will begin passive range of motion (PROM) and active assistive range of motion (AAROM) exercises within the patient's pain tolerance and hip precautions, if applicable, as determined by the treating surgeon (Table 71.1 and Figure 71.5). Other techniques—such as soft-tissue mobilization, active release techniques, and trigger point massage—are frequently used to maximize ROM restoration. The patient will progress from AAROM and active range of motion (AROM) exercises to progressive resistive exercises (PRE) of the lower extremity. Strengthening will begin with open-chain exercises and progress to closed-chain exercises as recommended by the surgeon and as tolerated by the patient. Arthroplasty patients are reminded of hip precautions.

Table 71.1 JOINT RANGE OF MOTION/ FLEXIBILITY EXAMPLES

Stretching into Hip	Exercise to Increase Flexibility
Flexion	Heel-slides, single knee to chest, hamstring stretch
Abduction	Butterfly stretch, standing groin stretch
Extension	Kneeling/standing hip flexor stretch, prone quad stretch
Adduction	Iliotibial band stretch, gluteus medius stretch
External rotation	Cross leg stretch, butterfly stretch
Internal rotation	Seated IR push, piriformis stretch

Note: Certain stretches should be avoided if postoperative hip precautions preclude such a maneuver. Joint mobilizations, soft-tissue mobilization, active release techniques, strain–counterstrain techniques are often used to maximize ROM restoration.

Phase II is also characterized with emphasis on eliminating recumbency and restoring ambulatory function. Depending on the surgical procedure performed, weight-bearing allowance will vary and the utilization of assistive devices will be necessary to return to ambulation. With progression to ambulation, the patient can avoid lower extremity and core musculature atrophy that is frequently observed with prolonged bed rest. Progression to full weight bearing ultimately depends on surgeon preferences, the surgical technique performed, and fracture healing when applicable (Table 71.2 and Figure 71.6). Femoral neck and intertrochanteric fractures are often healed by 3 months while subtrochanteric fractures may require up to 6 months, limiting tolerance to full weight bearing.

Weight bearing soon after surgical intervention can enhance the healing process at the fracture site while preserving muscle strength and balance (Table 71.3). Most patients, particularly the elderly, begin with partial weight bearing with a standard

Table 71.2 GAIT WEIGHT-BEARING PROGRESSION AND ASSISTIVE DEVICE

Weight-Bearing Status	Assistive Device
Non–Weight Bearing (0%)	Wheelchair
Toe-Touch Weight Bearing (0%–20%)	Crutches
Partial Weight Bearing (20%–50%)	Standard walker or crutches
Full Weight Bearing (>50%)	Rolling walker or crutches Quad cane Single-point cane

© 2018 American Academy of Orthopaedic Surgeons

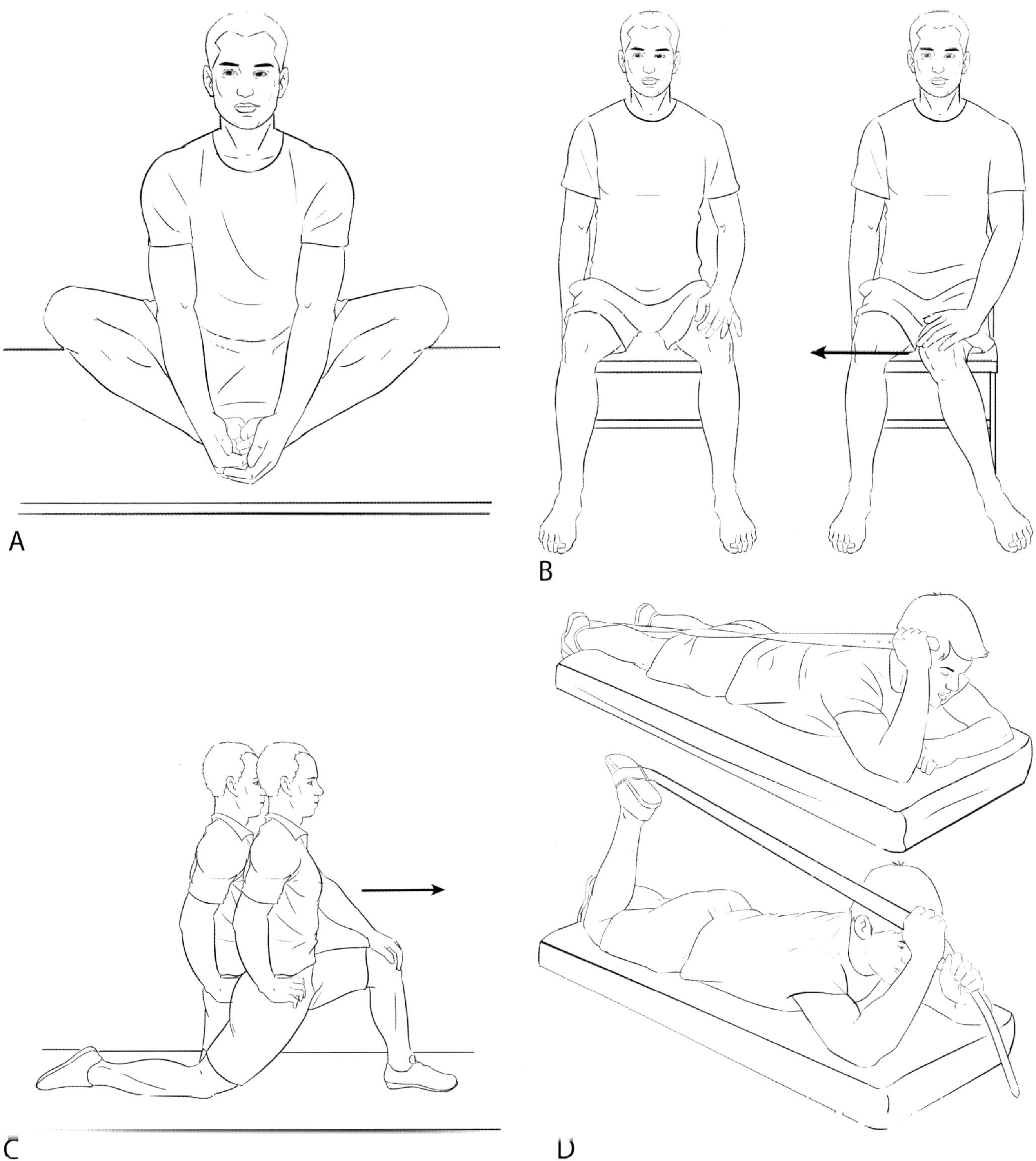

Figure 71.5 Illustrations of point range of motion and flexibility exercises. Note that all stretching durations range from 10 to 30 seconds per repetition. **A**, Butterfly stretch. **B**, Seated internal rotation stretch. **C**, Kneeling hip flexor stretch. **D**, Prone quadriceps stretch.

or rolling walker. If crutches can be tolerated, touch-down weight bearing can be initiated until partial weight bearing is more tolerable. As they become more comfortable ambulating with a walker, patients can move on to a cane in the contralateral hand for assistance until unassisted weight bearing is achieved. The physical therapist has methods to ensure that each phase of the gait cycle is achieved before progressing weight bearing in postoperative patients. Aqua therapy is often utilized to progress weight bearing on the affected extremity. It should be emphasized that aggressive progression off of assistive devices will often lead to compensatory mechanisms that will limit future functional recovery. Common

© 2018 American Academy of Orthopaedic Surgeons

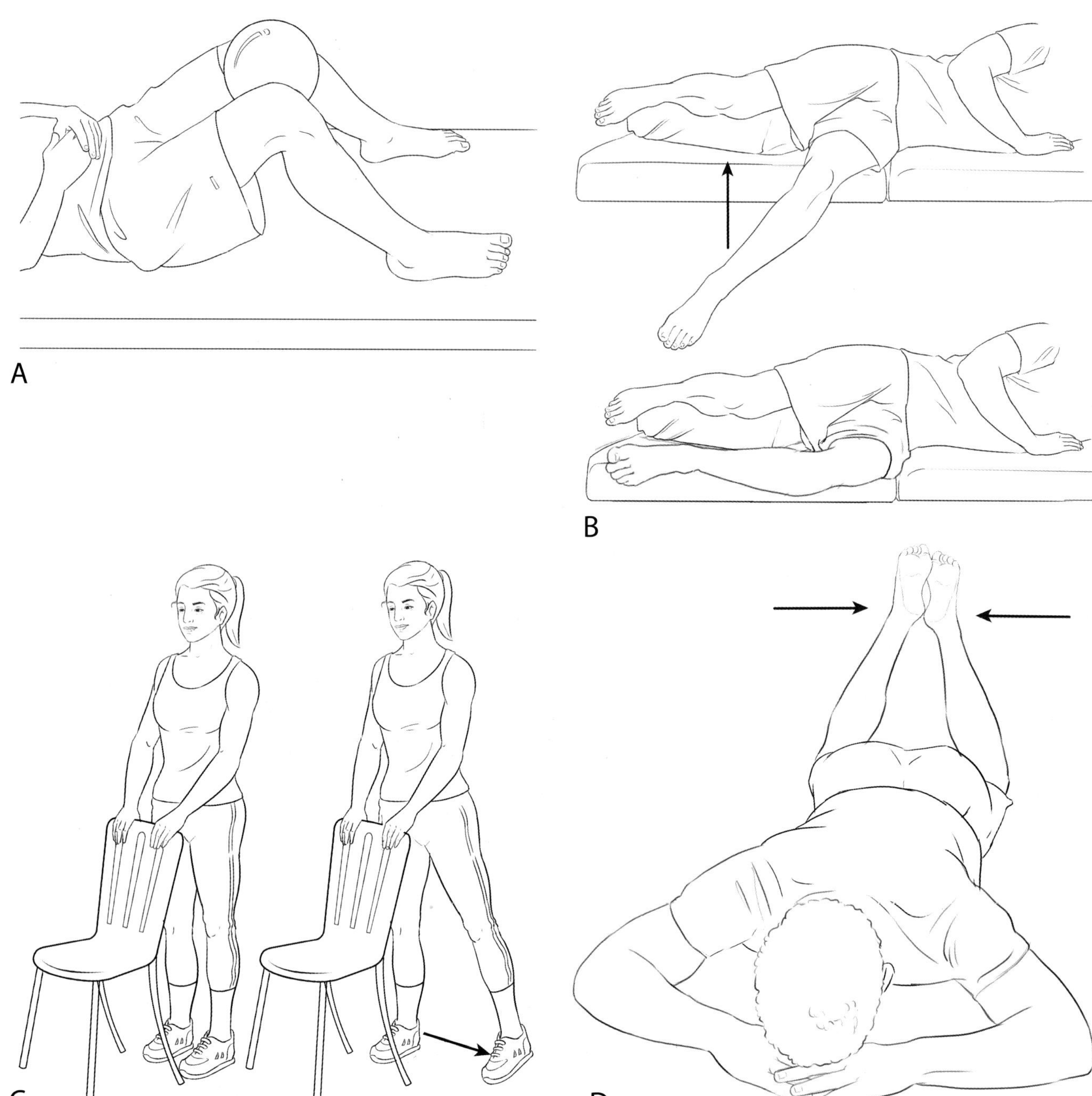

Figure 71.6 Illustrations of open- and closed-chain exercises. Note that sets and repetition of exercises vary from clinician to clinician. Three sets of 8–10 repetitions is common for the goal of increasing strength. **A**, Isometric ball squeeze. **B**, Active hip external rotation. **C**, Standing hip abduction. **D**, Prone internal rotation squeeze.

gait dysfunction after hip fracture repair and potential causes include the following.

- Trendelenberg gait: Ipsilateral gluteus medius weakness
- Waddling gait: Bilateral gluteus medius weakness
- Excessive trunk flexion: Gluteus maximus weakness, hip flexion contracture, lumbar stenosis
- Bouncing gait/toe walking: Achilles/gastrocnemius-soleus contracture
- Shuffling gait: Imbalance, weak hip extensors
- Bent knee ambulation: Imbalance, hamstring contracture
- Circumducted gait: Leg length discrepancy

Phase III: Restoration of Function (4–8 Weeks)

Once the surgical hip approaches normal ROM and ambulation is progressing nicely, the focus of the rehabilitative process is on maximizing functional recovery. Balance and proprioceptive activities, such as single-leg stance and vestibular training, will also be crucial to ensure full dynamic stability and to

© 2018 American Academy of Orthopaedic Surgeons

Table 71.3 OPEN-CHAIN AND CLOSED-CHAIN EXERCISE EXAMPLES

Open-Chain PRE Examples	Closed-Chain PRE Examples
Lower extremity isometrics, quad/hamstring sets	Weight shifts
Short-arc quad, long-arc quad, seated hip Flexion	Mini-squat
4 way hip straight-leg raises	Step-up/down (forward, lateral)
Standing hip abduction, flexion, extension	Leg press, bridging progression
Clam-shell (abduction/ external rotation)	Narrow Base of Support: tandem and single leg balance
Prone heel squeezes, resistance band internal/ external rotation	Shuffling activity, step tapping, monster walk

Note: A combination of eccentric and concentric training has proven to be effective for full strength recovery. For core strengthening, plank progression and transverse abdominal reeducation are often utilized.
PRE = progressive resistive exercises.

help avoid future falls and injuries. Core strengthening, such as co-contraction and abdominal reeducation, will reduce the patient's dependence on assistive devices and reduce compensatory functional movements. Closed-chain strengthening—such as squat training, lunges, hip hikes, and step-ups—will ensure lower extremity strength recovery and functional carryover to independent ADLs. Endurance training, such as use of a treadmill and stationary bike—will restore full body recovery, including cardiovascular efficiency. Once ROM, flexibility, strength, and gait approach normal levels, treatment will be progressed to a daily home exercise program.

Maximal recovery of strength, endurance, and balance may take up to 6 or 9 months depending on the extent of injury, comorbidities, and patient motivation to regain full function. In the elderly, it must be remembered that this injury is a marker of increased frailty with 1 year mortality approaching 20% to 30%. Another third of these patients will have a decrement in their ambulatory capacity by one level. The younger patient, barring associated injury, regains near full function.

PEARLS

- Rotational deformities after fixation of subtrochanteric fractures are occasionally discovered by the PT if missed by the treating surgeon. If this is the case, it is imperative that the PT alert the surgeon. This would be clearly exhibited by excessive intoeing or outtoeing during gait. This can be a fall risk and adversely affect gait in the long term. Early surgical correction while the patient is still in the hospital is typically much easier than late correction after the patient is following up in the office.
- A severe Trendelenberg gait may be indicative of a varus malreduction of the fracture. This is best avoided by the surgeon intraoperatively, as delayed revision can be challenging. It is helpful for the PT to alert the surgeon about this finding, particularly if it persists, as it can be a poor prognostic factor for functional outcome in a previously high-functioning patient. Varus malreduction also risks loss of fixation and nonunion, which frequently require additional surgical procedures.
- The rehabilitative phase after a proximal femur fracture in an elderly patient provides an opportunity to discuss formal evaluation and medical treatment for osteoporosis. Evaluation can be initiated with a DEXA scan or similar study, and appropriate referral to the primary care physician.
- Monitoring for signs of DVT and PE at each therapy session allows for early detection and initiation of treatment, which can ultimately minimize the effect that these complications have on progression through therapy. DVT and PE can occur weeks to months following the injury and subsequent surgical fixation; thus, it is important to maintain a high index of suspicion throughout the rehabilitation process.
- Fall prevention strategies are important to reduce future falls and injury.

BIBLIOGRAPHY

Binder EF, Brown M, Sinacore DR, Steger-May K, Yarasheski KE, Schechtman KB: Effects of extended outpatient rehabilitation after hip fracture: a randomized controlled trial. *JAMA* 2004;292(7):837–846.

Brauer CA, Coca-Perraillon M, Cutler DM, Rosen AB: Incidence and mortality of hip fractures in the United States. *JAMA* 2009;302(14):1573–1579.

Cuccurullo S, ed. *Physical Medicine and Rehabilitation Board Review.* New York, NY, Demos Medical Publishing, 2004. Available from: http://www.ncbi.nlm.nih.gov/books/NBK10277/

Haydel C, Rehman S. Femoral neck fractures. In Ilyas A, Rehman S, eds: *Contemporary Surgical Management of Fractures and Complications.* Ashland, OH, Jaypee Brothers Medical Pub, 2012, 588–630.

Lindskog DM, Baumgaertner MR: Unstable intertrochanteric hip fractures in the elderly. *J Am Acad Orthop Surg* 2004;12:179–190.

Lundy DW: Subtrochanteric femoral fractures. *J Am Acad Orthop Surg* 2007;15:663–671.

Probe R, Ward R: Internal fixation of femoral neck fractures. *J Am Orthop Surg* 2006;14:565–571.

Weinlein, JC: Fractures and dislocations of the hip. in Canale ST, Beaty JH, eds: *Campbell's Operative Orthopaedics.* ed 12. Philadelphia, PA, Mosby, 2013, pp 2725–2767.

Wilkins K: Health care consequences of falls for seniors. *Health Rep* 1999 Spring;10(4):47–55(ENG); 47–57(FRE).

© 2018 American Academy of Orthopaedic Surgeons

72 Femur and Tibial Shaft Open and Closed Fractures

Daniel J. Stinner, MD, and Alicia Faye White, PT, ATC, DPT

INTRODUCTION

The management of femur and tibial shaft fractures has made significant advances in recent decades, allowing safe, early postoperative mobilization of patients. These injuries can occur in isolation, but are also common in the polytrauma patient. Early stabilization of long-bone fractures is paramount to minimize the morbidity associated with these injuries, such as deep vein thrombosis (DVT) and pneumonia, as it allows patient mobilization. Modern techniques allow for early mobilization with rapid progression to full weight bearing in most circumstances. Comminuted, segmental, and severe open fractures can be exceptions to this rule. In addition, variations in surgical technique or time to definitive stabilization can alter a patient's rehabilitation. The common methods of surgical stabilization of diaphyseal femur and tibia fractures are discussed in this chapter with an explanation of the typical postoperative physical therapy regimen.

FEMUR FRACTURES

The overwhelming majority of femoral shaft fractures are stabilized with intramedullary (IM) nail fixation. As such, this section will focus primarily on femur fractures treated with an IM nail, but will offer a brief explanation of the indications, as well as variations in the surgical technique and postoperative rehabilitation for diaphyseal femur fractures managed with external fixation or plate fixation. It is important to note that in high-energy femoral shaft fractures, up to 6% of patients can have an ipsilateral femoral neck fracture, which would alter the postoperative rehabilitation. Some of these neck fractures are not visible on initial radiographs.

Surgical Procedure

Operative Treatment of Diaphyseal Femur Fractures: Intramedullary Nailing of the Femur (Antegrade or Retrograde)

Indications

Nonoperative management for a diaphyseal femur fracture is virtually nonexistent, and limited to nonambulators with limited function or those who cannot tolerate a surgical procedure, secondary to the morbidity associated with such treatment and the successful outcomes that can be achieved with operative management. As such, a diaphyseal femur fracture in an adult is an indication for operative management. Standard antegrade or retrograde IM nail fixation is indicated for the majority of diaphyseal femur fractures that occur more than 5 cm below the lesser trochanter and approximately 9 cm proximal to the knee joint. Refer to Chapters 71 and 73 for a more detailed explanation of the management of proximal and distal femur fractures.

Contraindications

Contraindications are limited to patients in extremis (life-threatening injuries) or who are medically unfit for anesthesia. Typically, these patients will undergo placement of temporary skeletal traction or external fixation, which can be performed safely at the bedside in the patient who is unfit for the operating room.

Procedure

Relevant anatomy: Knowledge of the anatomy of the hip, thigh, and knee are important when managing femur fractures. When performing antegrade IM nail fixation of a femur fracture, the hip abductors (gluteus medius and minimus), which insert on the greater trochanter, can be damaged during surgical dissection, reaming, and nail insertion. Damage to the abductors

Dr. Stinner or an immediate family member serves as a board member, owner, officer, or committee member of the American Academy of Orthopaedic Surgeons, the Orthopaedic Trauma Association, and the Society of Military Orthopaedic Surgeons. Neither Mrs. White nor any immediate family member has received anything of value from or has stock or stock options held in a commercial company or institution related directly or indirectly to the subject of this article.

© 2018 American Academy of Orthopaedic Surgeons

can lead to a Trendelenburg gait during the early postoperative period, but this rarely leads to a long-term functional deficit. Perhaps more important, if the starting point for the nail is too posterior, especially when using a piriformis starting point, the blood supply to the femoral head can be injured, increasing the risk of subsequent avascular necrosis. While rare occurrences of avascular necrosis have been reported in adults with the use of a piriformis starting point, cadaveric studies have demonstrated no difference in damage to the deep medial femoral circumflex artery when the piriformis starting point was compared to a trochanteric one. Distally, it is important to recognize the trapezoidal shape of the femur when placing interlocking bolts to ensure that they are not too long, which could lead to irritation of the soft tissues postoperatively. Finally, should the percutaneous placement of external fixator pins or reduction aids be needed, the anterolateral border of the thigh is a relatively safe zone for placement, as the significant neurovascular structures at risk when operating on the femur course medially and posterior in the thigh.

Techniques

Antegrade Nailing

There are a variety of surgical techniques associated with intramedullary nailing of the femur. It is often helpful to obtain rotational profiles of the well leg prior to positioning, especially if femoral rotation is going to be a concern based on the fracture type. The authors prefer the use of a fracture table for diaphyseal femur fractures; however, there are variations of this technique to include supine or lateral positioning on a radiolucent table with or without skeletal traction.

A 3- to 4-cm skin incision is made proximal to the tip of the greater trochanter following the trajectory of the femur. The gluteal fascia is split and if a piriformis entry nail is to be utilized, blunt dissection is carried down to the piriformis fossa, which is just medial to the greater trochanter. Once the guidewire is appropriately placed, an opening is made in the femur with a rigid reamer. The fracture is reduced using a variety of techniques, usually closed manipulation, but at times open reduction is required. A flexible guidewire is passed to the distal femur, and the canal is reamed, followed by insertion of an appropriately sized nail. The nail is adequately seated and appropriate rotation and restoration of length is confirmed. Interlocking bolts are placed percutaneously through the iliotibial band proximally using the insertion guide and distally using a freehand technique, to control the length and rotation of the femur.

Retrograde Nailing

Retrograde nailing can be performed for diaphyseal femur fractures with advantages in several clinical scenarios. Retrograde nailing may be preferred in morbidly obese patients in whom access to the starting point for an antegrade nail may be problematic, patients with a traumatic knee arthrotomy, patients with an ipsilateral femoral neck fracture that is stabilized prior to treatment of the femoral shaft fracture, and polytrauma patients for whom supine positioning on a radiolucent "flat-top" table is advantageous, that is, allowing for bilateral procedures to proceed simultaneously.

The patient is placed supine on a radiolucent table with a bump under the operative hip. A radiolucent triangle is positioned under the operative knee for access to the appropriate starting point. An incision is made over the patellar tendon. A medial, patellar tendon split, or lateral arthrotomy can be made to gain access to the knee joint. The guidewire is then inserted to the distal femur, centered on the anteroposterior (AP) fluoroscopic view and at the tip of Blumensaat's line on the lateral fluoroscopic view of the knee. This puts the optimal starting point just anterior to the femoral origin of the posterior cruciate ligament (PCL) and at the midpoint of the intercondylar sulcus. Once the canal is reamed and an appropriately sized femoral nail is inserted, appropriate rotation and restoration of length is confirmed and interlocking bolts are placed percutaneously in the distal femur through the iliotibial band and proximally in an anterior to posterior direction using the freehand technique through the quadriceps muscle (Figure 72.1).

Alternative treatments include plate and external fixation of the femur, which typically require variations of the physical therapy protocol. They are discussed in the next sections.

Plate Fixation of the Femur

Although commonly performed for proximal and distal femur fractures, plating of the femur is not commonly performed for diaphyseal (shaft) fractures due to the need to limit weight bearing postoperatively. Indications for plate fixation of a femoral shaft fracture include deformity or proximal or distal hardware that precludes placement of an IM nail, for example, total hip replacement. When plating of the femur is performed, an open technique may be used or a minimally invasive lateral, subvastus approach is employed. Care must be taken to ensure that adequate hemostasis is obtained, as there are a few large perforating vessels that must be ligated when elevating the vastus lateralis from the intermuscular septum. When reaching the femur, the fracture is reduced and the plate is applied to the lateral border of the femur just anterior to the intermuscular septum.

External Fixation of the Femur

External fixation of a femur fracture is commonly performed initially in the trauma patient as a bridge to IM nail fixation when the patient is too sick or unstable to undergo definitive fixation acutely (Figure 72.2). In exceptional cases, external fixation is used as definitive fixation of the femur. Skin conditions, such as severe burns, may also preclude safe placement of IM nails or plates. It may also be used in conjunction with a nail as a reconstructive tool to regain length.

External fixators are commonly placed in a uniplanar fashion and usually are not stable enough to allow weight bearing. As such, these are often not used for definitive fixation, but rather they are commonly converted to definitive internal fixation within 2 weeks, after the patient is more stable and able to tolerate such a procedure. Ringed external fixators, which provide multiplanar fixation, can be used for definitive fixation of diaphyseal fractures, but have a very specific set of indications,

© 2018 American Academy of Orthopaedic Surgeons

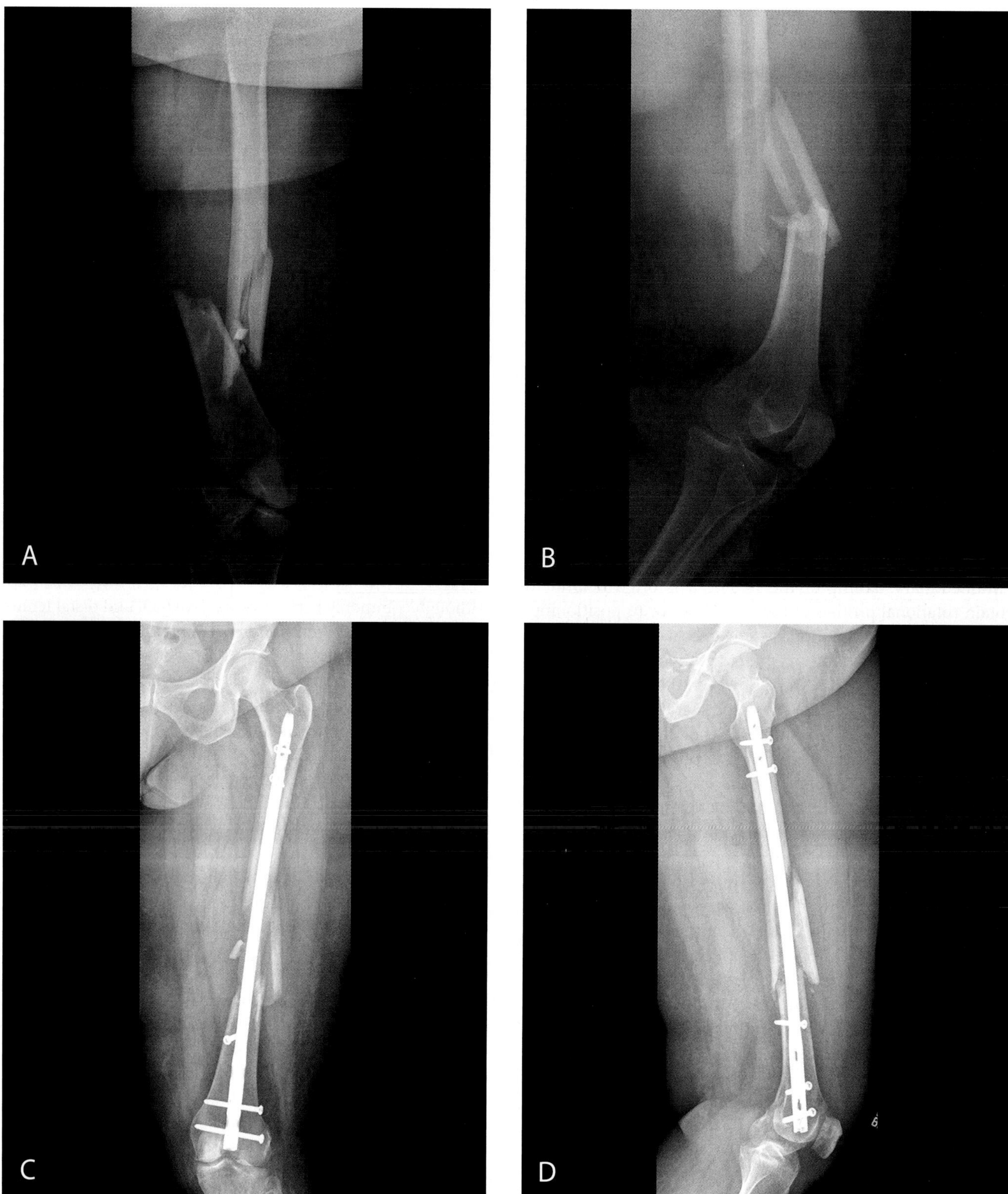

Figure 72.1 Anteroposterior (**A**) and lateral (**B**) radiographs demonstrate a midshaft femur fracture that underwent retrograde intramedullary nailing (**C** and **D**) through a traumatic knee arthrotomy.

 © 2018 American Academy of Orthopaedic Surgeons

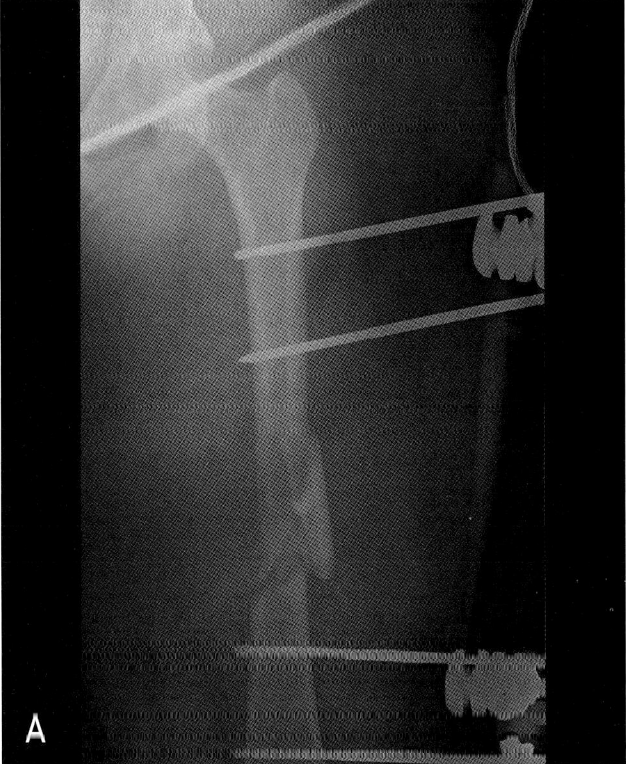

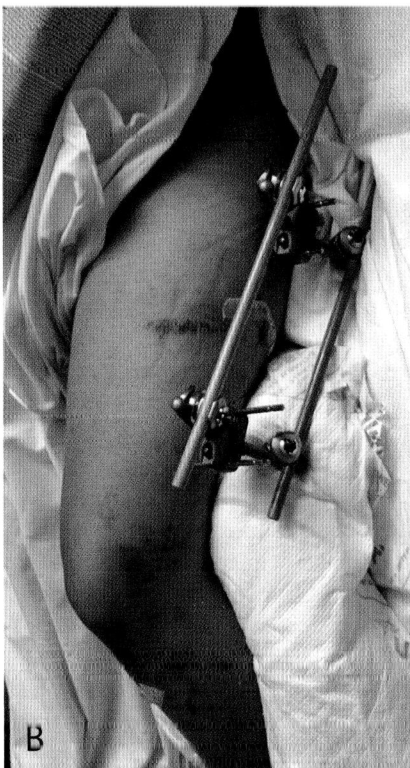

Figure 72.2 Both a radiograph (**A**) and a clinical photograph (**B**) are shown demonstrating placement of a uniplanar external fixator prior to definitive fixation.

as this treatment modality requires great technical skill and can be extremely burdensome on the patient. A benefit of this form of fixation is the ability to perform distraction osteogenesis to treat a large bony defect or correct angular deformities. It can also be used in the setting of infection or osteomyelitis, as the fixation can be distant to the zone of injury/infection while still providing rigid enough fixation to permit weight bearing during the postoperative period. Both forms of external fixation must contend with the entrapment of muscle by the pins or wires, which limit motion and risk infection. Additionally, patients contend with the external bulk of the frame.

Complications of Femur Fracture Fixation

- Infection
- Delayed union or nonunion
- Malunion
- Hip and/or knee pain
- Symptomatic hardware
- Heterotopic ossification
- Compartment syndrome
- Neurologic injury

TIBIA FRACTURES

The majority of tibia shaft fractures are also stabilized with intramedullary nail fixation, as this treatment modality commonly allows for early post-operative weightbearing. As such, this section will focus primarily on tibia fractures treated with an intramedullary nail, but will offer a brief explanation of the indications, as well as variations in the surgical technique and post-operative rehabilitation for diaphyseal tibia fractures managed with external fixation or plate fixation.

Surgical Procedure

Intramedullary Nailing of the Tibia

Indications

Length unstable, comminuted, and tibial shaft fractures whose alignment cannot be maintained in a cast are indicated for operative stabilization. It also offers the advantage of allowing motion at the knee and ankle, which may become stiff with casting. Modern techniques have greatly expanded the use of IM nails to even fractures in the proximal and distal metaphysic, potentially avoiding skin problems associated with plating.

Contraindications

Contraindications are limited to patients in extremis (life-threatening injuries) or are medically unfit for anesthesia. Typically, these patients can be temporarily stabilized in a splint or with the placement of temporary external fixation until they can be definitively managed with internal fixation.

Procedure

Relevant anatomy: The leg has four compartments. The anterior compartment, which is just lateral to the crest of the tibia, contains the tibialis anterior, extensor digitorum longus, extensor hallucis longus muscles, and the anterior tibial artery and deep peroneal nerve. The lateral compartment, which is located on the lateral side of the leg, contains the peroneus longus and brevis along with the superficial peroneal nerve. The superficial peroneal nerve can be injured during surgical management of tibia fractures, and is especially vulnerable when performing fasciotomies for compartment syndrome and lateral submuscular plating of the tibia. Damage to the anterior compartment and lateral compartment muscles or the common, superficial, or deep peroneal nerves, which can occur in severe injuries or compartment syndrome, can result in the inability to dorsiflex the ankle (foot drop). This can present a challenge during postoperative rehabilitation, requiring the use of bracing or modification of the patient's gait. There are two compartments in the back of the leg: the superficial and deep posterior compartments. The superficial posterior compartment contains the gastrocnemius–soleus complex, the soleus, the popliteus, and the plantaris muscles. The sural nerve and saphenous vein also course through this compartment. The deep posterior compartment contains the tibialis posterior, flexor digitorum longus, and flexor hallucis longus. The deep peroneal nerve and tibial nerve course through the deep posterior compartment.

Technique

The patient is placed supine on a radiolucent operating table with a bump under the operative hip so that the patella is pointing straight up toward the ceiling. This procedure can be performed with placement of the IM nail through a suprapatellar portal (skin incision is approximately 2 cm proximal to the proximal pole of the patella, with a quadricieps split), a parapatellar incision, or through an infrapatellar portal (insertion below the patella, either medial to, lateral to, or splitting the patellar tendon). While the skin incision varies, the insertion site on the bone of the proximal tibia remains constant, centered over the canal at the anterior corner of the plateau proximal to the tibial tubercle (Figure 72.3).

In the suprapatellar technique, a skin incision is made proximal to the superior pole of the patella. The quadriceps tendon is split in line with its fibers to the superior pole on the patella, which allows extension medially or laterally if additional patellofemoral excursion is needed for safe passage of the instrumentation. In the patellar tendon technique, the tendon is split and the knee flexed, allowing access to the start point. Obtaining the correct starting point is paramount to ensure that intra-articular structures are not damaged and to ensure that passage of the IM nail does not cause a fracture malreduction. As in the femur, a guidewire establishes the start point and the proximal tibia is opened. A flexible guidewire is passed across the reduced fracture. In addition to closed manipulation, techniques such as percutaneous clamps, strategically placed screws to guide or block the nail, and even small plates assist in obtaining and maintaining alignment. Once the tibia is reamed, an appropriately sized tibial nail is inserted

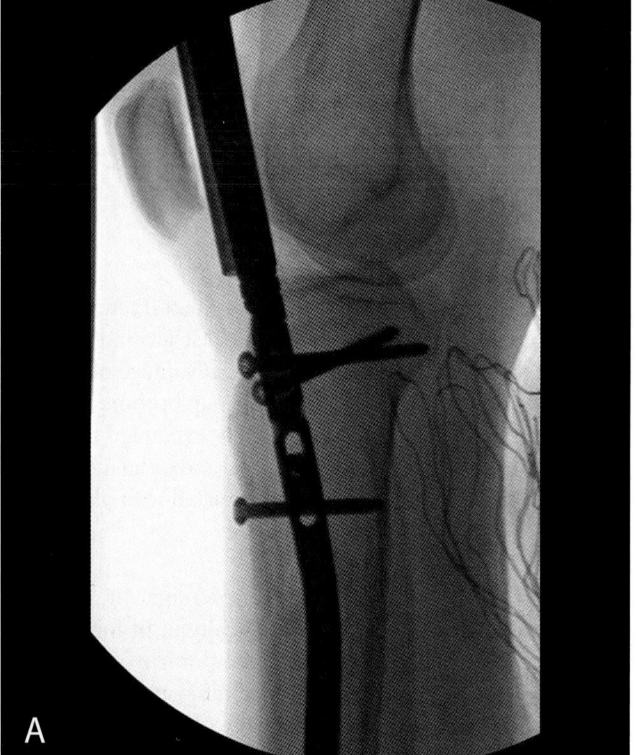

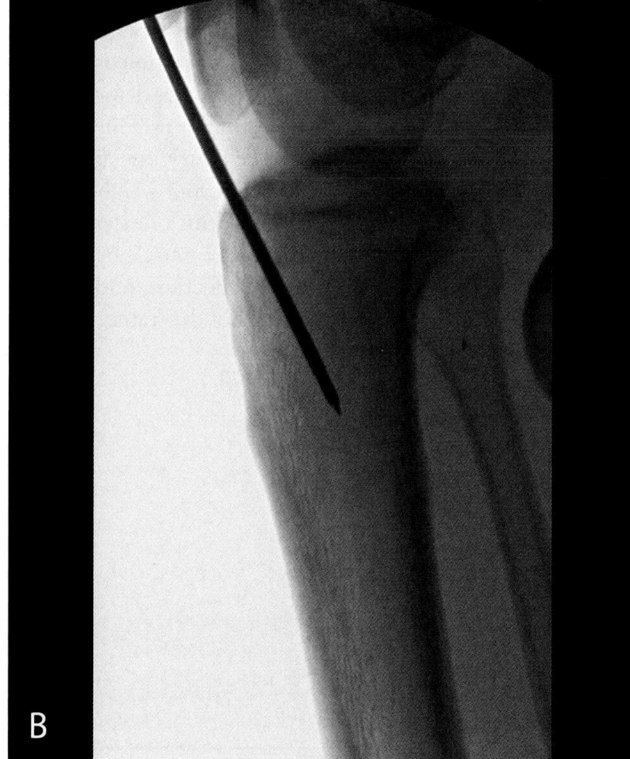

Figure 72.3 Lateral intraoperative fluoroscopic views of the knee demonstrate the difference between the suprapatellar nail technique (**A**), in which the instrumentation is placed within the knee joint behind the patella, and the infrapatellar technique (**B**), in which the instrumentation is placed inferior to the patella.

 © 2018 American Academy of Orthopaedic Surgeons

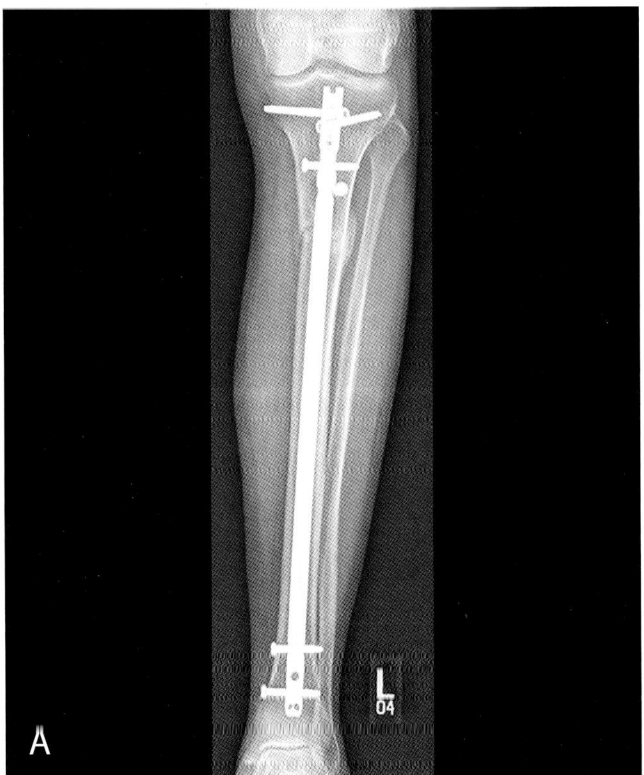

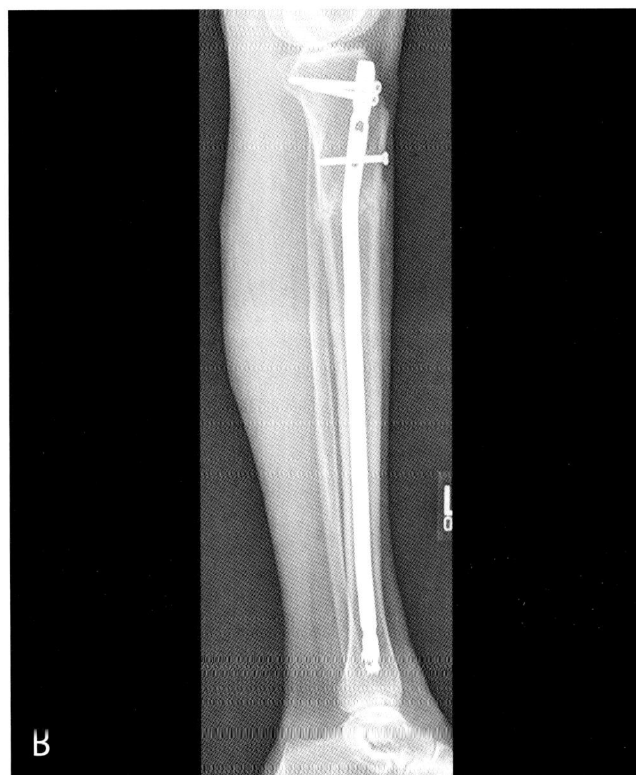

Figure 72.4 Anteroposterior (**A**) and lateral (**B**) radiographs following intramedullary nailing of a tibia fracture.

with placement of interlocking bolts proximally using the jig and distally using the freehand technique (Figure 72.4).

In open fractures, prior to performing IM nailing, the traumatic wound and bone ends are débrided. This typically requires extension of the traumatic wound to ensure that it is adequately débrided of all nonviable tissue and gross contamination. In some cases, definitive fixation can still be performed acutely after an adequate débridement and irrigation, but this depends on the level of contamination. For example, in severely contaminated open fractures, the extremity is often stabilized by external fixation with definitive fixation delayed until the wound is optimized for internal fixation or at the time of soft-tissue coverage, if a flap is needed, to minimize the risk of the patient developing an infection. The soft-tissue injury, especially in situations in which soft-tissue coverage is needed, can have a significant impact on postoperative rehabilitation.

Alternative treatments include plate and external fixation of the tibia, which typically require variations of the physical therapy protocol. They are discussed in the next subsections.

Plate Fixation of the Tibia

Plating of the tibia shaft is not commonly performed unless clinical scenarios preclude IM nail fixation because it may restrict the patient's weight bearing during the early postoperative period. For example, a common indication for plating a diaphyseal tibia fracture is a diaphyseal fracture that has extension into the tibial plateau proximally or tibial plafond distally, which is not amenable to treatment with an IM nail. Another indication for plating may be a previous deformity precluding nail fixation. The plate can be placed through standard open technique or minimally invasively. Medial or lateral plating may be used based on soft tissues and surgeon preference.

External Fixation of the Tibia

In hemodynamically unstable patients, the tibia can either be splinted or a temporary uniplanar external fixator applied to maintain length and alignment until the patient is able to undergo definitive fracture stabilization. The risk of infection begins to increase after an external fixator has been in place for more than 2 weeks when converting the patient to definitive stabilization with an IM nail. These temporary external fixators are commonly placed in a uniplanar orientation, restoring length and alignment. As such, these are rarely used for definitive fixation. Alternatively, ringed external fixators provide multiplanar fixation and can be used for definitive fixation of diaphyseal fractures (Figure 72.5), but have a very specific set of indications, as this treatment modality requires technical skill and can be burdensome on the patient. Nonetheless, careful patient selection is paramount for successful treatment in a ring fixator. They are typically reserved for patients with either large bony defects or significantly contaminated wounds or known deep infection/osteomyelitis, as the fixation can be distant to the zone of injury/infection while still providing rigid enough fixation to permit weight bearing.

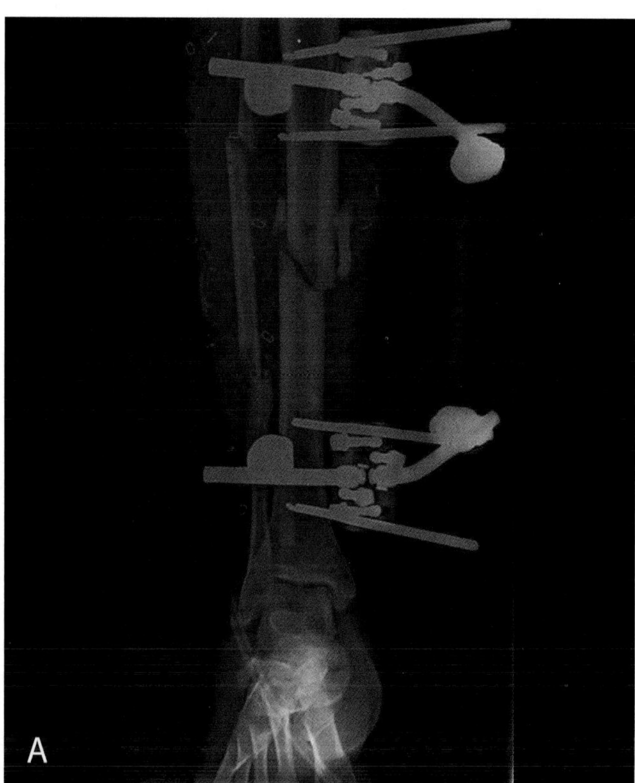

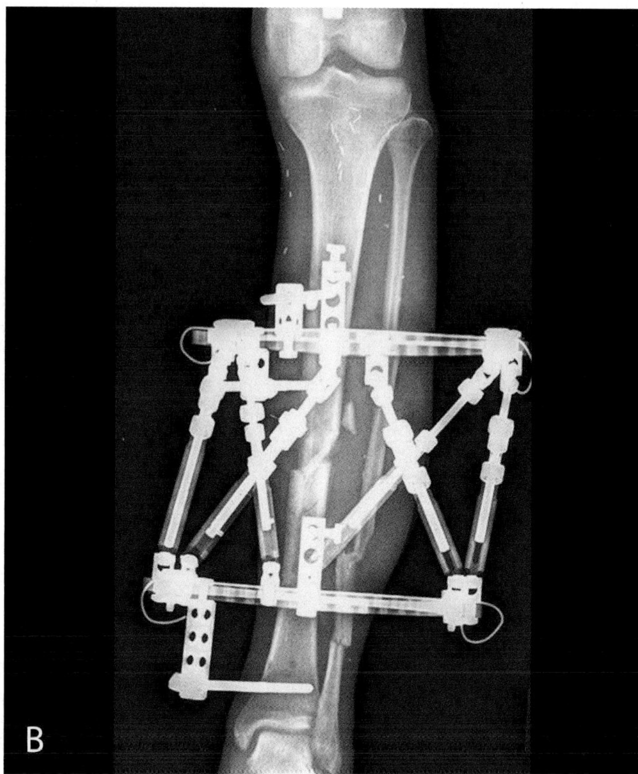

Figure 72.5 Anteroposterior radiographs of two tibial shaft fractures demonstrate the difference between a temporary uniplanar external fixator (**A**) and a definitive multiplanar ringed external fixator (**B**).

Complications of Tibia Fixation

- Infection
- Delayed union or nonunion
- Anterior knee pain
- Compartment syndrome
- Neurologic injury

POSTOPERATIVE REHABILITATION

Introduction

Most femoral and tibial shaft fractures in adults are treated with IM nail fixation. Surgical intervention will typically lessen the recovery time of the patient, but carries with it the risk of DVT, infection, knee pain, and nonunion. Fixation achieves accurate and stable alignment, allowing mobilization of adjacent joints. Standard postoperative rehabilitation precautions are weight bearing as tolerated, but it typically takes anywhere from 3 to 6 months for the femur or tibia to heal. However, weight bearing can be delayed based on surgeon preference in patients with more unstable fracture patterns as compared to those who undergo plate fixation or external fixation. Early weight bearing is beneficial, as it can not only decrease patient morbidity, but it can decrease hospital length of stay, total rehabilitation time, and time off from work. Physical therapy should focus on strengthening the joint above and below the surgical site as well as maintaining all joint range of motion (ROM). Ultimately, the patient should return to high levels of postoperative level of function in isolated fractures. Associated injuries may dictate rehabilitation potential. It is important to note that in patients with continued pain at the fracture site beyond the time in which the bone typically heals, the patient may be progressing to a nonunion, which might require additional surgical intervention. The authors' preferred protocol depends on the patient's tolerance of weight bearing. When the patient is unable to tolerate weight bearing or is not yet cleared to do so, rehabilitation treatment will begin in an un-weighted position, focusing on edema control and ROM, until the patient is cleared by the surgeon to bear weight.

Physical Therapy Goals

The general goals of any postoperative physical therapy intervention should begin with edema control and ROM. When tolerated by the patient and approved by the physician, the patient should progress through activities that will increase strength and improve proprioception. As the patient safely progresses, the program should focus on independence with activities of daily living (ADLs), proprioception, and agility to include required occupational skills and sports-specific drills. The following is a flow sheet with suggested exercises and their progressions as necessary to achieve these goals.

Edema Control

This phase can begin immediately following the surgery and will progress as necessary throughout the phases of

© 2018 American Academy of Orthopaedic Surgeons

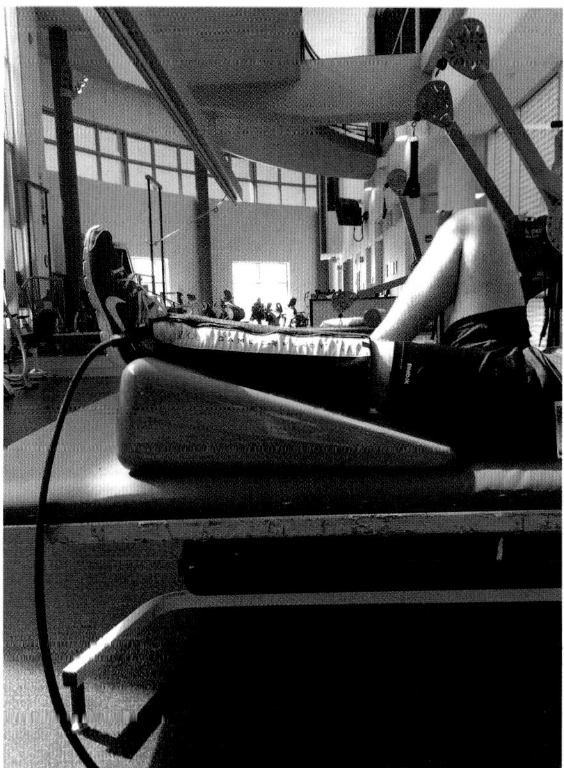

Figure 72.6 Photograph of devices to provide compression paired with cold which decreases edema and pain, promoting increased range of motion and function.

rehabilitation to prevent any possible increases in edema secondary to increased activity levels. Decreased edema will increase ROM and function of the limb. Methods of edema reduction include, but are not limited to:

- Ice bags/packs
- Compression garments
- Elastic compression wraps
- Cold and compression units (Figure 72.6)

Range of Motion

Therapists can begin to regain and/or maintain ROM of the joints immediately following the surgical procedure. Full available ROM of a joint will enhance functional movements and promote appropriate phases of gait. Progression of ROMs and examples of activities will include:

- Passive range of motion (PROM, completed entirely by the therapist or assistive device)
  - Prone hangs
  - Towel pulls
  - Contralateral limb assisted upright cycling
- Active assist range of motion (AAROM, completed by the patient with the support of the therapist)
  - Overpressure at end ranges
- Active range of motion (AROM, completed entirely by the patient)
  - Short arc quadriceps (SAQ)/long arc quadriceps (LAQ)/Heel slides
  - Terminal knee extensions
  - Upright cycling
  - Backward ambulation over ground (treadmill)
- Joint mobilizations as necessary to decrease any limitations in range

Strength

Muscle strength will decrease following musculoskeletal injuries and surgeries. It is the responsibility of the patient and therapist to return that strength to preoperative levels as quickly and as safely as possible to return to function. The following is a progression of strength training specific exercises which should be included, but are not limited to, the plan of care. When the patient is safely able to complete the first series of tasks without a severe increase in pain or edema, the patient can be progressed to the next series of strengthening activities.

- Body Weight
  - Mini squats
  - Lunges
  - Quad sets
  - Heel slides
  - SAQ and LAQ
  - Ankle plantar/dorsi/inversion/eversion
- Resistance Band
  - Ankle plantar/dorsi/inversion/eversion
  - Standing resisted hip strengthening on bilateral lower extremities (Figure 72.7)
  - Knee flexion and extension

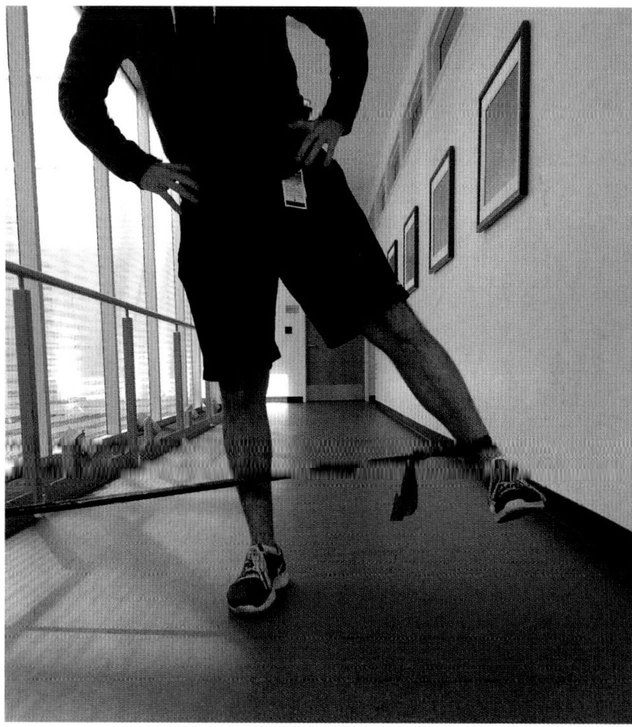

Figure 72.7 Photograph of standing resisted strengthening activities using a resistance band to increase hip strength and contralateral limb stability.

© 2018 American Academy of Orthopaedic Surgeons

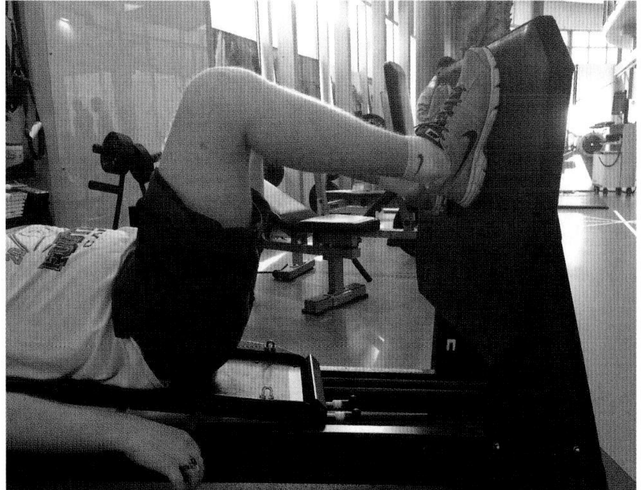

Figure 72.8 Photograph of a shuttle with the patient lying on a sliding platform, used to increase lower extremity strength and progress through jumping activities with the ability to control levels of weight bearing. This machine allows the therapist to educate the patient on proper forms of functional activities in an unweighted environment, which can be transitioned to traditional leg press for further strengthening.

- Weighted equipment
  - Calf raises
  - Leg press (Figure 72.8)
  - Squats
  - Hamstring curls
  - Standing hip fourflexion/extension/adduction/abduction

Proprioception

Postoperative consequences include a decrease in proprioception. Without including activities to improve this loss, the patient will be at an increased risk of reinjury. An appropriate treatment plan should include activities to increase proprioception in the limb. Advance through the following progression when the patient is able to maintain each stance for a minimum of 20 seconds.

- Bilateral lower extremity standing on even ground with eyes open
- Bilateral lower extremity standing on even ground with eyes closed
- Bilateral lower extremity standing on uneven ground with eyes open (Figure 72.9)
- Bilateral lower extremity standing on uneven ground with eyes closed
- Single limb standing on even ground with eyes open
- Single limb standing on even ground with eyes closed
- Single limb standing on uneven ground with eyes open
- Single limb standing on uneven ground with eyes closed

Agility and Return to Activity

When the patient is able to demonstrate full functional ROM and adequate strength, the patient should be progressed to more demanding activities as part of the plan of care. The final progression of any treatment plan should include agility activities, focusing on the patient's specific needs to return to previous levels of function. Educating patients on proper functional movement patterns necessary to complete ADLs, to include leisure or occupational activities, will assist with preventing injuries in the future. The plan of care should include education and training in each of the following areas:

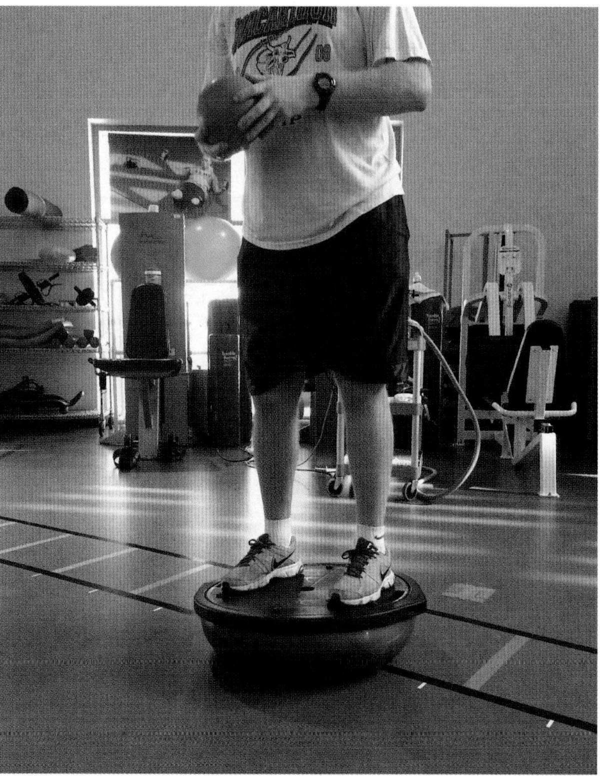

Figure 72.9 Proprioception activities include standing on uneven surfaces, to include a balance ball, as seen in this photograph, with eyes open and closed.

- ADLs
- Lateral movements
- Jumping drills
- Sport-specific drills/prerunning activities (Figure 72.10)

Outcomes

Modern treatment of femur and tibia shaft fractures generally have favorable outcomes. Femur fractures have union rates of 98% with index treatment while the tibia is slightly lower, around 90%. Delayed union and nonunion are related to higher-energy and open fractures, smoking, use of nonsteroidal anti-inflammatory drugs (NSAIDs), and other comorbidities. Continued pain at the fracture site should alert the surgeon and therapist to the potential of delayed union and nonunion. Pain may also be related to prominent hardware. Anterior knee pain may be present in up to 30% of tibia fractures treated with a nail. Focused programs to strengthen thigh musculature and maintain flexibility often alleviate these symptoms. In refractory cases, nail removal after fracture healing may be helpful in abating symptoms.

© 2018 American Academy of Orthopaedic Surgeons

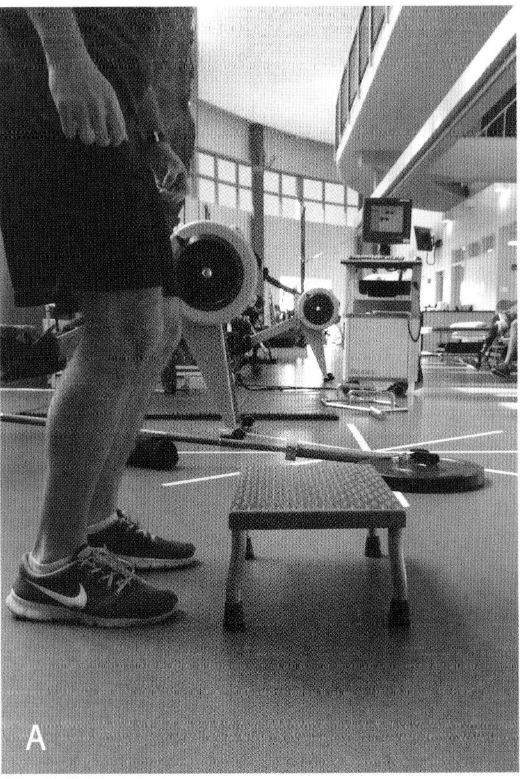

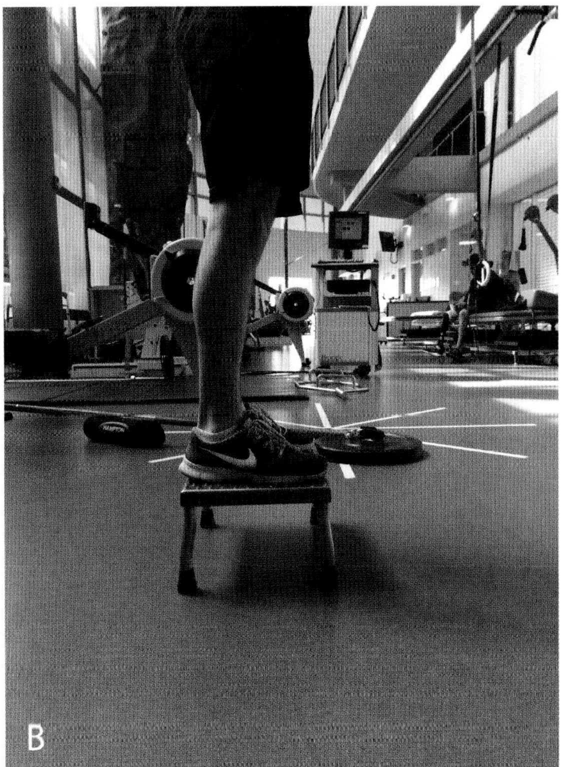

Figure 72.10 **A**, **B**, High-level functional activities and return to sport activities will include box jumps as necessary, as seen in these photographs, to improve explosive dynamic movements.

PEARLS

- Typically, knee extension, both active and passive, is more difficult to achieve postoperatively than flexion. Treatments should focus on attaining full extension with the expectation that flexion will return as edema is controlled.
- Modalities that combine compression with ice will see greater improvements that either one separately.
- Risk of reinjury increases without proper return of proprioception.

BIBLIOGRAPHY

Brumback RJ, Toal TR Jr, Murphy-Zane MS, Novak VP, Belkoff SM: Immediate weight-bearing after treatment of a comminuted fracture of the femoral shaft with a statically locked intramedullary nail. *J Bone Joint Surg Am* 1999;81(11):1538–1544.

Della Rocca GJ, Crist BD: External fixation versus conversion to intramedullary nailing for definitive management of closed fractures of the femoral and tibial shaft. *J Am Acad Orthop Surg* 2006;14(10 Spec No.):S131–S135.

Hooper GJ, Keddell RG, Penny ID: Conservative management or closed nailing for tibial shaft fractures. A randomised prospective trial. *J Bone Joint Surg Br* 1991;73(1):83–85.

Nyland J, Bealle DP, Kaufer H, Johnson DL: Long-term quadriceps femoris functional deficits following intramedullary nailing of isolated tibial fractures. *Int Orthop* 2001;24(6): 342–346.

Paterno MV, Archdeacon MT: Is there a standard rehabilitation protocol after femoral intramedullary nailing? *J Orthop Trauma* 2009;23(5 Suppl):S39–S46.

Paterno MV, Archdeacon MT, Ford KR, Galvin D, Hewett TE: Early rehabilitation following surgical fixation of a femoral shaft fracture. *Phys Ther* 2006;86(4):558–572.

© 2018 American Academy of Orthopaedic Surgeons

73 Postoperative Orthopaedic Rehabilitation of Distal Femur Fractures

H. Michael Frisch, MD

INTRODUCTION

Distal femur fractures encompass a wide spectrum of injuries with various characteristics that must be considered when developing a treatment plan with respect to both surgery and rehabilitation. On one end of the spectrum are the high-energy injuries, such as those seen in young patients after a motor vehicle crash. These are often open, comminuted, and intra-articular, but have better bone quality. On the other end of the spectrum are low-energy injuries that tend to occur in elderly patients after a fall. These are often closed and extra-articular, but with osteoporotic bone.

Distal femur fractures are classified based on the anatomy of the fracture pattern. The extra-articular group includes the supracondylar and periprosthetic types. The intra-articular group includes the unicondylar and the much more common bicondylar types. The AO/OTA classification system is most commonly used to further subdivide these fractures based on comminution. The surgical approach, extent of the exposure, and form of fixation are driven by the fracture pattern and its severity.

The location and severity of fracture comminution, as well as bone loss, all have a negative impact on the stability of the fracture fixation and must be taken into consideration when developing a rehabilitation plan. Signs of fracture healing usually dictate progression in strengthening and weight bearing.

When developing an operative and rehabilitation treatment plan, it is critical to consider other components of the injury rather than just the fracture pattern. The soft tissue envelope often dictates not only operative timing but also rehabilitation timing. Swelling, open wounds, and degloving injuries risk infection with definitive internal fixation necessitating the placement of a provisional external fixator until adequately resolved. Incisions and exposures must take open wounds into account. Rehabilitation may be delayed by wound healing considerations. Muscle injury and loss, most commonly the quadriceps, affect fracture coverage and time to union but also result in scaring and adhesions, which impact range of motion (ROM) and strength.

The patient's comorbidities must also be considered in the overall treatment plan. Underlying osteoporosis should be evaluated and treated, as it will affect fixation stability and rehabilitation progression. Nutritional deficiencies should be corrected to improve healing and muscle recovery. The overall medical condition of the patient and ability to compensate for the increased energy and oxygen consumption associated with weight bearing restrictions. The additional challenges and increased complications associated with obesity must also be taken into account, such as decreased ability to comply with weight bearing restrictions.

In the past, the operative treatment of distal femur fractures was associated with high complication rates, including nonunion, malunion, hardware failure, infection, and decreased ROM. Although these fractures remain a challenge, recent advances in surgical technique and implants have significantly improved clinical outcomes. Complete fracture exposure and precise fracture reduction, which resulted in significant stripping and devitalization of bone and tissue, has been replaced with less invasive techniques utilizing minimal exposures and indirect reductions. The use of precontoured plates with locking-screw technology and insertion guides has facilitated insertion, reduction, and alignment while improving fixation and decreasing hardware and fracture displacement.

SURGICAL PROCEDURE

Indications

The majority of distal femur fractures are treated with operative fixation. Nonoperative management in a hinged brace is limited to nondisplaced or impacted supracondylar fractures.

Contraindications

Operative fixation is contraindicated in patients whose medical condition precludes surgery. Fractures deemed not reconstructable secondary to comminution and osteoporosis

Neither Dr. Frisch nor any immediate family member has received anything of value from or has stock or stock options held in a commercial company or institution related directly or indirectly to the subject of this article.

© 2018 American Academy of Orthopaedic Surgeons

should be considered for a distal femoral replacement, otherwise known as a mega-prosthesis total knee arthroplasty (TKA).

Procedure: Knee Bridging External Fixation

Knee bridging external fixation is utilized primarily as provisional stabilization in damage control orthopedics if the patient requires further resuscitation or medical optimization prior to definitive fixation. It is also utilized in the treatment of open fractures that require serial débridements. The femoral half pins are placed percutaneously through the quadriceps, which may result in scaring and adhesions that limit motion and contribute to quadriceps dysfunction and atrophy.

Procedure: Lateral Plating

The majority of distal femur fractures can be addressed with a lateral plate for fixation. The major exception is medial condyle fractures.

A lateral incision is centered over the lateral femoral condyle. The iliotibial band is split in line with its fibers. The distal edge of the vastus lateralis is then elevated anteriorly to expose the femoral condyle. For supracondylar fractures and periprosthetic fractures, a closed reduction is performed over a bump. The plate is attached to the insertion guide and passed submuscularly between the vastus lateralis and periosteum. The plate is pinned distally to the condyles and proximally to the shaft while ensuring proper plate position, fracture reduction, and alignment. Particular attention is paid to varus valgus and flexion extension alignment. Proximal screw placement is performed percutaneously through the vastus lateralis using the insertion guide. If more proximal exposure is needed, the vastus lateralis can be elevated off the lateral intermuscular septum and retracted anteriorly. Great care should be taken to limit medial dissection and exposure to preserve vascularity.

The exposure can be extended distally for simple intra-articular fracture by curving the incision towards the tibial tubercle and making a lateral parapatellar arthrotomy. Fractures with articular comminution may require an anterior incision and lateral parapatellar arthrotomy. Anatomic reduction of the articular surface is ensured, then fixed with screws placed so as not to interfere with subsequent plate placement (Figure 73.1).

Procedure: Medial Plating

A medial buttress plate is placed to address medial condyle fractures and oblique supracondylar fractures that exit distally on the lateral cortex just before the articular surface. A medial incision is centered over the medial femoral condyle, the fascia is incised, and the vastus medialis is elevated off the intermuscular septum and adductor tendon to expose the medial condyle. Reduction and plating is performed in standard fashion.

Procedure: Retrograde Intramedullary Nail Fixation

Retrograde intramedullary nail fixation is predominantly utilized to address supracondylar and periprosthetic fractures, but may be used in select bicondylar fractures as well. The nail can be inserted percutaneously by splitting the patella tendon for supracondylar fractures. A medial parapatellar approach is utilized for periprosthetic fractures to ensure that the prosthesis is not damaged during reaming and bicondylar fractures to assess the articular reduction (Figure 73.2). As with plating, flexion extension alignment as well as varus valgus are important to maintain during fixation.

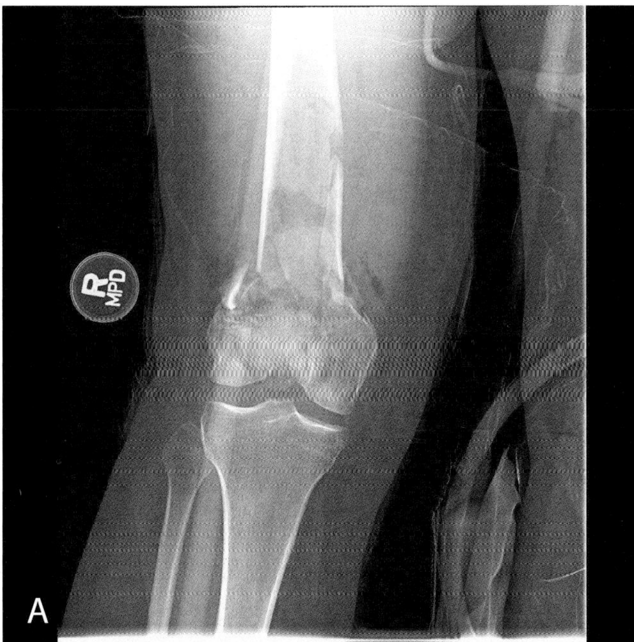

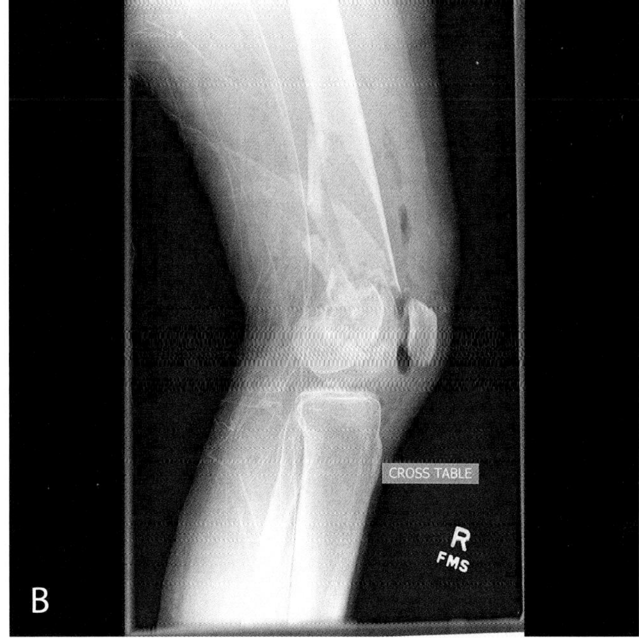

Figure 73.1 Young patient with open comminuted intercondylar distal femur fracture with Hoffa fragments after motor vehicle crash. **A**, Anteroposterior radiograph of injury. **B**, Lateral radiograph of injury. *(continued)*

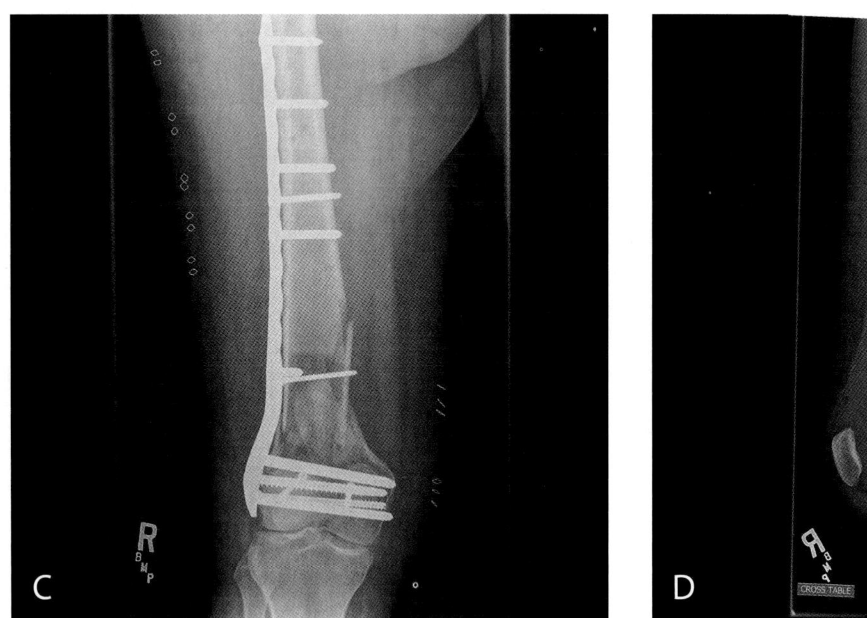

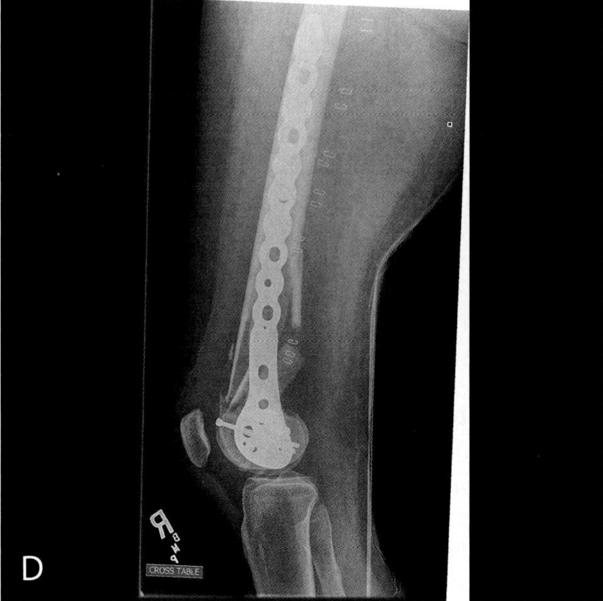

Figure 73.1 (*Continued*) **C**, Anteroposterior postoperative radiograph. **D**, Lateral postoperative radiograph.

Procedure: Distal Femoral Replacement

In select cases precluding stable functional reconstruction of the articular surface, a distal femoral replacement may be performed. Major articular or metadiaphyseal bone loss, particularly in an older patient, severe preexisting arthritis, and periprosthetic fracture with an unstable femoral component are indications to consider mega-prosthetic replacement. In this procedure, the entire distal femur is resected along with the ligament, and is replaced with a hinged knee replacement. Although these patients can weight bear immediately due to the stability of the implant, ROM may be more limited. In addition to wear of the components, infection is a major problem and may require amputation.

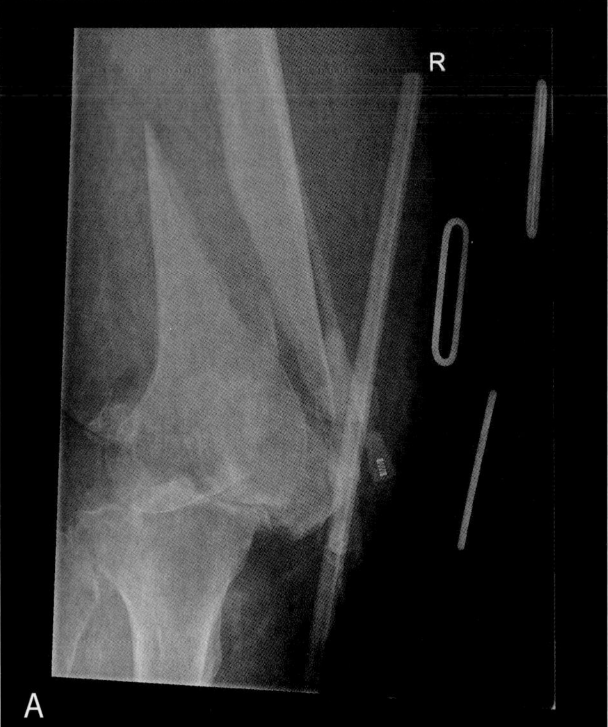

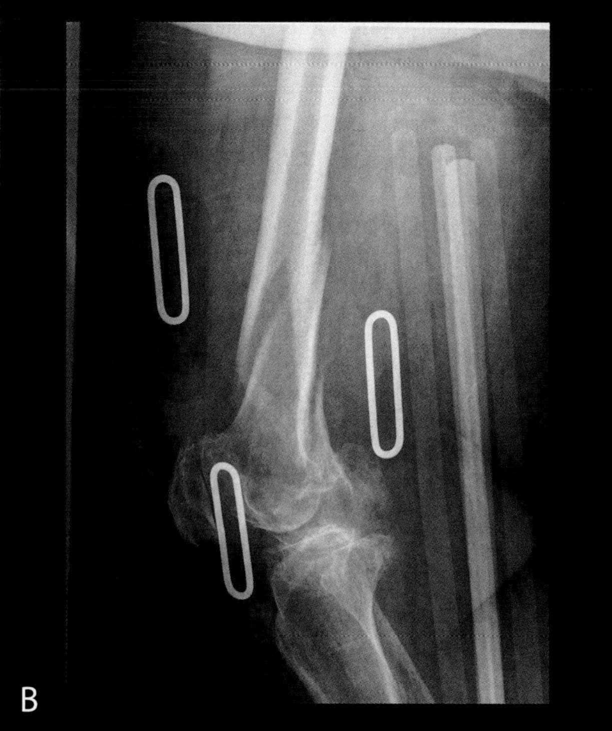

Figure 73.2 Elderly patient with closed intercondylar distal femur fracture after a fall. **A**, Anteroposterior radiograph of injury. **B**, Lateral radiograph of injury.

 © 2018 American Academy of Orthopaedic Surgeons

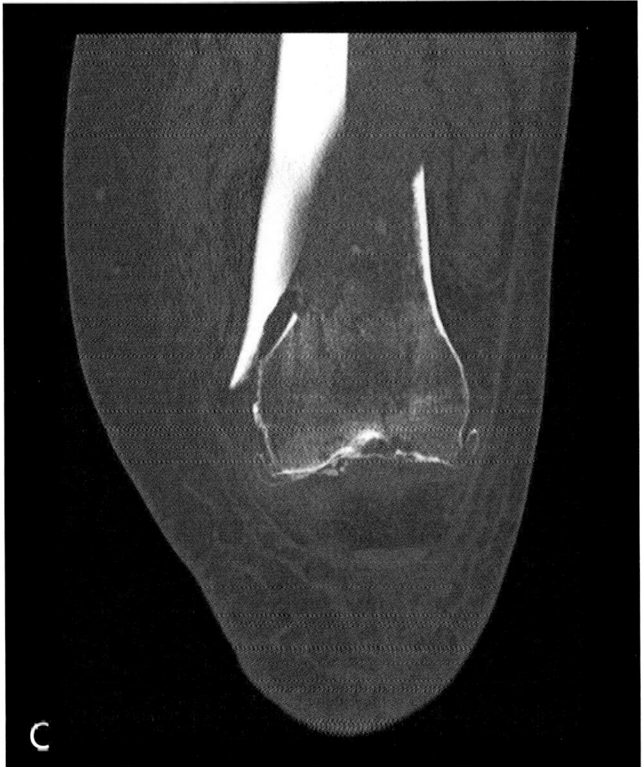

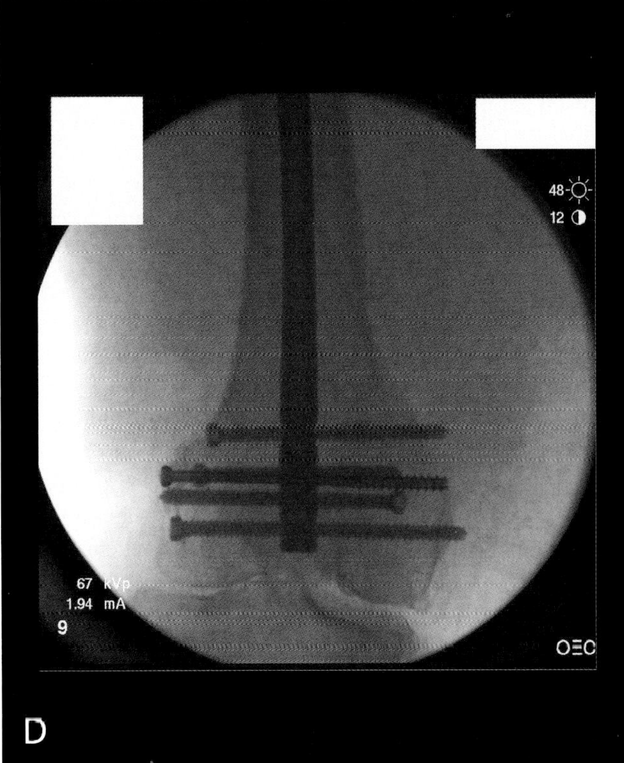

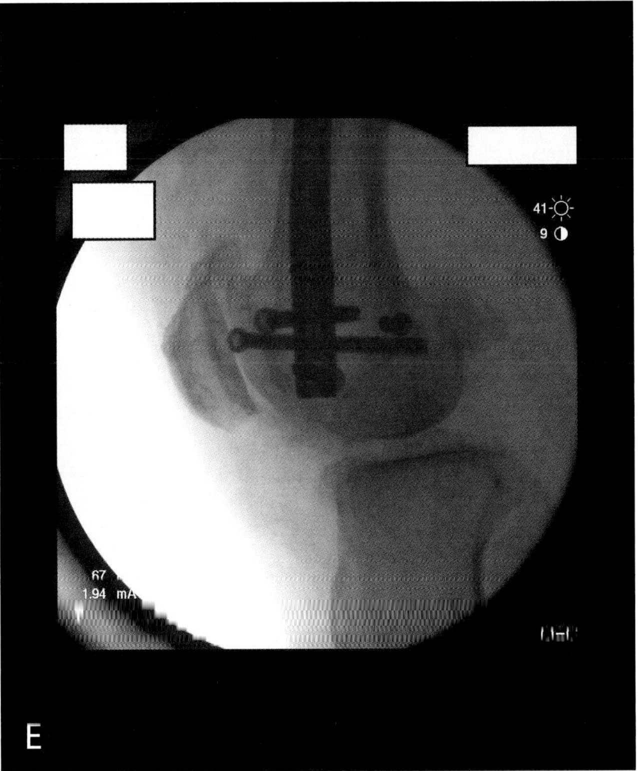

Figure 73.2 (*Continued*) **C**, CT scan of injury. **D**, Anteroposterior postoperative fluoroscopic image. **E**, Lateral postoperative fluoroscopic image.

Complications

Nonunion and delayed unions are common complications of distal femur fractures that will directly impact rehabilitation if weight-bearing progression is delayed. Symptomatic hardware may cause pain that interferes with therapy. Patients almost universally develop crepitus and a bursitis between the iliotibial band and the plate or screws on the lateral femoral condyle. Fortunately, this is usually asymptomatic or resolves.

© 2018 American Academy of Orthopaedic Surgeons

Conversely, prominent screw tips on the medial femoral condyle are often symptomatic and interfere with therapy. The surgeon must always be cognizant of the trapezoidal shape of the distal femur when measuring screw length.

POSTOPERATIVE REHABILITATION

Introduction

Rehabilitation of distal femur fractures is dictated by weight-bearing restrictions and progression focuses on quadriceps dysfunction and regaining knee ROM. However, controlled trials focusing on weight-bearing restrictions for distal femur fractures are not available to guide recommendations at this time. Clinical studies of distal femur fractures using modern techniques and implants have shown an average healing time of approximately 12 weeks, while implant failures have also been attributed to early weight bearing. Current recommendations for postoperative weight-bearing restrictions and progression restrict weight bearing until 8 to 12 weeks, although modifications may be made according to individual fracture, injury, and patient characteristics. Weight-bearing progression ultimately depends on fracture healing.

Quadriceps dysfunction and weakness after femur fractures is well recognized. The muscle damage to the quadriceps from the injury and operative procedure leads to dysfunction after distal femur fractures. Quadriceps weakness impacts both gait and functional recovery, thus should be a focus of rehabilitation.

Distal femur fractures are prone to knee stiffness and contractures. Intra-articular fractures promote intra-articular adhesions, scarring to the fracture site, and quadriceps contracture. Stable fixation is critical to initiating immediate postoperative ROM. Prolonged resting with a pillow under the knee is prohibited despite being the most comfortable position because it promotes contracture. The use of continuous passive motion (CPM) machines may also be considered. ROM and strengthening of the hip and ankle should also be incorporated into the program to prevent deconditioning and stiffness while under weight-bearing restrictions.

Patient compliance with the physical therapy program is critical for success. Ice and elevation to control swelling helps recovery between therapy sessions. Proper pain control and pharmacologic management has been shown to increase compliance with therapy.

Rehabilitation Protocol

- Phase I: Immediately postoperative until discharge
  - Weight-Bearing Restrictions
    - Non–weight bearing
  - Range of Motion
    - Passive (PROM) and active ROM (AROM) of hip, knee, and ankle
    - Patellar mobilization
    - Focus on terminal knee extension
      - Heel prop stretch
        - The heel is elevated on a rolled towel so that the back of the knee is elevated off the bed or floor. The quadriceps is contracted and the patient attempts to touch the back of the knee to the bed.
  - Strengthening
    - Knee
      - Static quadriceps contractions
    - Hip
      - Straight-leg raises
    - Ankle
      - Ankle pumps
      - Resistance bands
  - Proprioception
    - Transfer training
  - Gait
    - Walker or crutch training
  - Conditioning
    - Core, upper extremities, and opposite limb
  - Bracing
    - Hinged knee brace locked in extension for transferring and ambulation in select patients based on fracture and fixation
  - Modalities
    - Swelling
      - Cryotherapy and elevation
    - Pain management
- Phase II: 0 to 12 weeks
  - Weight-Bearing Restrictions
    - Non–weight bearing usually for 12 weeks, but may increase incrementally based on fracture healing
  - Range of Motion
    - PROM and AROM of hip, knee, and ankle
    - Continue focus on terminal knee extension
      - Hamstring and Achilles stretching
    - Goal: 90° of knee flexion by 6 weeks, 110° by 12 weeks
  - Strengthening
    - Knee
      - Isometric quadricep sets
      - Open-chain knee extension gradually progressing resistance
      - Goal: Straight-leg raise without lag by 6 weeks
    - Hip
      - Straight-leg raises
        - Four planes
          - Limit abduction if concern for fracture instability and varus collapse
    - Ankle
      - Ankle pumps
      - Resistance bands
  - Proprioception
  - Gait
    - Walker or crutch training
  - Conditioning
    - Gradually progress to stationary bike with resistance based on fracture healing
    - Pool therapy

© 2018 American Academy of Orthopaedic Surgeons

- Bracing
  - Wean from brace as quad control improves
- Modalities
  - Electric stimulation of quadriceps
  - Swelling
    - Cryotherapy and elevation
  - Pain management
- Phase III: After 12 weeks
  - Weight-Bearing Restrictions
    - Progress to weight bearing as tolerated, progression individualized to the patient
  - Range of Motion
    - PROM and AROM of hip, knee, and ankle
    - Consider knee manipulation under anesthesia if patient has failed to progress past 90° by 12 weeks
  - Strengthening
    - Knee
      - Closed -chain exercises: mini squats
    - Hip
      - Straight-leg raises with resistance bands
    - Ankle
      - Toe and heel raises
  - Proprioception
    - Balance board exercises
  - Gait
    - Gait training
    - Wean from assistive devices
  - Conditioning
    - Treadmill
    - Stationary bike
      - May also be used to regain flexion
  - Bracing
    - None
  - Modalities
    - Swelling
      - Cryotherapy and Elevation
    - Pain Management

Functional Goals and Restrictions

As patients progress through rehabilitation, it is important to be mindful of potential complications. Failure to improve ROM may result in contractures. Persistent or worsening pain and swelling can be an early sign of infections and nonunions. New swelling that extends down the leg could also be a sign of a deep vein thrombosis. If any of these conditions are suspected, the surgeon should be notified immediately.

OUTCOMES

The goal of orthopaedic surgery and rehabilitation of distal femur fractures is to return the patient to preinjury function and activities without restrictions. Patients with intra-articular fractures are counseled on the likelihood of future posttraumatic osteoarthritis, and that high-impact activities should be done in moderation to slow its progression. However, subsequent need for knee replacement is rare. The typical outcome following successful fracture repair is mild stiffness with some loss of terminal flexion. More complex fractures or a complicated postinjury course may have more limited results.

PEARLS

- Weight-bearing restrictions and progression are dependent on fracture fixation and healing.
- Immediate knee ROM exercises facilitated by stable fracture fixation with a particular focus on preventing flexion and extension contractures is optimal course of treatment.
- Rehabilitation of quadriceps is crucial to functional recovery.

BIBLIOGRAPHY

Bolhofner BR, Carmen B, Clifford P: The results of open reduction and internal fixation of distal femur fractures using a biologic (indirect) reduction technique. *J Orthop Trauma* 1996;10:372–377.

Button G, Wolinsky P, Hak D: Failure of less invasive stabilization system plates in the distal femur: A report of four cases. *J Orthop Trauma* 2004;18:565–570.

Gliatis J, Megas P, Panagiotopoulos E, Lambiris E: Midterm results of treatment with a retrograde nail for supracondylar periprosthetic fractures of the femur following total knee arthroplasty. *J Orthop Trauma* 2005;19:164–170.

Hustedat JW, Blizzard DJ, Baumgaertner MR, Leslie MP, Grauer JN: Effect of age on weight-bearing training. *Orthopedics* 2012;35:e1061–e1067.

Issa K, Banerjee S, Kester MA, Khanuja HS, Delanois RE, Mont MA: The effect of timing of manipulation under anesthesia to improve range of motion and functional outcomes following total knee arthroplasty. *J Bone Joint Surg Am* 2014;96:1349–1357.

Kregor PJ, Stannard JA, Zlowodzki M, Cole PA: Treatment of distal femur fractures using the less invasive stabilization system. *J Orthop Trauma* 2004;18:509–520.

Mira AJ, Markley K, Greer RB 3rd: A critical analysis of quadriceps function after femoral shaft fracture in adults. *J Bone Joint Surg Am* 1980;62:61–67.

Padua L, Aprile I, Cecchi F, Molino Lova R, Arezzo MF, Pazzaglia C; Don Carlo Gonocchi Pain-Rehab Group: Pain in postsurgical orthopedic rehabilitation: a multicenter study. *Pain Med* 2012;13:769–776.

Paterno MV, Archdeacon MT: Is there a standard rehabilitation protocol after femoral intramedullary nailing? *J Orthop Trauma* 2009;23:S39–S49.

Rademakers MV, Kerkhoffs GM, Sierevelt IN, Raaymakers EL, Marti RK: Intra-articular fractures of the distal femur: A long term follow-up study of surgically treated patients. *J Orthop Trauma* 2004;18:213–219.

© 2018 American Academy of Orthopaedic Surgeons

Ricci WM, Loftus T, Cox C, Borrelli J: Locked plates combined with minimally invasive insertion technique for the treatment of periprosthetic supracondylar femur fractures above a total knee arthroplasty. *J Orthop Trauma* 2006;20:190–196.

Vallier HA, Hennessey TA, Sontich JK, Patterson BM: Failure of LCP condylar plate fixation in the distal part of the femur: A report of six cases. *J Bone Joint Surg Am* 2006;88:846–853.

Waters RL, Campbell J, Perry J: Energy cost of three-point crutch ambulation in fracture patients. *J Orthop Trauma* 1987;1: 170–173.

Weight M, Collinge C: Early results of the less invasive stabilization system for mechanically unstable fractures of the distal femur (AO/OTA Types A2, A3, C2, and C3). *J Orthop Trauma* 2004;18:503–508.

© 2018 American Academy of Orthopaedic Surgeons

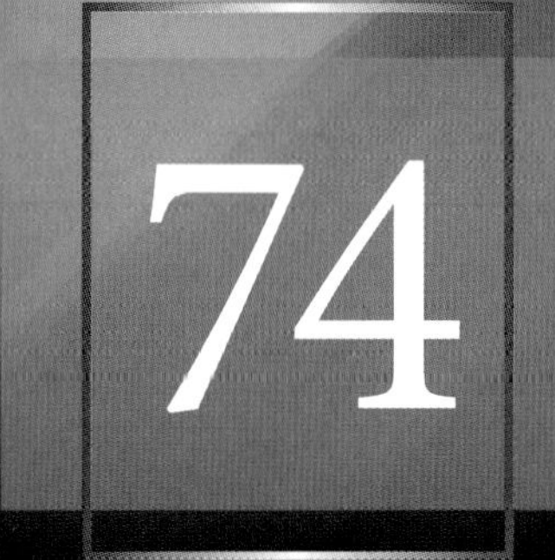

74 Tibial Plateau

Vivek Venugopal, MD, Madeline C. Rodriguez, PT, MS, DPT, John J. Wixted, MD, and Kempland C. Walley, BSc

INTRODUCTION

Tibial plateau fractures are serious injuries involving the articular portion of the proximal tibia and the proximal tibial metaphysis. They account for 1% of all fractures and up to 8% of fractures found in the elderly. As is often the case, the occurrence of tibial plateau fractures follows a typical bimodal demographic distribution: there is a peak of high-energy injuries among young, active patients and a secondary peak of low-energy injuries seen in the elderly. Just as the surgical management of these injuries will change based on the nature of the injury and the amount of energy involved in the fracture, the rehabilitation protocol must also be tailored to the patient's age and activity level.

The history of the injury itself can be helpful in determining surgical plans for repair and for determining the best plans for maximizing the patient's postoperative functional recovery. Historically, these injuries can largely be grouped into three types. First, there are low-energy falls in patients with osteoporosis, which typically cause lateral tibial plateau fractures. Second, younger patients can incur these fractures from either sports or falls. These types of fractures also tend to involve isolated portions of the tibial plateau, either laterally or medially; the prognosis with these types of fractures for functional recovery is quite good. Third, high-energy mechanisms such as major motor vehicle accidents, serious falls, or injuries occurring at high speed will cause the most serious problems and have the poorest outcomes. Knee fracture-dislocations, such as from logging accidents or motorcycle injuries, can be devastating and cause permanent loss of mobility and function.

ANATOMY AND CLASSIFICATION OF FRACTURES

The classification system used by surgeons for many years to describe these injuries was first proposed by Schatzker et al in 1979. This classification system is important because many surgeons use it to guide their operative interventions. While the system describes six characteristic fracture patterns, it is useful to understand that the fractures occur in this fashion largely based on the osseous anatomy of the tibial plateau. The lateral portion of the tibia is higher than the medial; as such, the lateral plateau forms an angle of 3° varus in regards to the tibial shaft. Furthermore, the lateral plateau is smaller and convex compared to the medial plateau, which is larger and concave. The shape of the plateaus, then, favors the medial portion of the tibia, which, in turn, bears 60% of the physiologic load. This asymmetric distribution of weight results in the medial portion of the tibia forming stronger, denser bone. As such, it requires less energy to fracture the lateral plateau, which often fails before the medial side; thus, low-energy mechanisms predispose to lateral plateau fractures. Since older patients are more likely to have osteoporosis, lateral plateau fractures are more commonly found in that demographic. Involvement of the medial side is more common in younger patients, while involvement of both the medial and lateral plateau requires a far greater amount of energy. Statistically, the majority of plateau fractures occur in the lateral side. Between 10% to 23% of fractures are isolated medial plateau injuries, and only 10% to 30% are bicondylar fractures.

More specifically, the Shatzker system describes six general patterns of fractures (Figure 74.1). While there is clearly overlap among the pattern of injury that cause the bone to fracture into any one of these general categories, most injuries occur in a fairly characteristic manner. Specifically, low-energy falls in the elderly would generally result in a Shatzker type II or Shatzker type III injury. While many younger, active patients may sustain Shatzker type II fractures, the vast majority of Shatzker types I and IV injuries occur in young patients with good bone quality. Last, Shatzker types V and VI fractures are usually a result of high-energy injuries, with potentially dramatic disruption of both the bone and associated soft-tissue structures.

Dr. Wixted or an immediate family member serves as a paid consultant to DePuy, A Johnson & Johnson Company, and has received research or institutional support from Merck. Neither of the following authors nor any immediate family member has received anything of value from or has stock or stock options held in a commercial company or institution related directly or indirectly to the subject of this article: Dr. Venugopal and Dr. Rodriguez.

© 2018 American Academy of Orthopaedic Surgeons

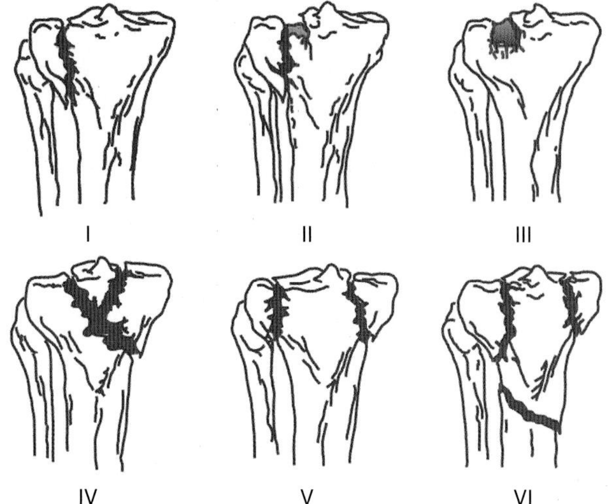

Figure 74.1 Illustration of the Schatzker classification system. Roman numeral assignments are defined as follows: I, split; II, split depression; III, central depression; IV, split fracture and medial plateau; V, bicondylar fracture; and VI, dissociation of metaphysis and diaphysis.

While injuries to ligaments and menisci also commonly occur in conjunction with tibial plateau fractures, treatment of the fracture generally takes precedence. The complications resulting from the fracture itself or poor recovery from such a fracture are often more significant impediments to the patient's recovery than any concomitant ligament or soft-tissue injury. Ligamentous injuries can occur in almost 30% of tibial plateau fractures, and meniscal tears occur in as much as 50% of these injuries. As the energy level of the mechanism of injury increases or the bone quality decreases, there is a greater likelihood of bicondylar fractures or fractures involving the tibial spines and potentially the cruciate ligaments. When ligamentous injuries to the knee occur in isolation, much of the treatment is directed toward addressing the instability caused by their loss. When such injuries occur in conjunction with a plateau fracture, an entirely opposite set of problems arises. In plateau fractures, even those associated with anterior cruciate ligament (ACL) or posterior cruciate ligament (PCL) ruptures, stiffness or loss of motion is a far more serious and common problem; instability from the associated ligamentous injury is rarely encountered and is only dealt with in delayed fashion, after the fracture has been treated and is well healed. Compartment syndrome and injury to neurovascular structures—namely, the peroneal nerve—may also occur with higher-energy mechanisms. Regardless of the mechanism, a tibial plateau fracture portends other concomitant injuries, and as such, almost 40% are polytraumas.

Overall, tibial plateau fractures occur due to direct axial and/or indirect coronal compressive forces. The location, comminution, and displacement are directly related to the bone quality and the degree of knee flexion, as well as the direction, force, and location of the impact. Typically, varus stress and compression will yield a medial plateau fracture and a valgus stress with compression will yield a lateral plateau fracture.

INITIAL ASSESSMENT

All patients with pain or tenderness around the knee after an injury should be assessed for a tibial plateau fracture. Often, a hemarthrosis may be present, but with enough damage to the surrounding tissue, the capsule can be disrupted, leading to its decompression to the surrounding area. Any lacerations should be assessed to ascertain if it communicates with the joint. In all patients, but especially in high-energy traumas, neurovascular status should be assessed and the popliteal, posterior tibial, and dorsalis pedis pulses should be palpated or found on Doppler. Patients should also be assessed for compartment syndrome. Initial radiographic investigation should start with anteroposterior and lateral views of the knee, 15° caudal, and two oblique views. CT scan with axial, sagittal, and coronal reconstruction can aid in surgical planning to assess the degree of comminution, and MRI has increasingly been used to assess for associated soft-tissue injury. One study that compared CT versus MRI found that while CT could be used to diagnose bony ligament avulsion, MRI analysis was necessary to detect ligament and meniscal injury.

CLASSIFICATION

There are two predominant methods in classifying tibial plateau fractures: the Schatzker classification and the AO/ASIF classification. The Schatzker classification subdivides these injuries into six types. In type I, there is a split fracture of the lateral tibial plateau, which can be displaced laterally and distally. This has a large incidence of ligamentous disruption and trapping of meniscus at the fracture site. Type II is a split depression fracture of the lateral plateau, in which the femoral condyle splits and depresses the lateral tibial plateau. A type III is a pure depression of the lateral articular surface without a split of the bone. Type IV is a fracture of the medial tibial plateau, and carries a poor prognosis. This injury pattern is frequently associated with cruciate and lateral ligament tears and a possible traction lesion of the peroneal nerve and popliteal artery. It is considered to be equivalent to knee dislocation. A type V is a bicondylar fracture of the medial and lateral tibial plateau. A type VI is a tibial plateau fracture with associated proximal shaft fracture. Types V and VI fractures have the highest incidence of compartment syndrome.

The AO/ASIF Classification first subdivides the injury pattern into whether the fracture is nonarticular, partial articular, or complete articular. 41-A1 is a nonarticular fracture with ligamentous avulsion. 41-B fractures are partially articular and 41-C injuries are complete articular with increasing decrees of comminution.

SURGICAL MANAGEMENT

Indications

As is the case with most fractures, some tibial plateau fractures can be treated nonoperatively with good expectations

 © 2018 American Academy of Orthopaedic Surgeons

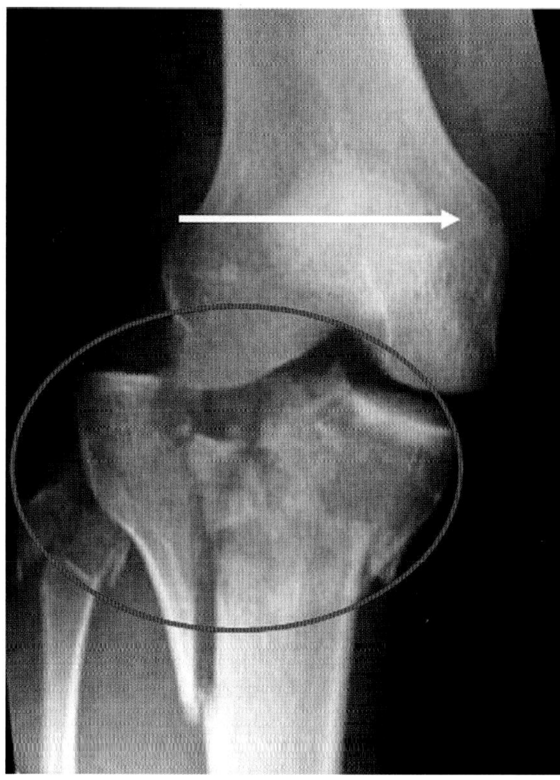

Figure 74.2 Radiograph of a Schatzker type VI dissociation of metaphysis and diaphysis tibial plateau fracture (*red circle*), which characteristically causes articular displacement of the knee joint medially (*white arrow*).

for full recovery, while others have a better chance of good long-term outcomes with surgery. Plateau fractures actually encompass a fairly broad range of injuries; as such, the rationale for operating on them will vary with the fracture pattern and mechanism of injury. Indications for surgery include:

- Articular displacement (Figure 74.2). This is the most common reason for patients and surgeons to pursue surgery. A step-off or widening of the articular surface not only leads to deformity of the joint but disrupts the weight-bearing surface. Left uncorrected, this will result in instability and premature arthritis. Depending on the fracture location and activity demands of the patient, 2 to 5 mm of displacement is typically addressed with surgery.
- Minor degrees of articular depression and very peripheral articular injuries may be considered for nonoperative management if the knee is considered stable and if the patient is older with lower demand.
- Limb alignment: In addition to restoring articular congruity to maximize knee function, many plateau fractures can cause malalignment of the lower extremity, another common surgical indication. When the lateral plateau alone is involved, this tends to cause genu valgum if left untreated. Isolated medial plateau involvement contributes to genu varum. In higher-energy injuries involving both medial and lateral portions of the joint line, both sides of the joint may require fixation; stabilizing one side and not the other may lead to some collapse on the side of the joint that was not addressed, causing malalignment in the coronal plane. Last, specific injuries to the medial side of the joint—namely, posterior shearing fractures of the medial side—may lead to loss of sagittal plane alignment if the posteromedial joint line is not reduced and fixed, another common indication for surgery.
- Extensor mechanism involvement: Although less common, higher-energy injuries may also involve the tibial tubercle; thus, the extensor mechanism may be compromised. Surgically, this requires a strategy to stabilize the mechanism sufficiently to allow for early ROM, which, in turn, may have implications for postoperative rehabilitation. Injuries of this magnitude almost never happen in isolation, and generally require restoration of limb alignment and joint congruity simultaneously.

Contraindications

There are few, if any, absolute contraindications to operative fixation of tibial plateau fractures. While some injuries may be more amenable to late reconstruction if the initial fracture is treated nonoperatively, in plateau fractures, the initial management is often a prerequisite for further surgery. While total knee arthroplasty is a good late-term but infrequently needed salvage for poor outcome after these injuries, successful knee replacement is predicated on restoration of bone stock and limb alignment; as such, it requires successful management of plateau fractures initially. However, in the face of preexisting symptomatic arthritis and mild deformity, definitive surgery may consist of knee arthroplasty following adequate healing of the fracture to avoid sequential surgery. Even those patients with major open injuries, severe ligamentous involvement, or extensive articular involvement will frequently require initial surgery to restore the extensor mechanism, rebuild bone stock, and ensure proper mechanical axis of the lower limb.

Procedure

Surgeons will typically use one of three approaches to reconstruct tibial plateau fractures. Soft-tissue considerations may have some impact on approach; however, the dominant factor is the location of the injury (Figure 74.2).

Low Energy Mechanisms: The Anterolateral Approach

The most common plateau fractures result in isolated lateral plateau injuries. By the Schatzker Classification system, these are typically types 1, 2, and 3. In these injuries, the lateral collapse of the joint line predisposes to valgus malalignment. A straight or posterior curving incision is made lateral to the patella tendon, extending proximally past the joint line and distally to the insertion of the tibialis anterior. The deep fascia anterior to the iliotibial (IT) tract is incised, and proximally the IT band may be split in line with its fibers, if necessary. In the distal extent of the wound, the fascia overlying the tibialis anterior is incised, and a portion of the tibialis anterior is released to allow for submuscular plating. The skin incision can be extended distally and the fascia over the tibialis anterior split as well to allow for access to holes in the plate.

© 2018 American Academy of Orthopaedic Surgeons

The joint capsule can then be incised, releasing the meniscotibial ligament, creating a submeniscal approach to directly visualize the joint. Frequently, the lateral meniscus is torn off its capsular insertion anteriorly and laterally, and sutures can be placed into the periphery of the meniscus for later repair. The sutures also facilitate retracting the meniscus proximally; in this manner, the split and depressed surface of the lateral plateau can be visualized.

The main reconstruction efforts should focus on elevating the depressed segments and restoring the proper width and alignment of this damaged lateral surface. If the fracture line extends anteriorly, this will facilitate access to the depressed segments of the joint. Once the joint has been restored as closely as possible to its correct location, there will often be a void underneath the surface, where the metaphyseal bone was compressed. This can be back filled with allograft bone or any number of bone substitutes. The joint surface can be supported with screws, and a lateral plate is frequently used to further support the lateral portion of the joint, helping to restore the proper width of the plateau and preventing any further collapse into valgus.

Rehabilitation Considerations Specific to the Anterolateral Approach

This approach does involve release of the tibialis anterior, which can result in weak ankle dorsiflexion. However, this release is fairly limited and should not result in profound weakness. Anterolateral plating should be anterior enough not to put the peroneal nerve at risk, but the presence of a new footdrop should alert the providers to potential injury to the peroneal nerve proximally. Some IT band irritation can also occur, as the plate may be prominent over the surface of the tibia. Typically, the fascia is closed over the plate and a prominent plate can cause some degree of local irritation.

Isolated Medial Plateau Fractures: Direct Medial Approach

Although uncommon, isolated medial plateau fractures do occur. In isolated fractures of the medial plateau, the denser bone on the medial side of the knee tends to split in the sagittal plane and result in a single simple fracture line.

A direct medial incision can be used to repair these injuries. Analogous to lateral collapse contributing to valgus malalignment, collapse on the medial side, particularly in the presence of an intact lateral plateau, can cause varus malalignment. The direct medial approach uses a medial, vertical incision and the dissection is largely superficial. The simple split can be reduced with large clamps, and a medial plate can be used to support the medial side of the knee and prevent varus collapse.

Rehabilitation Considerations Specific to the Direct Medial Approach

This approach, while far less common than anterolateral approaches, is useful for supporting the medial side of the knee. In general, varus malalignment at the knee is poorly tolerated. Even minimally or nondisplaced isolated medial plateau fractures are at significant risk for varus collapse because the time for healing is fairly prolonged. Thus, if nonoperative management is chosen for treatment, bracing is mandatory and providers must be vigilant in recognizing progressive varus deformity. When the medial plateau is plated, the plate typically sits on top of the medial collateral ligament (MCL) insertion. This can lead to medial irritation. Once the bone has healed and motion has been restored, the irritating hardware can readily be removed, typically 9 to 12 months postinjury. Therapists and patients may frequently encounter MCL or pes anserinus insertional irritation when treating isolated medial plateau injuries.

Higher-Energy Injuries: Combined Approaches Using the Posteromedial Approach

Higher-energy injuries involving both lateral and medial plateaus are common, and often require two surgical approaches. The lateral side can generally be fixed using an anterolateral approach, but the medial side may require separate posteromedial fixation. In distinction from isolated medial fractures, high-energy bicondylar fractures more commonly fracture medially in the coronal plane, causing a posterior shearing pattern on the medial side. This needs to be supported from below; reducing and plating this injury requires access to the back of the medial plateau. This can be readily gained by using the interval between the hamstrings and the medial head of the gastrocnemius muscle. An incision along the posterior margin of the hamstring incision is typically used and, if necessary, can be extended proximally and curved across the skin folds in the popliteal fossa. The hamstring tendons do not need to be individually dissected out, but can simply be retracted anteriorly as a group. Flexion of the knee facilitates this. The fascia overlying the medial head of the gastrocnemius is incised, and the medial border of this muscle can be readily identified under the proximally coursing hamstring tendons. Directly below the medial head of the muscle is the tibia, and dissection directly on the bone can be used to gain access to both the posterior and medial aspects of the proximal tibia. This allows for full access to the fracture fragments for reduction and plating. Typically, the medial side of combined injuries tends to be the more straightforward and is fixed first, followed by a separate anterolateral approach to address the lateral portion of the plateau fracture.

Rehabilitation Considerations Specific to the Posteromedial Approach

Injuries requiring the posteromedial approach typically are high energy, and it is unusual to perform this approach without also having to repair the lateral plateau through the anterolateral approach. Thus the soft tissues tend to be at higher risk for infection and wound complications, because of the need for dual approaches. Further, the fractures themselves are far more involved, and issues of stability, alignment, and the quality of the fixation may limit the amount and extent of motion and activity in the immediate postoperative period. This, in turn, can limit early motion and contribute to stiffness. This balance between early motion while maintaining the integrity of the

© 2018 American Academy of Orthopaedic Surgeons

repair should lead to individualized rehabilitation protocols and instructions in such cases.

The posteromedial approach itself gives access to the posterior aspect of the knee, and requires mobilization of the medial head of the gastrocnemius muscle. The extent of the injury, the higher-energy mechanism, and the surgical exposure behind the knee can all contribute to the posterior stiffness that is commonly seen after this approach. While isolated lateral injuries may result in loss of flexion, posteromedial approaches can lead to both loss of knee extension and equinus at the ankle.

Last, high-energy bicondylar injuries can suffer concomitant ligamentous injury. Early surgical treatment is largely focused on restoration of the osseous anatomy; frequently, the stiffness associated with these injuries after surgery and healing renders ligamentous issues moot. However, combined ligamentous and osseous injuries, as in the rare knee fracture-dislocation, can lead to significant heterotopic bone formation, particularly posterior to the knee. This can profoundly limit both extension from stiffness and flexion from mechanical blocking by the heterotopic bone.

Alternate Approaches

Although lateral and medial plating are by far the most common mode of fixation, certain circumstances may dictate an alternate approach. External fixation may be used as a preliminary form of stabilization in high-energy injuries to maintain length and alignment while the soft tissues recover. As a second procedure, open reduction and plating is performed. With very severe soft-tissue injury, external fixation may be the definitive form of treatment to avoid the risk of wound breakdown and infection, but may lead to knee stiffness. In fractures in the coronal plane, a posterior approach to the knee may be advantageous to directly support the displaced fragments.

Postoperative Rehabilitation

The major objectives of rehabilitation can be broken down into short- and long-term goals. Short-term goals should include decreasing edema, decreasing pain, increasing lower extremity ROM, improving patellar mobility, and allowing the patient to be independent in short-distance ambulation while non–weight bearing. Long-term goals should include regaining full ROM at the knee and ankle, restoring full strength, proprioception training, and functional or sports-specific training. Ultimately, the patient should strive to walk without an assistive device or limp.

As with all significant injuries, a rehabilitation program will be determined by a patient's age, preinjury functional status, and goals of the patient. Before a rehabilitation program begins, the physical therapist should be made aware of the type of approach used during reconstruction of the tibial plateau and any specific contraindications or special considerations that will impact the patient's rehabilitation process.

Early Phase Rehabilitation

The early phase of rehabilitation should focus on passive and active knee and ankle ROM exercises to combat stiffness. Continuous passive motion (CPM) machines are sometimes appropriate to begin early motion, thus combating stiffness and encouraging early mobility of the knee joint. Isometric exercises are begun, which include quadriceps setting exercises to ensure full active extension, vastus medialis oblique (VMO) reeducation to ensure proper patella tracking long term, and gluteal setting to encourage gluteal strengthening. Modalities such as ice should also be used to assist with pain control and edema. Gait training with either a walker or crutches is essential. Although slight knee flexion is often more comfortable, prolonged rest with a pillow under the knee should be avoided.

Early Phase Summary (Weeks 1 to 2)

- Gait training
- Ice for edema control
- Quadriceps sets
- Gluteal sets
- Ankle pumps
- CPM machine if indicated 0° to 30° to begin

After the first 2 weeks, exercises can gradually be increased as the patient tolerates them. For instance, active and active assisted knee exercises must be done with the goal of at least 90° of knee flexion unless repair of the tibial tubercle or extensor mechanism was performed. In the case of extensor mechanism repair, the degree of flexion and active knee extension may be limited. Obtaining proper ROM is the most important goal of the early rehabilitation phase. Open-chain exercises, such as straight-leg raises, can also begin to strengthen the hip musculature. Knee extension exercises can begin with a towel roll under the knee once pain is adequately controlled. Once the incision is healed, patella mobilization should begin to ensure proper patella tracking. Meniscal repair does not alter the rehabilitation course. Focus should also be on strengthening the uninjured side to improve the ability to maintain non–weight bearing status of the injured side.

In summary, exercises the patient can do include,:

- Active and active assistive range of motion (AROM and AAROM) as tolerated with the goal of at least 0° to 90° of flexion
- Straight-leg raises
- Heel slide
- Knee extension exercises
- Global strengthening exercises of the uninvolved side to improve tolerance of NWB status on the involved side
- Patella mobilization
- Hip abduction in supine with the brace on

Long-Term Rehabilitation

After 3 to 4 weeks of rehabilitation, if pain is well managed and the patient is able to tolerate, the following exercises can be added:

- ROM on a stationary bike without resistance with the goal of 90° of flexion
- Hip abduction

© 2018 American Academy of Orthopaedic Surgeons

- Once the patient is independent in AROM and AAROM exercises, the CPM can be discontinued.

By 4 to 6 weeks of rehabilitation, the patient can continue these exercises, then add the following:

- Heel slides, supine and sitting
- Standing hip abduction, if tolerated
- Standing hip extension, if tolerated

By 6 to 12 weeks of rehabilitation, exercise progression should focus on continued stretching and strengthening of the lower extremities. After 12 weeks, when full weight bearing is allowed, gait training should include proper heel–toe gait. The patient can add closed-chain progressive resistive exercises, such as:

- Heel raises
- Squats
- Hamstring curls
- Bridging

At 4 to 6 months of rehabilitation, functional activities or sports-specific rehabilitation should be the focus. Exercise progression will always depend on weight-bearing status, age and preinjury level of activity.

Rehabilitation Protocol (Figure 74.3)

The current standard for rehabilitation of an operative tibial plateau fracture calls for limiting weight bearing in the affected leg and promoting early ROM. This is done to prevent stiffness, which is amenable to physical therapy. By 4 weeks postoperative, 90° of flexion should be achieved. The average time to fracture union is 12 weeks, dictating non–weight bearing for the first 6 to 12 weeks followed by partial weight bearing until 12 weeks. Through the course of recovery, regular radiographs should be completed to observe for signs of fracture migration.

For patients who require operative fixation, any rehabilitation should also consider any concomitant injuries. Regardless, nonoperative and operative patients follow similar guidelines; acute management consists of early ROM and instruction on how to maintain non–weight bearing on the injured leg. At rest, patients may keep their leg at 0° of extension in order to allow the incisions to heal. A CPM machine can be prescribed, and set to 15° to 70° of flexion based on how the incision is healing. Patients should also be placed in a hinged knee brace to avoid any varus or valgus strain and to allow healing of any injured collateral ligaments. The patient should also begin AROM or AAROM as tolerated. Before discharge, patients should be instructed on how to maintain non–weight bearing and undergo gait training; any patients, regardless of operative status, unable to adequately maintain a non–weight bearing status or with altered mental status should be placed in a wheelchair to protect the fracture as it heals. For patients able to maintain a non–weight bearing status of the affected extremity, the decision to use a walker or crutches should be based up the patient's upper body strength and balance.

During the first 6 weeks of rehabilitation, all patients should initiate a lower extremity stretching program along with focusing on ROM exercises to gain 90° of flexion of the injured leg. Patients should also be counseled to extend their knee to 0° to prevent a flexion contracture. Furthermore, since the majority of the patient's weight will be on the uninvolved side, hip strengthening exercises of the uninjured side should be started to help with gait. The focus should be on regaining ROM, as up to 20% of patients report knee stiffness as a common complication.

Between 6 and 8 weeks, patients can begin partial weight bearing progressing up to 50% weight bearing as tolerated. Earlier weight bearing may result in fracture migration, a feared complication that can lead to early osteoarthritis. Regardless

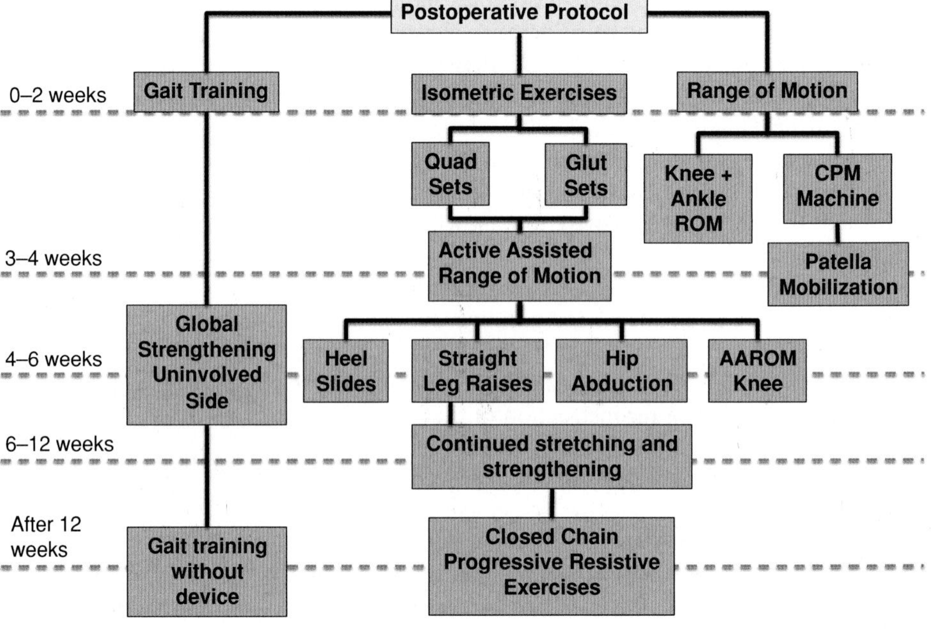

Figure 74.3 Flowchart of rehabilitation exercise protocol for tibial plateau fractures, weeks 0 to 12. Exercise protocol can be modified based on the patient's injury, surgical status, and preinjury functional status. Program should begin in the hospital but should be supplemented with an outpatient program at least two times per week.

© 2018 American Academy of Orthopaedic Surgeons

of weight-bearing status during weeks 6 to 8, patients should continue their ROM exercises and global stretching program.

At this point, muscle strengthening and proprioception exercises should become the primary focus. Muscle strengthening should target the quadriceps, hamstrings, gastrocnemius, abductors, adductors, and gluteus medius and maximus. While there are limited studies focused on rehabilitation of tibial plateau fractures, multiple studies have investigated rehabilitation models after ACL injury. In these studies, it has been shown that restoring quadriceps muscle strength correlates with better outcomes after knee surgery. Furthermore, contraction of the gastrocnemius and/or quadriceps has been shown to increase ACL strain and increase joint compression. Thus, it is clear that restoring muscle strength and function is critical in returning a patient to the highest level of function.

In addition to muscle strengthening, proprioception exercises should also be started. Proprioception is defined as a sensory modality that includes joint movement and joint position sense. Rehabilitation should focus on restoring motor control at three levels: spinal, cognitive programming, and brainstem activity. This can be done by performing exercises that focus on dynamic joint stabilization. Examples of this include balance training and joint repositioning exercises.

By 12 weeks, patients may wean off of any assistive devices as tolerated and, after radiographic assessment, assess fracture migration. A stationary bike or elliptical program may begin, but patients should avoid any impact activity.

Outcomes

Regardless of rehabilitation, some patients do not regain their full preinjury functionality. Unsurprisingly, this is largely related to the extent of the initial injury. Most lower-energy, isolated lateral plateau fractures do recover fully, while high-energy bicondylar plateau fractures or those with severe articular damage do not. A case series of 89 patients found that 88.8% of patients were engaged in a sporting activity preinjury, which decreased to 62.9% after recovery. Additionally, there was a decrease in the amount of sessions and hours of physical activity. Return to work depends significantly on the patient, as well as the patient's type of work. For those who can maintain a non–weight bearing status, they may return to work as soon as they feel able. For patients with professions that require more mobility, they may have to remain out of work for up to 6 months to a year. This requires negotiation between the physician and patient, and even the employer, and can be tailored to each patient's individual needs.

In summary, tibial plateau fractures are devastating injuries that not only require immediate intervention, but long-term rehabilitation. Coordination between the surgeon and the physical therapist is vital to help the patient achieve the best possible outcome. Physical therapists should be aware of the injury mechanism and fixation method, as well as the preinjury status of the patient, in order to target therapy and optimize the patient's functional status.

BIBLIOGRAPHY

Berkson EM, Virkus WW: High-energy tibial plateau fractures. *J Am Acad Orthop Surg* 2006;14(1):20–31.

Fenton P, Porter K: Tibial plateau fractures: A Review. *Trauma* 2011;13(3):181–187.

Hohl M: Fractures of the proximal tibia and fibula, in Rockwood C, Green D, Bucholz R, eds: *Fractures in Adults,* ed 3. Philadelphia, PA, J. B. Lippincott, 1991, pp 1725–1761.

Koval KJ, Helfet DL: Tibial plateau fractures: evaluation and treatment. *J Am Acad Orthop Surg* 1995;3(2):86–94.

Kraus TM, Martetschläger F, Müller D, et al: Return to sports activity after tibial plateau fractures: 89 cases with minimum 24-month follow-up. *Am J Sports Med* 2012;40(12):2845–2852.

Kvist J: Rehabilitation following anterior cruciate ligament injury: current recommendations for sports participation. *Sports Med* 2004;34(4):269–280.

Lachiewicz PF, Funcik T: Factors influencing the results of open reduction and internal fixation of tibial plateau fractures. *Clin Orthop Relat Res* 1990;(259):210–215.

Moore TM: Fracture–dislocation of the knee. *Clin Orthop* 1981; 156:128–140.

Mui LW, Engelsohn E, Umans H: Comparison of CT and MRI in patients with tibial plateau fracture: can CT findings predict ligament tear or meniscal injury? *Skeletal Radiol* 2007; 36(2):145–151.

Schatzker J, McBroom R, Bruce D: The tibial plateau fracture: the Toronto experience: 1968–1975. *Clin Orthop Relat Res* 1979; 138:94–104.

Watson J, Schatzker J: *Skeletal Trauma,* ed 2. Philadelphia, PA, W. B. Saunders Company, 1998.

© 2018 American Academy of Orthopaedic Surgeons

75 Ankle and Pilon Fractures

Kevin L. Kirk, DO, and Johnny Owens, MPT

INTRODUCTION

Ankle fractures involve the lateral malleolus of the fibula, or the medial or posterior malleolus of the tibia, either alone or in combination. These patterns are due to a rotational injury of the ankle. Fractures of the ankle are typically associated with lower-energy mechanisms, such as a twisting injury while descending from stairs or sports injury. Pilon fractures, on the other hand, result from an axial load and involve the disruption of the weight-bearing articular surface to varying degrees. Pilon fractures therefore carry a worse prognosis. Common mechanisms are falls from a height or motor vehicle crashes.

The ankle joint is a complex, three-bone joint. It consists of the tibial plafond, including the posterior malleolus articulating with the body of the talus, the medial malleolus, and the lateral malleolus. The joint is considered saddle-shaped, with a larger circumference of the talar dome circumference laterally than medially. The dome itself is wider anteriorly than posteriorly; as the ankle dorsiflexes, the fibula rotates externally through the tibiofibular syndesmosis to accommodate this widened anterior surface of the talar dome. The unique osseous anatomy of the talocrural joint, in which the talus is wider anteriorly than posteriorly, provides stability in dorsiflexion and relative mobility in plantarflexion. In standing, the relatively dorsiflexed ankle joint behaves like a true mortise, with stability conferred principally by articular contact. In the non–weight-bearing, plantarflexed position, ankle joint stability is mostly conferred from the ligamentous structures. It is this unique structure that can have implications for rehabilitation in that loss of dorsiflexion is much more common than loss of plantarflexion motion. Therefore, rehabilitation strategies should be developed to regain dorsiflexion motion as early as possible in the rehabilitation course.

Pilon fractures are intra-articular fractures of the distal end of tibia that involve a significant portion of the weight-bearing articular surface. Although the articular component will involve some combination of the medial, lateral, or posterior malleoli, the defining character of the tibial pilon fracture is the involvement of the superior weight-bearing articular area and the and metaphysis. The comminution of the articular surface, primary articular cartilage damage, and joint surface incongruity contribute to the generally worse outcome of these injuries compared to ankle fractures.

Specific knowledge of the mechanism of injury is an important aspect of the assessment of pilon fractures. The mechanisms of injury can either be high-energy, such as motor vehicle accidents, falls from heights, and industrial accidents, or low energy torsional injuries with an axial load component, such as skiing ("boot-top fracture"; Figure 75.1). The fracture pattern is influenced by the axial compression that occurs from the talus being driven into the tibial plafond. In addition, the shearing or rotational component produces variable degrees of separation of the fracture fragments and instability. Rehabilitation of tibial pilon fractures is influenced by the greater involvement of the articular surface and metaphyseal involvement, in which weight-bearing progression may be more delayed and full range of motion (ROM) of the ankle more difficult to achieve.

SURGICAL PROCEDURE: ANKLE FRACTURE

Indications

Any fracture that disrupts the ankle mortise may require open reduction and internal fixation (ORIF) of either the lateral, medial, and/or the posterior malleolus. Instability is present when the talus shifts laterally or medially from its position under the tibia. Fracture of the lateral malleolus and disruption of the deltoid ligament is a common unstable ankle fracture treated surgically. When two or more malleoli are fractured, the ankle is by definition unstable and usually also best treated with surgery as well. In addition, the syndesmosis—the joint between the distal tibia and fibula—may be disrupted, requiring fixation with either screws or suture button fixation.

Dr. Kirk or an immediate family member is a member of a speakers' bureau or has made paid presentations on behalf of Horizon Pharma; and serves as a board member, owner, officer, or committee member of the American Orthopaedic Foot and Ankle Society. Dr. Owens or an immediate family member serves as a paid consultant to Delfi Medical Innovations.

© 2018 American Academy of Orthopaedic Surgeons

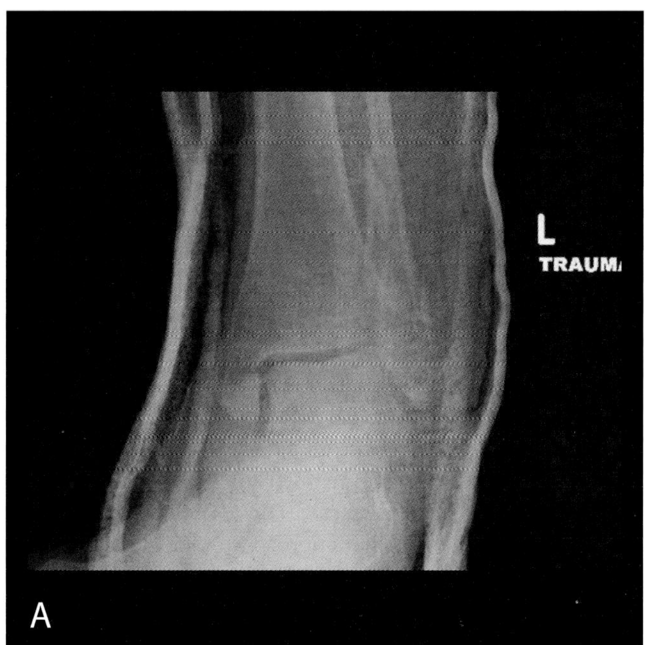

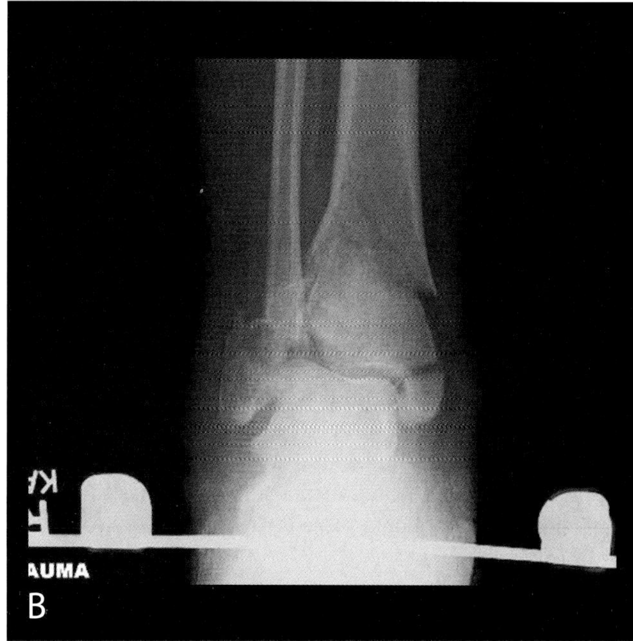

Figure 75.1 **A**, Ankle fracture radiograph. Note fracture of the medial and lateral malleolus. **B**, Pilon fracture radiograph. Note that, in addition to the fracture of the medial and lateral malleolus, the plafond or weight-bearing area is fractured.

The goal is to restore accurate joint alignment to limit the risk of arthritis, especially in the younger active patient.

Contraindications

While the decision for operative versus nonoperative treatment is frequently clear, for a group of patients such as diabetics and low-demand elderly, the treatment decision is more difficult. In these patients, closed reduction may be acceptable when considering the acute risk of anesthesia and soft-tissue breakdown compared to the late risk of arthritis. Specific contraindications to surgery include severe soft-tissue compromise, active infection, and medical instability that would prevent safe surgery.

Relevant Surgical Anatomy

The approach to the lateral or medial malleolus is generally straightforward; however, the superficial peroneal nerve on the lateral side and the saphenous nerve on the medial side can be encountered during dissection. Identification of the nerves and avoidance of trauma to the nerves can prevent any unnecessary complications.

Technique

Since the medial and lateral malleoli are subcutaneous, the approach is directly over these structures. Laterally, the dissection pays attention to the peroneal tendons and the superficial peroneal nerve. Once identified and protected, the fracture is reduced and the plate is applied laterally or posterolaterally. Careful closure is performed to ensure healing. Medially, the dissection secures the saphenous nerve. The fracture is reduced, then fixed with either screws, plates, or, in some cases with comminution, wires and pins. Attention is paid to the posterior tibial tendon to avoid injury.

The posterior malleolus, depending on its size and displacement, may require fixation. It may be indirectly reduced and fixed percutaneously. Many surgeons prefer to perform a direct reduction from a posterolateral approach. A vertical incision is made laterally between the lateral malleolus and the Achilles tendon. The deeper fascia posterior to the peroneals is split, exposing the flexor hallucis muscle, which is elevated off the posterior tibia, exposing the posterior malleolus. The posterior malleolus is then reduced and fixed with either screws or a plate. Following fixation of the malleoli, the syndesmosis is evaluated and fixed with screws or suture to ensure a stable mortise. Syndesmotic screws may also be useful in patients with poor bone stock to optimize fibular fixation in the absence of syndesmotic injury.

Complications

Wound Healing and Infection

The subcutaneous nature of the malleoli can lead to wound healing problems and infection. Diabetics, smokers, and noncompliant patients not vigilant with elevation instructions following injury and surgery are at particular risk. Initial surgery may be delayed to resolve severe swelling and blisters. Any wound dehiscence or drainage warrants prompt notification of the surgeon, who may institute wound care, antibiotics, and even surgical débridement.

Stiffness

Loss of motion, especially dorsiflexion, can be problematic following ankle fracture. If independent ROM exercises and

© 2018 American Academy of Orthopaedic Surgeons

stretching is not rapidly successful in restoring a functional ROM, early referral should be made to physical therapy. Rarely, a posterior, soft-tissue, capsular release, along with lengthening of the Achilles and other flexor tendons, may be indicated to improve severely restricted ankle dorsiflexion.

Hardware Prominence and Pain

Hardware prominence is fairly common in thin individuals following ankle fracture fixation due to the subcutaneous location of the hardware. This most commonly involves lateral fibular plates and screws. Symptomatic relief can usually be obtained with outpatient hardware removal after the fracture is adequately healed. Often, patients are encouraged to wait 1 year from the time of surgery before removing their hardware. Patients are permitted full weight bearing after hardware removal, but are cautioned against activities that could cause significant torsional force for 6 to 12 weeks following hardware removal.

Nerve Injury

The superficial peroneal and the saphenous nerves can be injured at the time of the event, during surgery, or postoperatively become entrapped in scar tissue. If symptomatic, desensitization and occasionally injections can ameliorate symptoms.

Complex Regional Pain Syndrome

An exaggerated response to injury of an extremity manifested by (1) intense or unduly prolonged pain, (2) vasomotor disturbances, (3) delayed functional recovery, and (4) various associated trophic changes. The exact pathophysiology is unknown. However, women are affected more than men, especially with the risk factor of smoking. Symptoms in the lower extremity are more refractory to intervention than those in the upper extremity. Early diagnosis and aggressive treatment with desensitization, edema control, ROM, pharmacologic treatment with gabapentinoids, and at times sympathetic nerve block can lead to successful outcomes.

SURGICAL PROCEDURE: TIBIAL PILON FRACTURE

Indications

Most surgeons agree that displaced tibial pilon fractures require accurate reduction of the articular surface, proper alignment between the articular segment with the metaphysis/diaphysis, and a stable construct to allow early motion. The ability to achieve these goals is directly related to the severity of the articular damage, displacement, and comminution of the metaphysis/ diaphysis, the quality of bone, and patient factors. Due to the high incidence of wound complications, most surgeons perform a two-stage approach in the management of these fractures, that is, initial temporary external fixation with or without internal fixation of the fibula followed by delayed internal fixation. In some cases, the interval may be 3 or more weeks in the event of severe soft-tissue compromise.

Contraindications

Specific contraindications to surgery are similar to those of displaced ankle fractures and include severe soft-tissue compromise, active infection, and medical comorbidities. However, the extent of soft-tissue compromise is usually much more severe in tibial pilon fractures.

Procedure

Several approaches may be useful in treating these complex fractures. The specific approach depends on the fracture configuration, soft-tissue constraints, and surgeon preference. Standard approaches include anteromedial, direct anterior, anterolateral, and posterolateral.

The classic anteromedial approach provides ready access to the medial and anterior tibia. The anterior of the ankle is accessed by releasing the retinaculum and capsule working under the tibialis anterior, the anterior tibial artery, and the toe extensors. The anterolateral approach is made anterior to the fibula generally in line with the fourth ray. The extensor retinaculum is released and the peroneus tertius and toe extensors are elevated, exposing the joint and the fracture. The posterolateral approach is performed as described in the ankle section. These approaches may be used alone or in combination to allow adequate exposure for reduction and rigid fixation with plates and screws. Careful closure is performed to include the retinaculum and skin to optimize skin healing.

Complications

Wound Complications

Soft-tissue compromise can occur in both ankle and tibial pilon fractures. However, due to the higher-energy mechanisms of injury in pilon fractures and the wider dissection, the risk of wound complications and infection is higher. Due to these higher risks of wound breakdown, active motion of the ankle may be delayed for several weeks to ensure adequate healing of the soft tissues.

Hardware Prominence and Pain

Hardware prominence and pain in tibial pilon fractures is similar to those in ankle fractures. In addition to lateral hardware complications, medial hardware prominence is more common in pilon fractures owing to the bulkier implants required for fixation of the articular segment to the metaphysis/diaphysis.

Malunion/Nonunion

Rates of malunion and nonunion in pilon fractures are much higher than ankle fractures mainly related to the more significant comminution of the fractures and intra-articular involvement. These complications may be related to degree of comminution, bone quality, and stability of the fixation; premature weight bearing may also have an influence. Most

© 2018 American Academy of Orthopaedic Surgeons

surgeons will delay weight bearing for 8 to 12 weeks to allow for adequate bone healing to minimize this complication.

Posttraumatic Arthritis/Stiffness

The combination of articular damage, immobilization, and soft-tissue scarring makes some degree of stiffness and posttraumatic arthritis unavoidable. Early non–weight bearing ankle and subtalar joint motion may help lessen this complication. The benefits of early motion must be weighed against the risk of a wound breakdown from instituting a too-aggressive approach to early motion.

External Fixation

Some cases of pilon fracture are treated definitively with external fixation. This technique involves smaller incisions with limited fixation of the joint with screws or small plates. A unilateral frame or circular frame is then applied across the joint to maintain alignment until healed. Some surgeons prefer this technique routinely, as it limits dissection. However, most surgeons reserve this for rare occasions when soft-tissue considerations and severe articular injury preclude safe restoration of the joint.

POSTOPERATIVE REHABILITATION

Ankle Fracture

Immediately after surgery, the patient will be placed in a bulky Jones dressing and will be non-weight bearing until the first follow-up visit with the surgeon. Typically, the consult for rehabilitation will not be placed until after the first postoperative visit, which is 7 to 10 days after surgery.

Postoperative swelling and pain can limit the patient's ability to participate in rehabilitation. The standard principles of the RICE regimen (rest, ice, compression, elevation) should be applied early. It is imperative that the patient understand all four elements of RICE. Too much activity early on can increase swelling and inflammation, slowing progress. Ice provides analgesia, and has the potential to constrict capillaries in the immediate area as well as diminish swelling. However, patients should be cautioned against ice use for more than 15 to 20 minutes because of the potential for vasodilation and a large reperfusion of fluid to the area, which could actually increase swelling. The use of elevation and compression will also help with the initial swelling and act somewhat as a buffer to any reperfusion. The patient is instructed to follow the RICE regimen for 10- to 15-minute intervals throughout the day until the postoperative swelling has subsided. The patient is instructed that swelling may take weeks to subside. If swelling reoccurs during later phases of rehabilitation, the patient should return to this regimen as well as potentially limit or stop activities. Commercial systems that provide compression and cold therapy are an excellent means to achieve swelling control (Figure 75.2). Although a compression sleeve can be beneficial, patients often struggle with pain attempting to apply or remove it when their ankle is too swollen. Continued use of an elastic wrap may be necessary until the swelling has subsided enough to tolerate the compression stocking.

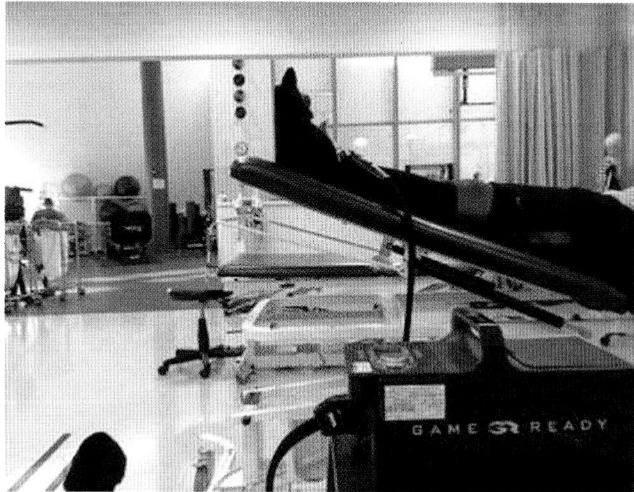

Figure 75.2 Photograph of an icing/compression system.

Early ROM has been shown to benefit ankle fractures. A systematic review of ankle fractures in adults concluded that using a removable brace or splint to allow ankle exercises may facilitate an earlier return to normal activities, reduce pain, and improve ankle movement. However, there is an increased risk of wound complications with early motion; the rehabilitation specialist should monitor for signs of this. Initially, the patient is instructed in gentle pain-free ROM of the ankle and subtalar joints as well as the foot and toes. Because the foot rests in plantarflexion, the patient is instructed to wear the controlled-ankle-motion (CAM) boot at all times, except when performing exercises or showering. If cleared by the surgeon, a dorsiflexion assist boot can be utilized to apply a low-load sustained stretch on the posterior leg (Figure 75.3). The patient is instructed to wear the dorsiflexion boot 30 minutes to an hour the first day and slowly increase time over the following days with the end goal of wearing the boot all night.

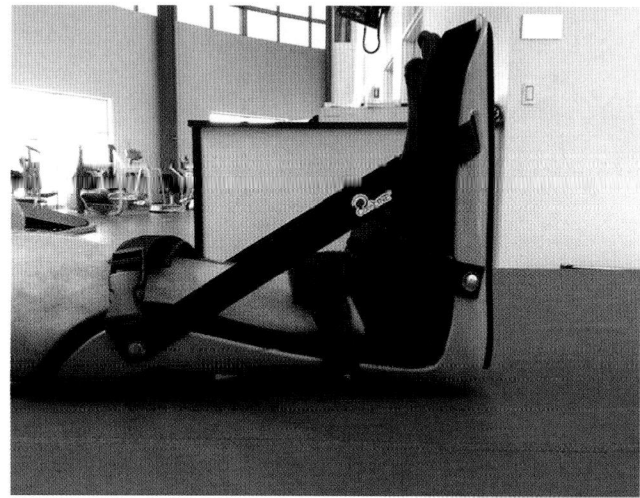

Figure 75.3 Photograph of a dorsiflexion assist boot.

© 2016 American Academy of Orthopaedic Surgeons

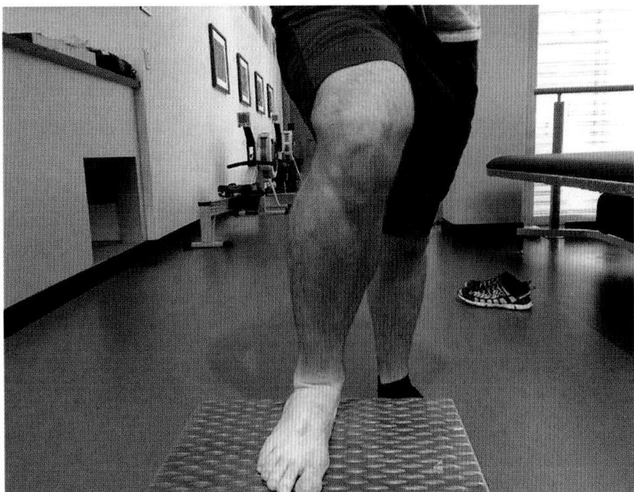

Figure 75.4 Photograph of an improper ankle stretch into pronation.

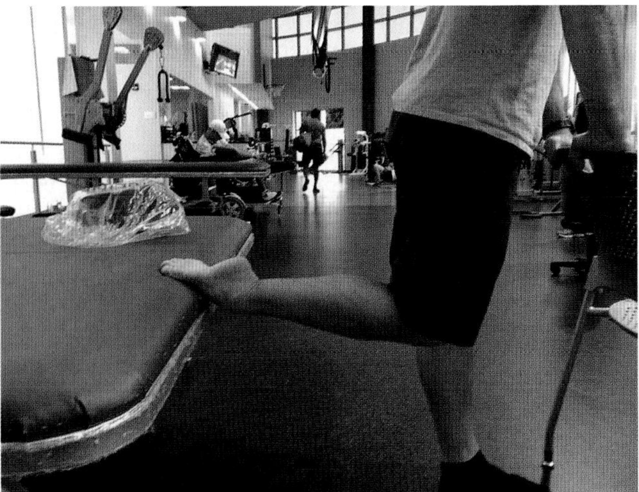

Figure 75.6 Photograph of self-plantarflexion stretch.

ROM should progress from gentle active range of motion (AROM) to passive range of motion (PROM) to therapist-assisted mobilizations, if needed. In particular, ankle dorsi flexion should be emphasized since this is the motion most often lost after ankle trauma. To help regain ankle dorsiflexion, the patient can use straps or towels to perform a heel cord stretch for about 1 minute 4 times throughout the day. Doing this with the knee straight and bent will stretch the gastrocnemius and soleus, respectively. The patient can also use a stool or chair and slowly advance the foot into dorsiflexion. The patient should be instructed to maintain a subtalar neutral position when doing closed-chain stretches to avoid a valgus collapse at the knee and ankle, thus stretching primarily into pronation (Figure 75.4). Doing the stretch barefoot can give visual feedback to the patient and a simple off-the-shelf orthotic can be placed under the foot to maintain a neutral position (Figure 75.5).

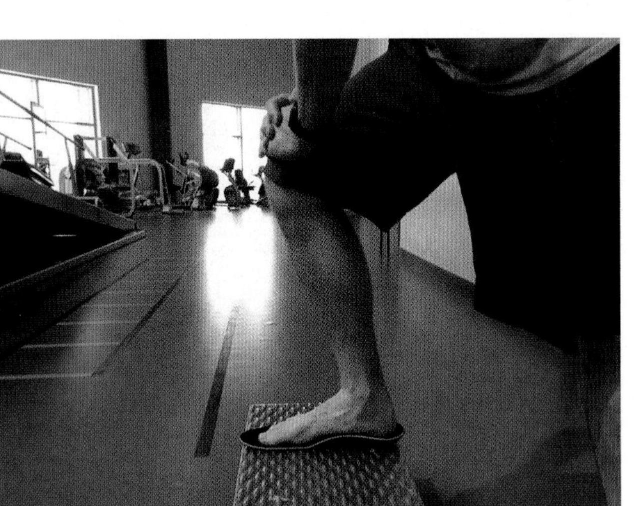

Figure 75.5 Photograph of use of an off-the-shelf orthotic to maintain the subtalar neutral during stretching.

Plantarflexion mobility can include the patient using the hand to self-mobilize the joint and progress to using a chair or stool (Figure 75.6). If motion is lacking into plantarflexion in the late stages of rehabilitation, the patient can perform a kneeling sustained stretch within the limits of pain (Figure 75.7).

If mobility is lacking, the rehabilitation specialist may apply joint mobilizations to regain accessory motion within the joints. As always, respect for the healing fracture and soft tissue is important, and communication with the surgeon about the timing and intensity of the mobilizations should always take place. Once the fracture has healed, and the patient is suffering from anterior impingement of the ankle, a mobilization with movement utilizing a belt and the patient in a weight-bearing position can be used. The goal of this mobilization is to glide the talus posteriorly by stabilizing it anteriorly with your hand and gliding the tibia anteriorly using the belt (Figure 75.8). These mobilizations should be done without causing pain; if pain is experienced, change hand/belt

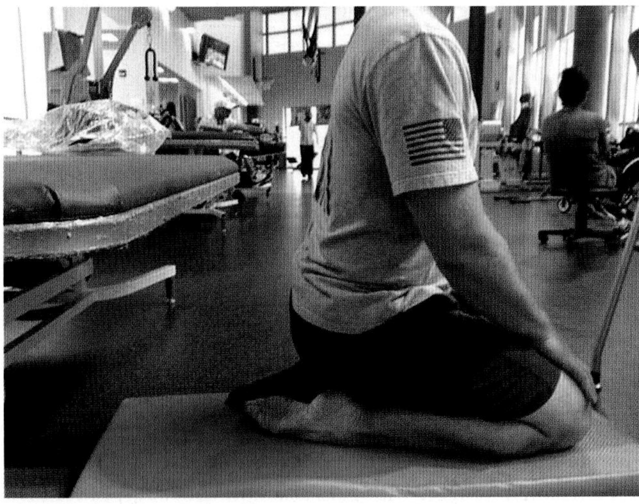

Figure 75.7 Photograph of an advanced plantarflexion stretch.

© 2018 American Academy of Orthopaedic Surgeons

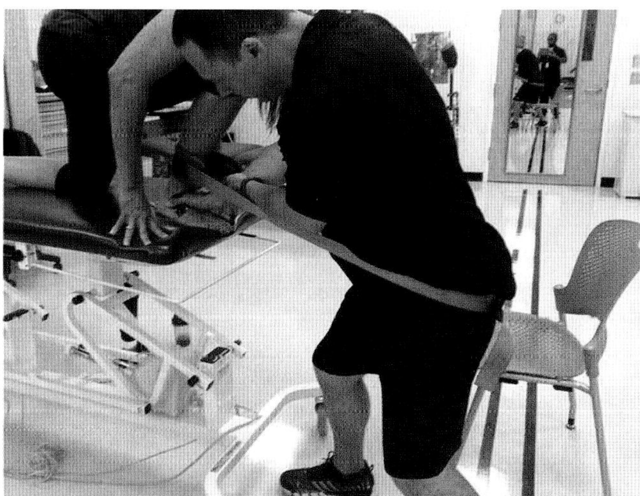

Figure 75.8 Photograph of mobilization with movement for dorsiflexion.

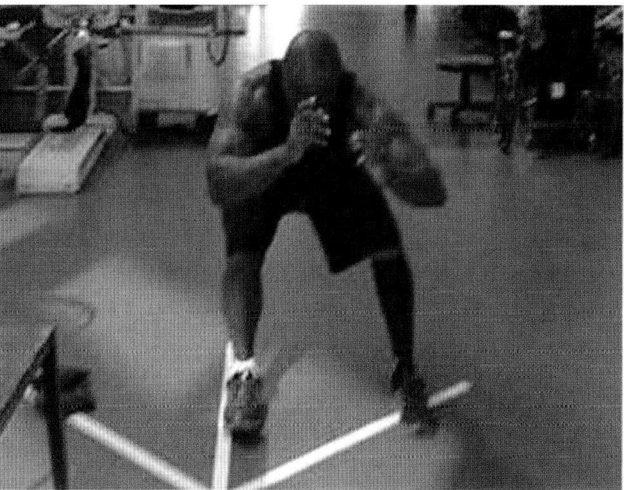

Figure 75.9 Photograph of a patient shifting weight away from the affected limb secondary to lost dorsiflexion range of motion.

positions or abandon the mobilization. As with any manual therapy, the patient should supplement the mobilization with a home program to restore the motion.

Weight-bearing guidance should always be addressed through the surgeon. In special circumstances, such as diabetic patients with neuropathy or patients with poor bone quality due to osteoporosis, weight bearing may be delayed to prevent hardware failure prior to adequate bone healing. Typically, patients are non–weight bearing the first 7 to 10 days while in the bulky Jones dressing. After this, partial weight bearing is allowed in a CAM boot to the patient's tolerance. Follow-up radiographs with the surgeon typically at the 6-week mark will guide the progression from partial to full weight bearing. It is generally expected that by the third month, all patients will be full weight bearing and ready to advance to sport-specific or functional rehabilitation.

Strengthening and functional exercise progression should respect the same weight-bearing applied loads as mentioned earlier. Progressions generally move from bilateral activities, such as weight shifts and squats, to split-stance exercises, such as a static lunge to single-leg stance variations.

Bilateral squatting can be started when the patient is at partial or 50% weight bearing. Often, the loss of dorsiflexion can lead to the patient shifting weight to the uninvolved side, externally rotating the involved foot, which emphasizes sagittal plane motion through the midfoot rather than the ankle, excessive forward trunk lean, and/or rotating the pelvis to compensate for lost ankle motion (Figure 75.9). To combat this, heel lifts of various sizes can be used to assist proper squat form. Through this, the patient works on a functional pattern (squatting) and self-mobilizes the ankle joint into dorsiflexion with each repetition (Figure 75.10). As the functional pattern and dorsiflexion return, the height of the heel lift can be lowered until the patient can complete a normal squat with the foot flat on the floor. Progressive loading can be utilized once proper mechanics have been achieved.

The next functional progression is loading the injured limb in a split stance. This allows an increased applied load to the limb while challenging leg, hip, and lumbar stability, and is a precursor to single-leg stance training. The patient should start with the affected foot flat on the ground in front of the body and both legs in a split squat position. The patient lowers into a lunge position with the goal of controlling the descent. Regaining control of the leg during eccentric movements such as this prepares the patient for the deceleration of the limb necessary for descending stairs, running, and cutting activities. Initially, the patient focuses on keeping the affected tibia on the front leg in a perpendicular position to the floor. This diminishes the deceleration moment at the ankle and provides more emphasis on the quadriceps and gluteal musculature to perform the movement (Figure 75.11). Over time, the patient progresses to advancing the tibia over the foot, increasing the deceleration moment of the lower leg (Figure 75.12). Eventually, the patient is expected to progress to a controlled single-leg squat. This mimics the mechanics of stair climbing and emphasizes the

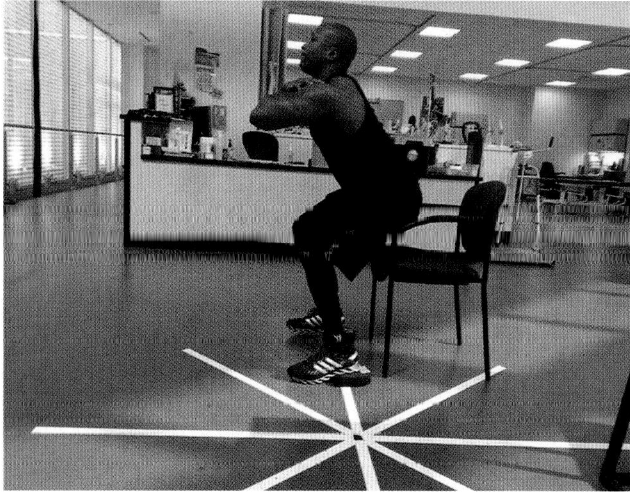

Figure 75.10 Corrected squat pattern using a heel wedge to assist lost dorsiflexion motion. Smaller heel lifts can be used each week until full range of motion and a correct squat is restored.

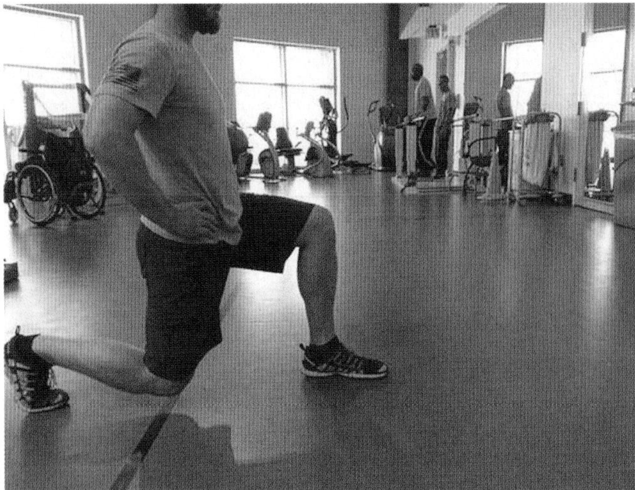

Figure 75.11 Photograph of a split squat without dorsiflexion.

single-leg control needed for most sports. The lunge can be performed in the sagittal, frontal, and transverse planes. Last, the patient will progress to single-limb training. The patient who has gone through the aforementioned progressions should have ample ROM, strength, and stability to start single-limb training (Figure 75.13). Moving to this phase too quickly can create unnecessary compensatory patterns for balancing and possibly anterior ankle impingement from dorsiflexion that has not yet been restored. Once the patient can perform a single-leg squat, we progress to sport-specific skills.

The advanced phases of rehabilitation work on running, cutting, and jumping skills. Devices that allow walking and running activities with reduced load can be used to begin running at a lower body weight. The pool can also be used for the early phases of running.

Power development is started in the horizontal plane using a sled for plyometrics (Figure 75.14). Progressions are the same as the functional exercises, in which the patient starts with a bilateral jump, an alternating leg bound, and a single-leg hop. It is important to emphasize a soft controlled landing in order for the muscle to store and release the energy and diminish the load on the bone/joint. The patient would then advance to ground-based plyometrics, such as box jumps and depth jumps, following the same progressions.

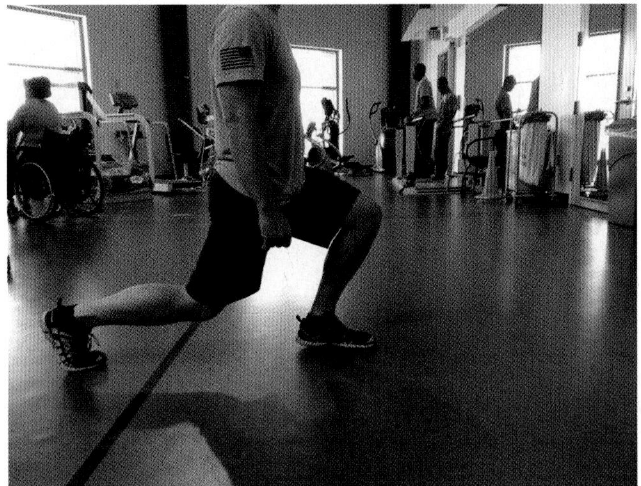

Figure 75.12 Photograph of a dynamic lunge onto the affected limb. The lower leg must decelerate the leg, similar to descending stairs, running, and cutting.

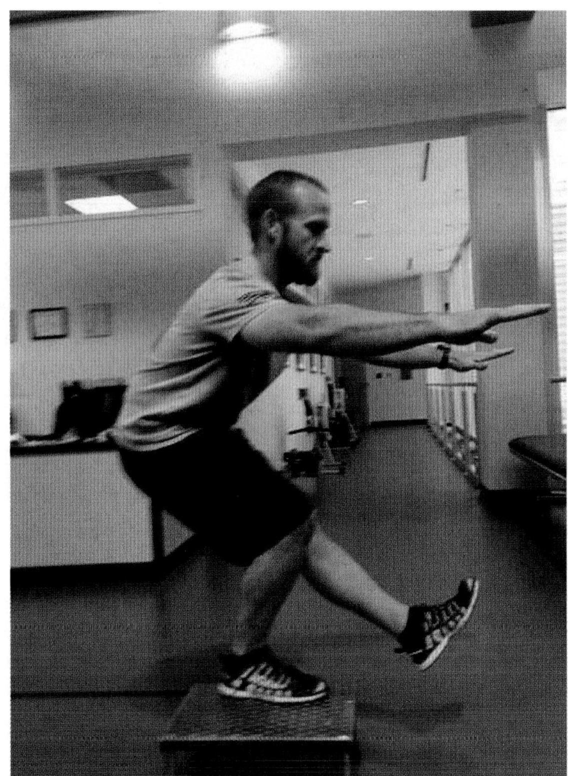

Figure 75.13 Photograph of single-leg squat training.

Cutting skills require the patient to be comfortable moving the leg outside of the patient's base of support (BOS). Until this point, the majority of the exercises have been done with the foot underneath the body. The lateral wall drill is an example of a technique that works on placing the foot outside the BOS for a cut. The patient jogs in place, then puts the affected leg outside the BOS to push the body laterally (Figure 75.15). Over time, the movement can become more dynamic by placing the foot further away from the body and/or the rehabilitation specialist calling out left or right, making it an open loop drill. Ladder drills are also an excellent means of addressing cut mechanics after ankle fracture.

Pilon Fracture

Although many of the same ankle fracture principles apply to the pilon fracture, there are significant differences that the rehabilitation specialist should be aware of. These injuries usually involve higher-energy trauma, and the bone and soft-tissue envelope are much more severely compromised. There should be careful attention paid to the incision for signs of dehiscence or infection in the early stages. Additionally, muscle flaps

© 2018 American Academy of Orthopaedic Surgeons

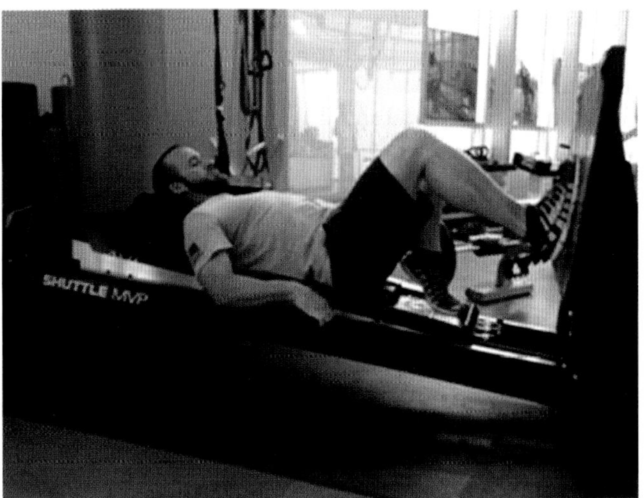

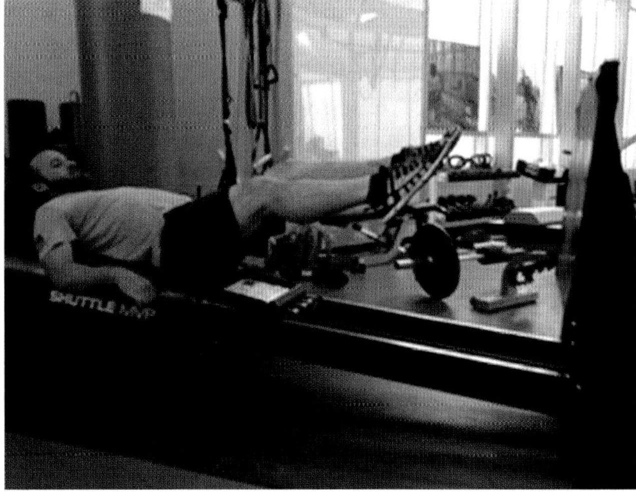

Figure 75.14 Photographs of jump training and power development using a horizontal shuttle.

and/or skin grafting may have been used for closure and will complicate the rehabilitative process.

ROM of the ankle, subtalar joint, foot, and toes follow the same general principles as ankle fractures. Because of the intra-articular injury from the fracture, motion at the ankle can be much more painful and needs to progress slowly and carefully. Toe mobility should be addressed early and aggressively. Contracture of the tendon sheath or compartment syndromes of the foot and lower leg can lead to clawing of the toes. The patient should be instructed early in self-mobilization of the toes, primarily into extension. In general, restoration of motion equal to the other ankle and foot is usually not obtained after a pilon fracture, and educating the patient can help ease expectations. Additionally, the patient should be educated in the progression of posttraumatic arthritis that can accompany these injuries, and that it may take a year to 18 months for symptoms to resolve.

Patients with pilon fractures often have hypersensitivity of the foot and lower leg, and the rehabilitation specialist should always be wary of complex regional pain syndrome. An early desensitization program that focuses on the use of varying textures can help reduce these symptoms.

Weight bearing will be significantly different between the pilon and ankle fracture. After a pilon fracture, the patient will typically be non–weight bearing for 6 to 12 weeks. Healing of the metaphysis will guide the decision-making process. Close communication with the surgeon is essential for the safe weight-bearing progression of these difficult fractures. A pool or unloading treadmill system can be used to help gradually progress weight bearing (Figure 75.16).

Figure 75.15 Photograph of dynamic wall drill. The patient jogs in place, then pushes laterally with his foot outside of his body to simulate a cutting moment.

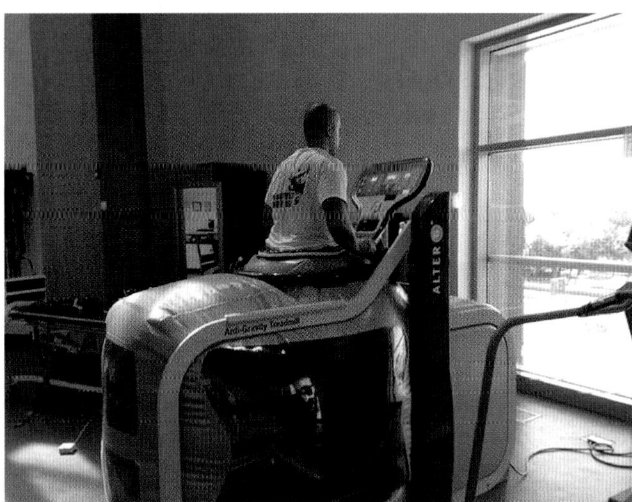

Figure 75.16 Photograph of a load-controlling treadmill.

© 2010 American Academy of Orthopaedic Surgeons

Often, the loss of ROM and power, as well as joint pain, that accompanies these fractures severely limits activities such as sports and the ability to return to work that requires physical labor. The medical team should make the patient aware of these potential limitations to help manage expectations. Patients are encouraged to find a nonimpact sport, such as cycling or swimming, to maintain fitness as well as a light-duty alternative for work if they are consistently on their feet.

OUTCOMES

Ankle and pilon fractures present as a spectrum of injuries. With accurate surgical restoration of ankle fractures, good outcomes can be expected. Although recovery may take 6 or even 12 months, many patients return to all activities, including sport. However, it is common to experience some residual symptoms, such as mild swelling and stiffness. If a patient experiences more debilitating symptoms, evaluation may reveal injuries to the tendons, especially the peroneal and tibialis posterior tendon, or chondral injury. These may benefit from further surgical treatment.

Pilon fractures, on the other hand, may develop radiographic signs of arthritis in up to half of cases. These often result in a decrease of physical activity and benefit from supportive care, such as bracing and anti-inflammatory medication. More severe cases, especially when associated with deformity, may be treated with surgical fusion to control symptoms.

BIBLIOGRAPHY

Brown OL, Dirschl DR, Obremskey WT: Incidence of hardware-related pain and its effect on functional outcomes after open reduction and internal fixation of ankle fractures. *J Orthop Trauma* 2001;15:271–274.

Dehghan N, McKee MD, Jenkinson RJ, et al: Early weightbearing and range of motion versus non-weightbearing and immobilization after open reduction and internal fixation of unstable ankle fractures: A randomized controlled trial. *J Orthop Trauma* 2016;30(7):345–352.

Lin CW, Moseley AM, Refshauge KM: Rehabilitation for ankle fractures in adults. *Cochrane Database Syst Rev* 2008;(3): CD005595. doi: 10.1002/14651858.CD005595.pub2

© 2018 American Academy of Orthopaedic Surgeons

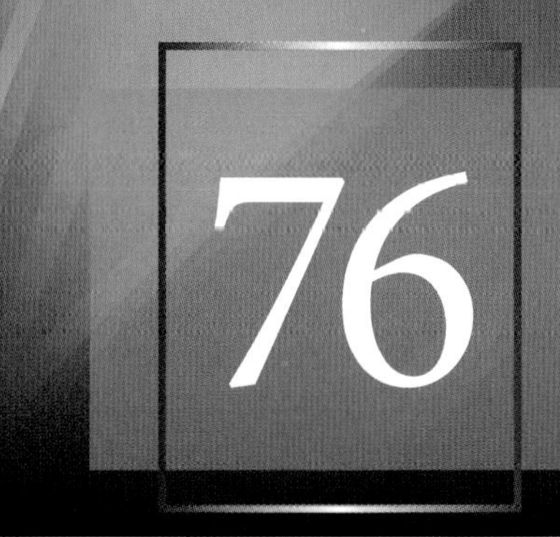

76 Humeral Shaft

Caleb Campbell, MD, Kathleen E. Snelgrove, OTR/L, CHT, and Christopher Got, MD

INTRODUCTION

Fractures of the humeral shaft are relatively common injuries of the upper extremity. These fractures comprise approximately 3% to 5% of all fractures annually and typically follow a bimodal age distribution. Younger patients are more likely to sustain these fractures secondary to high-energy trauma; older patients with osteoporotic bone may sustain humerus fractures after relatively minor trauma. Humeral shaft fractures are also frequently a component of high-energy polytrauma.

Fortunately, the majority of humerus fractures can be managed nonoperatively with a combination of acute closed reduction and splinting, followed by conversion to a functional brace. A custom-fabricated humerus cuff brace can be molded, which is especially helpful if the fit of the prefabricated Sarmiento brace is uncomfortable or inadequate in holding the humerus in a stable position.

Functional bracing may require a shoulder or elbow extension component for fractures of the proximal and distal thirds, respectively. Union rates using functional bracing exceed 90% in most published series.

SURGICAL TREATMENT

Isolated injuries of the humeral shaft most often require surgery if the fracture cannot be maintained in acceptable alignment with closed measures, if there is severe shortening of the fracture, or if there is a significant fracture gap predisposing nonunion. Generally accepted criteria for operative intervention include greater than 20° of sagittal angulation, greater than 30° of coronal angulation, and shortening of greater than 3 cm. Absolute indications for surgery include open injuries and concomitant vascular injuries. Frequently, humeral shaft fractures sustained in the setting of polytrauma are treated with operative fixation to maximize postoperative rehabilitation. If the extremity is needed for mobility, surgical stabilization of many humeral shaft fractures allows for weight bearing with crutches. Some controversy still exists regarding treatment in the presence of an ipsilateral radial nerve palsy, but most surgeons agree that a radial nerve palsy sustained at the time of injury is not a reason for surgical exploration and fracture repair.

Fracture patterns of the humeral shaft correspond to the forces applied to the bone during injury. Simple transverse patterns typically are the result of bending forces perpendicular to the long axis of the humerus. Spiral oblique fracture patterns are generally the result of torsional forces on the bone at the time of injury. Comminuted fractures are typically a combination of bending and torsional forces, and frequently have one or more large butterfly fragments between the 2 main fracture fragments. Methods of fixation and surgical approach are tailored to the specific clinical situation.

Open Reduction and Internal Fixation (ORIF)

The majority of humeral shaft fractures treated with ORIF use an anterolateral or posterior plating and the principles of absolute stability where severe comminution or bone loss is not present. Bridge plating incorporating the principles of relative stability may be required in the presence of significant bone loss or severe comminution. Fixation is achieved with 3.5- or 4.5-mm compression plates incorporating 6 to 8 cortices above and below the fracture, where space permits. Absolute stability is preferred in simple patterns. Transverse fractures are reduced and compression applied to the fracture site through the plating technique. Spiral oblique fractures can be compressed with lag screws perpendicular to the fracture plane with additional compression provided through the plating technique. Comminuted fractures that demonstrate large butterfly fragments may also be reduced and compressed with lag screws prior to compression plating.

The anterolateral approach to the humerus can be utilized for the majority of these fractures. This surgical approach is comprised of a distal extension of the deltopectoral interval.

Dr. Got or an immediate family member serves as a board member, owner, officer, or committee member of the American Society for Surgery of the Hand. Neither of the following authors nor any immediate family member has received anything of value from or has stock or stock options held in a commercial company or institution related directly or indirectly to the subject of this article: Dr. Campbell and Dr. Snelgrove.

© 2018 American Academy of Orthopaedic Surgeons

Most fractures can be treated using the midportion of the incision without requiring a proximal extension to the delto pectoral interval. The skin is divided sharply over the biceps, centered on the fracture site. The cephalic vein must be identified and mobilized to avoid injury. The fascia overlying the biceps is then divided in line with the skin incision to reveal the interval between the biceps (musculocutaneous nerve) and the brachialis (dual innervation) muscles. The biceps is then mobilized, typically in the medial direction. Care must be taken to avoid injury to the lateral antebrachial cutaneous nerve if the incision is carried distally within 5 cm of the antecubital fossa. The brachialis may then be divided longitudinally in its midline, as this muscle receives dual innervation (medially from the musculocutaneous nerve and laterally from the radial nerve). Reduction is obtained and anterolateral or lateral compression plating stabilizes the fracture.

Structures at risk during this approach include the cephalic vein, the lateral antebrachial cutaneous nerve and the radial nerve. The cephalic vein is generally easily visualized in the anterior subcutaneous tissue immediately after skin incision has been made. Blunt dissection will allow for mobilization and subsequent protection of the vascular structure during the remainder of the case. The radial nerve lies in the spiral groove of the posterior humerus in the middle third and courses later ally to pierce the lateral intermuscular septum approximately 10 cm from the radiocapitellar joint. Care must be taken to avoid overpenetration of drill bits and screws in the location of the spiral groove to avoid iatrogenic radial nerve injury during fixation. In the distal portion of the incision, the radial nerve may be identified laterally between the brachialis and brachioradialis muscles.

If a proximal extension must be utilized in order to provide fixation in the proximal third of the humerus, the deltopectoral interval may be utilized. The internervous plane between the deltoid (axillary nerve) and the pectoralis major (medial and lateral pectoral nerves) is utilized. Care must be taken in the deep dissection to incise the periosteum of the humeral shaft lateral to the long head biceps tendon and the pectoralis major insertion. A small portion of the anterior insertion of the deltoid may be sharply reflected, if necessary. Excessive retraction on the deltoid must be avoided to prevent traction injury of the axillary nerve. When proximal plate fixation extends to or past the level of the bicipital groove, the anterior humeral circumflex artery must be identified and ligated.

Occasionally, a direct lateral approach may be utilized for fixation of humeral shaft fractures in the distal third or if the radial nerve warrants direct exploration and visualization due to potential injury. Skin incision is centered over the lateral supracondylar ridge on the lateral portion of the arm. Deep dissection takes place between the brachioradialis anteriorly and the triceps posteriorly. Proximally, the radial nerve is encountered as it courses from posterior to anterolateral at the lateral intermuscular septum approximately 10 cm from the radiocapitellar joint. The nerve may be explored in a posterior and proximal direction as it approaches the spiral groove and distally in a lateral direction as it travels between the brachioradialis and brachialis muscles. If the incision must be carried distally, the interval between the anconeus muscle (radial nerve) and extensor carpi ulnaris is utilized.

A posterior approach to the humeral shaft may be required for distal third fractures or fractures extending into the metadiaphysis of the distal humerus (so-called Holstein-Lewis fractures). There is no internervous plane for this approach, as it utilizes muscle-splitting of the triceps or medial and lateral windows between the triceps and the respective intermuscular septa. A skin incision is centered posteriorly over the triceps muscle and tendon from 8 cm distal to the acromion to the tip of the olecranon. The spiral groove of the humerus lies in the middle third of the bone and will typically be located 14 to 15 cm from the lateral epicondyle. A sterile tourniquet is usually required to facilitate a surgical field conducive to identifying the radial nerve and profundi brachii vessels in the spiral groove. The incision is carried down sharply through skin and the fascia overlying the triceps. Proximally, the fascia between the long and lateral head of the triceps is divided and the long head is retracted medially while the lateral head is retracted laterally. Distally, the fibers of the triceps muscle and tendon can be split longitudinally in line with the incision. The radial nerve and profundi brachii vessels must be located in the spiral groove and traced distally and proximally to allow for protection during the case. Fixation is accomplished using a long posterior or posterolateral plate. As before, absolute stability is preferred using compression through the plate in combination with lag screws, where necessary. If absolute stability cannot be accomplished, bridge plating is then carried out. Once fixation is complete, it is helpful to provide documentation of where the radial nerve crosses the plate (i.e., which hole) following fixation in case revision surgery is required in the future.

The physician and therapist must communicate to determine the stability of the fracture and strength of the repair. Early gentle use of the hand and elbow can usually begin as soon as patient comfort allows, but strenuous use of the arm should be restricted.

Intramedullary Nail (IMN) Fixation

In certain cases, the surgeon may elect to proceed with intramedullary nail (IMN) fixation of a humeral shaft fracture as opposed to plate fixation. Relative indications for IMN fixation include polytrauma, elderly patients who are unlikely to tolerate prolonged operative procedures, pathologic fractures of the humerus, and fractures with extensive comminution or bone loss precluding plate fixation. IMN fixation is not the mainstay of treatment for humeral shaft fractures due to higher rates of nonunion in some published series and a significantly higher rate of shoulder pain postoperatively. However, IMN fixation does provide certain advantages: shorter operative time, smaller incisions, and fixation of the entire length of the bone (pathologic fractures or fractures with extensive communition/ bone loss).

IMN fixation is typically accomplished in an antegrade fashion, though retrograde techniques are described. The

 © 2018 American Academy of Orthopaedic Surgeons

proximal incision for antegrade nailing is located lateral to the acromion. Sharp dissection is carried out until the rotator cuff is visualized. The rotator cuff is then sharply divided to obtain access to the appropriate starting point medial to the greater tuberosity and lateral to the articular surface of the humeral head. Entry into the intramedullary canal is gained using a guide pin under fluoroscopy. An entry reamer opens the cortex while protecting the divided rotator cuff. A guidewire is then passed down the intramedullary canal with the fracture in a reduced position. Sequential reaming is carried out, then the nail is passed across the fracture. Proximal interlocking fixation is carried out through the jig. Distal interlocking is performed using fluoroscopic guidance. Care must be taken when placing these distal interlocking screws, as the radial nerve is at risk when placing lateral-to-medial screws and the musculocutaneous nerve is at risk during placement of anterior-to-posterior screws. The rotator cuff is then directly repaired using nonabsorbable suture. Postoperatively, shoulder ROM and strengthening is not limited and immediate weight bearing is allowed through the fracture.

Complications

Acute

In the immediate postoperative period, wound healing, infection, and nerve palsy are specifically monitored. Injury to the radial nerve specifically may occur at the time of the incident or as a result of the surgery, and may involve sensory and motor deficits. Those following surgery are most commonly traction injuries and resolve within weeks to months of surgery. Documentation of the deficit and its recovery, along with prevention of contracture with stretching and bracing, generally leads to full recovery.

Late

Late complications seen in the surgical treatment of humerus fractures are joint stiffness and nonunion. Fractures that are very distal or proximal in a patient who is unwilling or unable to move these joints are risk factors for clinically significant contracture. Nonunion is signaled by persistent pain and possibly recurrence of deformity. Radiographs with at least 2 views can confirm the diagnosis. Oblique views or computerized tomography may also be useful. In the case of nonunion, repeat surgery is often required.

Rehabilitation Program

Initial

- Performing exercises 4 to 6 times daily
- Active fist and extension of fingers
- Light grasp and squeeze of a large sponge or facecloth
- Holding a pencil or marker in a hook or claw fist, then moving into a "full fist" (Figure 76.1, A and B)
- Finger abduction/adduction
- Active wrist extension and flexion.
- Active elbow extension and flexion. This is best performed with the patient either supine with the humerus against a flat surface or seated or standing against a wall to support

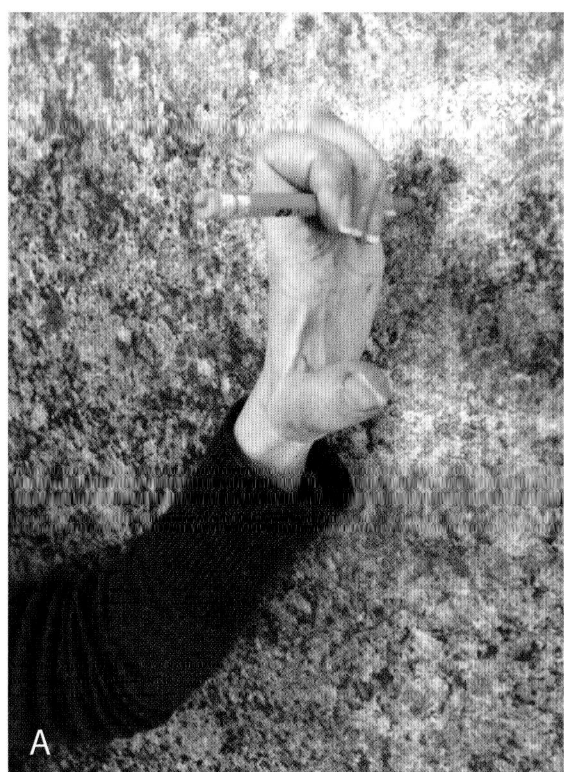

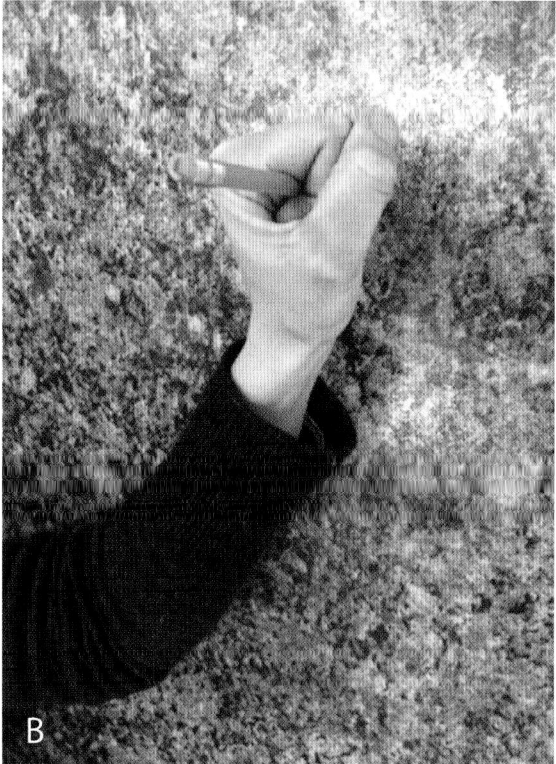

Figure 76.1 Hook fist into full fist facilitated by the use of a pencil is a helpful addition to a home exercise program. A, Hook or claw fist and B, full fist.

© 2018 American Academy of Orthopaedic Surgeons

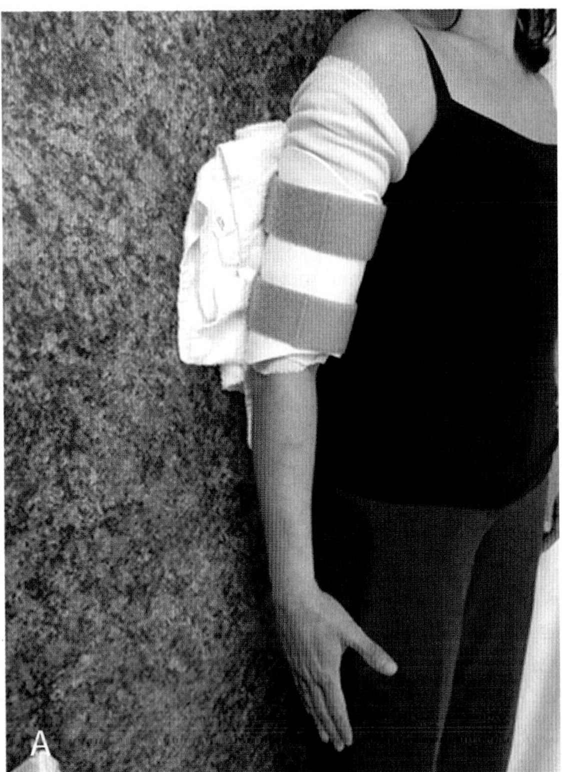

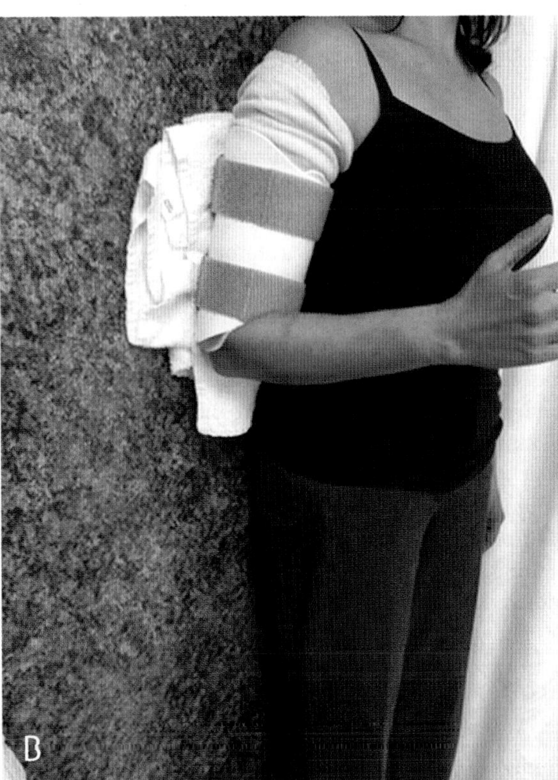

Figure 76.2 Elbow extension (**A**) and flexion (**B**) while standing. Note the position to support the humerus while ensuring pure elbow range of motion avoiding compensation.

the humerus and ensure pure elbow range of motion (ROM) without compensation (Figures 76.2–76.3).

- Pendulum exercises for 5 minutes 6 times a day.
- Instruct patient in retrograde massage and edema reduction.
- Weight-bearing restrictions may be implemented at the discretion of the surgeon depending on bone quality and the stability of the construct, and is progressed as the cone heals. In instances of polytrauma, weight-bearing is allowed at least for mobilization purposes. Fracture fixation constructs have limited torsional stability, leading to restrictions of aggressive rotational activities.
- In the case of radial nerve palsy symptoms, it can be helpful to perform a Semmes Weinstein monofilament testing and Tinel's test, and document the lack of active extension at the wrist, digits, and thumb to assist in tracking return. Patients should be instructed in passive extension exercises

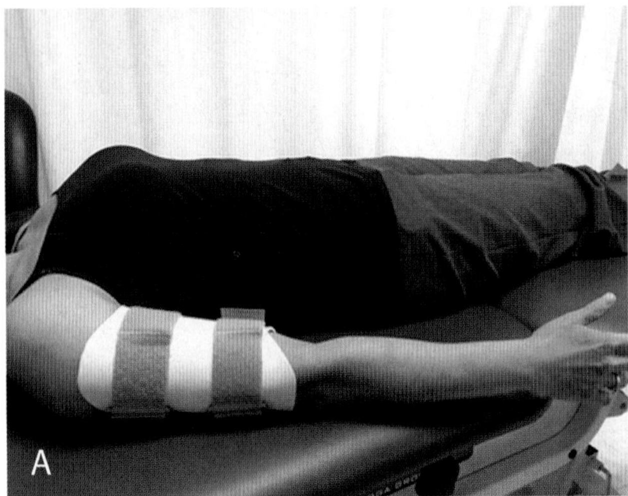

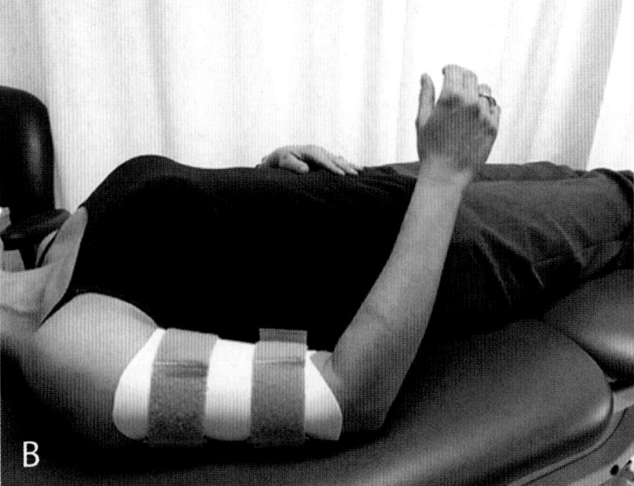

Figure 76.3 Elbow extension (**A**) and flexion (**B**) while supine. Note positioning to support the humerus while ensuring pure elbow range of motion without compensation.

 © 2018 American Academy of Orthopaedic Surgeons

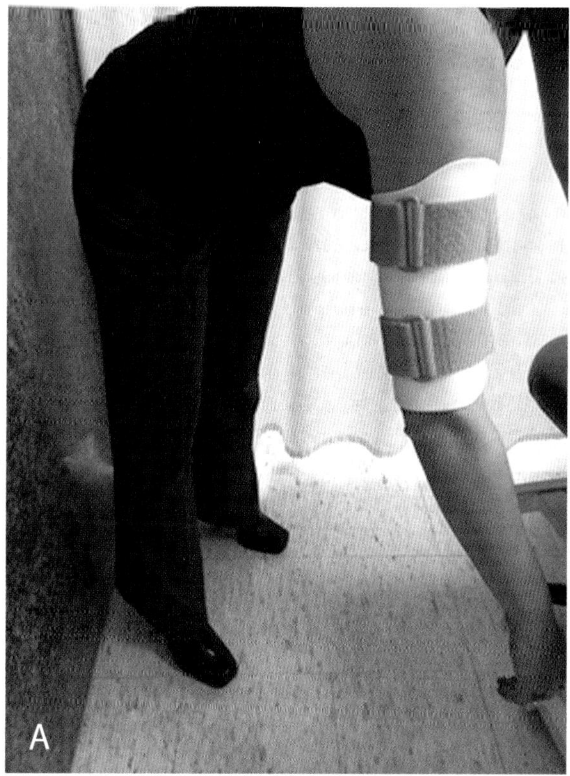

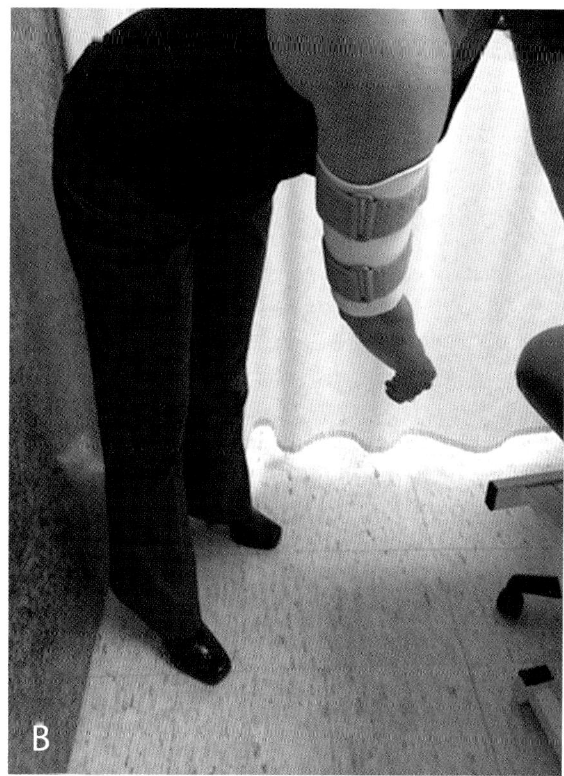

Figure 76.4 If the fracture is stable, pendulum exercises can be performed.

of the wrist and digits to prevent joint contraction while regeneration occurs. Bracing in extension also allows for use of the hand.

- Additional home program exercises include:
  - Pendulum exercises at first postoperative visit (Figure 76.4, A and B)
  - Active range of motion (AROM) and active-assistive range of motion (AAROM) shoulder flexion in the supine position at 1 to 2 weeks postoperatively. Progress to seated or standing AROM/AAROM shoulder flexion (Figures 76.5–76.7, A and B).
  - Patients are allowed to weight bear and perform light activities of daily living (ADLs) per pain tolerance.
  - A sample list of tasks allowed and discouraged is helpful for compliance.

Phase 1 (0–21 Days)

- Elbow, wrist, and hand AROM/AAROM
- Sling or cuff and collar sling when not exercising
- Begin pendulum exercises (clockwise and counter clockwise)
- AROM/AAROM of shoulder in the supine position. *It is important to avoid rotational stress.*

Phase 2 (3–6 Weeks)

- The sling or cuff and collar can be discontinued once wound healing is achieved and comfort level improves.
- The patient can begin light ADLs.
- Begin AROM of shoulder seated or standing.

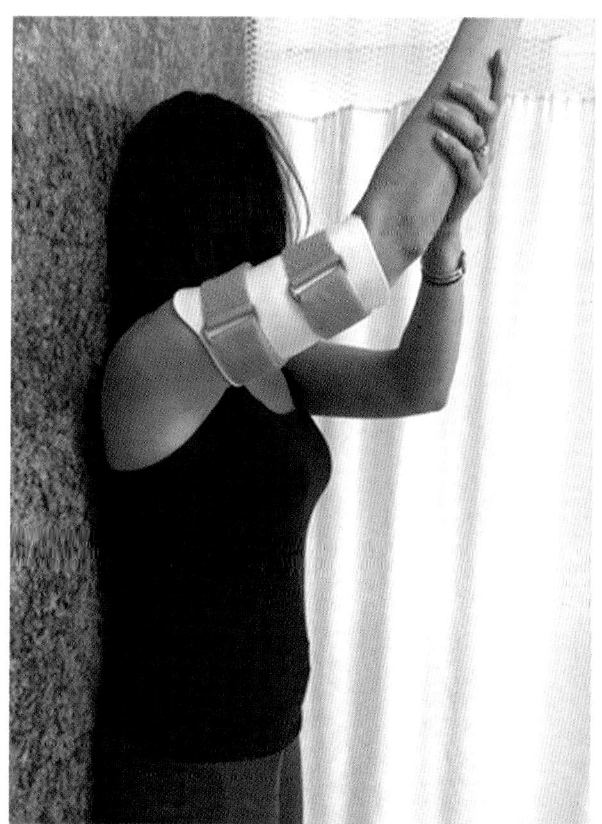

Figure 76.5 Seated or standing active range of motion/active-assisted range of motion shoulder flexion using self-assist.

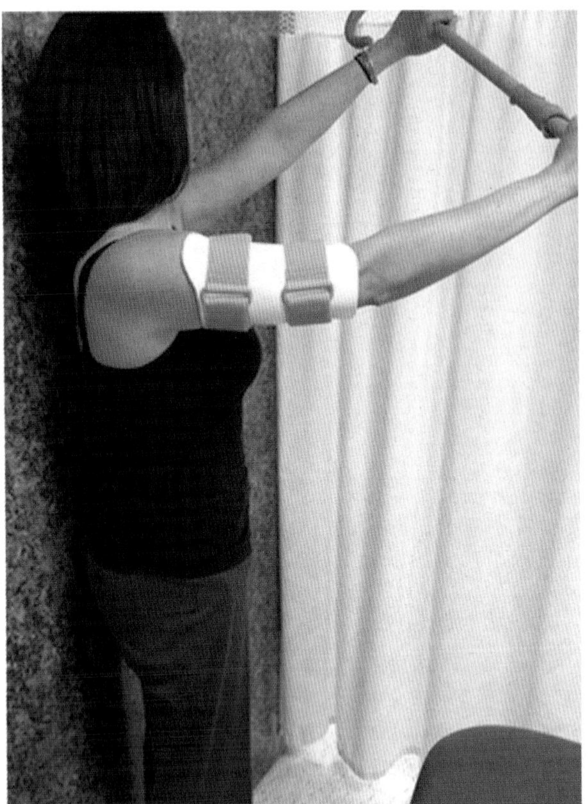

Figure 76.6 Seated or standing active range of motion/active-assisted range of motion shoulder flexion using a cane for assistance.

- AAROM of forward flexion with pulleys
- No resistive lifting, pulling, or pushing
- Instruct patient in isometric exercises for internal rotation, external rotation, extension, and abduction of the shoulder.

Phase 3 (7 Weeks to 2 Months)

- Light functional strengthening
- Self-care activities can increase
- Pulley exercises and addition of shoulder abduction and adduction AROM/AAROM
- Shoulder internal and external AROM/AAROM
- Discontinue functional brace/orthosis if used as healing allows per surgeon's order
- Strengthening exercises progressed as required depending on patient's functional demands
- Stretching if full ROM has not been achieved and surgeon indicates the fracture is stable
- Typically, by 10 to 12 weeks, full resistive exercises are permitted and light lifting can be started, provided radiographs demonstrate adequate fracture healing.

OUTCOMES

Fixation of humerus fractures results in union in around 95% of cases between 3 and 6 months. Similarly, a majority of associated radial nerve palsies resolve by 6 months, although mild weakness of wrist extension may persist. Typically, there is enough healing evident around the 6- to 8-week mark to allow

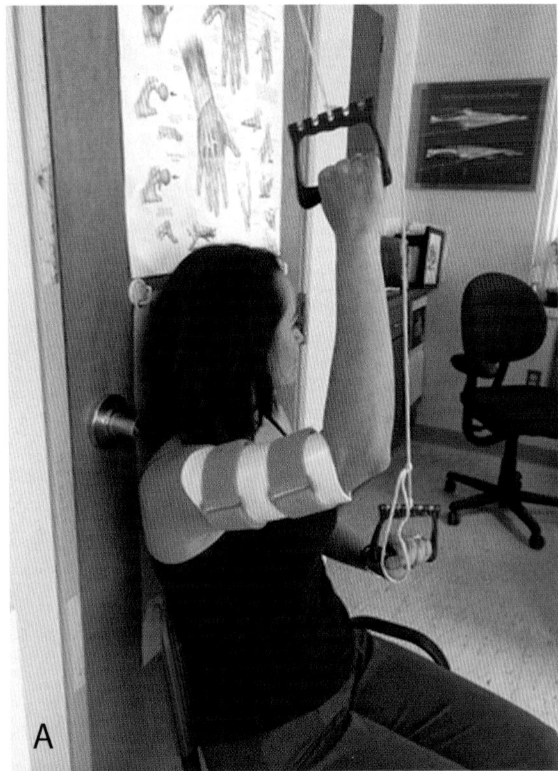

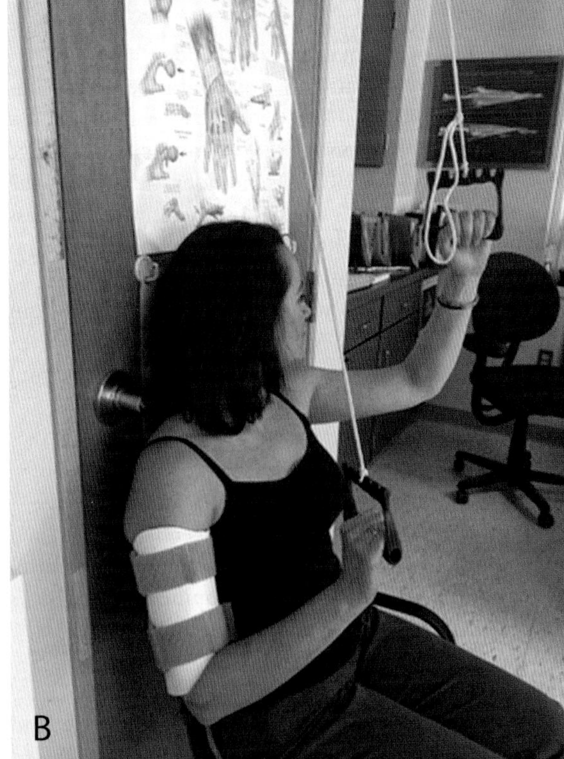

Figure 76.7 Seated active range of motion/active-assisted range of motion shoulder flexion with use of pulleys for assistance.

© 2018 American Academy of Orthopaedic Surgeons

for increasing activities. However, in the setting of fixation for a nonunion, longer durations of time to healing can be expected up to 3 months or more. Should a patient experience a change in alignment or a prominence of hardware, this may represent a hardware failure. Along the same lines, should a patient have persistent pain at the fracture site even in the setting of making gains with therapy, this should be followed both clinically and radiographically for signs of obvious union or nonunion.

Restoration of full arm strength and endurance to allow sport or heavy labor activity may require more time, but is generally achieved. It should be noted that fractures with more proximal extension benefit from a greater focus on shoulder motion and strength as the healing progresses, and may behave more like proximal humerus fractures in terms of functional results.

BIBLIOGRAPHY

Hoppenfeld S, deBoer P: *Surgical Exposures in Orthopaedics: The Anatomic Approach,* ed 2. Philadelphia, PA, J. B. Lippincott, 1994, pp 51–82.

Koch PP, Gross DF, Gerber C: The results of functional (Sarmiento) bracing of humeral shaft fractures. *J Shoulder Elbow Surg* 2002;11(2):143–150.

Tytherleigh-Strong G, Walls N, McQueen MM: The epidemiology of humeral shaft fractures. *J Bone Joint Surg Br* 1998; 80:249–253.

Van Houwelingen A, McKee MD: Management and complications of humeral shaft fractures. *University of Toronto Medical Journal* 2004;81:96–102.

© 2018 American Academy of Orthopaedic Surgeons

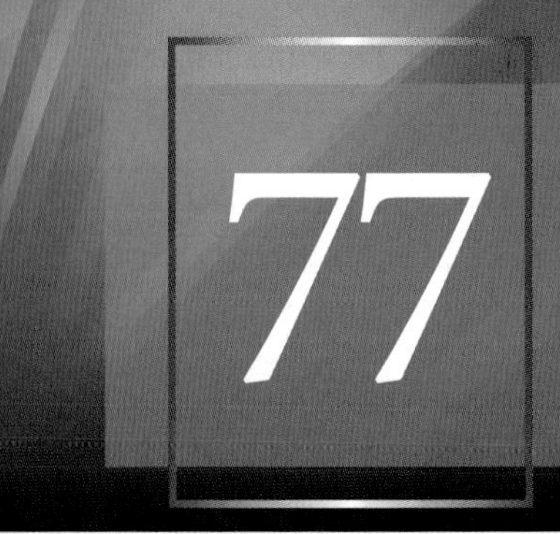

77 Amputation

Benjamin K. Potter, MD, and Bradley M. Ritland, MD

INTRODUCTION

Loss of a limb(s) represents a life-changing physical, functional, social, and psychological event for any patient. While the need for sound psychosocial support, care, and well-being following major extremity amputation cannot be overemphasized, physical therapy and rehabilitation concerns remain crucial to successful outcomes. In addition to restoring mobility and/or function, a thorough and complete rehabilitation process may improve the self-esteem, body image, personal and societal acceptance, and independence of persons with limb loss. Depending on premorbid function, medical comorbidities, indication for amputation(s), amputation level(s), and patient goals, desired outcomes range widely from wheelchair mobility with functional independence to near-complete recovery of function with aggressive pursuit of recreational or competitive athletics through adaptive or conventional means. Developing practical goals and a roughly targeted timeline shortly after amputation, in collaboration with the patient, the patient's family, and the surgical and rehabilitation team can address early expectations while providing necessary hope and encouragement. Specific advanced training in rehabilitation of the upper or lower extremity amputee is useful in achieving optimal results.

SURGICAL PROCEDURE

Given the myriad conventional and described major amputation levels and technical variations, a detailed description of each is beyond the scope of this chapter. Furthermore, distinct therapeutic and surgical amputation considerations vary greatly based on the indication for major extremity amputation, be it trauma, oncologic, infectious, congenital, or dysvascular and/or diabetic. The ideal residual limb preserves a mobile joint where possible, is cylindrical in shape with a durable and sensate skin, and is free of neuromas and deep skin invaginations. However, a few general principles are broadly applicable to upper and lower amputations that are extremely important.

First, all diseased tissue, whether traumatized and contaminated, dysvascular, infectious, or neoplastic, must be removed to avoid recurrence of the disease process, amputation failure, and early revision. All large and named vessels should be securely ligated. As all cut nerves form neuromas, named nerves should transected distally and buried proximally to avoid symptomatic neuromata without deinnervating functionally important proximal muscle groups or those useful for myoelectric control.

Next, the goal of amputation surgery is to provide a robust, healthy soft-tissue envelope that can biologically heal and provide a durable, ideally painless, terminal residual limb that can tolerate the functional demands of the patient—most commonly the pressure and shear of regular prosthesis utilization. As such, the soft-tissue envelope remains at least as important as the underlying osseous platform in achieving these goals. A stable myodesis and (secondary) myoplasty are important for achieving these goals, particularly for transfemoral amputations: both techniques improve terminal residual limb control, stabilize and anchor distal padding, and thus prevent soft-tissue retraction. Amputation level and bone cut selection should thus be based on the available soft tissue in addition to functional considerations. Skin grafts are variably tolerated depending on the location on the residual limb, the amputation level, and the underlying soft tissue. Grafts are generally manageable over healthy underlying muscle and padding, but are prone to breakdown and late revision if performed directly over bone or marginal soft tissue, particularly on the terminal aspect of the lower extremity amputation. Free-tissue transfers may be indicated to salvage a functional knee or elbow joint, and can sometimes be innervated to provide protective sensation. With the exception of well-conceived and padded

Dr. Potter or an immediate family member serves as an unpaid consultant to Biomet; and serves as a board member, owner, officer, or committee member of Clinical Orthopaedics and Related Research, *the* Journal of Orthopaedic Trauma, *the* Journal of Surgical Orthopaedic Advances, *and the Society of Military Orthopaedic Surgeons. Neither Dr. Ritland nor any immediate family member has received anything of value from or has stock or stock options held in a commercial company or institution related directly or indirectly to the subject of this article.*

© 2018 American Academy of Orthopaedic Surgeons

disarticulations, adequate space should be left for functional prosthetic components. Extra-long, or novel, amputation levels are to be avoided, as these often lack adequate soft-tissue padding and provide little space for prosthetic components; as such, these levels tend to offer the limitations of both the more proximal and distal amputation levels without conferring the full benefits of either.

Last, some form of rehabilitation is indicated following any major extremity amputation. The intensity of this rehabilitation may vary based on the indication for amputation, associated injuries or medical comorbidities, and functional potential and wishes of the patient with limb loss. For some diabetic or dysvascular patients with multiple amputations or severe cardiovascular disease, simply improved transfer capacity and independence may be the full extent of the rehabilitation potential and goals. The remainder of this chapter is directed largely at patients with at least some ambulatory potential (following major lower extremity amputation) or prosthetic use potential for assisting with activities of daily living (ADLs) following major upper extremity amputation. Fortunately, most patients with adequate blood supply to heal a major amputation(s) will also have adequate skin tolerance to be able to tolerate at least limited prosthesis wear at those levels.

Complications and anatomic difficulties are common following major amputation. In addition to physical and occupational therapist and prosthetist care, regular orthopaedic surgery and physiatrist follow-up is essential in order to minimize secondary morbidity due to complications. These visits can identify both overt surgical complications and persistently symptomatic residual limbs with correctable problems such as wound or residual limb breakdown, infection, myodesis failure, heterotopic ossification, and symptomatic neuromata. Diligent attention to, and correction of, these concerns can make the crucial difference between a content and functional amputee and a dissatisfied and truly disabled one.

POSTOPERATIVE REHABILITATION

Similar to any surgical procedure, there are protocols that guide the rehabilitation process for patients sustaining major limb loss. Each patient is unique and will progress differently following the amputation; thus, each rehabilitation program should be individualized. The comprehensive rehabilitation program should commence as soon as practicable—in some cases, prior to performing the amputation or wound closure—and progress each patient aggressively, but as individually tolerated, through each phase.

Regardless of the indication for amputation, the limb(s) involved, or the number of joint levels lost, the primary goal of the rehabilitation team should be to return the patient to the highest level of achievable and desired function. The rehabilitation team members should be the primary advocates for the patient and should develop an individualized rehabilitation program to help the patient achieve his or her goals. Be open minded with the patient's goals and aspirations [illegible] time, the patient will gain a better understanding of achievable function and limitations. Conversely, providers should not overpromise a patient and the patient's family with regard to potential function. Encouraging the patient to have realistic goals and expectations early will set up the patient for success throughout the rehabilitation program. The rehabilitation team should utilize appropriate, evidence-based techniques to optimize the functional recovery of the patient and goals should be continuously updated throughout rehabilitation.

Initial Management/Preprosthetic Training

The goal of initial management is to thoroughly evaluate, educate, and adequately manage the patient perioperatively, generally in preparation for a prosthesis. A thorough evaluation of the entire patient, not just the limb(s) lost, is critical. Assessing the surgical location, sensation, pain/sensitivity, strength, flexibility, endurance, and functional capabilities of the patient will lay the foundation for the entire rehabilitation program. Once the evaluation is complete, specific focus areas include educating the patient and family members, reducing pain/edema, promoting residual limb healing, wheelchair management and/or ambulation with appropriate assistive devices, preventing loss of motion/strength/functional status, and optimizing core strength and cardiovascular fitness (Table 77.1).

Following the initial assessment and introductory therapy sessions with the patient, the provider progresses every aspect of the rehabilitation program. The focus is on optimally preparing the patient for the prosthesis and mitigating any factors that may limit progression (e.g., contractures, atrophy, deconditioning).

Rigid dressings (e.g., casting) can be useful for wound protection in patients at high risk for falling as well as for contracture prevention. This modality is generally utilized in patients who have difficulty complying with early rehabilitation or in whom delayed wound healing is anticipated. The rigid dressing may also be fitted with an immediate postoperative prosthesis. These casts, although useful, must be meticulously and adequately padded to prevent skin breakdown, particularly over osseous prominences (e.g., the patella).

Exercises should be continuously modified to challenge the patient to prepare the muscles important for gait and physical functioning, even when patients remain on bed rest or are wheelchair bound. The rehabilitation program should continue to incorporate flexibility, strengthening, balance, and cardiovascular exercises. Patient motivation and focus on performing the exercises with proper form and technique are critical. Functional training and multiplanar activities should be implemented as soon as appropriate based on the injury pattern.

Patient/Family Member Education

The patient must be educated on the injury/amputation, expectations in rehabilitation, general timelines of expected milestones, and the anticipated rehabilitation course of action. These are described by all members of the medical team, who must engage the patient and family members in the [illegible] New amputees should also be encouraged to look at,

© 2018 American Academy of Orthopaedic Surgeons

Table 77.1 INITIAL MANAGEMENT/PREPROSTHETIC TRAINING

	Upper Extremity	Lower Extremity
Pain Management	Pharmaceutical interventions (NSAIDs, narcotic, gabapentinoids, tricyclics), patient controlled anesthesia, sciatic catheter, transcutaneous electrical nerve stimulation (TENS), heat, cold, desensitizing/tapping techniques, mirror therapy	
Core Exercises	Lumbar stabilization program, plank exercises, prone extension exercises	
Strengthening	Shoulder: flexion, extension, abduction, adduction Elbow: flexion, extension Intact limb strengthening, as tolerated	Hip: flexion, extension, abduction, adduction Knee: flexion, extension Intact limb strengthening, as tolerated
Stretching	Avoid contractures. Chest, scapular protractors/retractors, shoulder flexors, abductors, rotators	Avoid contractures. Hip flexor/abductor, hamstring, abdominal, lumbar
Cardiovascular	Upper body ergometer, ergo skier, rope-pull machine, rock wall treadmill, rowing, cycling, elliptical, treadmill	
Balance	Perform seated and standing, as indicated. Alter surface, provide resistance/perturbations, and conduct additional tasks/movements as indicated.	
Ambulation	Begin in parallel bars, then transition to assistive device (crutches or walker), as indicated	

NSAIDs = nonsteroidal anti-inflammatory drugs, TENS = transcutaneous electrical nerve stimulation.

touch, and massage their residual limb(s). This can improve patient comfort with and acceptance of the amputation, as well as helping to desensitize the residual limb in the early postsurgical period.

Early Functional Training

Encourage early independence with bed mobility, transfers, ADLs, and any mobility assistive device. Pay special attention to protecting the residual limb during this functional training. Falls resulting in contusions, fractures, frank wound dehiscence, or even simply loss of patient confidence and security substantially slow rehabilitation progress. Using appropriate adaptive devices or techniques will help build the patient's confidence with these activities and prevent or mitigate setbacks.

Edema Control

Following an amputation, compression is arguably the most important method of edema control because of the effect it has on the shape and size of the residual limb and on the integrity of the incision. Compression techniques and dressing types can vary. A compressive wrap applied in a figure-of-eight pattern or a stump shrinker are commonly used. Whether using rigid or soft dressings, it is important to fit the patient with the desired compression device over the residual limb as soon as possible, ensuring distal-to-proximal compression. Compression should be aggressively progressed to mitigate postoperative swelling and to assist with residual limb shaping. Inappropriate application leads to proximal constriction and a bulbous limb, which is difficult to fit with a prosthesis. Icing techniques are also appropriate, but pay close attention to areas of decreased sensation to avoid thermal injury and skin compromise. Avoid keeping, or allowing the patient to maintain, the residual limb in dependent positions for extended periods.

Skin/Wound Care

Frequent skin checks are important to mitigate skin breakdown and monitor early wound problems. Patient education, especially for those with decreased sensation, in repositioning all limbs to prevent pressure sores is critical. Sutures following an amputation are typically removed around 17 to 21 days postsurgery.

The patient can be fitted for a silicone liner, the final step prior to prosthetic socket casting and fitting, shortly after the sutures are removed provided the swelling is controlled and pain is controlled to allow donning the liner. Liners should be worn for limited periods initially to develop skin tolerance. The patient should initially check the skin of the residual limb every 45 to 60 minutes to avoid early folliculitis or wound problems secondary to sweating and maceration, and to ensure proper progression of liner wear time. The patient should adjust liner wear time based on skin tolerance with the goal of wearing the liner all day, except when sleeping, to prepare for prosthesis wear. Wound care should be performed as needed on soft-tissue injuries. A dedicated team of wound care experts can be invaluable in this regard. Begin scar mobilization shortly after suture removal as well to avoid invaginations or deep adhesions, which can lead to late irritation and ulceration due to skin immobility and friction.

Desensitization

Desensitization techniques should be introduced to the patient as early as possible in the postoperative period, generally prior

 © 2018 American Academy of Orthopaedic Surgeons

to suture removal through the dressing or shrinker. Commonly utilized techniques include rubbing/tapping the residual limb with varying objects and textures, soft-tissue mobilization, introducing heat/cold modalities, and electrical stimulation to the residual limb. The patient should perform the desensitization as tolerated throughout the day outside of formal therapy sessions.

Phantom limb pain refers to painful sensations within the absent portion of the limb(s). It is very common, if not ubiquitous. Generally, its severity decreases as the patient progresses through rehabilitation, but in some cases may be a barrier to recovery. In addition to other desensitization techniques and medical therapy, mirror therapy, a treatment technique in which the patient looks at the reflection of the intact limb in a mirror while imagining performing the same actions with the amputated limb, has been shown to reduce phantom limb pain in some patients Mirror therapy can also be effectively utilized by bilateral amputees working alongside another person willing to physically act as the limb(s) of the patient. The authors recommend performing this therapy for 15 minutes, 2 to 3 times a day while the phantom limb pain is bothersome. The patient should be educated that wearing a prosthesis, when appropriate, and subsequent increases in duration and activity level, can also decrease phantom limb pain.

General Postsurgical Guidelines

Surgeons may have preferred methods and guidelines following their procedures. The rehabilitation team should be aware of these guidelines in order to optimize recovery while not compromising surgical aspects of the amputation, such as tenuous skin healing, myodeses, or a bridge synostosis. Many amputation closures are, by anatomic necessity, somewhat unique; thus, clear communication between the surgeon and the rehabilitation provider is essential prior to initiating and throughout rehabilitation. The general guidelines utilized at our center are outlined in Table 77.2.

Stretching

Strive to maintain a functional range of motion (ROM) in both the affected and unaffected limbs. The authors recommend an aggressive daily stretching program but are not partial to a specific stretching technique, and often mix modalities based on patient tolerance and progress. The main consideration is where to apply pressure on the residual limb. Because the patient often has increased sensitivity on the residual limb, the patient will likely inform the provider where it is comfortable to apply the pressure; thus, naturally, the incision line or myodesis site is avoided initially. Ask for this feedback to optimize the stretch while respecting the comfort of the patient.

Contracture Avoidance

It is imperative to avoid contractures in this patient population. The shorter the residual limb, the more prone it is to contracture. The most common contracture following transfemoral amputation is that of hip flexion, external rotation, and abduction. Encourage the patient to avoid prolonged periods in this position and educate the patient to maintain a neutral hip position in bed by placing a sandbag or similar object along the lateral residual limb. Placing a pillow under

Table 77.2 GENERAL POSTSURGICAL GUIDELINES

Amputation Level	Weight Bearing	Exercise Restrictions
Partial foot	Immediate heel WBAT; full WBAT with heel–toe gait at 6 wk for transmetatarsal amputations, 8 wk for Lisfranc or Chopart amputations	None; prevent equinas contracture
Symes	NWB for 5–6 wk, progress to WBAT at 8 wk	None
Transtibial	NWB for 4–6 wk; delay to 6–8 wk for patients with tenuous closure/soft-tissue envelope; delay to 6 wk for Modified Ertl (bridge synostosis) procedure	Hamstring stretching restricted for 2 wk with tenuous myodesis
Knee disarticulation	NWB for 4 wk	No restrictions to hip abduction/adduction
Transfemoral	NWB for 5–6 wk	No active hip abduction strengthening past neutral for 2 wk (abduction to neutral is permissible), no resisted hip flexion for 2 wk, no resisted hip adduction for 4 wk
Hip disarticulation	NWB for 4 wk	None
Transradial Transhumeral	Limited WB for 4 wk Soft tissue permitting, initial prosthetic fitting when sutures have been removed	None: Begin MyoSite testing as soon as possible (common wrist flexors/extensors for below-elbow amputations and biceps/triceps for above-elbow amputations)

NWB = non–weight bearing, WB = weight bearing, WBAT = weight bearing as tolerated.

© 2018 American Academy of Orthopaedic Surgeons

the thigh for elevation following the amputation should be avoided. Periodic prone lying can be beneficial, and focused hip flexor stretching and abdominal stretching are helpful in all patients with lower extremity amputations. Knee and elbow flexion contractures are also common following transtibial and transradial amputations, respectively. The primary culprit in both instances is frequently dependent positioning and a flexed resting posture, which is to be avoided despite the fact that this is nearly always the most comfortable position for the patient. Likewise, stretching the shoulder muscle groups (with particular emphasis on flexion, external rotation, and abduction) for upper extremity amputees is imperative.

Strengthening

Strengthening exercises should also be performed daily independent of amputation level(s). In general, hip and core strengthening should be initiated as early as possible following a lower extremity amputation. Hip strengthening, commonly started with isometrics, can be conducted on a mat utilizing a bolster/stool and additional weight, as indicated. The patient is encouraged to maintain a neutral spine and conduct abdominal bracing while performing the four basic hip movements (abduction, adduction, flexion, extension) into the bolster/stool. While all hip-strengthening exercises are important, extra emphasis is placed on the hip abductors for their role in single-leg stance during standing balance exercises and ambulation. Patients with transtibial amputations should also initiate knee flexion/extension exercises at this time. Upper extremity amputees should begin elbow, shoulder, and posture exercises. For unilateral upper and lower amputation, we recommend continuing to perform exercises as tolerated on the nonamputated side. All amputees should begin a lumbar stabilization program that strengthens the transverse abdominals and multifidus muscles, along with other core-stabilizing muscles, to prevent deconditioning, improve posture, and ostensibly decrease the risk of low back pain. Progress the upper extremity exercises, the lower extremity exercises, and core stabilization program as aggressively as tolerated and overall patient condition permits.

Balance

Balance training is initiated immediately, as the patient's center of mass has been altered. Begin with seated balance, shifting balance, and sit-to-stand transfers, then progress to standing balance, as indicated. Key components to balance training include altering the surface, providing resistance to the patient, and/or conducting additional tasks/movements during balance drills.

Cardiovascular Exercises

Cardiovascular exercise is crucial and should be encouraged throughout the entire rehabilitation program. Varying upper body and lower body aerobic exercises allows the patient to maintain, restore, or build cardiovascular endurance, and limits the propensity for undesired weight gain. Exercises may include upper body ergometer, ergo skier, continuous rope-pull, rock wall treadmill, rowing, cycling, and so forth. Modifications or adaptations are often necessary for the patient to utilize these devices properly.

Ambulation Assistance

The degree and type of assistive device necessary is always dependent on amputation level(s). Most patients with a lower extremity amputation will need a wheelchair, either manual or powered, at some point following their amputation. Therefore, educate the patient on advanced wheelchair skills (performing a wheelie, ascend/descend curbs, remounting after a fall, and so on) as necessary. In addition, providers should be familiar with different types of available wheelchairs and wheelchair modifications (e.g., elevated limb rest/residual limb holders, anti-tippers). For unilateral lower extremity amputees, begin early ambulation with appropriate assistive device (crutches/walker) or on parallel bars.

Prosthetic Training

Prosthetic training (Table 77.3) can begin when the surgeon clears the patient for prosthetic fitting and weight bearing, full or partial. Upon clearance from the surgeon, a prosthetist will cast and fit the patient for the initial socket and discuss component options. For upper extremity amputations, this often occurs once the sutures are removed. Early upper extremity prosthesis fitting may decrease developing single-limb adaptive strategies and improve long-term prosthesis use/acceptance. For lower extremity amputations, the timing will depend on the surgical procedure performed. Generally speaking, below-knee amputation patients can begin prosthetic training 4 to 8 weeks following final closure of the amputation and above-knee patients can begin prosthetic training 6 to 8 weeks following final closure of the amputation (refer to Table 77.2 for more specifics). While the prosthetist is the subject matter expert, rehabilitative providers and surgeons should have a general understanding of upper and lower extremity prosthesis components. This knowledge will allow the provider to train the patient appropriately based on the specifications of the prosthesis, and allow the surgeon to appropriately constrain (or not) certain activities. Once the patient is fit with the initial prosthesis, training begins.

During this phase, the patient will learn proper techniques for mobility, gait, and other functional tasks. The focus initially is getting the patient comfortable with weight shifting and equally distributing the weight across both legs while standing, and/or using the upper extremity prosthesis to perform simple tasks. The patient should begin with parallel bars or using an appropriate assistive device. It is important to introduce a variety of balance and proprioception exercises that progressively improve the confidence and quality of movement from the patient. Concentrated gait training is implemented to build the foundation for optimal gait symmetry and efficiency. The provider should offer feedback to the patient regarding the patient's kinematics, including stride length, width, cadence, trunk rotation, and arm swing. Trunk rotation and arm swing training can be conducted with and without prostheses. Aside

© 2018 American Academy of Orthopaedic Surgeons

Table 77.3 PROSTHETIC TRAINING

Activity	Training
Donning/doffing prosthesis	Educate on proper sequence and wear progression.
Transfer training	Sit to stand, stand to sit with prosthesis.
Standing tolerance/weight shifting	Begin with stable surface in parallel bar, progress to unsupported positions, add upper extremity/trunk movement
Balance training	Progress to unsupported position, add upper extremity/trunk movements, add resistance, implement uneven surfaces, transition to single-leg balance, cone drills, standing with feet at different heights.
Ambulation/gait training	Begin in parallel bars, educate loading/activating prosthesis appropriately, provide feedback on stride length, width, cadence, trunk rotation, and arm swing, perform training forwards, backwards, side-stepping, and multidirectional.
Fall training/recovery	Start with fall/recover distances close to patient (can use plyometric boxes or plinths). Progress through 24-, 18-, 12-, and 6-inch boxes, and use assistive devices, as needed.
Ramp/stair training	Activating the prosthesis properly for ascend and descend
Uneven terrain/obstacles	Modify terrain, add different height/width obstacles to walk over
Strengthening	Focus on "functional" strengthening exercises (squats, lunges, resisted walking, and so on)
Agility training	Implement low-impact agility training, dynamic/multiplanar exercises, agility ladder exercises, change of speed/direction exercises. Progress to higher-impact activities, when appropriate.

from this basic gait training, low-impact agility and multiplanar exercises can be gradually introduced.

Patients who sustain bilateral knee disarticulation or transfemoral amputations often begin prosthesis training with just the foot component attached directly to the socket. These modified prostheses are often called "shorties" or "stubbies" (Figure 77.1). This practice allows the patient to adjust to wearing bilateral prostheses, establish the base of support, and develop functional strength and confidence prior to learning how to operate the knee components. Consequently, this practice appears to reduce the frequency of falls with these patients. The patient's confidence, performance, and desire dictate the progressive lengthening of the pylon length to a more functional and practical height, with the graduated incorporation of drop-lock short knees. The patient should be able to ambulate independently, ideally without nonprosthetic assistive device(s), and perform most functional activities (i.e., return to standing after a fall, transfers, and so on) before increasing the length of the pylon. The transition to knee components typically occurs when the patient has reached this proficiency and has achieved a standing height providing enough clearance for a conventional knee component under the socket. Most patients stop increasing their height when they are around their original height or slightly shorter. It is practical and achievable to have most healthy patients with bilateral transfemoral amputations, with reasonable residual limb length, become a proficient ambulator without the need for an additional assistive device. Continued advancements in lower extremity prosthetic components help make this level of function a reality, but ultimately it is the patient, not the prosthesis, who walks.

The goal of this phase is to reach a point at which the patient has achieved near-normal biomechanics when ambulating and can complete all ADLs in the prosthesis. This ambulation may be achieved with an appropriate assistive device, if necessary. Ideally, most patients will utilize their prostheses all day or nearly all day.

High Impact/Activity-Specific Training

The rehabilitation program should meet the needs of the patient, to include returning to higher-impact activities (running, jumping, return to sport, and so on). Even for patients who do not desire or who are not medical candidates for high-level activities, a targeted maintenance fitness program is indicated to prevent further core or cardiovascular deconditioning. This helps maintain general fitness and stable body weight in an effort to prevent loss of function over time and socket fitting problems due to weight and volume fluctuation, respectively.

In addition to looking at the clinical snapshot of the patient, our program requires bone mineral density (BMD) scans prior to initiating this phase of rehabilitation. Profound decreases in BMD can occur following major lower extremity amputation, placing patients at increased risks for fragility or insufficiency fractures. For patients with severe BMD loss, pharmacologic intervention (e.g., supplemental calcium and vitamin D, bisphosphonates) may be instituted along with a slowed progression to higher impact activities, as well as more time ambulating or performing weight bearing exercise

© 2018 American Academy of Orthopaedic Surgeons

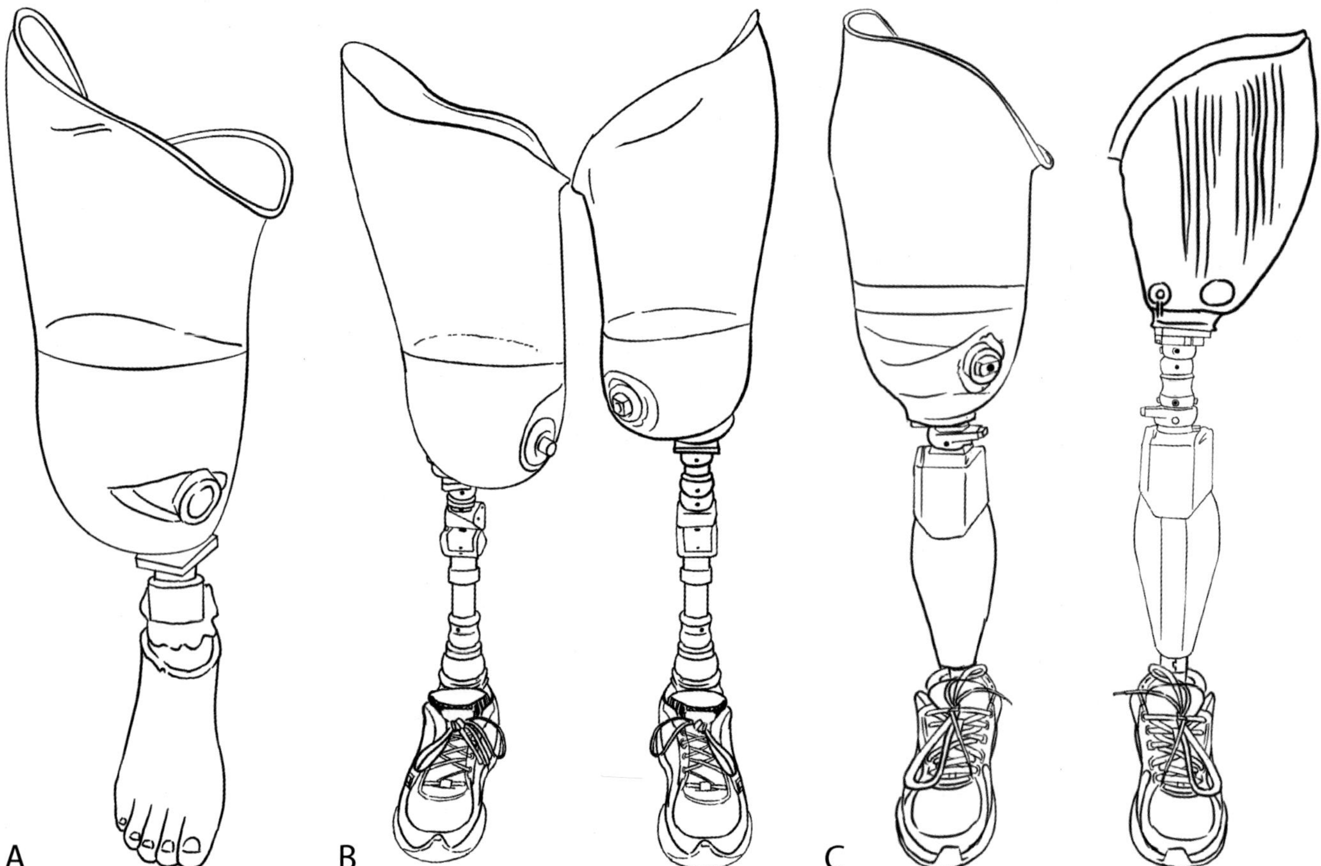

Figure 77.1 **A**, Illustration of the initial socket with "shortie" prosthesis: minimal prosthetic limb with a foot attached to the socket. **B**, Illustration of interval lengthening of the pilon to include drop-lock knees: passively flexed when sitting or utilizing a wheelchair. **C**, Illustration of the final prosthesis with microprocessor knees and reestablishment of premorbid patient height.

Once the patient is cleared, the rehabilitation program should naturally implement higher agility/impact/plyometric exercises and return-to-run training as desired by the patient. The prosthetist should be aware of when these exercises are being introduced so that the socket is made with highly durable material (likely carbon fiber) to mitigate the risk of prosthesis failure that can lead to falls or injury.

We recommend a return-to-run regimen that gradually progresses both running distance and time. Like other prosthetic components, there are numerous running-specific devices to choose from. Consequently, the training can differ depending on the specific component that the patient and/or prosthetist have chosen. The prosthetist should ensure that the running prosthesis is properly aligned to optimize the patient's running mechanics. Unilateral below-knee patients can initiate return-to-run training with a "regular" foot prosthesis prior to getting fit for a formal running prosthesis. If needed, initial run training can be performed in a harness system for added security. Patients with bilateral above-knee amputations often begin training in "shorty" running sockets attached directly to the running foot. The patient's height will progress to the patient's desired height and running/mechanical knees can be added as per initial ambulation progression. Running drills and techniques (e.g., high knee drills, butt kicks, skipping, quick feet, bounding) should be implemented based off the individual patient need. Once the patient is able to run independently and perform high-impact activities, it is important to educate the patient on proper self-care measures and proper independent progression of the program prior to discharge to avoid overuse injuries or skin breakdown.

PEARLS

- Patient and family education is particularly important early in the recovery process, concurrent with expectation management and establishing challenging, but realistic, goals. Managing expectations and outlining general timelines of expected milestones can substantially mitigate the fear and concerns associated with an amputation. These initial interactions also foster a trusting bond with the therapist, surgeon, and other providers.
- Rehabilitation and recovery after a major limb loss can be an emotional experience for the patient. Patients commonly oscillate between emotional highs and lows during this process. The first day that the patient is fit with the prosthesis is commonly an emotionally high day for the patient and the patient's family. This is typically the first time that

 © 2018 American Academy of Orthopaedic Surgeons

the patient and the patient's family members observe the patient stand, walk, or use the arm since prior to the injury/amputation. Conversely, there can be stressful days when the patient is not progressing as quickly as anticipated or when the patient has setbacks. It is important to be supportive at all times and to focus on the patient's accomplishments. Mental health consultants should be informed of patients struggling with their injury or their progression. Behavioral health and psychosocial support can assist with acceptance and coping strategies and posttraumatic stress disorder, as well as managing the understandable anger, fear, or regret that can accompany traumatic limb loss.

- Socket fit is extremely important for a successful outcome. It is common for patients to receive new sockets as their residual limb adjusts size, especially within the first 12 months post-amputation. A poorly fit socket can significantly negatively affect the progression of rehabilitation. We highly encourage that a patient receive a new socket when needed to avoid rehabilitation setbacks and/or prosthesis abandonment.
- Pursue an objective, outcome-based approach when managing patients with limb loss. Some common outcome measures and evaluation tests utilized with this patient population include the Functional Independence Measure, Jebsen-Taylor hand function evaluation, Minnesota Rate of Manipulation Test, Boxes and Blocks, Nine-Hole Peg tests, Timed Up and Go (TUG) test, 2- or 6-minute walk tests, and the Comprehensive High-Level Activity Mobility Predictor (CHAMP). Depending on the level of amputation(s), some outcome measures may or may not be appropriate. Utilize these outcome measures, along with other simple objective findings such as strength and ROM, to monitor progress, as this offers providers an objective means of monitoring progress and establishes intermediary goals for patients.
- People who sustain limb loss have an increased risk of multiple additional secondary comorbidities, including arthritis, lower back pain, obesity, cardiovascular disease, and ongoing skin ailments. Reducing potential risk factors for these sequelae should be considered when developing a rehabilitation program. The provider should educate the patient about these risk factors and encourage an active and healthy lifestyle outside the clinic in an effort to avoid them.
- Adaptive sport and recreation programs are an important part of the rehabilitation process and encourage the return to an active, fun lifestyle following an amputation. These programs are designed to introduce ways that the patient can continue to participate in sports and can have a significant positive impact on the recovery of the patient. Such activities can provide significant physical and mental benefits by allowing patients to move past their disability and enable them to participate through an appropriate adapted method. In addition, this helps reintegrate the patient back into the community after the amputation and allow development of relationships with patients with similar conditions. Peer-to-peer interaction is invaluable throughout the rehabilitation process. Consequently, many amputee rehabilitation programs have developed peer mentorship programs in which patients can communicate directly with people with similar conditions. These peer programs are an excellent resource for newer patients and allow previous patients to "give back" to the community of amputees.
- Last, while this chapter focuses on the surgical and rehabilitative team members caring for patients with major limb loss, the value and need for an engaged, multidisciplinary medical team cannot be overemphasized. Communication and respect between all members of this team is invaluable to successful patient outcomes. As managing patients with complex injuries and multilimb involvement can be overwhelming, utilizing the relative strengths of each member of the medical team is critical. Following the basic surgical and rehabilitative guidelines outlined in this chapter should provide the fundamentals of treating any patient with major limb loss.

BIBLIOGRAPHY

Bosse MJ, Mackenzie EJ, Kellam JF, et al. An analysis of outcomes of reconstruction or amputation after leg-threatening injuries. *N Engl J Med* 2002;347:1924–1931.

Harvey ZT, Loomis GA, Mitsch S, Murphy IC, Griffin SC, Potter BK, Pasquina P: Advanced rehabilitation techniques for the multi-limb amputee. *J Surg Orthop Adv* 2012;21(1):50–57.

Mackenzie EJ, Bosse MJ, Pollak AN, et al: Long-term persistence of disability following severe lower-limb trauma: Results of a seven-year follow-up. *J Bone Joint Surg Am* 2005;87:1801–1809.

Pierce RO Jr, Kernek CB, Ambrose TA 2nd: The plight of the traumatic amputee. *Orthopedics* 1993;16:793–797.

Ramachandran VS, Rogers-Ramachandran D. Synaesthesia in phantom limbs induced with mirrors. *Proc Biol Sci* 1996;263:377–386.

Smurr LM, Gulick K, Yancosek K, Ganz O: Managing the upper extremity amputee: a protocol for success. *J Hand Ther* 2008;21:160–175; quiz 176.

Tintle SM, Baechler MF, Nanos GP 3rd, Forsberg JA, Potter BK: Traumatic and trauma-related amputations: part II: upper extremity and future directions. *J Bone Joint Surg Am* 2010;92:2934–2945.

Tintle SM, Baechler MF, Nanos GP, Forsberg JA, Potter BK: Reoperation following combat-related upper extremity amputations. *J Bone Joint Surg Am* 2012;94(16):e1191–e1196.

Tintle SM, Keeling JJ, Shawen SB, Forsberg JA, Potter BK: Traumatic and trauma-related amputations: part I: general principles and lower-extremity amputations. *J Bone Joint Surg Am* 2010;92:2852–2868.

Tintle SM, Shawen SB, Forsberg JA, Gajewski DA, Keeling JJ, Andersen RC, Potter BK: Re-operation following combat-related major lower extremity amputations. *J Orthop Trauma* 2014;28:232–237.

© 2018 American Academy of Orthopaedic Surgeons

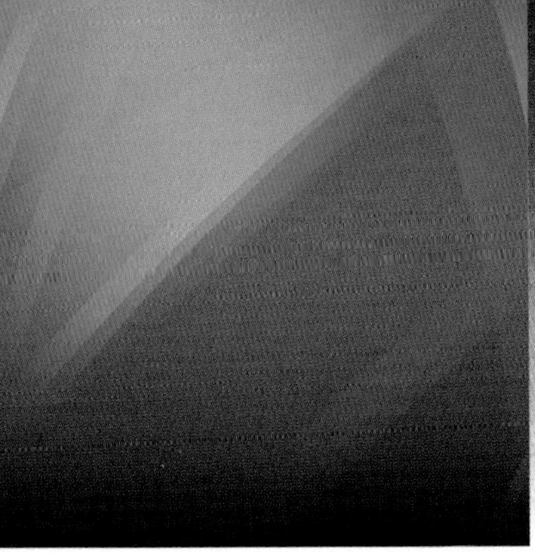

Index

Note: Page numbers followed by *f* and *t*, respectively, indicate figures and tables.

A

© 2018 American Academy of Orthopaedic Surgeons

B

C

D

E

 © 2018 American Academy of Orthopaedic Surgeons

F

© 2018 American Academy of Orthopaedic Surgeons

M

N

O

P

© 2018 American Academy of Orthopaedic Surgeons

Q

R

S

© 2018 American Academy of Orthopaedic Surgeons

T

© 2018 American Academy of Orthopaedic Surgeons

 © 2018 American Academy of Orthopaedic Surgeons

© 2018 American Academy of Orthopaedic Surgeons

W

X

Z

RRS1705

© 2018 American Academy of Orthopaedic Surgeons